Oxford Textbook of

Clinical Nephrology

Project Administration Newgen Imaging Systems (P) Ltd
Project Manager Kate Martin
Indexer Newgen Imaging Systems (P) Ltd
Design Manager Andrew Meaden
Publisher Helen Liepman

Editors

Alex M. Davison

Emeritus Professor of Renal Medicine, St James's University Hospital, Leeds, UK

J. Stewart Cameron

Emeritus Professor of Renal Medicine, Guy's, King's and St Thomas' School of Medicine, London, UK

Jean-Pierre Grünfeld

Professor of Nephrology, Hôpital Necker, Faculté de Médecine de Paris 5, Paris, France

Claudio Ponticelli

Professor and Director, Division of Nephrology and Dialysis, Istituto Scientifico Ospedale Maggiore Milano, Milan, Italy

Eberhard Ritz

Emeritus Professor of Nephrology, Department of Internal Medicine, Division of Nephrology, Heidelberg, Germany

Christopher G. Winearls

Consultant Nephrologist, Oxford Radcliffe Hospital, Oxford, UK

Charles van Ypersele

Professor of Medicine, Universite Catholique de Louvain, Cliniques Universitaires Saint-Luc, Brussels, Belgium

Subject Editors

Martin Barratt

Emeritus Professor of Paediatric Nephrology, Institute of Child Health, University College London, London, UK

James M. Ritter

Professor of Clinical Pharmacology, Guy's, King's and St Thomas' School of Medicine, London, UK

Jan Weening

Professor of Renal Pathology, University of Amsterdam, The Netherlands

volume **1**

Oxford Textbook of Clinical Nephrology

Third Edition

Edited by
Alex M. Davison
J. Stewart Cameron
Jean-Pierre Grünfeld
Claudio Ponticelli
Eberhard Ritz
Christopher G. Winearls
and Charles van Ypersele

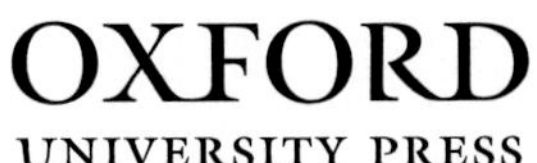
UNIVERSITY PRESS

OXFORD
UNIVERSITY PRESS

Great Clarendon Street, Oxford OX2 6DP

Oxford University Press is a department of the University of Oxford.
It furthers the University's objective of excellence in research, scholarship,
and education by publishing worldwide in

Oxford New York

Auckland Cape Town Dar es Salaam Hong Kong Karachi
Kuala Lumpur Madrid Melbourne Mexico City Nairobi
New Delhi Shanghai Taipei Toronto

With offices in

Argentina Austria Brazil Chile Czech Republic France Greece
Guatemala Hungary Italy Japan South Korea Poland Portugal
Singapore Switzerland Thailand Turkey Ukraine Vietnam

Oxford is a registered trade mark of Oxford University Press
in the UK and in certain other countries

Published in the United States
by Oxford University Press Inc., New York

First edition published 1992
Reprinted (with corrections) 1992
Second edition published 1998
Third edition published 2005

British Library Cataloguing in Publication Data

Data available

Library of Congress Cataloging in Publication Data

ISBN 0 19 856796 0 (volume 1)
0 19 856797 9 (volume 2)
0 19 856798 7 (volume 3)
0 19 850824 7 (set)
available as a set only

10 9 8 7 6 5 4 3 2 1

Typeset by Newgen Imaging Systems (P) Ltd, Chennai, India
Printed in Italy
on acid-free paper by Lego

Summary of contents

Contents

Volume 1

Section 1 Assessment of the patient with renal disease

Section 2 The patient with fluid, electrolyte, and divalent ion disorders

Section 3 The patient with glomerular disease

Index

Volume 2

Section 4 The kidney in systemic disease

Section 8 The patient with renal stone disease

Section 9 The patient with renal hypertension

Section 10 Acute renal failure

Index

Volume 3

Section 11 The patient with failing renal function

Section 12 The patient on dialysis

Section 13 The transplant patient

Preface to the third edition

Seven years after the publication of the second edition of this clinical text many advances in clinical practice justify the publication of a third edition. The text remains primarily a reference for the practising clinician. The chapters of the second edition have been carefully and critically reviewed. The overall framework of the book has been retained. Several previous chapters have been changed and some additions have been made. In line with our previous policy, the Editors have also modified the authorship of several chapters so as to keep the text as fresh as possible. As with previous editions we have, wherever possible, limited authors to two for each chapter. It is not surprising that a new view on a subject brings a different approach but this maintains vitality. In addition, where new concepts develop and new information becomes available, we have included such material—as illustrated by the information about the influence of smoking on renal diseases.

In this edition we have encouraged authors to add appropriate illustrations and to include pathological illustrative material. Wherever possible we have tried to avoid duplication in text, tables, and figures in an effort to maintain a reasonable overall size to the text. Some repetitions are unavoidable, but they have been included to avoid unnecessary cross-references.

In the production of a text of this size there are a number of people to thank for their hard work and devotion. There has been a change in Editors in that Claudio Ponticelli and Charles van Ypersele have joined the Editorial Board in place of David Kerr who has retired. We would like to thank David Kerr most sincerely for his encouragement in the production of this third edition and his invaluable help with the first two editions. Once again thanks go to the Subject Editors who have provided much useful critical advice which has gone a long way in securing authority and currency. Finally our thanks to the production team at Oxford University Press for all they have done towards launching this third edition.

Alex M. Davison
J. Stewart Cameron
Jean-Pierre Grünfeld
Claudio Ponticelli
Eberhard Ritz
Christopher G. Winearls
Charles van Ypersele
October 2004

Preface to the second edition

We have been gratified by the sales and published reviews of the first edition of our clinical text, published in 1992. During the preparation of this second edition all chapters in the first edition were subjected to review by practising nephrologists who were given the specific task of critically commenting on the content and practical value of each chapter. The authors were asked to revise their chapters in the light of the comments and the advances in clinical science since the production of the first edition. In some areas, such as molecular medicine, there have been very significant advances in our understanding of renal disease while in other areas there have been few changes. The challenge was readily accepted by the contributors and we hope that the final result is a thoroughly revised and up-to-date text.

We have retained the prime aim of the first edition—to produce a text of value to those with clinical responsibility for patients with renal disease. The changes we have introduced have been made in order to keep the text fresh; as a matter of policy we have introduced some new chapters and some new authors for existing chapters. The overall structure is unchanged: each section is centred on the patient with a particular disease or syndrome but the order of the sections has been slightly changed to a more logical sequence.

A major change has been the introduction of colour illustrations throughout the text, wherever possible. We greatly appreciate the efforts of chapter authors in finding suitable clinical and pathological illustrative material. We hope that the clinical illustrations will be of particular value to those in training.

It is with great sadness that we record the deaths of four distinguished authors, Professor Claude Amiel of Paris, Dr Ross R. Bailey of Christchurch, New Zealand, Dr A. Gordon Leitch of Edinburgh, and Professor Tony Raine of London. Claude and Tony died after tragic illnesses borne with supreme courage, Ross while swimming, and Gordon suddenly by drowning while trying to save the life of a fellow holiday-maker. Their chapters are a fitting memorial to their lives. We are all diminished by their loss.

The revision of the text could not have been undertaken without the enthusiastic support of a number of people. We would like to record our thanks to our Subject Editors, Martin Barratt (paediatrics), Michael Dunnill (pathology), Rainer Greger (physiology), and James Ritter (pharmacology) and to our Associate Editors, Claudio Ponticelli, Andy Rees, and Charles van Ypersele de Strihou without whose help and expertise this revised text would not have been completed. In addition our thanks are due to Marion Davison for secretarial support and to the staff of Oxford University Press for their devotion in seeing this venture to conclusion.

Alex M. Davison
J. Stewart Cameron
Jean-Pierre Grünfeld
David N.S. Kerr
Eberhard Ritz
and Christopher Winearls
June 1997

Preface to the first edition

Why another large text of nephrology? Because this one is *different*. It begins not with the anatomy of the nephron, but with the approach to the renal patient. It is intended as a text on *clinical nephrology*, of primary use to those caring for patients with renal disease. Not that we do not value the science that underlies our clinical practice—far from it. In each section the basic science relevant to the problem under discussion will be found incorporated at the appropriate point in the text for the clinician. In this area we have had the assistance of one of the foremost renal physiologists.

We deal in this book with many of the rarer renal problems and renal manifestations of systematic disease that are not dealt with in other texts—as a glance at the index and that of other similar volumes will show. A unique feature of the book is that at the end we have provided a guide to the book from the point of view of other specialist physicians—gastroenterologists, rheumatologists, neurologists, and so on—so that both they and generalists can enter the complex world of nephrology more easily. We have paid special attention to the handling of drugs by the kidney, and to the effects of drugs upon the kidney and renal tract. In this we have been assisted by our distinguished editor in clinical pharmacology.

We have tried to look at nephrology in a global context, remembering that the great majority of patients with renal diseases live in the developing world. Several chapters deal specifically with nephrology as it is seen in the tropics. We have also included chapters which deal with renal disease at the extremes of life. Paediatric nephrology has been blended into the text throughout with the assistance of our able paediatric editor, and several chapters deal with the special problems of the growing number of elderly patients with renal disease.

Finally, we hope that these volumes will be, as well as for day-to-day use when needed, a useful and pleasurable source for browsing when the pressure is off. Above all we hope that these volumes will be a literate as well as a comprehensive guide to diseases of the kidney, and diseases affecting the kidney. We thank our Associate Editors Luis Hernando, Claudio Ponticelli, Andy Rees, Charles van Ypersele de Strihou, and C.J. Winearls without whom these volumes could never have been completed.

Stewart Cameron
Alex M. Davison
Jean-Pierre Grünfeld
David Kerr
Eberhard Ritz

Contributors

Daniel Abramowicz Departement Medico-Chirurgical de Nephrologie, Dialyse et Transplantation, Hopital Erasme, Brussels, Belgium
13.2.2 Immunosuppression for renal transplantation

Horacio J. Adrogué Chief, Renal Section, The Methodist Hospital, Professor of Medicine, Baylor College of Medicine, Houston, Texas, USA
2.1 Hypo–hypernatraemia: disorders of water balance
5.4 Renal tubular acidosis

Dwomoa Adu Department of Nephrology, University Hospital Birmingham, Birmingham, UK
4.9 The patient with rheumatoid arthritis, mixed connective tissue disease, or polymyositis
6.3 Non-steroidal anti-inflammatory drugs and the kidney

J.-R. Allenberg Department of Vascular Surgery, University of Heidelberg School of Medicine, Heidelberg, Germany
9.7 Renovascular hypertension

Alessandro Amore Professor of Nephrology, Nephrology Dialysis Transplantation Unit, Ospedale Regina Margherita, Turin, Italy
4.5.2 The nephritis of Henoch–Schönlein purpura
11.3.11 Effect on the immune response

Corinne Antignac INSERM U574 and Department of Genetics, Hôpital Necker—Enfants Malades, Paris, France
16.3 Nephronophthisis

Pierre Aucouturier INSERM E209, Hopital Saint-Antoine, Batiment Raoul Kourilsky 184, Paris, France
4.3 Kidney involvement in plasma cell dyscrasias

Manuel Urrutia Avisrror Professor of Urology, Department of Surgery, University of Salamanca, Salamanca, Spain
18.1 Renal carcinoma and other tumours

Giovanni Banfi Vice-Director, Division of Nephrology, Instituto Scientifico, Ospedale Maggiore di Milano, Milan, Italy
4.7.2 Systemic lupus erythematosus (clinical)

Rashad S. Barsoum Professor of Internal Medicine, Cairo Kidney Center, Antikhana, Bab-El-Louk, Cairo, Egypt
7.4 Schistosomiasis

Chris Baylis Professor of Physiology and Medicine, University of Florida, Gainsville, Florida, USA
15.1 The normal renal physiological changes which occur during pregnancy
15.3 Pregnancy in patients with underlying renal disease

Michel Beaufils Department of Internal Medicine, Hopital Tenon, Paris, France
10.7.2 Pregnancy

Gordon M. Bell Consultant Nephrologist and Clinical Director of Nephrology, Royal Liverpool University Hospital, Liverpool, UK
4.12.1 Substance misuse, organic solvents and kidney disease

Rinaldo Bellomo Department of Intensive Care, Austin & Repatriation Medical Centre, Heidelberg, Victoria, Australia
10.4 Renal replacement methods in acute renal failure

Jo H.M. Berden Professor of Nephrology, Department of Nephrology 545, University Medical Center St Radboud, Nijmegen, The Netherlands
1.8 Immunological investigation of the patient with renal disease

Jaap J. Beutler Consultant Nephrologist, Department of Nephrology and Hypertension, University Medical Centre Utrecht, Utrecht, The Netherlands
1.6.1.vii Isotope scanning

Daniel G. Bichet Professor of Medicine, Universite de Montreal, Canada Research Chair, Genetics in Renal Diseases, Director, Clinical Research Unit, Hospital du Sacre-Coeur de Montréal, Montréal, Québec, Canada
5.6 Nephrogenic diabetes insipidus

Carol M. Black Professor of Rheumatology, Centre for Rheumatology, Royal Free & University College London Medical School, Royal Free Campus, London, UK
4.8 The patient with scleroderma—systemic sclerosis

Guillaume Bobrie Unite d'hypertension arterielle, Hopital Europeen Georges Pompidou, Paris, France
16.4.3 Nail-patella syndrome and other rare inherited disorders with glomerular involvement

Paola Boccardo Mario Negri Institute for Pharmacological Research, Bergamo, Italy
11.3.12 Coagulation disorders

Jürgen Bommer Klinikum der Universitat Heidelberg, Sektion Nephrologie, Heidelberg, Germany
11.3.3 Sexual disorders

Michael Boulton-Jones Renal Unit, Walton Building, Royal Infirmary, Glasgow, UK
4.2.1 Amyloidosis

J. Douglas Briggs 48 Kingsborough Gardens, Glasgow, UK
13.3.3 Long-term medical complications

J. Trevor Brocklebank Reader in Paediatric Nephrology, Department of Paediatrics, Clinical Science Building, St James's University Hospital, Leeds, UK
10.7.1 Infants and children

Nilufer Broeders Hopital Erasme, Brussels, Belgium
13.2.2 Immunosuppression for renal transplantation

Alison L. Brown Consultant Nephrologist, Freeman Hospital, High Heaton, Newcastle-upon-Tyne, UK
9.2 Clinical approach to hypertension

Michael Broyer Group Hospitalier, Hopital Necker-Enfants Malades, Paris, France
16.5.1 Cystinosis

Vincenzo Cambi Cattedra di Nefrologia, Ospedale Maggiore, Parma, Italy
12.1 Dialysis strategies

J. Stewart Cameron Emeritus Professor of Renal Medicine, Guy's, King's, and St Thomas' School of Medicine, London, UK
1.5 The ageing kidney
3.3 The patient with proteinuria and/or haematuria
3.4 The nephrotic syndrome: management, complications, and pathophysiology
6.4 Uric acid and the kidney
14.2 Chronic renal failure in the elderly
16.5.3 Inherited disorders of purine metabolism and transport
16.7 Some rare syndromes with renal involvement
17.5 Medullary sponge kidney

José M. Campistol Renal Transplant Unit, Hospital Clinic, University of Barcelona, Barcelona, Spain
10.6.4 Acute renal failure in liver disease

Marco Cappelletti Radiologist, Viale Scarampo, Milan, Italy
1.6.2.v Living donor workup

Ruggero Caputo Director, Institute of Dermatological Sciences, University of Milan, IRCCS Osperdale Maggiore, Milan, Italy
11.3.13 Dermatological disorders

Andrés Cárdenas Instructor in Medicine, Division of Gastroenterology and Hepatology, Beth Israel Deaconess Medical Center, Harvard Medical School, Boston, Massachusetts, USA
10.6.4 Acute renal failure in liver disease

D.J.S. Carmichael Consultant Nephrologist, Southend General Hospital, Pricklewood Chase, Westcliff on Sea, Essex, UK
19.2 Handling of drugs in kidney disease

Ralph Caruana Professor of Medicine, Vice Dean for Clinical Affairs, Medical College of Georgia, Augusta, Georgia, USA
4.11 The patient with sickle-cell disease

Michael J.D. Cassidy Clinical Director, Renal and Transplant Unit, Nottingham City Hospital NHS Trust, Nottingham, UK
11.2 Assessment and initial management of the patient with failing renal function

W.R. Cattell 30 Tavistock Terrace, London, UK
7.1 Lower and upper urinary tract infections in the adult

Daniel Cattran University Health Network, Toronto General Hospital, Toronto, Ontario, Canada
3.7 Membranous nephropathy

Dominique Chauveau Service de Néphrologie, Hôpital Necker, Paris, France
16.2.2 Autosomal-dominant polycystic kidney disease

Paramit Chowdhury Department of Nephrology, King's College London, London, UK
9.5 Ischaemic nephropathy
10.6.5 Ischaemic renal disease

Y. Chrétien Radiotherapie, Hopital europeen Georges-Pompidou, Paris, France
1.6.1.iii Percutaneous nephrostomy and ureteral stenting

Kirpal S. Chugh Emeritus Professor of Nephrology, National Kidney Clinic and Research Centre, Chandigarh, India
3.14 Glomerular disease in the tropics
10.7.3 Acute renal failure in the tropical countries

Pierre Cochat Professor of Pediatrics/Head Renal Unit, Department of Pediatrics, Hopital Edouard Herriot, Universite Claude-Bernard, Lyon, France
16.5.2 The primary hyperoxalurias

Fredric L. Coe Professor of Medicine and Physiology, University of Chicago School of Medicine, Chicago, Illinois, USA
8.2 The medical management of stone disease

Eric P. Cohen Professor of Medicine, Nephrology Division, Medical College of Wisconsin, Milwaukee, Wisconsin, USA
6.6 Radiation nephropathy

Rosanna Coppo Ospedale Regina Margherita, Nefrologia, Dialisi e Trapianto, Turin, Italy
3.6 IgA nephropathies
4.5.2 The nephritis of Henoch–Schönlein purpura
11.3.11 Effect on the immune response

Catherine M. Corbishley Consultant Histopathologist, Department of Cellular Pathology, St George's Hospital, London, UK
7.3 Renal tuberculosis and other mycobacterial infections

François Cornud Consultant Radiologist, Hospital Cochin, Paris, France
1.6.1.iii Percutaneous nephrostomy and ureteral stenting

Jean-Michel Correas Vice Chairman, Service de Radiologie, Hôpital Necker, Paris, France
1.6.1.i Ultrasound
1.6.2.ii Hypertension and suspected renovascular disease
1.6.2.iv Renal masses
1.6.2.vi Transplant dysfunction

J.P. Cosyns Professor of Clinical Pathology, Department of Pathology, Medical School, Cliniques Universitaires Saint-Luc, Universite Catholque de Louvain, Brussels, Belgium
6.7 Balkan nephropathy
6.8 Chinese herbs (and other rare causes of interstitial nephropathy)

Malcolm G. Coulthard Department of Paediatric Nephrology, Royal Victoria Infirmary, Newcastle-upon-Tyne, UK
7.2 Urinary tract infections in infancy and childhood

Vincenzo D'Intini Divisione Nefrologia, Ospedale San Bortolo, Vicenza, Italy
10.4 Renal replacement methods in acute renal failure

André Noël Dardenne Associate Professor of Radiology, Universite Catholique de Louvain, Cliniques Universitaires Saint-Luc, Brussels, Belgium
1.6.1.v CT scanning and helical CT

Markus Daschner Pediatric Nephrologist, University Children's Hospital, Heidelberg, Germany
11.3.2 Endocrine disorders

Andrew Davenport Consultant Nephrologist/Honorary Senior Lecturer, Centre for Nephrology, Royal Free Campus, Royal Free and University College Medical School, London, UK
11.3.14 Neuropsychiatric disorders

Salvatore David Cattedra di Nefrologia, Ospedale Maggiore, Parma, Italy
12.1 Dialysis strategies

Alex M. Davison Emeritus Professor of Renal Medicine, St James's University Hospital, Leeds, UK
1.1 History and clinical examination of the patient with renal disease
3.12 Infection related glomerulonephritis
3.13 Malignancy-associated glomerular disease

John M. Davison School of Surgical and Reproductive Sciences, Department of Obstetrics & Gynaecology, Medical School, Newcastle-upon-Tyne, UK
15.1 The normal renal physiological changes which occur during pregnancy
15.2 Renal complications that may occur in pregnancy
15.3 Pregnancy in patients with underlying renal disease

Marc E. De Broe Department of Nephrology, University Hospital Antwerp, Edegem/Antwerp, Belgium
6.2 Analgesic nephropathy
6.5 Nephrotoxic metals
19.1 Drug-induced nephropathies

John M.H. De Klerk Consultant in Nuclear Medicine, Department of Nuclear Medicine, University Centre Utrecht, Utrecht, The Netherlands
1.6.1.vii Isotope scanning

Rita De Smet Department of Nephrology, University Hospital, Ghent, Belgium
11.3.1 Uraemic toxicity

Peter R.F. Dear Regional Neonatal Intensive Care Unit, St James's University Hospital, Leeds, UK
1.4 Renal function in the newborn infant

Christopher P. Denton Clinical Research Fellow, Academic Unit of Rheumatology, Royal Free Hospital School of Medicine, University of London, London, UK
4.8 The patient with scleroderma—systemic sclerosis

Robert J. Desnick Professor and Chairman, Department of Human Genetics, Mount Sinai School of Medicine, New York, USA
16.4.2 Fabry disease

Olivier Devuyst Division of Nephrology, UCL Medical School, (Universite Catholique de Louvain), Brussels, Belgium
16.2.2 Autosomal-dominant polycystic kidney disease

Ralf Dikow Sektion Nephrologie, Heidelberg, Germany
4.1 The patient with diabetes mellitus
9.6 Hypertension and unilateral renal parenchymal disease
9.8 Malignant hypertension
11.3.4 Hypertension
14.3 The diabetic patient with impaired renal function

John H. Dirks Chair, ISN COMGAN, President, The Gairdner Foundation, Senior Fellow, Massey College, University of Toronto, Toronto, Ontario, Canada
2.5 Hypo–hypermagnesaemia

Ciaran Doherty Regional Nephrology Unit, Belfast City Hospital, Belfast, UK
10.1 Epidemiology of acute renal failure
11.3.6 Gastrointestinal effects

Raymond A.M.G. Donckerwolcke Professor and Chairman, Department of Paediatrics, University Hospital Maastricht, Maastricht, The Netherlands
3.4 The nephrotic syndrome: management, complications, and pathophysiology

Sven Dorph Department of Radiology, Helsingor Hospital, Helsingor, Denmark
1.6.2.i Haematuria, infection, acute renal failure, and obstruction

Dominique Droz Service d'Anatomie Pathologique, Hopital Saint-Louis, Paris, France
10.6.2 Acute tubulointerstitial nephritis

Tilman B. Drüeke INSERM Unit 507 and Division of Nephrology, Hopital Necker, Paris, France
11.3.9 Skeletal disorders

I. Dulau-Florea Schwabing General Hospital, Ludwig Maximilians University, Munich, Germany
9.7 Renovascular hypertension

John B. Eastwood Consultant Renal Physician and Reader in Medicine, Department of Renal Medicine, and Transplantation, St George's Hospital, London, UK
7.3 Renal tuberculosis and other mycobacterial infections

Kai-Uwe Eckardt Department of Nephrology and Medical Intensive Care, Charité, Campus Virchow Klinikum, Berlin, Germany
11.3.8 Haematological disorders

Lisette El Hajj Hôpital de Rangueil, Service Central d Radiologie, Toulouse, France
1.6.1.iv Renal arteriography

A. Meguid El Nahas Professor of Nephrology, Sheffield Kidney Institute, Sheffield teaching Hospitals NHS Trust, Northern General Hospital, Sheffield, UK
11.1 Mechanisms of experimental and clinical renal scarring

Marlies Elger Abteilung Nephrologie, Forschungszentrum der Medizinischen Hochschule, am Oststadtkrankenhaus, Hannover, Germany
3.1 The renal glomerulus—the structural basis of ultrafiltration

Paul Emery ARC Professor of Rheumatology, Molecular Medicine Unit, School of Medicine, Leeds, UK
4.9 The patient with rheumatoid arthritis, mixed connective tissue disease, or polymyositis

Karlhans Endlich Assistant Professor, Department of Anatomy and Cell Biology, University of Heidelberg, Heidelberg, Germany
9.1 The structure and function of blood vessels in the kidney

John Feehally Department of Nephrology, Leicester General Hospital, Leicester, UK
3.2 Glomerular injury and glomerular response

Terry Feest The Richard Bright Renal Unit, Southmead Hospital, Westbury-on-Trym, Bristol, UK
1.9 The epidemiology of renal disease

J.D. Firth Consultant Physician and Nephrologist, Addenbrooke's Hospital, Cambridge, UK
10.3 The clinical approach to the patient with acute renal failure

Maggie Fitzpatrick Consultant Paediatric Nephrologist, Department of Paediatrics Nephrology, St James's Hospital, Leeds, UK
1.1 History and clinical examination of the patient with renal disease
10.7.1 Infants and children

Jürgen Floege Medizinische Klinik II der RWTH, Aachen, Germany
3.2 Glomerular injury and glomerular response

Giovanni B. Fogazzi Divisione di Nefrologia e Dialisi, Oespadele Maggiore, IRCCS, Milan, Italy
1.2 Urinalysis and microscopy

Robert N. Foley Department of Medicine, Hennepin County Medical Center, Minneapolis, Minnesota, USA
11.3.5 Cardiovascular risk factors

Gérard Friedlander Professor and Chief, INSERM U 426, Department of Physiology, Xavier Bichat Medical Faculty, Paris, France
1.3 The clinical assessment of renal function
2.4 Hypo–hyperphosphataemia

Marie-France Gagnadoux Pediatric Nephrologist, Necker-Enfants Malades, Paris, France
16.2.1 Polycystic kidney disease in children

Gillian Gaskin Renal Section, Division of Medicine, Faculty of Medicine, Imperial College, Hammersmith Hospital, London, UK
4.5.3 Systemic vasculitis

Pere Ginès Associate Professor of Medicine, Liver Unit, Institut de Malalties Digestives, Hospital Clinic, University of Barcelona, Barcelona, Spain
10.6.4 Acute renal failure in liver disease

Matthias Girndt Assistant Professor of Internal Medicine and Nephrology, Medical Department IV, University of Saarland, Homburg, Germany
11.3.7 Liver disorders

Sven Glaesker Department of Nephrology, Clinics of the Albert Freiburg University, Freiburg, Germany
16.6 Renal involvement in tuberous sclerosis and von Hippel–Lindau disease

Griet Glorieux Nephrology Department, University Hospital Ghent, Ghent, Belgium
11.3.1 Uraemic toxicity

Ram Gokal Consultant Nephrologist, Honorary Professor of Medicine, Manchester Royal Infirmary, Manchester, UK
12.4 Peritoneal dialysis and complications of technique

David S. Goldfarb Associate Professor of Medicine and Physiology, New York University School of Medicine, Nephrology/111G, NY Department of Veterans Affairs Medical Centre, New York, USA
8.2 The medical management of stone disease

John M. Grange Visiting Professor, Royal Free and University College Medical School, Windeyer Institute for Medical Science, London, UK
7.3 Renal tuberculosis and other mycobacterial infections

Ian A. Greer Deputy Dean—Faculty of Medicine, Regius Professor—Obstetrics and Gynaecology, University of Glasgow, Glasgow Royal Infirmary, Glasgow, UK
15.4 Pregnancy-induced hypertension

Rainer Greger Physiologisches Institut, Albert-Ludwigs-Universität, Freiburg, Germany
19.3 Action and clinical use of diuretics

Jean-Pierre Grünfeld Professor of Nephrology, Hôpital Necker, Faculté de Médecine de Paris 5, Paris, France
1.1 History and clinical examination of the patient with renal disease
16.4.1 Alport's syndrome
16.4.2 Fabry disease
16.4.3 Nail-patella syndrome and other rare inherited disorders with glomerular involvement
16.7 Some rare syndromes with renal involvement

Marie-Claire Gubler INSERM U574, Hôpital Necker—Enfants Malades, Paris, France
16.3 Nephronophthisis
16.5.1 Cystinosis

Sanjeev Gulati Department of Nephrology, Sanjay Gandhi Postgraduate Institute of Medical Sciences, Lucknow, India
3.8 Mesangiocapillary glomerulonephritis

Krishan Lal Gupta Additional Professor of Nephrology, Postgraduate Institute of Medical Education and Research, Chandigarh, India
7.5 Fungal infections and the kidney

Suresh K. Gupta 46 Glebe Avenue, Grappenhal, Warrington, UK
8.3 The surgical management of renal stones

Kenneth R. Hallows Assistant Professor, Renal-Electrolyte Division, Department of Medicine, University of Pittsburgh School of Medicine, Pittsburgh, Pennsylvania, USA
2.2 Hypo–hyperkalaemia

Neveen A.T. Hamdy Head Clinic Section, Department of Endocrinology & Metabolic Diseases, Leiden University Medical Center, Leiden, The Netherlands
2.3 Hypo–hypercalcaemia

Barrie Hartley Department of Pathology, St James's University Hospital, Leeds, UK
3.13 Malignancy-associated glomerular disease

George B. Haycock Consultant in Paediatrics, Guy's, King's, and St Thomas' Hospital, London, UK
5.2 Isolated defects of tubular function

August Heidland Department of Internal Medicine, University of Wurzburg, Kuratorium für Dialysis und Nierentransplantation, Wurzburg, Germany
19.3 Action and clinical use of diuretics

Olivier Hélénon Chairman, Service de Radiologie, Hôpital Necker, Paris, France
1.6.1.i Ultrasound
1.6.1.iii Percutaneous nephrostomy and ureteral stenting
1.6.2.ii Hypertension and suspected renovascular disease
1.6.2.iv Renal masses
1.6.2.vi Transplant dysfunction

Udo Helmchen Department of Pathology, Universitätsklinikum Hamburg-Eppendorf, Hamburg, Germany
9.4 The effects of hypertension on renal vasculature and structure

Elizabeth Petri Henske Fox Chase Cancer Center, 7701 Burholme Avenue, Philadelphia, Pennsylvania, USA
16.6 Renal involvement in tuberous sclerosis and von Hippel–Lindau disease

Lukas B. Hilbrands University Medical Centre Nymegen, Department of Nephrology, Nijmegen, The Netherlands
13.1 Selection and preparation of the recipient

Friedhelm Hildebrandt Professor of Pediatrics and Human Genetics, Huetwell Professor for the Cure and Prevention of Birth Defects, Department of Pediatrics, University of Michigan, Ann Arbor, Michigan, USA
16.1 Strategies for the investigation of inherited renal disease

Andries J. Hoitsma Division of Nephrology, University Medical Center St Radboud, Nijmegen, The Netherlands
13.1 Selection and preparation of the recipient

Christer Holmberg Hospital for Children and Adolescents, University of Helsinki, Helsinki, Finland
16.4.4 Congenital nephrotic syndrome

Matthew L.P. Howse Link 6C, Royal Liverpool University Hospital, Liverpool, UK
4.12.1 Substance misuse, organic solvents and kidney disease

Othon Iliopoulos MGH Cancer Center, Massachusetts General Hospital, Boston, Massachusetts, USA
16.6 Renal involvement in tuberous sclerosis and von Hippel–Lindau disease

Enrico Imbasciati Director, Division of Nephrology, Ospedale Maggiore di Lodi, Lodi, Italy
1.7 Renal biopsy: indications for and interpretation

David A. Isenberg Centre for Rheumatology, Royal Free and University College Hospital, London, UK
4.7.1 The pathogenesis of systemic lupus erythematosus

Claude Jacobs Groupe hospitalier Pitié-Salpêtrière, Service de nephrologie, Paris, France
12.6 Medical management of the dialysis patient

Michel Jadoul Cliniques Universitaires St Luc, Department of Nephrology, Brussels, Belgium
11.3.10 β2M Amyloidosis

Hannu Jalanko Hospital for Children and Adolescents, University of Helsinki, Helsinki, Finland
16.4.4 Congenital nephrotic syndrome

Vivekanand Jha Associate Professor, Department of Nephrology, Postgraduate Institute of Medical Education and Research, Chandigarh, India
3.14 Glomerular disease in the tropics
10.7.3 Acute renal failure in the tropical countries

Francis G. Joffre Hôpital de Rangueil, Service Central d Radiologie, Toulouse, France
1.6.1.iv Renal arteriography

Kate Verrier Jones KRUF Children's Kidney Centre for Wales, University of Wales, College of Medicine, Heath Park, Cardiff, UK
17.2 Vesicoureteric reflux and reflux nephropathy

Nicola Joss Renal Unit, Walton Building, Royal Infirmary, Glasgow, UK
4.2.1 Amyloidosis

Islam Junaid Consultant Urologist and Transplant Surgeon, Department of Renal Medicine & Transplantation, The Royal London Hospital, Whitechapel, London, UK
17.3 The patient with urinary tract obstruction

Brian Junor Consultant Nephrologist, Renal Unit, Western Infirmary, Glasgow, UK
13.3.5 Outcome of renal transplantation

Cees G.M. Kallenberg Department of Clinical Immunology, University Hospital Groningen, Groningen, The Netherlands
4.5.1 Pathogenesis of angiitis

John A. Kanis Sheffield Metabolic Bone Unit, Sheffield, UK
2.3 Hypo–hypercalcaemia

Alexandre Karras Service de Néphrologie et Transplantation Rénale, Hopital Saint-Louis, Paris, France
10.6.2 Acute tubulointerstitial nephritis

Akira Kawashima Professor of Radiology, Mayo Clinic College of Medicine, Department of Radiology, Mayo Clinic, Rochester, Minnesota, USA
1.6.1.ii Plain radiography, contrast radiography, and excretion radiography
1.6.1.vi Magnetic resonance imaging

Vijay Kher Department of Nephrology, Indraprastha Apollo Hospitals, New Delhi, India
3.8 Mesangiocapillary glomerulonephritis

Bernard F. King, Jr. Mayo School of Graduate Medical Education, Department of Radiology, Mayo Clinic, Rochester, Minnesota, USA
1.6.1.vi Magnetic resonance imaging

Bertrand Knebelmann Hôpital Necker, Paris, France
16.4.1 Alport's syndrome

Nine V.A.M. Knoers University Hospital Nijmegen, Nijmegen, The Netherlands
5.5 Hypokalaemic tubular disorders

Karl-Martin Koch Medizinische Hochschule Hannover, Zentrum Innere Medizin und Dermatologie, Abteilung Nephrologie, NHH, Hannover, Germany
12.3 Haemodialysis, haemofiltration, and complications of technique

Hans Köhler Universitätskliniken des Saarlandes, Medizinische Klinik und Poliklinik, Medical Department IV, University of Saarland, Homburg, Germany
11.3.7 Liver disorders

Hein A. Koomans Professor of Nephrology and Head of Department of Nephrology and Hypertension, Department of Nephrology, University Centre Utrecht, Utrecht, The Netherlands
1.6.1.vii Isotope scanning

Stephen M. Korbet Professor of Medicine, Rush University Medical Center, Chicago, Illinois, USA
4.2.2 Fibrillary and immunotactoid glomerulopathy

Wilhelm Kriz Professor and Chairman, Institute of Anatomy and Cell Biology, University of Heidelberg, Heidelberg, Germany
3.1 The renal glomerulus—the structural basis of ultrafiltration

B. Krumme Department of Nephrology, Deutsche Klinik fur Diagnostick, Wiesbaden, Germany
9.7 Renovascular hypertension

Heather J. Lambert Department of Paediatric Nephrology, Royal Victoria Infirmary, Newcastle-upon-Tyne, UK
7.2 Urinary tract infections in infancy and childhood

Norbert Hendrik Lameire Renal Division, University Hospital Ghent, Ghent, Belgium
10.2 Acute renal failure: pathophysiology and prevention
10.7.4 The elderly
11.3.1 Uraemic toxicity

Florian Lang Department of Physiology, University of Tubingen, Tubingen, Germany
19.3 Action and clinical use of diuretics

Andrew J. LeRoy Associate Professor of Radiology, Mayo Clinic College of Medicine, Department of Radiology, Mayo Clinic, Rochester, Minnesota, USA
1.6.1.ii Plain radiography, contrast radiography, and excretion radiography

Philippe Lesavre Service de Nephrologie, Hôpital Necker, Paris, France
3.12 Infection related glomerulonephritis

Jeremy Levy Consultant Nephrologist and Physician, Imperial College, Hammersmith Hospital, London, UK
3.10 Crescentic glomerulonephritis

Edmund J. Lewis Professor of Medicine, Rush University Medical Center, Chicago, Illinois, USA
4.2.2 Fibrillary and immunotactoid glomerulopathy

Gerhard Lonnemann Department of Nephrology, Medical School, Hannover, Germany
12.3 Haemodialysis, haemofiltration, and complications of technique

Iain C. Macdougall The Renal Unit, King's College Hospital, London, UK
11.3.8 Haematological disorders

Nicolaos E. Madias Chairman, Department of Medicine, Caritas St Elizabeth's Medical Center and Professor of Medicine, Tufts University School of Medicine, Boston, Massachusetts, USA
2.1 Hypo–hypernatraemia: disorders of water balance
5.4 Renal tubular acidosis

J.F.E. Mann Krankenhaus Monchen Schwabing, Munich, Germany
9.7 Renovascular hypertension

A.M. Marinaki Purine Research Unit, Guy's Hospital, London Bridge, London, UK
16.5.3 Inherited disorders of purine metabolism and transport

Frank Martinez Service de Néphrologie et Transplantation Rénale, Hopital Saint-Louis, Paris, France
10.6.2 Acute tubulointerstitial nephritis

Angelo Valerio Marzano Assistant Dermatologist, Institute of Dermatological Sciences, University of Milan, IRCCS Osperdale Maggiore, Milan, Italy
11.3.13 Dermatological disorders

L.J. Mason Research Assistant, Centre for Rheumatology, University College London, Windeyer Institute of Medical Sciences, London, UK
4.7.1 The pathogenesis of systemic lupus erythematosus

Philip D. Mason Consultant Nephrologist, Oxford Kidney Unit, Churchill Hospital, Headington, Oxford, UK
10.6.1 Glomerulonephritis, vasculitis, and the nephrotic syndrome

Arnaud Méjean Service d'Urologie, Paris, France
1.6.2.iv Renal masses
1.6.2.vi Transplant dysfunction

Jean-Philippe Méry 59 rue Madame, Paris, France
4.4 The patient with sarcoidosis

Alain Meyrier Hôpital Europeen Georges-Pompidou, Paris, France
3.5 Minimal change and focal–segmental glomerular sclerosis

Michael J. Mihatsch Director, Institute for Pathology, University of Basel, Basel, Switzerland
1.7 Renal biopsy: indications for and interpretation

Robert D. Mills Consultant Urologist, Norfolk & Norwich University Hospital, Norwich, UK
18.4 Tumours of the bladder

Christopher Mitchell Paediatric Haematology/Oncology Unit, The John Radcliffe Hospital, Headington, Oxford, UK
18.2 Wilms' tumour

Leo A.H. Monnens Department of Pediatrics, University Hospital Nijmegen, Nijmegen, The Netherlands
5.5 Hypokalaemic tubular disorders

Emmanuel Morelon Department on Transplantation, Hôpital Necker, Universite Paris V, Paris, France
1.6.2.vi Transplant dysfunction

Stephen H. Morgan Basildon Hospital, Nether Mayne, Basildon, UK
16.4.2 Fabry disease

Gabriella Moroni Assistant Nephrologist, Division of Nephrology, Instituto Scientifico, Ospedale Maggiore di Milano, Milan, Italy
4.7.2 Systemic lupus erythematosus (clinical)

Béatrice Mougenot Pathologist, Hôpital Tenon, Paris, France
4.3 Kidney involvement in plasma cell dyscrasias

Claudia A. Müller Section Transplantation Immunology, ZMF, Tubingen, Germany
6.1 Mechanisms of interstitial inflammation

Gerhard A. Müller Universitätsklinikum/Innere Medizin, Abteilung für Nephrologie und Rheumatologie, Göttingen, Germany
6.1 Mechanisms of interstitial inflammation

Robert G. Narins Director of Postgraduate Education, American Society of Nephrology, Washington, DC, USA
2.6 Clinical acid–base disorders

Guy H. Neild Institute of Urology and Nephrology, Middlesex Hospital, London, UK
10.6.3 Acute renal failure associated with microangiopathy (haemolytic–uraemic syndrome and thrombotic thrombocytopenic purpura)

Hartmut P.H. Neumann Medizinische Universitätsklinik, Freiburg im Breisgau, Germany
16.6 Renal involvement in tuberous sclerosis and von Hippel–Lindau disease

Simon J. Newell Regional Neonatal Intensive Care Unit, St James's University Hospital, Leeds, UK
1.4 Renal function in the newborn infant

Chas G. Newstead Department of Renal medicine, St James's University Hospital, Leeds, UK
13.3.4 Recurrent disease and de novo disease

Patrick Niaudet Nephrologie Paediatrique, Hospital Necker-Enfants Malades, Paris, France
3.5 Minimal change and focal–segmental glomerular sclerosis

Michael Nicholson Division of Transplant Surgery, Leicester General Hospital, Leicester, UK
13.3.1 Surgery and surgical complications

Juan F. Macías-Núñez Unidad de Hipertension, Hospital Universitario de Salamanca, Salamanca, Spain
1.5 The ageing kidney
14.2 Chronic renal failure in the elderly

Christopher Olbricht Klinik fur Nieren-und Hochdruckkrankheiten, Katharine Hospital, Stuttgart, Germany
12.3 Haemodialysis, haemofiltration, and complications of technique

Stephan R. Orth Dialysis Centre Schwandorf, Schwandorf, Germany
4.12.2 Smoking and the kidney

Kazuo Ota Director, Ota Medical Research Institute, Chouo-ku, Tokyo, Japan
12.2 Vascular access

Edgar Otto Research Investigator, Department of Pediatrics, University of Michigan, Ann Arbor, Michigan, USA
16.1 Strategies for the investigation of inherited renal disease

Biff F. Palmer Professor of Internal Medicine, Department of Internal Medicine, Division of Nephrology, University of Texas Southwestern Medical School, Dallas, Texas, USA
2.6 Clinical acid–base disorders

Vicente Arroyo Pérez Institute of Digestive Diseases, Hospital Clinic 1 Provincial de Barcelona, Barcelona, Spain
10.6.4 Acute renal failure in liver disease

Phuong-Chi T. Pham Assistant Clinical Professor of Medicine, Division of Nephrology, Department of Medicine, David Geffen School of Medicine at UCLA, Los Angeles, California, USA
13.3.2 The early management of the recipient

Phuong-Thu T. Pham Assistant Clinical Professor of Medicine, Division of Nephrology, Kidney Transplant Program, David Geffen School of Medicine at UCLA, Los Angeles, California, USA
13.3.2 The early management of the recipient

Yves Pirson Department of Nephrology, University of Louvain Medical School, Cliniques Universitaires St Luc, Faculté de médecine, Brussels, Belgium
16.2.2 Autosomal-dominant polycystic kidney disease

Wolfgang Pommer Director, Department of Internal Medicine—Nephrology, Vivantes Humboldt Klinikum, Berlin, Germany
6.2 Analgesic nephropathy

Claudio Ponticelli Professor and Director, Division of Nephrology and Dialysis, Istituto Scientifico Ospedale Maggiore Milano, Milan, Italy
1.6.2.iii Renal biopsy—procedure and complications
1.6.2.v Living donor workup
1.7 Renal biopsy: indications for and interpretation
4.7.2 Systemic lupus erythematosus (clinical)
11.3.13 Dermatological disorders

Dominique Prié Assistant Professor INSERM U 426, Department of Physiology, Xavier Bichat Medical Faculty, Paris, France
1.3 The clinical assessment of renal function

Charles D. Pusey Renal Section, Division of Medicine, Imperial College, Hammersmith Hospital, London, UK
3.10 Crescentic glomerulonephritis

Uwe Querfeld Director, Pediatric Nephrology, Department of Pediatric Nephrology, Charité Campus, Virchow Klinkum Children's Hospital, Berlin, Germany
14.1 Chronic renal failure in children

Wolfgang Rascher Professor of Pediatrics, Head and Chairman, Department of Pediatrics, Erlangen, Germany
9.9 The hypertensive child
17.4 Congenital abnormalities of the urinary tract

Andrew J. Rees Regius Professor of Medicine, University of Aberdeen, Institute of Medical Sciences, Foresterhill, Aberdeen, UK
3.11 Antiglomerular basement disease

Giuseppe Remuzzi Division of Nephrology and Dialysis, Ospedali Riuniti di Bergamo, Mario Negri Institute for Pharmacological Research, Bergamo, Italy
11.3.12 Coagulation disorders

Eberhard Ritz Emeritus Professor of Nephrology, Department of Internal Medicine, Division of Nephrology, Heidelberg, Germany
4.1 The patient with diabetes mellitus
9.8 Malignant hypertension
11.3.4 Hypertension
11.3.5 Cardiovascular risk factors
11.3.9 Skeletal disorders
14.3 The diabetic patient with impaired renal function

Paul J. Roderick Senior Lecturer in Public Health Medicine, Applied Clinical Epidemiology Group, Community Clinical Sciences Research Division, School of Medicine, University of Southampton, Southampton, UK
1.9 The epidemiology of renal disease

Bernardo Rodríguez-Iturbe Professor of Medicine and Chief of Nephrology, Hospital Universitario, Universidad del Zulia and Director, Instituto de Investigaciones Biomedicas, Maracaibo, Venezuela
3.9 Acute endocapillary glomerulonephritis

Marie-Odile Rolland Laboratoire de Biochimie Pediatrique, Hospitalk Debrousse, Lyon, France
16.5.2 The primary hyperoxalurias

Claudio Ronco Director, Department of Nephrology, St Bortolo Hospital, Vicenza, Italy
10.4 Renal replacement methods in acute renal failure

Pierre M. Ronco Renal Department and INSERM, Unité 489, Hôpital Tenon, Paris, France
4.3 Kidney involvement in plasma cell dyscrasias

Wolfgang H. Rösch Kinderurologische Abteilung der Universität Regensburg, In der Klinik St Hedwig, Regensburg, Germany
17.4 Congenital abnormalities of the urinary tract

Luis M. Ruilope Univdad de Hipertension, Hospital 12 de Octubre, Madrid, Spain
9.3 The kidney and control of blood pressure

Rémi Salomon INSERM U574 and Department of Pediatric Nephrology, Hôpital Necker—Enfants Malades, Paris, France
16.3 Nephronophthisis

John Savill Professor of Medicine, Vice Principal and Head of the College of Medicine & Veterinary Medicine, University of Edinburgh, Edinburgh, UK
3.2 Glomerular injury and glomerular response

Franz Schaefer Division of Pediatric Nephrology, University Children's Hospital, Heidelberg, Germany
11.3.2 Endocrine disorders

Francesco Paolo Schena University of Bari, Renal Unit, Policlinico, Bari, Italy
3.6 IgA nephropathies

Michael Schömig Sektion Nephrologie, Heidelberg, Germany
9.6 Hypertension and unilateral renal parenchymal disease

Melvin M. Schwartz Professor of Pathology, Rush University Medical Center, Chicago, Illinois, USA
4.2.2 Fibrillary and immunotactoid glomerulopathy

John E. Scoble Department of Renal Medicine and Transplantation, Guy's Hospital, London, UK
9.5 Ischaemic nephropathy
10.6.5 Ischaemic renal disease

Katarina Sebekova Institute of Preventive and Clinical Medicine, Bratislava, Slovakia
19.3 Action and clinical use of diuretics

Günter Seyffart Head, Dialysis Center, Bad Homburg, Germany
10.5 Dialysis and haemoperfusion treatment of acute poisoning

David G. Shirley Research Fellow and Honorary Reader, Royal Free & University College Medical School, London, UK
5.1 The structure and function of tubules

Caroline Silve Senior Investigator, INSERM U 426, Department of Physiology, Xavier Bichat Medical Faculty, Paris, France
2.4 Hypo–hyperphosphataemia

H. Anne Simmonds Purine Research Unit, Guy's Hospital, London Bridge, London, UK
6.4 Uric acid and the kidney
16.5.3 Inherited disorders of purine metabolism and transport

Visith Sitprija Director, Queen Saovabha Memorial Institute, Thai Red Cross Society, Patumwan, Bangkok, Thailand
10.7.3 Acute renal failure in the tropical countries

Philip H. Smith 2 Creskeld Lane, Bramhope LS16 9AW, UK
18.5 Tumours of the prostate

John S. Smyth Department of Renal Medicine, Guy's, St Thomas' NHS Trust, London, UK
10.6.5 Ischaemic renal disease

Patrick G.J.F. Starremans Department of Paediatrics & Cell Physiology, University of Nijmegen, Nijmegen, The Netherlands
5.5 Hypokalaemic tubular disorders

Vladisav Stefanović Professor of Medicine, Institute of Nephrology and Haemodialysis, University School of Medicine, University of Niš, Niš, Yugoslavia
6.7 Balkan nephropathy

Coen A. Stegeman Associate Professor of Nephrology, Department of Nephrology, University Hospital Groningen, Groningen, The Netherlands
4.5.1 Pathogenesis of angiitis

Henk Stevens Consultant in Nuclear Medicine, Department of Nuclear Medicine, University Centre Utrecht, Utrecht, The Netherlands
1.6.1.vii Isotope scanning

Terry B. Strom Professor of Medicine, Harvard Medical School, Chief, Division of Immunology, BI-Deaconess Medical Center, Boston, Massachusetts, USA
13.2.1 The immunology of transplantation

Frank Strutz Universitätsklinikum/Innere Medizin, Abteilung für Nephrologie und Rheumatologie, Göttingen, Germany
6.1 Mechanisms of interstitial inflammation

Manikkam Suthanthiran Chief, Nephrology and Transplantation Medicine, Stanton Griffis Distinguished Professor of Medicine, Cornell University Medical College, New York, USA
13.2.1 The immunology of transplantation

Dante Tagliavini Cattedra di Nefrologia, Ospedale Maggiore, Parma, Italy
12.1 Dialysis strategies

Richard L. Tannen University of Pennsylvania School of Medicine, Philadelphia, Pennsylvania, USA
2.2 Hypo–hyperkalaemia

Antonio Tarantino Divisione Di Nefrologia, Ospedale Maggiore, IRCCS, Milan, Italy
4.6 The patient with mixed cryoglobulinaemia and hepatitis C infection

James Tattersall Department of Nephrology, St James's University Hospital, Leeds, UK
12.5 Adequacy of dialysis

C. Mark Taylor Department of Nephrology, Birmingham Children's Hospital, Birmingham, UK
10.6.3 Acute renal failure associated with microangiopathy (haemolytic–uraemic syndrome and thrombotic thrombocytopenic purpura)

Hans-Göran Tiselius Professor of Urology, Department of Urology, Huddinge University Hospital, Stockholm, Sweden
8.1 Aetiological factors in stone formation

Wai Y. Tse Department of Nephrology, Derriford Hospital, Plymouth, UK
6.3 Non-steroidal anti-inflammatory drugs and the kidney

A. Neil Turner Professor of Nephrology, University of Edinburgh, Renal & Autoimmunity Group, Royal Infirmary, Edinburgh, UK
3.2 Glomerular injury and glomerular response
3.11 Antiglomerular basement disease

William H. Turner Consultant Urologist, Addenbrooks NHS Trust, Cambridge, UK
18.4 Tumours of the bladder

Robert J. Unwin St Peter's Professor of Nephrology, Centre for Nephrology, Royal Free and University College Medical School, London, UK
5.1 The structure and function of tubules

Seppo Vainio Department of Biochemistry, University of Oulu, Linnanmaa, Finland
17.1 The development of the kidney and renal dysplasia

Bernard E. Van Beers Professor of Radiology, Universite Catholique de Louvain, Cliniques Universitaires Saint-Luc, Brussels, Belgium
1.6.1.v CT scanning and helical CT

Nele Van Den Noortgate Department of Internal Medicine, Division of Geriatric Medicine, Ghent University Hospital, Ghent, Belgium
10.7.4 The elderly

Charles van Ypersele Professor of Medicine, Universite Catholique de Louvain, Cliniques Universitaires Saint-Luc, Brussels, Belgium
6.8 Chinese herbs (and other rare causes of interstitial nephropathy)
10.6.6 Hantavirus infection
11.3.10 β2M Amyloidosis

William G. van't Hoff Consultant Paediatric Nephrologist, Great Ormond Street Hospital for Children, NHS Trust, London, UK
5.3 Fanconi syndrome
8.5 Renal and urinary tract stone disease in children

Raymond Camille Vanholder Nephrology Department, University Hospital Ghent, Ghent, Belgium
10.2 Acute renal failure: pathophysiology and prevention
10.7.4 The elderly
11.3.1 Uraemic toxicity

Patrick J.W. Venables Kennedy Institute of Rheumatology, Faculty of Medicine, The Charing Cross Hospital Campus, Arthritis Research Campaign Building, London, UK
4.10 The patient with Sjögren's syndrome and overlap syndromes

Christoph Wanner Department of Medicine, Division of Nephrology, University Hospital, Würzburg, Germany
11.3.4 Hypertension

Richard P. Wedeen Professor of Medicine, Professor of Preventive Medicine and Community Health, UMDNJ—New Jersey Medical School and Associate Chief of Staff for Research and Development, Department of Veterans Affairs New Jersey Health Care System, East Orange, New Jersey, USA
6.5 Nephrotoxic metals

Pieter M. Ter Wee Department of Nephrology, Vrije Universiteit Academic Medical Center, Amsterdam, The Netherlands
11.2 Assessment and initial management of the patient with failing renal function

Richard B. Weiner Clinical Assistant Professor of Psychiatry, SUNY Health Sciences Center at Brooklyn and Director, Children's Psychiatric Impatient Unit, Division of Child and Adolescent Psychiatry, Kings County Hospital Center, Brooklyn, New York, USA
12.7 Psychological aspects of treatment for renal failure

Ulrich Wenzel Department of Medicine, Division of Nephrology, Universitätsklinikum Hamburg-Eppendorf, Hamburg, Germany
9.4 The effects of hypertension on renal vasculature and structure

Jack F.M. Wetzels University Medical Center St Radboud, Division of Nephrology 545, Nijmegen, The Netherlands
1.8 Immunological investigation of the patient with renal disease

Peter Whelan Department of Urology, St James's University Hospital, Leeds, UK
18.3 Tumours of the renal pelvis and ureter

Hugh Whitfield Department of Urology, Battle Hospital, Reading, Berkshire, UK
8.3 The surgical management of renal stones

Alan H. Wilkinson Professor of Medicine, Director Kidney & Kidney/Pancreas Transplantation, David Geffen School of Medicine, University of California at Los Angeles, Los Angeles, California, USA
13.3.2 The early management of the recipient

Robert Wilkinson Department of Nephrology, The Freeman Hospital, High Heaton, Newcastle-upon-Tyne, UK
9.2 Clinical approach to hypertension

K. Martin Wissing Departement Medico-Chirurgical de Nephrologie, Dialyse et Transplantation, Hopital Erasme, Brussels, Belgium
13.2.2 Immunosuppression for renal transplantation

Oliver Wrong University College London, Department of Nephrology, Middlesex Hospital, London, UK
8.4 Nephrocalcinosis

Muhammad Magdi Yaqoob Professor and Lead Consultant in Nephrology, Department of Renal Medicine & Transplantation, The Royal London Hospital, Whitechapel, London, UK
17.3 The patient with urinary tract obstruction

Jerry Yee Division Head, Division of Nephrology and Hypertension, Department of Medicine, Henry Ford Hospital, Detroit, Michigan, USA
2.6 Clinical acid–base disorders

Michael Zellweger Nephrology Fellow, Research Center, Hôpital du Sacré-Coeur de Montréal, Montréal, Québec, Canada
5.6 Nephrogenic diabetes insipidus

Carla Zoja Mario Negri Institute for Pharmacological Research, Bergamo, Italy
11.3.12 Coagulation disorders

1

Assessment of the patient with renal disease

1.1 History and clinical examination of the patient with renal disease

Alex M. Davison, Jean-Pierre Grünfeld, and Maggie Fitzpatrick

Introduction

Effective management of patients with renal disease is dependent upon establishing an accurate diagnosis. The clinician must be aware of the possible presentations of renal diseases and the constellation of symptoms and signs that form recognized disease syndromes. It is essential to obtain a detailed history relating to the presenting symptoms, past history, family history, and social history. The need for specific, detailed documentation of exposure to environmental factors, such as chemicals, which may be encountered at work or during recreation, is being increasingly recognized and full details of all recent medications must be obtained. Following this, a thorough examination should be undertaken, paying particular attention to those clinical signs that are known to reflect underlying renal disease. Finally, a structured investigative approach should be formulated to obtain maximum information with minimum inconvenience to the patient. In this way, unnecessary investigations are avoided and the most cost-effective use is made of available resources. Thereafter a plan can be formulated for effective management and follow-up.

The nephrologist is particularly privileged because, unlike other organs, the kidney can be effectively replaced by dialysis or transplantation. This, however, poses unique problems as it raises social and ethical issues, which have to be considered in the integrated management of the patient. This chapter, devoted to history and clinical examination of the patient, is not intended to be comprehensive, but rather an overview, and the reader is referred throughout to the relevant chapters for a detailed discussion of individual syndromes.

Clinical presentation of renal disease

The patient with renal disease may come to the attention of the clinician for one of several reasons.

1. The patient is asymptomatic, but an abnormality has been detected on clinical or laboratory examination.
2. The patient complains of a symptom or has physical signs which directly or indirectly indicates underlying renal disease.
3. The patient has a systemic disease that is known to be associated with renal involvement.
4. The patient has a family history of an inherited renal disorder.

Asymptomatic patients

Asymptomatic patients are most commonly detected following routine investigations such as urine analysis, blood pressure measurement, biochemical analyses following hospital admission, or as part of a health screening programme (see Chapter 3.3). In some patients, renal disease is detected during clinical examination for health insurance, occupational purposes, or during pregnancy. In a small number of instances, there is regular screening in view of a known association between an employment and development of renal disease, for example, aniline dye workers have a greater than normal incidence of urothelial tumours. Asymptomatic patients may be detected as a result of investigation of family members following the diagnosis of a familial renal disease. It will be appreciated therefore that the detection of asymptomatic patients depends on many factors, including the policy with respect to regular medical screening in particular age groups, such as at school entry and/or school leaving. It will also depend to a certain extent on chance, as not all occupations require pre-employment medical examinations and not all patients undergo medical examinations for insurance purposes. To some extent, this may well explain purported differences in the incidence of various forms of renal disease reported from different countries.

Symptomatic patients

Symptomatic renal disease most commonly presents as a disorder of micturition, urine volume or composition, pain, oedema, or symptoms related to impairment of renal function.

Disorders of micturition

The most common disorder of micturition is frequency, a term used to indicate that the bladder is emptied more often than normal. This may be associated with an increased urine volume (polyuria; see below) or with a normal urine volume. The latter results from irritation of the bladder by inflammation, stone, or tumour; from a reduction in the bladder capacity as a consequence of fibrotic contraction, as, for example, fibrosis following radiotherapy to pelvic organs; or external pressure from a pelvic mass or gravid uterus. In many, frequency will be accompanied by nocturia. In patients with frequency, it is important to determine whether there is a normal volume of urine at each bladder emptying, or whether only small quantities are passed. The former indicates increased urine formation; the latter indicates bladder dysfunction. Nocturia may arise from sleep disturbances, normally sleep stimulates antidiuretic hormone (ADH) secretion, with a consequent diminution in urine volume. Patients who lie awake at night do not have increased ADH secretion, and in the recumbent position, have increased renal blood flow with consequent increased urine volume and subsequent nocturia.

Men past middle age frequently have prostatic enlargement, which characteristically causes the urinary stream to be poor. There may also be some difficulty in initiating micturition (hesitancy) or in stopping (terminal dribbling). Eventually, the enlargement may cause complete urethral obstruction resulting in urinary retention. In a number of patients with prostatic hypertrophy, there is retention and back pressure, reducing flow in the nephrons, thus interfering with the ability of the medulla to maintain a concentration gradient. This results in impairment of urinary concentration, and consequently, increased urine volume. Paradoxically, therefore, some patients with developing obstruction may present with increased urine output, and this may falsely reassure the patient and clinician, resulting in late diagnosis (see Chapter 17.3).

Dysuria is pain or discomfort during micturition. This is usually described as a burning or tingling sensation felt in the urethra or in the suprapubic area during or immediately after micturition. It is usually a consequence of bladder, prostatic, or urethral inflammation (see Section 7). When associated with frequency and urgency of micturition, it indicates cystitis, particularly common in young women and often related to sexual activity. In older women or in men, there is usually an underlying condition, such as a structural abnormality of the bladder or prostate. In men, perineal or rectal pain suggest inflammation of the prostate.

Disorders of urine volume

Disorders of urinary volume consist of polyuria, where the volume is increased, oliguria, where the urine volume is diminished, and anuria, where there is an absence of urine.

Polyuria may be due to: (a) an excess intake of fluid such as in compulsive water drinking; (b) an increase in tubular solute load, as with urea in chronic renal failure, glucose from hyperglycaemia, or low molecular weight proteins in myeloma; (c) a diminution in ADH production, which may occur following trauma to the head or tumours or infections of the hypothalamus or pituitary; (d) disordered medullary concentration gradient as a consequence of medullary disease such as nephrocalcinosis, analgesic nephropathy, renal papillary necrosis, medullary cystic disease, or sickle cell disease; or (e) conditions that impair the tubular response to ADH, such as hypercalcaemia, potassium depletion, and a rare inherited form of tubular insensitivity to ADH, called congenital nephrogenic diabetes insipidus (see Chapter 5.5).

Oliguria describes a reduction in urine volume to less than that required for the excretion of the residues from normal daily metabolic functions. Under extreme conditions, homeostasis can usually be maintained with a daily urine output of 500 ml, thus in the adult a urinary output of less than 400 ml per day would constitute oliguria. This usually indicates an underlying acute renal failure whether from prerenal causes, vascular, glomerular, tubular, or interstitial diseases.

Anuria, the absence of any urine output, indicates obstruction of the urinary tract, although rarely it may arise from renal infarction or cortical necrosis. In a patient with anuria, there must be careful examination of the lower abdomen; rectal examination and abdominal ultrasound are mandatory investigations. Patients with pelvic malignancies, such as carcinoma of the cervix or rectum, may present with anuria due to the tumour spreading laterally to the pelvic wall, causing external compression of the lower ureter.

Alteration in urinary composition (see also Chapter 1.2)

Visible haematuria may arise from any part of the renal tract from the glomerulus to the urethra and may be due to conditions such as glomerulonephritis, infection, calculi, or tumours. However, it may indicate thrombocytopenia, disordered coagulation, or may occur as a result of anticoagulant drugs. Not all discoloured urine is due to the presence of blood (Table 1), and factitious causes must be considered.

In some patients, haematuria is detectable only on microscopic examination or by chemical testing (microscopic haematuria); in others, it is visible to the naked eye (macroscopic haematuria) and may be even sufficient to produce clots. Blood arising from the glomerulus frequently gives rise to a red-brown discolouration of the urine, which is sometimes described as 'smokey' or likened to tea or coca cola. In some patients, macroscopic haematuria is only intermittent; such recurrent haematuria is common in IgA nephropathy where episodes are closely associated with mucosal inflammation (frequently of the respiratory tract), and may last for 1–3 days. Between episodes, microscopic haematuria is usually present, although in children the urine may clear completely. Blood arising from the urethra is dislodged by the urinary flow and appears only in the initial urinary stream. Bleeding from the bladder and prostatic bed is, however, more commonly noticed at the end of micturition and described as terminal haematuria. Transient haematuria is common in people following extensive jogging and is almost universal during marathon running. Some patients present with haemospermia, and this is usually indicative of a prostatic problem or a bleeding diathesis. Overall, however, the most common cause of haematuria, both micro- and macroscopic, is infection in the urinary tract (see Section 7).

Proteinuria is usually determined chemically, although some patients will have noticed that their urine appears frothy. A small amount of protein is normally present (up to 150 mg/24 h, or a urinary protein/creatinine ratio of <130) and more than 50 per cent of this is tubular in origin (see Chapter 3.3). Urine screening for protein is usually undertaken by a 'stix' test, but it must be remembered that this test does not detect light chains. In such patients, a negative test in the presence of a positive sulfosalicylic acid test is a useful diagnostic aid. In some patients, minor degrees of proteinuria may be present (1 g/24 h), without being of any pathological significance. In others, proteinuria is related to posture, being absent in the urine passed immediately on

Table 1 Differential diagnosis of red/brown urine

Haematuria
Haemoglobinuria
Myoglobinuria
Urates
Porphyria
Alkaptonuria (homogentisic acid)
Drugs[a] Analgesics: phenacetin, antipyrine Antibiotics: rifampicin, metronidazole, nitrofurantoin Anticoagulants: phenindione, warfarin Anticonvulsants: phenytoin
Vegetable dyes Beetroot and some berries (anthocyanins) Paprika Food colouring materials

[a] Many more have been described in occasional case reports.

rising in the morning, but being present after the subject has been up and about for some time. This is described as orthostatic or postural proteinuria and is usually benign. In some subjects, proteinuria is only present following exercise or associated with hypertension.

Pathological proteinuria may indicate glomerular or interstitial disease. Generally, that arising from interstitial disease is mild, up to 2 g daily (although rarely nephrotic range proteinuria has been described), that from glomerular disease is variable, up to 10 g or more daily. In some instances, the type of proteinuria is diagnostic, for example 'selective' proteinuria in minimal lesion glomerulonephritis (see Chapter 3.5), Bence Jones proteinuria in myeloma (see Chapter 4.3).

Bacteriuria may be symptomatic or asymptomatic. Bladder urine is normally sterile, but the urethra, and particularly the urethral meatus is not sterile, and urine may become contaminated during micturition. For this reason, bacteriuria is usually only considered significant if the number of bacteria in a midstream specimen of properly collected urine exceed 105 organisms per millilitre (see Section 7).

Leucocyturia—the presence of white blood cells in the urine—occurs in a number of conditions such as nephrocalcinosis, papillary necrosis, and analgesic nephropathy. Eosinophils may be detected in the urine in tubulointerstitial nephritis of immunoallergic origin.

Pyuria is always considered significant and indicative of infection. Sterile pyuria should always raise the possibility of underlying tuberculosis, but this also occurs in chlamydial infections.

Occasionally, small pieces of tissue may be passed in the urine and these may arise from papillary necrosis or tumours. Other patients may pass small pieces of material which have entered the bladder as a consequence of a vesicocolonic fistula.

Pneumaturia indicates a communication between the urinary and alimentary tracts, most commonly as a consequence of diverticular disease or carcinoma of the colon.

Pain

Pain is an inconsistent symptom of renal disease, but when present, most commonly represents inflammation or obstruction. Inflammation of the kidney, in the form of pyelonephritis, causes pain localized to the renal angle on the side of the affected kidney. It develops gradually and is variable in severity but is usually constant in nature. A perirenal abscess can give symptoms related to diaphragmatic irritation if the abscess tracks upwards and to psoas muscle irritation if it tracks downwards. Glomerular inflammation is usually asymptomatic, but may be associated with a dull lumbar ache, particularly in acute glomerulonephritis and IgA-associated nephropathy.

Some patients present with an intermittent dull aching loin pain, variable in severity, and associated with visible haematuria. This has been termed the loin pain haematuria syndrome. Renal biopsy yields unremarkable findings apart from complement (C3) deposition in the walls of afferent arterioles (Fig. 1) (Naish *et al.* 1975), the significance of which is not clear. In addition, renal angiography may reveal focal or generalized vascular lesions of tortuosity, beading, stenosis, or occlusion, sometimes associated with cortical infarcts (Burden *et al.* 1975).

Pain arising from an acute obstruction is usually sudden in onset, severe and colicky in nature, radiating to the groin or scrotum. Chronic obstruction may, however, be remarkably asymptomatic. It is important to emphasize that significant renal destruction can occur without any pain or discomfort and in many patients the first symptoms relate to the metabolic consequences of severely impaired kidney function (Fig. 2).

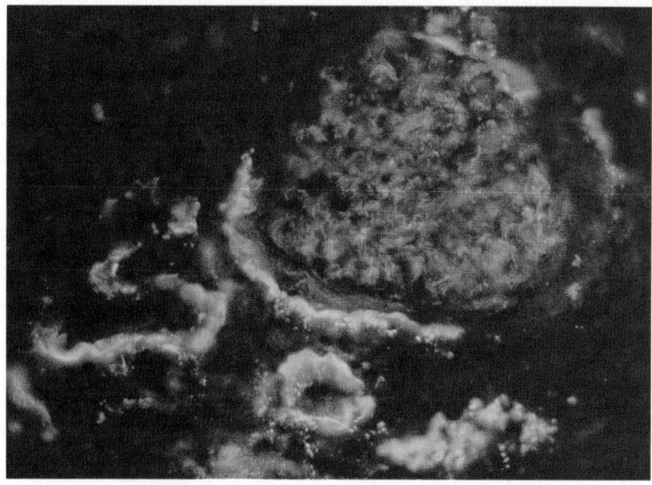

Fig. 1 Complement (C3) deposition in the afferent arteriole of a renal biopsy from a patient with loin pain and haematuria syndrome. (Immunofluorescence with FITC labelled antiserum to complement C3.) Kindly provided by Dr P.F. Naish.

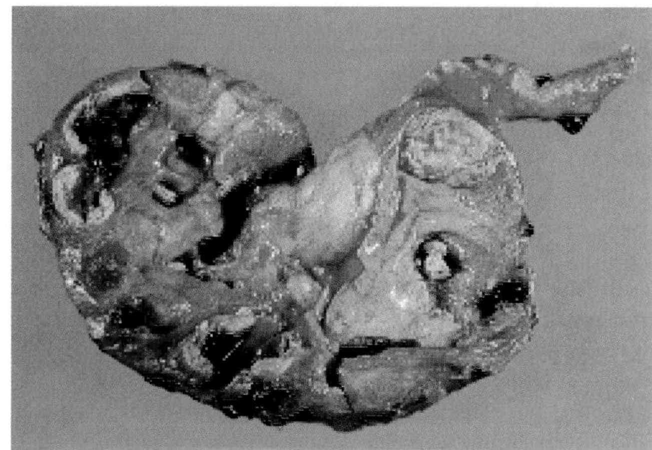

(a)

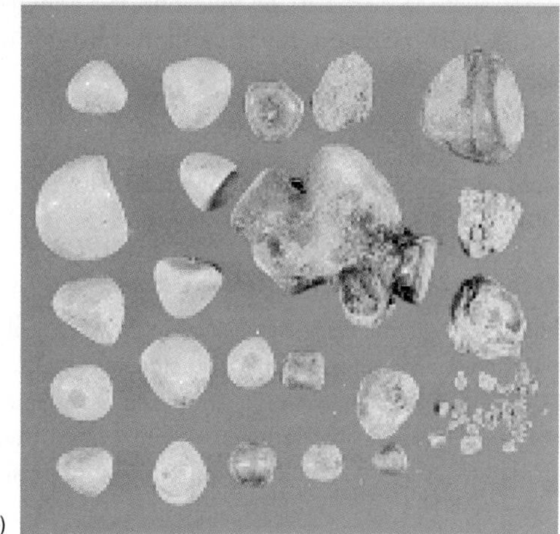

(b)

Fig. 2 (a) Autopsy specimen of a kidney from a patient who died in terminal renal failure from systemic oxalosis and who was asymptomatic and working as a heavy goods vehicle driver until one week prior to death from a cardiac arrest. (b) The multiple stones recovered from one of the kidneys of the patient described in (a).

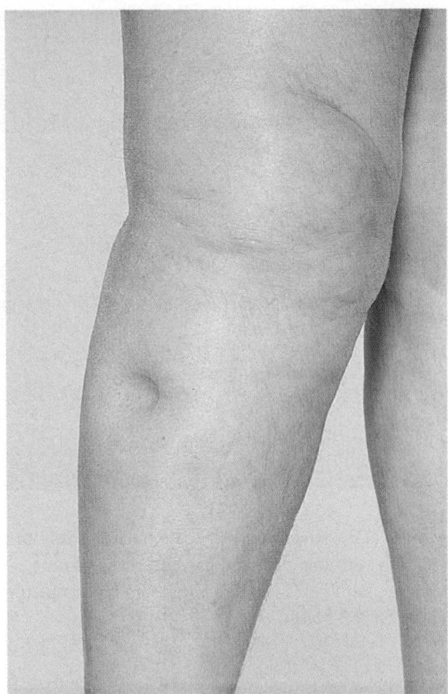

Fig. 3 Marked peripheral oedema of the lower limb. The pitting oedema is obvious distal to the knee.

Oedema

Oedema may arise due to the hypoproteinaemia, which is a consequence of significant proteinuria (in adults the prolonged daily excretion of 3.5 g). This is termed the nephrotic syndrome (see Chapters 3.3 and 3.4) and the oedema is usually most noticeable around the eyes in the morning, and in the feet and ankles in the evening. With increasing severity, this diurnal change is lost and the patient notices more generalized swelling throughout the day (Fig. 3).

Oedema may occur as a consequence of salt and water retention in patients with chronic renal failure, congestive cardiac failure, chronic hepatic disease such as cirrhosis, or following the administration of certain drugs, such as non-steroidal anti-inflammatory drugs or calcium-channel antagonists.

Impairment of renal function

Some patients present with symptoms of uraemia due to chronic impairment of renal function (see Sections 10 and 11).

Renal disease associated with systemic disease

Many patients with systemic disease (see Section 4) have renal disease, and this may become manifest before, coincidentally with, or subsequent to the diagnosis of the systemic condition. As a general rule, however, the occurrence or development of renal impairment in a patient with systemic disease is indicative of a worse prognosis.

Specific clinical syndromes

Asymptomatic proteinuria

This is the chance detection of proteinuria during a medical examination such as, for example, at school, for life insurance purposes, or for employment. Protein excretion is usually less than 3.5 g daily and may represent 'physiological' proteinuria, which is either orthostatic or exercise-induced, or pathological proteinuria due to glomerular, tubular, or interstitial disease.

The nephrotic syndrome

This is a consequence of hypoproteinaemia, which develops as a result of prolonged heavy proteinuria (see Chapters 3.4 and 3.5).

Acute nephritic syndrome

Haematuria, proteinuria, oliguria, and hypertension are diagnostic of this syndrome. Poststreptococcal glomerulonephritis is one example and occurs some 10–20 days following infection (see Chapter 3.9). It may also be due to an acute exacerbation of a chronic glomerular disease such as IgA nephropathy. The syndrome is due to immune complex formation with consequent activation of the complement and coagulation systems, giving rise to an inflammatory response.

Microscopic haematuria

This is usually detected at routine clinical examination and may be due to bleeding from any part of the renal tract. Red cells originating from the glomerulus usually have a dysmorphic appearance and/or are present as red cell casts. The more normal the microscopic appearance of red cells the more likely it is that bleeding originates from the lower tract.

Recurrent haematuria

Intermittent episodes of macroscopic haematuria are referred to as recurrent haematuria. Commonly, this occurs at the time of mucosal inflammation in patients with IgA nephropathy, or rarely in patients with Alport's syndrome, but it may be the result of intermittent bleeding from a structural lesion such as a tumour or polycystic kidney disease.

Hypertension

Patients with glomerular disease are frequently hypertensive; raised blood pressure is seen less frequently in tubular or interstitial conditions. Accelerated or severe hypertension may be a feature of systemic sclerosis (see Chapter 4.8). Severe hypertension is particularly common, but not invariable, in the late stages of chronic renal failure (see Section 9).

Acute renal failure

An acute reduction in renal function may be prerenal, renal, or postrenal in origin (see Section 10).

Chronic renal failure

A host of non-specific symptoms is usually present, none of which individually indicates an underlying renal problem. When taken together, however, the symptoms point to a widespread metabolic abnormality (see Section 11).

Clinical history

History of presenting complaint

The first step in a clinical interview should be to elicit the patient's symptoms in a clear, chronological order. Many patients, particularly when being interviewed for the first time, are anxious and tense and it is worth spending some time making the patient feel at ease prior to starting the interview. Patients should be encouraged to describe their symptoms in their own words and if they use diagnostic terms, they should be asked to explain in detail what they mean; for example, a patient may use the term 'cystitis' to indicate dysuria, frequency, nocturia, or foul-smelling urine. In some instances, the patient will previously have sought medical opinion and will reiterate the previously postulated diagnosis, which may or may not be correct. It is sometimes only with the most careful probing that the exact nature of the underlying symptom is determined. Wherever possible, precise dates should be obtained, but many have a poor recall for chronological events.

Enquiry must be made relating to associated symptoms, but frequently patients will omit what they consider to be insignificant unless asked directly, for example, the presence of upper respiratory tract symptoms at the time of macroscopic haematuria. It is thus important to ask patients about any activity being undertaken at the time of or immediately before the development of symptoms, to establish relationships between, for example, exercise and haematuria, or sexual activity and dysuria. It should be remembered, however, that patients may falsely attribute symptoms with an associated event, and caution must be undertaken when interpreting the information gained.

Pain is possibly the most common reason for a patient seeking medical opinion. It is important to determine the site of the pain and whether it is localized, or is diffuse. The mode of onset is important; a gradually increasing pain is suggestive of inflammation whereas sudden severe onset suggests ureteric obstruction. In addition, the clinician must determine whether the pain radiates and, if so, whether this follows any recognized pathway. The character of the pain should be determined, although many patients find this difficult to describe. A pain that waxes and wanes may be indicative of a colic and may cause the patient to be restless, whereas a steady pain such as that from pyelonephritis may cause the patient to remain still to avoid aggravation by movement. Factors that are known to precipitate or aggravate the pain should be determined, as well as those measures which cause relief. Although enquiry is frequently made regarding severity of pain, it is usually very difficult for the patient to describe this.

In patients with haematuria and/or proteinuria, it is important to establish whether previous urine analyses have been undertaken. In some instances, the patients will know the results; if not, a careful review of the records of prior hospital attendances may well provide much useful information. In any event, it is important to obtain the results of any previously arranged investigations, as these can be of value in dating the onset of a particular illness.

A history of hypertension may be closely related to renal disease and it is important to document the date of diagnosis and subsequent complications, as well as efficacy, tolerance, and patient compliance with prescribed therapy.

The rate of progression of various forms of renal disease is variable, and can frequently only be assessed by retrospective analysis. Slowly progressive renal failure may extend over years or decades, in contrast to the rapid deterioration, which may be due to crescentic glomerulonephritis. Patients with chronic renal failure may have an acute deterioration related to dehydration, urinary tract obstruction, drug toxicity, the development of an accelerated phase of hypertension, or to hypotension induced by excessive antihypertensive therapy.

Thus, in obtaining the history of the present complaint, it is important to determine all the factors surrounding the particular illness and care should be taken to ensure that each symptom is fully described and documented in a proper chronological order.

Past history

In many renal diseases, and particularly in chronic renal failure, the past history is of particular relevance. Wherever possible, this should be documented in as much detail as can be obtained and should include childhood as well as adolescence and all major illnesses and hospital admissions.

A large number of conditions may be associated with renal involvement, directly, indirectly, or as a complication of treatment. In this introductory text, it is impossible to cover all of them, and a few examples will be used for illustrative purposes. A long-standing condition, such as lupus erythematosus, may initially be confined to skin or joints and only later affect the kidneys. Other conditions, such as chronic sepsis from either bronchiectasis or osteomyelitis, may be complicated by amyloidosis. Finally, patients with rheumatoid arthritis may be treated with a variety of agents such as analgesics, gold, or penicillamine, all of which may result in renal damage.

A number of metabolic diseases may eventually cause renal problems. For instance, hyperparathyroidism may manifest as unexplained abdominal pain and bone problems; these may precede the development of renal calculi. Similarly, diabetes mellitus of either type may be associated with the development of diabetic glomerulosclerosis. This most commonly develops after 10 years of known diabetes mellitus, but can occur surprisingly early following diagnosis, particularly of the maturity-onset type (see Chapter 4.1).

When constructing the past history, it is not uncommon to find that the patient's memory is unreliable, and every effort should be made to resort to previous medical notes, whether from the family physician or from hospital attendances. The past history is not only important with respect to achieving a diagnosis, but is also of value when drug treatment is being considered. For instance, in hypertensive patients it is important to avoid the use of β-blockers in patients with a history of asthma. Similarly, centrally acting antihypertensive drug should be avoided in patients with a history of depression. In other circumstances, therapy can only be introduced with the concomitant use of prophylactic drugs: for example, H:2-receptor blocking drugs such as ranitidine should be given to patients with a history of peptic ulceration who require steroid therapy.

Gynaecological and obstetric history (see Section 15)

In women, it is important to obtain details of menstrual history, contraception, and pregnancy. The menarche may be delayed in patients with impaired renal function. Some with renal failure may develop amenorrhoea, although in some, particularly older patients, menorrhagia may occur due to abnormalities of coagulation and/or platelet function. Heavy and prolonged menstrual bleeding, a common aggravating factor of anaemia, may be considerably improved by progesterone treatment. Underlying renal disease significantly increases the risk of hypertension with the combined oestrogen–progesterone contraceptive; this may not be reversible.

Pregnancy may be associated with aggravation or initiation of renal disease. Hypertension may develop, while pre-existing hypertension may be exacerbated. In obtaining a history, therefore, the course of blood pressure throughout pregnancy should be ascertained, together with details of drug therapy and whether or not hypertension was complicated by proteinuria and whether the pregnancy proceeded to term. Commonly, patients with proteinuria have increased urinary protein excretion during pregnancy, and this may be sufficient to produce a nephrotic syndrome. In such patients, it is difficult to differentiate between pre-eclampsia and previously asymptomatic glomerular disease.

Pregnancy predisposes to urinary tract infection, particularly of the upper tract. Bacteriuria is common, but symptomatic upper urinary tract infections usually indicate a structural abnormality requiring detailed investigations after delivery.

Recurrent fetal loss may indicate the presence of antiphospholipid antibodies (lupus anticoagulant) and should raise the possibility of underlying systemic lupus erythematosus. Details of parturition should be obtained, particularly with respect to the term and circumstances of delivery and the weight and Apgar score of the neonate. Acute renal failure developing shortly after delivery may indicate a form of haemolytic–uraemic syndrome, which is sometimes irreversible (Robson *et al.* 1968).

Drug history

Recent drug intake should be carefully noted with respect to the first day of administration, dosage, and duration. A single tablet or dose of a large variety of drugs may be sufficient to induce an acute allergic interstitial nephritis. In contrast, interstitial nephritis induced by ingestion of non-steroidal anti-inflammatory agents may develop after several months of administration. Elderly patients, who often use non-steroidal anti-inflammatory drugs to relieve articular pain, are highly susceptible to the adverse effects on the kidney. Furthermore, these patients are at risk of drug toxicity for many reasons, including the reduction of renal function with age, changes in pharmacokinetics, the common association of other organ impairment (such as borderline heart failure), and the frequent use of several drugs which may interact.

Hypoproteinaemia may reduce drug binding to plasma proteins resulting in an increased availability of 'free' drug and increasing the potential for toxicity. It must also be remembered that corticosteroids, particularly in pulse form, may affect drug binding plasma to proteins resulting in an increase in the free or unbound portion.

Hypotensive drugs may cause a deterioration in renal function, particularly in patients with renovascular disease or when the blood pressure is lowered precipitously. In addition, angiotensin-converting enzyme inhibitors may produce profound renal failure in patients with undiagnosed bilateral renovascular disease or vascular disease, such as severe atheroma, in a solitary kidney.

Information on chronic drug intake is important. Long-term renal and tubulointerstitial toxicity of analgesics has been clearly demonstrated, and similar nephrotoxicity has been described with regard to lithium. Other drugs (gold salts or D-penicillamine) may induce reversible glomerular changes.

In addition to exerting direct toxic effects on the kidney, some drugs elevate blood pressure (Table 2). The possibility of drug-induced or aggravated hypertension should be considered in all hypertensive patients (Grossman and Messerli 1995). Hypertension is most frequently associated with oestrogen–progesterone compounds (hypertension may be moderate, accelerated, or associated with the haemolytic–uraemic syndrome), corticosteroids, cyclosporin, and liquorice. With regard to the last, hypertension is probably not related to the mineralocorticoid activity of liquorice *per se*, but to its inhibition of 11-hydroxysteroid dehydrogenase activity (Stewart *et al.* 1987).

Table 2 Drug-induced hypertension

1. Steroid-mediated hypertension
   - Corticosteroids (mainly in patients with pre-existent renal failure)
   - Oestroprogestative pills or oestrogens (oral administration)
   - Mineralocorticoids (9α-fluoroprednisolone by nasal spray or antihaemorrhoid cream)
   - Androgen derivatives (danazol)
   - Liquorice intoxication
2. Hypertension mediated by sympathomimetic drugs
   - Isoproterenol
   - Various sympathomimetic drugs in nasal or eye drops or in anorectic preparations (such as phenylpropanolamine)
   - Monoamineoxidase inhibitor associated with sympathomimetic drug or tyramine-rich food
   - Sulpiride, metoclopramide, haloperidol, methylergometrine, tricyclic derivatives (such as imipramine) in very rare cases
3. Cyclosporin-associated hypertension (increased incidence in patients also receiving steroids)
4. Erythropoietin
   - In dialysis patients, particularly those with a history of previous hypertension

Finally, it should be emphasized that the extrarenal side-effects of many drugs are increased in patients with renal diseases and caution should be exercised in the use of any recent drug for which medical experience is limited. In some cases, a toxic effect may be predicted on a pathophysiological basis. For example lovastatin, an HMG-CoA reductase inhibitor may induce rhabdomyolysis, particularly in patients treated with cyclosporin or gemfibrozil. Lovastatin-induced myositis may severely aggravate hyperkalaemia in diabetic patients with mild renal failure receiving an angiotensin converting enzyme inhibitor (Edelman and Witztum 1989).

Many patients do not relate medicines that they can buy without prescription, commonly referred to as 'over-the-counter drugs', to drugs that are prescribed by medical practitioners. Careful enquiry about use of non-prescription drugs, particularly analgesics and non-steroidal anti-inflammatory drugs is always useful. Similarly, details need to be obtained regarding herbal remedies, particularly Chinese herbs, as some may contain contaminants that may cause interstitial nephritis (see also Chapter 6.8).

Clinicians should also be aware of covert drug intake, especially of laxatives or diuretics, or surreptitious vomiting in emotionally labile women. These patients experience severe potassium depletion or recurrent oedema on drug withdrawal, leading to the incorrect belief that diuretics are required for the so-called 'idiopathic oedema syndrome' and resulting in a perpetuation of drug intake (MacGregor *et al.* 1975; MacGregor and de Wardener 1988).

Dietary history

A dietetic history can be of diagnostic value as well as being of importance in patient management, particularly in the presence of renal failure. The help and advice of a skilled dietitian is frequently required.

Excessive sodium intake may account for resistance to antihypertensive therapy or for recurrent pulmonary oedema in patients with advanced renal failure. In contrast, sudden and excessive sodium restriction or increased sodium loss through the skin or gastrointestinal tract may precipitate severe hypovolaemia in a patient with salt-losing nephropathy.

Idiopathic stone formers ingest more animal protein than normal subjects; such a diet is associated with increased urinary excretion of calcium, oxalate, and uric acid, known risk factors for calcium stone formation (see Chapter 8.1). The prevalence of stones in vegetarians is less than half of that in the general population. Inadequate fluid intake may explain the frequent recurrence of urinary stones in certain patients. In patients with absorptive hypercalciuria, stone recurrence may also be favoured by the ingestion of calcium-rich water. Some patients have a high intake of milk and alkali, which can lead to both nephrolithiasis and nephrocalcinosis. Patients with a history of food allergy may develop a nephrotic syndrome (Lagrue *et al.* 1989).

Alcohol intake should also be estimated: excessive consumption induces an increase in blood pressure and is responsible for a substantial percentage of cases of essential hypertension (Saunders *et al.* 1981; Lang *et al.* 1987). It may also account for poor compliance with therapy.

Some patients have a particular desire for acidic foods such as fruit juices and rhubarb, many of which have a high oxalate content and may result in calcium oxalate precipitation in the kidney. Other patients may consume large quantities of strong tea or coffee every day, leading both to extrasystoles and polyuria, depending upon the methyl xanthine content.

Vegetarian patients may be prone to vitamin B_{12} deficiency, depending upon the strictness of their diet. Ethnic diets contain either very large amounts of sodium (Japanese, Indian) or potassium (Indian). The use of unleavened bread, such as chapatis, results in a high phosphate intake, calcium binding, and acceleration of osteomalacia or the rachitic component of renal osteodystrophy.

Factitious history

Self-induced or factitious disease may also be encountered, and commonly involves the addition of material, such as blood, protein, or sugar, to a normal urine specimen. On occasions, patients with Munchausen's syndrome will focus their symptoms on the renal tract (Duffy 1992; Ifudu *et al.* 1992). The lengths to which adult patients will go in falsifying information are surprising: intravenous injection of metaraminol or isoprenaline has been used to produce hypertension (Lurvey *et al.* 1973; Portioli and Valcavi 1981); the intravenous injection of milk, tetanus toxoid, or faeces producing immune complex nephritis (Boulton-Jones *et al.* 1974); 'stones' which clearly could not originate in the renal tract (e.g. date stones), and physical signs, such as temperature, may be altered to mislead the attending physician. In the majority, a clue may be obtained from the willingness of the patients to go along with prolonged, frequently repetitive investigations, the bizarre nature of the symptoms/sign complex, or the inexplicable laboratory findings, for example, *Mycobacterium smegmatis* from sputum or Lactobacillus from blood. On confrontation, most patients will deny any possibility of factitious illness and will frequently seek medical attention and investigation elsewhere.

Social history

Socioeconomic and educational status influence the incidence and mode of presentation of many renal diseases and may also give an indication as to the required degree of follow-up. The frequency of bacteriuria is much greater in multiparous patients and in pregnant women of low socioeconomic status (Turck *et al.* 1962). Poor compliance with therapy is common in hypertensive patients of low socioeconomic class, and this may explain in part the relatively high incidence of accelerated hypertension in this group of patients. Idiopathic calcium stone formation is more common in men of higher social class, which may relate to the increased protein intake of affluence.

Details of tobacco consumption should be obtained, since this represents a significant risk factor (see Chapter 4.12.2). Smoking contributes to the development of artherosclerosis in dialysis patients and it is also a risk factor for renovascular hypertension (MacKay *et al.* 1979), accelerated hypertension (Isles *et al.* 1979), Goodpasture's syndrome in young males, and for the development of diabetic nephropathy (Rossing *et al.* 1995). Drug addiction exposes the patient to a number of renal complications, such as acute renal failure due to rhabdomyolysis, amyloidosis, vasculitis, proliferative glomerulonephritis, and septicaemia. In addition, these patients are at risk from a number of infections, including HIV, which may be associated with a focal and segmental glomerulosclerosis (see Chapter 3.13).

Occupational history

A number of occupational factors are important in the development of renal disease. Working in hot atmospheres with increased insensible fluid loss increases the incidence of urinary stone formation. Certain workers are exposed to toxins and chemicals, and hydrocarbon inhalation may play a role in triggering glomerulonephritis, although convincing evidence has been reported only for Goodpasture's syndrome. It may be that solvent exposure does not cause glomerulonephritis, but rather delays its resolution or renders the patient more susceptible (see Chapter 4.12.1). Exposure to a number of agents has been identified as a risk factor for chronic renal failure (Nuyts *et al.* 1995). Certain chemicals are associated with the induction of renal disease; for example, the increased incidence of urothelial tumours in aniline dye workers.

Infections with a predilection for the kidney may also be contracted by certain occupational groups. Acute renal failure due to leptospirosis is more common in miners, sewage workers, and farm labourers; Hantavirus infection may arise in laboratory workers handling animals such as rats, or in farmers from endemic areas. Occupational details should be recorded, particularly in patients who handle chemicals or are exposed to toxic vapours. Exposure to lead, particularly in a vaporized form, such as occurs during welding lead pipes or in using oxyacetylene to cut metal previously covered with a lead-based paint, may result in lead nephropathy and subsequent chronic renal failure.

Ethnic and geographical factors

Ethnic factors may be important in various renal diseases. Amyloidosis complicates familial Mediterranean fever in Arabs from the Mediterranean area, Turks, and Sephardic Jews, whereas Sephardic Jews from Baghdad, Southern Russia, and the Balkans, Ashkenazic Jews, and Armenians are rarely affected. The incidence of IgA nephropathy is greater in White populations and in some Asian countries (Japan, Singapore, and China) than in Black populations in North America and Africa or in North African patients. Mesangioproliferative glomerulonephritis is common in Navajo and Zuni Indians in the United States, whereas the incidence of renal disease due to non-insulin dependent diabetes mellitus is increased in Zuni and Pima Indians. Systemic lupus erythematosus is several times more common in oriental and Black populations than amongst Caucasians, and within the latter group it is more common in the Middle East and India than in Europe.

Sickle-cell disease is widespread amongst African, Middle Eastern, and Indian populations and both severe hypertension and diabetes mellitus with renal failure are more common in Black patients. Black and Indian patients may develop tuberculosis during immunosuppressive treatment for systemic disease or following transplantation. Patients from the tropics may have positive treponemal serology due to previous exposure to yaws, and the incidence of a positive antinuclear factor is much greater. Finally, it must be remembered that there are ethnic differences in enzymes involved in the handling of drugs, such as the reduced oxidoreductase activity of oriental patients.

Travel abroad exposes many patients to diseases that may affect the kidneys. It is not uncommon for patients to neglect proper prophylactic antimalarial therapy, and details of foreign travel, even years previously, may be important. For instance, fulminant and disseminated strongyloidiasis may develop in immunosuppressed transplant patients who visited endemic tropical areas even up to 30 years previously. In such patients, a prophylactic course of thiabendazole or mebendazole is justified before surgery, this should be repeated 2–3 weeks after transplantation.

Table 3 Classification of the main groups of inherited kidney diseases

1. Cystic kidney disease (Section 16.2)
2. Alport's syndrome and variants (Chapter 16.4.1)
3. Inherited metabolic diseases with kidney involvement
   - With non-glomerular involvement—such as cystinosis primary hyperoxaluria (Chapter 16.5.2) or inherited urate nephropathy (Chapter 6.4)
   - With glomerular involvement—such as Fabry's disease or lecithin-cholesterol acyltransferase deficiency (Section 16.2), and also associated with diabetes mellitus, defects of the complement system, genetic amyloidosis etc.
4. Other inherited diseases with glomerular or non-glomerular involvement
   - With glomerular involvement, such as the congenital nephrotic syndrome (Chapter 16.4.4) or the nail–patella syndrome and other syndromes with extrarenal defects (Chapter 16.4.3)
   - With non-glomerular involvement, such as nephronophthisis (Chapter 16.3)
   - With cystic kidney disease (Section 16.2), tuberous sclerosis with renal angiomyolipoma and von Hippel–Lindau's disease with renal cell carcinoma (Chapter 16.1, Section 16.2, and Chapter 18.1)
5. Primary immune glomerulonephritis, occasionally familial such as in IgA nephropathy, or more rarely in other primary glomerular diseases (Section 3)
6. Inherited tubular disorders such as cystinuria (Section 8) and various inherited tubular defects described in Section 5
7. Various renal diseases with 'genetic influence' such as calcium nephrolithiasis, vesicoureteric reflux and related nephropathy, haemolytic uraemic syndrome
8. Unclassified cases

Family history

It is important to obtain medical information on the spouse, children, parents, siblings, and other relatives. The family pedigree should be established in as much detail as possible; this may involve obtaining medical notes and interviewing and examining relatives. This is obviously essential in hereditary renal diseases (the main groups of which are listed in Table 3 and described in Section 16), although it may be time-consuming to collect precise data on unaffected as well as affected family members. Some families show psychological reluctance to undergo genetic investigation and considerable care and tact are required. Genetic predisposition is observed in other renal diseases in addition to the well-established inherited disorders. The familial predisposition to systemic lupus erythematosus and other autoimmune diseases is well known. Familial occurrence has been documented in primary immune glomerulonephritis and in IgA nephropathy.

Genetic heterogeneity should also be kept in mind: renal diseases that are similar on clinical grounds (on the basis of our current knowledge) may have different modes of inheritance in different families. This is well substantiated in Alport's syndrome (see Chapter 16.4.1) and in nephronophthisis and medullary cystic disease (see Chapter 16.3). Genetic susceptibility to diabetic nephropathy has been demonstrated, and it has also been suggested that patients with insulin-dependent diabetes mellitus and a family history of hypertension are more prone to diabetic nephropathy than those without such a family history (see Chapter 4.1). On occasions, it is difficult to differentiate between genetic and environmental factors.

Systematic enquiry

Even when the patient interview has proceeded along the previously described lines, there may still be areas which have not been covered, or a reluctance of the patient to reveal details. There is, therefore, a need for a systematic enquiry which should cover all aspects of general health including changes in weight and appetite. Enquiries should always be made to determine whether the patient has at any time suffered from dysuria, frequency, nocturia, or haematuria. In patients with chronic renal failure, it is important to document whether the patient has suffered from pruritus, breathlessness, peripheral oedema, sleep disturbance, restless legs, visual changes, or gritty eyes. The duration of nocturia may give a valuable clue to the duration and rate of progression of the disease. The majority of patients are reluctant to discuss, particularly at a first interview, problems related to sexual function but it is important to enquire about libido and impotence in males. These factors can cause considerable anxiety in a patient and are commonly only discussed once the examining clinician has introduced the subject.

Clinical examination in adults

Examination of the kidneys and urinary tract

Clinical examination of the urinary tract follows the standard pattern of inspection, palpation, percussion, and auscultation. On abdominal inspection, it may be possible to see one or both kidneys, particularly if advanced polycystic kidney disease is present. Occasionally, chronic obstructive uropathy may cause such distension of the ureters that they become visible. Obstruction to the bladder outflow track results in bladder distension, which may be readily visible in patients, particularly those who are thin.

Palpation of the kidneys is best carried out with the patient in the recumbent position with the head slightly raised on a pillow and the arms resting at the side of the body. The right kidney is palpated by placing the left hand posteriorly in the loin and the right hand horizontally on the anterior abdominal wall to the right of the umbilicus. By pushing forward with the left hand and asking the patient to take a deep breath, the lower pole of the kidney is commonly palpable in thin patients by pressing the right hand inwards and upwards. To palpate the left kidney, the left hand should be placed posteriorly in the left loin and the right hand on the anterior abdominal wall to the left of the umbilicus. The left kidney is not as readily palpable as the right. Care should be taken to distinguish kidney from spleen. On palpation, an estimate of the size and shape of the kidney should be made if possible, although this may be difficult except in those who are very thin. In normal patients, the surface of the kidney is smooth and relatively hard, but in those with cystic disease an irregular surface may be detected. Any tenderness on palpation should be recorded.

Abdominal percussion may be of value if there is difficulty distinguishing between an enlarged left kidney and splenomegaly or in patients with hepatomegaly. Percussion is also of value in determining the presence and degree of ascites.

Auscultation of the abdomen is essential in all patients with hypertension; the stethoscope should be placed posteriorly in the loin, laterally in the flank, and anteriorly and in each area the examiner should listen carefully for the presence of a bruit. In addition, auscultation is mandatory in any patient who has had a renal biopsy and who subsequently develops hypertension, in view of the possibility of the development of a postbiopsy arteriovenous fistula.

Examination of the urinary tract is incomplete without a carefully conducted rectal examination and, where indicated, a vaginal examination. Prostatic hypertrophy is common and, when present, may aggravate impaired renal function. In females, carcinoma of the cervix may extend laterally and result in a 'frozen' pelvis. On occasions, an unexpected finding, such as a villous adenoma of the large bowel giving rise to profound hypokalaemia, will be detected.

Measurement of blood pressure

The measurement of blood pressure is an important step in the clinical examination of a renal patient. It is worth recalling the main precautions to prevent artefacts in these measurements (Frohlich *et al.* 1988). The patient should be supine or sitting, then standing, in a quiet environment with an arm resting at heart level. An appropriately sized cuff should be selected: the width should be at least 40 per cent of arm circumference, and length at least 80 per cent of arm circumference. For example, for an arm circumference of 30 cm and a bladder width of 12 cm, blood pressure readings will be correct; in contrast, for an arm circumference of 40 cm, using the same cuff, systolic blood pressure will be overestimated by 10 mm Hg. Cuff errors are of great importance in obese individuals with thick arms and lead to overestimation of blood pressure. A cuff that is too wide causes less error than one that is too narrow. The use of a wide bladder (15 cm) is recommended for all adults except those with thin arms that are out of the cuff range. The use of mercury manometers should be encouraged; aneroid apparatus should be calibrated at least once every 6 months with a mercury gravity manometer. In adults, cessation of sound (Phase V) rather than muffling (Phase IV) corresponds to diastolic blood pressure. However, in certain subjects, including those with aortic valvular insufficiency or high cardiac output (as in anaemia, thyrotoxicosis, or pregnancy) the Korotkoff sounds do not disappear. In such conditions, Phase IV is the only reliable index of diastolic blood pressure. In patients with cardiac dysrhythmias, such as atrial fibrillation, multiple readings are needed and blood pressure values should be considered only as approximations.

Overestimation of systolic blood pressure is common in elderly patients with hard, calcified vessels. This may be detected clinically when the radial artery is palpable even when the cuff is inflated above systolic blood pressure (positive Osler's manoeuvre, suggesting pseudohypertension). Bias in reading on the part of the observer may be overcome by devices that 'blind' to the actual pressure values (e.g. the Hawksley Random-Zero Device and the London School of Hygiene Sphygmomanometer).

In addition to casual blood pressure measurements, two other modes of monitoring have recently been developed. Home blood pressure measurements (Hunt *et al.* 1985) can be obtained with either the usual manometers or with electronic manometers, whose accuracy is difficult to assess. This technique may be useful in some patients who are willing to participate in their own management. It is particularly useful to reassure patients taking antihypertensive medications that the prescribed dose is effective and furthermore, it affords the prescribing physician the opportunity of not altering therapy on the basis of single outpatient blood pressure readings in patients with 'white coat' hypertension. However, in those who have a tendency to become easily alarmed by minor changes in blood pressure it can have deleterious effects. Ambulatory blood pressure measurements can be performed with various devices (Winslow *et al.* 1986).

General examination

In any patient with renal disease, it is important to undertake a full clinical examination and carefully document all detected abnormalities. It is important to remember that the absence of certain findings may be as important as the presence of a diagnostic sign. Each clinician develops his/her own particular examination technique and therefore, there is no standardized 'correct' method. The most important fact to remember is that the patient must be fully examined.

The skin of patients with renal disease may reveal a number of interesting abnormalities. Patients with uraemia frequently have pallor and pigmentation, and the skin is dry and flaky. There may be evidence of purpura and frequently, scratch marks will indicate pruritus. Palpable subcutaneous nodules may be present, indicating dystrophic calcification. In terminal renal failure, uraemic frost may be visible, particularly on the face. Purpura may be the presenting feature of Henoch–Schönlein purpura (Fig. 4) and in patients with malignancy there may

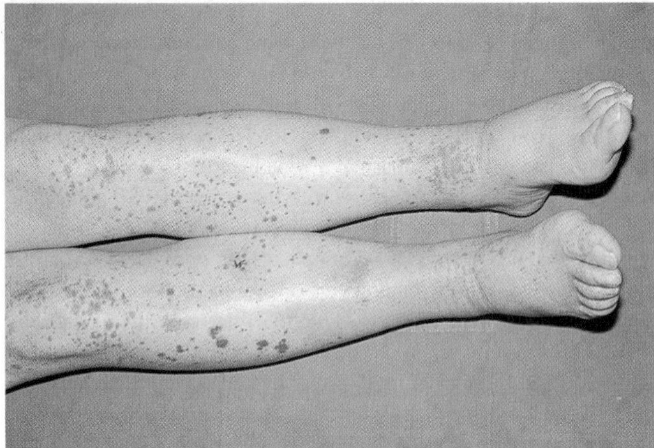

Fig. 4 Purpura of the lower limbs in a patient with Henoch–Schönlein nephritis.

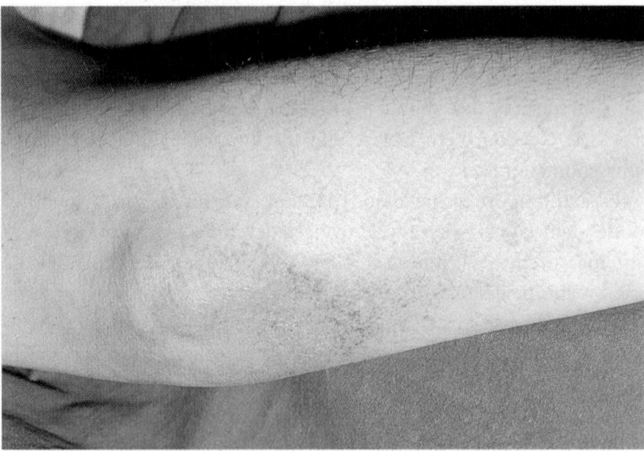

Fig. 5 Acanthosis nigrans with typical discolouration and thickening of the skin in the region of the elbow of a patient with renal failure who also had a carcinoma of the lung.

be acanthosis nigrans (Fig. 5). In Fabry's disease, small dark red hyperkeratotic papules are visible, most commonly in the groin area, and are more marked in males than in females (Fig. 6). In transplant recipients, manifestations of steroid side-effects, such as mooning of the face (Fig. 7), a central redistribution of body fat, purpura, and acne are common. Long-term immunosuppression is also associated with hyperkeratotic lesions (Fig. 8), which can progress to keratoacanthoma and undergo malignant change.

The general appearance of the patient may also be diagnostic. In some patients with type II mesangiocapillary glomerulonephritis, there is a partial lipodystrophy, where there is a loss of subcutaneous fat in the upper part of the body with a normal or increased distribution in the lower part (Fig. 9) (see Chapter 3.8). A number of inherited conditions are associated with typical facial appearances. Skin turgor is also an important sign: lax and slowly collapsing skin tension is indicative of salt and water depletion, whereas a plastic consistency may be indicative of water intoxication.

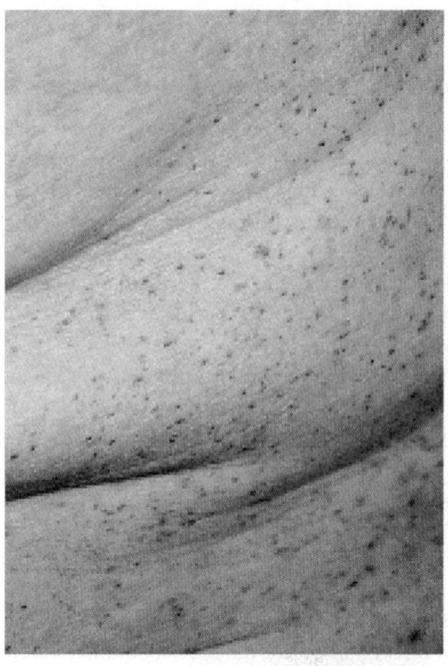

Fig. 6 Angiokeratoma in a patient with Fabry's disease.

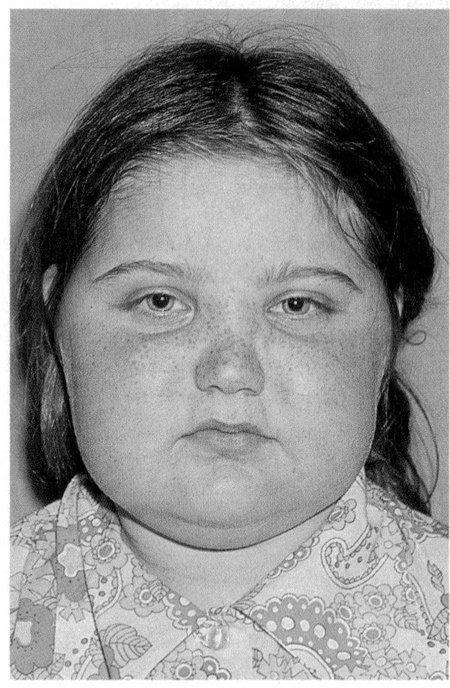

Fig. 7 Typical steroid facies in a young patient receiving corticosteroids following renal transplantation.

Examination of the eyes may reveal perilimbal calcification in patients with long-standing uraemia, subconjunctival haemorrhages in patients with vasculitis (Fig. 10), and lenticonus in Alport's syndrome (Fig. 11). Fundoscopic examination may reveal the changes typical of hypertension, diabetes mellitus, or vasculitis. In some patients, the fundus is particularly difficult to visualize, due to the presence of cataracts,

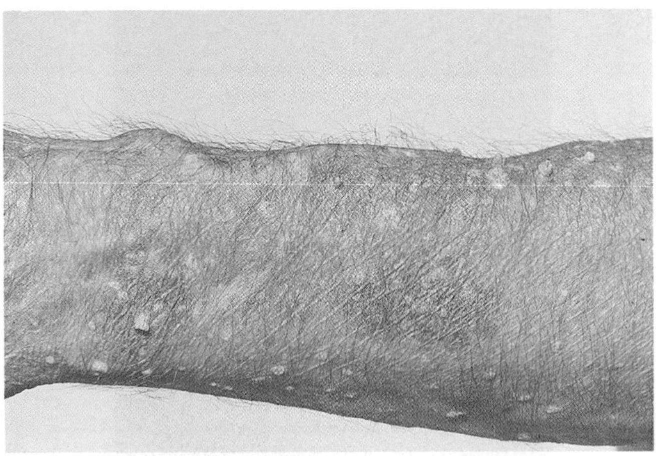

Fig. 8 Multiple hyperkeratotic lesions of the forearm of a patient on long-term immunosuppression following renal transplantation.

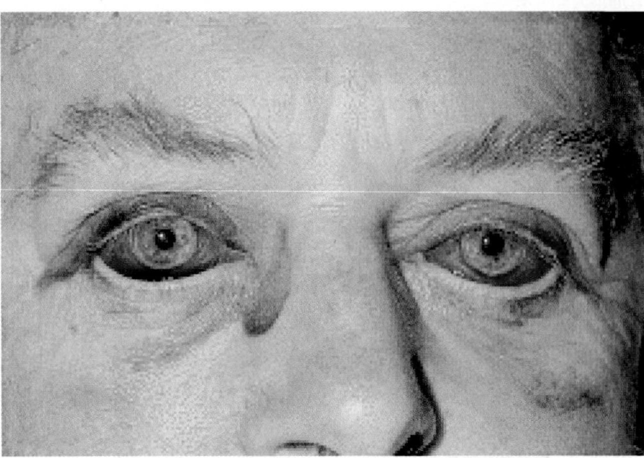

Fig. 10 Bilateral subconjunctival haemorrhage in a patient with microscopic polyarteritis.

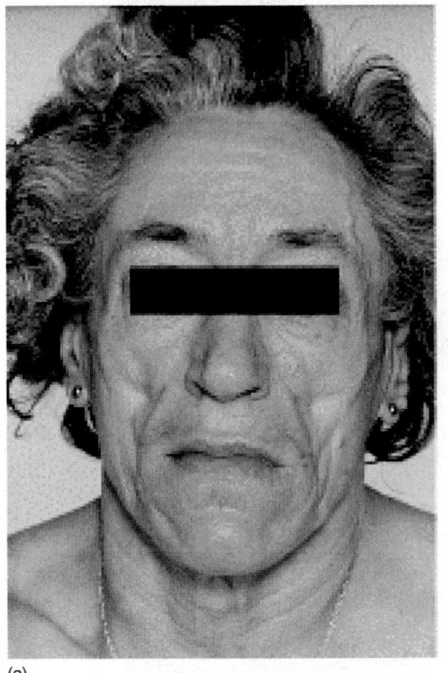

(a)

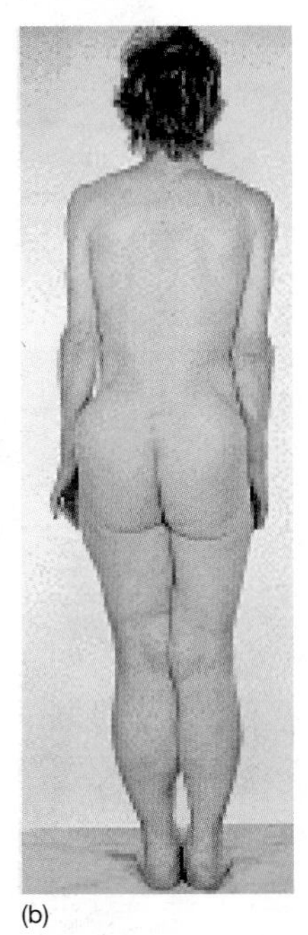

(b)

Fig. 9 (a) Facial appearance in a patient with mesangiocapillary glomerulonephritis of the dense deposit form and partial lipodystrophy. Note the loss of the buccal pad of fat. (b) Partial lipodystrophy showing the loss of subcutaneous fat from the upper half of the body with a normal or slightly increased lipid deposition in the lower half.

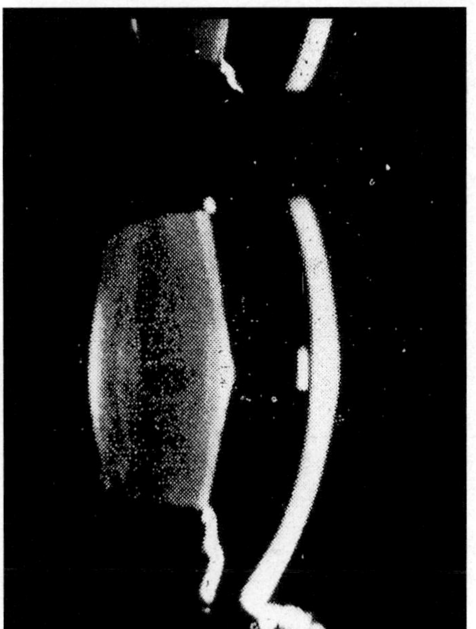

Fig. 11 Lenticonus.

particularly common in patients who have received high-dose corticosteroids.

The facial appearance may be suggestive of an underlying disease, for instance, the thickening and rigidity of the skin in systemic sclerosis, which may be associated with multiple telangiectasia (Fig. 12). Patients with systemic lupus erythematosus may present the typical butterfly facial rash (Fig. 13). In Wegener's granulomatosis, there may be loss of the nasal cartilaginous septum giving a typical facial appearance (Fig. 14). Hearing may be abnormal in patients with Alport's syndrome and also in patients with impaired renal function who have been exposed to excessive doses of aminoglycosides. During examination of the mouth, it is important to document the state of the teeth, the condition of the palate and gums, and the presence of any fungal infections (Fig. 15).

On examination of the praecordium, particular attention should be paid to murmurs and the presence of a pericardial rub. Any murmurs should be carefully documented—as a changing murmur is particularly suggestive of infective endocarditis. Flow murmurs are particularly common in patients with uraemic anaemia. Uraemic pericarditis is now rarely encountered, except in patients who have not been followed-up, and present in terminal uraemia. It may also arise from infection and vasculitis. Additional heart sounds may indicate fluid overload. In examining the chest, particular attention should be paid to the presence of crepitations, pleural fluid, and pleuritic rubs.

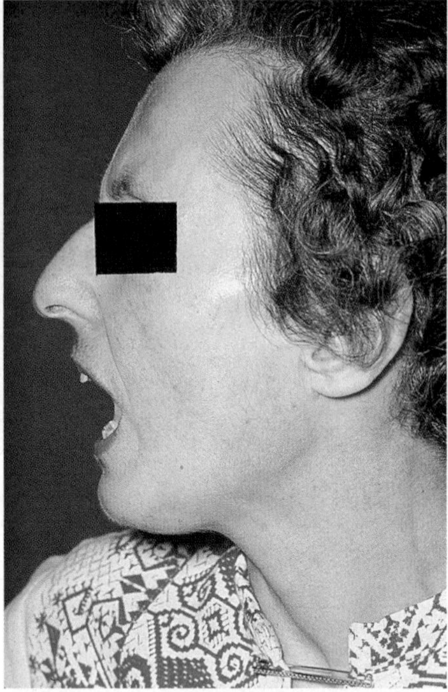

Fig. 12 Scleroderma.

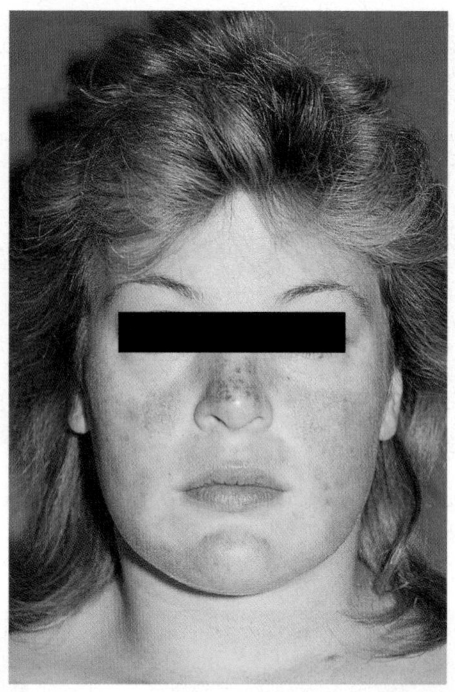

Fig. 13 Extensive butterfly rash in a patient with systemic lupus erythematosus.

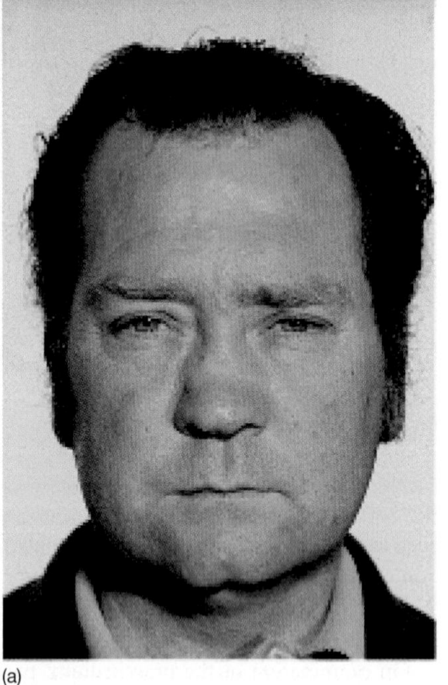

(a)

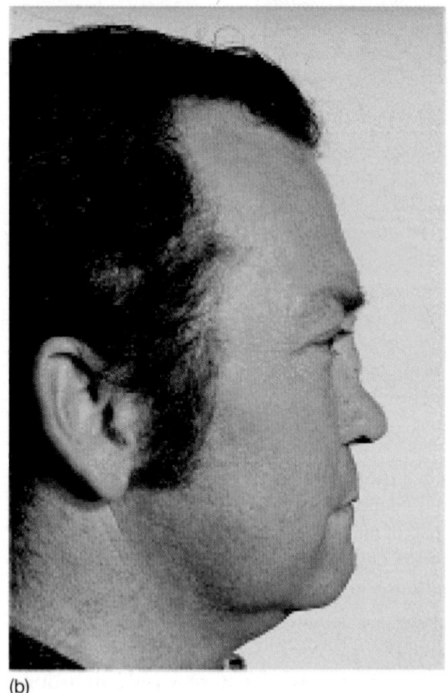

(b)

Fig. 14 Facial appearance in a patient with loss of the cartilaginous part of the nasal septum as a consequence of Wegener's granulomatosis.

Abdominal examination mainly involves an estimation of kidney size, but the presence of any other organomegaly or tumours should be determined. Lymphadenopathy may indicate an underlying lymphoproliferative disease. Testicular examination should be undertaken to determine whether atrophy or tumour is present. In patients in chronic renal failure, who may subsequently require chronic ambulatory peritoneal dialysis, it is necessary to exclude inguinal or umbilical hernias which may not be evident with the patient lying down.

During examination of the limbs, attention should be paid to the hands, with specific reference to the nails. Transverse ridges (Beau's lines)

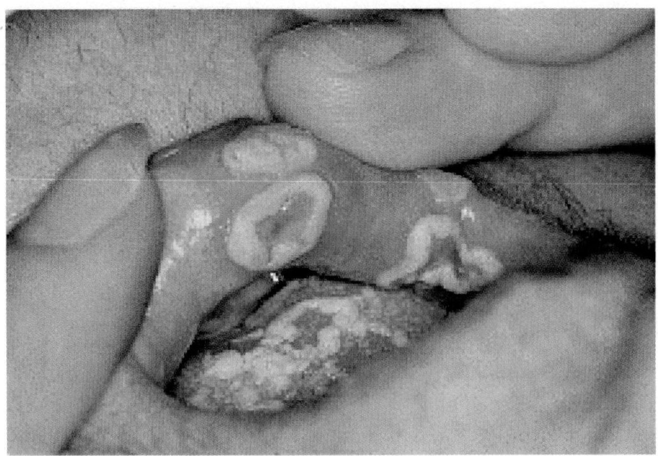

Fig. 15 Severe candida albicans infection of the mouth of a patient on immunosuppressive therapy for systemic disease.

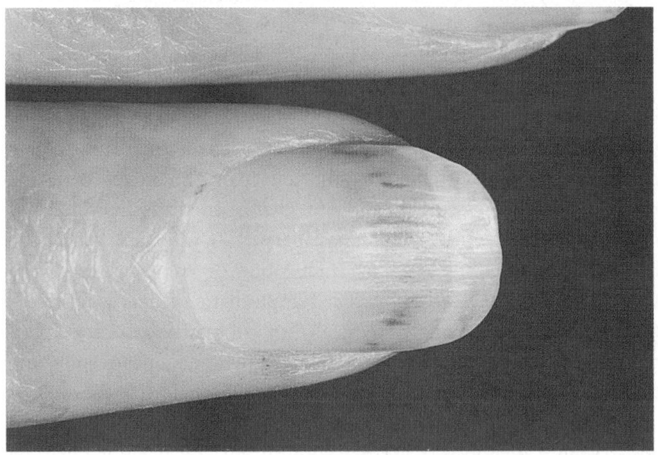

Fig. 16 Splinter haemorrhages in a patient with bacterial endocarditis.

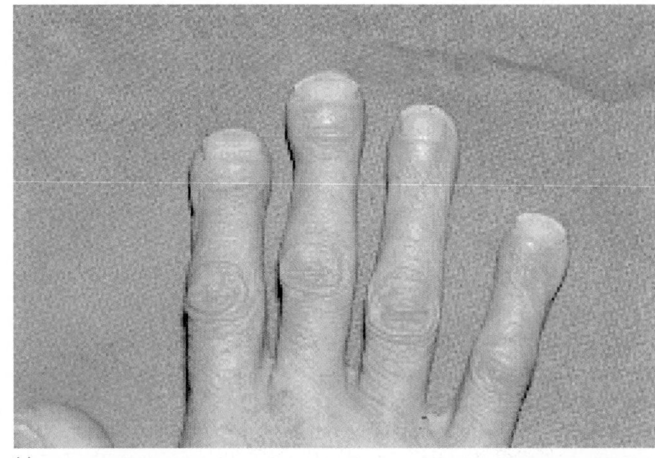

(a)

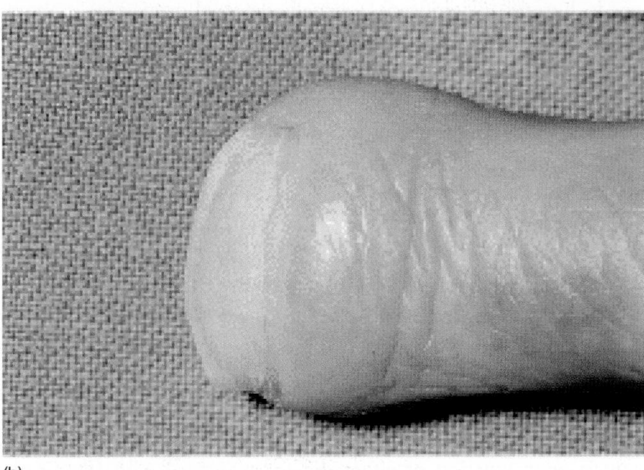

(b)

Fig. 17 (a) Hand showing pseudoclubbing due to loss of the terminal phalanges as a consequence of severe secondary hyperparathyroidism in a patient with chronic renal failure. (b) Enlargement to illustrate the loss of the terminal phalange.

may indicate serious preceding illness. In a nephrotic syndrome, the nails are pale and opaque, whereas splinter haemorrhages may be visible in patients with vasculitis and endocarditis (Fig. 16). In patients with long-standing renal failure, there may be evidence of secondary hyperparathyroidism with reduction and loss of the terminal phalange giving the appearance of clubbing (Fig. 17). In the lower limbs, oedema may be obvious and (particularly in older patients) examination should be made of the vascular supply, as atherosclerosis is particularly frequent in long-standing renal failure. The presence of proximal myopathy can be assessed by asking the patient to rise from a chair without using the upper limbs. The patella should be examined for the abnormalities of the nail–patella syndrome.

Examination should include the central, peripheral, and autonomic nervous systems. Motor and sensory function should be tested and the integrity of the autonomic nervous system can be tested by measuring the increase in blood pressure with sustained hand grip or the changes in the R–R interval during a Valsalva manoeuvre. Clinical neuropathy is particularly likely to be manifest in patients with diabetes mellitus.

A full examination in patients with renal disease is mandatory and while particular attention should be paid to the urinary tract and the clinical signs indicative of underlying renal disease, all systems should be examined thoroughly, so that the degree of systemic involvement is carefully documented.

Particular aspects of the neonate and child with renal disease

In paediatric practice, a carefully taken medical and family history are of vital importance. The history should emphasize the parents' worries and reasons for bringing the child to medical attention. It is important to allow the parents and child to tell the history in their own words. Parents are, in the main, excellent observers of their children and make good interpreters of their problems when they are unwell. With older children, it is very useful to ask questions about comparison with relatives, friends, and schoolmates of the same age.

Obstetric, neonatal, and past medical history

Past history should include details of the mother's health during pregnancy, the place of the child's birth, the gestational age, mode of delivery, birth weight, and any problems occurring around the time of the birth. It is important to document the historical milestones and any previous illnesses. Details of immunizations should be obtained and any infectious disease contacts noted. Any allergies or drug hypersensitivities should be detailed. All medicines recently taken, including any prescribed for the presenting illness, should be listed including dose, frequency, and duration. If the child has been in hospital elsewhere, it is important to obtain a copy of the notes to ensure complete information. It is often useful to check details of the pregnancy and perinatal history from obstetric notes.

Routine ultrasound screening during pregnancy has resulted in prenatal detection of urological disorders such that currently the incidence in Europe of significant prenatally detected uropathies is about 1 in 500–600 pregnancies. Neonatal ultrasound scanning has led to a predictable increase in the detection of urinary tract abnormalities, the most common of which is hydronephrosis. Neonatal management of urinary tract abnormalities includes a thorough assessment of the fetus for other anomalies and counselling the parents regarding the prenatal and long-term implications. Specific problems such as multicystic dysplasia and duplex kidneys are easily managed postnatally. Multicystic kidneys require postnatal confirmation of diagnosis with a DMSA scan, further investigation should assess the function and any abnormalities of the contralateral kidney. A micturating cystourethrogram is indicated only when there is pre- or postnatal dilatation of the contralateral kidney and/or ureter or a bladder abnormality. Duplex kidneys with dilatation of either moeity without a ureterocele benefit from prophylactic antibiotics and surgery is only indicated where there is poor function of either moeity associated with significant dilatation. The presence of an associated large ureterocele justifies early intervention to prevent serious sepsis. Fifty per cent of prenatally diagnosed urinary tract anomalies are simple upper tract dilatation which may be consistent with a radiological diagnosis of pelviureteric junction obstruction. The challenge is to prospectively differentiate between an obstructed hydronephrosis and a dilatation which is insignificant. Good functioning kidneys (>40 per cent on DTPA/MAG3) with varying degrees of hydronephrosis pose the greatest challenge. Long-term follow-up has shown that less than 30 per cent eventually warrant surgery and these derive from the more severe end of the spectrum where renal pelvic dilatation is 50 mm or greater. Postnatal investigation for prenatally diagnosed urinary tract anomalies needs to achieve a balance between early surgery for appropriate cases that would otherwise deteriorate whilst avoiding excessive investigations for those who have an anomaly of no clinical significance. Vesicoureteric reflux is clearly familial in some kindreds. This is not only of theoretical interest, but may be clinically relevant; recurrent febrile illnesses in a child of a woman with reflux nephropathy requires urological investigation.

Abnormalities of amniotic fluid volume may indicate renal dysfunction in the newborn. Oligohydramnios may be caused by reduced fetal urine production, which is very severe in renal agenesis, and may be present with renal dysplasia and obstructive uropathy such as posterior urethral valves. Polyhydramnios may result from an increase in fetal urine volume as occurs in nephrogenic diabetes insipidus and Bartter's syndrome. A large placenta, defined as more than 25 per cent of birth weight, is associated with the Finnish type of congenital nephrotic syndrome (see Chapter 16.4.4). A single umbilical artery may be associated with a variety of renal morphological abnormalities including dysplasia, duplex systems, obstructive uropathy, and bladder extrophy.

Severe birth asphyxia may be complicated by renal venous thrombosis in the newborn, which is characterized by macroscopic haematuria, thrombocytopenia, and an enlarged firm kidney. Umbilical arterial catherization may be complicated by vascular damage with later renal impairment and possible hypertension.

Family history

A detailed family history is essential. It is important to be aware of consanguinity which may be relevant to recessively inherited conditions and is much more common in certain racial and religious groups. Genetic factors are of increasing relevance in a wide variety of renal diseases (see Section 16).

General medical history

A general systems review must be undertaken as renal disease in childhood may present as part of a multisystem disorder or metabolic disease. This includes a history of any hearing or visual problems that may suggest Alport's syndrome, Bardet–Biedl syndrome, or familial juvenile nephronophthisis. A detailed micturition history is essential with information about urinary frequency, pain on micturition, force and continuity of urinary stream, loin pain, character of urine including smell and colour, and any change in urine habit, clearly documented. In young children, urinary tract infection should be considered if the child cries on micturition or has an unexplained fever. A history suggestive of earlier symptomatic urinary tract infections with the child being systemically unwell may be associated with the later development of reflux nephropathy and upper respiratory, throat, or skin infections may precede glomerulonephritic illnesses.

A review of nutrition and any feeding problems may be helpful in elucidating a diagnosis. Children with chronic renal failure may be losing salt and this can be associated with increased salt intake and a preference for savoury rather than sweet foods. Children who have high obligatory water losses, as occurs in nephrogenic diabetes insipidus and Fanconi syndrome, often present with constipation, and failure to thrive as a reduced calorie intake often accompanies a high fluid intake.

Factitious history

In some instances, a parent will provide false symptoms and signs, or will tamper with the child's urine or other laboratory samples, resulting in excessive and unnecessary investigations (frequently invasive) being undertaken: this has been called 'Munchausen by proxy' (Meadow 1977).

Clinical examination

Clinical features associated with acute renal impairment in childhood, as in adult practice, include a significantly reduced urine output, less than 200 ml/day (<0.5/kg body weight/h), oedema, and fluid overload. The child may have acidotic breathing, an impaired level of consciousness, and be hypertensive.

Blood pressure measurement in children can be one of the most difficult aspects of the physical examination and demands both experience and care. It is essential that an appropriate size cuff is used, one which ensures that the inflatable bladder encircling the circumference of the arm is wide enough to cover more than 40 per cent of the distance from the acromion to the olecranon. Ideally, the length of the cuff should fully encompass the arm, a cuff that is too small for the child may result in a falsely elevated reading leading to potentially unnecessary investigations and/or treatment. Sustained severe hypertension, however, in a child usually indicates underlying renal disease.

The onset of symptoms in chronic renal failure in childhood is generally insidious, but acute deterioration may be precipitated by intercurrent infections or by episodes of dehydration. As the glomerular filtration rate (GFR) falls to 20–25 per cent, the child may develop polyuria and polydipsia which can be associated with episodes of enuresis and early signs of failing to thrive. As the GFR declines to less than 20 per cent, children and infants become more anorexic, develop a metabolic acidosis; normal growth and development are impeded, and the child may experience bone pain or problems with mobility as a consequence of developing renal osteodystrophy. A proper assessment of the child's growth requires accurate measurement of height with a stadiometer and weight with scales with reference to charts of height and weight percentiles appropriate for age, race, and sex.

The state of hydration can be assessed from the anterior fontanelle in infants, and from the eyes, mouth, and skin in older children, and over time by measuring urine volume and osmolality. There is no simple clinical way to estimate total body water, although some clues may be obtained from reviewing recent changes in body weight which largely reflect changes in total body water. Dehydration in children is defined as being mild when associated with approximately 5 per cent loss in body weight and severe when this approaches a 15 per cent loss in body weight.

If a rash is present, this may be helpful diagnostically, for example, Henoch–Schönlein disease is associated with a characteristic maculopapular rash on the buttocks and back of the legs, and systemic lupus erythematosus with a butterfly rash across the nose and cheeks, but the majority of skin lesions in childhood are less specific, such as the rash associated with polyarteritis nodosa. In children, oedema always seems to be more noticeable in the face (Fig. 18).

The abdomen in toddlers and young children is often protruberant in the upright posture, which may be related to an exaggerated lordosis. Respiration is abdominal in preschool children, and small umbilical hernias relatively common. Intra-abdominal masses are occasionally visible and Wilm's tumours may be detected by parents when bathing their child. Kidneys are not easily palpable in infants and children, and are best palpated bimanually. In the neonate, the left kidney is more easily palpable than the right, even if of normal size. Fetal lobulation of the newborn kidney is not clinically appreciable. If kidneys are easily palpable in children, they are probably enlarged. Enlargement of the kidney in the newborn period may be bilateral or unilateral. If unilateral, this may be associated with a congenital mesonephroma/nephroblastoma, a multicystic dysplastic kidney, hydronephrosis, or renal venous thrombosis when the kidney is also very hard on palpation. If the enlargement is bilateral, then this may indicate autosomal recessive polycystic kidney disease, severe bilateral obstructive uropathy with hydronephroses secondary to posterior urethral valves, or the congenital nephrotic syndrome. Absent abdominal wall musculature (prune belly) (Fig. 19) is associated with cryptorchidism and urological abnormality, and is probably the consequence of transient urethral obstruction in fetal life. The bladder can be palpated in the neonate and infant as it is at this stage an abdominal organ, and it is also easily percussable when full. A very full bladder

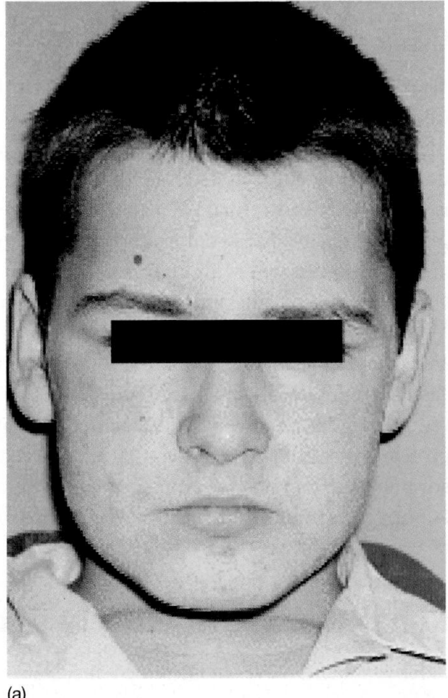

(a)

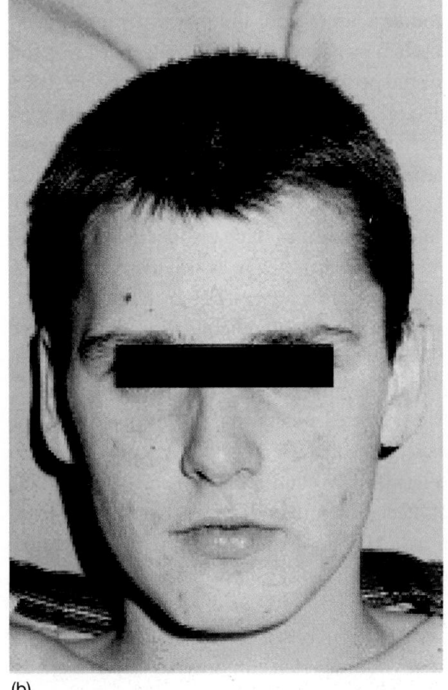

(b)

Fig. 18 (a) Facial oedema in a young adult with nephrotic syndrome. (b) Same patient after resolution of oedema. The extent of facial swelling is more obvious once an oedema free state is achieved.

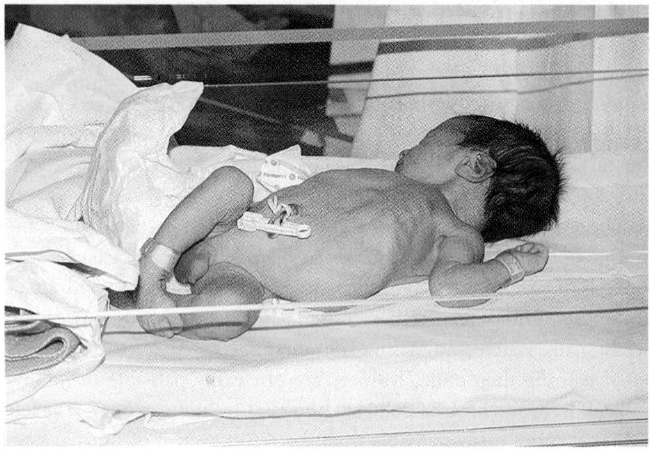

Fig. 19 Prune belly.

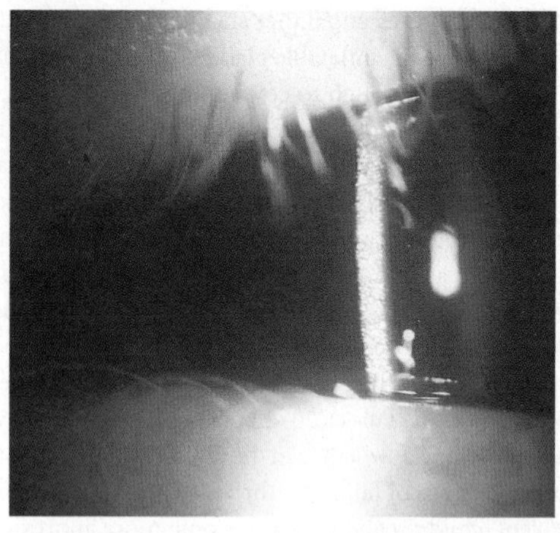

Fig. 20 Nephropathic cystinosis. Slit lamp biomicroscopy shows cystine crystals throughout the corneal stroma in this 5-year-old patient.

in these situations may sometimes be visible and this is particularly so with neuropathic bladders. Ascites in children with renal disease is most commonly seen in nephrotic syndrome, and if gross, may be obvious on inspection and be associated with scrotal and penile oedema. A fluid thrill is an unreliable sign to detect ascites and can easily be elicited incorrectly in obese children, far more reliable is the sign of shifting dullness. The distribution of ascitic dullness is horseshoe shaped, and the child should be allowed to lie on his side for 30–60 s before checking for dullness. Ascites in the newborn may be a transudate as in the hydropic infant or an exudate as occurs in peritonitis. Urinary ascites may occur spontaneously or be associated with a severe obstructive uropathy and rupture of the bladder and/or renal capsule.

Inspection and examination of the genitalia are a routine part of the examination of infants, toddlers, and school children, and more is generally learnt by inspection than by palpation. In the male, one looks for normality/abnormality of the penis, scrotum, and testes. The presence of the foreskin in a male and the position of the urethral meatus in both sexes should be ascertained as anomalies are common. Bilateral undescended testes are a feature of the prune belly syndrome which is also associated with lax abdominal musculature, bilateral ureteric/pelvicalyceal dilatation, and a neuropathic-type bladder. Male pseudohermaphroditism with undescended testes is associated with Wilm's tumour and a nephropathy in the Denys–Drash syndrome (see Chapter 18.2) and female pseudohermaphroditism may suggest adrenal hyperplasia with salt wasting. The vulva is usually inspected in females as adhesions of the labial mucosa are not infrequent. Vaginal palpation is not usually performed unless there is clear cut clinical indication such as suspected sexual abuse or a foreign body. The clitoris is prominent in preterm infants and a bloody postnatal vaginal discharge can be normal. Rectal examination can be helpful in assessing a pelvic mass, such as a rhabdomyosarcoma and a very dilated ureter may be felt rectally as well as by careful anterior abdominal examination.

A thorough neurological examination is always necessary, particularly when children present with hypertension or renal impairment as part of a multisystem disorder. Hypertension may present as a facial palsy or result in cerebral haemorrhage, and if blood pressure is reduced too quickly, visual pathway infarction, blindness, and abnormalities of pupillary response may occur. Ophthalmological examination may be helpful diagnostically: cystinosis is associated with cystine deposition in the cornea, best detected by slit-light examination (Fig. 20), and Alport's disease is associated with lenticonus or a macular abnormality (Fig. 11). Cataracts may be associated with long-term steroid therapy and are also found in children affected by Bardet–Biedl and Lowe's syndrome. Tapito retinal degeneration may be present in familial juvenile nephronophthisis and retinitis pigmentosa is characteristic of Bardet–Biedl syndrome (Fig. 21).

A careful examination of the spine is important, particularly when looking for a sacral pit. Anal tone, perianal sensation, and neurological assessment of the lower limbs is mandatory to exclude any neurological problems that may be associated with a neuropathic bladder such as spinal cord tethering.

Urine analysis

The dipstick nitrite test is a useful screening test for urinary tract infection in children as most gram-negative urinary tract pathogens have the ability to break down urinary nitrate to nitrite. This test is usually done with the leucocyte esterase reaction used to assess whether there is associated leucocyturia. A positive test for nitrite and leucocyte esterase is reliable for a coliform urinary tract infection, but this must always be confirmed with culture and microscopy. Leucocyturia in children is not specific and may be caused by many factors including fever, dehydration, local irritation, and recent immunizations. When assessing the degree of proteinuria in infants and children, it is often easier and potentially more accurate to measure the protein/creatinine ratio in an early morning urine, rather than attempting to measure protein in a difficult to collect 24 h specimen. This has the added advantage of removing the possible contribution of orthostatic proteinuria, which may exaggerate the degree of proteinuria.

Renal disease in elderly patients

Elderly patients have an increased incidence of certain conditions (Table 4). The changes in renal function that occur with age (see Chapter 1.5) must be taken into account when assessing the results of investigations. Care must also be exercised in the use of therapeutic agents and appropriate adjustments of dosage must be made (see Chapter 19.2).

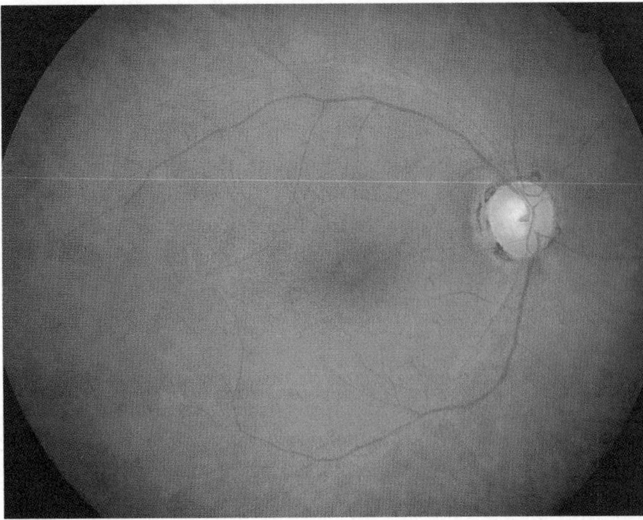
(a)

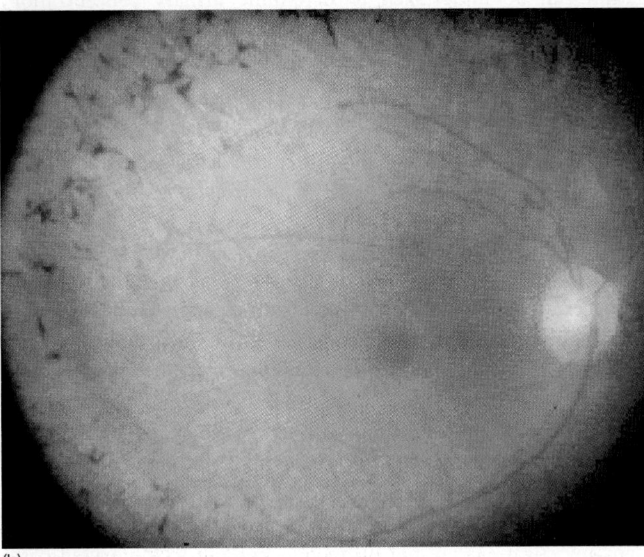
(b)

Fig. 21 Bardet–Biedl syndrome in sibs. (a) Photoreceptor degeneration in an 15-year-old child with visual loss to 0.3. Note attenuated retinal vessels, a pale optic disc, and mild pigmentary abnormalities. (b) His 24-year-old sister is nearly blind, and her fundus shows retinitis pigmentosa with retinal atrophy and migration of pigment into the overlying retina in a bone-spicule pattern, marked attenuation of retinal vessels, and optic atrophy. Note also two haemorrhages associated with arterial hypertension and end-stage renal disease.

Table 4 Main renal disorders having relatively high incidence in elderly patients

Glomerular
Membranous nephropathy (with nephrotic syndrome)
Crescentic glomerulonephritis (with rapidly progressive renal failure)
Anti-GBM nephritis (in women)
Amyloidosis
Tubulointerstitial
Analgesic nephropathy
Obstructive uropathy (e.g. prostate obstruction, retroperitoneal fibrosis, pelvic cancer)
Multiple myeloma and related diseases
Vascular
Nephrosclerosis
Diabetic nephropathy (mainly type II diabetes, with vascular and glomerular involvement)
Renal atheromatous disease (including renal artery stenosis or thrombosis, associated or not with abdominal aorta aneurysm, and multiple cholesterol emboli disease)
Vasculitis (Wegener's granulomatosis; microscopic polyarteritis)
Drug-induced
Cystic
Solitary or multiple renal cysts
Autosomal dominant polycystic disease
Malignant
Renal adenocarcinoma
Transitional cell carcinoma of urinary tract
Water and electrolyte disorder

Adapted from Macías-Núñez and Cameron (1987).

Table 5 Emergencies in the renal patient

Malignant or severe hypertension
Acute renal failure with oligoanuria
Acute glomerulonephritis (in childhood)
Severe water and electrolyte disorders, particularly hyperkalaemia
Renal colic and any acute urinary tract obstruction
Cardiovascular and respiratory emergencies: not only myocardial infarction, acute pulmonary oedema, aortic dissection, etc., but also uraemic pericarditis, pulmonary embolism in the nephrotic patient, severe haemoptysis in a patient with the Goodpasture's syndrome etc.
Acute thrombosis of arteriovenous fistula
Severe haemorrhage such as gastrointestinal bleeding in patients with acute renal failure, severe bleeding after renal biopsy or from arteriovenous fistula, acute rupture of a transplanted kidney, intracranial haemorrhage due to ruptured aneurysm in polycystic kidney disease
Fever such as that due to upper urinary tract infection or to septicaemia of any other origin; or fever in immunodepressed patients

Emergencies in patients with renal diseases

A number of renal diseases and complications of renal disease present as acute medical emergencies requiring urgent action. Some, such as hyperkalaemia, require immediate treatment, whereas in others, there is time to undertake certain specific investigations to confirm the diagnosis, for example, renal biopsy and serological testing for anti-GBM antibodies in Goodpasture's syndrome (Table 5).

In patients with primary renal disease, the major acute emergencies involve rapidly progressing glomerulonephritis, Goodpasture's syndrome, vasculitis, mesangiocapillary glomerulonephritis, and rarely, IgA nephropathy. In such situations, urgent investigations, including renal biopsy, should be undertaken so that appropriate therapy may be undertaken at the earliest opportunity. In many instances, if the glomerular disease has progressed to the stage of oliguria, the prognosis for recovery of renal function is poor.

In patients with acute renal failure, the most common medical emergencies involve disorders of fluid and electrolytes, and sepsis. Pulmonary oedema, particularly of acute onset, may have few physical signs other than breathlessness and tachypnoea. Hyperkalaemia is asymptomatic and can be life-threatening; children seem to tolerate hyperkalaemia better than adults. In patients with prolonged acute renal failure, particularly if associated with hypotension, there is always the risk of gastrointestinal haemorrhage from multiple small areas of mucosal infarction.

Fluid and electrolyte disorders are also common in chronic renal failure but they tend to be more insidious in progression. Pericarditis may occur and give rise to cardiac tamponade.

In patients with end-stage renal failure receiving dialysis, a number of medical emergencies may arise such as fluid overload, hyperkalaemia, hypertensive crises, and septicaemia from infected vascular access. The nephrologist must be aware of their presentations and management.

The nephrologist may therefore be faced with many diverse acute medical emergencies, and must be aware of their presentations and management.

Structured investigation

Having obtained a full history and undertaken a careful clinical examination, the clinician will be in a position to formulate a differential diagnosis with respect to the underlying disease. The investigations that are subsequently undertaken should be structured in such a way as to confirm or refute the postulated diagnosis.

A number of basic investigations are essential in any patient who is known to have or suspected of having an underlying renal disease. Urine analysis should be performed at each clinic visit and the results carefully recorded in the patient's notes. As a minimum, the urine pH and the presence of blood, protein, and glucose should be documented. Urine should also be obtained for microscopy; particular attention should be paid to the presence and type of casts and, if haematuria is detected, the morphology of red cells. Urine culture should also be undertaken; where appropriate, this should include investigation for anaerobic organisms and *Mycobacterium tuberculosis*. All patients should also have blood urea, serum creatinine, and electrolytes determined and a full blood count should be performed.

If a 'stix' examination reveals proteinuria, then further investigations to determine its type and extent are indicated. Since it is difficult to obtain an accurate 24-h urine collection for protein quantitation in outpatients, it has been suggested that determination of protein–creatinine ratio in a single sample is adequate; this is particularly helpful in children, and is probably sufficient for patient follow-up. However, it should be remembered that there is a diurnal variation in urinary protein and creatinine excretion, and samples should be collected at approximately the same time of day so that reasonable comparisons can be made. The type of protein being excreted in the urine can be determined by electrophoresis.

In the presence of urinary abnormalities, particularly proteinuria and haematuria, consideration should be given to more detailed investigation of the urinary tract and kidney histology. In most circumstances, the first investigation should be a renal ultrasound examination. If investigation of the urine reveals the presence of red cell casts, or dysmorphic red cells, then it is more appropriate to proceed to renal biopsy than to undertake an intravenous pyelogram. Before biopsy, it is important to determine that the patient has two kidneys of a reasonable size, and this can best be undertaken by ultrasound examination just prior to the biopsy procedure, which may be ultrasound guided. Material obtained on renal biopsy should be placed in appropriate fixative so that subsequent examination can include light microscopy, immunological investigation, and electron microscopy.

In hypertensive patients, renal perfusion should be investigated particularly if renovascular disease is suspected; abnormal results should be followed by either digital vascular imaging or arteriography. In patients with vascular abnormalities, it may be necessary to proceed to the estimation of renal vein renin concentrations.

In patients suspected of having renal tubular defects, specific investigation can be undertaken to determine urinary concentration, acidification, and urinary amino-acid excretion.

In a properly structured investigative plan, tests are undertaken in a sequential fashion, commencing with simple screening tests and proceeding to specific diagnostic tests.

Conclusion of initial interview

After obtaining the relevant clinical history and undertaking a full clinical examination, it is possible to formulate a differential diagnosis from cognitive associations. In some instances, this diagnosis will be obvious at this stage, as in patients with gross adult type polycystic kidney disease, but in many it will only be obtained following the results of specific investigations such as renal biopsy. The nature of the investigations should be explained in full to the patient and, where appropriate, to the relatives. This is particularly important for the so-called invasive investigations such as biopsy and arteriography. Many investigations are not diagnostic, but add to the overall basic data base and increase the ability to predict prognosis. Failure to explain this to the patient may subsequently result in considerable confusion. Some conditions, such as Goodpasture's syndrome, require rapid invasive investigations, but many can be treated in a more considered way and patients should be given the opportunity of considering the advice offered before committing themselves to potentially hazardous investigations. At all times, the patient should be encouraged to raise questions, although many, particularly the elderly, are reluctant to trouble the 'busy' physician. Finally, the patient should be advised how long the investigation will take and also how long it will take for laboratory studies to be completed and for the results to become available. It is sometimes worth documenting this advice in the patient's notes so that important information is not 'lost'.

It is worth remembering that the most important points to emerge may only come at the conclusion of the interview, when a patient may remark 'while I am here may I ask you about . . . '. Sometimes, it takes this much time for the patient to pluck up courage to ask about something which is a major cause for concern. Commonly, patients believe they have an illness of a more serious nature than reality and much anxiety may develop. To avoid mentioning certain diagnoses, such as malignancy, may only serve to reinforce the patient's mistaken belief, and time must be spent in explaining the nature of investigations and the results obtained together with the details of treatment and prognosis.

Planning follow-up

The aim of patient follow-up is:

(1) to measure the effectiveness of therapy;

(2) to detect any change in the clinical condition, particularly with respect to deteriorating renal function; and more rarely

(3) to gain experience of a particular clinical condition or the effects of newly introduced therapeutic measures.

Such follow-up should inconvenience the patient as little as possible, while ensuring that these aims are properly achieved.

Planning of a follow-up programme should consider who is to undertake the observations, the intervals at which the patient should be seen and the measurements that should be taken.

In many conditions, follow-up can be undertaken adequately by the family physician, with advice as and when required from the specialist centre. In some patients, particularly those who live some distance from the specialist centre, follow-up is best achieved by a local physician with a specific interest in renal disease. For patients with conditions that require treatment with potentially hazardous medications, such as the combination of corticosteroids and immunosuppressive drugs, and for patients whose clinical status is likely to change rapidly, observation by a nephrologist is advisable.

If follow-up is to be undertaken outside a specialist centre, the clinician must be provided with adequate information. This should include the diagnosis and details regarding the natural history of the condition, outlining what could be expected to happen to a particular patient. Full details relating to specific therapy should be clearly documented, along with specific advice relating to when the patient should be referred back to the specialist centre.

The frequency of follow-up visits should be reviewed at regular intervals. Initially, review is required at short intervals to determine the adequacy of therapy and to detect deterioration in renal function. Even in apparently homogeneous conditions such as membranous glomerulonephritis, the rate of progression of renal functional impairment is very variable; the only means of determining this at present is through regular follow-up visits at which renal function is estimated. Fortunately, for many conditions the rate of progression in an individual is relatively constant, and it is possible to lengthen the time between clinic visits for those patients with stable or only slowly deteriorating disease, whilst increasing the frequency in those in whom function is deteriorating more rapidly.

References

Boulton-Jones, J. M., Sissons, J. G. P., Naish, P. F., Evans, D. J., and Peters, D. K. (1974). Self induced glomerulonephritis. *British Medical Journal* **3**, 387–390.

Burden, R. P., Booth, L. J., Ockenden, B. G., Boyd, W. N., Higgins, P. McR., and Aber, G. M. (1975). Intrarenal vascular changes in adult patients with recurrent haematuria and loin pain—a clinical, histological and angiographic study. *Quarterly Journal of Medicine* **44**, 433–474.

Duffy, T. P. (1992). The Red Baron. *New England Journal of Medicine* **327**, 408–411.

Edelman, S. and Witztum, J. L. (1989). Hyperkalaemia during treatment with HMG-CoA reductase inhibitor. *New England Journal of Medicine* **320**, 1219–1220.

Frohlich, E. D., Grim, C., Labarthe, D. R., Maxwell, M. H., Perloff, D., and Weidman, W. H. (1988). Recommendations for human blood pressure determination by sphygmomanometers; report of a special task force appointed by the Steering Committee. *American Heart Association Circulation* **77**, 502A–514A.

Grossman, E. and Messerli, F. H. (1995). A side effect of drugs, poisons, and food. *Archives of Internal Medicine* **155**, 450–460.

Hunt, J. C., Frohlich, E. D., Moser, M., Roccella, E. J., and Keighley, E. A. (1985). Devices used for self-measurement of blood pressure. Revised statement of the National High Blood Pressure Education Programme. *Archives of Internal Medicine* **145**, 2231–2234.

Ifudu, O., Kolasinski, S. L., and Friedman, E. A. (1992). Kidney-related Munchausen's syndrome. *New England Journal of Medicine* **327**, 388–389.

Isles, C. *et al.* (1979). Excess smoking in malignant phase hypertension. *British Medical Journal* **1**, 579–581.

Lagrue, G., Laurent, J., and Rostoker, G. (1989). Food allergy and idiopathic nephrotic syndrome. *Kidney International* **27** (Suppl.), S147–S151.

Lang, T., Degoulet, P., Aime, F., Devries, C., Jacquinet-Salord, M. C., and Fouriaud, C. (1987). Relationship between alcohol consumption and hypertension prevalence and control in a French population. *Journal of Chronic Diseases* **40**, 713–720.

Lurvey, A., Ysin, A., and Dequattro, V. (1973). Pseudopheochromocytoma after self-administered isoproterenol. *Journal of Clinical Endocrinology and Metabolism* **36**, 766–769.

MacGregor, G. A., Tasker, P. R. W., and de Wardener, H. E. (1975). Diuretic induced oedema. *Lancet* **i**, 489–492.

MacGregor, G. A. and de Wardener, H. E. (1988). Idiopathic oedema. In *Diseases of the Kidney* 4th edn. (ed. R. W. Schrier and C. W. Gottsshalk), pp. 2743–2753. Boston: Little Brown and Co.

MacKay, A., Brown, J. J., Cumming, A. M. M., Isles, C., Lever, A. F., and Robertson, J. I. S. (1979). Smoking and renal artery stenosis. *British Medical Journal* **2**, 770.

Meadow, R. (1977). Munchausen syndrome by proxy. The hinterland of child abuse. *Lancet* **ii**, 343–345.

Naish, P. F., Aber, G. M., and Boyd, W. N. (1975). C3 deposition in the renal arterioles in the loin pain and haematuria syndrome. *British Medical Journal* **3**, 746.

Nuyts, G. D., Van Vlem, E., Thys, J., De Leernjider, D., D'Haese, P. C., Elseviers, M. M., and De Broe, M. E. (1995). New occupational risk factors for chronic renal failure. *Lancet* **346**, 7–11.

Portioli, I. and Valcavi, R. (1981). Factitious phaeochromocytoma: a case for Sherlock Holmes. *British Medical Journal* **283**, 1660–1661.

Robson, J. S., Martin, A. M., Ruckley, V. A., and MacDonald, M. K. (1968). Irreversible post-partum renal failure: a new syndrome. *Quarterly Journal of Medicine* **37**, 423–435.

Rossing, P., Rossing, K., Jacobsen, P., and Parving, H. H. (1995). Unchanged incidence of diabetic nephropathy in IDDM patients. *Diabetes* **44**, 739–743.

Saunders, J. B., Beevers, D. G., and Paton, A. (1981). Alcohol-induced hypertension. *Lancet* **ii**, 653–656.

Stewart, P. M., Valentino, R., Wallace, A. M., Burt, D., Shackleton, C. H. L., and Edwards, C. R. W. (1987). Mineralocorticoid activity of licorice: 11-beta-hydroxysteroid dehydrogenase deficiency comes of age. *Lancet* **ii**, 821–823.

Turck, M., Goffe, B. S., and Petersdorf, R. G. (1962). Bacteruria of pregnancy. Relation to socioeconomic factors. *New England Journal of Medicine* **266**, 857–860.

Winslow, C. M. *et al.* (1986). Automated ambulatory blood pressure monitoring. *Annals of Internal Medicine* **104**, 275–278.

1.2 Urinalysis and microscopy

Giovanni B. Fogazzi

Introduction

Urinalysis is one of the basic tests for the evaluation of patients with renal disease. This chapter describes basic urinalysis, which includes the physicochemical features of urine and urine microscopy. Moreover, it deals with microalbuminuria, enzymuria, and the instruments for the automated analysis of urine sediments.

Physical and chemical examination

Preanalytical aspects

The preanalytical phase is an important aspect of urinalysis because the timing of collection, the preparation of the patient, and the storage of specimens can affect the accuracy of the results.

Collection of specimens

Written instructions describing the procedure should be given to the subject (Kouri *et al.* 2000). These should suggest avoiding strenuous physical exercise (e.g. marathon, jogging, a soccer match) in the hours preceding the collection, since these activities may cause proteinuria and/or haematuria; avoiding the collection of urine during menstruation because this can contaminate the urine with blood; preceding urine collection by washing of the hands with water and the washing of external genitalia with clean wet paper towels, which in females is best done after the spreading of the labia and in males after the withdrawing of the foreskin of the penis; collecting the urine after discarding the first portion of micturition (Kouri *et al.* 2000).

Depending on the type of investigation, a timed urine collection (e.g. 24 h for proteinuria) or a spot urine collection (this aspect is dealt with in the sections about urine protein–creatinine ratio—see section on 'Proteins' and 'Urine microscopy') may be needed. In case, a spot sample is requested, this should be of at least 50 ml.

Urine should be collected in a container supplied by the laboratory or bought in a pharmacy. It should have a capacity of at least 50–100 ml and a diameter opening of at least 5 cm to allow easy collection by both females and males (Kouri *et al.* 2000).

Storage of specimens

To avoid alterations in physical or chemical features, urine should ideally be analysed within 1 h of voiding. Several means of preservation, such as addition of thymol, borate, formalin, toluene, etc. to urine or refrigeration at 4°C, have been proposed. Some of these can, however, cause some interfering chemical reactions. For instance, formalin may precipitate protein and thymol interferes with the acid precipitation test for proteins. Thus, there is no definitive substitute for the study of fresh urine.

Physical features

Colour

The colour of the urine must be evaluated in optimal conditions, under good lighting with the specimen in a transparent container and viewed against a white background. The colour of normal urine ranges from pale to dark yellow and amber, depending on the concentration of urochrome.

Gross haematuria is the most frequent cause of altered colour. In this condition, the urine is pink to black, the factors that influence the final colour being the number of erythrocytes or the amount of haemoglobin, the pH, and the duration of contact between the haemoglobin and urine. The lower the pH and the longer the contact, the darker the colour (Berman 1977). Urine is also of a variable red colour in haemoglobinuria, myoglobinuria, after eating beetroot by some genetically susceptible people, or after rifampicin or other drugs.

Jaundice and all other states associated with increased concentrations of conjugated bilirubin are also frequent causes of hyperpigmented urine (dark yellow to brown).

In other conditions, urine may be normal in colour when fresh, but darkens upon standing. This occurs in porphyria because of urinary porphobilinogen, in melanoma because of melanogen, and in alkaptonuria because of homogentisic acid. Therefore, when such diseases are suspected the urine must be exposed to light for some time.

Drugs may also influence the colour of urine. Urine containing nitrofurantoin is dark yellow to brown and that containing levodopa is brown to black; amitryptyline and methylene blue colour urine green or blue-green. Imipenem–cilastatin can cause a brown urine, very similar to that due to bilirubin, upon standing.

Turbidity

Normal, freshly voided urine is usually clear or transparent. High concentrations of leucocytes, erythrocytes, epithelial cells, bacteria, crystals, or contaminants such as candida can all be associated with a cloudy specimen.

A clear, fresh urine may cloud after standing, especially when kept in a refrigerator, because of the precipitation of phosphates or urates.

A rare cause of urine turbidity and colour abnormality at the same time is represented by chyluria. This is characterized by a 'milky' or even 'cheese-like' appearance, due to a mixture of lipids (especially triglycerides), erythrocytes, leucocytes, and fibrin. When allowed to stand, chylous urine forms three layers: a white top layer that contains fatty material, a middle pinkish layer often containing clots, a bottom layer containing cells and debris. Turbidity may be intermittent, and may be precipitated by fatty meals.

The microscopic examination of chylous urine reveals large amounts of fat globules, lymphocytes, and erythrocytes.

Chyluria is due to a fistulous connection between the lymphatic and urinary system. In most instances this is caused by the obstruction of the lymphatic system by the parasite *Filaria bancrofti*, which is endemic in several tropical regions. However, very rarely, chyluria may have non-parasitic causes, such as trauma, tuberculosis, neoplasms, or renal surgery (Diamond and Schapira 1985; Campieri *et al.* 1996; Tuck *et al.* 2000).

Another peculiar and rare abnormality of urine is pneumaturia. This consists of the passage of gas, which is usually odourless, in the urine. In most instances, pneumaturia is seen in patients with a fistulous connection between the bowel and the urinary tract. However, it may also be associated with urinary tract infection including emphysematous pyelonephritis, especially in diabetic patients. In such cases, it is thought that the production of gas derives from bacterial proteolysis or, in patients with diabetes mellitus, from glucose fermentation. When urinary infection reverses pneumaturia also disappears (Synhaivsky and Malek 1985; Jain *et al.* 2001).

Odour

The most common cause of abnormal urine odour is urinary tract infection, which confers a pungent smell. Ketones, instead, cause a sweet or fruity odour.

Some rare diseases confer a characteristic smell to the urine. These are maple syrup urine disease, which confers a 'maple syrup' odour, which is due to a substance called sotolone (Podebrad *et al.* 1999); phenylketonuria, which is associated with a 'mousy' odour; isovaleric acidaemia, which comes with a 'sweaty feet' odour; fish odour syndrome, which confers to the urine and other body secretions the odour of rotten fish (Rehman 1999).

Relative density

This variable may be measured by four methods: specific gravity, refractometry, osmolality, and dry chemistry (dipsticks).

Specific gravity

The specific gravity of a solution refers to the ratio of its weight to that of an equal volume of water at the same temperature. For urine, the specific gravity is a function of the number and weight of the dissolved solute particles. It is usually measured with a hydrometer, commonly called a 'urinometer', which is a weighted float marked with a scale for specific gravities from 1.000 to 1.060. The urinometer is simple and quick to use, but has some drawbacks: it requires a volume of urine not always available in spot samples; there may be difficulty in reading the meniscus; and there may be a tendency for the device to cling to the side of the container. Moreover, specific gravity varies with temperature and urinometers may be inaccurately calibrated. Urine specific gravity should be corrected for protein and glucose, if either is present (Strasinger 1985). Proteins increase the specific gravity by 0.001 for each 0.4 g/dl and glucose by 0.001 for each 0.27 g/dl. When specific gravities in excess of 1.040 are recorded and there is no glycosuria or proteinuria, the presence of abnormal substances in the urine, such as radiographic contrast media, should be considered.

Refractometry

This method is based on measurement of the refractive index, which is related to the weight of solutes per unit volume of urine. Several types of refractometers are available, which are very simple to use and require only one drop of urine. Because of the interdependence between refractive index and temperature, the refractometer should be of the temperature-compensating type. Refractometry is affected by proteins (0.005/g protein/dl), radiopaque contrast media, and glucose.

Osmolality

Osmolality is a function of the number of particles in solution and is usually measured through the effect of colligative properties on the freezing point of the solution. Numerous manual or fully automated osmometers are available commercially. Measurement of osmolality offers definite advantages over other methods. These include: (a) temperature correction is not necessary; (b) only small volumes of urine are required; and (c) there is no interference from proteins or other macromolecules. However, high glucose concentrations contribute significantly to the measured osmolality (10 g/l of glucose = 55.5 mOsm).

Dry chemistry

The chemical principle of the reagent-strip reaction is based on the pK_a change of pretreated polyelectrolytes in relation to the ionic concentration of the urine in the presence of an indicator (Burkhardt *et al.* 1983). This method is incorporated into dipsticks, therefore it is widely used. However, it does not strictly correlate with the findings obtained by refractometry (Dorizzi and Caputo 1998).

False-negative results. Reduced values occur in the presence of glucose, urea, or alkaline urine.

False-positive results. Increased values are found in the presence of ketoacids or proteins greater than 1 g/l.

Chemical features

pH

In the normal individual, urinary pH ranges from 4.5 to 8.0. It usually averages from 5.0 to 6.0, with variations mainly caused by food intake. The pH is generally evaluated by dipsticks utilizing two indicators, methyl red and bromothymol blue, which cover the values between pH 5 and 9. In most cases, the dipsticks for pH are sufficiently reliable, although they deviate significantly from the true pH when this is less than 5.5 or greater than 7.5. Therefore, when a more accurate measurement of the pH is needed, a pH meter with a glass electrode must be used.

False-negative results. Reduced values are observed in the presence of formaldehyde.

False-positive results are not reported.

Haemoglobin

Haemoglobin is detected by a dipstick. This is based on peroxidase activity that catalyzes the reaction of a peroxide and a chromogen to produce a coloured product. The presence of haemoglobin is expressed either as spots or as a homogeneous pattern. Spots occur in the presence of intact erythrocytes, while the homogeneous pattern is caused by free haemoglobin. Most often this derives from the lysis of erythrocytes favoured by standing, alkaline pH or low relative density/osmolality. The dipsticks for haemoglobin are sensitive, showing positive reactions at concentrations as low as 0.1–0.6 mg/l.

False-negative results may occur with a high concentration of urinary ascorbic acid (Brigden *et al.* 1992). In an attempt to reduce interference from this substance, some manufacturers have incorporated oxidants into the reagent strip that promote oxidation of ascorbic acid into dehydroascorbate acid. However, even with this improvement, potentially dangerous false-negative results can occur. Other false-negative results may be caused by high nitrite concentration, high urine density, and formaldehyde (0.5 g/l).

False-positive results may be seen in urine containing oxidizing agents, large numbers of bacteria (Lam 1995), or myoglobin, which is found in the urine after muscle damage. The pattern caused by myoglobin is homogeneous and is identical to that caused by haemoglobin.

Myoglobin and haemoglobin can be distinguished by dissolving 2.8 g of ammonium sulfate in 5 ml of urine, followed by filtration or centrifugation. In the presence of ammonium sulfate, haemoglobin precipitates, while myoglobin does not. Thus, haemoglobin gives a clear filtered solution or supernatant, while myoglobin gives a pigmented solution or supernatant. The two pigments can also be distinguished by spectrophotometry, electrophoresis, ultracentrifugation, or immunochemical methods.

Glucose

Under normal conditions, glucose is not detectable in urine. Urinary glucose is commonly estimated with dipsticks by a coupled, two-stage, enzyme-catalyzed reaction. Glucose is oxidized, with glucose oxidase as catalyst, to gluconic acid and hydrogen peroxide. Then, a peroxidase catalyzes the reaction between hydrogen peroxide and a reduced, colourless chromogen to form a coloured product. This test is highly specific and is sensitive to concentrations of 1–20 g/l. Some commercial sticks are more sensitive (0.5 g/l or less) and have a greater value for detecting glucosuria (Dyerberg *et al.* 1976).

False-negative results. Ascorbic acid at concentrations greater than 4000 μmol/l abolishes the reaction that reveals glucose. Another cause of false-negative results is urinary tract infection.

False-positive results. Strong oxidizing substances, such as hypochlorite and chlorine bleach, can produce a positive reaction.

The best quantitative methods for the routine measurement of urinary glucose are enzymatic, in particular, hexokinase. They overcome the disadvantages of the coupled glucose oxidase assays, with which several compounds, such as bilirubin, uric acid or ascorbic acid, can be oxidized by the hydrogen peroxide produced by the glucose oxidase reaction.

Proteins

Under physiological conditions, urinary protein excretion does not exceed 150 mg/day for adults and 140 mg/m^2 of body surface for children. The daily physiological proteinuria contains mucoprotein (e.g. Tamm–Horsfall glycoprotein; 70 mg), blood group-related substances (35 mg), albumin (16 mg), immunoglobulins (6 mg), mucopolysaccharides (16 mg), and very small amounts of other proteins such as hormones and enzymes (King and Boyce 1963).

There are four categories of pathological proteinuria: 'glomerular', 'tubular', 'overload', and 'benign' (Abuelo 1983).

Glomerular proteinuria is due to increased glomerular permeability to proteins and occurs in primary and secondary glomerulopathies.

Tubular proteinuria is due to decreased tubular reabsorption of proteins normally present in the glomerular filtrate. It is seen in tubular and interstitial disorders, including those which develop in the course of chronic glomerular diseases.

Overload proteinuria is secondary to increased production, or release, of low-molecular weight proteins which are usually reabsorbed by the proximal tubular cells, such as immunoglobulin light chains (which are increased in monoclonal gammopathies), lysozyme (which is increased in some leukaemias), or myoglobin (which is increased in rhabdomyolysis).

Benign proteinuria includes functional proteinuria, as seen in fever or after exercise, idiopathic transient proteinuria, and orthostatic proteinuria.

Once pathological proteinuria has been detected, it must be quantified and submitted to qualitative analysis to discover to which of the above four categories it belongs.

Detection

Dipsticks Proteinuria is usually detected by dipsticks. Dipsticks for proteins are based on the principle of 'the protein error of indicators'. With increasing concentrations of protein in urine the dye indicators undergo sequential colour changes from pale green to green and blue. The binding of a protein to the indicators, which are structurally similar to bromocresol green, is highly pH dependent. Albumin binds to indicators at pH between 5 and 7. Other proteins bind at lower pH, but with a lower affinity than albumin, while Bence Jones protein does not bind at any pH.

The results are expressed on a scale from 0 to +++ or ++++, at each of which correspond approximate protein concentrations, which vary according to the manufacturer.

False-negative results. Dipsticks almost exclusively detect albumin, the sensitivity being for concentrations as low as 250 mg/l. Therefore microalbuminuria is not detected by dipsticks as also are globulins, tubular proteins or Bence Jones protein. Therefore, dipsticks must not be used whenever a tubular proteinuria or a Bence Jones proteinuria are suspected. Underestimation of albuminuria can also occur in diluted urine.

False-positive results occur in heavily alkaline urine, since the buffer contained in the pad is insufficient to achieve the optimal pH for the indicator to function adequately. In addition, deeply pigmented urine and urine containing quaternary ammonium compounds or phenazopyridine tend to give false-positive results.

Precipitation methods These evaluate the turbidity occurring after proteins are precipitated by sulfosalicylic acid, trichloracetic acid or by heat and acetic acid–sodium acetate buffer. Turbidimetric methods detect all urinary proteins, but α_1-acid glycoprotein and Tamm–Horsfall mucoprotein are not precipitated by sulfosalicylic acid (Shiba *et al.* 1985). Turbidimetric methods are very sensitive and may detect protein concentrations as low as 2.5 mg/l. With these methods too the protein concentration is expressed on a semiquantitative scale, from 0 to +++ or ++++.

Many drugs can cause positive interference, for example, large amounts of penicillin or cephalosporin analogues, miconazole, tolbutamide, or sulfonamide metabolites. False-positive results can also be caused by the presence in the urine of radiographic contrast media.

Quantitative evaluation

Urine proteins can be quantified by several methods (Table 1), but as urine can contain a large range of proteins and also many interfering substances, all the available methods are imperfect.

Turbidimetric methods These methods, which are based on sulfosalicylic acid, tricholoracetic acid, or benzethonium chloride in alkaline medium, are among the most used. However, since they suffer from major drawbacks, other methods should be preferred.

The sulfosalicylic procedure is more sensitive to albumin than to other proteins, and it also causes the precipitation of significant quantities of polypeptides. This method, moreover, does not detect some glycoproteins and is affected by an inhibitor in urine that decreases the analytical recovery of proteins (Nakamura and Yakata 1982).

Trichloroacetic acid is unaffected by protein composition provided it is used at low concentrations and the urine temperature ranges between 20 and 25°C. However, numerous drugs can interfere with this method (Lorentz and Weiss 1986).

The method based on benzethonium chloride gives a stable turbidity and is less dependent on temperature than the previous methods. However, it produces 11–31 per cent less turbidity for gammaglobulins than for albumin, and gives unevenly dispersed aggregates in the presence of large protein concentrations, with consequent falsely low protein estimates (McElderry *et al.* 1982; Lacher and DeBeukelaer 1986).

Dye-binding techniques These are based on the interaction between proteins and a dye, which causes a shift in the absorption maxima (measured photometrically) of the dye.

Coomassie brilliant blue G250 (Bradford 1976) is very sensitive, but with diluted samples significant deviations from linearity are possible. Moreover, underestimation of tubular proteinuria and interference from various metabolites, drugs, and preservative compounds have been observed. The method is somewhat improved by the addition of sodium dodecylsulfate. Ponceau S, introduced by Pesce and Strande (1973), is equally sensitive to albumin and globulins, but falsely low values can result from the loss of precipitate during the decantation step while falsely high values may derive from the contamination of the precipitate by unbound dye. Modifications have been proposed to circumvent these problems (Meola *et al.* 1977; Lievens and Celis 1982), but these affect the practicability of the method. Aminoglycoside antibiotics interfere positively.

Biuret methods These methods are based on the interaction between copper ions and the carbamide group of proteins, and are at present the methods of choice (Lorentz and Weiss 1986). They have the same sensitivity for all proteins. The protein in the urine must be concentrated before the biuret reaction and Tsuchiya reagent (ethanolic hydrochloride–phosphotungstic acid) is the best precipitating compound. Interference from drugs, radiographic contrast media, and coloured metabolites is minimal (Bradford 1976; Lorentz and Weiss 1986). A modification of the biuret method, which is now the reference method recommended by the American Association for Clinical Chemistry, utilizes gel filtration to exclude small interfering compounds.

The Folin–Lowry procedure is a variant of biuret methods in that copper ions bind not only to peptide bonds, but also to the amino acids tyrosine and tryptophan. This method is 100 times more sensitive than the biuret method, but is non-specific and suffers from numerous interferences. These can partially be removed by the pretreatment of the urine by dialysis, precipitation, and ultrafiltration.

The protein–creatinine ratio

The 24-h urine collection is considered as the 'gold standard' for the quantitative evaluation of proteinuria. However, it is time-consuming, subject to error, and is frequently associated with significant collection

Table 1 The quantitative methods for proteinuria

Method	Analytical sensitivity (mg/l)	Linearity (mg/l)	Distinctive features
Turbidimetric			
Sulfosalicylic acid	10–20	10–3000	Albumin overestimation; some glycoproteins are not detected
Trichloroacetic	20	20–2400	Same sensitivity for albumin and globulins; many drugs can interfere
Benzethonium chloride	10	10–1600	Albumin overestimation; underestimation of increased protein concentrations
Dye binding			
Coomassie brilliant blue	2.5	5–1500	High sensitivity; underestimation of tubular proteins
Ponceau	20	100–1600	Same sensitivity for albumin and globulins; positive interference with aminoglycoside antibiotics
Biuret			
Precipitation with Tsuchiya reagent	5–17	5–270[a] 5–2000[b]	Same sensitivity to all proteins; very few interferences
Folin–Lowry	10	10–700	Interference by tyrosine and tryptophan

[a] Sample volume, 0.2 ml.

[b] Sample volume, 2.0 ml.

The figures for linearity indicate measurement intervals that do not require predilution of the samples.

errors, which are mainly due to improper timing and missed samples. The calculation of protein–creatinine ratio on spot urine samples, which corrects for variations in urinary concentration due to hydration, is an alternative to the 24-h collection (Ginsberg *et al.* 1983).

In the experience of Ginsberg *et al.* (1983) the measurements obtained with this method correlated well with those obtained in the classical way. In fact, all patients with proteinuria of greater than 3.5 g/24 h had a ratio of greater than 3.5 in single voided samples, and all patients with a proteinuria of less than 0.2 g/24 h had a ratio of less than 0.2. The applicability and reliability of this method has been confirmed by several investigators (Schwab *et al.* 1987; Rodby *et al.* 1995; Ruggenenti *et al.* 1998), and is now recommended by recent American Guidelines (K/DOQI clinical practice guidelines for chronic kidney diseases: evaluation, classification and stratification 2002).

The protein–creatinine ratio is preferably calculated on the first morning urine. This avoids the possible variations caused by the circadian rhythm of protein excretion, which is maximal during the day and minimal during the night, compared to the urinary excretion of creatinine, which is rather constant over the day (Koopman *et al.* 1989).

Qualitative analysis

Several methods are available for the qualitative analysis of proteinuria.

Electrophoresis Electrophoresis on cellulose acetate or agarose after protein concentration or using very sensitive staining (silver or gold stains) is one of the most widely used method. Better resolution is obtained by sodium dodecylsulfate-polyacrylamide gel electrophoresis (SDS-PAGE), which detects urinary proteins on the basis of their molecular weight. This technique allows the identification of proteins of tubular origin with low molecular weight (e.g. 10 kDa). The identification of these proteins may be of importance, since in nephrotic patients they have been found to be an indicator of poor prognosis (Bazzi *et al.* 1997).

Specific proteins Another way to distinguish the different types of proteinuria is based on the measurement of specific proteins. For instance, the measurement of tubular proteins such as β_2-microglobulin, retinol-binding protein, or α_1-microglobulin is used to diagnose and follow-up tubulointerstitial diseases. These are also used to investigate the involvement of the tubulointerstitial compartment in nephrotic syndrome caused by membranous nephropathy (Reichert *et al.* 1995).

A possible approach is based on the simultaneous measurement in the same specimen of different proteins both of glomerular (albumin and IgG) and tubular origin [α_1-microglobulin, and *N*-acetyl-β-D-glucosaminidase (NAG)]. This method has been found to be more sensitive than dipsticks for albumin in revealing a renal disease (Hofmann *et al.* 1992). A similar approach, based on the simultaneous measurement of IgG and α_1-microglobulin, may be used to evaluate the course and response to treatment in glomerular diseases such as membranous nephropathy (Bazzi *et al.* 2001).

Selectivity of proteinuria Classically, this is evaluated by the ratio of the clearance of IgG (molecular weight 160,000) to the clearance of transferrin (molecular weight 88,000). When the ratio is less than 0.1 the proteinuria is defined as selective (Cameron and Blandford 1966). In children with nephrotic syndrome, this indicates the presence of minimal change disease responsive to corticosteroids.

Newer approaches are based on the use of SDS-PAGE coupled with the fractional excretion of α_1-microglobulin (Bazzi *et al.* 2000) or the ratio of the clearance of IgM to that of albumin (Bakoush *et al.* 2001).

For proteinuria due to the excretion of monoclonal light-chain, electrophoresis reveals the presence of a homogeneous band in the pattern, and immunofixation electrophoresis is used to characterize the monoclonal component (Merlini *et al.* 2001). Today immunofixation is the gold standard technique, however, it can occasionally give misleading 'pseudo-oligoclonal' patterns in urine specimens that contain polyclonal immunoglobulin (Harrison *et al.* 1992).

Microalbuminuria

Microalbuminuria is defined as a urine albumin concentration greater than normal but negative by dipstick testing. According to the American Diabetes Association (1994) this corresponds to an albumin excretion rate of approximately 30–300 mg/24 h.

Besides diabetes mellitus, a number of other conditions have been found to be associated with microalbuminuria, including high blood pressure (Rosa and Palatini 2000), obesity and hypertriglyceridaemia (Pannacciulli *et al.* 2001), smoking (Gambaro *et al.* 2001), oral contraceptive use and hormone replacement therapy (Monster *et al.* 2001), female gender, old age, etc. (Jones *et al.* 2002).

The most common methods to measure microalbuminuria are radioimmunoassay (Woo *et al.* 1978), enzyme immunoassay (Fielding *et al.* 1987), nephelometric (Stamp 1988), and turbidimetric (Shukla *et al.* 1988).

Test strips are also available, which can be used in screening procedures. These detect albumin at concentration of 10–20 mg/l, and have a 70–90 per cent specificity (Mogensen *et al.* 1997; Pugia *et al.* 1997; Gerber *et al.* 1998). It is recommended that a positive strip test is followed by a quantitative determination (American Diabetes Association 1994).

The 24-h urine collection is considered the 'gold standard' method for the measurement of microalbuminuria. However, the urine albumin–creatinine ratio on random urine samples can also be used (Assadi 2002). With this method microalbuminuria is defined as a ratio of 30–300 μg albumin/mg creatinine.

Leucocyte esterase

This dipstick is based on the esterase activity of granulocytes; 3-hydroxy-5-phenyl-pyrrole esterified with an amino acid or indoxyl carbonic acid ester is used as substrate. Hydrolysis of these esters by the esterase releases 3-hydroxy-5-phenyl-pyrrole and indoxyl, which react with a diazonium salt, yielding an azo dye.

The method is very specific for lysed leucocytes (Scheer 1987). Thus, in urine with alkaline pH or low specific gravity, dipsticks for esterase may be positive, while microscopic examination for leucocytes may be negative.

False-negative results. Glucose at concentrations of 20 g/l or more inhibits the trace reaction. A decreased sensitivity is also observed in isotonic urine. False-negative results may also occur in the presence of increased concentrations of proteins (>5 g/l), or in presence of cephalexin, cephalotin, nitrofurantoin, tetracycline, and tobramycin.

False-positive results occur in the presence of oxidizing detergents, formaldehyde (0.4 g/l), sodium azide, coloured urine due to beet ingestion, or bilirubin.

Nitrites

The presence of bacteria in the urine may be revealed by the reduction of nitrates to nitrites, which are shown by a dipstick containing an aromatic amine that reacts with nitrites to form a coloured diazonium compound. This test has a low sensitivity and a high specificity

(Pfaller *et al.* 1985; Wilkins *et al.* 1985). In some instances, however, the nitrite test may be more sensitive than urine culture. This happens especially when urine cultures based on cystine–lactose electrolyte-deficient (CLED) agar are used, which fail to grow organisms such as haemophili.

False-negative tests may occur in alkaline urine, when the retention of urine in the bladder is too short, or also when the urinary nitrate concentration is too low. Moreover, some bacteria, such as *Pseudomonas* spp., *Staphylococcus albus*, *Staph. saprophyticus*, and *Streptococcus faecalis*, may be mild nitrate reducers or express no nitrate-reducing capacity.

False-positive results are seen with coloured urine, which hamper the correct reading of the pad.

Ketones

Ketones are usually detected by dipsticks based on the reaction of acetone and acetoacetate with nitroprusside in a strongly alkaline medium, with glycine as the nitrogen source. The dipsticks are more sensitive to acetoacetate than to acetone, with a detection limit for acetoacetate of the order of 50–100 mg/l.

False-negative results may be seen if the urine has improperly been stored.

False-positive findings are seen in the presence of drugs such as phenylketones, phthalein derivatives, levodopa metabolites, and captopril or other substances containing sulfydryl groups.

Bilirubin–urobilinogen

In some countries, these measurements are included in routine urinalysis. Recent European guidelines consider these parameters as useless in screening urinalysis (Kouri *et al.* 2000).

Enzymuria

Normal individuals excrete small amounts of enzymes located in the cells of the renal tubules in their urine [see Pesce and First (1979) for a detailed listing]. Increased excretion of these enzymes is a sensitive index of renal damage (Marhun 1979; Price 1982). These measurements have the advantage of being easily made and have great sensitivity, but unfortunately are non-specific so far as disease processes are concerned. Thus, they are not very useful for diagnostic purposes, and their main value lies in screening populations at risk for renal damage, examining the detailed nephrotoxicity of agents used clinically or commercially, or in investigating consecutively the activity of processes already identified.

A number of brush-border enzymes have been studied in normal and pathological urines, including alkaline phosphatase (EC 3.1.3.1) (Hartman *et al.* 1985), leucine aminopeptidase (EC 3.4.11.2) (Hartman *et al.* 1985; Cavaliere *et al.* 1987), γ-glutamyltransferase (EC 2.3.2) (Hartman *et al.* 1985; Cavaliere *et al.* 1987), α-glucosidase (EC 3.2.1.20) (Hartman *et al.* 1985), trehalase (EC 3.2.1.28) (Hartman *et al.* 1985), dipeptidyl aminopeptidase IV (EC 3.4.14.5) (Wolf *et al.* 1990), and neutral endopeptidase (EC 3.4.24.11) (Vlaskou *et al.* 2000) all located in the brush border of the proximal tubule. Most data, however, relate to NAG (EC 3.2.1.30), a 130 kDa hydrolytic enzyme present in lysosomes (Sherman *et al.* 1983).

The excretion of tubular enzymes or NAG increases in a large variety of conditions, for example aminoglycoside antibiotics (Mondorf *et al.* 1984), prolonged rifampicin therapy (Kumar *et al.* 1992), cisplatin (Rojanasthien *et al.* 2001), contrast media (Erley *et al.* 1999), heavy metals and organic solvents (Meyer *et al.* 1984; Ng *et al.* 1993; Tassi *et al.* 2000), glomerulonephritis (Valles *et al.* 2000), acute interstitial nephritis (Wolf *et al.* 1990), extracorporeal shock-wave lithotripsy (Weichert-Jacobsen *et al.* 1998), and protein malnutrition (Yazzie *et al.* 1998).

Thus, the assay of urinary NAG or other tubular enzymes may detect minimal degrees of renal dysfunction, which is both an advantage and disadvantage for clinical use. The problem in using these assays diagnostically is that, for example, modest renal insults, intercurrent urinary tract infections, increased urinary flow, and therapeutic doses of aminoglycosides will all increase urinary enzyme excretion. Thus, the clinical value of urinary NAG estimations in patients is limited.

Urine microscopy

Urine collection and handling

The second urine of the morning is the most suitable for microscopy, since it is still acidic and concentrated but without the overnight stay in the bladder, which is detrimental to the preservation of formed elements (Aas 1961).

The hands and the urethral meatus must be cleaned as for the physicochemical analysis (Kouri *et al.* 2000). Mid-stream collection is an advisable and well-accepted procedure that prevents contamination from the genitalia and the urethral meatus. Strenuous activity must be avoided for several hours before the collection of urine for microscopy, because it can cause transient haematuria and cylindruria (Fasset *et al.* 1982b), while heavy meals can be followed by the so-called alkaline tide, which can cause the precipitation of phosphates. During menstruation, the urine is almost invariably contaminated with blood, which makes microscopic analysis unreliable. The use of bladder catheters to collect the sample for urine microscopy should be avoided, since they can cause mild microscopic haematuria (Hockberger *et al.* 1987). In selected cases, suprapubic bladder puncture may be appropriate.

The container for urine should be provided by the laboratory or bought in a pharmacy. It should be clean and have a capacity of at least 50–100 ml, with a diameter opening of at least 5 cm to allow easy collection by both females and males. It should also have a wide base to avoid accidental spillage and should be capped (Kouri *et al.* 2000).

The collected urine should be used as soon as possible, since especially in the presence of either alkaline pH or low specific gravity, elements such as erythrocytes and especially leucocytes can lyse (Triger and Smith 1966). To prevent cell lysis, the samples may be kept in the refrigerator at +2 to +8°C, but phosphates and urates at these temperatures may precipitate, which makes the samples difficult to examine. Alternatively, formaldehyde-based fixatives, such as CellFIX, can be used (Van der Snoek and Koene 1997).

Standardized methods for the handling of urine must be used. These include the use of measured samples, well-defined duration and speed of centrifugation, removal of a fixed volume of supernatant (avoiding pouring off), gentle and thorough resuspension of the sediment, transfer to the slide of fixed volumes of sediment, and the application of coverslips with a defined surface (Table 2). It is only by adopting such procedures that unacceptable, quantitative intersample variability can be avoided (Gadeholt 1964).

Microscopic examination

Before analysing the sample, one should know both its pH and osmolality (or relative density), since these variables can influence the findings. For instance, at higher pH the number of casts tends to decrease (Burton *et al.* 1975), and neutrophils tend to lyse (Triger and Smith 1966). At low osmolalities, erythrocytes tend to lose their haemoglobin content (Rath *et al.* 1992), thus becoming less identifiable. At osmolalities of less than 360 mOsm/l (relative density of approximately 1.010), the sample is no longer reliable since erythrocytes and leucocytes tend to lyse. For this reason, it is advisable to couple microscopy with dipsticks for haemoglobin and leucocyte esterase, cell lysis being suggested by the finding of positive dipstick and negative microscopy results.

Counting chambers are suggested to quantify the observed elements (Kessom *et al.* 1978), which are then expressed as number per unit time or per unit volume. Instead, if conventional slides and coverslips are used, the elements are semiquantitated as mean numbers or ranges per field (low-power field for casts, high-power field for cells). Provided that the samples are prepared according to a standardized procedure, the latter method can also give reproducible results between samples (Alwall 1973; Fogazzi *et al.* 1989).

The phase-contrast microscope is recommended for urine microscopy (NCLLS 1995; Kouri *et al.* 2000). Compared to the conventional bright-field microscope it allows a better visualization of all the elements, and makes the use of general stains unnecessary. Phase-contrast microscopy with polarizing filters is mandatory for identifying lipids and crystals when these have unusual appearances (NCLLS 1995; Kouri *et al.* 2000). Two magnifications are needed: 100× or 160× for an overview of the whole sample, and 400× to pick up details.

For special clinical or research purposes, other techniques such as immunofluorescence (Fairley *et al.* 1983; Fogazzi *et al.* 1991), electron microscopy (Mandal *et al.* 1985), or monoclonal antibodies (Segasothy *et al.* 1989; Dooper *et al.* 1991) may be employed.

Table 2 Procedures for the preparation and examination of the urine sediments used in the author's laboratory

Written instructions to the patients for urine collection
Collection in disposable containers of the second urine of the morning after discarding the first few millilitres of urine
Sample handling and analysis within 2 h from collection
Centrifugation of a 10 ml aliquot of urine at 400*g* for 10 min
Removal by suction of 9.5 ml of supernatant urine
Gentle but thorough resuspension with a pipette of the sediment in the remaining 0.5 ml of urine
Transfer by a pipette of 50 μl of resuspended urine to a slide
Covering of sample with a 24 × 32 mm coverslip
Examination of the urine sediment by a phase contrast microscope at 160× and 400× (objectives: 16× and 40× binocular 10×)
Use of polarized light to identify doubtful lipids and crystals
Match of the microscopic findings with dipstick for pH, density, haemoglobin, and leucocyte esterase
Cells quantitated as lowest–highest number seen/high-power field, casts as number/low-power field, all the other elements on a scale from 0 to ++++

The formed elements

Cells

Several types of cells can be found in the urine, some of which come from the blood and others from the different types of epithelium that line the urinary tract. The following are the cells that can be identified by conventional techniques (Table 3).

Erythrocytes

Erythrocytes may be found in the urine due to bleeding occurring at any point of the urinary tract or a contamination of the urine, as frequently happens in women during menstruation.

When true haematuria occurs, the examination of erythrocyte morphology can be used to differentiate the source of the bleeding. If the erythrocytes come from the excretory system they have a regular shape (Fig. 1a), while if they come from the glomeruli, they have irregular shapes and contours (Fig. 1b) (Fairley and Birch 1982).

According to some investigators (Fasset *et al.* 1982a) haematuria is defined as 'non-glomerular' when at least 80 per cent of the erythrocytes show a regular (or 'isomorphic') appearance and 'glomerular' when a similar proportion of erythrocytes are changed (or 'dysmorphic'). The haematuria is 'mixed' when the two types of cells are approximately in the same proportion. Instead, other investigators define, haematuria as glomerular when more than two (Koene 1999) or three (Crompton *et al.* 1993) different forms of erythrocytes are found. Still others have demonstrated that haematuria is glomerular when at least 5 per cent of erythrocytes are acanthocytes of G1 cells (Köhler *et al.* 1991; Kitamoto *et al.* 1993; Lettgen and Wohlmuth 1995; Dinda *et al.* 1997). Compared to generically defined dysmorphic erythrocytes, acantocythes/G1 cells have the advantage of being easily identifiable due to their shape, which is characterized by one or more blebs of different shapes and sizes protruding from a ring-shaped cell body (Fig. 1c). For this reason they are worth looking for. However, they are

Table 3 The cells which can be identified by microscopy in the urine sediment. Other cells such as macrophages, platelets, or podocytes have been described, but their identification requires special techniques

Type	Subtypes
Erythrocytes	Isomorphic Dysmorphic ± acanthocytes Others (sickle cells, anisopoikilocytes)
Leucocytes	Neutrophils Lymphocytes Eosinophils
Tubular cells	Different shapes and sizes according to the tubular segment
Uroepithelial cells	Deep (from basal layers of urothelium) Superficial (from superficial layers of urothelium)
Squamous cells	—

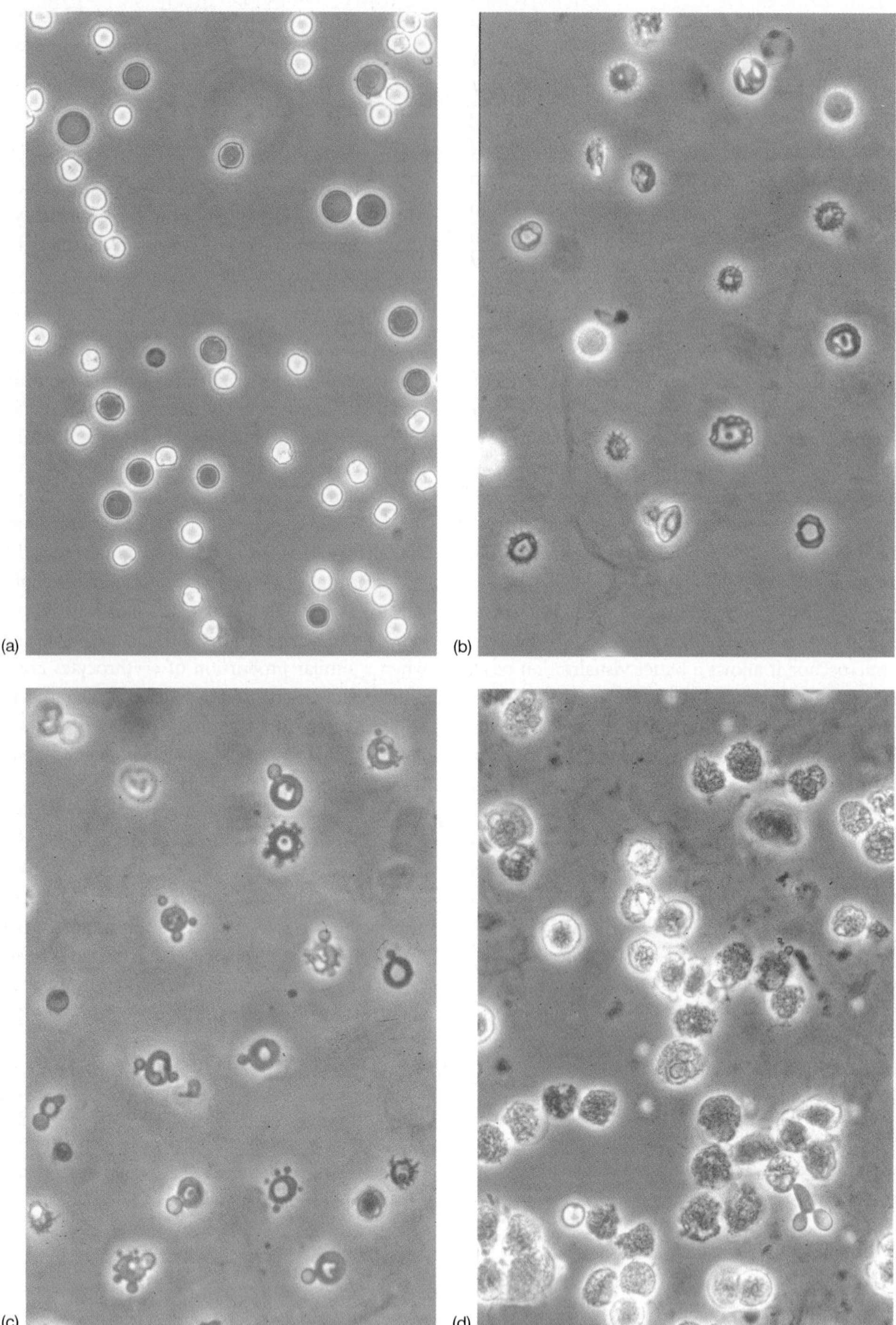

Fig. 1 (a) Isomorphic erythrocytes (dark cells have lost their haemoglobin content). (b) Different types of dysmorphic erythrocytes. (c) Different types of acanthocytes or G1 cells. (d) Neutrophils with their lobulated nucleus and granular cytoplasm (phase-contrast microscopy, original magnification 400×).

not always found in patients with haematuria caused by a glomerular disorder, their sensitivity varying in different studies from 52 to 100 per cent (specificity 98–100 per cent) (Köhler *et al.* 1991; Kitamoto *et al.* 1993; Lettgen and Wohlmuth 1995; Dinda *et al.* 1997).

The evaluation of erythrocyte morphology is an important tool in the management of patients with isolated microscopic haematuria of unknown origin. In fact, it allows an early orientation of the diagnostic work-up towards a nephrological or a urological disorder, which avoids unnecessary and often invasive investigation (Schrameck *et al.* 1989a).

When I have a patient with isolated microscopic haematuria of unknown origin, I do examine red cell morphology. I do this by evaluating 100 erythrocytes/sample, and first I look for acanthocytes or G1 cells. If they are not found or are less than 5 per cent of total erythrocytes,

I look for other dysmorphic erythrocytes and use the cut-off of 80 per cent to discriminate between a glomerular and a non-glomerular bleeding. When I come across a mixed haematuria, I consider this, similarly to others (Rizzoni *et al.* 1983; Rath *et al.* 1990), as the expression of glomerular bleeding. In addition, since in occasional cases, I found a change in the type of haematuria in the same patient over time, I examine at least three consecutive samples for each patient before establishing the origin of haematuria. Using these criteria, I found, at renal biopsy, a clear-cut glomerular disease in 10 of 12 patients (83 per cent) whose isolated microscopic haematuria, I had classified as glomerular on the basis of red-cell morphology (data unpublished).

The cause of red-cell dysmorphism is not entirely clear. However, clinical observations and experimental findings suggest that dysmorphism is the result of a dual injury—passage through gaps in the glomerular basement membrane and exposure within the tubular lumen to different osmolalities, pH, and haemolytic substances (Schramek *et al.* 1989b; Briner and Reinhart 1990; Rath *et al.* 1992).

It is worth remembering that the appearance of erythrocytes in the urine may also reflect the appearance they have in the blood. Thus, patients with haematuria caused by sickle-cell disease may have sickled erythrocytes in their urine (Fogazzi *et al.* 1996), and patients with peripheral anisopoikilocytosis may have poikilocytes in the urine (personal observation).

Leucocytes

Neutrophils These are the most frequently found leucocytes in the urine. They appear as cells with an average diameter of about 10 μm, and a granular cytoplasm surrounding a lobulated nucleus (Fig. 1d). When, degenerated, however, the differentiation between cytoplasm and nucleus may no longer be evident.

Neutrophils are a typical finding in urinary tract infections. However, they are also found in patients with active proliferative glomerulonephritis, acute or chronic interstitial nephritis, and urological disorders. Especially in women, neutrophils are frequently found as a consequence of urine contamination from genital secretions. In such cases, they are associated with large amounts of squamous epithelial cells and bacteria.

Lymphocytes These are usually identified by general or specific stains, such as methyl green pyronin, even though the experienced urine microscopist can identify them by phase contrast alone.

The gradual or abrupt appearance of lymphocyturia in renal graft recipients is an early and sensitive marker of acute cellular rejection (Sandoz *et al.* 1986).

Eosinophils These too can be identified only by stains; the most sensitive available today being Hansel's stain (Nolan *et al.* 1986; Corwin *et al.* 1989).

Eosinophiluria was in the past considered as a marker of acute interstitial nephritis caused by drugs such as methycillin. However, it is now known that they can be found in several disorders such as extracapillary glomerulonephritis, atheroembolic renal disease, urinary tract infection, prostatitis, urinary schistosomiasis, etc. (Ruffing *et al.* 1994). Therefore, the finding of eosinophiluria must carefully be considered in the clinical context.

Renal tubular cells

The most frequently found tubular cells in the urine are round to ovoid mononucleated cells, which have an average diameter of about 13 μm. Other less frequently found tubular cells are rectangular, polygonal, or even columnar (Fig. 2a).

Tubular cells are a typical finding in acute tubular necrosis, in which case they may occur in clumps and with variable morphological changes (Mandal *et al.* 1985). They are also found in acute interstitial nephritis, acute cellular allograft rejection (Eggensperger *et al.* 1988), and acute nephritic or nephrotic syndrome.

Urothelial cells

These come from the urothelium, which is a multilayered epithelium lining the urinary excretory tract from the calyces to the bladder in the female and to the proximal urethra in the male. Two main types of urothelial cells can be found in the urine: those deriving from the deep layers, which have a club-like or ovoid appearance, a thin cytoplasm, and a mean diameter of about 18 μm (Fig. 2b), and those deriving from the superficial layers, which are round to oval and are much larger having a mean diameter of about 30 μm (Fig. 2c).

These two types of cells have different clinical significances. The cells of the deep layers, when greater than or equal to 1/high-power field, are typical of conditions such as urolithiasis, bladder cancer, hydronephrosis, or are associated with the presence of ureteric stents or prolonged bladder catheterization (Fogazzi *et al.* 1995; Fogazzi *et al.* 1999). In contrast, the superficial cells are a frequent finding in urinary tract infection.

Squamous cells

These cells have abundant cytoplasm with few granules and a small, central nucleus (Fig. 2d). They are the largest cells found in the urine, with a mean diameter of about 55 μm.

They are found routinely in small numbers, being exfoliated from the urethra. When found in large numbers, they indicate a contamination of urine from vaginal discharge.

Lipids

Lipids are present in urine mainly as droplets. These can be either free—isolated or in aggregates (Fig. 3a)—or within casts and cells. In the latter case, they can form the so-called 'oval fat bodies', which are tubular cells or macrophages (Hotta *et al.* 2000) gorged with lipids (Fig. 3b).

Lipid droplets may have different diameters, and have a typical appearance, being round and distinctly translucent. Under polarized light, when containing free cholesterol and cholesterol esters, they appear as 'Maltese crosses', which are bright particles cut by symmetrical crosses (Fig. 3c).

Less frequently, lipids can also appear as cholesterol crystals, which are thin and transparent plates with straight edges (Fig. 3d).

Lipids are a typical finding in the urine of patients with nephrotic syndrome or heavy proteinuria, even though they may occasionally also be found in the urine of patients with polycystic kidney disease or with non-glomerular diseases (Duncan *et al.* 1985; Braden *et al.* 1988). Lipids are also found in the urine of patients with primary abnormalities of lipid metabolism, such as Fabry's disease (Desnick *et al.* 1971; Chatterjee *et al.* 1984). The lipid droplets seen in this condition resemble large fat droplets, which are also birefringent under polarized light. However, they show a membrane protrusion on one side and, using electron microscopy, myelin bodies, which are not found in other lipid particles.

In patients with a glomerular disease, lipiduria is the result of abnormal glomerular ultrafiltration. Once within the tubules, it is hypothesized that lipids are reabsorbed by proximal tubular cells and transported for hydrolysis into lysosomes. Then, they re-enter the

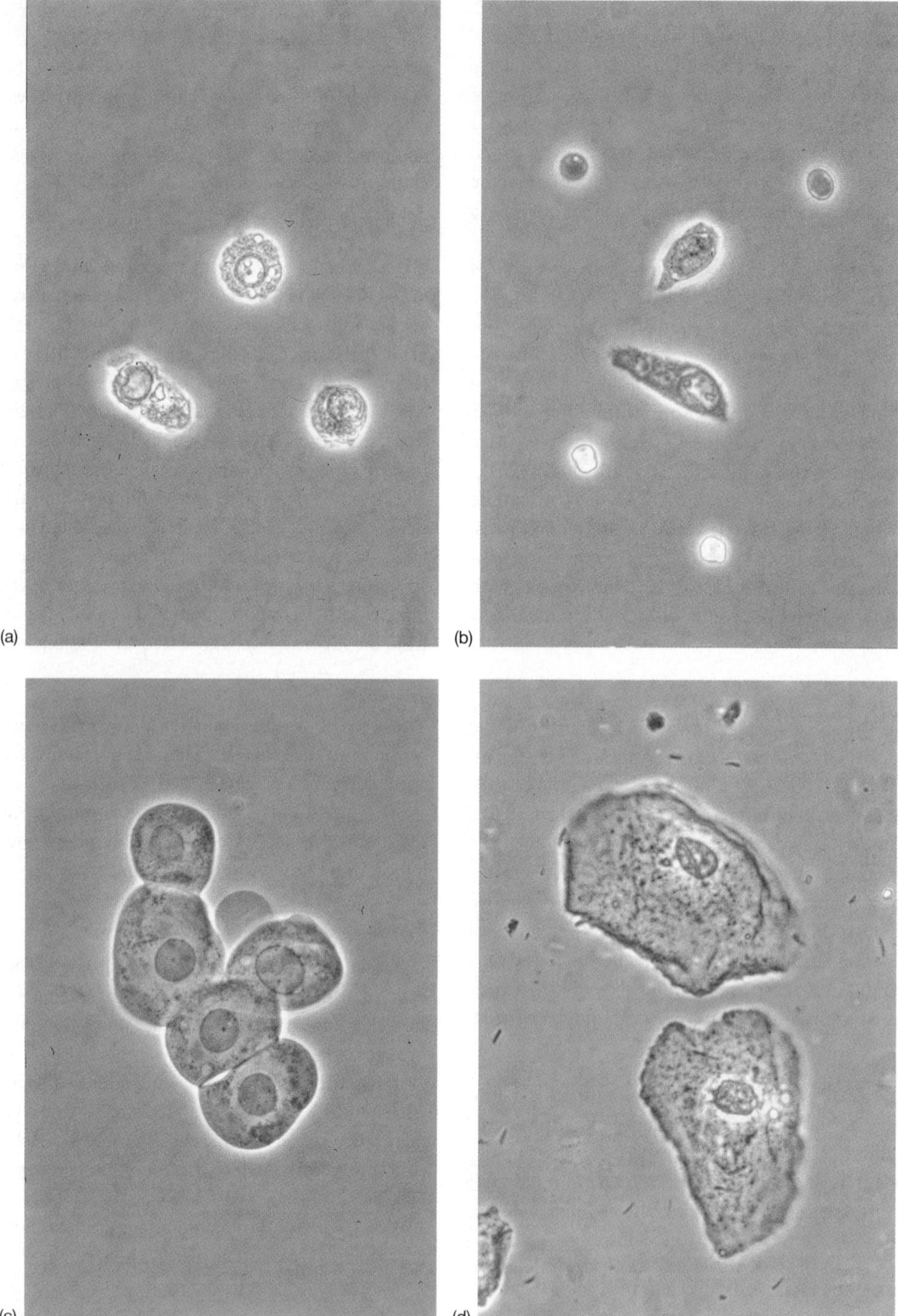

Fig. 2 (a) Different types of tubular cells. (b) Urothelial cells from the deep cell layers of the urothelium. (c) An aggregate of urothelial cells from the superficial cell layers of the urothelium. (d) Squamous cells surrounded by bacteria (rods) (phase-contrast microscopy, original magnification 400×).

tubular urine via active cellular expulsion or as the consequence of cellular breakdown (Blackburn *et al.* 1998).

Casts

Casts are elongated elements with a basic cylindrical shape that has some possible variation due to bending, wrinkling, and irregular edges. They form within the distal tubules and the collecting ducts of the kidneys from the aggregation and transformation into a gel of the fibrils of Tamm–Horsfall glycoprotein (Lindner and Haber 1983), which is the matrix of casts (McQueen 1966) and is produced by the cells of the thick ascending limb of Henle's loop and of the early distal convoluted tubules. Cast formation is favoured by all the factors that promote the aggregation of Tamm–Horsfall protein—increased urinary concentration of electrolytes, hydrogen ions, and ultrafiltered proteins—or by the

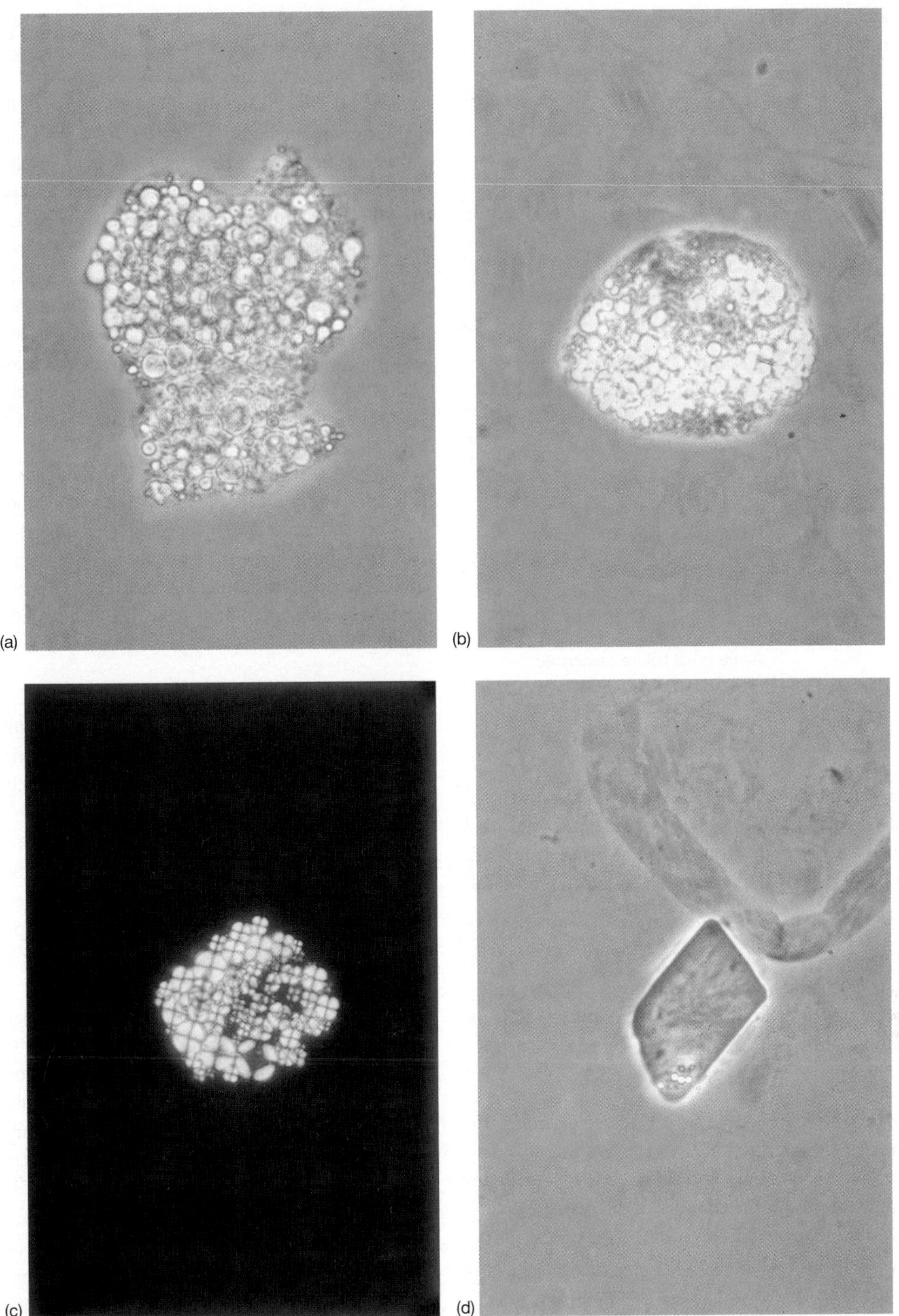

Fig. 3 (a) A large aggregate of lipid droplets. (b) A macrophage partly gorged with lipid droplets (a so-called 'oval fat body'). (c) An aggregate of lipid droplets as seen under polarized light. Note the symmetrical 'Maltese crosses' (400×). (d) A plate of cholesterol crystal (on its lowest corner, a few small lipid droplets; on the background, a hyaline cast) (phase-contrast microscopy, original magnification 400×).

interaction between the protein and haemoglobin or myoglobin, Bence Jones protein or radiocontrast media (Hoyer and Seiler 1979). When cells, granules, lipids, crystals, microorganisms, and the like are transported along the nephron by the tubular fluid and come across the forming cast they are entrapped, with the consequent appearance in the urine of a large variety of casts (Table 4).

Hyaline casts

These contain Tamm–Horsfall protein only, have a low refractive index (Fig. 4a), and can easily escape detection if the bright-field microscope is used.

They are present in variable number in the normal individual, but are increased in renal diseases, where they are usually associated

Table 4 The main types of urinary casts with their main clinical associations

Cast	Main clinical associations
Hyaline	Normal subject Renal disease
Hyaline–granular	Normal subject Renal disease
Granular	Renal disease
Waxy	Renal insufficiency either acute or chronic
Fatty	Nephrotic syndrome
Erythrocyte/haemoglobin	Glomerular bleeding Proliferative/necrotizing glomerulonephritis
Leucocyte	Acute pyelonephritis Acute interstitial nephritis Proliferative glomerulonephritis
Epithelial	Acute tubular necrosis Acute interstitial nephritis Glomerulonephritis
Myoglobin	Acute renal failure associated with rhabdomyolysis

with other casts. Larger numbers of hyaline casts may also be observed in patients with acute cardiac failure or fever but without renal diseases, in those receiving furosemide (frusemide) or ethacrynic acid (Imhof *et al.* 1972), or in normal people after strenuous physical exercise.

Hyaline–granular casts

These are hyaline casts containing variable amounts of fine granules (Fig. 4b). In my experience, they are the most frequent casts seen in patients with glomerulonephritis.

Granular casts

These casts can contain either fine (Fig. 4c) or coarse granules. In patients with proteinuria, the granules of the casts are due to lysosomes containing ultrafiltered proteins (Rutecki *et al.* 1971), while in patients with acute tubular necrosis the granules of the casts are probably due to degenerated tubular cells (Orita *et al.* 1977). Coarse granules too, probably, derive from degenerated cells.

Granular casts are found in patients with renal disease.

Waxy casts

These owe their name to their appearance, which is similar to that of melted wax (Fig. 4d). Other distinguishing morphological features of these casts are large size and clear-cut edges, which are often indented.

Waxy casts are found in patients with renal insufficiency, either chronic or rapidly progressive.

Cellular casts

There are three types of cellular casts:

Erythrocyte casts These are casts which contain variable amounts of erythrocytes embedded in the matrix of the cast (Fig. 5a).

They are usually considered as a highly specific marker of glomerular bleeding with only a 25–30 per cent sensitivity (Rizzoni *et al.* 1983; Rath *et al.* 1990; Köhler *et al.* 1991). However, recent studies suggest that, if examined carefully, they can be found in up to 85 per cent of patients with haematuria caused by glomerulonephritis (Koene 1999).

The search for erythrocyte casts is of particular value in patients with isolated microscopic haematuria of unknown origin in whom their presence indicates the glomerular origin of the bleeding.

When the erythrocytes embedded in the matrix of cast undergo degenerative processes *haemoglobin casts* are formed, which have a typical brownish hue and a granular appearance (Fig. 5a inset). Therefore, in such instances haemoglobin casts have the same clinical significance as erythrocyte casts. However, haemoglobin casts can be found without haematuria. This may happen as a consequence of free haemoglobinuria in patients with intravascular haemolysis.

Leucocyte casts These contain variable amounts of neutrophils (Fig. 5b), and indicate the renal origin of leucocytes.

Therefore, the search for these elements is of particular value in patients with urinary tract infection, since their presence suggests the involvement of the renal parenchyma. However, they may also be found in acute interstitial nephritis and proliferative active glomerulonephritis.

Epithelial casts These contain tubular epithelial cells (Fig. 5c), and can be found in all conditions associated with tubular damage such as acute tubular necrosis, acute interstitial nephritis, acute renal allograft cellular rejection, acute nephritic syndrome, nephrotic syndrome, etc.

Fatty casts

These contain variable amounts of lipids (Fig. 5d).

They are a typical finding, with lipid droplets and oval fat bodies, in patients with nephrotic syndrome or heavy proteinuria.

Casts containing crystals

These can contain crystals such as calcium oxalate, uric acid, amorphous urates, or phosphates, or even crystals due to drugs.

They indicate that precipitation of crystals or salts occurred in the tubular lumen which, in most instances, happens without clinical consequences. However, in other cases intratubular precipitation of crystals is associated with acute renal failure, and crystal-containing casts may be a marker of this condition (Fogazzi 1996).

Casts containing microorganisms

These may contain bacteria or fungi (Lindner *et al.* 1980; Gregory *et al.* 1984). They indicate that there is a bacterial or fungal infection in the renal parenchyma.

Pigmented casts

In addition to haemoglobin casts described above, pigmented casts encompass myoglobin and bilirubin casts.

Myoglobin casts have a brownish colour due to myoglobin, which makes them often hardly distinguishable from haemoglobin casts. However, myoglobin casts are found in a totally different clinical situation, which is acute renal failure associated with rhabdomyolysis.

Bilirubin casts are all types of casts (hyaline, granular, etc.), which have taken the typical yellow colour of bilirubin. They are a feature of patients with jaundice due to increased conjugated bilirubinaemia.

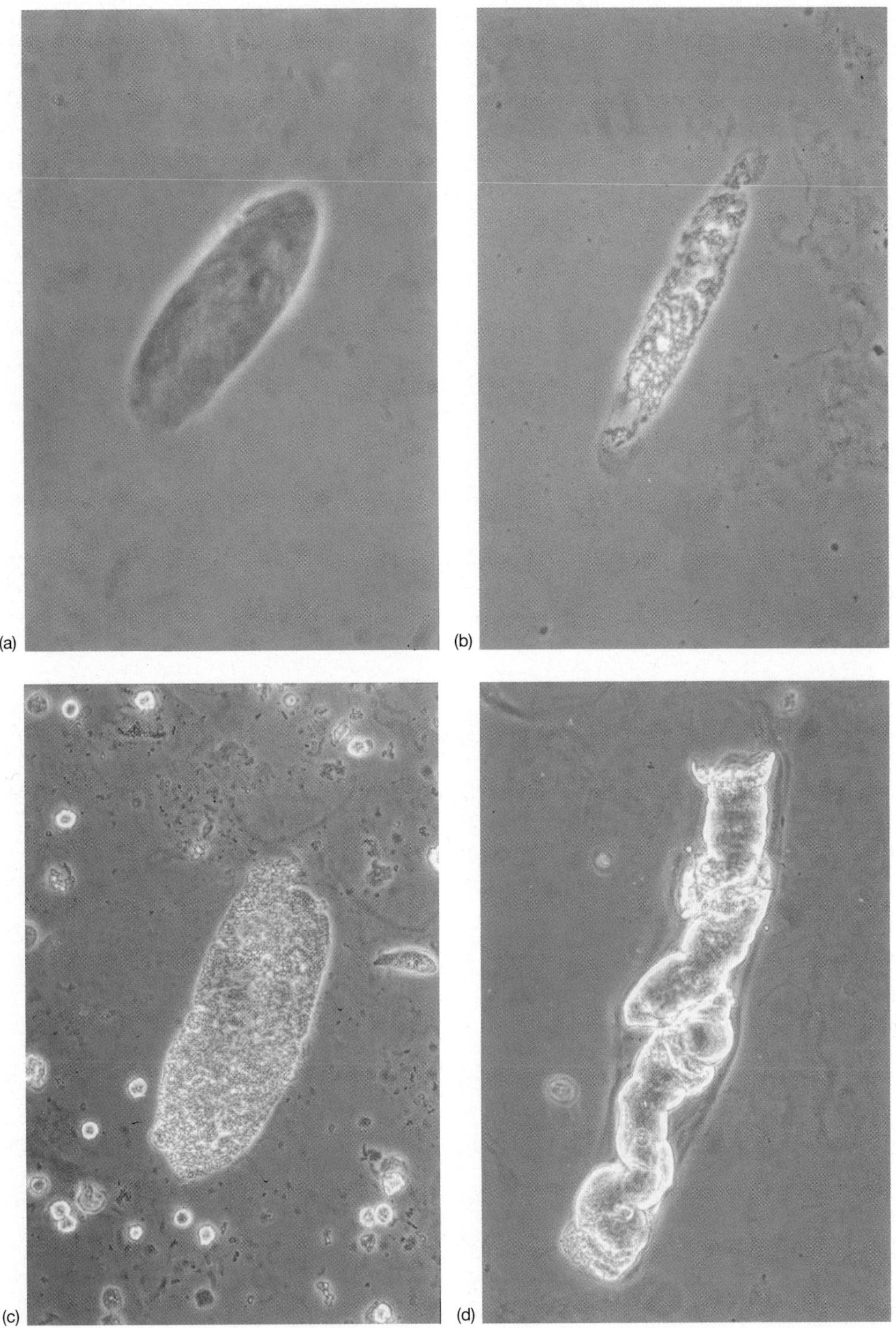

Fig. 4 (a) A hyaline cast with a 'fluffy' appearance due to the fibrillary substructure of Tamm–Horsfall glycoprotein. (b) A hyaline–granular cast. (c) A finely granular cast. (d) A waxy cast (phase-contrast microscopy, original magnification 400×).

Mixed casts

These contain two or more of the constituents of casts described above. Thus, besides hyaline–granular casts, a large variety of mixed casts can be seen such as granular–waxy casts, granular–epithelial casts, etc.

The clinical significance of mixed casts varies according to their composition. Thus, granular–waxy casts are typical of renal insufficiency, granular–epithelial casts indicate tubular damage, etc.

Cylindroids

There is no agreement on the definition of cylindroids. However, if one defines them as elements similar to casts but for one end, which is not rounded but resembles a mucus thread, in my experience these elements are nothing but casts. In fact, they can contain all particles found in casts including erythrocytes, and by immunofluorescence they appear to have a matrix made of Tamm–Horsfall glycoprotein.

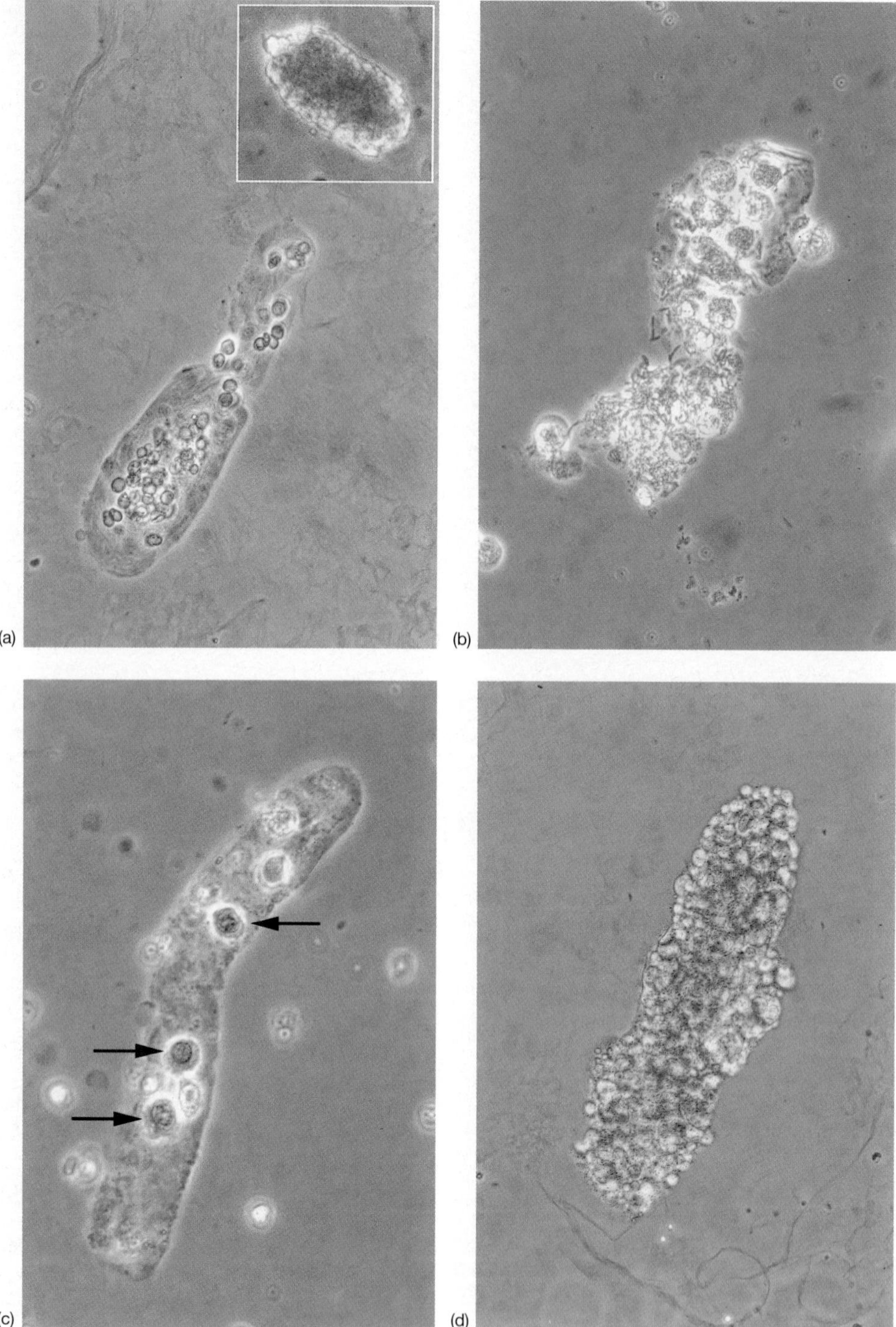

Fig. 5 (a) An erythrocyte cast. Inset: a haemoglobin cast. (b) A leucocyte cast containing packed neutrophils. (c) An epithelial cast. The tubular cells are indicated by the arrows. (d) A fatty cast made of packed lipid droplets (phase-contrast microscopy, original magnification 400×).

Pseudocasts

These are elements of various nature, mostly contaminants, with an appearance that may mimic those of casts. They are not important *per se*, but the urine microscopist must be able to differentiate them from true casts to avoid misdiagnoses.

Mucus

Mucus in the urine appears as ribbon-like threads of variable width and length, or as large masses, which can entrap cells or other elements. In the last case, mucus contributes largely to the irregular distribution of particles throughout the specimen.

Mucus derives from the secretion of accessory glands, such as Littré (urethral) glands in men and Skene (para-urethral) ducts in women. It is a normal constituent of urine, its quantity varying according to urine density, being absent or scarce in low density urine and abundant in urine of high density.

Crystals

Urine can contain several types of crystals. Some of which are found only or predominantly in acid urine while others prevail in alkaline urine. In addition, some crystals are birefringent under polarized light while others are not. Thus, by knowing crystal morphology, urine pH, and polarizing features, most urine crystals can be identified using a conventional equipment. However, in some instances this is not sufficient and more sophisticated techniques such as infrared spectroscopy are necessary (Daudon *et al.* 1991). This is especially useful to identify crystals due to drugs or even common crystals when they come with unusual appearances.

The most important crystals in urine are as follows.

Uric acid

These crystals precipitate at a pH less than or equal to 5.4. They may have a wide range of shapes. However, they appear mostly as lozenges (Fig. 6a), which have a typical amber colour. Under polarized light they show a beautiful polychromatic birefringence (Fig. 6a inset).

Calcium oxalate

There are two main types of calcium oxalate crystals: the mono- and the bihydrated, either of which is mainly found in acidic pH. The former appear as ovoid particles or as dumb-bell or as biconcave/biconvex discs, while the latter have a typical bipyramidal shape (Fig. 6b). Monohydrated calcium oxalate crystals are birefringent, while the bihydrated are not.

Calcium phosphate

This salt appears in alkaline urine either as crystals, the appearance of which includes prisms, needles, and star-like aggregates (Fig. 6c) or as plates with a granular surface. While the crystals polarize light, the plates do not.

Triple phosphate

The crystals of triple phosphate are birefringent prisms which precipitate at a pH greater than or equal to 7.0. Most frequently they have a 'coffin lid' appearance (Fig. 6d).

Amorphous urates and phosphates

These appear as granular material, often in clumps, and are morphologically undistinguishable. However, urates are found in acid urine and are birefringent, while phosphates precipitate only in alkaline urine and do not polarize light.

Cystine

These crystals are thin, hexagonal, birefringent plates with irregular sides. They can be isolated, heaped upon one another, or in clumps (Fig. 7a). They are a marker of cystinuria, and are found mostly in acid urine.

2,8-Dihydroxyadenine (see Chapter 16.5.3)

These crystals are round to reddish-brown, with dark outlines and central spicules (Fig. 7b), and polarize light.

They are caused by 2,8-dihydroxyadeninuria, which is a condition associated with the homozygous deficiency of the enzyme adenine phosphoribosyltransferase, which catalyzes the conversion of adenine to adenosine monophosphate. Patients suffer from stone formation or acute renal failure caused by intratubular precipitation of 2,8-dihydroxyadenine.

The finding of 2,8-dihydroxyadenine crystals is a clue to the diagnosis of the disease (Edvardsson *et al.* 2001).

Cholesterol

Cholesterol crystals appear as brownish and transparent thin plates, with sharp edges and corners (see Fig. 3d). They are found, with other lipid particles, in the urine of patients with nephrotic syndrome or heavy proteinuria.

Crystals due to drugs

Many drugs can cause transient crystalluria (Fogazzi 1996). Among these are the sulfonamide sulfadiazine, the antiviral agents acyclovir and indinavir (Kopp *et al.* 1997), the diuretic triamterene, the coronary dilator piridoxylate, the barbiturate primidone, the vasodilator naftidrofuryl oxalate, vitamin C (Wong *et al.* 1994), and the antibiotic amoxycillin (Boffa *et al.* 2000), etc.

Drug crystals may have a special appearance, as with acyclovir (i.e. birefringent needles) or indinavir (i.e. flat rectangular plates with internal layering), or amoxycillin (Fig. 7c and d). Others may come as monohydrated calcium oxalate crystals, as with naftidrofuryl oxalate or vitamin C.

Clinical significance of crystals

The finding of few crystals of uric acid, calcium oxalate, and calcium phosphate is usually irrelevant, their precipitation being the consequence of unremarkable events such as the intake of foods or changes in urine temperature and pH occurring upon standing.

However, in a minority of cases, crystalluria may be associated with intratubular precipitation of crystals and acute renal failure. This has been observed mainly in acute uric acid nephropathy, ethylene glycol poisoning, and after the administration of high dosages of drugs such as sulfadiazine, acyclovir, indinavir, naftidrofuryl oxalate, vitamin C, amoxycillin, etc.

These circumstances are suggested by the finding of either massive or atypical crystalluria, including crystalline casts.

Some crystals are always pathologic. This is the case with cystine which is a marker of cystinuria; 2,8-dihydroxyadenine, which is a marker of homozygotic deficiency of the enzyme adenine phosphoribosyltransferase; cholesterol, which is found in patients with marked proteinuria.

The study of crystalluria may also be used to monitor the patients with recurrent metabolic urolithiasis. These patients have been found to have in their urine larger crystals and more crystal aggregates than normal subjects. However, special methodology and equipment are necessary to evaluate these features properly. Thus, this type of investigation can be carried out only in specialized laboratories.

Microorganisms

Bacteria

These are frequently seen in urine sediments, either as rods or cocci (Fig. 8a). However, since urine is usually not collected and handled under sterile conditions, bacteria may be due to contamination rather than infection. The presence of leucocytes increases the probability of a real infection, especially in women, but leucocytes and bacteria may contaminate urine from genitalia. In patients with acute pyelonephritis, bacterial casts have been described (Lindner *et al.* 1980).

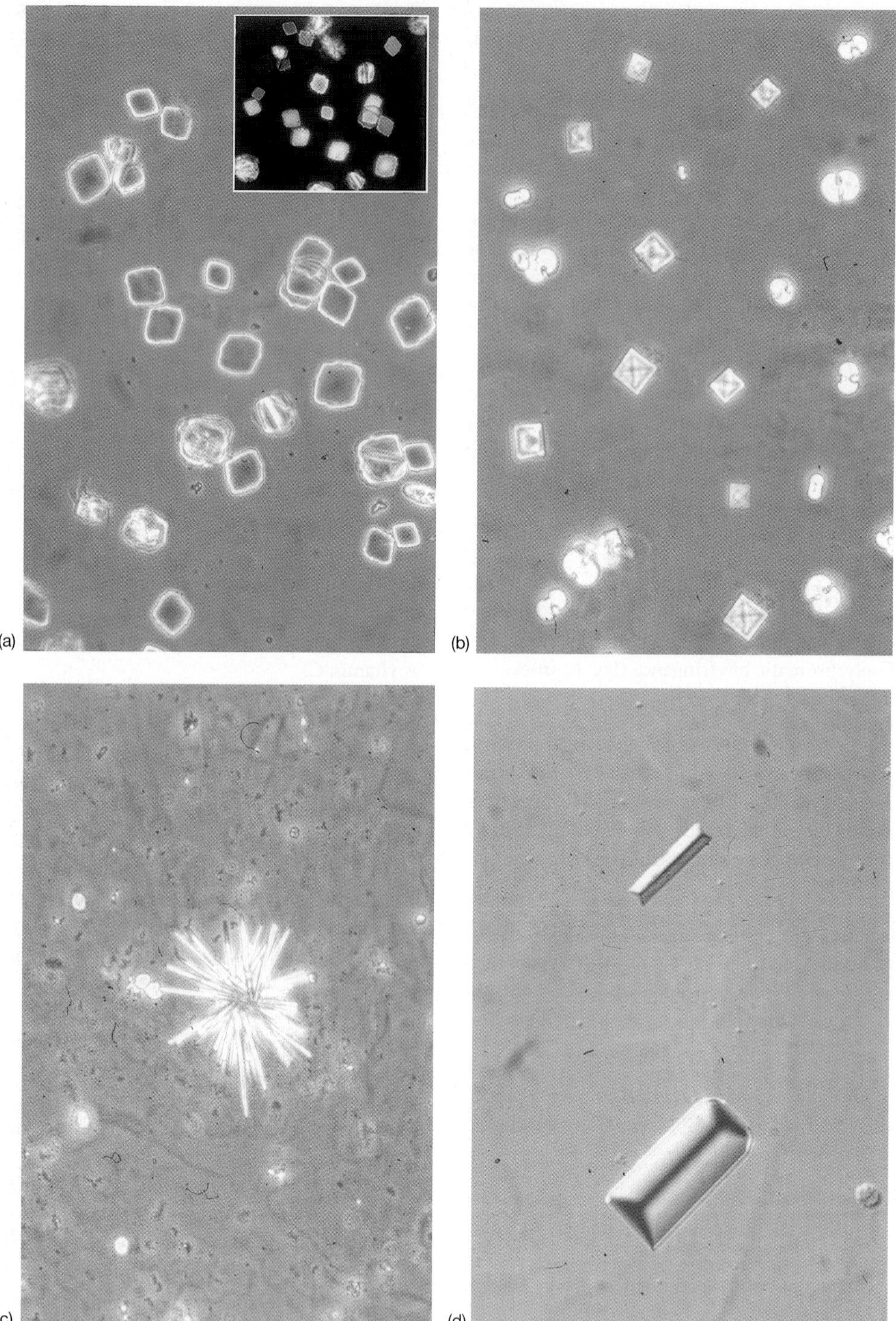

Fig. 6 (a) Uric acid crystals (lozenge variety). Inset: the same under polarized light. (b). Monohydrated (biconvex disc) and bihydrated (bipyramidal) calcium oxalate crystals. (c) A star-like calcium phosphate crystal resulting from the aggregation of needle-like crystals. Typical triple phosphate crystals (a–c phase-contrast microscopy; (d) interference contrast microscopy, original magnification 400×).

Fungi

Candida is the most frequent yeast found in urine. Candidae appear as refractile, pale-green cells, often nucleated and with smooth and well-defined walls. Depending on the species they may be elongated, ovoid, or spherical. One common morphological feature is the presence of buds (Fig. 8b).

The most frequent cause of candida in the urine is contamination from the genitalia, but candida can also grow in the urinary tract, mostly in patients with diabetes mellitus, structural abnormalities, indwelling catheters, prolonged antibiotic treatment or immunosuppression. Candidal casts have been found in the urine of patients with renal candidiasis (Gregory *et al.* 1984).

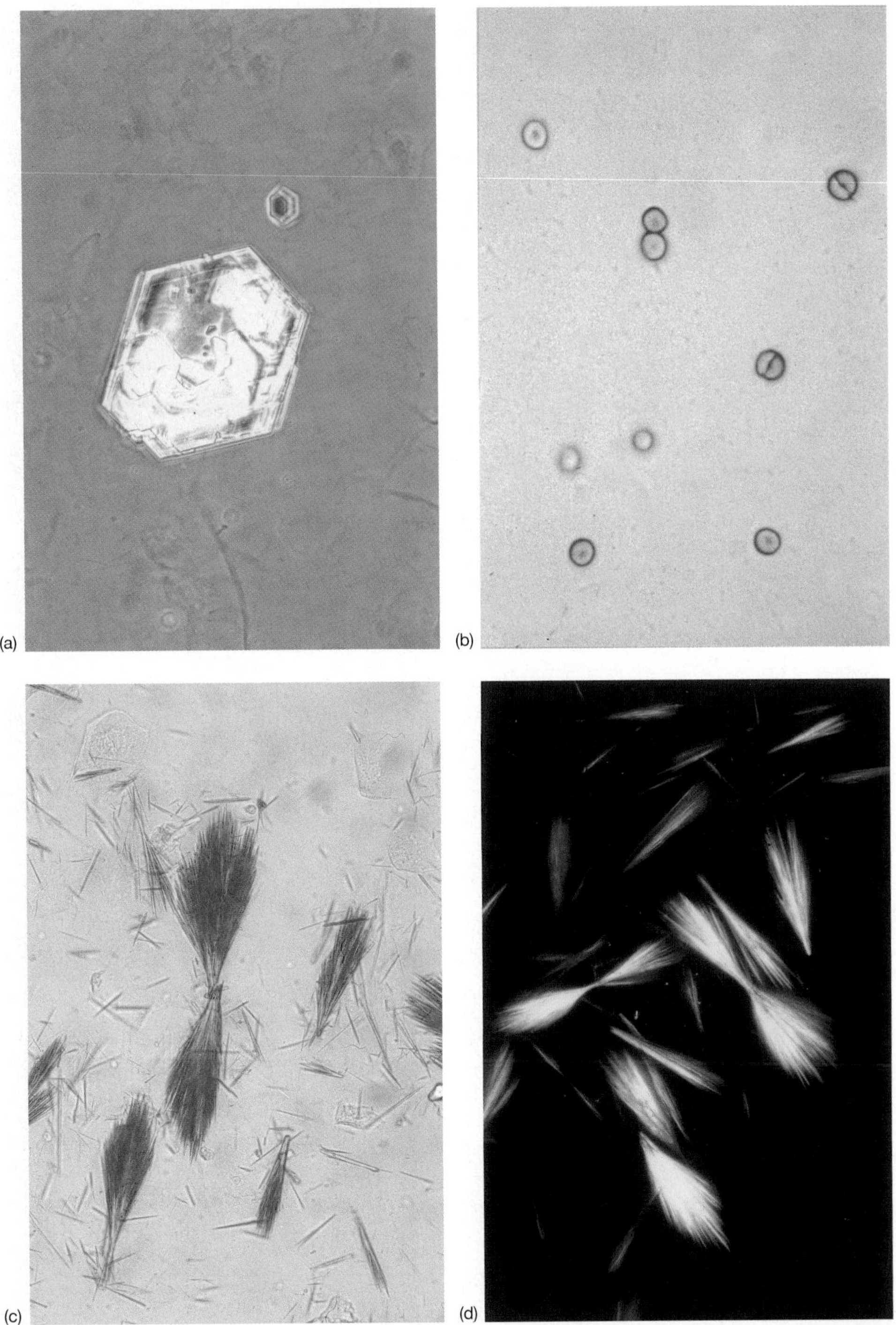

Fig. 7 (a) Aggregated cystine crystals. (b) 2,8-Dihydroxyadenine crystals (courtesy of Dr Simona Barberi, Roma). (c) Amoxycillin trihydrate crystals. (d) Amoxycillin trihydrate crystals under polarized light (400×). Their nature was confirmed by infrared spectroscopy. [(a) phase-contrast microscopy, original magnification 400×; (b and c): light microscopy, original magnification 400×].

Protozoa

Trichomonas vaginalis It has four flagella, is round or pear shaped (Fig. 8c), and is slightly larger than a neutrophil. When alive, it is identified by the motility of the flagella and the rapid and irregular movements of the body. When dead, *T. vaginalis* is very similar to neutrophils.

This protozoan is found in the urine of both sexes, mostly as a consequence of genital contamination.

Parasites

Schistosoma haematobium This parasite, which in the adult form lives and lays the eggs in the vesical plexus and veins draining the ureters, is endemic in several geographic areas such as Nile valley, West Africa,

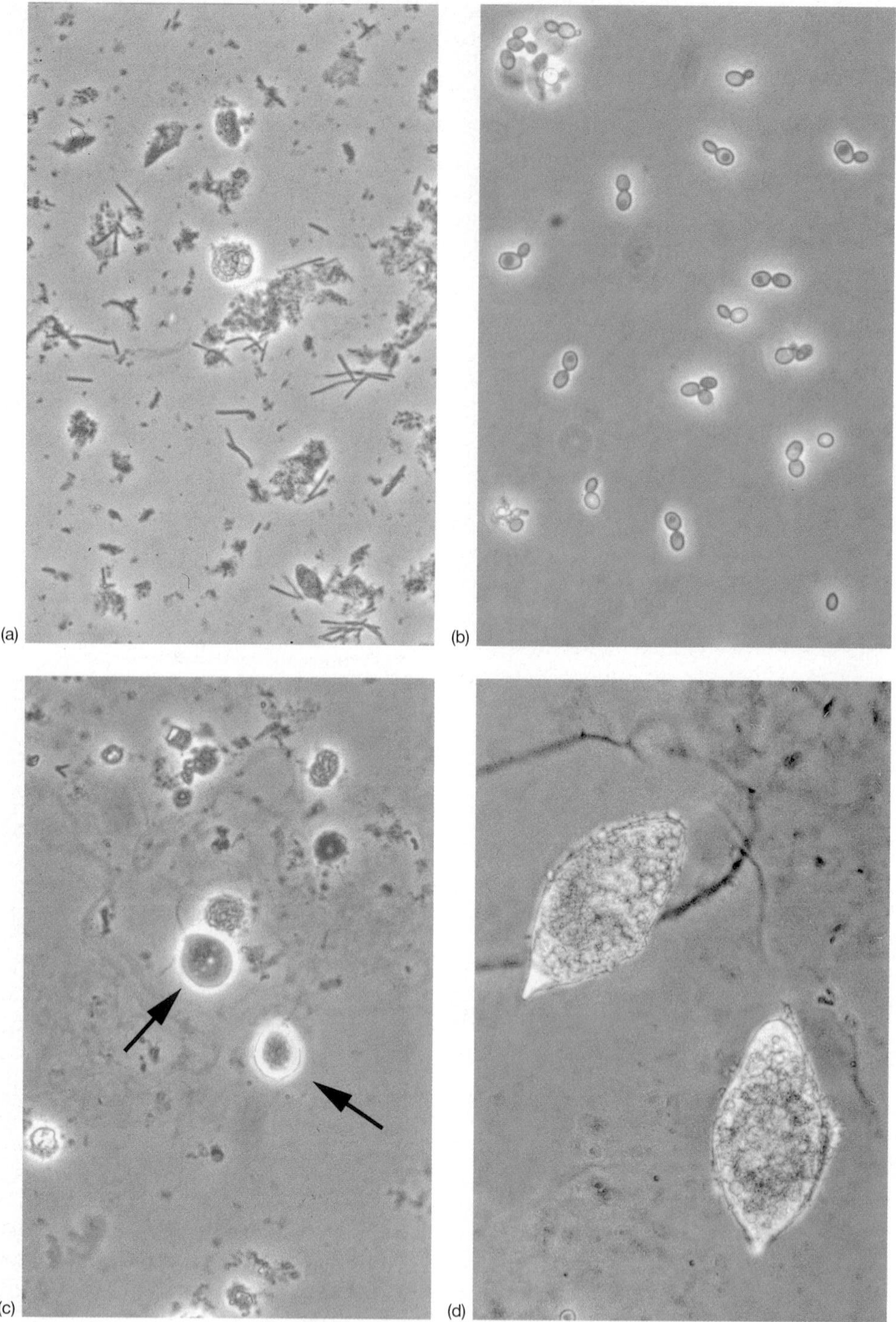

Fig. 8 (a) A 'dirty' urine background showing many bacteria (rods) and debris. (b) *Candida albicans.* (c) *Trichomonas vaginalis* (arrows) (note the flagella). (d) Two eggs of *Schistosoma haematobium* (phase-contrast microscopy, original magnification 400×).

Arabia, etc. It is responsible for haematuria, chronic renal failure due to obstructive uropathy, glomerulonephritis, or bladder cancer.

The diagnosis heavily relies on the observation of the eggs in the urine after filtration (Peters *et al.* 1976) or, more simply, centrifugation. To increase the shedding of the eggs, urine collection should be performed between 12 and 2 p.m. and after a physical exercise such as bending or running (Colucci and Fogazzi 1999).

Eggs of *S. haematobium* measure about 140 × 50 μm and are spindle shaped, with a rounded anterior and a conical posterior end tapering into a delicate terminal spine (Fig. 8d).

Contaminants

Several types of contaminants can be found in the urine sediments. They may originate from the patient (e.g. blood from menstruation;

leucocytes, bacteria, candida, *T. vaginalis*, or spermatozoa from genital secretions; pubic hair, faeces, talcum, etc.), the laboratory (e.g. starch from gloves used by the laboratory personnel), or the environment (e.g. pollen granules, plant cells, fungal spores, etc.) (Fogazzi *et al.* 1999).

Some of these particles may be prevented by adopting proper urine collection and working conditions. Their correct identification is important in order to avoid mistaking them for true particles of the urine sediment.

The urine sediment of the normal individual

Although there is a general agreement that the urine sediment of the normal person contains only a 'few' erythrocytes and leucocytes, there is no consensus at all about their number. This may partly be explained by the fact that different methods have been used for the collection, handling, and scanning of the urine. Moreover, there are interindividual differences in the excretion of cells and casts among normal people and, within a population, there may also be differences related to age (Loh *et al.* 1990).

In my laboratory, with the method reported in Table 2, we found that the urine of 70 adults of both sexes contained on the average, 5.8 ± 5.7 erythrocytes (range 0–26) and 3.1 ± 3.5 (range 0–17) leucocytes in 20 high-power fields at 400× (Fogazzi *et al.* 1989). Therefore, I consider a urine sample as normal when it contains up to one erythrocyte per high-power field and up to one leucocyte every two high-power fields. I did not observe differences between sexes, but these have been found in children (Loh *et al.* 1990).

The urinary erythrocytes in normal individuals are usually dysmorphic (Fairley and Birch 1982; Loh *et al.* 1990; Köhler *et al.* 1991), although isomorphic erythrocytes were also found by Fasset *et al.* (1982b).

As to casts, it is commonly accepted that variable amounts of hyaline casts and even some hyaline–granular casts may be found in the urine of the normal subject. However, no reliable recent data are available on this aspect.

Other features accepted as normal are the presence of 'some' squamous epithelial cells, especially in women, and mucus.

The interpretation of main urine sediment findings

Urine microscopy, *integrated with physicochemical urine findings and blood tests*, contributes to the diagnosis of the diseases of the kidneys and is also useful in evaluating their activity and in identifying complications or superimposed conditions. Some major patterns can be identified, which reflect different clinical conditions. All nephrologists should be familiar with these patterns.

The nephrotic sediment

The typical nephrotic sediment is characterized by large amounts of lipids (appearing as free droplets, oval fat bodies, fatty casts, and, much less frequently, cholesterol crystals) associated with tubular cells, and variable amounts of hyaline, granular, or epithelial casts. Erythrocytes are absent or only a few, mostly up to 10/high-power field. Neutrophils are also absent.

This sediment is associated with non-proliferative glomerular diseases such as minimal-change disease, focal segmental glomerulosclerosis, membranous nephropathy, diabetic nephropathy, amyloidosis, light-chain deposition disease, etc.

Some urinary differences may exist between one disease and another. For instance, microscopic haematuria is absent in about 50 per cent of patients with minimal-change disease, while it is almost always present in membranous nephropathy (Fogazzi and Ponticelli 1996), and lipiduria is more marked and frequent in membranous nephropathy than in minimal-change disease (Ravigneaux *et al.* 1991). In spite of these differences, however, by no means can one diagnose a disease on the basis of the urinary findings alone.

Occasionally, the course of a nephrotic syndrome can be complicated by acute events. The study of urine sediment may be very useful in these circumstances. In minimal-change disease, a nephrotic sediment may transform into a sediment with abundant haematuria and leucocyturia with the occurrence of an acute interstitial nephritis due to antibiotics or diuretics. A transformation into a nephritic sediment (see below) may occur in membranous nephropathy from a superimposed extracapillary proliferation, in diabetic nephropathy from a superimposed proliferative glomerulonephritis, and in membranous lupus nephritis during transformation into a proliferative form.

The nephritic sediment

The distinguishing feature of the nephritic sediment is the presence of abundant erythrocyturia associated with erythrocyte/haemoglobin casts. In this context, the finding of greater than or equal to 100 erythrocytes/high-power field is in my experience almost invariably associated with extracapillary/necrotizing glomerulonephritis. Neutrophils are also frequent, however, in low numbers (usually ≤10/high-power field). Leucocyte casts are possible, but they are rare. Other findings are: tubular cells, hyaline, granular, epithelial, and waxy casts.

The nephritic sediment is typically found in patients with active proliferative glomerulonephritis and impairment of renal function. As a general rule there is a loose positive correlation between the intrarenal changes and the severity of the urinary changes and of haematuria (Leaker *et al.* 1987), but with striking exceptions as demonstrated by cases of 'silent lupus nephritis' (Eiser *et al.* 1979) and by patients with acute glomerulonephritis and no urinary abnormalities (Goorno *et al.* 1967).

Monitoring the urinary sediment in patients with proliferative glomerulonephritides is important because the sediment reflects to some extent the progressive changes in the kidneys. Thus, a clearing of the urinary abnormalities, especially when confirmed by repeated examinations, indicates a decrease in the activity of the renal disease, either from healing or transformation into a chronic disease, while the reappearance of a nephritic sediment is usually associated with a relapse. Such monitoring is of particular value for patients with renal diseases that can wax and wane, such as lupus nephritis (Hebert *et al.* 1995) or systemic vasculitis with renal involvement (Fujita *et al.* 1998).

The nephrotic and nephritic sediment

In conditions such as mesangiocapillary glomerulonephritis, lupus nephritis with both proliferative and membranous changes, Henoch–Schönlein purpura, cryoglobulinaemic glomerulonephritis, the combination of nephrotic and nephritic sediment can be found.

This is characterized by the co-existence of lipiduria with abundant erythrocyturia and cylindruria which also encompasses erythrocyte/haemoglobin casts.

The sediment of acute tubular necrosis

This is characterized by variable amounts of tubular cells, which often appear damaged (Mandal *et al.* 1985). In most severe cases also fragments of tubular epithelium can be found. Epithelial and granular casts are another typical finding.

The presence of additional elements depends on the cause of acute tubular necrosis. Thus, in renal damage due to rhabdomyolysis, myoglobin casts may be seen, while erythrocytes may be present in acute interstitial nephritis, and crystals in crystalluric forms of acute tubular necrosis such as that caused by hyperoxaluria or drugs.

The sediment containing crystals

See section titled 'Crystals'.

The sediment of urinary tract infection

The typical finding is represented by the association of bacteriuria with leucocyturia. Several studies have shown that there is a good correlation between urine culture and urine sediment findings (Vickers *et al.* 1991). However, with urine sediment false negative results may occur due to the lysis of leucocytes upon standing especially at alkaline pH, while false-positive results may be caused by leucocyturia and bacteriuria secondary to urine contamination from genitalia.

The instruments for the automated analysis of the urine sediments

Bioindustry has recently proposed two instruments for the automated analysis of urine sediments. One is based on automated intelligent microscopy, the other on flow cytometry (Fenili 1999).

Automated intelligent microscopy has been incorporated into an instrument (Deindorfer *et al.* 1985), which has not yet gained a large diffusion and needs further technological development. In contrast, flow cytometry is today in use in many laboratories.

The instrument based on flow cytometry analyses uncentrifuged urine samples, which are first stained with dyes for nucleic acids and cell membranes and are subsequently irradiated with laser light. The results appear on a screen as both 'scattergrams' and numeric data (Delanghe *et al.* 2000; Regeniter *et al.* 2001). With this instrument most urine sediment particles are correctly identified and quantified, and it is also possible to distinguish between glomerular and non-glomerular erythrocytes based on their different size (Apeland *et al.* 2001). However, the instrument does not recognize lipids and some types of crystals, casts, and epithelial cells (transitional cells and renal tubular cells being all classified as 'small round cells') (Delanghe *et al.* 2000; Regeniter *et al.* 2001). As a partial remedy to this limit, the instrument is programmed to point out the samples of particular complexity for which a microscopic analysis is preferable.

Today, flow cytometry is used especially in large generalized laboratories to screen large numbers of samples in a short time. This approach greatly reduces the number of samples to be analysed by microscopy, with obvious advantages on the quality of the results.

References

Aas, K. (1961). The cellular excretion in the urine of normal newborn infants. *Acta Paediatrica* **50**, 361–370.

Abuelo, J. G. (1983). Proteinuria: diagnostic principles and procedures. *Annals of Internal Medicine* **98**, 186–191.

Alwall, N. (1973). Pyuria: deposit in high power microscopic field—WBC/HPF—versus WBC/mm^3 in counting chamber. *Acta Medica Scandinavica* **194**, 637–640.

American Diabetes Association (1994). Consensus development conference on the diagnosis and management of nephropathy in patients with diabetes mellitus. *Diabetes Care* **17**, 1357–1361.

Apeland, T., Mestad, O., and Hetland, Ø. (2001). Assessment of haematuria: automated urine flowmetry versus microscopy. *Nephrology, Dialysis, Transplantation* **16**, 1615–1619.

Assadi, F. K. (2002). Quantitation of microalbuminuria using random urine samples. *Pediatric Nephrology* **17**, 107–110.

Bakoush, O. *et al.* (2001). High proteinuria selectivity index based upon IgM is a strong predictor of poor renal survival in glomerular diseases. *Nephrology, Dialysis, Transplantation* **16**, 1357–1363.

Bazzi, C. *et al.* (1997). Characterization of proteinuria in primary glomerulonephritides. SDS-PAGE patterns: clinical significance and prognostic value of low molecular weight ('tubular') proteins. *American Journal of Kidney Diseases* **29**, 27–35.

Bazzi, C. *et al.* (2000). A modern approach to selectivity of proteinuria and tubulointerstitial damage in nephrotic syndrome. *Kidney International* **58**, 1732–1741.

Bazzi, C. *et al.* (2001). Urinary excretion of IgG and α_1-microglobulin predicts clinical course better than extent of proteinuria in membranous nephropathy. *American Journal of Kidney Diseases* **38**, 240–248.

Berman, L. B. (1977). When the urine is red. *Journal of the American Medical Association* **237**, 2753–2754.

Blackburn, V., Grignani, S., and Fogazzi, G. B. (1998). Lipiduria as seen by transmission electron microscopy. *Nephrology, Dialysis, Transplantation* **13**, 2682–2684.

Boffa, J. J. *et al.* (2000). Insuffisance rénale aiguë par cristallisation d'amoxicilline. *La Presse Médicale* **29**, 699–701.

Braden, L. *et al.* (1988). Urinary doubly refractile lipid bodies in non-glomerular diseases. *American Journal of Kidney Diseases* **11**, 332–337.

Bradford, M. M. (1976). A rapid and sensitive method for the quantitation of microgram quantities of protein utilizing the principle of protein–dye binding. *Analytical Biochemistry* **72**, 248–254.

Brigden, M. L. *et al.* (1992). High incidence of significant urinary ascorbic acid concentrations in a West Coast population—implication for routine urinalysis. *Clinical Chemistry* **38**, 426–431.

Briner, V. A. and Reinhart, W. H. (1990). *In vitro* production of 'glomerular red cells': role of pH and osmolality. *Nephron* **56**, 13–18.

Burkhardt, A. E. *et al.* (1983). A reagent strip for measuring the specific gravity of the urine. *Clinical Chemistry* **28**, 2068–2072.

Burton, J. R. *et al.* (1975). Quantitation of casts in urine sediment. *Annals of Internal Medicine* **83**, 518–519.

Cameron, J. S. and Blandford, G. (1966). The simple assessment of selectivity in heavy proteinuria. *Lancet* **ii**, 242–247.

Campieri, C. *et al.* (1996). Posttraumatic chyluria due to lymphorenal fistola regressed after somatostatin therapy. *Nephron* **72**, 705–707.

Cavaliere, G. *et al.* (1987). Tubular nephrotoxicity after intravenous urography with ionic high-osmolal and nonionic low-osmolal contrast media in patients with chronic renal insufficiency. *Nephron* **46**, 128–133.

Chatterjee, S. *et al.* (1984). Immunohistochemical localization of glycosphingolipid in urinary renal tubular cells in Fabry's disease. *American Journal of Clinical Pathology* **82**, 24–28.

Colucci, P. and Fogazzi, G. B. (1999). The Sudanese immigrant with recurrent gross haematuria—diagnosis at a glance by examination of urinary sediment. *Nephrology, Dialysis, Transplantation* **14**, 2249–2251.

Corwin, L. C. *et al.* (1989). The detection and interpretation of urinary eosinophils. *Archives of Pathology and Laboratory Medicine* **113**, 1256–1258.

Crompton, C. H., Ward, P. B., and Hewitt, I. K. (1993). The use of red cell morphology to determine the source of hematuria in children. *Clinical Nephrology* **39**, 4–9.

Daudon, M. *et al.* (1991). Investigation of urinary crystals by Fourier transformed infrared microscopy. *Clinical Chemistry* **37**, 83–87.

Deindorfer, F. H. *et al.* (1985). 'The yellow IRIS™' Urinalysis Workstation—the first commercial application of 'automated intelligent microscopy'. *Clinical Chemistry* **31**, 1491–1499.

Delanghe, J. R. *et al.* (2000). The role of automated urine particle flow cytometry in clinical practice. *Clinica Chimica Acta* **301**, 1–18.

Desnick, R. J. *et al.* (1971). Diagnosis of glycosphingolipidoses by urinary sediment analysis. *New England Journal of Medicine* **284**, 739–744.

Diamond, E. and Schapira, H. E. (1985). Chyluria—a review of the literature. *Urology* **26**, 427–431.

Dinda, A. K. *et al.* (1997). Diagnosis of glomerular haematuria: role of dysmorphic red cell, G1 cell and bright field microscopy. *Scandinavian Journal of Clinical & Laboratory Investigation* **57**, 203–208.

Dooper, I. M. *et al.* (1991). Immunocytology of urinary sediments as a method of differentiating acute rejection from other causes of declining renal graft function. *Transplantation* **52**, 266–271.

Dorizzi, R. and Caputo, M. (1998). Measurement of urine relative density using refractometer and reagent strips. *Clinical Chemistry and Laboratory Medicine* **36**, 925–928.

Duncan, K. A. *et al.* (1985). Urinary lipid bodies in polycystic kidney diseases. *American Journal of Kidney Diseases* **49**, 49–53.

Dyerberg, J. *et al.* (1976). Evaluation of a dipstick test for glucose in urine. *Clinical Chemistry* **22**, 205.

Edvardsson, V. *et al.* (2001). Clinical features and genotype of adenine phosphoribosyltransferase deficiency in Iceland. *American Journal of Kidney Diseases* **38**, 473–480.

Eggensperger, D. *et al.* (1988). The utility of cytodiagnostic urinalysis for monitoring renal allograft injury. *American Journal of Nephrology* **8**, 27–34.

Eiser, A. R. *et al.* (1979). Clinically occult diffuse proliferative lupus nephritis. *Archives of Internal Medicine* **139**, 1022–1025.

Erley, C. M. *et al.* (1999). Prevention of radiocontrast-media-induced nephropathy in patients with pre-existing renal insufficiency by hydration in combination with the adenosine antagonist theophylline. *Nephrology, Dialysis, Transplantation* **14**, 1146–1149.

Fairley, K. F. and Birch, D. (1982). Hematuria: a simple method for identifying glomerular bleeding. *Kidney International* **21**, 105–108.

Fairley, K. F. *et al.* (1983). Protein composition of urinary casts from healthy subjects and patients with glomerulonephritis. *British Medical Journal* **287**, 1834–1840.

Fasset, R. G. *et al.* (1982a). Detection of glomerular bleeding by phase-contrast microscopy. *Lancet* **i**, 1532–1534.

Fasset, R. G. *et al.* (1982b). Urinary red-cell morphology during exercise. *British Medical Journal* **285**, 1455–1457.

Fenili, D. Automated systems for urinary sediment analysis. In *The Urinary Sediment. An Integrated View* 2nd edn. (ed. G. B. Fogazzi, C. Ponticelli, and E. Ritz), pp. 175–181. Oxford: Oxford University Press, 1999.

Fielding, B. A. *et al.* (1987). Enzyme immunoassay for urinary albumin. *Clinical Chemistry* **29**, 355–357.

Fogazzi, G. B. (1996). Crystalluria: a neglected aspect of urinary sediment analysis. *Nephrology, Dialysis, Transplantation* **11**, 379–387.

Fogazzi, G. B. and Ponticelli, C. (1996). Microscopic haematuria diagnosis and management. *Nephron* **72**, 125–134.

Fogazzi, G. B., Ponticelli, C., and Ritz, E. *The Urinary Sediment. An Integrated View*, 2nd edn., pp. 50–55. Oxford: Oxford University Press, 1999.

Fogazzi, G. B. *et al.* (1989). Use of high power field in the evaluation of formed elements of urine. *Journal of Nephrology* **2**, 107–112.

Fogazzi, G. B. *et al.* (1991). Utility of immunofluorescence of urine sediment for identifying patients with renal disease due to monoclonal gammopathies. *American Journal of Kidney Diseases* **17**, 211–217.

Fogazzi, G. B. *et al.* (1995). The cells of the deep layers of the urothelium in the urine sediment: an overlooked marker of severe diseases of the excretory urinary system. *Nephrology, Dialysis, Transplantation* **10**, 1918–1919.

Fogazzi, G. B. *et al.* (1996). Don't forget sickled cells in the urine when investigating a patient for haematuria. *Nephrology, Dialysis, Transplantation* **11**, 723–725.

Fujita, T. *et al.* (1998). Level of red blood cells in the urinary sediment reflects the degree of renal activity in Wegener's granulomatosis. *Clinical Nephrology* **50**, 284–288.

Gadeholt, H. (1964). Quantitative estimation of urinary sediment, with special regard to sources of errors. *British Medical Journal* **1**, 1547–1549.

Gambaro, G. *et al.* (2001). Cigarette smoking is a risk factor for nephropathy and its progression in type 2 diabetes mellitus. *Diabetes Nutrition and Metabolism* **14**, 337–342.

Gerber, L. M., Johnston, K., and Alderman, M. H. (1998). Assessment of a new dipstick test in screening for microalbuminuria in patients with hypertension. *American Journal of Hypertension* **11**, 1321–1327.

Ginsberg, J. M. *et al.* (1983). Use of single voided urine samples to estimate quantitative proteinuria. *New England Journal of Medicine* **309**, 1543–1546.

Goorno, W. *et al.* (1967). Acute glomerulonephritis with absence of abnormal urinary findings. *Annals of Internal Medicine* **66**, 345–353.

Gregory, M. C. *et al.* (1984). The clinical significance of candidal casts. *American Journal of Kidney Diseases* **4**, 179–184.

Harrison, H. H. *et al.* (1992). Comparison of microheterogeneity patterns of purified monoclonal light chains (Bence Jones proteins) and polyclonal free light chains that produce the pseudo-oligoclonal ('ladder light chain') pattern in immunofixation studies of urine. *Clinical Chemistry* **38**, 963.

Hartman, H. G. *et al.* (1985). Detection of renal tubular lesions after abdominal aortography and selective arteriography by quantitative measurements of brush-border enzymes in the urine. *Nephron* **39**, 95–101.

Hebert, L. A. *et al.* (1995). Relationship between appearance of urinary red blood cell/white blood cell casts and the onset of renal relapse in systemic lupus erythematosus. *American Journal of Kidney Disease* **26**, 432–438.

Hockberger, R. S. *et al.* (1987). Hematuria induced by urethral catheterization. *Annals of Emergency Medicine* **16**, 550–552.

Hofmann, W. *et al.* (1992). A new strategy for characterizing proteinuria and haematuria from single pattern of defined proteins in urine. *European Journal of Clinical Chemistry and Clinical Biochemistry* **30**, 707–712.

Hoyer, J. R. and Seiler, M. W. (1979). Pathophysiology of Tamm–Horsfall protein. *Kidney International* **16**, 279–289.

Hotta, O. *et al.* (2000). Urinary macrophages as activity markers of renal injury. *Clinica Chimica Acta* **297**, 123–133.

Imhof, P. R. *et al.* (1972). Excretion of urinary casts after administration of diuretics. *British Medical Journal* **2**, 199–202.

Jain, H., Greenblatt, J. M., and Albornoz, A. M. (2001). Emphysematous pyelonephritis: a rare cause of pneumaturia. *The Lancet* **357**, 194.

Jones, C. A. *et al.* (2002). Microalbuminuria in the US population: Third National Health and Nutrition Examination Survey. *American Journal of Kidney Diseases* **39**, 445–459.

K/DOQI clinical practice guidelines for chronic kidney disease: evaluation, classification, and stratification (2002). *American Journal of Kidney Diseases* **39** (Suppl. 1), S93–S102.

Kessom, A. M. *et al.* (1978). Microscopic examination of urine. *Lancet* **ii**, 809–812.

King, J. S. and Boyce, W. H. *High Molecular Weight Substances in Human Urine.* Springfield IL: Thomas, 1963.

Kitamoto, Y. *et al.* (1993). Differentiation of hematuria using a uniquely shaped red cell. *Nephron* **64**, 32–36.

Koene, R. A. P. (1999). Unexplained haematuria. *Nephrology, Dialysis, Transplantation* **14**, 2025–2027.

Köhler, H. *et al.* (1991). Acanthocyturia. A characteristic marker for glomerular bleeding. *Kidney International* **40**, 115–120.

Koopman, M. G. *et al.* (1989). Circadian rhythm of proteinuria: consequences of the use of urinary protein : creatinine ratios. *Nephrology, Dialysis, Transplantation* **4**, 9–14.

Kopp, J. B. *et al.* (1997). Crystalluria and urinary tract abnormalities associated with indinavir. *Annals of Internal Medicine* **127**, 119–125.

Kouri, T. *et al.* (2000). European urinalysis guidelines. *Scandinavian Journal of Clinical & Laboratory Investigation* **60** (Suppl. 231), 1–96.

Kumar, B. D. *et al.* (1992). Detection of rifampicin-induced nephrotoxicity by *N*-acetyl-3-D-glucosaminidase. *Journal of Tropical Medicine and Hygiene* **95**, 424–427.

Lacher, D. A. and De Beukelaer, M. (1986). Falsely low value for total protein in urine as measured in the Du Pont Automatic Clinical Analyzer (ACA). *Clinical Chemistry* **32**, 203.

Lam, M. O. (1995). False 'hematuria' due to bacteriuria. *Archives of Pathology and Laboratory Medicine* **119**, 717–721.

Leaker, B. *et al.* (1987). Lupus nephritis: clinical and pathological correlation. *Quarterly Journal of Medicine* **62**, 163–179.

Lettgen, B. and Wohlmuth, A. (1995). Validity of G1-cells in the differentiation between glomerular and non-glomerular haematuria in children. *Pediatric Nephrology* **9**, 435–437.

Lievens, M. M. and Celis, P. J. (1982). Drug interference in turbidimetry and colorimetry of proteins in urine. *Clinical Chemistry* **28**, 23–28.

Lindner, L. E. and Haber, M. H. (1983). Hyaline casts in the urine: mechanisms of formation and morphologic transformations. *American Journal of Clinical Pathology* **80**, 347–352.

Lindner, L. E. *et al.* (1980). A specific cast in acute pyelonephritis. *American Journal of Clinical Pathology* **73**, 809–811.

Loh, E. H. *et al.* (1990). Blood cells and red cell morphology in the urine of healthy children. *Clinical Nephrology* **34**, 185–187.

Lorentz, K. and Weiss, T. (1986). Protein bestimmung intramuscular Urin—Eine kritische Uebersicht. *Journal of Clinical Chemistry and Clinical Biochemistry* **24**, 309–323.

McElderry, L. A. *et al.* (1982). Six methods for urinary protein compared. *Clinical Chemistry* **28**, 2294–2296.

McQueen, E. G. (1966). Composition of urinary casts. *Lancet* **i**, 397–399.

Mandal, A. K. *et al.* (1985). Transmission electron microscopy of urinary sediment in human acute renal failure. *Kidney International* **28**, 58–63.

Marhun, D. (1979). Evaluation of urinary enzyme patterns in patients with kidney diseases and primary benign hypertension. *Current Problems in Clinical Biochemistry* **9**, 135–139.

Meola, J. M. *et al.* (1977). Simple procedure for measuring total protein in urine. *Clinical Chemistry* **23**, 975–977.

Merlini, G. *et al.* (2001). The Pavia approach to clinical protein analysis. *Clinical Chemistry and Laboratory Medicine* **39**, 1025–1028.

Meyer, B. R. *et al.* (1984). Increased urinary enzyme excretion in workers exposed to nephrotoxic chemicals. *American Journal of Medicine* **76**, 989–996.

Mogensen, C. E. *et al.* (1997). Multicenter evaluation of the Micral-Test II test strip, an immunologic rapid test for the detection of microalbuminuria. *Diabetes Care* **20**, 1642–1646.

Mondorf, A. W. *et al.* Brush border enzymes and drug nephrotoxicity. In *Acute Renal Failure* (ed. K. Solez and A. Wellthon), pp. 281–298. New York: Dekker, 1984.

Monster, T. B. *et al.* (2001). Oral contraceptive use and hormone replacement therapy are associated with microalbuminuria. *Archives of Internal Medicine* **161**, 200–205.

Nakamura, J. and Yakata, M. (1982). Urine contains an inhibitor for turbidimetric determinations of protein. *Clinical Chemistry* **28**, 356–360.

NCCLS (1995). Urinalysis and collection, transportation and preservation of urine specimens; approved guidelines. NCCLS Document GP16A.

Ng, T. P. *et al.* (1993). Further evidence of human silica nephrotoxicity in occupationally exposed workers. *British Journal of Industrial Medicine* **50**, 907–912.

Nolan III, C. R. *et al.* (1986). Eosinophiluria—a new method of detection and definition of the clinical spectrum. *New England Journal of Medicine* **315**, 1516–1519.

Orita, Y. *et al.* (1977). Immunofluorescent studies of urinary casts. *Nephron* **19**, 19–25.

Pannacciulli, N. *et al.* (2001). Urinary albumin excretion is independently associated with C-reactive protein levels in overweight and obese nondiabetic premenopausal women. *Journal of Internal Medicine* **250**, 502–507.

Pesce, A. J. and First, R. M. (1979). *Proteinuria. An Integrated Review.* New York: Dekker, 1979.

Pesce, A. J. and Strande, C. S. (1973). A new micromethod for determination of protein in cerebrospinal fluid and urine. *Clinical Chemistry* **19**, 1265–1267.

Peters, A. *et al.* (1976). Field studies of a rapid accurate means of quantifying *Schistosoma haematobium* eggs in urine samples. *Bulletin of the World Health Organization* **54**, 159–162.

Pfaller, M. A. *et al.* (1985). Laboratory evaluation of leucocyte esterase and nitrite test for the detection of bacteriuria. *Journal of Clinical Microbiology* **21**, 840–842.

Podebrad, F. *et al.* (1999). 4,5-Dimethyl-3-hydroxy-2[5H]-furanone (sotolone)—the odour of maple syrup urine disease. *Journal of Inherited Metabolic Diseases* **22**, 107–114.

Price, R. G. *et al.* (1982). Urinary enzymes, nephrotoxicity and renal disease. *Toxicology* **26**, 99–134.

Pugia, M. J. *et al.* (1997). Comparison of urine dipsticks with quantitative methods for microalbuminuria. *European Journal of Clinical Chemistry and Clinical Biochemistry* **35**, 693–700.

Rath, B. *et al.* (1990). Evaluation of light microscopy to localise the site of haematuria. *Archives of Disease in Childhood* **65**, 338–340.

Rath, B. *et al.* (1992). What makes red cells dysmorphic in glomerular haematuria? *Pediatric Nephrology* **6**, 424–427.

Ravigneaux, M.-H. *et al.* (1991). Signification d'une cytolipidurie dans le cadre d'un syndrome nephrotique. *Néphrologie* **12**, 12–16.

Regeniter, A. *et al.* (2001). Urine analysis performed by flow cytometry: reference range determination and comparison to morphological findings, dipstick chemistry and bacterial culture results—a multicenter study. *Clinical Nephrology* **55**, 384–392.

Rehman H. U. (1999). Fish odour syndrome. *Postgraduate Medical Journal* **75**, 451–452.

Reichert, L. J. M. *et al.* (1995). Urinary excretion of β_2-microglobulin predicts renal outcome in patients with idiopathic membranous nephropathy. *Journal of the American Society of Nephrology* **6**, 1666–1669.

Rizzoni, G. *et al.* (1983). Evaluation of glomerular and nonglomerular hematuria by phase-contrast microscope. *Journal of Pediatrics* **103**, 370–374.

Rodby, R. A. *et al.* (1995). The urine protein to creatinine ratio as a predictor of 24-hour urine protein excretion in type 1 diabetic patients with nephropathy. The Collaborative Study Group. *American Journal of Kidney Diseases* **26**, 904–909.

Rojanasthien, N. *et al.* (2001). Protective effects of fosfomycin on cisplatin-induced nephrotoxicity in patients with lung cancer. *International Journal of Clinical Pharmacology and Therapy* **39**, 121–125.

Rosa, T. T. and Palatini, P. (2000). Clinical value of microalbuminuria in hypertension. *Journal of Hypertension* **18**, 645–654.

Ruffing, K. A. *et al.* (1994). Eosinophils in urine revisited. *Clinical Nephrology* **41**, 163–166.

Ruggenenti, P. *et al.* (1998). Cross sectional longitudinal study of spot morning urine protein : creatinine ratio, 24 urine protein excretion rate, glomerular filtration rate, and end stage renal failure in chronic renal disease in patients without diabetes. *British Medical Journal* **316**, 504–509.

Rutecki, G. J. *et al.* (1971). Characterization of proteins in urinary casts. *New England Journal of Medicine* **284**, 1049–1052.

Sandoz, P. F. *et al.* (1986). Value of urinary sediment in the diagnosis of interstitial rejection in renal transplants. *Transplantation* **41**, 343–348.

Scheer, W. D. (1987). The detection of leukocytes esterase activity in urine with a new reagent. *American Journal of Clinical Pathology* **87**, 856–893.

Schramek, P. *et al.* (1989a). Value of urinary erythrocyte morphology in assessment of symptomless microhaematuria. *Lancet* **ii**, 1316–1319.

Schramek, P. *et al.* (1989b). *In vitro* generation of dysmorphic erythrocytes. *Kidney International* **36**, 72–77.

Schwab, S. J. *et al.* (1987). Quantitation of proteinuria by the use of protein : creatinine ratios in single urine samples. *Archives of Internal Medicine* **147**, 943–944.

Segasothy, M. *et al.* (1989). Immunoperoxidase identification of nucleated cells in urine in glomerular and acute tubular disorders. *Clinical Nephrology* **31**, 281–291.

Sherman, R. L. *et al.* (1983). *N*-acetyl-β-glucosaminidase and β_2-microglobulin: their urinary excretion in patients with parenchymatous renal diseases. *Archives of Internal Medicine* **143**, 1183–1185.

Shiba, K. S. *et al.* (1985). A cause of discrepancy between values for urinary protein as assayed by the Coomassie Brilliant Blue G-250 method and the sulphosalycilic acid method.*Clinical Chemistry* **31**, 1215–1218.

Shukla, P. S. *et al.* (1988). Effects of five different antisera on the immunoturbidimetric determination of urinary albumin. *Clinical Chemistry* **34**, 430.

Stamp, R. J. (1988). Measurement of albumin in urine by end-point immunonephelometry. *Annals of Clinical Biochemistry* **245**, 442–445.

Strasinger, S. K. *Urinalysis and Body Fluids.* Philadelphia: Davis, 1985.

Synhaivsky, A. and Malek, R. S. (1985). Isolated pneumaturia. *The American Journal of Medicine* **78**, 617–620.

Tassi, C. *et al.* (2000). Activity and isoenzyme profile of *N*-acetyl-beta-D-glucosaminidase in urine from workers exposed to cadmium. *Clinica Chimica Acta* **299**, 55–64.

Triger, D. R. and Smith, J. W. C. (1966). Survival of urinary leucocytes. *Journal of Clinical Pathology* **19**, 443–447.

Tuck, J., Pearce, I., and Pantelides, M. (2000). Chyluria after radical nephrectomy treated with n-butyl-2-cyanocrylate. *Journal of Urology* **164**, 778–779.

Valles, P. *et al.* (2000). Follow-up of steroid-resistant nephrotic syndrome: tubular proteinuria and enzymuria. *Pediatric Nephrology* **15**, 252–258.

Van der Snoek, B. E. and Koene, R. A. P. (1997). Fixation of urinary sediment. *The Lancet* **350**, 933–934.

Vickers, D., Ahmad, T., and Coulthard, M. G. (1991). Diagnosis of urinary tract infection in children: fresh urine microscopy or culture? *The Lancet* **338**, 767–770.

Vlaskou, D. *et al.* (2000). Human neutral brush border endopeptidase EC 3.4.24.11 in urine, its isolation, characterisation and activity in renal diseases. *Clinica Chimica Acta* 297, 103–121.

Weichert-Jacobsen, K. *et al.* (1998). Urinary leakage of tubular enzymes after shock wave lithotripsy. *European Urology* **33**, 104–110.

Wilkins, E. *et al.* (1985). Leucocyte esterase-nitrite screening method for pyuria and bacteriuria. *Journal of Clinical Pathology* **38**, 1342–1345.

Wolf, G. *et al.* (1990). Urinary excretion of dipeptidyl aminopeptidase IV in patients with renal diseases. *Clinical Nephrology* **33**, 136–142.

Wong, K. *et al.* (1994). Acute oxalate nephropathy after a massive intravenous dose of vitamin C. *Australian and New Zealand Journal of Medicine* **24**, 410–411.

Woo, J. *et al.* (1978). Radioimmunoassay for urinary albumin. *Clinical Chemistry* **24**, 1464–1467.

Yazzie, D. *et al.* (1998). Lysosomal enzymuria in protein energy malnutrition. *American Journal of Nephrology* **18**, 9–15.

1.3 The clinical assessment of renal function

Dominique Prié and Gérard Friedlander

In this chapter, we will present the methods that can be used in clinical practice to evaluate the various aspects of renal function. We will consider the measurement of renal blood flow (RBF), glomerular filtration rate (GFR), and the methods to assess proximal tubule functions, the ability of kidney to dilute or concentrate urine, and to adapt H^+, K^+, and calcium excretion. We will also deal briefly with the endocrine functions of the kidney.

Renal blood flow measurement

Under resting conditions, about one-fifth of the cardiac output is delivered to the kidneys. In humans, these organs represent about 0.4 per cent of the total body weight, thus the perfusion flow of the kidneys is 4 ml/g/min. Although renal oxygen consumption is high, this enormous blood flow largely exceeds the energy requirement for the tubular reabsorption or secretion of solute but is essential to allow an efficient GFR. However, RBF is not homogeneous throughout the kidney; in the inner stripe of the renal medulla the supply of the metabolic needs can be limited by medullary perfusion in pathological conditions. In clinical practice, the physician is mainly interested in total RBF measurement, that is, the flow of blood that enters and leaves the kidney. We will not detail here the experimental methods to assess blood repartition within the kidney.

Classical methods of measurement of renal blood flow

Para-aminohippurate clearance

The classical method to measure the RBF is based on clearance techniques using a marker that is completely extracted from plasma during a single pass through the kidney and eliminated in urine without any modifications (Smith 1951; Back *et al.* 1989; Hirata-Dulas *et al.* 1994; Toto 1995). Under these conditions, during a given period of time, the quantity of the non-toxic marker that enters the kidney with the arterial blood is equal to the quantity of marker appearing in urine during the same period. This relationship is expressed mathematically by the following equation:

$$\dot{Q} \times A = U \times \dot{V} \quad \text{or} \quad \dot{Q} = \frac{U \times \dot{V}}{A},$$

where $\dot{Q}$ is the renal plasma flow (RPF) rate, A the concentration of indicator in arterial plasma, U the concentration of indicator in urine, and V the urine flow rate.

RBF is obtained from RPF as follows:

$$\text{RBF} = \frac{\text{RPF}}{1 - \text{Ht}},$$

where Ht stands for haematocrit value expressed in fractional form (0.37–0.49 in normal adults).

The complete clearance of the indicator from the plasma is obtained by filtration in the glomeruli and active secretion by the tubules. However, because the markers bind proteins, their extraction ratio is less than 1. The most commonly used marker of RPF is *p*-aminohippuric acid (PAH). Its extraction ratio varies from 0.7 to 0.9, provided PAH plasma concentrations do not exceed maximal tubule capacity of extraction (Aurell *et al.* 1978). The PAH extraction ratio differs from one subject to another and may be modified by pharmacological treatment. This parameter cannot be calculated easily since the difference of the marker concentration between the renal artery and the renal vein is unknown. Conventionally, RPF is estimated from PAH clearance by assuming an extraction ratio of 1, giving the effective renal plasma flow (ERPF) value.

In practice, a loading dose of PAH is intravenously injected followed by a constant infusion of the indicator. PAH plasma concentration reaches a steady state within an hour, then urine and venous blood samples are collected over successive time-controlled periods (Hirata-Dulas *et al.* 1994; Visscher *et al.* 1995; Hollenberg *et al.* 1999). This method assumes that renal arterial and peripheral venous plasma concentrations are identical. When urine collection is difficult, a metabolic clearance rate is used to calculate the PAH clearance on the assumption that in the steady state, the rate of PAH infusion equals its rate of excretion.

Related indicators

PAH clearance is considered as the gold standard to measure ERPF, but many other markers have also been studied. The most often used markers are: *ortho*-iodo-hippuran, a radioiodine labelled PAH analogue that exhibits an extraction ratio of 0.8 (Russell *et al.* 1989; Nakashima *et al.* 1996; Akutsu *et al.* 1998) and ^{99m}Tc-mercapto-acetyl-triglycerine (^{99m}Tc-MAG3) (Russell *et al.* 1996; Itoh 2001) which provides renal scintigraphy images of high quality and is used to measure ERPF despite high protein binding and relatively low extraction efficiency (<0.6). Combining renal imaging with functional data gives additional information regarding the relative contribution of each kidney to the global function.

The serotonin metabolite 5-hydroxyindoleacetic acid has also been proposed as an endogenous index of RPF (Hannedouche *et al.* 1989).

To avoid continuous infusions of radiomarkers and urine collections, alternative methods have been developed to measure RPF. These are based upon the administration of a single intravenous dose of tracer followed by multiple blood samplings. The calculation of ERPF rests on the analysis of one- or two-compartment models of plasma clearance of the marker (Hirata-Dulas *et al.* 1994; Kotzerke *et al.* 1997; Kanazawa *et al.* 1998; Werner *et al.* 1998). Double- and single-blood sample methods have also been proposed but these give less accurate results. The reproducibility of these various methods has been measured for different markers, essentially in subjects with normal renal function (Piepsz *et al.* 1996; Kotzerke *et al.* 1997; Kanazawa *et al.* 1998; Werner *et al.* 1998). The coefficient of variation is about 12 per cent between successive periods for continuous infusion of PAH and is similar for plasma clearance of *ortho*-iodo-hippuran or ^{99m}Tc-MAG3 measured after different intervals of time.

Interpretation of renal plasma flow variation

A low PAH clearance may reflect an actual diminution of RPF or it may be due to a decrease in the extraction ratio, in particular, either when drugs are used or in kidney diseases (Carriere and Friborg 1969; Aukland and Loyning 1970; Battilana *et al.* 1991). In general, PAH clearance decreases at the same rate as GFR and it does not give further information on the mechanism of GFR decline. Thus, the interpretation of isolated changes of the PAH clearance should be done cautiously.

Non-invasive methods

^{99m}Tc-MAG3 has been used to measure ERPF without blood sampling in patients with renal disorders (Itoh 2001). This method is based on ^{99m}Tc-MAG3 gamma-camera renography and a theoretical modelling of the pharmacokinetics of the marker. Further studies will determine the place of this method in patient investigation. Similar studies have been conducted with *ortho*-iodo-hippuran (Schlegel *et al.* 1979) but have shown limited accuracy and reproducibility (Oriuchi *et al.* 1996).

The measurement of RBF by colour Doppler sonography, a non-invasive and safe method, has been recently evaluated in children and shows interesting results (Scholbach 1999; Strandness 2000). However, in adults, the study of renal perfusion is often more difficult and less reproducible than in children.

Different techniques based on magnetic resonance (MR) imaging or computed tomography have been used for measuring RBF (Roberts *et al.* 1995; Debatin 1998; de Haan *et al.* 2000; Romero and Lerman 2000), especially in patients with suspicion of renal artery stenosis (Binkert *et al.* 1999, 2001). The injection of a contrast medium such as gadolinium-DTPA (DTPA = diethylene triamine penta-acetic acid) can improve the accuracy of the measurements (Dumoulin *et al.* 1994; Vallee *et al.* 2000). MR velocity mapping showed correlation with PAH clearance in healthy volunteers (Sommer *et al.* 1998) and in patients with impaired renal functions (Cortsen *et al.* 1996). These methods do not provide functional information but merely measure the renal blood supply.

Glomerular filtration rate assessment

Inulin clearance

Renal insufficiency is defined as the decrease of the GFR. Consequently it is necessary to have an accurate, reliable, and reproducible method to measure the GFR. The method of reference to measure GFR is based on the clearance concept (Smith *et al.* 1943; Smith 1951; Harvey 1980). Let us consider a substance that is freely filtered at the glomeruli and is neither reabsorbed nor secreted by the renal tubules, nor is it modified after filtration. The quantity of substance that appears in urine per unit time equals the quantity of substance that is filtered at the glomeruli. Mathematically, this can be expressed as follows:

$$C \times \mathrm{Pi} = \mathrm{Ui} \times V \quad \text{or} \quad C = \frac{\mathrm{Ui} \times \dot{V}}{\mathrm{Pi}},$$

where C is the volume of plasma filtered at the glomeruli per unit time and also represents the volume of plasma that is completely cleared of the indicator per unit of time, Pi the substance concentration in plasma, Ui the urinary concentration of the substance, and $\dot{V}$ the urinary flow rate.

If the substance meets the criteria defined above, then C = GFR.

Two non-toxic substances fulfil these criteria and are currently in use in humans: inulin and polyfructosan. Both these substances are fructose polymers that are extracted from plants. Nowadays the polyfructosans (Inutest®) are preferred to inulin since they are easily soluble in water at room temperature. These substances are not endogenously present in humans and must be intravenously infused throughout the GFR measurement. In practice, after a bolus injection, the dose of which is calculated according to the patient's body weight, the marker is infused at a constant rate to obtain a stable plasma concentration. This is achieved within 1 h. To ensure a urine flow rate above 2 ml/min throughout the investigation, the patients are hydrated with an oral water load, and additional water is given periodically. Once the steady state for plasma marker concentration has been achieved, the patients are asked to empty their bladder completely and several urine samples are collected at regular intervals (generally 30 or 60 min). The indicator plasma concentration is serially measured either at the middle or at the beginning and at the end of each period of urine collection. To minimize error, an average of three to five determinations are made. Polyfructosan and inulin determinations in the plasma are based upon hydrolysis of the polymer and measurement of the resultant free fructose with colorimetric assay. High-performance liquid chromatography (HPLC) techniques can also be used. Glucose may interfere with the colorimetric dosages, so plasma samples should be treated with glucose oxydase whenever plasma glucose concentrations are above 10 mM. The coefficient of variation of polyfructosan or inulin clearance between consecutive periods or between measurements on different days is about 7 per cent (Levey 1989). This means that for an initial GFR value of 40 ml/min, a variation of 6 ml/min in a subsequent investigation predicts a real modification of GFR at an alpha error less than 5 per cent.

Radionuclide markers such as ^{51}Cr-labelled ethylenediaminetetraacetic acid (^{51}Cr-EDTA), technecium-radiolabelled DTPA (^{125m}Tc-DTPA) or ^{125}I-iothalamate can be used in renal clearance studies. However, in order to avoid high radiation exposures, sustained infusions of these radioisotope-labelled compounds are rarely performed.

Creatinine clearance

To avoid marker infusion, an endogenous substance is often used—creatinine. This marker, however, does not meet all the criteria defined above for an acute measurement of GFR. Creatinine is a metabolic product of creatine and phosphocreatine, two substances found almost exclusively in the muscle (Wyss and Kaddurah-Daouk 2000).

The other source of creatine is meat (Jacobsen *et al.* 1979; Hoogwerf *et al.* 1986). Thus, the serum creatinine level is proportional to muscle mass and depends on dietary protein intake (Crim *et al.* 1975; Heymsfield *et al.* 1983; Lew and Bosch 1991). Its production rate is decreased in patients with hepatic diseases (Cocchetto *et al.* 1983). Creatinine is a small molecule of molecular weight (MW) 113 Da that does not bind plasma proteins and is mainly eliminated by the kidney in patients with normal renal function. Creatinine is freely filtered by the glomerulus and is almost never reabsorbed throughout the tubules. However, it has long been known that in the renal tubule, a saturable process secretes creatinine (Wyss and Kaddurah-Daouk 2000). The relative contribution of tubule secretion to creatinine excretion increases when serum creatinine concentration increases. Thus, creatinine clearance exceeds inulin clearance especially in patients with decreased GFR (Levey 1990). The secretion process can be inhibited by some commonly used drugs such as cimetidine, trimethoprim, pyrimethamine, or dapsone (Berglund *et al.* 1975; McElligott 1978; Burgess *et al.* 1982; Opravil *et al.* 1993). Some authors tried to use cimetidine to improve the accuracy of GFR measurement by the creatinine clearance (van Acker *et al.* 1992; Payne 1993; Zaltzman *et al.* 1996; Hellerstein *et al.* 1998; Walser 1998; Serdar *et al.* 2001). However, these attempts did not give convincing results because the inhibition of secretion varies between individuals. Similarly, the basal tubular secretion of creatinine is not constant over time for a given subject and differs between individuals. Another pitfall is the increase of extra renal elimination of creatinine when its serum concentration increases (Wyss and Kaddurah-Daouk 2000).

Despite these limitations, the creatinine clearance is still widely used and can give a good but not accurate estimate of GFR (Fig. 1). This is a simple technique that can be performed easily in ambulatory (out)patients (Herget-Rosenthal *et al.* 1999).

Since serum creatinine concentration does not vary significantly during the day, its value can be obtained from a single blood sample. At the beginning of the investigation the patient takes an oral water load then empties his bladder. Urine is collected by spontaneous voiding at 1-h intervals. Increasing the number of urine collections improves the accuracy of the results. Urine can also be collected over longer periods of time; 24 h, for example. However, this method is responsible for 'lost samples' of urine that are not mentioned by the patient, leading to inaccurate values of $U \times \dot{V}$.

The major disadvantage of the classical clearance techniques is the requirement of accurate urine collection, a problem that can be difficult to deal with especially in children and elderly people. Two methods circumvent this problem: the infusion-equilibrium technique and the measurement of the plasma clearance of a single bolus injection of a marker.

Infusion-equilibrium technique

The infusion-equilibrium technique is based on the assumption that when the infusion rate of a marker equals its urinary excretion ($U \times \dot{V}$), the plasma concentration of the marker is stable. The marker must fulfil the same criteria as those described for classical clearance techniques. A loading dose of marker is injected, followed by an infusion through a very accurate pump. Several consecutive blood samples are drawn to check that the marker plasma concentration is constant. The urinary excretion rate is not measured but is taken to equal the quantity of marker delivered through the pump. The amount delivered is obtained from the concentration of the marker × the infusion rate (Cole *et al.* 1972; Holliday *et al.* 1993; van Acker *et al.* 1995; van Guldener *et al.* 1995). The principal disadvantage of this method is the long time of infusions.

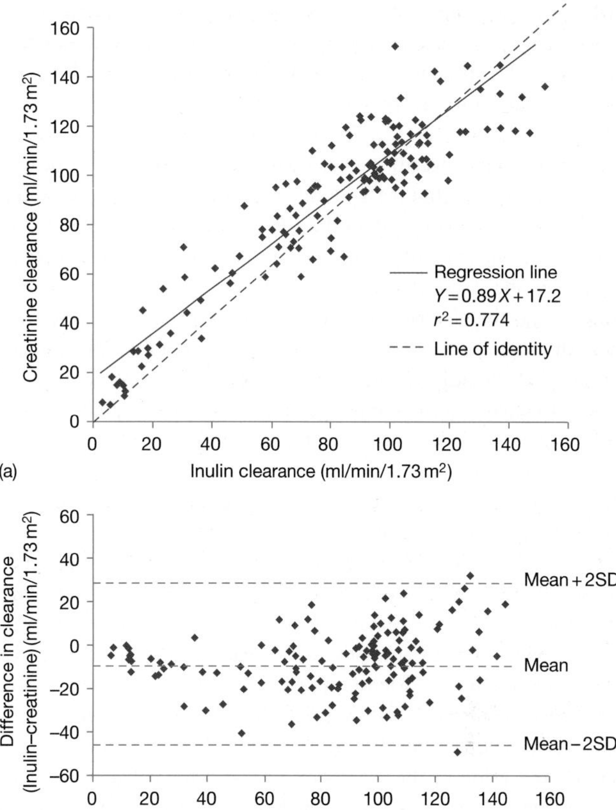

Fig. 1 Comparison of the clearance of creatinine and inulin measured in 144 patients with normal or impaired glomerular filtration rate (Prié and Friedlander, unpublished data). Panel (a) shows the correlation of the two methods of measurement. Panel (b) shows the agreement of the two methods of measurements (Bland and Altman 1986).

Plasma clearance techniques

The measurement of GFR using a single injection technique is based on assumptions of critical importance. At any time, the quantity of indicator excreted by the kidney is $dQ = \text{GFR} \cdot C(t)\, dt$ where $C(t)$ is the plasma concentration of the indicator at time t. When the total amount of marker injected (Q_0) has been excreted by the kidney, this equation gives:

$$\text{GFR} = \frac{Q_0}{\int_0^{\infty} C(t)\, dt} \tag{1}$$

where the denominator represents the area under the plasma concentration–time curve (Chantler *et al.* 1969; Brochner-Mortensen 1972). An accurate measurement of this parameter requires a large number of blood samples (Gaspari *et al.* 1995, 1997, 1998). Mathematical models have been developed to describe the decline of the marker plasma levels over time using a limited number of samples (Picciotto *et al.* 1992; Gaspari *et al.* 1996). All the models used to estimate plasma clearance assume that the volume distribution of the marker and its renal excretion are constant over time. One- and two-compartment models have been used to calculate GFR (Chantler *et al.* 1969). The plasma disappearance curve of the indicator can be fitted by the sum of two exponential functions of the form $C = Ae^{-at} + Be^{-bt}$ (Fig. 2). This means that when plasma concentration is plotted on a logarithmic scale against time this curve appears as the sum of two straight lines with different slopes. These values can be substituted in Eq. (1) to obtain the GFR: $\text{GFR} = Q_0/[(A/a) + (B/b)]$. In the two-compartment model, both slopes are used to calculate the area under the curve and the GFR. The first compartment can be thought of as the plasma pool and the second one as the extracellular fluid. Although the two-compartment model is oversimplified, since it assumes that the indicator distributes between only two pools, it still requires frequent plasma sampling (Gaspari *et al.* 1995). In this model, the first exponential corresponds to the equilibrium of the indicator between the two compartments and the second one represents its renal excretion. In the one-compartment model, only the data obtained during the elimination phase are used to calculate the second exponential and the GFR (Hagstam *et al.* 1974). This phase generally begins 120 min after injection. Since, in the one-pool system, the area under the curve is approximate, a correction is applied to obtain the GFR value. The most frequently used equation for correction is that defined by Brochner-Mortensen (1972). To ensure accurate measurements, several samplings are required to get the regression line during the elimination phase. Ideally, the higher the sample number the most accurate the value of the regression line and the calculation of the GFR. Some authors have used methods based on a single blood sample obtained between 60 and 240 min after injection. These techniques can give a reasonable estimate of the GFR (Groth and Aasted 1981; Jacobsson 1983; Brown and O'Reilly 1991; Rydstrom *et al.* 1995; Gaspari *et al.* 1996). Nevertheless, multiple sampling yields a more accurate determination of GFR (Picciotto *et al.* 1992). Four samples drawn every hour from 2 to 5 h after the indicator injection are

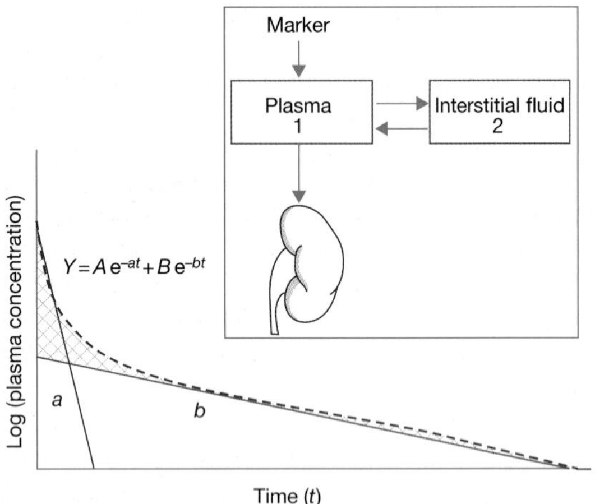

Fig. 2 The top panel represents a two-compartment model. The bottom panel shows a typical plasma disappearance curve after single intravenous injection of a marker of GFR. This curve can be expressed as a double exponential function. The first exponential corresponds to the marker equilibration between compartments 1 and 2, and the second function corresponds to the renal elimination phase. The straight lines represent the least-square best fit with slopes *a* and *b*, respectively. In a one-compartment model, the hatched area is not considered for calculating the GFR.

enough in patients with normal or slightly decreased renal function (usually serum creatinine $< 130\ \mu\text{M}$). When the decline of the GFR is more pronounced, the sampling time must be adapted. In these cases, samples obtained as late as 24 h after injection are suitable (Brochner-Mortensen 1985; Frennby *et al.* 1995). These methods used to measure GFR have been validated in adults and show good precision and correlation with inulin clearance (Garnett *et al.* 1967; Chantler *et al.* 1969; Chantler and Barratt 1972; Hagstam *et al.* 1974; Rehling *et al.* 1984; Brown and O'Reilly 1991; Isaka *et al.* 1992; Gaspari *et al.* 1995, 1998), however, there is still some controversy over their applicability in children, and further study is required (Chantler 1973; Geva and Spitzer 1995).

Another limitation to the use of plasma clearance technique is the presence of a third compartment. For example, in patients with ascites the assumptions made to calculate the GFR from a one- or a two-compartment model are not met, so other mathematical models should be used (Henriksen *et al.* 1980).

Two types of markers can be used to calculate plasma clearance: radiolabelled markers or non-radioactive markers (Gaspari 1997). The most frequently used radionuclide-labelled agents are: ^{51}Cr-EDTA, ^{125m}Tc-DTPA, or ^{125}I-iothalamate. ^{51}Cr-EDTA and ^{125}I-iothalamate have been extensively studied and they give GFR values very close to those measured with the 'gold standard' method—the clearance of inulin (Garnett *et al.* 1967; Brochner-Mortensen *et al.* 1969; Hagstam *et al.* 1974; Perrone *et al.* 1990; Brown and O'Reilly 1991) except in advanced renal insufficiency (Jagenburg *et al.* 1978) and in some patients with cardiac dysfunction (Motwani *et al.* 1992). ^{51}Cr-EDTA is a small molecule (MW: 292 Da) with little binding to plasma proteins that is freely filtered by the glomerulus. ^{125}I-iothalamate is a high osmolar ionic radiocontrast agent, in which ^{127}I has been replaced by its isotope ^{125}I. Its MW is 614 Da. The relatively long half-life of ^{125}I (60 days) makes it easy to use. The main advantages of the radiolabelled indicators are the ease and the accuracy of measurements. Their drawback is the delivery of radioactivity. In adults, the total dose delivered is less than the amount received during standard X-ray procedures. However, these radioisotopes are excreted and concentrated in urine, exposing the bladder and the gonads to higher levels of radiation. Furthermore, in many patients, the measurement of GFR is controlled repeatedly throughout their lifetime increasing the cumulative dose irradiation. The use of these radiomarkers is also problematical in women before menopause, since in most cases the physician cannot be sure that they are not pregnant. Similarly, the use of radioisotope in children should be avoided. In Europe and the United States, the regulatory agencies maintain a strict control over the storage, the dispensation, and the disposal of radioactive products and the use of isotopes is limited to specific departments. To avoid using radiolabelled compounds, several techniques have been developed especially to measure non-radioactive radiocontrast agent concentration in plasma. Two molecules have been used: iothalamate sodium, and more recently, iohexol (omnipaque), which has become the most popular non-radioactive marker used to calculate GFR with the plasma clearance technique (Effersoe *et al.* 1990; Brown and O'Reilly 1991; Isaka *et al.* 1992; Frennby *et al.* 1995; Gaspari *et al.* 1995, 1998; Brandstrom *et al.* 1998). Iohexol (MW: 821 Da) is a non-ionic low osmolar contrast medium with few adverse effects that fulfils all the criteria for a marker of the GFR. Extrarenal clearance of iohexol is low, so it has been used to determine residual renal function in patients on peritoneal or haemodialysis (Marx *et al.* 1995; Swan *et al.* 1996; Sterner *et al.* 2000).

Only few millitres of radiocontrast media are injected for the GFR determination; a dose lower than that used in radiographic imaging. The GFR determination can also be measured during standard urography. These agents carry a risk of allergic reactions and should not be administered to patients who are allergic to iodine. The dosage techniques of iothalamate and iohexol are based either on the ability of the carbon–iodine bond to absorb ultraviolet or on the capacity of iodine atoms to emit a characteristic X-ray fluorescence when excited with high-energy photons (Brown and O'Reilly 1991). In the first method, iothalamate or iohexol are separated from other plasmatic compounds by HPLC before detection (Isaka *et al.* 1992; Gaspari *et al.* 1995). HPLC is a time-consuming technique but is now used routinely in most biochemistry or pharmacological department in hospitals. In the second method, plasma samples are directly used for measurement, avoiding complex manipulations. However, this technique requires a specific and expensive device dedicated to the measure of contrast medium concentration.

Iothalamate concentrations can also be measured in urine by HPLC, hence, continuous infusion of iothalamate can be used to measure GFR by renal clearance technique (Prueksaritanont *et al.* 1986; Reidenberg *et al.* 1988; Agarwal 1998). Since low concentration of marker can be accurately measured in plasma and urine, single subcutaneous bolus of either ^{125}I-iothalamate or non-radiolabelled iothalamate have been used to measure renal clearance (Levey 1989; Levey *et al.* 1993). The marker is injected alone or together with epinephrine. After an equilibration period of at least 1 h, serum and urine samples are obtained. This method gives an acceptable estimation of the GFR.

Other markers of glomerular filtration rate

Most of the methods described above require sophisticated investigation and cannot be performed easily in outpatients. For many years, the physicians have been seeking for an endogenous marker, the plasma concentration of which would be related to the renal filtration levels and would be readily measured. For this purpose, three molecules have been used: urea, creatinine, and cystatin C.

Urea was the first marker of renal dysfunction, and renal failure is still referred to as uraemia. Urea is a small molecule (MW: 60 Da) produced from the metabolism of amino acid. Its daily production varies largely with protein intake and is also dependent on protein degradation in the intestine as this can be observed during gastrointestinal bleeding (Cottini *et al.* 1973; Maroni *et al.* 1985; Chalasani *et al.* 1997). It is freely filtered by the glomeruli, however, it is also easily reabsorbed by the tubules. The tubular reabsorption of urea depends on water reabsorption, hence plasma urea (also referred to as blood or serum urea nitrogen) and urea renal excretion can be modified by many parameters in addition to the decrease of GFR (Chasis and Smith 1938). When water reabsorption is increased in renal tubules, or when intravascular volume is depleted, urea reabsorption is augmented leading to high urea serum concentration. Adversely, liver diseases reduce urea plasma levels. For these reasons, plasma urea cannot be used for the assessment of the GFR (Rickers *et al.* 1978).

As described above, serum creatinine concentration is dependent on GFR and was employed by Rehberg (1926) as a marker of the rate of filtration in clinical medicine. The limits of measuring creatinine clearance to assess GFR have already been exposed. However, since serum creatinine concentration can be easily measured routinely, many authors have tried to find mathematical formulae taking into account the various causes of variation of serum creatinine to deduce the glomerular filtration level. Some of these formulae are reported in Table 1. Sex gender, age, body weight, race, and nutritional state are some of the parameters considered. In large populations, these methods show correlations with the gold standard, however, they can lead to inaccuracy in individuals. This can be partially due to the fact that the characteristics of the populations used to derive the formulae differ from those of some of the individuals or subpopulations studied. These formulae are not accurate enough to allow precise follow-up of renal impairment but they give a reasonable account of renal filtration and help the physician to select the patients who should undergo more sophisticated investigations.

Recently, in 1985, cystatin C has been proposed as an alternative endogenous marker of GFR (Grubb 1992). Cystatin C is an unglycosylated polypeptide member of the cysteine proteinase inhibitor superfamily, encoded by a housekeeping gene expressed in most nucleated cells (Brzin *et al.* 1984; Abrahamson *et al.* 1990; Saitoh *et al.* 1991). Its rate of production *in vivo* seems to be independent of body mass, age, sex, inflammation, and malignancy (Dworkin 2001). Cystatin (MW $\approx$ 13 kDa) is freely filtered at the glomerulus and reabsorbed and metabolized by proximal tubular cells. Urinary cystatin C concentrations are very low precluding the use of this marker to measure GFR by clearance techniques (Dworkin 2001). Serum cystatin C concentration have been studied in various clinical settings in adults, children, and the elderly. There are still some controversies regarding the utility of this marker compared to creatinine, but it does not represent a major step forward in the determination of GFR (Chantrel *et al.* 2000; Laterza *et al.* 2002). No mathematical formulae including serum cystatin C concentration have been developed so far in order to improve the predictive value of GFR by serum cystatin C.

Definition of normal values of glomerular filtration rate and normalization

Renal insufficiency is defined as the decrease in the GFR, consequently it is necessary to define normal range values from data obtained in healthy individuals of various ages. Only few studies, which are also old, have been devoted to this issue (Smith *et al.* 1943; Barnett *et al.* 1948; Smith 1951; Edelmann and Bernstein 1968; Wibell and Bjorsell-Ostling 1973; Rowe *et al.* 1976b). The physiologic variability of GFR is important in healthy individuals of different ages and sizes (Rowe *et al.* 1976c). To take these parameters into account and reduce interindividual variations, it was suggested to normalize GFR and RPF according to body surface area. Body surface area can be calculated by various formulae using power functions of height and weight. These formulae are inappropriate to calculate body surface area in infants, young children, and in the elderly. It has become conventional to correct GFR and RPF to a body surface area of 1.73 m^2. This indexing practice assumes that GFR and RPF increase as a linear function of body surface area. Hence, the indexed values should no longer vary as a function of body size. Obesity, the presence of oedema, and anorexia perturb this relationship leading to under- or overestimation of renal functional data. It has been proposed to substitute ideal weight for height. However, this notion requires more accurate validations. Some authors checked the validity of adjusting GFR and RBF to body surface area in healthy adults (Masarei 1975; Turner and Reilly 1995) and concluded that this method should be abandoned even in subjects with normal nutritional status and should be replaced by use of the

Table 1 Some of the formulae used to estimate GFR from serum creatinine concentration

Males	Females	Children	Units	Reference
$(100/\text{Pcr}) - 12$	$(80/\text{Pcr}) - 7$		GFR, ml/min/1.73 m^2; Pcr, mg/dl	Jelliffe (1971), Jelliffe and Jelliffe (1971)
$\frac{98 - [16 \times (\text{age} - 20)/20]}{\text{Pcr}}$	Male × 0.9		GFR, ml/min/1.73 m^2; Pcr, mg/dl	Jelliffe (1973)
		$\frac{0.43 \times \text{Ht (cm)}}{\text{Pcr}}$	ml/min/1.73 m^2; Pcr, mg/dl	Counahan *et al.* (1976)
		$\frac{38 \times \text{Ht (cm)}}{\text{Pcr}}$	ml/min/1.73 m^2; Pcr, mM	Counahan *et al.* (1976)
$\frac{(140 - \text{age}) \times \text{Wt}}{72 \times \text{Pcr}}$	Male × 0.85		ml/min; Pcr, mg/dl	Cockcroft and Gault (1976), Gault *et al.* (1992)
$\frac{1.2 \times (140 - \text{age}) \times \text{Wt}}{\text{Pcr}}$	Male × 0.85		ml/min; Pcr, mM	Cockcroft and Gault (1976), Gault *et al.* (1992)
$\frac{27 - (0.173 \times \text{age})}{\text{Pcr}}$	$\frac{25 - (0.175 \times \text{age})}{\text{Pcr}}$		ml/min; Pcr, mg/dl	Bjornsson *et al.* (1983)
$\frac{7.57}{\text{Pcr}} - (0.103 \times \text{age}) + (0.096 \times \text{Wt}) - 6.66$ Only when Pcr > 0.177 mM	$\frac{6.05}{\text{Pcr}} - (0.08 \times \text{age}) + (0.08 \times \text{Wt}) - 4.81$ Only when Pcr > 0.177 mM		ml/min/3 m^2 (of Ht^2); Pcr, mM	Walser *et al.* (1993)
$\frac{7.58}{\text{Pcr}} - 4.29$ Only when Pcr > 0.177 mM	$\frac{6.11}{\text{Pcr}} - 3.8$ Only when Pcr > 0.177 mM		ml/min/3 m^2 (of Ht^2); Pcr, mM	Walser *et al.* (1993)
$\frac{86}{\text{Pcr}} - 4.29$ Only when Pcr > 2 mg/dl	$\frac{6.11}{\text{Pcr}} - 3.8$ Only when Pcr > 2 mg/dl		ml/min/3 m^2 (of Ht^2); Pcr, mg/dl	Walser *et al.* (1993)
$170 \times (\text{Pcr})^{-0.999} \times (\text{age})^{-0.176} \times (\text{SUN})^{-0.17} \times (\text{Alb})^{0.318} \times 1.18$ if Black	$170 \times (\text{Pcr})^{-0.999} \times (\text{age})^{-0.176} \times (\text{SUN})^{-0.17} \times (\text{Alb})^{0.318} \times 0.762$		ml/min/1.73 m^2; Pcr, mg/dl	Levey *et al.* (1999)
$186 \times (\text{Pcr})^{-1.154} \times (\text{age})^{-0.203} \times 1.212$ if Black	$186 \times (\text{Pcr})^{-1.154} \times (\text{age})^{-0.203} \times 0.742$		ml/min/1.73 m^2; Pcr, mg/dl	Levey *et al.* (2000)
$198 \times (\text{Pcr})^{-0.858} \times (\text{age})^{-0.167} \times (\text{SUN})^{-0.293} \times (\text{UUN})^{0.249} \times 1.178$ if Black	$198 \times (\text{Pcr})^{-0.858} \times (\text{age})^{-0.167} \times (\text{SUN})^{-0.293} \times (\text{UUN})^{0.249} \times 0.822$		ml/min/1.73 m^2; Pcr, mg/dl	Levey *et al.* (1999)

Pcr, serum creatinine; Ht, height; Wt, body weight (kg); SUN, serum urea nitrogen (mg/dl); Alb, serum albumin (g/dl); UUN, urine urea nitrogen (g/day).

An evaluation of the predictive performance of these equations can be found in Manjunath *et al.* (2001) and Bostom *et al.* (2002).

regression method. In practice, the clinician should always consider both non-normalized and normalized values.

Other methods of normalization have been proposed, for example, the regression method (Turner and Reilly 1995), the extracellular fluid volume (White and Strydom 1991; Peters *et al.* 1994, 1995), or the height only method. However, these methods require further validations.

Choice of a method for assessing glomerular filtration rate in practice

The various methods described above to estimate the GFR differ in their accuracy, convenience for the patient, technical difficulty (which can depend on the access to hospital facilities), and cost. The choice of a method will depend on the information requested by the physician. When the clinician wishes only to check whether GFR of a patient is in the normal range, the measurement of serum creatinine concentration and the use of one of the formulae reported in Table 1 is useful. If the GFR values are found in the lower normal value its estimation can be improved by measuring the creatinine clearance over short periods of time (Herget-Rosenthal *et al.* 1999). These methods are safe, reliable, easy to perform, and sufficiently inexpensive to allow screening of large populations of patients.

When a decrease in the GFR is likely, a precise measurement is important to detect further alteration at an early stage and manage the therapy (Levey 1989, 1990; Bostom *et al.* 2002). This is also the case in clinical trials, since the accuracy of GFR measurement determines the number of patients to be included and the decrease of the GFR with time may be an end point of the study (Levey *et al.* 1993). Renal or plasma clearance technique should be used in these conditions (Bostom *et al.* 2002); the choice of one of these methods being usually determined by the access to laboratory facilities. To date, there is no available study comparing the rate of decline of GFR assessed with different methods.

Measurement of tubular functions

The main role of glomeruli is to permit plasma filtration, a function that can be assessed by the measurement of the filtration rate. The tubule functions are more complex and differ along the nephron. Tubule functions cannot be studied as a whole, but must be divided into different parts. Some functions take place in one specific tubular segment but others involve different regions of the nephron. Most of the investigations of the tubule functions are accompanied by an accurate measurement of the GFR.

Investigating proximal tubule functions

The first postglomerular segment of the nephron is the proximal tubule. This segment reabsorbs about 60 per cent of the water filtered at the glomerulus and the solutes in an inhomogeneous manner. Some functions are specific of the proximal tubule; their alterations indicate proximal tubule dysfunction.

Glucose reabsorption

Glucose is completely and specifically recovered from the primitive urine in this segment. Glucose reabsorption through the epithelium requires two steps. Under physiological conditions, the limiting step is located at the apical pole of the proximal cells where two sodium-dependent glucose transporters are expressed, namely SGLT2 and SGLT1 (Hediger and Rhoads 1994; Wright 2001). SGLT2 is exclusively expressed in the kidney; SGLT1 is also present in the intestine. SGLT2 is a low-affinity high-capacity glucose transporter and is expressed in the first two-thirds of the proximal tubule (convoluted part). SGLT1 is a high-affinity low-capacity transporter present in the pars recta of the proximal tubule. Glucose exits from the proximal tubular cells via two facilitative carriers: GLUT2 (pars convoluta) and GLUT1 (pars recta) (Hediger and Rhoads 1994) (Fig. 3). Renal glucose reabsorption is a saturation process, which means that glucose reabsorption in the proximal tubule is complete and consequently urine glucose concentration is nil, provided that the amount of glucose delivered to the proximal tubule is maintained below the maximal capacity of tubule to transport glucose (Smith *et al.* 1943; Deetjen *et al.* 1992). The presence of glucose in urine can be due to the increase in the filtered load of glucose, secondary to an increase in plasma glucose concentration, or to a decrease in the ability of proximal tubule to transport glucose. The maximal capacity of proximal tubule to reabsorb glucose (Tm_{Glu}) can be measured in clinical practice (McPhaul and Simonaitis 1968; Pontoglio *et al.* 2000). Plasma glucose concentration is progressively increased by a priming dose of glucose followed by a continuous venous perfusion of glucose. Time-controlled urine collections are recovered every 15 or 30 min and venous plasma glucose concentrations are measured at the beginning and the end of each period. In parallel, GFR is measured using a renal or a plasma clearance technique permitting the construction of a titration curve as initially described by Smith (1943) and Smith *et al.* (1943). The quantity of glucose reabsorbed by the proximal tubule (T_{Glu}) is given by the difference between the filtered load of glucose minus the rate of urinary glucose excretion that can be mathematically expressed as:

$$T_{Glu} = (GFR \times P_{Glu}) - (U_{Glu} \times \dot{V})$$

where GFR is the glomerular filtration rate, P_{Glu} the plasma concentration of glucose, U_{Glu} the urinary concentration of glucose, and $\dot{V}$ the urine flow rate.

As long as the filtered load of glucose is below the Tm_{Glu}, glycosuria equals zero and T_{Glu} equals the filtered load of glucose. When P_{Glu} increases T_{Glu} reaches a maximal value, Tm_{Glu}, leading to significant urinary excretion of glucose with a linear relationship with P_{Glu} (see Fig. 4). The transition from complete glucose reabsorption to

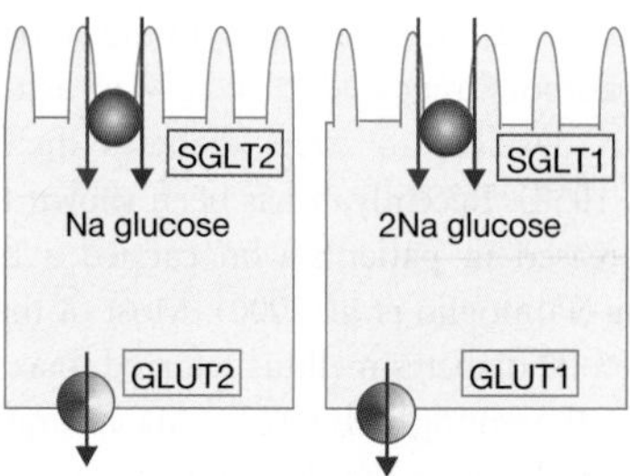

Fig. 3 Schematic representation of transepithelial glucose reabsorption in the renal proximal tubule. Left: early proximal tubule segment S1 (pars convoluta). Right: late proximal tubule segment S3 (pars recta). Glucose enters at the apical side via a sodium-dependent cotransporter (SGLT1 or SGLT2) and exits the basolateral side via a facilitated carrier (GLUT1 or GLUT2).

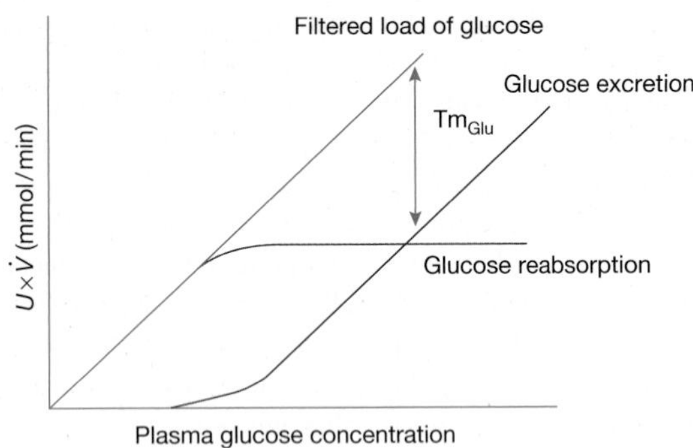

Fig. 4 Curves of renal filtration, urinary excretion, and renal reabsorption of glucose as a function of plasma glucose concentration.

Table 2 Normal values of the Tm glucose and Tm glucose/GFR (mean ± SD)

Tm mmol/min/1.73 m^2	Tm/GFR mmol/l/1.73 m^2	Reference
1.80 ± 0.2	13 ± 1.15	McPhaul and Simonaitis (1968)
1.84 ± 0.2		De Marchi *et al.* (1993)
1.37 ± 0.2	12.4 ± 0.98	Pontoglio *et al.* (2000)

significant excretion of glucose in urine is curvilinear; this phenomenon is referred to by the term splay and may be due to nephron heterogeneity. This includes the heterogeneity between nephrons and within the proximal tubule because of the presence of several glucose transporters with different affinities for glucose. The threshold of glucose reabsorption refers to the plasma concentration of glucose above which glycosuria appears. It is often difficult to determine the real threshold for glucose in humans, however, when the rate of urinary glucose excretion is plotted against glycaemia, the plasma concentration of glucose above which the transport of glucose is maximum, is obtained at the intercept of the regression straight line with the X-axis (Fig. 4) allowing comparison between subjects. This value is referred to as the renal threshold glucose concentration.

Since Tm_{Glu} can be modified by GFR, it is normalized for this parameter (Tm_{Glu}/GFR). This ratio is expressed as a concentration and is equivalent to the renal threshold glucose concentration defined above. Tm_{Glu} is also sensitive to extracellular volume expansion; extracellular volume should be stable during the determination of Tm_{Glu}. Renal glucosuria can be due to a decrease of Tm_{Glu} or to an increase in the splay of the glucose reabsorption curve (McPhaul and Simonaitis 1968). The first pattern was referred to as type A and the second one as type B. Type A renal glucosuria has been described in patients with reduced expression of SGLT2 (Pontoglio *et al.* 2000) and type B is observed in patients with glucose–galactose malabsorption who lack SGLT1. However, the molecular basis of renal glucosuria have been established only in a few cases. Defects in GLUT1 function have been reported (OMIM 138140) but the consequences on Tm_{Glu} are unknown.

Renal glucosuria has been thought to be a benign condition although some authors reported that it was associated with an increased risk to develop an overt diabetes mellitus with time (Ackerman *et al.* 1958). Recently, it has been shown that Tm_{Glu}/GFR dramatically decreased in patients who carried a mutation in the HNF1 alpha gene (Pontoglio *et al.* 2000). Most of these patients will develop a non-ketotic diabetes mellitus referred to as type 3 maturity onset diabetes of the young (MODY3). An accurate measurement of Tm_{Glu}/GFR may facilitate the detection of these patients among subjects with isolated glucosuria or with diabetes mellitus and abnormally high glucose excretion in urine. The determination of Tm_{Glu}/GFR is suitable whenever a renal glucosuria is suspected, in order to confirm the diagnostic and measure the importance of the defect. Other proximal tubule functions should be assessed to determine whether this trouble is isolated or is a part of larger tubular defects.

Normal values of Tm_{Glu} and Tm_{Glu}/GFR have been published by several authors and are summed up in Table 2.

Renal handling of phosphate

Phosphate is almost exclusively reabsorbed in the proximal tubule. The limiting step to phosphate reabsorption is located in the proximal tubule. The mechanisms and regulation of renal phosphate reabsorption are described in Chapter 2.4. Briefly, phosphate is taken back from the initial urine through the type 2a sodium-dependent phosphate transporter (NPT2a). The mechanism whereby phosphate exits the proximal tubular cells at the basolateral membrane is unknown. Contrary to glucose, renal reabsorption of phosphate is hormonally regulated. Parathyroid hormone decreases NPT2a expression at the apical membrane of proximal tubular cells and increases urinary excretion of phosphate. Under physiological conditions in adult, phosphate is excreted in urine; its fractional excretion is about 20 per cent. As described for glucose, during phosphate infusion the excretion rate of phosphate varies linearly with plasma phosphate concentration above a given concentration. The difference between the filtered load and the excretion rate is constant and represents the maximum reabsorption rate of phosphate (Tm_{Pi}) (Bijvoet 1969; Bijvoet *et al.* 1969). Because phosphate infusion procedures cannot be easily performed in routine, Walton and Bijvoet (1975) developed a nomogram that permits calculation of Tm_{Pi}/GFR from plasma and urine concentrations of phosphate and creatinine (or polyfructosan). Kenny and Glen (1973) derived an equation from these data, see Table 3. The calculation of Tm_{Pi}/GFR with these methods requires that blood and urine samples be collected from overnight fasting patients. The methods described above can be used in infants and children to calculate Tm_{Pi}/GFR (Thalassinos *et al.* 1970; Brodehl *et al.* 1988). Tm_{Pi}/GFR value is the main determinant of plasma phosphate levels. This parameter is essential in the investigation of patients with hypophosphataemia. It must always be accompanied by the measurement of plasma parathyroid hormone (PTH) concentration. Normal range values according to age and gender are presented in Table 4. A low Tm_{Pi}/GFR with normal plasma PTH values and hypophosphataemia is observed in various familial hypophosphataemic rickets, in Fanconi syndrome, in oncogenic hypophosphataemic osteomalacia in some patients with urolithiasis or bone demineralization (Prié *et al.* 1998, 2001) and in patients with mutations in the NPT2a gene (Prié *et al.* 2002). The aetiologies and the

Table 3 Calculation of Tm_{Pi}/GFR (Kenny and Glen 1973; Payne 1998)

Validity assumption	Equation
TRP > 0.86	$Tm_{Pi}/GFR = TRP \times Pi$
TRP ≤ 0.86	$Tm_{Pi}/GFR = \frac{0.30 \times TRP}{1 - (0.8 \times TRP)} \times Pi_p$ mmol/l

TRP, fractional tubular reabsorption of phosphate; Pi_P, plasma phosphate concentration; TRP, 1 − FE, where FE is the fractional excretion of phosphate.

FE is calculated as follows: $FE = (U/P)_{phosphate}/(U/P)_{creatinine\ or\ inulin}$, where U and P stand for urinary and plasma concentrations, respectively.

Table 4 Normal ranges for Tm_{Pi}/GFR

	Range (mmol/l)	Reference
Children		
Birth to 3 months	1.43–3.43	Bistarakis *et al.* (1986)
6 months to 18 years	1.15–2.60	Bistarakis *et al.* (1986), Kruse *et al.* (1982), Shaw *et al.* (1990)
Adults		
Male: 25–75 years	0.8–1.35	Minisola *et al.* (1993)
Female: 25–75 years	0.80–1.44	Minisola *et al.* (1993)

physiopathology of hypophosphataemia are described by Silve and Friedlander in Chapter 2.4.

Amino acids reabsorption

Ninety-five per cent of filtered amino acids are reabsorbed by the proximal tubule through various carriers and a Tm can be defined for each amino acid. However, in clinical practice only the fractional excretion of amino acids and the amino acid to creatinine ratio in urine are used for the diagnosis of aminoacidurias. The transport defect may affect one or several categories of amino acids. The causes of aminoaciduria are developed in Chapters 5.1 and 5.3.

Uric acid transport

Urate transport takes place in the proximal tubule; however, it is a more complex process than the transport of glucose or phosphate described above. Urate is both reabsorbed and secreted in the proximal tubule (Maesaka and Fishbane 1998; Roch-Ramel and Guisan 1999) resulting in a fractional excretion (clearance of urate/GFR) ranging between 9 and 15 per cent. A reduction in the tubular reabsorption of urate occurs in Fanconi syndrome or as an isolated defect and is responsible for hypouricaemia. In these cases, the diagnostic of renal hypouricaemia is based on the measurement of the fractional excretion of urate that largely exceeds the normal upper value of 15 per cent (Munoz Sanz *et al.* 1983). Hypouricaemia can also be due to volume expansion, to a decrease in urate production or an increase in urate secretion in proximal tubule. In some patients, it has been described that a diminution in the fractional excretion of urate below 8 per cent, due to a decrease in urate secretion, induces hyperuricaemia (Calabrese *et al.* 1990; Moro *et al.* 1991; McBride *et al.* 1997, 1998). Various drugs interfere with the transport of urate in the proximal tubule and have been used to characterize the defects observed in patients (Garcia Puig *et al.* 1983). Hence, pyrazinamide is considered as an inhibitor of urate secretion or a stimulator of urate reabsorption, and probenecid, benzbromarone, and tienilic acid stimulate urate secretion (Colussi *et al.* 1987; Diamond 1989).

Sodium reabsorption—the lithium clearance

Sodium reabsorption occurs along the entire nephron by various mechanisms. In the proximal tubule, 60 per cent of the filtered sodium is recovered from the initial urine by active transcellular movements and passive paracellular pathway. In the first mechanism, sodium enters the apical pole of proximal cells coupled to organic (glucose, aminoacids, etc.) or inorganic (phosphate) solutes via specific sodium-dependent carriers or is exchanged with H^+ ion. In all tubule segments, sodium is actively pumped out of the cells via the basolateral Na^+,K^+-ATPase. The passive paracellular sodium flux is due to osmotic water flow from lumen to blood that entrains sodium through the lateral intercellular space (Moe *et al.* 2000). The thick ascending limb reabsorbs about 30 per cent of the sodium filtered at the glomerulus. Sodium is transported across the apical membranes via the $Na^+/K^+/2Cl^-$ cotransporter and the Na/H^+ exchanger. The K^+ recycling at the apical membrane generates a lumen positive transepithelial voltage driving additional paracellular sodium reabsorption. Furosemide and bumetanide inhibit the $Na^+/K^+/2Cl^-$ transporter and sodium absorption in the thick ascending limb. The distal convoluted tubule reabsorbs about 10 per cent of the filtered sodium load via the apical thiazide-sensitive sodium chloride transporter (Moe *et al.* 2000). This transporter is also expressed in the apical membrane of the collecting duct principal cells together with the amiloride sensitive sodium channel (ENaC) (Kim *et al.* 1998). In this segment, sodium reabsorption is regulated by the mineralocorticoid hormone aldosterone and coupled to K^+ secretion.

A global measurement of sodium absorption by the tubules is obtained by measuring the fractional excretion of sodium (FE_{Na}) which is expressed as the ratio of the sodium excretion rate to the sodium filtered load:

$$FE_{Na} = \frac{U_{Na} \times \dot{V}}{P_{Na} \times GFR},$$

where U_{Na} is the urinary concentration of sodium, $\dot{V}$ the urine flow rate, P_{Na} the plasma concentration of sodium, and GFR the glomerular filtration rate.

Since

$$GFR = \frac{U_{creat} \times \dot{V}}{P_{creatinine}} \quad \text{or} \quad \frac{U_{inulin} \times \dot{V}}{P_{inulin}},$$

$$FE_{Na} = \frac{(U/P)_{Na}}{(U/P)_{creatinine}} \quad \text{or} \quad \frac{(U/P)_{Na}}{(U/P)_{inulin}}.$$

In various clinical conditions, physicians are interested in knowing what proportion of sodium is being reabsorbed in the proximal and distal parts of the nephron. The measurement of sodium absorption in the proximal tubule is based on the assumption that lithium is absorbed to the same extent as sodium in this segment but is not handled in the distal parts of the nephron (Thomsen 1990).

If these criteria are fulfilled, since sodium and water reabsorption are iso-osmotic in the proximal tubule, the lithium clearance measures the rate of fluid delivery to the distal segments. The lithium clearance is expressed as follows:

$$C_{Li} = \frac{U_{Li} \times \dot{V}}{P_{Li}}.$$

—The reabsorption of sodium in the proximal tubule equals the quantity of sodium filtered at the glomerulus × minus the quantity delivered to the distal parts of the nephron: (GFR − C_{Li}) × P_{Na}.
—The reabsorption of water in the proximal tubule is GFR − C_{Li}.
—The reabsorption of water beyond the proximal tubule is $C_{Li} - \dot{V}$.
—The reabsorption of sodium beyond the proximal tubule is $(C_{Li} - C_{Na}) \times P_{Na}$.

The physicochemical characteristics of lithium resemble those of sodium, however, it does not imply that lithium can substitute for sodium on proximal tubule carriers. The affinity of the Na/H^+ exchanger is higher for lithium than for sodium (Greger 1990). Amiloride-sensitive sodium channel and $Na^+/K^+/Cl^-$ transporter are able to transport lithium with an affinity lower than that for sodium. Furthermore, lithium may be reabsorbed paracellularly in the thick ascending limb (Greger 1990). On the contrary, sodium–glucose and sodium–amino acid transporters and Na^+,K^+-ATPase are specific for sodium under physiological conditions. For these reasons, lithium is rather a marker of sodium absorption via the paracellular pathway in the proximal tubule and lithium clearance may be a valid marker of proximal sodium reabsorption only in sodium- and water-repleted patients, in the absence of osmotic diuresis (Atherton *et al.* 1990; Greger 1990; Thomsen 1990).

The calculation of lithium clearance requires the measurement of lithium concentration in plasma and urine. These concentrations are very low and require a load of lithium to achieve detectable values when lithium is measured by flame photometry. Twelve hours before the investigation, 250 or 500 mg of lithium carbonate is given orally (Colussi *et al.* 1990).

Plasma lithium concentration increases but remains within the non-toxic range and then decreases slowly. An alternative reliable but expensive method uses atomic absorption spectrophotometry. This method is very sensitive and avoids the necessity of lithium load (Durr *et al.* 1990).

Concentrating and diluting urine

The kidney plays a central role in water homeostasis by its ability to concentrate or dilute urine according to water intake and extrarenal losses (Valtin and Schafer 1995). Water is absorbed in the proximal tubule, the thin descending limb, and the collecting tubule. In the proximal tubule water movement from lumen to blood is iso-osmotic and driven by active solute transports: solutes accumulate at the external side of basolateral cell membranes, generating a transepithelial osmotic pressure difference that drives water flow. Consequently, when an osmotically active solute is present in the tubular fluid and cannot be reabsorbed, water reabsorption in the proximal tubule is decreased leading to an osmotic diuresis. In the proximal tubule transepithelial water transport uses two routes: transcellular and paracellular. Water crosses proximal cell membranes through the type 1 aquaporin, which is constitutively expressed at the apical and basolateral sides of the cells. The relative importance of these two pathways depends on species. In knock-out mice for aquaporin 1 gene, the proximal tubule permeability is decreased, activating the tubuloglomerular feedback responsible for the diminution in the GFR indicating that the transcellular pathway is predominant in this species (Schnermann *et al.* 1998). On the contrary, humans with complete deficiency of aquaporin 1 exhibit a very mild phenotype (King *et al.* 2001) suggesting that the paracellular route is preponderant.

In the thick ascending limb and the distal convoluted tubule no net water reabsorption occurs; only solutes are retrieved from the urine. The loop of Henle creates the countercurrent multiplication process and the corticomedullary osmotic gradient (Morello and Bichet 2001). In the distal convoluted tubule, the lumen osmolality decreases to 60 mOsm/kg H_2O. The collecting duct has extremely low water permeability in the absence of the antidiuretic hormone vasopressin. Under this condition, no water transport is observed along the collecting duct and the final urine is maximally diluted. In the presence of vasopressin, transepithelial movements of water occur across the principal cells. Three types of aquaporins are involved in water transport in the principal cells. Aquaporin 3 and 4 expressions are restricted to the basolateral plasma membrane and are not regulated by vasopressin. They provide the pathways that permit water to enter the interstitium. Aquaporin 2 is expressed at the apical plasma membrane exclusively in the presence of vasopressin, thus increasing the water permeability. The transepithelial difference in osmolality drives water from the lumen to the interstitium. When the level of vasopressin in plasma is high enough, water reabsorption occurs along the entire collecting duct and the final urine is maximally concentrated (Nielsen *et al.* 2002).

Testing the concentrating ability

The concentrating ability of the kidney depends not only on the action of vasopressin but also on the presence of the osmotic corticomedullary gradient. This gradient is altered at the early stage of renal insufficiency, and is profoundly reduced in particular in pathology with medullary damages such as polycystic kidneys, sickle cell disease, reflux nephropathy, tubular necrosis, or transplanted kidneys. The assessment of the concentrating capacity of the kidney is based on the measurement of the urine osmolality. Plasma osmolality must be measured simultaneously for a better interpretation of the results. Urine and plasma osmolalities are measured by the depression of the freezing point. The study of the maximal capacity of kidney to concentrate urine is important whenever a diabetes insipidus is suspected. This defect can be of genetic origin or can be acquired. It can be located in the kidney (nephrogenic diabetes insipidus) or due to the lack of vasopressin secretion. The causes of diabetes insipidus are presented in Table 5. The maximal concentrating capacity of the kidney is determined by a fluid restriction test (Davis and Zenser 1993). The patient has to stop all fluid and food intake from 6:00 p.m., the day prior to the investigation. The next morning, plasma and urine osmolalities are measured. In normal subjects, plasma osmolality ranges between 280 and 295 mOsm/kg H_2O and urine osmolality is above 600 mOsm/kg H_2O. The maximal urine concentration, that usually exceeds 1000 mOsm/kg H_2O, is achieved after water deprivation from 18 to 24 h (Miles *et al.* 1954; Isaacson 1960; Rowe *et al.* 1976a). The maximum concentrating ability is lower in infants and elderly people (Edelmann *et al.* 1967; Rowe *et al.* 1976a; Monnens *et al.* 1981; Aperia *et al.* 1983; Davis and Davis 1987). During the investigation, the urinary flow falls below 0.4 ml/min, blood pressure and urine osmolality are controlled every hour and plasma osmolality every 2 h. The test is usually stopped when urine osmolality

Table 5 Principal causes of diabetes insipidus

1. Nephrogenic diabetes insipidus = resistance to vasopressin
Acquired
Hypercalcaemia
Hypokalaemia
Drugs: Lithium, Amphotericin B, Diphenylhydantoin, Methoxyflurane
Toxic: Alcohol
Sickle-cell disease
Sarcoidosis
Sjögren syndrome
Post obstructive nephropathy
Hereditary
Mutation of the type 2 vasopressin receptor (X-linked transmission)
Mutation of the aquaporin 2 (autosomal transmission)
2. Central diabetes insipidus = defect of AVP secretion
Acquired: Trauma, tumor, infection, granuloma, autoimmune disease
Congenital: Mutation in vasopressin gene, dysplasia

exceeds 800 mOsm/kg H_2O, which excludes major defects in the urine concentrating process, or when plasma osmolality is above the upper normal values (296 mOsm/kg H_2O). In this case, the intravenous or subcutaneous injection of 4 μg of the vasopressin analogue, dDAVP (1-desamino-8-D-arginine vasopressin) permits the distinction between nephrogenic diabetes insipidus and central deficiency of vasopressin secretion. In central diabetes insipidus, dDAVP increases urine osmolality above 750 mOsm/kg H_2O within the first 2 h following the injection (Rado *et al.* 1976; Curtis and Donovan 1979; Moses *et al.* 1985; Williams *et al.* 1986). In nephrogenic diabetes insipidus, dDAVP injection does not increase urine osmolality further. A blood sample is usually drawn before dDAVP injection to allow plasma vasopressin concentration measurement in case of central deficiency. This test can be used in infants and children (Edelmann *et al.* 1967; Monnens *et al.* 1981). In compulsive water drinkers, urine osmolality rises above 600 mOsm/kg H_2O. Surreptitious water ingestions induce a fall in urine osmolality between two successive collections accompanied by an increase in urinary flow rate.

Testing the diluting capacity

The diluting capacity of the kidney can also be tested. This investigation is useful in patients who present unexplained hyponatraemia. The lowest urinary osmolality is obtained when vasopressin secretion is completely suppressed. The diuretics, by decreasing sodium reabsorption especially in the distal convoluted tubule (thiazide), impair the diluting capacity. The diluting capacity requires normal solute intake. At the beginning of the investigation, plasma and urinary osmolality are measured, then the patients drink a water load of 20 ml/kg body weight in 20 min (Derubertis *et al.* 1971; Davis and Zenser 1993). In normal subjects, the plasma osmolality remains within the normal range after the water load and urine osmolality rapidly decreases below 100 mOsm/kg H_2O within 2 h and 80 per cent of the ingested water are excreted within 4 h. An alteration of the diluting capacity can be due to an incomplete inhibition of vasopressin secretion, or to adrenal insufficiency, hypothyroidism, potassium depletion, or liver disease.

Osmolar clearance and free-water clearance

The quantitative ability of the kidney to excrete or retain water can be estimated by the calculation of osmolar and free-water clearance. Conceptually, the rate of water excreted in urine can be divided into two components. One contains all the urinary solutes and the amount of water required to obtain a solution iso-osmotic to plasma. This defines the osmolar clearance:

$$C_{osm} = \frac{U_{osm}}{P_{osm}} \times \dot{V}.$$

The other component is made of solute-free water and is called free-water clearance (C_{H_2O}). This theoretical flow is positive when urine is hypotonic to plasma (water has been 'added in excess' to osmoles in urine) and negative when final urine is hypertonic to plasma (water has been 'substracted in excess' to osmoles to concentrate urine).

The rate of water excreted is the sum of these two components:

$$\dot{V} = C_{H_2O} + C_{osm}.$$

$$C_{H_2O} = \dot{V} - C_{osm}$$

$$C_{H_2O} = \dot{V}\left(1 - \frac{U_{osm}}{P_{osm}}\right)$$

The amount of water reabsorbed per unit of time is noted $T_{C_{H_2O}}$, and equals $-C_{H_2O}$. The contribution of urea to water excretion and the use of urea concentration to calculate osmolality are detailed in Soroka *et al.* (1997).

Investigation of hydrogen ion excretion

Hydrogen ions are continuously produced by metabolism and immediately buffered to maintain constant pH. The role of the kidney in the acid–base homeostasis is to reclaim the filtered load of HCO_3^- and regenerate the HCO_3^- decomposed by the H^+ buffering, to secrete H^+ in tubular fluid and to produce buffers to eliminate H^+. All these processes take place in different parts of the nephron.

Bicarbonate reabsorption

Most of the HCO_3^- filtered at the glomerulus are reclaimed in the proximal tubule. This reabsorption is mediated by the type 3 neutral Na^+/H^+ exchanger (NHE3) located at the apical plasma membrane. Sodium enters the cells along its electrochemical gradient and is exchanged with an H^+ that is secreted in the tubular fluid. A proton is also secreted via an apical H^+-ATPase. Hydrogen ions react in the tubular fluid with HCO_3^- to produce H_2CO_3 that is rapidly dehydrated by the type 4 luminal carbonic anhydrase to form H_2O and CO_2, which freely diffuse into the cell. The type 2 cytoplasmic carbonic anhydrase catalyzes the formation of H_2CO_3 from CO_2 and H_2O. H_2CO_3 dissociates to H^+ and HCO_3^-. HCO_3^- exits the cells across the basolateral plasma membrane via an electrogenic $Na^+/3HCO_3^-$ symporter or a Cl^-/HCO_3^- exchanger. Sodium leaves the cell via the Na^+,K^+-ATPase. When the filtered load of HCO_3^- increases, its reabsorption by the proximal tubule reaches a plateau and HCO_3^- appears in urine in parallel. By progressively increasing the plasma bicarbonate concentration, the threshold and the Tm for bicarbonate reabsorption can be measured using a procedure similar to that described for glucose. Patients are infused with sodium bicarbonate 4.2 per cent (3 ml/min), arterial and venous blood samples and urine recovered under oil are collected every 30 min; pH, HCO_3^-, and P_{CO_2} are measured. Type 2 renal tubular acidosis is characterized by a decrease in the ability of the proximal tubule to reabsorb HCO_3^-. In this condition, bicarbonate plasma concentration diminishes until it reaches the renal threshold; bicarbonaturia is absent under basal condition and the urinary pH is normally low. The kidney can still challenge an acid load since proton secretion is maintained but with low plasma bicarbonate concentration. When the bicarbonate plasma concentration exceeds the threshold, urine becomes alkaline. In normal adults, bicarbonates are detected in urine only when the bicarbonate plasma concentration is above 20 mM; these values are higher in infants (Soriano *et al.* 1967). Proximal tubular acidosis can occur as part of the Fanconi syndrome, as an isolated defect, or can be associated with specific tubular deficiencies. The causes of this defect are detailed in Chapters 5.1 and 5.4.

An average of 50–80 meq of protons are produced every day by an adult as a result of protein catabolism and must be excreted in urine. The pH of urine cannot be lower than 4.5, which corresponds to $10^{-4.5}$ meq/l of free H^+ ions. The great majority of protons are buffered before being excreted in urine. Under basal conditions 30 per cent of H^+ are linked to phosphate ions, which represents the titratable acid and 70 per cent to ammonium ions (NH_4^+). The renal net acid excretion equals NH_4^+ + titratable acid − HCO_3^- in urine.

Ammonia (NH_3) is generated by the proximal tubule mostly from glutamine and is converted to NH_4^+ in the cell or in the lumen. Production of NH_3 is stimulated by acidosis and by chronic K^+ depletion. The measurement of NH_4^+ excretion in urine is valuable in patients with acidosis of unclear mechanism. Because the technique is not available in all hospitals, some authors have suggested that NH_4^+ concentration in urine can be assessed by calculating the urinary anion gap as follows: $Cl^- - (Na^+ + K^+)$ provided that the anion gap in plasma is normal (hyperchloraemic metabolic acidosis) (Batlle *et al.* 1988).

A default of NH_4^+ production participates in the genesis of acidosis in chronic renal failure and in chronic hyperkalaemia due to mineralocorticoid deficiency, for instance. The urinary pH is acid, but the net acid excretion is diminished. Similarly, in hyperkalaemic distal renal tubular acidosis the capacity of the distal tubule to secrete H^+ and K^+ is impaired and typically the urine pH is greater than 5.5; however, this sign can be absent until serum concentration of K^+ is decreased close to normal values.

H^+ secretion by the distal tubule

The thick ascending limb, the convoluted distal tubule and the collecting duct secrete H^+ in lumen via Na^+/H^+ exchangers, H^+ and H^+,K^+-ATPases by mechanisms similar to those described for the proximal tubule. These processes permit the reabsorbtion of the remainder of the filtered bicarbonate and the excretion of the protons generated by metabolism. In the collecting duct, H^+ ions are secreted by the alpha intercalated cells, which intensely express carbonic anhydrase. The ability of distal tubules to secrete proton can be estimated by comparing the plasma and urine $P\text{CO}_2$ (U-B $P\text{CO}_2$) during bicarbonate loading. When the filtered load of bicarbonate overwhelms the capacity of proximal tubule reabsorption, the amount of bicarbonate delivered to the distal tubule increases and then it combines with proton leading to the formation of carbonic acid that slowly dehydrates in CO_2 in the collecting duct and cannot diffuse into the blood. The higher the distal proton secretion the higher the $P\text{CO}_2$ in the urine. The bicarbonate load is delivered orally or intravenously; urine samples are recovered every 30 min under oil, and blood samples are obtained simultaneously. The urine pH must exceed the blood pH whilst making the measurement. The threshold for appearance of bicarbonate in the urine can be measured in parallel. In distal (type 1) renal tubular acidosis, the urinary $P\text{CO}_2$ tension does not significantly exceed blood values (Halperin *et al.* 1974) and the Tm for bicarbonate is normal. During chronic renal failure, bicarbonate infusion fails to raise the urinary $P\text{CO}_2$ above the arterial $P\text{CO}_2$ (Fillastre *et al.* 1968a,b, 1969).

Assessment of renal potassium excretion

Potassium reabsorption in the proximal tubule occurs through the paracellular pathway and follows that of sodium. No significant regulation of potassium transport has been described in this segment, but osmotic diuresis and bicarbonaturia decrease proximal reabsorption of K^+.

In the thick ascending limb, K^+ is actively reabsorbed by the $Na^+/K^+/2Cl^-$ cotransporter, but is partially recycled in the lumen and generates a positive transepithelial voltage. The site of regulation of K^+ excretion is the collecting duct, which is sensitive to dietary K^+ intake. Three cell types contribute to K^+ homeostasis in this segment: the principal cells and the intercalated cells alpha and beta. The principal cells, the most numerous (70 per cent) in the collecting duct, are responsible for K^+ secretion. Potassium is actively transported across the basolateral membrane via the Na^+,K^+-ATPase and exits the cell at its apical domain via specific channels. Potassium secretion is coupled to Na^+ reabsorption. Sodium enters the cell at the apical membrane through the epithelial amiloride sensitive channel (ENaC) and exits the cell via the Na^+,K^+-ATPase. Sodium reabsorption induces a lumen negative voltage, which facilitates the K^+ exit. Mineralocorticoids increase Na^+ reabsorption (by increasing the opening probability and the number of ENaC units) and stimulate K^+ secretion.

In contrast to the principal cells, the intercalated cells (alpha and beta) reabsorb luminal K^+ and secrete H^+ via an apical H^+/K^+-ATPase.

Since the kidney plays a major role in K^+ homeostasis, the rate of K^+ excretion in urine should be examined in patients with dyskalaemia: when the renal handling of K^+ is normal, its fractional excretion is low in hypokalaemia and high in hyperkalaemia. If the excretion rate of K^+ is abnormal, the transfer of K^+ in the collecting duct can be estimated by calculating the transtubular K^+ gradient (TTKG) defined as:

$$\text{TTKG} = \frac{(U/P)_K}{(U/P)_{\text{osm}}},$$

where U and P represent the urine and plasma concentrations, respectively, of K^+ or osmoles.

TTKG estimates the ratio of K^+ concentration between urine and plasma in the collecting duct and is based upon numerous assumptions. In the presence of vasopressin, osmolality of the fluid in the end of cortical collecting duct equals that of plasma. Consequently, K^+ concentration in the collecting duct can be assessed by correcting K^+ urinary concentration by water reabsorption in this segment, which is measured by the ratio of osmolality between urine and plasma (West *et al.* 1986). The use of this index is restricted to situations where the urine is not hypotonic and distal nephron sodium delivery is not limiting for potassium secretion (>25 mM). In hypo- and hyperkalaemia due to non-renal causes, TTKG is lower than 2 and higher than 10, respectively (Halperin and Kamel 1998). TTKG may be useful to assess

K^+ secretion but does not provide better information than the fractional excretion of K^+ which is calculated as:

$$FE_K = \frac{(U/P)_K}{(U/P)_{\text{inulin or creatinine}}}.$$

The investigation of dyskalaemia with inappropriate K^+ renal handling also requires the measurements of other parameters as renin and aldosterone plasma concentrations, and blood pH and $P\text{CO}_2$.

Calcium and magnesium transport in the nephron

About 60 per cent of the filtered calcium and magnesium are recovered from initial urine in the proximal tubule; this mechanism follows the reabsorption of water and other solutes. In the thick ascending limb, the divalent cation absorption depends on the $Na^+/K^+/2Cl^-$ transporter activity. As described earlier in this chapter, the recycling of K^+ in this segment is responsible for a lumen positive transepithelial voltage that drives the divalent cations across the epithelium through the paracellular pathway (Friedman 2000). Hence, in this segment, calcium absorption parallels that of sodium (Friedman 1998). Inhibition of $Na^+/K^+/2Cl^-$ transporter activity by furosemide, or by a mutation, or a mutation of a K^+ channel (ROMK) (Bartter's syndrome) induces hypercalciuria and hypermagnesuria (Friedman 2000). Mutations of paracellin, a renal tight junction protein, can also result in renal magnesium and calcium wasting (Simon *et al.* 1999). Two physiological factors control calcium reabsorption in the thick ascending limb: the plasma level of PTH and the plasma ionized calcium concentration. PTH stimulates the $Na^+/K^+/2Cl^-$ transporter, thus increasing calcium reabsorption (Friedman 1998). Conversely, binding of plasma ionized calcium to the calcium sensor expressed at the basolateral plasma membrane of the tubular cells inhibits the $Na^+/K^+/2Cl^-$ carrier, thereby decreasing calcium reabsorption (Brown *et al.* 1998).

In the distal convoluted tubule, in contrast to transport by proximal tubules and thick ascending limbs, calcium and sodium absorptions are characterized by a reciprocal relation. Calcium crosses the apical plasma membrane through the epithelial calcium channel ECaC and exits cells at the basolateral plasma membrane via a sodium calcium exchanger or a calcium ATPase (Friedman 1998). Inhibition of the amiloride sensitive channel ENaC or of the NaCl transporter with thiazide diuretics or by a mutation (Gitelman's syndrome) hyperpolarizes membrane voltage augmenting the driving for diffusional calcium entry at the apical pole and calcium efflux through the calcium exchanger at the basolateral membrane. PTH stimulates calcium reabsorption by hyperpolarizing membrane voltage. Calcitriol augments ECaC and calbindin-D_{28k} expressions and increases calcium reabsorption (Hoenderop *et al.* 2001).

Two parameters measure urinary calcium excretion. The daily urine calcium excretion depends on calcium ingestion, intestinal absorption rate, and renal reabsorption, consequently its normal range is very large from 1 to 7.5 mmol/24 h. Values above 0.1 mmol/kg of body weight are usually considered abnormal. Calcium excretion is also measured in morning urine samples in fasting subjects and normalized for urine creatinine concentration. The calcium to creatinine ratio is lower than 0.5 (mmol/mmol) in normal subjects.

Calcium excretion should be interpreted in the light of other biological factors in plasma: ionized calcium concentration, PTH, vitamin D, and calcitriol levels. The kidney contributes to the regulation of ionized calcium concentration in plasma. When plasma calcium concentration increases, renal calcium reabsorption diminishes and a decrease in plasma calcium level is normally associated with low calcium excretion rate. Mutations in the calcium sensing-receptor (CaSR) gene alter this relationship. Inhibiting mutations in the CaSR are responsible for hypocalciuric hypercalcaemia (Pollak *et al.* 1993), and activating mutation of this receptor cause hypercalciuric hypocalcaemia (Pollak *et al.* 1994). About 30–50 per cent of patients with kidney stones have hypercalciuria (Bushinsky 2002). The genetic basis of this hypercalciuria is unknown; in particular it is not associated with genetic variants in CaSR gene (Petrucci *et al.* 2000).

When plasma calcium concentration is normal, high fasting urinary calcium in patients maintained on a low calcium diet, consisting usually of avoidance of dairy products for 3 days, indicates an impairment in the renal tubular reabsorption of calcium or an excessive skeletal mobilization of calcium (Pak *et al.* 1974, 1975). The measurement of markers of bone remodelling may help distinguish these two possibilities.

The diagnosis of hypercalciuria secondary to intestinal hyperabsorption of calcium is obtained after an oral calcium load (Pak *et al.* 1974, 1975). In absorptive hypercalciuria, fasting urinary calcium is normal on a low calcium diet, daily excretion of calcium in urine is high on normal calcium diet, and the increase in the ratio of urinary calcium to creatinine after oral calcium load is exaggerated (Pak *et al.* 1974, 1975).

Endocrine functions of the kidney

Calcitriol synthesis

The kidney plays a central role in calcium and phosphate homeostasis not only by controlling ion reabsorption but also by synthesizing 1,25-dihydroxyvitamin D_3 (1,25$(OH)_2D_3$), the most active metabolite of vitamin D. Vitamin D_3 is obtained from 7-dehydrocholesterol by action of sunlight on the skin or is derived from the diet, then it is hydroxylated in the liver in 25-hydroxyvitamin D whose circulating levels are commonly used as indicators of vitamin D status (Brown *et al.* 1999). This step is not regulated. Under physiological conditions the formation of 1,25$(OH)_2D_3$ occurs exclusively in the renal proximal tubule. The activity of the 1α-hydroxylase is regulated by PTH and plasma phosphate concentration. High levels of PTH and hypophosphataemia stimulate 1,25$(OH)_2D_3$ production; hypoparathyroidism and hyperphosphataemia blunt renal 1α-hydroxylase activity even in the presence of hypocalcaemia. Vitamin D and its hydroxylated metabolites are transported in the plasma bound to the vitamin D-binding protein. The vitamin D-binding protein complex is filtered through the glomerulus and reabsorbed by the proximal tubule by the endocytic receptor megalin (Nykjaer *et al.* 1999).

To estimate the ability of the kidney to synthesize 1,25$(OH)_2D_3$ the plasma levels of several parameters should be determined: 1,25$(OH)_2D_3$, 25-hydroxyvitamin D, PTH, phosphate, and also GFR. Low circulating concentration of 1,25$(OH)_2D_3$ may be due to low vitamin D storage, hypoparathyroidism, hyperphosphataemia, or advanced renal insufficiency. Although plasma calcitriol concentration is usually within the normal range in mild and moderate renal failures, the decrease of calcitriol synthesis is an early event (Portale *et al.* 1984; Wilson *et al.* 1985; Llach and Velasquez Forero 2001). Megalin-null mice are unable to retrieve vitamin D from urine and hence develop vitamin D deficiency; it is unknown if a similar defect exists in humans. Increased levels of $1,25(OH)_2D_3$ are observed in granulomatous disorders (sarcoidosis, tuberculosis, etc.) because of the expression of extrarenal non-regulated 1α-hydroxylase, and in most chronic hypophosphataemia.

Erythropoietin production

Erythropoietin is mandatory for erythropoiesis (Moritz *et al.* 1997). About 90 per cent of the circulating levels of this hormone are produced by the kidney. Erythropoietin is synthesized by interstitial cells in the cortex, in the vicinity of proximal tubule (Eckardt *et al.* 1989; Liapis *et al.* 1995). During chronic renal failure, erythropoietin production is variably altered depending on the cause of kidney destruction and anaemia can be secondary to diverse mechanisms: iron, folate or vitamin B_{12} deficiencies, blood loss, and decrease in erythropoietin production. If, even after investigating the classical causes of anaemia, the reason for erythropoietin production remains doubtful in the genesis of anaemia, then the blood concentration of this hormone can be measured.

Renin secretion

Almost all circulating renin is produced by the kidney. Renin, the primary determinant of activity of the renin–angiotensin system, is secreted by the granular cells of the juxtaglomerular apparatus. Renin production is controlled by the renal vascular baroreceptor in the afferent arteriole, the delivery of sodium chloride at the macula densa, the renal sympathetic nerve activity, and various humoral agents including angiotensin II, nitric oxide, adenosine, atrial natriuretic peptide, and prostaglandins. Renin secretion is inhibited by high renal perfusion pressure and high sodium chloride delivery to the macula densa. The measurement of plasma renin activity and the investigation of renin angiotensin system are described in other chapters of this book (Section 9).

References

Abrahamson, M. *et al.* (1990). Structure and expression of the human cystatin C gene. *Biochemical Journal* **268**, 287–294.

Ackerman, I. P., Fajans, S. S., and Conn, J. W. (1958). The development of diabetes mellitus in patients with non diabetic glycosuria. *Clinical Research Proceedings* **6**, 251.

Agarwal, R. (1998). Chromatographic estimation of iothalamate and *p*-aminohippuric acid to measure glomerular filtration rate and effective renal plasma flow in humans. *Journal of Chromatography. B, Biomedical Sciences and Applications* **705**, 3–9.

Akutsu, T. *et al.* (1998). Modification of measurement of effective renal plasma flow from blood pool clearance curve of I-123-orthoiodohippurate using single blood sampling. *Radiation Medicine* **16**, 245–250.

Aperia, A. *et al.* (1983). Postnatal control of water and electrolyte homeostasis in pre-term and full-term infants. *Acta Paediatrica Scandinavica. Supplement* **305**, 61–65.

Atherton, J. C. *et al.* (1990). Lithium clearance in healthy humans: effects of sodium intake and diuretics. *Kidney International. Supplement* **28**, 36–S38.

Aukland, K. and Loyning, E. W. (1970). Intrarenal blood flow and para-aminohippurate (PAH) extraction. *Acta Physiologica Scandinavica* **79**, 95–108.

Aurell, M. *et al.* (1978). Renal extraction of *p*-aminohippurate: physiological and clinical observations. *Contributions to Nephrology* **11**, 14–18.

Back, S. E. *et al.* (1989). Age dependence of renal function: clearance of iohexol and *p*-amino hippurate in healthy males. *Scandinavian Journal of Clinical and Laboratory Investigation* **49**, 641–646.

Barnett, H. L. *et al.* (1948). Measurement of glomerular filtration rate in premature infants. *Journal of Clinical Investigation* **27**, 691.

Batlle, D. C. *et al.* (1988). The use of the urinary anion gap in the diagnosis of hyperchloremic metabolic acidosis. *New England Journal of Medicine* **318**, 594–599.

Battilana, C. *et al.* (1991). PAH extraction and estimation of plasma flow in diseased human kidneys. *American Journal of Physiology* **261**, F726–F733.

Berglund, F., Killander, J., and Pompeius, R. (1975). Effect of trimethoprim-sulfamethoxazole on the renal excretion of creatinine in man. *Journal of Urology* **114**, 802–808.

Bijvoet, O. L. M. (1969). Relation of plasma phosphate concentration to renal tubular reabsorption of phosphate. *Clinical Science* **37**, 23–36.

Bijvoet, O. L. M., Morgan, D. M., and Fourman, P. (1969). The assessment of phosphate reabsorption. *Clinica Chimica Acta* **26**, 15–24.

Binkert, C. A. *et al.* (1999). Characterization of renal artery stenoses based on magnetic resonance renal flow and volume measurements. *Kidney International* **56**, 1846–1854.

Binkert, C. A. *et al.* (2001). Can MR measurement of renal artery flow and renal volume predict the outcome of percutaneous transluminal renal angioplasty? *Cardiovascular and Interventional Radiology* **24**, 233–239.

Bistarakis, L. *et al.* (1986). Renal handling of phosphate in the first six months of life. *Archives of Disease in Childhood* **61**, 677–681.

Bjornsson, T. D. *et al.* (1983). Nomogram for estimating creatinine clearance. *Clinical Pharmacokinetics* **8**, 365–369.

Bland, J. M. and Altman, D. G. (1986). Statistical methods for assessing agreement between two methods of clinical measurement. *Lancet* **1**, 307–310.

Bostom, A. G., Kronenberg, F., and Ritz, E. (2002). Predictive performance of renal function equations for patients with chronic kidney disease and normal serum creatinine levels. *Journal of the American Society of Nephrology* **13**, 2140–2144.

Brandstrom, E. *et al.* (1998). GFR measurement with iohexol and 51Cr-EDTA. A comparison of the two favoured GFR markers in Europe. *Nephrology, Dialysis, Transplantation* **13**, 1176–1182.

Brochner-Mortensen, J. (1972). A simple method for the determination of glomerular filtration rate. *Scandinavian Journal of Clinical and Laboratory Investigation* **30**, 271–274.

Brochner-Mortensen, J. (1985). Current status on assessment and measurement of glomerular filtration rate. *Clinical Physiology (Oxford, England)* **5**, 1–17.

Brochner-Mortensen, J., Giese, J., and Rossing, N. (1969). Renal inulin clearance versus total plasma clearance of 51Cr-EDTA. *Scandinavian Journal of Clinical and Laboratory Investigation* **23**, 301–305.

Brodehl, J., Krause, A., and Hoyer, P. F. (1988). Assessment of maximal tubular phosphate reabsorption: comparison of direct measurement with the nomogram of Bijvoet. *Pediatric Nephrology* **2**, 183–189.

Brown, A. J., Dusso, A., and Slatopolsky, E. (1999). Vitamin D. *American Journal of Physiology* **277**, F157–F175.

Brown, E. M., Pollak, M., and Hebert, S. C. (1998). The extracellular calcium-sensing receptor: its role in health and disease. *Annual Review of Medicine* **49**, 15–29.

Brown, S. C. and O'Reilly, P. H. (1991). Iohexol clearance for the determination of glomerular filtration rate in clinical practice: evidence for a new gold standard. *Journal of Urology* **146**, 675–679.

Brzin, J. *et al.* (1984). Human cystatin, a new protein inhibitor of cysteine proteinases. *Biochemical and Biophysical Research Communications* **118**, 103–109.

Burgess, E. *et al.* (1982). Inhibition of renal creatinine secretion by cimetidine in humans. *Renal Physiology* **5**, 27–30.

Bushinsky, D. A. (2002). Recurrent hypercalciuric nephrolithiasis—does diet help? *New England Journal of Medicine* **346**, 124–125.

Calabrese, G. *et al.* (1990). Precocious familial gout with reduced fractional urate clearance and normal purine enzymes. *Quarterly Journal of Medicine* **75**, 441–450.

Carriere, S. and Friborg, J. (1969). Intrarenal blood flow and PAH extraction during angiotensin infusion. *American Journal of Physiology* **217**, 1708–1715.

Chalasani, N., Clark, W. S., and Wilcox, C. M. (1997). Blood urea nitrogen to creatinine concentration in gastrointestinal bleeding: a reappraisal. *American Journal of Gastroenterology* **92**, 1796–1799.

Chantler, C. (1973). The measurement of renal function in children: a review. *Guy's Hospital Reports* **122**, 25–41.

Chantler, C. and Barratt, T. M. (1972). Estimation of glomerular filtration rate from plasma clearance of 51-chromium edetic acid. *Archives of Disease in Childhood* **47**, 613–617.

Chantler, C. *et al.* (1969). Glomerular filtration rate measurement in man by the single injection methods using 51Cr-EDTA. *Clinical Science* **37**, 169–180.

Chantrel, F. *et al.* (2000). Comparison of cystatin C versus creatinine for detection of mild renal failure. *Clinical Nephrology* **54**, 374–381.

Chasis, H. and Smith, H. W. (1938). The excretion of urea in normal man and in subjects with glomerulonephritis. *Journal of Clinical Investigation* **17**, 347–358.

Cocchetto, D. M., Tschanz, C., and Bjornsson, T. D. (1983). Decreased rate of creatinine production in patients with hepatic disease: implications for estimation of creatinine clearance. *Therapeutic Drug Monitoring* **5**, 161–168.

Cockcroft, D. W. and Gault, M. H. (1976). Prediction of creatinine clearance from serum creatinine. *Nephron* **16**, 31–41.

Cole, B. R. *et al.* (1972). Measurement of renal function without urine collection. A critical evaluation of the constant-infusion technic for determination of inulin and para-aminohippurate. *New England Journal of Medicine* **287**, 1109–1114.

Colussi, G. *et al.* (1987). Pharmacological evaluation of urate renal handling in humans: pyrazinamide test vs combined pyrazinamide and probenecid administration. *Nephrology, Dialysis, Transplantation* **2**, 10–16.

Colussi, G. *et al.* (1990). Lithium clearance in humans: effects of acute administration of acetazolamide and furosemide. *Kidney International. Supplement* **28**, S63–S66.

Cortsen, M. *et al.* (1996). MR velocity mapping measurement of renal artery blood flow in patients with impaired kidney function. *Acta Radiologica* **37**, 79–84.

Cottini, E. P., Gallina, D. L., and Dominguez, J. M. (1973). Urea excretion in adult humans with varying degrees of kidney malfunction fed milk, egg or an amino acid mixture: assessment of nitrogen balance. *Journal of Nutrition* **103**, 11–19.

Counahan, R. *et al.* (1976). Estimation of glomerular filtration rate from plasma creatinine concentration in children. *Archives of Disease in Childhood* **51**, 875–878.

Crim, M. C., Calloway, D. H., and Margen, S. (1975). Creatine metabolism in men: urinary creatine and creatinine excretions with creatine feeding. *Journal of Nutrition* **105**, 428–438.

Curtis, J. R. and Donovan, B. A. (1979). Assessment of renal concentrating ability. *British Medical Journal* **1**, 304–305.

Davis, B. B. and Zenser, T. V. (1993). Evaluation of renal concentrating and diluting ability. *Clinics in Laboratory Medicine* **13**, 131–134.

Davis, P. J. and Davis, F. B. (1987). Water excretion in the elderly. *Endocrinology and Metabolism Clinics of North America* **16**, 867–875.

de Haan, M. W. *et al.* (2000). Renal artery blood flow: quantification with breath-hold or respiratory triggered phase-contrast MR imaging. *European Radiology* **10**, 1133–1137.

De Marchi, S. *et al.* (1993). Renal tubular dysfunction in chronic alcohol abuse—effects of abstinence. *New England Journal of Medicine* **329**, 1927–1934.

Debatin, J. F. (1998). MR quantification of flow in abdominal vessels. *Abdominal Imaging* **23**, 485–495.

Deetjen, P., von Baeyer, H., and Drexel, H. Renal glucose transport. In *The Kidney: Physiology and Pathophysiology* (ed. D. W. S. A. G. Giebisch), pp. 2873–2888. New York NY: Raven Press, 1992.

Derubertis, F. R., Jr. *et al.* (1971). Impaired water excretion in myxedema. *American Journal of Medicine* **51**, 41–53.

Diamond, H. S. (1989). Interpretation of pharmacologic manipulation of urate transport in man. *Nephron* **51**, 1–5.

Dumoulin, C. L. *et al.* (1994). Noninvasive measurement of renal hemodynamic functions using gadolinium enhanced magnetic resonance imaging. *Magnetic Resonance in Medicine* **32**, 370–378.

Durr, J. A., Miller, N. L., and Alfrey, A. C. (1990). Lithium clearance derived from the natural trace blood and urine lithium levels. *Kidney International. Supplement* **28**, S58–S62.

Dworkin, L. D. (2001). Serum cystatin C as a marker of glomerular filtration rate. *Current Opinion in Nephrology and Hypertension* **10**,+- 551–555.

Eckardt, K. U. *et al.* (1989). Erythropoietin in polycystic kidneys. *Journal of Clinical Investigation* **84**, 1160–1166.

Edelmann, C. M. and Bernstein, J. *Paediatrics*, New York NY: Appleton-Century-Crofts, 1968.

Edelmann, C. M., Jr. *et al.* (1967). A standarized test of renal concentrating capacity in children. *American Journal of Diseases of Children* **114**, 639–644.

Effersoe, H. *et al.* (1990). Measurement of renal function with iohexol. A comparison of iohexol, 99mTc-DTPA, and 51Cr-EDTA clearance. *Investigative Radiology* **25**, 778–782.

Fillastre, J. P., Ardaillou, R., and Richet, G. (1968a). Bicarbonate excretion in response to an increased alkaline load in chronic renal insufficiency. *Nephron* **5**, 437–453.

Fillastre, J. P., Ardaillou, R., and Richet, G. (1968b). Renal response to alkaline overload during chronic renal insufficiency. *Journal d'urologie et de nephrologie* **74**, 682–685.

Fillastre, J. P., Ardaillou, R., and Richet, G. (1969). Urinary pH and $P\text{CO}_2$ in response to an increased alkaline load during chronic renal insufficiency. *Nephron* **6**, 91–101.

Frennby, B. *et al.* (1995). The use of iohexol clearance to determine GFR in patients with severe chronic renal failure—a comparison between different clearance techniques. *Clinical Nephrology* **43**, 35–46.

Friedman, P. A. (1998). Codependence of renal calcium and sodium transport. *Annual Review of Physiology* **60**, 179–197.

Friedman, P. A. (2000). Mechanisms of renal calcium transport. *Experimental Nephrology* **8**, 343–350.

Garcia Puig, J. *et al.* (1983). Renal handling of uric acid in normal subjects by means of the pyrazinamide and probenecid tests. *Nephron* **35**, 183–186.

Garnett, E. S., Parsons, V., and Veall, N. (1967). Measurement of glomerular filtration-rate in man using a 51Cr-edetic-acid complex. *Lancet* **1**, 818–819.

Gaspari, F. *et al.* (1995). Plasma clearance of nonradioactive iohexol as a measure of glomerular filtration rate. *Journal of the American Society of Nephrology* **6**, 257–263.

Gaspari, F. *et al.* (1996). Glomerular filtration rate determined from a single plasma sample after intravenous iohexol injection: is it reliable? *Journal of the American Society of Nephrology* **7**, 2689–2693.

Gaspari, F., Perico, N., and Remuzzi, G. (1997). Measurement of glomerular filtration rate. *Kidney International. Supplement* **63**, S151–S154.

Gaspari, F. *et al.* (1998). Precision of plasma clearance of iohexol for estimation of GFR in patients with renal disease. *Journal of the American Society of Nephrology* **9**, 310–313.

Gault, M. H. *et al.* (1992). Predicting glomerular function from adjusted serum creatinine. *Nephron* **62**, 249–256.

Geva, P. and Spitzer, A. (1995). Special considerations for the evaluation of renal function in the pediatric patient. *Current Opinion in Nephrology and Hypertension* **4**, 525–530.

Greger, R. (1990). Possible sites of lithium transport in the nephron. *Kidney International. Supplement* **28**, S26–S30.

Groth, S. and Aasted, M. (1981). 51Cr-EDTA clearance determined by one plasma sample. *Clinical Physiology (Oxford, England)* **1**, 417–425.

Grubb, A. (1992). Diagnostic value of analysis of cystatin C and protein HC in biological fluids. *Clinical Nephrology* **38** (Suppl. 1), S20–S27.

Hagstam, K. E. *et al.* (1974). Comparison of different methods for determination of glomerular filtration rate in renal disease. *Scandinavian Journal of Clinical and Laboratory Investigation* **34**, 31–36.

Halperin, M. L. and Kamel, K. S. (1998). Potassium. *Lancet* **352**, 135–140.

Halperin, M. L. *et al.* (1974). Studies on the pathogenesis of type I (distal) renal tubular acidosis as revealed by the urinary PCO_2 tensions. *Journal of Clinical Investigation* **53**, 669–677.

Hannedouche, T. *et al.* (1989). Plasma 5-hydroxyindoleacetic acid as an endogenous index of renal plasma flow. *Kidney International* **35**, 95–98.

Harvey, A. M. (1980). Classics in clinical science: the concept of renal clearance. *The American Journal of Medicine* **68**, 6–8.

Hediger, M. A. and Rhoads, D. B. (1994). Molecular physiology of sodium–glucose cotransporters. *Physiological Reviews* **74**, 993–1026.

Hellerstein, S. *et al.* (1998). Creatinine clearance following cimetidine for estimation of glomerular filtration rate. *Pediatric Nephrology* **12**, 49–54.

Henriksen, J. H. *et al.* (1980). Over-estimation of glomerular filtration rate by single injection [51Cr]EDTA plasma clearance determination in patients with ascites. *Scandinavian Journal of Clinical and Laboratory Investigation* **40**, 279–284.

Herget-Rosenthal, S. *et al.* (1999). Two by two hour creatinine clearance—repeatable and valid. *Clinical Nephrology* **51**, 348–354.

Heymsfield, S. B. *et al.* (1983). Measurement of muscle mass in humans: validity of the 24-hour urinary creatinine method. *American Journal of Clinical Nutrition* **37**, 478–494.

Hirata-Dulas, C. A. *et al.* (1994). Evaluation of two intravenous single-bolus methods for measuring effective renal plasma flow. *American Journal of Kidney Diseases* **23**, 374–381.

Hoenderop, J. G. *et al.* (2001). Calcitriol controls the epithelial calcium channel in kidney. *Journal of the American Society of Nephrology* **12**, 1342–1349.

Hollenberg, N. K. *et al.* (1999). Age, renal perfusion and function in island-dwelling indigenous Kuna Amerinds of Panama. *Nephron* **82**, 131–138.

Holliday, M. A. *et al.* (1993). Serial measurements of GFR in infants using the continuous iothalamate infusion technique. Southwest Pediatric Nephrology Study Group (SPNSG). *Kidney International* **43**, 893–898.

Hoogwerf, B. J., Laine, D. C., and Greene, E. (1986). Urine C-peptide and creatinine (Jaffe method) excretion in healthy young adults on varied diets: sustained effects of varied carbohydrate, protein, and meat content. *American Journal of Clinical Nutrition* **43**, 350–360.

Isaacson, L. C. (1960). Urine osmolarity in thirsting subjects. *Lancet* **275**, 467–468.

Isaka, Y. *et al.* (1992). Modified plasma clearance technique using nonradioactive iothalamate for measuring GFR. *Kidney International* **42**, 1006–1011.

Itoh, K. (2001). 99mTc-MAG3: review of pharmacokinetics, clinical application to renal diseases and quantification of renal function. *Annals of Nuclear Medicine* **15**, 179–190.

Jacobsen, F. K. *et al.* (1979). Pronounced increase in serum creatinine concentration after eating cooked meat. *British Medical Journal* **1**, 1049–1050.

Jacobsson, L. (1983). A method for the calculation of renal clearance based on a single plasma sample. *Clinical Physiology (Oxford, England)* **3**, 297–305.

Jagenburg, R. *et al.* (1978). Determination of glomerular filtration rate in advanced renal insufficiency. *Scandinavian Journal of Urology and Nephrology* **12**, 133–137.

Jelliffe, R. W. (1971). Estimation of creatinine clearance when urine cannot be collected. *Lancet* **1**, 975–976.

Jelliffe, R. W. (1973). Letter: creatinine clearance: bedside estimate. *Annals of Internal Medicine* **79**, 604–605.

Jelliffe, R. W. and Jelliffe, S. M. (1971). Estimation of creatinine clearance from changing serum-creatinine levels. *Lancet* **2**, 710.

Kanazawa, T. *et al.* (1998). Reproducibility of 99Tcm-MAG3 clearance in normal volunteers with the two-sample method: comparison with 131I-OIH. *Nuclear Medicine Communications* **19**, 899–903.

Kenny, A. P. and Glen, A. C. (1973). Tests of phosphate reabsorption. *Lancet* **2**, 158.

Kim, G. H. *et al.* (1998). The thiazide-sensitive Na–Cl cotransporter is an aldosterone-induced protein. *Proceedings of the National Academy of Sciences of the United States of America* **95**, 14552–14557.

King, L. S. *et al.* (2001). Defective urinary-concentrating ability due to a complete deficiency of aquaporin-1. *New England Journal of Medicine* **345**, 175–179.

Kotzerke, J. *et al.* (1997). Reproducibility of a single-sample method for 99Tcm-MAG3 clearance under clinical conditions. *Nuclear Medicine Communications* **18**, 352–357.

Kruse, K., Kracht, U., and Gopfert, G. (1982). Renal threshold phosphate concentration (TmPO4/GFR). *Archives of Disease in Childhood* **57**, 217–223.

Laterza, O. F., Price, C. P., and Scott, M. G. (2002). Cystatin C: an improved estimator of glomerular filtration rate? *Clinical Chemistry* **48**, 699–707.

Levey, A. S. (1989). Use of glomerular filtration rate measurements to assess the progression of renal disease. *Seminars in Nephrology* **9**, 370–379.

Levey, A. S. (1990). Measurement of renal function in chronic renal disease. *Kidney International* **38**, 167–184.

Levey, A. S. *et al.* (1993). Glomerular filtration rate measurements in clinical trials. Modification of Diet in Renal Disease Study Group and the Diabetes Control and Complications Trial Research Group. *Journal of the American Society of Nephrology* **4**, 1159–1171.

Levey, A. S. *et al.* (1999). A more accurate method to estimate glomerular filtration rate from serum creatinine: a new prediction equation. Modification of Diet in Renal Disease Study Group. *Annals of Internal Medicine* **130**, 461–470.

Levey, A. S. *et al.* (2000). A simplified equation to predict glomerular filtration rate from serum creatinine. *Journal of the American Society of Nephrology* **11**, A0828 (abstract).

Lew, S. W. and Bosch, J. P. (1991). Effect of diet on creatinine clearance and excretion in young and elderly healthy subjects and in patients with renal disease. *Journal of the American Society of Nephrology* **2**, 856–865.

Liapis, H. *et al.* (1995). *In situ* hybridization of human erythropoietin in pre- and postnatal kidneys. *Pediatric Pathology and Laboratory Medicine* **15**, 875–883.

Llach, F. and Velasquez Forero, F. (2001). Secondary hyperparathyroidism in chronic renal failure: pathogenic and clinical aspects. *American Journal of Kidney Diseases* **38**, S20–S33.

Maesaka, J. K. and Fishbane, S. (1998). Regulation of renal urate excretion: a critical review. *American Journal of Kidney Diseases* **32**, 917–933.

Manjunath, G., Sarnak, M. J., and Levey, A. S. (2001). Prediction equations to estimate glomerular filtration rate: an update. *Current Opinion in Nephrology and Hypertension* **10**, 785–792.

Maroni, B. J., Steinman, T. I., and Mitch, W. E. (1985). A method for estimating nitrogen intake of patients with chronic renal failure. *Kidney International* **27**, 58–65.

Marx, M. A. *et al.* (1995). Plasma iohexol clearance as an alternative to creatinine clearance for CAPD adequacy studies. *Kidney International* **48**, 1994–1997.

Masarei, J. R. (1975). Validity of corrections for creatinine excretion and creatinine clearance. *New Zealand Medical Journal* **82**, 197–198.

McBride, M. B., Simmonds, H. A., and Moro, F. (1997). Familial renal disease or familial juvenile hyperuricaemic nephropathy? *Journal of Inherited Metabolic Disease* **20**, 351–353.

McBride, M. B. *et al.* (1998). Presymptomatic detection of familial juvenile hyperuricaemic nephropathy in children. *Pediatric Nephrology* **12**, 357–364.

McElligott, M. (1978). Impaired creatinine clearance after cimetidine. *Lancet* **1**, 99.

McPhaul, J. J., Jr. and Simonaitis, J. J. (1968). Observations on the mechanisms of glucosuria during glucose loads in normal and nondiabetic subjects. *Journal of Clinical Investigation* **47**, 702–711.

Miles, B. E., Paton, A., and de Wardener, H. E. (1954). Maximum urinary concentration. *British Medical Journal* **2**, 901–905.

Minisola, S. *et al.* (1993). Serum ionized calcium, parathyroid hormone and related variables: effect of age and sex. *Bone Miner* **23**, 183–193.

Moe, O. W., Berry, C. A., and Rector, F. C. J. Renal transport of glucose, aminoacids, sodium, chloride and water. In *The Kidney* (ed. B. M. Brenner), pp. 375–415. Philadelphia PA: W.B. Saunders Company, 2000.

Monnens, L. *et al.* (1981). DDAVP test for assessment of renal concentrating capacity in infants and children. *Nephron* **29**, 151–154.

Morello, J. P. and Bichet, D. G. (2001). Nephrogenic diabetes insipidus. *Annual Review of Physiology* **63**, 607–630.

Moritz, K. M., Lim, G. B., and Wintour, E. M. (1997). Developmental regulation of erythropoietin and erythropoiesis. *American Journal of Physiology* **273**, R1829–R1844.

Moro, F. *et al.* (1991). Familial juvenile gouty nephropathy with renal urate hypoexcretion preceding renal disease. *Clinical Nephrology* **35**, 263–269.

Moses, A. M., Scheinman, S. J., and Schroeder, E. T. (1985). Antidiuretic and PGE2 responses to AVP and dDAVP in subjects with central and nephrogenic diabetes insipidus. *American Journal of Physiology* **248**, F354–F359.

Motwani, J. G., Fenwick, M. K., and Struthers, A. D. (1992). Comparison of three methods of glomerular filtration rate measurement with and without captopril pretreatment in groups of patients with left ventricular dysfunction. *European Heart Journal* **13**, 1195–1200.

Munoz Sanz, A. *et al.* (1983). Hypouricemia and renal tubular urate secretion. *Archives of Internal Medicine* **143**, 1633–1634.

Nakashima, R. *et al.* (1996). Measurement of effective renal plasma flow (ERPF) with 123I-orthoiodohippurate (I-123-OIH). *Radiation Medicine* **14**, 147–150.

Nielsen, S. *et al.* (2002). Aquaporins in the kidney: from molecules to medicine. *Physiological Reviews* **82**, 205–244.

Nykjaer, A. *et al.* (1999). An endocytic pathway essential for renal uptake and activation of the steroid 25-(OH) vitamin D3. *Cell* **96**, 507–515.

Opravil, M., Keusch, G., and Luthy, R. (1993). Pyrimethamine inhibits renal secretion of creatinine. *Antimicrobial Agents and Chemotherapy* **37**, 1056–1060.

Oriuchi, N. *et al.* (1996). Evaluation of gamma camera-based measurement of individual kidney function using iodine-123 orthoiodohippurate. *European Journal of Nuclear Medicine* **23**, 371–375.

Pak, C. Y. *et al.* (1974). The hypercalciurias. Causes, parathyroid functions, and diagnostic criteria. *Journal of Clinical Investigation* **54**, 387–400.

Pak, C. Y. *et al.* (1975). A simple test for the diagnosis of absorptive, resorptive and renal hypercalciurias. *New England Journal of Medicine* **292**, 497–500.

Payne, R. B. (1993). Creatinine clearance with cimetidine for measurement of GFR. *Lancet* **341**, 187.

Payne, R. B. (1998). Renal tubular reabsorption of phosphate (TmP/GFR): indications and interpretation. *Annals of Clinical Biochemistry* **35** (Pt 2), 201–206.

Perrone, R. D. *et al.* (1990). Utility of radioisotopic filtration markers in chronic renal insufficiency: simultaneous comparison of 125I-iothalamate, 169Yb-DTPA, 99mTc-DTPA, and inulin. The Modification of Diet in Renal Disease Study. *American Journal of Kidney Diseases* **16**, 224–235.

Peters, A. M., Allison, H., and Ussov, W. (1994). Measurement of the ratio of glomerular filtration rate to plasma volume from the technetium-99m diethylene triamine pentaacetic acid renogram: comparison with glomerular filtration rate in relation to extracellular fluid volume. *European Journal of Nuclear Medicine* **21**, 322–327.

Peters, A. M., Allison, H., and Ussov, W. (1995). Simultaneous measurement of extracellular fluid distribution and renal function with a single injection of 99mTc DTPA. *Nephrology, Dialysis, Transplantation* **10**, 1829–1833.

Petrucci, M. *et al.* (2000). Evaluation of the calcium-sensing receptor gene in idiopathic hypercalciuria and calcium nephrolithiasis. *Kidney International* **58**, 38–42.

Picciotto, G. *et al.* (1992). Estimation of chromium-51 ethylene diamine tetra-acetic acid plasma clearance: a comparative assessment of simplified techniques. *European Journal of Nuclear Medicine* **19**, 30–35.

Piepsz, A. *et al.* (1996). Reproducibility of technetium-99m mercaptoacetyltriglycine clearance. *European Journal of Nuclear Medicine* **23**, 195–198.

Pollak, M. R. *et al.* (1993). Mutations in the human Ca(2+)-sensing receptor gene cause familial hypocalciuric hypercalcemia and neonatal severe hyperparathyroidism. *Cell* **75**, 1297–1303.

Pollak, M. R. *et al.* (1994). Autosomal dominant hypocalcaemia caused by a Ca(2+)-sensing receptor gene mutation. *Nature Genetics* **8**, 303–307.

Pontoglio, M. *et al.* (2000). HNF1alpha controls renal glucose reabsorption in mouse and man. *EMBO Reports* **1**, 359–365.

Portale, A. A. *et al.* (1984). Effect of dietary phosphorus on circulating concentrations of 1,25-dihydroxyvitamin D and immunoreactive parathyroid hormone in children with moderate renal insufficiency. *Journal of Clinical Investigation* **73**, 1580–1589.

Prié, D. *et al.* (1998). Dipyridamole decreases renal phosphate leak and augments serum phosphorus in patients with low renal phosphate threshold. *Journal of the American Society of Nephrology* **9**, 1264–1269.

Prié, D. *et al.* (2001). Frequency of renal phosphate leak among patients with calcium nephrolithiasis. *Kidney International* **60**, 272–276.

Prié, D. *et al.* (2002). Nephrolithiasis and osteoporosis associated with hypophosphatemia caused by mutations in the type 2a sodium phosphate cotransporter. *New England Journal of Medicine* **347**, 983–991.

Prueksaritanont, T. *et al.* (1986). Renal and non-renal clearances of iothalamate. *Biopharmaceutics & Drug Disposition* **7**, 347–355.

Rado, J. P. *et al.* (1976). The antidiuretic action of 1-deamino-8-D-arginine vasopressin (DDAVP) in man. *International Journal of Clinical Pharmacology and Biopharmacy* **13**, 199–209.

Rehberg, P. (1926). Studies on kidney function. I: The rate of filtration and reabsorption in the human kidney. *Biochemistry Journal* **20**, 447–460.

Rehling, M. *et al.* (1984). Simultaneous measurement of renal clearance and plasma clearance of 99mTc-labelled diethylenetriaminepenta-acetate, 51Cr-labelled ethylenediaminetetra-acetate and inulin in man. *Clinical Science (London, England: 1979)* **66**, 613–619.

Reidenberg, M. M. *et al.* (1988). A nonradioactive iothalamate method for measuring glomerular filtration rate and its use to study the renal handling of cibenzoline. *Therapeutic Drug Monitoring* **10**, 434–437.

Rickers, H., Brochner-Mortensen, J., and Rodbro, P. (1978). The diagnostic value of plasma urea for assessment of renal function. *Scandinavian Journal of Urology and Nephrology* **12**, 39–44.

Roberts, D. A. *et al.* (1995). Renal perfusion in humans: MR imaging with spin tagging of arterial water. *Radiology* **196**, 281–286.

Roch-Ramel, F. and Guisan, B. (1999). Renal transport of urate in humans. *News in Physiological Sciences* **14**, 80–84.

Romero, J. C. and Lerman, L. O. (2000). Novel noninvasive techniques for studying renal function in man. *Seminars in Nephrology* **20**, 456–462.

Rowe, J. W., Shock, N. W., and DeFronzo, R. A. (1976a). The influence of age on the renal response to water deprivation in man. *Nephron* **17**, 270–278.

Rowe, J. W., Andres, R., and Tobin, J. D. (1976b). Age-adjusted standards for creatinine clearance. *Annals of Internal Medicine* **84**, 567–569 (letter).

Rowe, J. W. *et al.* (1976c). The effect of age on creatinine clearance in men: a cross-sectional and longitudinal study. *Journal of Gerontology* **31**, 155–163.

Russell, C. D., Dubovsky, E. V., and Scott, J. W. (1989). Estimation of ERPF in adults from plasma clearance of 131I-hippuran using a single injection and one or two blood samples. *International Journal of Radiation Applications and Instrumentation. Part B, Nuclear Medicine and Biology* **16**, 381–383.

Russell, C. D., Taylor, A. T., and Dubovsky, E. V. (1996). Measurement of renal function with technetium-99m-MAG3 in children and adults. *Journal of Nuclear Medicine* **37**, 588–593.

Rydstrom, M. *et al.* (1995). Measurement of glomerular filtration rate by single-injection, single-sample techniques, using 51Cr-EDTA or iohexol. *Scandinavian Journal of Urology and Nephrology* **29**, 135–139.

Saitoh, E. *et al.* (1991). The human cystatin gene family: cloning of three members and evolutionary relationship between cystatins and Bowman–Birk type proteinase inhibitors. *Biomedica Biochimica Acta* **50**, 599–605.

Schlegel, J. U., Halikiopoulos, H. L., and Prima, R. (1979). Determination of filtration fraction using the gamma scintillation camera. *Journal of Urology* **122**, 447–450.

Schnermann, J. *et al.* (1998). Defective proximal tubular fluid reabsorption in transgenic aquaporin-1 null mice. *Proceedings of the National Academy of Sciences of the United States of America* **95**, 9660–9664.

Scholbach, T. (1999). Color Doppler sonographic determination of renal blood flow in healthy children. *Journal of Ultrasound in Medicine* **18**, 559–564.

Serdar, M. A. *et al.* (2001). A practical approach to glomerular filtration rate measurements: creatinine clearance estimation using cimetidine. *Annals of Clinical Laboratory Science* **31**, 265–273.

Shaw, N. J., Wheeldon, J., and Brocklebank, J. T. (1990). Indices of intact serum parathyroid hormone and renal excretion of calcium, phosphate, and magnesium. *Archives of Disease in Childhood* **65**, 1208–1211.

Simon, D. B. *et al.* (1999). Paracellin-1, a renal tight junction protein required for paracellular Mg^{2+} resorption. *Science* **285**, 103–106.

Smith, H. W. *The Kidney: Structure and Function in Health and Disease.* New York NY: Oxford University Press, 1951.

Smith, H. W. *et al.* (1943). The application of saturation methods to the study of glomerular and tubular function in the human kidney. *Journal of Mount Sinai Hospital* **10**, 59.

Sommer, G. *et al.* (1998). Renal blood flow: measurement *in vivo* with rapid spiral MR imaging. *Radiology* **208**, 729–734.

Soriano, J. R., Boichis, H., and Edelmann, C. M., Jr. (1967). Bicarbonate reabsorption and hydrogen ion excretion in children with renal tubular acidosis. *Journal of Pediatrics* **71**, 802–813.

Soroka, S. D. *et al.* (1997). Minimum urine flow rate during water deprivation: importance of the nonurea versus total osmolality in the inner medulla. *Journal of the American Society of Nephrology* **8**, 880–886.

Sterner, G. *et al.* (2000). Assessing residual renal function and efficiency of hemodialysis—an application for urographic contrast media. *Nephron* **85**, 324–333.

Strandness, D. E. (2000). Doppler and ultrasound methods for diagnosis. *Seminars in Nephrology* **20**, 445–449.

Swan, S. K. *et al.* (1996). Determination of residual renal function with iohexol clearance in hemodialysis patients. *Kidney International* **49**, 232–235.

Thalassinos, N. C. *et al.* (1970). Urinary excretion of phosphate in normal children. *Archives of Disease in Childhood* **45**, 269–272.

Thomsen, K. (1990). Lithium clearance as a measure of sodium and water delivery from the proximal tubules. *Kidney International. Supplement* **28**, S10–S16.

Toto, R. D. (1995). Conventional measurement of renal function utilizing serum creatinine, creatinine clearance, inulin and para-aminohippuric acid clearance. *Current Opinion in Nephrology and Hypertension* **4**, 505–509; discussion 03–04.

Turner, S. T. and Reilly, S. L. (1995). Fallacy of indexing renal and systemic hemodynamic measurements for body surface area. *American Journal of Physiology* **268**, R978–R988.

Vallee, J. P. *et al.* (2000). Absolute renal blood flow quantification by dynamic MRI and Gd-DTPA. *European Radiology* **10**, 1245–1252.

Valtin, H. and Schafer, J. A. *Renal Function/Mechanisms Preserving Fluid and Solute Balance in Health.* Boston MA: Little, Brown, and Co., 1995.

van Acker, B. A., Koomen, G. C., and Arisz, L. (1995). Drawbacks of the constant-infusion technique for measurement of renal function. *American Journal of Physiology* **268**, F543–F552.

van Acker, B. A. *et al.* (1992). Creatinine clearance during cimetidine administration for measurement of glomerular filtration rate. *Lancet* **340**, 1326–1329.

van Guldener, C., Gans, R., and ter Wee, P. (1995). Constant infusion clearance is an inappropriate method for accurate assessment of an impaired glomerular filtration rate. *Nephrology, Dialysis, Transplantation* **10**, 47–51.

Visscher, C. A. *et al.* (1995). Drug-induced changes in renal hippurate clearance as a measure of renal blood flow. *Kidney International* **48**, 1617–1623.

Walser, M. (1998). Assessing renal function from creatinine measurements in adults with chronic renal failure. *American Journal of Kidney Diseases* **32**, 23–31.

Walser, M., Drew, H. H., and Guldan, J. L. (1993). Prediction of glomerular filtration rate from serum creatinine concentration in advanced chronic renal failure. *Kidney International* **44**, 1145–1148.

Walton, R. J. and Bijvoet, O. L. (1975). Nomogram for derivation of renal threshold phosphate concentration. *Lancet* **2**, 309–310.

Werner, E., Blasl, C., and Reiners, C. (1998). Reproducibility of technetium-99m-MAG3 clearance using the Bubeck method. *Journal of Nuclear Medicine* **39**, 1066–1069.

West, M. L. *et al.* (1986). New clinical approach to evaluate disorders of potassium excretion. *Mineral and Electrolyte Metabolism* **12**, 234–238.

White, A. J. and Strydom, W. J. (1991). Normalisation of glomerular filtration rate measurements. *European Journal of Nuclear Medicine* **18**, 385–390.

Wibell, L. and Bjorsell-Ostling, E. (1973). Endogenous creatinine clearance in apparently healthy individuals as determined by 24 hour ambulatory urine collection. *Upsala Journal of Medical Sciences* **78**, 43–47.

Williams, T. D. *et al.* (1986). Antidiuretic effect and pharmacokinetics of oral 1-desamino-8-D-arginine vasopressin. 1. Studies in adults and children. *Journal of Clinical Endocrinology and Metabolism* **63**, 129–132.

Wilson, L. *et al.* (1985). Altered divalent ion metabolism in early renal failure: role of $1,25(OH)_2D$. *Kidney International* **27**, 565–573.

Wright, E. M. (2001). Renal Na(+)-glucose cotransporters. *American Journal of Physiology. Renal Physiology* **280**, F10–F18.

Wyss, M. and Kaddurah-Daouk, R. (2000). Creatine and creatinine metabolism. *Physiological Reviews* **80**, 1107–1213.

Zaltzman, J. S. *et al.* (1996). Accurate measurement of impaired glomerular filtration using single-dose oral cimetidine. *American Journal of Kidney Diseases* **27**, 504–511.

1.4 Renal function in the newborn infant

Peter R.F. Dear and Simon J. Newell

Introduction

The transition from intrauterine to extrauterine life is perhaps most remarkable for the ease with which it is usually accomplished. Those few observers who stop to ponder the process are generally most impressed with the extraordinary cardiorespiratory events relating to the onset of breathing and the transition from placenta to lung as the organ of gas exchange. Less obviously dramatic but no less remarkable, or vital, are the changes that must occur in the kidney as the fetus moves from an aquatic to a terrestrial environment and simultaneously takes over responsibility for its biochemical homeostasis from the placenta and the maternal kidneys. Some familiarity with these adaptational processes is essential for the understanding and interpretation of renal function in the newborn and the management of sick infants.

Renal function in the fetus

The metanephros or definitive kidney appears at about 5 weeks of gestation with the appearance of nephrons and the onset of renal function at about 10 weeks. Fetal kidneys can be recognized on ultrasound by week 18 and nephrogenesis is complete by 36 weeks.

The principal function of the fetal kidney is to maintain the volume of the fluid in the amniotic cavity, and to this end about 1000 ml of fetal urine are passed daily by the end of gestation (Rabinowitz *et al.* 1989). Amniotic fluid contains microproteins of fetal origin and changes in the concentrations of these (especially α-1 microglobulin) through gestation provide a way to assess the maturation of tubular function (Cagdas *et al.* 2000). A normal volume of amniotic fluid is necessary for fetal lung growth and to allow the fetus to exercise its joints and muscles. Significant fetal oliguria may be associated with pulmonary hypoplasia, joint contractures, and other postural deformities.

The role of the fetal kidney in maintaining fluid, electrolyte, and acid–base status is far less vital as biochemical homeostasis is maintained by the placenta and ultimately the maternal kidneys. As a result, even the anephric fetus is born with respectable serum biochemistry. In fact, such babies usually die of respiratory failure secondary to pulmonary hypoplasia before they develop signs of renal failure! This lack of fetal autonomy also means that if the pregnant woman has significantly abnormal renal function, the fetus will be unable to maintain homeostasis. However, in practice, if maternal serum biochemistry cannot be kept under reasonable control, successful pregnancy is unlikely (see also Chapter 15.3).

Another well-recognized consequence of this lack of fetal autonomy is seen when maternal serum electrolyte concentrations are rendered abnormal by inappropriate fluid and electrolyte intake during labour. The obstetric practice of infusing large volumes of dextrose to treat maternal ketoacidosis is less common than it used to be, but the occasional birth of a baby with a serum sodium concentration of 125 mmol/l provides a reminder of just how dependent the fetus is.

Renal vascular resistance in the fetus is high (Andriani *et al.* 2001), and the kidneys receive only 2–3 per cent of the cardiac output compared with 15–18 per cent in the newborn and around 20–25 per cent in the adult. In contrast, the placenta, across which the fetus receives constant haemodialysis, receives about 50 per cent of the cardiac output. Thus the renal filtration fraction is low and the fetal glomerular filtration rate (GFR) is in the region of 30 ml/min/1.73 m^2.

Tubular function in the fetal kidney shows progressive maturation in preparation for its postnatal role. Towards the end of gestation there is evidence of a mature secretory pathway for potassium, a high renal plasma threshold for glucose, rapidly improving excretion rates of titratable acid and ammonia (Kesby and Lumbers 1986), and the secretion of organic bases (Elbourne *et al.* 1990). A pronounced difference between pre- and postnatal tubular function is in the rate of absorption of filtered sodium. Fractional excretion of sodium (FE_{Na}) is a measure of the kidney's ability to reabsorb sodium, and after birth this figure is usually less than 1 per cent. In the fetus at mid-gestation, FE_{Na} is high and may exceed 10 per cent. The pattern of tubular sodium reabsorption is also different, with much of the filtered load being reabsorbed in the distal tubule rather than the proximal tubule where 70–80 per cent of reabsorption occurs in the child and the adult (Lumbers 1988). The reasons for this high rate of sodium excretion are not yet fully understood but probably include relative insensitivity to aldosterone, the influence of circulating natriuretic factors, and the large extracellular fluid compartment. The fractional excretion of sodium gradually declines as gestation progresses, but even at term is up to 3.5 per cent.

In terms of concentrating capacity, the fetus behaves as if it is trying to excrete a water load and produces urine with an osmolality of less than 180 mOsm/kg H_2O, approximately 25 per cent of the maternal urine osmolality. However, the fetus is able to reduce its free-water clearance in response to maternal dehydration or when there is a decrease in net transplacental fluid transport from mother to fetus. Indeed, when there is significantly impaired placental function, the fetal urine volume decreases and its osmolality increases (Wintour *et al.* 1985). The reduction in urine volume and consequent diminution in amniotic fluid volume can be detected by ultrasound and provides the obstetrician with one of the more sensitive ways of diagnosing fetal compromise and poor pregnancy outcome (Hackett *et al.* 1987; Casey *et al.* 2000).

A relationship between low birth weight and later susceptibility to renal disease has recently been described (Hoy *et al.* 1999; Lackland *et al.* 2000; Lackland *et al.* 2001; Spencer *et al.* 2001). This appears to be a new dimension to the so-called 'Barker hypothesis'. The mechanism is believed to be reduced renal growth and development secondary to poor nutrition and a diminution in glomerular number and size has been reported in low birth weight babies (Manalich *et al.* 2000).

Changes in renal function at birth

After birth, the newborn baby's kidneys must adapt rapidly to conserve water, to excrete the waste products of metabolism, and to regulate the acid–base and electrolyte composition of the body fluids. Fortunately, the kidneys of the healthy full-term infant can take on these new roles with remarkable efficiency.

There is no instantaneous augmentation of renal blood flow following birth, but there is a marked increase during the first few weeks of life (Lin and Cher 1997; Pokharel *et al.* 1997) as a consequence of increases in cardiac output and systemic arterial pressure and a decrease in renal vascular resistance. This increase is accompanied by a gradual redistribution of flow within the kidney towards the outer cortical nephrons. Effective renal plasma flow (by *p*-aminohippurate) increases from around 80 ml/min/1.73 m^2 at term to around 300 ml/min/1.73 m^2 at 3 months of age. However, the lower renal extraction of *p*-aminohippurate in the newborn may slightly exaggerate the size of the change as measured by this method.

In the term infant, GFR increases rapidly after birth, approximately doubling by 2 weeks of age. As there is no postnatal increase in the number of nephrons after term, the increase in GFR must be explained by an increase in the filtration rate of individual nephrons. Much of this increase in filtration rate relates to improved renal perfusion after birth, particularly of the numerous outer cortical nephrons near the zone of nephrogenesis, which are relatively poorly perfused before birth. This is reflected in the fall in blood creatinine concentration over the first weeks (Rudd *et al.* 1983). The serum concentration of cystatin C can be used to follow changes in GFR in newborns and infants (Bokenkamp *et al.* 1998; Finney *et al.* 2000; Harmoinen *et al.* 2000).

Tubular function also shows marked changes during the early weeks of life, although to some extent it initially lags behind glomerular function. In the rodent, a tubuloglomerular feedback mechanism, aimed at producing a constant rate of water and solute delivery to the distal tubule, is present from a very early stage (Muller-Suur 1983), and such a mechanism may also be important in the human.

The fractional excretion of sodium declines sharply after birth, falling from 3.5 to 1.5 per cent within hours (Smith and Lumbers 1989). Subsequently it continues to decline more slowly, and after a few days a state of positive balance is reached with retention of at least 70 per cent of the sodium intake (Forbes 1987). Sodium and water intake is initially low in the first days of breast feeding, and it is essential that high sodium retention is achieved in order to maintain hydration. Equally, it is important to retain sodium in large amounts for the growth of tissue (Chevalier 2001). Most of the improvement in the tubular reabsorption of sodium takes place in the proximal tubule as might be expected. Positive potassium balance is also important for growth and the normal infant achieves this by about 10 days of age (Engle 1985). Retention of potassium is contributed to by low renal potassium excretion (Aizman *et al.* 1998).

Perhaps the greatest challenge to the newborn's kidneys during the early days of postnatal life relates to the need to conserve water. During fetal life, water is available in abundance, with a net fluid flux between mother and fetus of about 3500 ml/day. After birth, the infant will receive very little fluid for several days and thereafter a relatively fixed intake of around 150 ml/kg/day. If the concentrating capacity does not improve swiftly, the infant will enter a state of hypertonic dehydration in response to quite minor reductions in fluid intake or increases in fluid loss. In the mature human kidney, water conservation is dependent upon interstitial hypertonicity in the medulla, which may exceed 1000 mOsm/kg H_2O. Water absorption from the tubule into the hypertonic medulla is then controlled by the permeability of the tubular membrane to water, which is increased in the presence of antidiuretic hormone (ADH). ADH-regulated water channels are expressed in the collecting ducts of the newborn but to a lesser extent than in adults (Tsukahara *et al.* 1998). The main factor preventing urine concentration in the collecting tubules of the kidney of the newborn is the relatively low tonicity of the medullary interstitium, providing a poor osmotic gradient across the tubular membrane. Thus, even in the presence of adequate ADH, as is often the case (Wiriyathian *et al.* 1986), the maximum urine osmolality is initially no more than 350 mOsm/kg H_2O. There is a rapid increase in the concentration of both urea and sodium in the renal medulla following birth which is paralleled by an increase in the maximum urine osmolality that can be achieved. A urine osmolality of 650 mOsm/kg H_2O is possible by 1 week of age, and by 1 month the maximum urine osmolality has increased to about 900 mOsm/kg H_2O. Not all of this improvement can be related to increased tonicity of the medulla, and it is likely that increasing tubular sensitivity to ADH is also important (Edwards 1982; Liu *et al.* 2001).

Another urgent task for the neonatal kidney is to take over the responsibility for acid–base balance from the placenta, and this is managed quite efficiently, at least in the term infant. Term babies respond appropriately to a NH_4Cl load (Svenningsen 1974). However, the renal threshold for bicarbonate is lower than in older infants and adults, and term babies typically have serum bicarbonate concentrations of around 20 mmol/l (Arant 1987). It is not known whether the low threshold relates mainly to tubular immaturity or to extracellular fluid volume expansion.

Growth, diet, and the excretory load

Postnatal renal adaptation in the healthy breast-fed infant is aided by the fact that the kidneys are presented with a relatively low solute load. This is partly because the solute content of human milk is low (of the order of 14 mOsm/100 kcal compared with 46 mOsm/100 kcal in cow's milk; Fomon and Ziegler 1999) but mainly because such infants grow rapidly and produce less in the way of waste products of metabolism than older children or adults. For example, in healthy newborn infants the efficiency of protein gain has been estimated to be in the range 0.65–0.75. This means that 65–75 per cent of the absorbed amino acid is retained as tissue protein and only 25–35 per cent is oxidized. As a result, the urea load presented to the neonatal kidney is usually low. However, if the infant is rendered catabolic, urea production can easily outstrip excretory capacity, and most sick infants have elevated blood urea concentrations compared with their healthy counterparts. This can also be seen in infants made catabolic by dexamethasone administered to treat chronic lung disease (Brownlee *et al.* 1992). This important effect of growth in reducing the demands placed on the kidney has led to growth's being referred to as the 'third kidney'.

Sodium is a necessary, permissive factor for normal growth. Breast milk provides only 1 mmol/kg/day, and growth is maintained because the term fetus is able to retain almost all this sodium (Haycock and Aperia 1991).

Renal function in the preterm infant

The fact that the fetal kidneys have such a limited role in maintaining homeostasis has provided no evolutionary stimulus for the development of the excretory or secretory functions of the kidney until late in gestation, in preparation for birth at term. Now that advances in neonatal medicine are allowing less and less mature babies to survive, the problems associated with immature renal function are more apparent. As well as having poor renal function, preterm infants are usually rendered markedly catabolic by the stress of their many adaptational difficulties, and this leads to a particularly challenging combination of problems. The group of infants who have the greatest problem with renal function are those born at less than 30 weeks gestation and weighing less than 1500 g. These are classified as very low birth weight (VLBW) infants and it is their problems that will be highlighted in this section.

Nephrogenesis is not completed until about 34 weeks gestation and prior to that blood flow to the renal cortex is low. At the end of the second trimester, most nephrons are juxtaglomerular with short loops of Henle, and it is the more cortical nephrons with greater concentrating power that develop by 34 weeks (Potter 1965). GFR of the VLBW infant is less than 25 per cent of that found in the term infant when adjusted for surface area (Arant 1978). Values as low as 0.70 ml/min/kg have been reported for babies of 26 weeks gestation rising to 0.84 ml/min/kg at 33 weeks (Wilkins 1992). The rapid postnatal increase in GFR seen in term infants is not seen in the VLBW baby (Gallini *et al.* 2000). Substantial improvements in GFR must await the completion of nephrogenesis (Engle and Arant 1983) and improvements in renal blood flow (Kusuda *et al.* 1999), advancing with gestational age irrespective of postnatal age (Coulthard 1985). In infants below 30 weeks gestation, there is a temporary and dramatic rise in creatinine in the first 48 h after birth, even in the absence of any other evidence of renal failure (Miall *et al.* 1999) (Fig. 1).

In addition to this primary inadequacy of renal function, sepsis, hypoxia, hypotension, persisting patency of the ductus arteriosus and mechanical ventilation, acidosis, and catabolism impose additional burdens on clearance in the sick infant (Vanpee *et al.* 1993; Toth-Heyn *et al.* 2000; Kluckow and Evans 2001). As a result it is impossible for the sick VLBW infant to excrete the waste products of metabolism sufficiently rapidly to avoid substantial increases in serum urea and creatinine concentrations after birth. Many of these babies will experience elevations of their serum urea concentrations to at least 15–20 mmol/l despite every effort to meet their fluid needs. The serum creatinine concentration will usually peak at about 200 μmol/l. The low GFR also has important implications for prescribing and makes careful monitoring for drug toxicity essential, for example, when using aminoglycosides, such as gentamicin, or other agents, such as vancomycin (van den Anker 1996). Low doses of dopamine (6 mg/kg/min) have been shown to improve renal blood flow and urine output (Seri *et al.* 1998) but some prescribed agents such as indomethacin and high-dose dopamine have an adverse effect upon renal perfusion and GFR. Ibuprofen seems no better than indomethacin in this respect (Chamaa *et al.* 2000).

Dexamethasone is currently in common use for the treatment of chronic lung disease in VLBW babies (the condition known as bronchopulmonary dysplasia). The catabolic effect of this drug provides a good illustration of the limited ability of the preterm kidney to excrete the waste products of metabolism (Brownlee *et al.* 1992). Figure 2 shows the increase in blood urea caused by dexamethasone therapy in these infants.

As far as tubular handling of filtered sodium is concerned, the situation in the VLBW infant mirrors that in the fetus. Urinary sodium

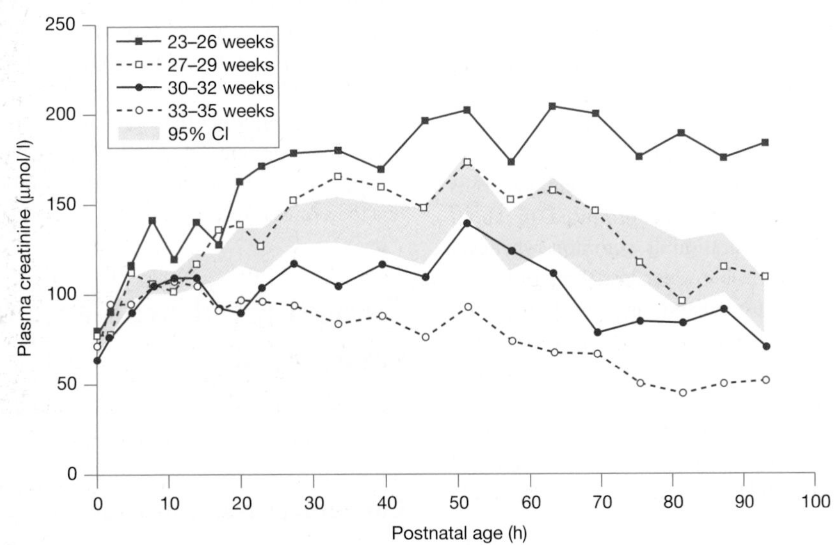

Fig. 1 Mean plasma creatinine against postnatal age for different gestational age groups. The shaded area represents 95% confidence intervals for the mean plasma creatinine of all infants (reproduced with permission from Miall *et al.* 1999).

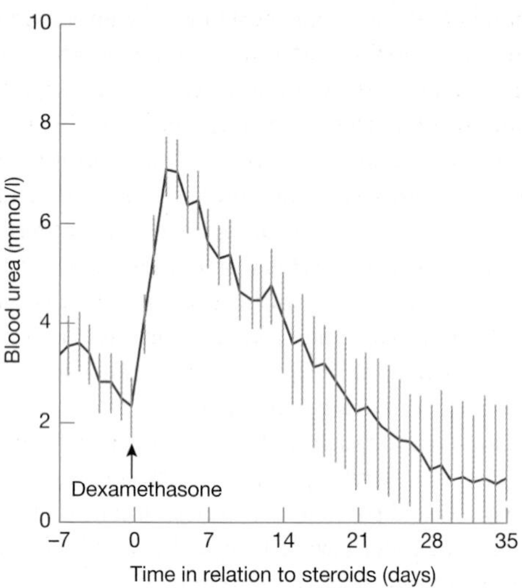

Fig. 2 Percentage change in blood urea concentration of 44 babies plotted against time in relation to the start of steroid treatment. The bars show the 95% confidence intervals.

losses are high, at least partly as a result of low sodium/potassium ATPase activity (Bistritzer *et al.* 1999), with fractional excretion values of around 3–6 and up to 10 per cent in sick infants (Siegel and Oh 1976). Unless the serum sodium concentration is monitored very carefully and appropriate sodium replacement is given, serious hyponatraemia can develop during the course of a few days. Sodium intakes of up to 10 mmol/kg/day may sometimes be required. It is probably advisable, though, to delay sodium supplementation until the normal physiological postnatal water loss has occurred, especially in babies with respiratory problems (Hartnoll *et al.* 2000a,b, 2001). The problem of hyponatraemia can be, and in practice often is, aggravated by excessive water intake, although the ability of the preterm baby's kidney to excrete a water load is relatively good. During intensive care, most VLBW infants require 4–6 mmol/kg/day of sodium. Once the VLBW infant has recovered from the initial problems of adaptation to life outside the womb, the next priority is rapid growth. Continuing excessive urinary losses of sodium prevent normal growth rates from being achieved unless the dietary sodium intake is adequate. Breast milk contains insufficient sodium for many growing VLBW babies and often needs to be supplemented. Special formula feeds for VLBW babies, which contain extra sodium, are in common use.

The concentrating capacity of the VLBW baby's kidney limits the maximum urine osmolality that can be produced to about 300 mOsm/kg and hypertonic dehydration is common whenever excess fluid losses occur. Large insensible water loss through poorly keratinized immature skin is a major predisposing factor to hypernatraemia, exacerbated by infusions and drugs containing sodium (Flenady and Woodgate 2000). In practice, very careful balancing of fluid and electrolyte intake guided by the results of frequent laboratory tests are necessary if VLBW infants are to maintain normal serum electrolyte concentrations (Henderson and Dear 1993). Fluid and electrolyte input and, if possible, fluid losses and weight change should be monitored closely.

Maintaining normal acid–base balance is major problem for the VLBW infant. The renal threshold for HCO_3 is low (Svenningsen 1974), and a typical value for plasma bicarbonate concentration among healthy VLBW babies is between 15 and 20 mmol/l. The ability of the kidney to produce ammonia and to buffer titratable acid is also limited. These are particular problems for a group of infants who often experience lactic acidosis secondary to tissue hypoxia and hypercarbia secondary to respiratory failure. To avoid a detrimental degree of acidosis, the maintenance of adequate ventilation, haemoglobin concentration, tissue perfusion, and arterial oxygenation are paramount. Sodium bicarbonate infusion is a last resort, but the dangers of giving it have been overestimated and the evidence that it can cause intraventricular haemorrhage is very poor. In order to minimize the impact on extracellular fluid osmolality, sodium bicarbonate is best given by slow infusion at about 1 mmol/kg/h titrated against frequent estimations of blood acid–base status. Sodium bicarbonate infusion is contraindicated when there is significant hypernatraemia or hypercarbia. A late metabolic acidosis is seen in many preterm babies once established on enteral feeds. This is because the acid load in the diet exceeds the renal acidification capacity (Manz *et al.* 1997). This may respond to dietary manipulation (Kalhoff *et al.* 1997a) or can be treated with sodium bicarbonate supplementation (Kalhoff *et al.* 1997b).

Renal calcium excretion is reported to be greater in VLBW babies than in more mature infants, and this predisposes to both inadequate bone mineralization, nephrocalcinosis (Jones *et al.* 1997; Saarela *et al.* 1999; Schell-Feith *et al.* 2000; Narendra *et al.* 2001) and stone formation (Shukla *et al.* 2001). Bone mineral content can best be improved by close attention to the supply of phosphate and the ratio of calcium to phosphate in the diet. As long as calcium and phosphate are incorporated into bone at a satisfactory rate, renal losses are minimized. Excess renal losses may be aggravated by the use of diuretics and respiratory stimulant drugs such as caffeine.

About 8 per cent of VLBW babies are reported to enter a state of acute renal failure during intensive care (Stapleton *et al.* 1987). Renal failure is defined by oliguria (<0.5 ml/kg/h) and an increasing blood creatinine concentration (Brocklebank 1988). Renal failure in this group of infants is commonly secondary to impaired renal perfusion as a result of systemic hypotension. The prognosis is generally good if the situation is recognized at an early stage and measures are taken to improve renal perfusion and to control fluid and electrolyte intake. The most acute danger is from cardiac arrhythmia secondary to hyperkalaemia and acidosis, particularly in babies who are very bruised and have been asphyxiated during birth. This problem is seen much less commonly than previously, probably as a consequence of better obstetric care. In our practice, we treat about 140 VLBW babies annually and have to resort to peritoneal dialysis or haemofiltration less than once a year.

Clinical renal problems in the term infant

Severe primary renal disease is rare compared with compromised renal function or acute renal failure secondary to other illnesses.

Congenital renal disease

The recognition of renal problems in the fetus has been revolutionized by fetal ultrasound. Routine ultrasound examination, usually performed at about week 18 of gestation, is now expected to detect most major problems of urinary tract morphology. Bilateral renal agenesis, or complete obstruction to urinary flow with secondary renal dysplasia, results in oligohydramnios with characteristic sequelae: Potter's facies with low-set ears and flattening of the nose and facial features, accompanied by joint and limb contractures. Associated pulmonary hypoplasia makes this condition lethal. Other forms of renal dysplasia may result from abnormal interaction of the two components of the embryonic kidney. In health, early in embryogenesis, the mesonephros (destined to become the collecting tubules, calyces, pelvis, and ureter) forms a ureteric bud, which invades the metanephros and divides. This process appears to be important in inducing normal nephronogenesis in the metanephros from weeks 20 to 36 of gestation (Thomas 1990). Failure of this process may result in renal tissue with little or no function. The most common form, unilateral multicystic dysplasia, results in a non-functional kidney which characteristically shows progressive atrophy in the fetus and in early childhood. Occasionally, these kidneys may become cystic and require surgical removal.

Fetal ultrasound also detects dilatation of the upper or lower renal tract. Urethral valves occur in the male fetus and cause bladder enlargement and hypertrophy, and often hydronephrosis. Clinically, the picture of renal function in the boy varies from one of renal failure to intense polyuria once obstruction is overcome by catheterization. The management is surgical. Associated renal dysplasia is common. Fifty per cent of boys with valves will develop chronic renal failure in childhood, a prognosis that is not altered by the choice of surgical management (Reinberg *et al.* 1992).

On antenatal ultrasound, pelviureteric obstruction may be suggested by renal pelvic dilatation, while vesicoureteric reflux is suggested by the presence of hydroureter. These conditions characteristically do not produce symptoms in the neonatal period. Their detection allows immediate investigation and presymptomatic surgical intervention when indicated and medical treatment to minimize the adverse effects of urinary tract infection. Initial enthusiasm for fetal intervention has been tempered by poor results and it is rarely indicated. The true impact of prenatal detection upon long-term natural history has yet to be established.

Overall, about 60 per cent of fetuses noted to have a urological 'abnormality' prove to have a normal renal tract. Amongst this group, many have a moderately dilated extrarenal pelvis, whilst in others the high urinary flow rates in fetal life produce dilatation that is not seen after birth. The most common significant lesions are unilateral cystic dysplasia, vesicoureteric reflux, and pelviureteric obstruction (Newell *et al.* 1990). Attempts to define the sensitivity of fetal renal ultrasound suggest great variation according to diagnosis: less than 50 per cent of significant vesicoureteric reflux, but up to 95 per cent of pelviureteric obstruction, are detected (Atkins and Hey 1991).

Other rare congenital renal conditions, not always amenable to fetal diagnosis, include polycystic disease, nephrogenic diabetes insipidus, congenital nephrotic syndrome, renal tubular acidosis, and other conditions associated with abnormal patterns of excretion and inborn errors of metabolism (Modi *et al.* 1999). Congenital renal disease should prompt a search for extrarenal anomalies.

Acquired renal disease

Acquired severe renal problems are almost always the consequence of hypotension, circulatory collapse, or hypoxia. This pattern of acute renal failure is particularly well recognized in association with hypoxic ischaemic encephalopathy following a period of birth asphyxia. Here, renal function over the first day is closely related to the magnitude of the insult and is one of the clinical features that can be used to predict eventual neurological outcome (Perlman and Tack 1988). Acute renal failure following hypotension or hypoxia also occurs in a wide spectrum of other illnesses, notably the severe neonatal infections.

The clinical picture of acute renal failure is characterized by oliguria with a urine output less than 1 ml/kg/h, uraemia, hyperkalaemia, metabolic acidosis, and often haematuria. The sick infant is characteristically catabolic, has increased circulating amino acids, and requires full intensive care, all adding to the clinical problem of managing the renal failure. Management is principally supportive. A fluid challenge may be given initially with or without frusemide. If there is no response, total daily fluid intake is reduced, while at the same time circulating volume and peripheral perfusion are maintained with colloid and inotropes as indicated clinically. Low-dose dopamine at 2–5 μg/kg/min may improve renal perfusion.

The neonatal kidney has a remarkable ability to recover, even after a period of sustained anuria, and in most cases close attention to fluid and electrolyte intake and circulatory support is all that is required. Acidosis may require the judicious use of bicarbonate. Hyperkalaemia can be managed with dextrose insulin infusions, intravenous salbutamol, or ion exchange resins but ECG changes are unusual in the newborn with potassium levels less than 8 mmol/l. Dialysis is indicated when fluid and electrolyte homeostasis cannot be maintained in an infant who has the potential for recovery. Fortunately, it is rarely needed.

Urinary tract infection can be treated successfully with antibiotics and is an indication for ultrasound assessment of renal anatomy. Renal vein thrombosis is an unusual but important acquired condition that may occur spontaneously in the term or preterm infant, but is well recognized for its association with congenital heart disease, polycythaemia, maternal diabetes, or other conditions leading to increased serum osmolality. Renal vein thrombosis results in the clinical triad of an abdominal mass, haematuria, and thrombocytopenia with renal dysfunction. Again, the management is usually conservative, although heparin may be beneficial to long-term outcome and underlying thrombophilic disorders should be considered (Lawson *et al.* 1999; Zigman *et al.* 2000).

Assessment of renal function in the newborn

Formal evaluation of renal function is undertaken relatively rarely during the first month of life, partly because many conventional tests are difficult to perform or evaluate and partly because most renal problems at this age are either gross or undetectable until the child is older.

Glomerular filtration rate

The GFR is usually assessed by endogenous creatinine clearance, and this method is reasonably reliable, even in preterm infants (Falcao *et al.* 1999), as long as the collection of urine is performed efficiently. There is a good correlation between GFR as measured by creatinine and inulin clearance (Brion *et al.* 1986). Beyond the first week of life, when the initial decline from the maternal serum creatinine concentration is complete, the baby's serum creatinine concentration correlates quite well with the GFR. Blood urea concentration is a poor guide to GFR but quite a good guide to the state of hydration and of metabolism. GFR in the newborn is better expressed in relation to weight than to surface area (Coulthard and Hey 1984).

Fractional excretion of sodium

The FE_{Na} is calculated as

$$FE_{Na} = U_{Na} \times S_{Cr} S_{Na} \times U_{Cr} \times 100$$

where S_{Cr} and S_{Na} are the serum concentrations of creatinine and sodium, respectively, and U_{Cr} and U_{Na} are their respective urine concentrations. The same methodology can be used to derive the fractional excretion of other substances. Figure 3 shows the FE_{Na} and phosphate at different gestations. The values for the least mature infants should be interpreted with some caution because of the influence of disease and therapy.

The urinary sodium–potassium ratio is a useful index of the renal response to aldosterone. During infancy urinary sodium usually exceeds urinary potassium, but this relationship may be changed in a situation of sodium deficiency prior to a reduction in the serum sodium. In response to sodium deficit aldosterone increases, enhancing sodium reabsorption and tubular potassium excretion. Therefore, a urinary sodium–potassium ratio that is less than unity suggests a state of sodium depletion. In the early neonatal period, serum aldosterone is greater than it is in adults and children, and urinary sodium–potassium ratios may be greater than unity. In the preterm infant, the ratio tends to be greater (Aperia *et al.* 1979). However, the interpretation of urinary electrolyte results is often difficult, and may not be possible for a spot urine sample taken outside the steady state, particularly in the presence of agents that may be natriuretic.

Urinary calcium excretion

Urinary calcium excretion can be estimated in terms of the calcium–creatinine ratio on spot samples of urine. The ratio is generally greater in infants than in older children or adults and is higher in preterm than in term infants (Karlén *et al.* 1985). Normal values are shown in Fig. 4.

Concentrating capacity

Urine osmolality can be measured following intranasal administration of an ADH analogue (Svenningsen and Aronson 1974). The test is rarely employed in the newborn. Figure 5 shows some interesting data on the development of urine concentrating capacity.

Urinary acidification

Urine pH changes in response to plasma bicarbonate concentration (Torrado *et al.* 1974), and urinary acidification can be assessed by simultaneously measuring urine pH and plasma bicarbonate concentration (Guignard 1987) under stable conditions.

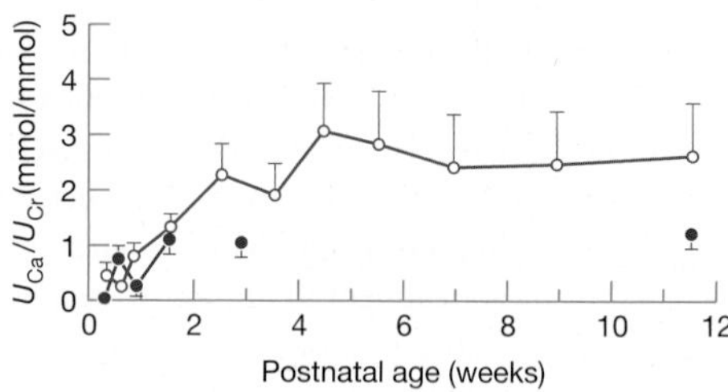

Fig. 4 Urinary calcium–creatinine ratio in preterm (○) and full-term (●) infants. The bars represent ±SEM (reproduced with permission from Karlén *et al.* 1985).

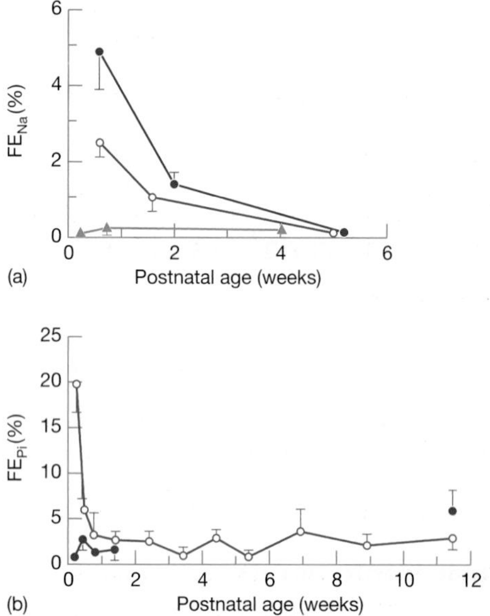

Fig. 3 Fractional urinary sodium in infants with a gestational age of 25–30 weeks (●), 31–34 weeks (○) and full-term infants (▲) in relation to postnatal age. The bars represent ±SEM (reproduced with permission from Vanpee *et al.* 1993).

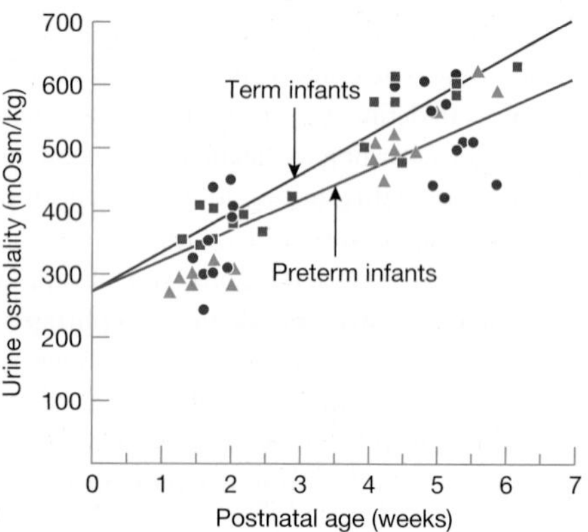

Fig. 5 Postnatal development of renal concentrating capacity, that is, maximum response after DDAVP test, during the first 6 weeks of life: (■) term infants (group I); (●) preterm infants (group II); (▲) asphyxiated infants (group III) (reproduced with permission from Svenningsen and Aronson 1974).

References

Aizman, R., Grahnquist, L., and Celsi, G. (1998). Potassium homeostasis: ontogenic aspects. *Acta Paediatrica* **87** (6), 609–617.

Andriani, G., Persico, A., Tursini, S., Ballone, E., Cirotti, D., and Lelli, C. P. (2001). The renal-resistive index from the last 3 months of pregnancy to 6 months old. *BJU International* **87** (6), 562–564.

Aperia, A., Broberger, O., Herin, P., and Zetterström, R. (1979). Sodium excretion in relation to sodium intake and aldosterone excretion in newborn preterm and full-term infants. *Acta Paediatrica Scandinavica* **68**, 813–817.

Arant, B. S., Jr. (1978). Developmental patterns of renal functional maturation compared in the human neonate. *Journal of Pediatrics* **92** (5), 705–712.

Arant, B. S. (1987). Postnatal development of renal function during the first year of life. *Paediatric Nephrology* **1**, 308–313.

Atkins, A. F. J. and Hey, E. N. The northern region fetal anomaly survey. In *Antenatal Diagnosis of Fetal Anomalies* (ed. J. O. Drife and D. Donnai), pp. 13–34. London: Springer Verlag, 1991.

Bistritzer, T., Berkovitch, M., Rappoport, M. J., Evans, S., Arieli, S., Goldberg, M., Tavori, I., and Aladjem, M. (1999). Sodium potassium adenosine triphosphatase activity in preterm and term infants and its possible role in sodium homeostasis during maturation. *Archives of Diseases in Childhood. Fetal and Neonatal Edition* **81** (3), F184–F187.

Bokenkamp, A., Domanetzki, M., Zinck, R., Schumann, G., and Brodehl, J. (1998). Reference values for cystatin C serum concentrations in children. *Pediatric Nephrology* **12** (2), 125–129.

Brion, L. P., Fleischman, A. R., McCarton, C., and Schwartz, G. J. (1986). A simple estimate of glomerular filtration rate in low birthweight infants during the first year of life: non-invasive assessment of body composition and growth. *Journal of Pediatrics* **109**, 698–707.

Brocklebank, J. T. (1988). Renal failure in the newly born. *Archives of Diseases in Childhood* **63**, 991–994.

Brownlee, K. G., Ng, P. C., Henderson, M. H., Smith, M., Green, J. H., and Dear, P. R. F. (1992). The catabolic effect of dexamethasone in the preterm baby. *Archives of Disease in Childhood* **67**, 1–4.

Cagdas, A., Aydinli, K., Irez, T., Temizyurek, K., and Apak, M. Y. (2000). Evaluation of the fetal kidney maturation by assessment of amniotic fluid alpha-1 microglobulin levels. *European Journal of Obstetrics, Gynecology and Reproductive Biology* **90** (1), 55–61.

Casey, B. M., McIntire, D. D., Bloom, S. L., Lucas, M. J., Santos, R., Twickler, D. M., Ramus, R. M., and Leveno, K. J. (2000). Pregnancy outcomes after antepartum diagnosis of oligohydramnios at or beyond 34 weeks' gestation [see comments]. *American Journal of Obstetrics & Gynecology* **182** (4), 909–912.

Chamaa, N. S., Mosig, D., Drukker, A., and Guignard, J. P. (2000). The renal hemodynamic effects of ibuprofen in the newborn rabbit. *Pediatric Research* **48** (5), 600–605.

Chevalier, R. L. (2001). The moth and the aspen tree: sodium in early postnatal development. *Kidney International* **59** (5), 1617–1625.

Coulthard, M. G. (1985). Maturation of glomerular filtration in preterm and mature babies. *Early Human Development* **11** (3–4), 281–292.

Coulthard, M. G. and Hey, E. N. (1984). Weight as the best standard for glomerular filtration in the newborn. *Archives of Diseases in Childhood* **59** (4), 373–375.

Edwards, B. R. Postnatal development of urinary concentrating ability in rats. Changes in renal anatomy and neurohypophysial hormones. In *The Kidney during Development: Morphology and Function* (ed. A. Spitzer), pp. 223–240. New York: Masson, 1982.

Elbourne, I., Lumbers, E. R., and Hill, K. J. (1990). The secretion of organic acids and bases by the ovine fetal kidney. *Experimental Physiology* **75**, 211–221.

Engle, W. D. (1985). Sodium balance in the growing preterm infant. *Pediatric Research* **19**, 376.

Engle, W. D. and Arant, B. S. (1983). Renal handling of beta-2 microglobulin in the human neonate. *Kidney International* **24**, 358.

Falcao, M. C., Okay, Y., and Ramos, J. L. (1999). Relationship between plasma creatinine concentration and glomerular filtration in preterm newborn infants. *Revista do Hospital das Clinicas* **54** (4), 121–126.

Finney, H., Newman, D. J., Thakkar, H., Fell, J. M., and Price, C. P. (2000). Reference ranges for plasma cystatin C and creatinine measurements in premature infants, neonates, and older children. *Archives of Diseases in Childhood* **82** (1), 71–75.

Flenady, V. J. and Woodgate, P. G. (2000). Radiant warmers versus incubators for regulating body temperature in newborn infants. *Cochrane Database of Systematic Reviews* **2**, CD000435 (review with 6 references).

Fomon, S. J. and Ziegler, E. E. (1999). Renal solute load and potential renal solute load in infancy. *Journal of Pediatrics* **134** (1), 11–14.

Forbes, G. B. *Human Body Composition—Growth, Ageing, Nutrition and Activity.* New York: Springer-Verlag, 1987, pp. 23–27.

Gallini, F., Maggio, L., Romagnoli, C., Marrocco, G., and Tortorolo, G. (2000). Progression of renal function in preterm neonates with gestational age < or = 32 weeks. *Pediatric Nephrology* **15** (1–2), 119–124.

Guignard, J. P. Neonatal nephrology. In *Paediatric Nephrology* 2nd edn. (ed. M. A. Holliday, T. M. Barratt, and R. L. Vernier), pp. 921–944. Baltimore, MD: Williams and Wilkins, 1987.

Hackett, G. A., Nicolaides, K. H., and Campbell, S. (1987). Doppler ultrasound assessment of fetal and uteroplacental circulations in severe second trimester oligohydramnios. *British Journal of Obstetrics and Gynaecology* **94**, 1074–1077.

Harmoinen, A., Ylinen, E., Ala-Houhala, M., Janas, M., Kaila, M., and Kouri, T. (2000). Reference intervals for cystatin C in pre- and full-term infants and children. *Pediatric Nephrology* **15** (1–2), 105–108.

Hartnoll, G., Betremieux, P., and Modi, N. (2000a). Randomised controlled trial of postnatal sodium supplementation on body composition in 25 to 30 week gestational age infants. *Archives of Diseases in Childhood. Fetal and Neonatal Edition* **82** (1), F24–F28.

Hartnoll, G., Betremieux, P., and Modi, N. (2000b). Randomised controlled trial of postnatal sodium supplementation on oxygen dependency and body weight in 25–30 week gestational age infants. *Archives of Diseases in Childhood. Fetal and Neonatal Edition* **82** (1), F19–F23.

Hartnoll, G., Betremieux, P., and Modi, N. (2001). Randomised controlled trial of postnatal sodium supplementation in infants of 25–30 weeks gestational age: effects on cardiopulmonary adaptation. *Archives of Diseases in Childhood. Fetal and Neonatal Edition* **85** (1), F29–F32.

Haycock, G. B. and Aperia, A. (1991). Salt and the newborn kidney. *Pediatric Nephrology* **5** (1), 65–70.

Henderson, M. J. and Dear, P. R. F. (1993). Role of the clinical biochemistry laboratory in the management of very low birthweight infants. *Annals of Clinical Biochemistry* **30**, 341–354.

Hoy, W. E., Rees, M., Kile, E., Mathews, J. D., and Wang, Z. (1999). A new dimension to the Barker hypothesis: low birthweight and susceptibility to renal disease. *Kidney International* **56** (3), 1072–1077.

Jones, C. A., King, S., Shaw, N. J., and Judd, B. A. (1997). Renal calcification in preterm infants: follow up at 4–5 years. *Archives of Diseases in Childhood. Fetal and Neonatal Edition* **76** (3), F185–F189.

Kalhoff, H., Diekmann, L., Hettrich, B., Rudloff, S., Stock, G. J., and Manz, F. (1997a). Modified cow's milk formula with reduced renal acid load preventing incipient late metabolic acidosis in premature infants. *Journal of Pediatric Gastroenterology and Nutrition* **25** (1), 46–50.

Kalhoff, H., Diekmann, L., Kunz, C., Stock, G. J., and Manz, F. (1997b). Alkali therapy versus sodium chloride supplement in low birthweight infants with incipient late metabolic acidosis. *Acta Paediatrica* **86** (1), 96–101.

Karlén, J., Aperia, A., and Zetterström, R. (1985). Renal excretion of calcium and phosphate in preterm and term infants. *Journal of Paediatrics* **106**, 814–819.

Kesby, J. G. and Lumbers, E. R. (1986). Factors affecting renal handling of sodium, hydrogen ions and bicarbonate by the fetus. *American Journal of Physiology* **251**, F226–F231.

Kluckow, M. and Evans, N. (2001). Low systemic blood flow and hyperkalemia in preterm infants. *Journal of Pediatrics* **139** (2), 227–232.

Kusuda, S., Kim, T. J., Miyagi, N., Shishida, N., Iitani, H., Tanaka, Y., and Yamairi, T. (1999). Postnatal change of renal artery blood flow velocity and its relationship with urine volume in very low birth weight infants during the first month of life. *Journal of Perinatal Medicine* **27** (2), 107–111.

Lackland, D. T., Bendall, H. E., Osmond, C., Egan, B. M., and Barker, D. J. (2000). Low birth weights contribute to high rates of early-onset chronic renal failure in the Southeastern United States. *Archives of Internal Medicine* **160** (10), 1472–1476.

Lackland, D. T., Egan, B. M., Fan, Z. J., and Syddall, H. E. (2001). Low birth weight contributes to the excess prevalence of end-stage renal disease in African Americans. *Journal of Clinical Hypertension (Greenwich.)* **3** (1), 29–31.

Lawson, S. E., Butler, D., Enayat, M. S., and Williams, M. D. (1999). Congenital thrombophilia and thrombosis: a study in a single centre. *Archives of Diseases in Childhood* **81** (2), 176–178.

Lin, G. J. and Cher, T. W. (1997). Renal vascular resistance in normal children—a color Doppler study. *Pediatric Nephrology* **11** (2), 182–185.

Liu, W., Morimoto, T., Kondo, Y., Iinuma, K., Uchida, S., and Imai, M. (2001). 'Avian-type' renal medullary tubule organization causes immaturity of urine-concentrating ability in neonates. *Kidney International* **60** (2), 680–693.

Lumbers, E. R. (1988). Proximal and distal tubular activity in chronically catheterised fetal sheep compared with the adult. *Canadian Journal of Physiology and Pharmacology* **66**, 697.

Manalich, R., Reyes, L., Herrera, M., Melendi, C., and Fundora, I. (2000). Relationship between weight at birth and the number and size of renal glomeruli in humans: a histomorphometric study. *Kidney International* **58** (2), 770–773.

Manz, F., Kalhoff, H., and Remer, T. (1997). Renal acid excretion in early infancy. *Pediatric Nephrology* **11** (2), 231–243.

Miall, L. S., Henderson, M. J., Turner, A. J., Brownlee, K. G., Brocklebank, J. T., Newell, S. J., and Allgar, V. L. (1999). Plasma creatinine rises dramatically in the first 48 hours of life in preterm infants. *Pediatrics* **104** (6), e76.

Modi, N., Mouriquand, P., and Wilcox, D. Disorders of the kidneys and urinary tract. In *Textbook of Neonatology* 3rd edn. (ed. J. M. Rennie and N. R. C. Roberton), pp. 1009–1050. Edinburgh. Churchill Livingstone, 1999.

Muller-Suur, R. (1983). Evidence for tubuloglomerular feedback in juxtamedullary nephrons of young rats. *American Journal of Physiology* **224**, F425–F427.

Narendra, A., White, M. P., Rolton, H. A., Alloub, Z. I., Wilkinson, G., McColl, J. H., and Beattie, J. (2001). Nephrocalcinosis in preterm babies. *Archives of Diseases in Childhood. Fetal and Neonatal Edition* **85** (3), F207–F213.

Newell, S. J. *et al.* (1990). Clinical significance of antenatal calyceal dilatation detected by ultrasound. *Lancet* **336**, 372.

Perlman, J. M. and Tack, E. D. (1988). Renal injury in the asphyxiated newborn infant: relationship to neurologic outcome. *Journal of Pediatrics* **113**, 875–879.

Pokharel, R. P., Uetani, Y., Tsuneishi, S., and Nakamura, H. (1997). Neonatal renal artery blood flow velocities using color Doppler ultrasonography. *The Kobe Journal of Medical Sciences* **43** (1), 1–12.

Potter, E. L. (1965). Development of the human glomerulus. *Archives of Pathology* **80**, 241–255.

Rabinowitz, R., Peters, M. T., Vyas, S., Campbell, S., and Nicolaides, K. H. (1989). Measurement of fetal urine production in normal pregnancy by real-time ultrasonography. *American Journal of Obstetrics and Gynecology* **161**, 1264–1266.

Reinberg, Y., de Castano, I., and Gonzalez, R. (1992). Prognosis for patients with prenatally diagnosed posterior urethral valves. *Journal of Urology* **148** (1), 125–126.

Rudd, P. T., Hughes, E. A., Placzek, M. M., and Hodes, D. T. (1983). Reference ranges for plasma creatinine during the first month of life. *Archives of Diseases in Childhood* **58** (3), 212–215.

Saarela, T., Vaarala, A., Lanning, P., and Koivisto, M. (1999). Incidence, ultrasonic patterns and resolution of nephrocalcinosis in very low birthweight infants. *Acta Paediatrica* **88** (6), 655–660.

Schell-Feith, E. A., Kist-Van Holthe, J. E., Conneman, N., van Zwieten, P. H., Holscher, H. C., Zonderland, H. M., Brand, R., and van der Heijden, B. J. (2000). Etiology of nephrocalcinosis in preterm neonates: association of nutritional intake and urinary parameters. *Kidney International* **58** (5), 2102–2110.

Seri, I., Abbasi, S., Wood, D. C., and Gerdes, J. S. (1998). Regional hemodynamic effects of dopamine in the sick preterm neonate. *Journal of Pediatrics* **133** (6), 728–734.

Shukla, A. R., Hoover, D. L., Homsy, Y. L., Perlman, S., Schurman, S., and Reisman, E. M. (2001). Urolithiasis in the low birth weight infant: the role and efficacy of extracorporeal shock wave lithotripsy. *Journal of Urology* **165** (6 Pt 2), 2320–2323.

Siegel, S. R. and Oh, W. (1976). Renal function as a marker of human fetal maturation. *Acta Paediatrica Scandinavica* **65**, 481.

Smith, F. G. and Lumbers, E. R. (1989). Comparison of renal function in term fetal sheep and newborn lambs. *Biology of the Neonate* **55** (4–5), 309–316.

Spencer, J., Wang, Z., and Hoy, W. (2001). Low birth weight and reduced renal volume in Aboriginal children. *American Journal of Kidney Diseases* **37** (5), 915–920.

Stapleton, F. B., Jones, D. P., and Green, R. S. (1987). Acute renal failure in neonates: incidence, etiology and outcome. *Pediatric Nephrology* **1**, 314–320.

Svenningsen, N. W. (1974). Renal acid–base titration studies in infants with and without metabolic acidosis in the neonatal period. *Pediatric Research* **8**, 659–665.

Svenningsen, N. W. and Aronson, A. S. (1974). Postnatal development of renal concentrating capacity as estimated by DDAVP-test in normal and asphyxiated neonates. *Biology of the Neonate* **25**, 230–41.

Thomas, D. F. M. (1990). Fetal uropathy. *British Journal of Urology* **66**, 225–231.

Torrado, A., Guignard, J. P., Prod'hom, L. S., and Gautier, E. (1974). Hypoxaemia and renal function in newborns with respiratory distress syndrome. *Helvetica Paediatrica Acta* **29**, 399–403.

Toth-Heyn, P., Drukker, A., and Guignard, J. P. (2000). The stressed neonatal kidney: from pathophysiology to clinical management of neonatal vasomotor nephropathy. *Pediatric Nephrology* **14** (3), 227–239.

Tsukahara, H., Hata, I., Sekine, K., Miura, M., Kotsuji, F., and Mayumi, M. (1998). Renal water channel expression in newborns: measurement of urinary excretion of aquaporin-2. *Metabolism* **47** (11), 1344–1347.

van den Anker, J. N. (1996). Pharmacokinetics and renal function in preterm infants. *Acta Paediatrica* **85** (12), 1393–1399.

Vanpee, M., Ergander, U., and Aperia, A. (1993). Renal function in sick, very low birthweight infants. *Acta Paediatrica* **82** (9), 714–718.

Wilkins, B. H. (1992). Renal function in sick very low birthweight infants: 1. Glomerular filtration rate. *Archives of Diseases in Childhood* **67** (10), 1140–1145.

Wintour, E. M., Bell, R. J., Congui, M., Macisaac, R. J., and Wang, X. (1985). The value of urine osmolality as an index of stress in the ovine fetus. *Journal of Developmental Physiology* **7**, 347–354.

Wiriyathian, S., Rosenfeld, C. R., Arant, B. S., Porter, J. C., Faucher, D. J., and Engle, W. D. (1986). Urinary arginine vasopressin: pattern of excretion in the neonatal period. *Pediatric Research* **20**, 103–108.

Zigman, A., Yazbeck, S., Emil, S., and Nguyen, L. (2000). Renal vein thrombosis: a 10-year review. *Journal of Pediatric Surgery* **35** (11), 1540–1542.

1.5 The ageing kidney

Juan F. Macías-Núñez and J. Stewart Cameron

Years steal Fire from the mind as vigour from the limb

Lord Byron: *Childe Harold's Pilgrimage*, 1812–1818

Old age isn't so bad when you consider the alternative

Maurice Chevalier, 1960

Introduction

As the proportion of elderly citizens in Western populations increases, so a greater and greater proportion of patients seen in nephrological services can be described as either 'young-elderly' (over 65 years) or 'elderly-elderly' (over 75–80 years). However, senescence must never be equated with illness. Ageing has been described as a universal, intrinsic, progressive, multifactorial, multiform, heterogeneous, and asynchronous physiological process, modulated by racial, inherited, environmental, dietetic, and health-care factors (Grimley Evans and Bond 1997). The asynchrony is of particular interest due to its importance in the interpretation of many of the physiological and biochemical aspects of ageing. For example, in aged animals, the activity of medullary collecting tubule (MCT) Na^+,K^+ATPase is 37 per cent lower than in young animals, but the activity of H^+,K^+ATPase in MCT and cortical collecting tubule (CCT) is markedly *increased* in the aged (Eiam-Ong *et al.* 2002).

Moreover, the relationship between 'normal' and 'abnormal' in the elderly—and in turn, the relationship of these alterations in function to pathology—is a complex one. For example, although the mean glomerular filtration rate (GFR) in all cross-sectional studies of elderly individuals decreases with age, this is shown by longitudinal studies (Lindeman 1990) to be the result of a range of individual profiles, some of which show retention of renal function appropriate in the young into great age, others declining steeply, as an example of the increasing heterogeneity of the elderly mentioned above. In general, those individuals whose GFR declines have, in general, higher mean blood pressures, and often vascular pathology. Is this to be regarded as part of 'normal' ageing, despite the strong evidence that this rise in mean blood pressure with age is in fact the result of cultural and dietary factors? Thus, the definition of what constitutes 'normal' elderly subjects for studies of function becomes blurred and controversial.

A number of hypotheses have been put forward which attempt to explain ageing in whole or in part. Among them are the exogenous or environmental hypotheses, based on the action of free radicals, accumulation of advanced glycosylation products (AGEs), or accumulation of damaged macromolecules. Others claim that ageing is principally programmed by genetic information. The ageing process is regulated by certain genes, but there are other hypotheses that postulate that genes themselves are damaged by external factors that will induce codon restriction, inactivation of sequential iterative genes, and telomere shortening or apoptotic unbalance (López-Novoa and Rodríguez-Puyol 1997). These two possibilities have been studied recently by Melk *et al.* (2000), Arnel and Gollapudi (2001), and Benetos *et al.* (2001).

The major characteristic of ageing physiology is that renal function is adequate to maintain equilibrium under normal circumstances, but shows a progressive inability to achieve a maximum response when faced with a challenge, compounded by a slower rate of adaptation (Fuiano *et al.* 2001). Although there is a widespread belief that *all* renal functions in the aged inexorably decline, again there is heterogeneity. For example, in healthy aged humans, the renal vascular response to an upright posture seems impaired with increasing age, but does not differ from the young under conditions of normal sodium intake and euvolaemia (Adachi *et al.* 2001). In contrast, medullary oxygenation after furosemide administration increases in the young, but is blunted in aged women (Epstein and Prasad 2000). The GFR of only some aged individuals declines (Lindeman *et al.* 1985; Fliser *et al.* 1997a,b, and see below) although the mean value for the population may fall.

Since the first morphological description in aged accident victims dating from 1933 (De Leon *et al.* 1933), numerous studies have addressed the anatomy, physiology, and function of the ageing kidney in humans (Epstein 1996; Fliser *et al.* 1997a,b; Van den Noortgate *et al.* 2001) or in animals (Baylis and Corman 1998).

Anatomy of the ageing kidney (McLachlan 1987)

Macroscopic changes

The normal aged kidney has a smooth or a sometimes finely granular surface. Renal weight decreases 20–30 per cent between the age of 30 and 90 years, from between 200 and 270 g to between 180 and 200 g (De Leon *et al.* 1933; Tauchi *et al.* 1971; Brown *et al.* 1986), whilst renal length diminishes by 2 cm between the age of 50 and 80 years, which represents an equivalent loss of volume of around 40 per cent (McLachlan 1987). The loss of substance affects the cortex more than the medulla. Fat in the renal sinus increases with age.

Glomeruli

Although the total number of glomeruli diminishes from the usual figure of about 1.3 million per kidney to half or two-thirds this number in the seventh decade as the kidney ages (McLachlan *et al.* 1977) (Fig. 1), the scatter of data at all ages is very large, and thus many aged

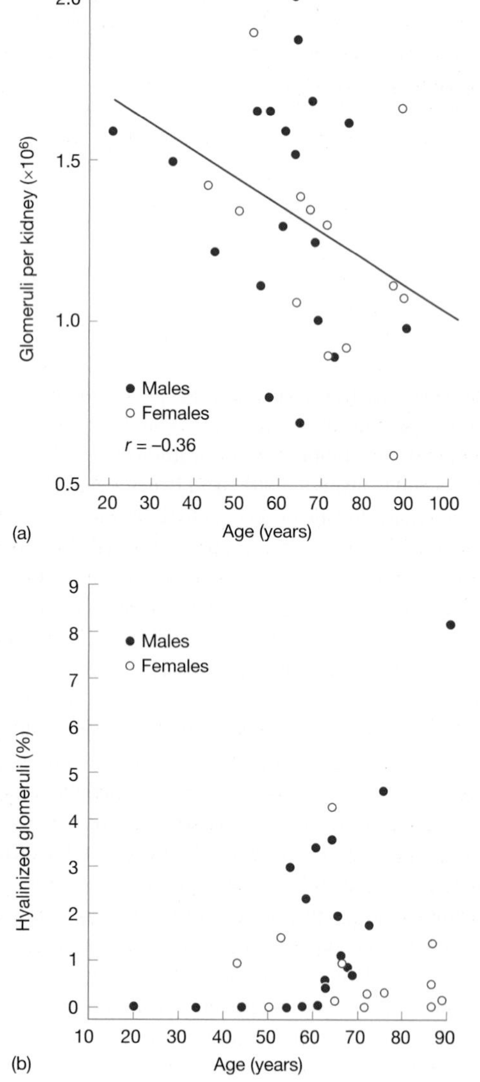

Fig. 1 (a) The number of glomeruli in human kidneys [reproduced with permission from McLachlan *et al.* (1977)]. There is very wide scatter, but the number of surviving glomeruli tends to decline with age. (b) The proportion of sclerosed glomeruli in the kidney as a function of age (see text for comment).

individuals are within the normal range for younger adults. Some remaining glomeruli appear partially or totally hyalinized or sclerosed. Glomerular sclerosis appears at approximately 30 years of age, the fraction of obsolete glomeruli varying between 1 and 30 per cent in persons aged 50 years or more (Kaplan *et al.* 1975; McLachlan *et al.* 1977; Smith *et al.* 1989; Nyengaard and Bendtsen 1992; Neugarten *et al.* 1999) with no difference with gender, race, or ethnicity. One can calculate the 90th percentile of totally sclerosed glomeruli as follows (Smith *et al.* 1989):

$$\text{90th percentile of obsolete glomeruli} = (\text{patient's age}/2) - 10.$$

Glomerular basement membranes are patchily reduplicated in older kidneys and, in general, thicker than in the young (but see Steffes *et al.* 1983 for a contrary view). On microangiographic examination, there is an obliteration particularly of juxtamedullary nephrons, but not of those sited more peripherally, with the formation of a direct channel between afferent and efferent arterioles in this area of the kidney (Takazakura *et al.* 1972). This differential loss of juxtamedullary glomeruli may play some part in both the impairment of the countercurrent multiplier in aged individuals (see below) and the increase in filtration fraction with age (see below). The mesangium, which accounts for 8 per cent of glomerular volume at 45 years of age, increases to nearly 12 per cent at the age of 70 (Sorensen 1977). At the same time, however, the glomerular cross-sectional area decreases (McLachlan *et al.* 1977), which may account, at least in part, for these data. The lobularity and complexity of the tuft decrease. In any case, the area of filtering surface per surviving glomerulus declines with age.

Protein intake in excess may play some role in the progression of glomerulosclerosis, but this does not mean that low protein intake necessarily prevents glomerular sclerosis in healthy elderly persons, as Lindeman (1991) found no differences in creatinine clearance among healthy vegetarians (low protein intake) and non-vegetarians. Obviously, the marked vascular changes with age could play a part (see below), but a primary involution of the glomeruli, as suggested by Jean Oliver (McLachlan 1987), may also take place; there is only a poor correlation between vascular changes and glomerulosclerosis.

Tubular changes

Tubular cells undergo fatty degeneration with age, showing an irregular thickening of their basal membrane. By microdissection, the existence of diverticula arising from the distal and convoluted tubules becomes more frequent with age. Mean proximal tubular volume decreases with age, from 0.136 to 0.061 mm^3 at the age of 84 years (Darmady *et al.* 1973). In general, as the kidney ages, the reduction in proximal tubular volume closely parallels that of the glomerular volume, so that anatomical glomerulotubular balance is preserved into old age (Darmady *et al.* 1973). As will be seen later, this is not true of all renal functions.

The interstitium

Interstitial changes consist mainly of increasing zones of tubular atrophy and fibrosis (Kappel and Olsen 1980; Fuiano *et al.* 2001), which may relate to the defects in concentration and dilution observed as part of the normal ageing process in the kidney (see below). There is a variable interstitial infiltrate of mononuclear cells; whether these are damaging agents or a reparative mechanism (or both) is unknown. Interstitial volume, as noted above, increases with age as a proportion of renal volume.

Renal vessels

The age-related changes in renal vessels have been well documented (Darmady *et al.* 1973). In apparently normal, aged individuals (McLachlan *et al.* 1977), prearterioles, from which afferent arterioles arise, show subendothelial deposition of hyaline and collagen fibres, resulting in an intimal thickening. Changes in arterioles are similar, except that fibrous material is less common. Small arteries exhibit a thickening of the intima due to proliferation of the elastic tissue. In vessels larger than arterioles, there is general agreement that progressive reduplication of elastic tissue and thickening of the intima are predominantly age related. In radiographic studies (Davidson *et al.* 1969) there is increasing tortuosity of the interlobular arteries and abnormalities in the arcuate arteries. As many as one-third of individuals with arteriosclerotic disease over the age of 50 develop clinical hypertension and autopsy studies show significant atherosclerotic stenosis of the main renal arteries (often without associated hypertension) in 49 per cent of individuals (Holley *et al.* 1964). Fuiano *et al.* (2001), in a study in young and old kidney donors found that arteriosclerotic lesions in interlobular and arcuate arteries were statistically greater in the aged, but arteriolar hyalinosis and glomerulosclerosis did not reach a statistically significant difference.

Functional changes in the ageing kidney

Renal plasma flow

Diodrast clearance, as a measure of renal plasma flow decreased from a mean of 613 to 290 ml/min in the ninth decade of life (Davies and Shock 1950), which implies a renal blood flow of about 1150 ml/min declining to 650 ml/min. Wesson (1969) analysed all the then available literature, and showed a reduction of approximately 10 per cent per decade of age in renal plasma flow. *Para*-aminohippurate (PAH) clearance studies such as those of Hollenberg *et al.* (1974) in prospective living kidney donors and Fuiano *et al.* (2001), confirmed these figures (361 ml/min/1.73 m^2 in the aged versus 618 in the young). There is an increase in calculated renal vascular resistance with age (Fliser *et al.* 1997a,b; Adachi *et al.* 2001) and, although the anatomical site of this is not known precisely in humans, it is well known that the calculated filtration fraction increases with age (Davies and Shock 1950). To what extent the reduction in renal perfusion is fixed as a result of anatomical changes or depends on functional changes has been examined by McDonald *et al.* (1951) and Hollenberg *et al.* (1974): response to vasoconstrictor stimulus (angiotensin) was unimpaired in aged individuals, whereas vasodilatation in response to pyrogen or acetylcholine (an endothelium-dependent vasodilator) was blunted, although that in reponse to infusion of aminoacids plus dopamine in 'renal' doses was less so (Fuiano *et al.* 2001).

It should be noted that all these studies depend upon the assumption that the renal tubular extractions of diodrast or PAH do not change with age. If this assumption is untrue, then the fall-off of clearances may exceed the actual fall-off in renal blood flow with age, and calculations of filtration fraction become suspect. Hollenberg *et al.* (1974) also showed a decrease in cortical blood flow, analysed by wash-out curves of radioactive xenon. Medullary flow, in contrast, was relatively well preserved. This decline in renal perfusion could, of course, result totally or in part from a decrease in cardiac output with age, but findings on this point are controversial. Some studies show a reduction in cardiac output in aged persons, whereas some do not (Rodeheffer *et al.* 1984; Lakatta 1987). Danziger *et al.* (1990) found no correlation of either blood pressure or cardiac output in ageing individuals with the reduction in GFR.

Glomerular filtration rate

It has been widely accepted that the GFR declines with age, regardless of the marker used to assess it. However, some recent studies question that the decline in GFR is either universal or inevitable. First, the few longitudinal studies (see below) have revealed some individuals whose GFR remains constant with age, even though the mean GFR of the whole population falls away; and recently Kimmel *et al.* (1996) showed that nutritional situation was of paramount importance at the time of measuring GFR, at least using creatinine clearances. Elderly subjects eating more than 1 g/day of protein/kg had a creatinine clearance in the range of 90–100 ml/min/1.73 m^2, whilst those with a lower protein intake had a lower creatinine clearance.

Inulin clearance

In cross-sectional data (Davies and Shock 1950), the decline in inulin clearance with ageing was from a mean of 122 to a mean of 65 ml/min between 30 and 90 years of age. Wesson (1969) summarized the available literature, from which Fig. 2 is derived, demonstrating the reduction in renal function from age 30 onwards; note that this graph is entirely derived from cross-sectional, not sequential studies; and that the lower limit of inulin clearance (mean − 2SD) for a population of apparently normal 80-year-olds is only 40 ml/min/1.73 m^2. In elderly people, as in prepubertal children, there is no gender difference in GFR.

This reduction in GFR parallels the anatomical changes described in the previous section. The remaining nephrons will thus contain a hyperperfused and hyperfiltering group. Anderson *et al.* (1987) have speculated as to the role of this group in progressive glomerulosclerosis (see Chapter 11.1).

Creatinine clearance, creatinine excretion, and plasma creatinine in the elderly

Using the creatinine clearance as an index of GFR, Kampmann *et al.* (1974) and Rowe *et al.* (1976a) among others (Laine *et al.* 1977) made the same observation in cross-sectional studies that this declines with age (Table 1). One problem is that similar populations were not studied: Rowe *et al.* (1976a) examined apparently healthy aged individuals in the community, whilst Kampmann *et al.* (1974) studied a hospital

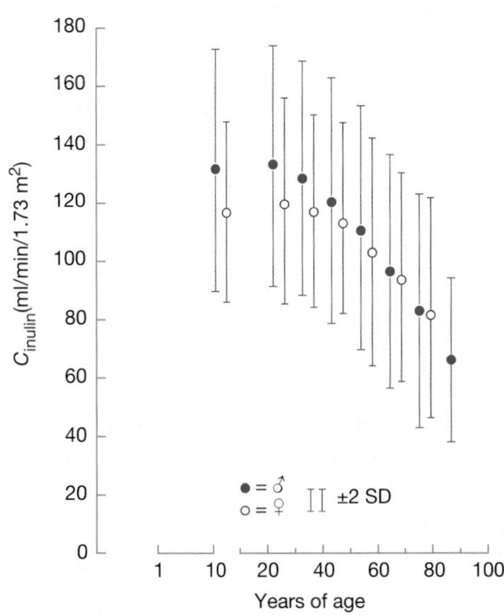

Fig. 2 The inulin clearance in healthy individuals at various ages. Graphical representation of data collected from the literature by Wesson (1969). Note that in older individuals not only does the inulin clearance decline, but the difference between the sexes seen in the young also disappears. [Modified from Macías-Núñez and Cameron (1987) with permission.]

Table 1 The mean creatinine clearance at different ages (ml/min/1.73 m^2)

Age (years)	Denmark (n = 249) ($\bar{x} \pm 2$ SD)	France (n = 1979) ($\bar{x} \pm 2$ SD)	Spain (n = 23) ($\bar{x}$)
20–29	110	107	
30–39	97	104	126
40–49	88	100	
50–59	81	95	
60–69	72	86	91
70–79	64	77	
80–89	47	73	
90–99	34		

Data of Kampmann *et al.* (1974), Laine *et al.* (1977), and Macías-Núñez *et al.* (1981).

population—but they excluded any patient with an increased plasma creatinine. Cockroft and Gault (1976), in deriving their formula (see below) also used hospital patients, but included all individuals, whatever their renal function.

Also, all these studies are cross-sectional (except for some data in the study of Rowe *et al.* 1976a), and not longitudinal. Lindeman *et al.* (1985) have since published an important extended longitudinal study of old people in Baltimore, some of whom were followed with repeat measurements for more than 30 years. Despite a *mean* calculated reduction in creatinine clearance of 0.75 ml/min/year for the whole group, 92 of the 254 individuals studied showed no reduction in creatinine clearance, and a few even increased their clearances (Lindeman 1990). Larsson *et al.* (1986) also found no decline in GFR in individuals between the ages of 70 and 79, although plasma creatinine increased from 91 to 96 μmol/l in women and from 100 to 107 μmol/l in men.

An important practical point is that despite the usual decline in creatinine clearance in otherwise healthy individuals, in the majority of studies, in contrast, there is *no corresponding increase in plasma creatinine with age* (Rowe *et al.* 1976a). Thus, the normal values for plasma creatinine are substantially the same at the ages of 20 and 80 years (Kampmann *et al.* 1974; Rowe *et al.* 1976a) (Table 1), so that the normal plasma creatinine in an aged individual often conceals a profound physiological reduction in GFR. This apparent paradox arises because the production of creatinine, and hence the urinary creatinine output, decreases steadily with age in relation to the decreasing muscle mass and total body weight. The significance of a modestly elevated plasma creatinine in an aged person is thus even greater than in a younger one.

It is clear that plasma creatinine is an inadequate method to estimate GFR in elderly people, since it will systematically overestimate it, in addition to the other factors discussed in Chapter 1.4. Because of this, it is necessary to also take into account age and body weight, and in middle-aged people, gender. Kampmann *et al.* (1974), Cockroft and Gault (1976), and Rowe *et al.* (1976a) have all constructed nomograms that allow a better estimate of GFR in clinical practice from plasma creatinine concentrations. The nomogram of Cockroft and Gault (1976) is the most reliable and most used, although it has been recently questioned due to the fact that it overestimates the decline in GFR, at least in persons aged over 80 years. However, Nicoll *et al.* (1991) found a good correlation in 18 individuals aged 66–82 years with the clearance of [^{99}Tc^{m}] diethylenetriamine penta-acetic acid (DTPA) as the reference.

Keller (1987), using the data of Kampmann *et al.* (1974), pointed out that the simplest formula to estimate the expected normal mean creatinine clearance in ml/min from 25 to 100 years of age is [130 − age (years)]. Although this is true, in general, for older persons, individual variation obtained with any of these formulae may be considerable (Duraković 1986). Despite the reduction in creatinine clearance and GFR in elderly people, the ability to respond with an increase to a protein load ('renal reserve') is relatively undiminished with age, at least up to 80 years (de Santo *et al.* 1991; Böhler *et al.* 1993; Fliser *et al.* 1993).

Plasma β_2-microglobulin and cystatin C concentrations

Unlike creatinine, the plasma concentration of β_2-microglobulin does increase as renal function declines with age (Evrin and Wibell 1972). Even so, there is a great deal of overlap and this method, despite the increased availability of β_2-microglobulin assays, has not been used in clinical practice to any extent in aged people.

Using *cystatin C* as a marker (see Chapter 1.4), Fliser and Ritz (2001) found that cystatin C was higher in the elderly, interpreting this as reflecting a diminished GFR. These data should be treated with caution because as yet there are few data concerning cystatin C in the elderly, but are of great interest because, in several other clinical situations (see Chapter 1.4), the serum concentration of cystatin C is capable of distinguishing decreases of much less than 50 per cent in the GFR.

Radioisotopic methods of GFR measurement

The only radioisotopic method that has been used in the aged is the [^{51}Cr] edetate method, apart from the 18 patients studied by Nicholl *et al.* (1991) using [^{99}Tc ^{m}] DTPA. Granerus and Aurell (1981) give reference values for the single injection method using [^{51}Cr] edetate for young and elderly individuals, which show the expected reduction with age. This decline has been confirmed by Macías-Núñez *et al.* (1981), but Larsson *et al.* (1986) were unable to show any decline in GFR in elderly people between 70 and 79 years of age with this measure of GFR. The mean (±2SD) for GFR in 79-year-olds in this study was 46–94 ml/min/1.73 m^2.

Tubular function

In general, the aged kidney is capable of maintaining plasma electrolyte concentrations (Refoyo and Macías-Núñez 1991) as well as pH (see below) constant under normal circumstances. The functional deficits appearing with age usually relate to a reduction in the total capacity of the kidney to change under stress, and the rate of change in response. Thus, electrolyte disturbances and deterioration of GFR are common in elderly patients admitted to general medical wards (Table 2). These disorders are made more likely by the tendency of elderly people to select a diet low in both sodium and in potassium and the general deterioration in GFR. The importance of nutrition and protein intake in the deterioration of GFR has been documented by Van den Noortgate *et al.* (2001) in patients admitted to an acute ward.

Table 2 Clinical and electrolyte disturbances in elderly patients admitted to a general medical ward

State	Number out of 106 patients[a]
Hyponatraemia	33
Hypokalaemia	33
Hypernatraemia	8
Hyperkalaemia	20
Worsening of pre-existing CRF	51
ARF	29
CRF	20
Obstructive uropathy	18
Glomerulonephritis	6

[a] $n = 106$, mean age 80 (76–93 years); 61 men and 45 women. CRF, chronic renal failure; ARF, acute renal failure. Data of Dr C. Musso.

Table 3 Sodium excretion and plasma sodium on a low sodium diet

	Young ($n = 6$)	Elderly ($n = 6$)	*p*
Plasma Na (mmol/l)	139.5 + 2.0	139.0 ± 2.2	NS
$U_{Na}V$ (mmol/24 h)	66.4 + 42.0	165.5 ± 97.6	<0.05
FE_{Na} (1%)	0.93 + 0.33	1.58 ± 0.71	<0.05

Data of Macías-Núñez *et al.* (1980).

Data after 9 days on a 50 mmol Na^+ diet (mean ± SD).

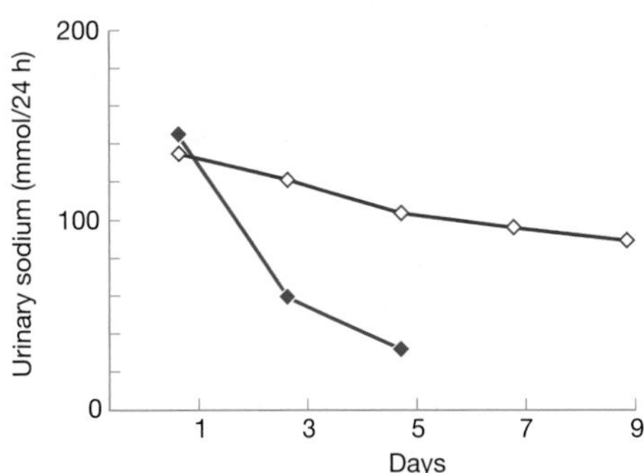

Fig. 3 Effect of a 50 mmol/24 h sodium diet on urinary excretion of sodium of young (closed diamonds) and elderly (open diamonds) individuals. The younger individuals adapted quickly and reached sodium balance within 5 days; the elderly ones failed to reach balance within the 9 days of the study, continuing to excrete more than 100 mmol of sodium per 24 h. [Data of Macías-Núñez et *al.* (1983), reproduced from Macías-Núñez et *al.* (1987) with permission.]

Sodium handling in the aged

In healthy elderly people, the plasma sodium concentration is the same as in younger subjects. As with younger subjects, there is no universal 'normal' urinary sodium output for healthy aged persons, since this depends so much on salt intake which is generally low in the West. Thus, in the elderly in the region of Iwate (Japan), the mean urinary Na output was as high as 236 ± 22 mmol/l/24 h (Adachi 2001), whilst in a collaborative study between the Universities of Catanzaro (Italy) and Oslo (Norway), Fuiano *et al.* (2001) found an excretion of only 115 ± 5.3. In the region of Buenos Aires, under the care of Hospital Italiano, similarly, it was 110 ± 35 mmol (Musso *et al.* 2000) whilst in the province of Salamanca it was 165 ± 97 (Macías-Núñez *et al.* 1980).

Acute studies

Renal responses to acute changes in sodium intake, especially to sodium depletion but also sodium loading, are both blunted. As a result of these slow adaptations, both hypernatraemia (Solomon and Lye 1990) and hyponatraemia (Solomon *et al.* 1992; Roberts and Robinson 1993) are frequent findings in patients on geriatric wards (Tables 2 and 3) (Epstein and Hollenberg 1976; Macías-Núñez *et al.* 1978, 1980). One study, however, showed no difference with age in renal handling of sodium (Karlberg and Tolagen 1977).

The renal response to mild acute sodium restriction differs substantially between young and elderly, well-nourished, healthy people (Fig. 3). The mean half-time for a reduction of Na^+ excretion in response to acute reduction in intake is 17.7 h in persons less than 30 years of age, but extends to 30.9 h in persons older than 60 (Meyer 1989), apparently mediated by the concomitant reduction in GFR. Under basal conditions, plasma sodium was similar in both groups. As the GFR was less in the aged, the amount of filtered sodium would also be less than in young people (Davies and Shock 1950; Sourander 1983). In spite of the decreased sodium tubular load, 24-h urinary sodium output and fractional excretion of sodium were significantly greater in elderly persons (Table 3). This suggests that the renal tubule of the elderly individual is unable to retain sodium adequately, either in absolute terms or when corrected for glomerular filtration.

There are minor discrepancies between studies of acute sodium loading in the elderly, but most researchers suggest that either under basal conditions or during volume expansion, the reponse diminishes with age (Yamada *et al.* 1979; Bengelé *et al.* 1981; Hiraide 1981; Hackbarth and Harrison 1982; Myers *et al.* 1982). The aged take much longer to eliminate the overload than the young, probably due to the diminution of GFR from reduction in glomerular surface area in the aged, in turn as a result of glomerulosclerosis. These differences in sodium handling by the elderly kidney can lead to confusion, for example, when some workers describe hypertension in the aged as 'salt dependent' or 'salt sensitive', because they find that when giving the same amount of salt to young and elderly hypertensive patients, the latter group takes longer to eliminate the extra salt. This is, however, not the result of increased 'avidity' of the ageing renal tubule for salt.

Chronic adaptation to a low sodium diet in the elderly

The capacity of the ageing kidney to adapt chronically to a low salt intake (50 mmol/24 h) is also clearly blunted (Epstein and Hollenberg 1976; Macías-Núñez *et al.* 1978). In the latter study, young people reached sodium balance in 5 days, whereas the elderly participants were unable to reach sodium balance, in spite of a mean loss of 1.3 kg of body weight during the 9 days of 50 mmol/24 h sodium diet (Fig. 3).

Site of loss of sodium regulatory capacity within the nephron

From studies on lithium clearance (which is mainly reabsorbed in the proximal tubule to an extent comparable with the reabsorption of sodium and water, see Chapter 1.4), it is probable that fractional delivery of sodium from the proximal tubule does not alter significantly with age (Schou *et al.* 1986). We measured the sodium excretion when healthy elderly subjects were challenged with a saline load (Macías Núñez *et al.* 1978). This test is believed to be able to discriminate the functional capacity of the 'proximal nephron' from that of the 'distal nephron' (thick ascending limb of the loop of Henle) (see Chapter 1.4 for discussion).

Table 4 shows, in agreement with the data of Schou *et al.* (1986), that the 'proximal nephron' behaved similarly in the young and the elderly participants, whereas in the 'distal nephron' a clear-cut difference in the handling of sodium in the elderly was evident, with a significantly lower percentage of sodium reabsorption at a distal site when compared with younger individuals. These results have since been confirmed by Abreu *et al.* (1999) and Fliser *et al.* (1997a,b).

Sodium handling in the elderly-elderly

In a recent study on the increasingly important group of the 'elderly-elderly', using the same technique as we used in the younger elderly (Table 4), Musso *et al.* (2000) compared a saline load in a group of five healthy young and five apparently healthy individuals aged 80–87 years, after ruling out detectable pathology by means of clinical examination, blood biochemistry, and cardiac ultrasonography. Total urinary Na^+ output was diminished in the elderly-elderly, most probably as a result of the low sodium usually chosen by this group (Table 5). Whilst the 'proximal nephron' was capable of reabsorbing almost all filtered sodium, the 'distal nephron' (ascending limb of the loop of Henle) produced less free water than in the young.

Apart from the 'intrinsic' incompetence of the ascending limb of the loop of Henle already mentioned, other factors contributing to the different handling of Na^+ by the aged kidney are the lower plasma and urine concentrations in stable conditions of aldosterone, which acts on the distal nephron (Ceruso *et al.* 1970), and the blunted response of the renin–aldosterone system following salt restriction in the elderly (Tables 6 and 7) (Macías-Núñez *et al.* 1978). Interstitial fibrosis, peritubular forces, or the action of sex hormones could all contribute to the defect as well, but definitive evidence is lacking for any of these (Epstein and Hollenberg 1979).

This diminished capacity to reabsorb sodium by the ascending limb of the loop of Henle of healthy elderly persons has two direct important consequences: first, the amount of sodium arriving at most distal segments of the nephron (distal convoluted and collecting tubules) increases with a concomitant decrease in free water, and second, the capacity to concentrate the medullary interstitium is also diminished. As a consequence, elderly individuals exhibit both decreased ability to regulate sodium excretion, and an inability to concentrate and dilute the urine maximally.

Table 4 Study of the segmental handling of sodium in different parts of the nephron in young and young-elderly individuals

	C_{Na} (ml/min)	'Proximal' nephron (ml/min)	'Distal' nephron (ml/min)
Young ($n = 10$)	3.20 ($p < 0.05$)	18.3 ± 7.2 NS	83.0 ± 6.3 ($p < 0.05$)
Elderly ($n = 12$)	6.52 ± 2.35	18.9 ± 5.9	59.1 ± 7.9

Participants were studied during zero ADH secretion during saline loading; all figures are mean ± SD.

Data of Macías-Núñez *et al.* (1978).

Potassium handling in aged individuals

Despite the spontaneous ingestion of lower amounts of potassium by the elderly (<60 mmol/24 h) because of a diet low in meat, fruit and vegetables, *plasma potassium concentrations* in aged persons do not differ from those of the younger population in any of many studies (Burini *et al.* 1973). However, when diuretics are taken, the elderly develop hypokalaemia much more rapidly and frequently than do the young. As might be expected from intake, the basal *urinary excretion of potassium* is also lower than in the young, although the FE_K is actually increased as a result of diminished GFR (Macías-Núñez 1980; Kirkland *et al.* 1983). Biswas and Mulkerrin (1997) obtained similar results and postulated that physiological changes such as low aldosterone and tendency to retain K associated with age would tend to predispose the elderly to hyperkalaemia, especially if angiotensin converting enzyme inhibitors are used (Rodríguez-Puyol 1998).

Measurements of *total exchangeable body potassium* by various isotopic dilution methods all agree that total body potassium is 15 per cent lower in elderly than young people (Hiraide 1981; Lye 1981), 2500 mmol versus ~3000 mmol, but administration of extra potassium does not raise the body potassium (Kromhout *et al.* 1977). The reasons for these differences are not altogether clear: muscle mass is a major site for potassium, and is diminished in the aged. Studies of red cell potassium exchange as a surrogate for muscle cell membrane activity have given conflicting results, and may not be relevant to muscle.

Water balance and handling in elderly people

Water balance is controlled by the regulation of thirst, neurohypophyseal function, and the renal capacity for water excretion (Shannon *et al.* 1984). Both perception of thirst and spontaneous intake of liquids

Table 5 Study of the segmental handling of sodium in different parts of the nephron in young and elderly-elderly individuals

	Na clearance	Free water clearance	Proximal	Distal
Young ($n = 5$)	2.6 ± 1.14	15.32 ± 2.63	17.93 ± 3.11	85.72 ± 4.51
Elderly-elderly ($n = 5$)	1.64 ± 0.31	5.92 ± 0.71*	7.82 ± 0.81*	75.64 ± 4.47*

* $p > 0.05$ with respect to young controls.

Participants were studied during zero ADH secretion during saline loading; all figures are mean ± SD.

Differences in Na clearance is due to different basal salt content in the diet chosen by groups. See text for comments.

Data of Musso *et al.* (2000).

Table 6 Blood and urinary aldosterone concentrations in young and elderly individuals on a normal diet and during sodium restriction

Blood		**Urine**	
Young ($n = 6$)	**Elderly ($n = 6$)**	**Young ($n = 6$)**	**Elderly ($n = 6$)**
Normal diet			
19.6 ± 9.6	5.6 ± 4.21	10.95 ± 8.8	4.2 ± 2.81
Sodium restriction			
30.6 ± 4.8	8.6 ± 3.91	29.3 ± 19.6*	9.61 ± 3.81

* $p < 0.05$ normal diet versus salt restriction; $p < 0.05$ young versus elderly.

All data expressed as mean SD in pg/ml (blood and ng/24 h urine).

Data of Macías-Núñez *et al.* (1978).

Table 7 Plasma renin concentrations in young and elderly individuals on a normal diet and sodium restricted diet, and at rest and walking

Rest		**Walking**	
Young	**Elderly**	**Young**	**Elderly**
Normal diet			
4.55 ± 0.36*	0.79 ± 0.601	7.06 ± 4.00*	0.98 ± 0.851
Sodium restriction			
6.20 ± 4.70*	1.75 ± 1.801	8.10 ± 4.20*	3.77 ± 3.771

* $p < 0.05$ between resting and walking; $p < 0.05$ between young and elderly.

All data are mean ± SD expressed in ng angiotensin l/ml per hour.

Data of Macías-Núñez *et al.* (1978).

diminish with age (Goldman 1981). When healthy active elderly volunteers were water-restricted for 24 h, the threshold for thirst was increased and water intake was reduced in comparison to a control group of younger individuals. Despite the reduction in water intake and thirst, a considerable increase in blood osmolality, plasma sodium concentration, and in circulating vasopressin occurred during water deprivation (Phillips *et al.* 1984). Osmotic release of arginine vasopressin (AVP) in response to intravenous hypertonic saline in elderly people is, in fact, greater than in the young, but the AVP response to volume depletion is blunted (Rowe *et al.* 1982). In the aged rat (Bengelé *et al.* 1983), there is insensitivity of the cortical collecting duct to AVP rather than a reduced medullary hyperosmolality, with a reduced generation of cAMP.

This lack of a sensation of thirst in elderly people, despite an increase in plasma tonicity, remains unexplained. Dryness of the mouth and a decrease of taste with age may contribute to the diminution of the thirst (Hugonot *et al.* 1978); another mechanism might be an alteration in mental capacity (Seymour *et al.* 1980) or cortical cerebral dysfunction (Miller *et al.* 1982). It has also been suggested that a reduction in the sensitivity of the osmoreceptors responsible for thirst regulation may play a part in water-handling alterations in elderly persons. A contrary view has arisen from the studies of Helderman *et al.* (1978), in which an *increase* in the sensitivity of the osmoreceptors that regulate the release of vasopresssin release was observed. Thirst diminution may also result from an inappropriate response to hypovolaemia. Age diminishes the sensitivity of the baroreceptors and the release of vasopressin mediated by them (Rowe *et al.* 1982). Finally, plasma concentration of angiotensin, a powerful generator of thirst, is diminished in elderly people. Therefore, stimulation of thirst requires a severe hypovolaemia and/or hypotension (Robertson 1984). There is no difference in the plasma concentration of vasopressin between young and elderly persons before or after water deprivation (Shannon *et al.* 1984).

Immobility syndrome (Musso et al. *2000)*

This syndrome of immobility together with instability and falling on movement, incontinence, and mental impairment constitutes one the major geriatric syndromes and is very frequent in aged persons. Water metabolism in this state has not been explored fully. In 40 elderly nursing-home patients (>64 years old), 20 of them with immobility syndrome had a significantly higher total body water (BW) than aged controls without it, which could influence the distribution volume and consequently the pharmacokinetics of water-soluble drugs (see below).

Urinary concentration and dilution

Ageing reduces the capacity of the kidney maximally to *concentrate the urine* (Dontas *et al.* 1972; Rowe *et al.* 1976b) by 5 per cent with every 10 years of age (Lewis and Alving 1938) from a maximum urinary specific gravity of 1030 at 40 years of age to only 1023 at 89 years of age. Rowe *et al.* (1976b) found a mean maximum osmolality of 1109 mOsm/kg in individuals aged 20–39 years, with a minimum urine flow rate of 0.49 ± 0.03 ml/min, 1051 mOsm/kg in 40–59-year-olds, and only 882 mOsm/kg in those aged 60–79 years, in whom minimum urinary flow rate was more than double that of the young at 1.03 ml/min. The data of Lindeman *et al.* (1960) are similar. Kirkland *et al.* (1983) noted that even healthy individuals aged 60– 80 years showed a greater excretion of water, sodium, and potassium during the night than younger controls, with complaints of nocturia in a high proportion. This alteration in circadian rhythm does not depend upon inability to concentrate the urine alone, but upon the defects in sodium handling and aldosterone secretion, and sensitivity already mentioned.

The origin of the diminution in concentration is also complex; the small differences between the amount of liquid taken by young and elderly individuals cannot completely explain the differences in solutes and urinary elimination observed during water deprivation (Rowe *et al.* 1976b). The diminution of the concentrating ability has been related to the decrement in GFR that occurs with age with induction of an osmotic diuresis in the remaining nephrons (Lindeman *et al.* 1960; Kleeman 1972). Despite this, some data do not reveal a close relation between the reduction in the GFR and the capacity to concentrate urine in elderly persons (Rowe *et al.* 1976b). The relative increase in medullary blood flow noted above could contribute to the impairment of renal concentration capacity (Takazakura *et al.* 1972; Hollenberg *et al.* 1974).

Nevertheless, data supporting this suggestion are not available. Inappropriately low ADH is not, as already discussed, a factor in the genesis of the defect. The defect in sodium chloride reabsorption in the ascending limb of the loop of Henle, which is the basic mechanism for the operation of the countercurrent concentration mechanism, may be an important factor for the decrease in the capacity to concentrate urine seen in aged individuals; this is also discussed above.

There are only a few reports dealing with the capacity of the ageing kidney to *dilute urine*, but generally it has been found to be decreased (Lindeman *et al.* 1960; Dontas *et al.* 1972; Editorial 1984; Phillips *et al.* 1984). Dontas *et al.* (1972) found a minimum urine concentration of only 92 mOsm/kg in elderly individuals compared with 52 mOsm/kg in the young. Maximum free water clearance (C_{H_2O}) was also reduced in elderly individuals from 16.2 to 5.9 ml/min. This is probably dependent in the main upon the reduced GFR, but the C_{H_2O}/GFR was, even so, somewhat reduced in the older participants (9.1 versus 10.2 per cent). Again, the functional impairment of the diluting segment of the thick ascending limb described above seems to account for the remainder of the diminution in the capacity to dilute urine observed in aged persons (Macías-Núñez *et al.* 1978).

Urinary acidification in elderly people

Table 8(a) shows that only four authors so far have studied the response to an *acute acid overload* in the elderly, but assessment of nutritional status, blood electrolytes previous to the test, and collection time were not uniform, and so the results are difficult to compare. The posture of the patients during the collection time is also very important, as has been recently confirmed by Adachi (2001): standing from a supine position is associated with significant decrease ($p < 0.001$) in creatinine clearance from 125 ± 18 to 117 ± 19 ml/min. It is known that standing is an excellent stimulus for aldosterone secretion, with its influence on potassium excretion, which in turn modifies ammonium synthesis.

Although resting pH and pCO_2 were not different between elderly individuals and younger control individuals in basal conditions, in response to a challenge with acid the reduction in blood pH and pCO_2 was greater and longer lasting in older individuals (Shock and Yiengst 1948). Adler *et al.* (1968) noted that elderly people excreted only 19 per cent of the acid load given within a mean of 5 days (variable collection periods were used) compared with 35 per cent in younger individuals. More recently, Frassetto *et al.* (1996), in a study performed in normal subjects aged 17–74 years examined the behaviour of blood H^+, $(HCO_3)^-$, and GFR, and found that steady-state blood acidity and $P_b\,CO_2$ (index of respiratory set-point) correlated positively with age, and negatively with $(HCO_3)^-$ and GFR, but had no correlation with net renal acid excretion.

The effect of ageing on *ammonium ion production* remains controversial (Adler *et al.* 1968; Agarwal and Cabebe 1980) probably because of different study conditions. We (Macías-Núñez *et al.* 1983) found no differences in the capacity for renal ammonium elimination with age in a carefully studied and controlled group of elderly individuals (mean age 72 years) in whom the study was prolonged to 8 h. The elderly participants, however, took longer to reach peak excretion, and the same dose of ammonium chloride induced a greater decline in blood bicarbonate [Table 8(b)].

There is almost a complete consensus that elderly individuals are able to eliminate the same (Agarwal and Cabebe 1980; Macías-Núñez *et al.* 1983), or even an increased (Schück and Nádvorníková 1987) amount of titratable acid in response to an acute acid load as younger

Table 8 Ageing and renal tubular acidification

(a) Methodology in published studies

Authors	Sex	Nutritional status (plasma albumin g/l)	Health assessment	Urine collection time	Subject position	Plasma electrolytes	Δ^a Blood CO_3HNa
Schock and Yiengst (1948)	M	Not given	Not given	Not given	Not given	Not given	Not given
Alder *et al.* (1968)	M/F	Not given	Bladder catheter	Variable	Not given	Not given	4.6
Agarbal and Cabebe (1980)	M/F	Not given	Not given	Variable	Not given	NS	2.5
Macías-Núñez *et al.* (1983)	M/F	E. 42.6 ± 0.7 Y. 42.6 ± 0.8	Healthy	8 h	Recumbent	NS	5.9
Schück and Nádvomilkova (1987)	M/F	Not given	Not given	5 h	Sitting, standing, or walking	Not given	Not given

(b) Results of published studies

Authors	Urinary pH	NH_4^+ elimination	Titratable acid	CO_3HNa threshold
Alder *et al.* (1968)	NS	Diminished	NS	Not given
Agarbal and Cabebe (1980)	NS	Diminished	NS	Not given
Macías-Núñez *et al.* (1983)	NS	NS	NS	NS
Schück and Nádvomilkova (1987)	NS	Impaired above 50[b]	Increased impaired above 60[b]	Not given

[a] Δ denotes diminution of blood bicarbonate (mmol/l) after acid overload.

[b] Corrected per 100 ml of GFR. NS = no statistical differences (<0.05) between young and elderly subjects after acute acid overload.

E, subjects aged 65 years and over; Y, young controls.

individuals. Equally, there is agreement that urinary pH can be lowered as effectively in age as in youth (Adler *et al.* 1968; Agarwal and Cabebe 1980; Macías-Núñez *et al.* 1983; Schück and Nádvorníková 1987). The only study that has examined bicarbonate handling by the ageing renal tubule (Macías-Núñez *et al.* 1983) found no differences for bicarbonate threshold between young controls and healthy aged subjects. There exist no data concerning bicarbonate 'Tm' in the aged.

In sum, of only four comprehensive studies available, it was found that after an acid load, urinary pH and titratable acid behave similarly in the aged and the young, but that plasma pH and pCO_2 together with ammonium ion excretion in the aged take longer to respond, rather than cause an absolute deficit in function.

Calcium, phosphate, and magnesium

Bone problems in elderly people are frequent, but alterations in renal function play only a small part in their genesis. A relatively reduced blood calcium and increased phosphate are usual clinical findings, with hypocalciuria and hyperphosphaturia (Galinsky *et al.* 1987). Phosphate Tm is less in the aged than in young individuals.

These changes in the metabolism of calcium and phosphate may be related to the diminished plasma 1,25-dihydroxyvitamin D found in elderly people, probably as a result not only of poor exposure to sunlight, but also of a deficit of renal 1α-hydroxylase during ageing, which is known to be present in the rat. This could also explain the increased parathyroid hormone (PTH) that accompanies ageing, although retention of PTH fragments with decreasing GFR may play a part. Serum concentrations of 24,25-dihydroxyvitamin D are also low in elderly people (Galinsky *et al.* 1987). The response of the 1α-hydroxylase to PTH and forskolin *in vitro* is reduced in ageing rats, and presumably in humans also.

Although diet and medicines may influence the negative balance of magnesium, the kidney is the major controller (see Chapter 2.5). Approximately 80 per cent of plasma magnesium is filtered and reabsorbed—25 per cent by proximal tubules, 65 per cent by the thick ascending limb of the loop of Henle—and the remaining 5 per cent eliminated in urine. Consequently, a diminution of the reabsorptive capacity of the ascending limb, as has been described (at least for sodium handling) in healthy aged individuals, may account for the magnesium wasting and negative balance if oral intake is lower than desirable, as is often the case. Since, in addition, intestinal absorption is poor, supplements are often necessary (Seeling and Preuss 1994). To make things even worse, many medicines taken by elderly persons, particularly digoxin, diuretics, laxatives, and aminoglycosides may aggravate magnesium deficiency.

Glucose

Glucose has been shown to have a normal threshold in elderly people, although Butterfield *et al.* (1967) had earlier suggested an increase; but a reduced apparent $Tm_{glucose}$ has been demonstrated in parallel with the reduction in glomerular filtration rate (Miller *et al.* 1952). The decline in the apparent $Tm_{glucose}$ averaged 359 mg/min/1.73 m^2 in the third decade, and only 219 mg/min/1.73 m^2 in the ninth. This peculiarity of the ageing kidney has some interest in everyday clinical practice, given the frequency of diabetes mellitus in the elderly population. With hyperglycaemia, elderly persons are more prone to develop glycosuria, which, however, does not mean that they are diabetic.

Body water and plasma volume in the elderly

Total body water is slightly diminished with age, so that it comprises only 54 per cent of total body weight (Edelman and Leibman 1959), probably because old people have a greater proportion of their body weight as fat than the young. The diminution seems to be predominantly intracellular (Edmonds *et al.* 1975). Cross-sectional and longitudinal studies have revealed that plasma and blood volume do not alter as a result of age alone in healthy adults (Cohn and Shock 1949; Chien *et al.* 1966), although Wörum *et al.* (1984) found that elderly women had a significantly greater plasma volume than young women. We have found that plasma and blood volume measurements using radiolabelled albumin do not differ between young and elderly healthy volunteers. Males have a greater volume than females, regardless of age. Thus, a diminished plasma volume in an elderly individual is almost always the result of disease.

Psychiatric disturbances and electrolytes in elderly people

In elderly untreated patients with psychiatric pathological changes, alterations of the intracellular, extracellular, and total body water have been found (Cox and Orme 1973). Deterioration of verbal learning is associated with an increase in body water, intracellular and extracellular fluid, and exchangeable sodium and potassium in relation to dry body weight. The diminution in verbal ability was associated with a shift of water from the extracellular to the intracellular compartments and diminution of the interchangeable sodium in relation to lean body weight. In addition, there may be effects of lithium or other drugs on water and electrolyte handling (see following text and Chapter 6.6). The importance of checking plasma electrolytes and urea in confused elderly individuals scarcely requires mention. In spite of this, we did not find significantly different water metabolism in a group of demented elderly patients (Musso *et al.* 2000), although results did show a tendency towards higher body water in the group with dementia.

Renal pharmacokinetics in elderly people

The ageing process is accompanied not only by modifications in renal function, but also in the function of other organs important in drug absorption, distribution, and disposal such as the intestine and liver, and by reduced serum albumin concentrations (Cohen 1986; Abernethy 1999). These changes can lead to severe adverse effects, and hence to increased costs (Scharf and Christophidis 1991; Swift 1994; Hippius *et al.* 2001). Although prescribing for elderly people is one of the most common tasks for physicians, guidelines for avoiding drug misuse in the elderly are often forgotten (Ferris and Menyah 2001), perhaps because it is difficult to control every factor that can modify pharmacokinetics apart from the frequent concomitant diseases, each with their own drug therapy. Hence, multiple drug ingestion and an even poorer compliance than usual with prescriptions is observed in elderly people (Claesson *et al.* 1999).

Absorption and distribution of drugs in the elderly

Ingested drugs are subject to gastrointestinal absorption and hepatic action (first-pass hepatic metabolism). Since age delays gastric emptying time, the speed and quantity of absorption will vary. Diminished gastric acid secretion and consequent increased gastric pH also occur with age. This may affect drug handling, either to enhance or diminish blood concentrations of the active drug. Splanchnic bloodflow is decreased 30–40 per cent in the aged, and as a consequence, there is an increase in the systemic availability of some drugs that are normally extracted in the liver.

The proportion of adipose tissue is increased in elderly individuals, more so in females, and lean body mass, total body water, and especially intracellular water are diminished. Therefore, lipid-soluble drugs show an increased volume of distribution. Plasma proteins, in particular albumin, are diminished from 40 to 35 g/l at the age of 80, which accounts for the decrement in protein binding of drugs in elderly people, with a corresponding increase in the free fraction of the drug.

Elimination of drugs in the elderly

Since both GFR and renal blood flow usually diminish as the individual ages, drugs excreted by the kidney exclusively or predominantly by filtration have slower rates of elimination, increased half-lives in the plasma, and many accumulate leading to undesirable side-effects, including nephrotoxicity (Goldberg *et al.* 1987). In addition to excretion by filtration, many drugs are secreted by the renal tubules, which in some cases may be the dominant mode to excretion.

Because of all these factors, it is neccessary to modify the intervals of administration, and sometimes also the priming dosage, of such drugs. In addition, states of dehydration, cardiac failure, and occult renal disease, such as prostatic or renal vascular obstruction in elderly individuals, may reduce renal drug elimination even further, temporarily, or in the long term. Bearing all this in mind, it is essential to calculate the approximate GFR using the actual or the calculated creatinine clearance derived drom the plasma creatinine measurement. Despite its inaccuracies and disadvantages discussed in Chapter 1.4, the formula of Cockroft and Gault (1976) is the best validated. In addition, drug elimination is a very complicated process of which renal excretion is only one component. Metabolism, with the potential for accumulation of metabolites as well as (or instead of) the parent drug and hepatic (biliary) as well as renal excretion present further complications (Vestal 1997).

Therefore, numerous drugs require modified dosage regimens in elderly patients, particularly digoxin, aminoglycosides, lithium, practolol, quinidine, tetracycline, procainamide, and methotrexate, all well-known examples of those with reduced rates of renal elimination in elderly people (Chutka *et al.* 1995). In addition, the potential extra delterious effects of non-steroidal anti-inflammatory drugs (NSAIDs), angiotensin converting enzyme (ACE) inhibitors, and drugs affecting release of AVP mentioned throughout this chapter must not be forgotten.

The use of kidneys from the elderly for transplantation

Until recently, potential kidney donors over the age of 50 years were rarely considered, largely because of the sclerosis and diminished renal function and reserve outlined in this chapter. However, given the continuing shortage of cadaver donors, more and more elderly donors are now being considered and used. In some highly productive donor programmes such as that in Spain, almost half the heart-beating cadaver donations were from subjects over the age of 60–65 years in 1999 (see Chapter 14.2).

However, in every major study of outcomes, a steady decline in long-term graft survival with increasing age of the donor is seen (Takemoto and Terasaki 1988; Opeltz 1998 and see Chapter 14.2) as well as an increased incidence of delayed function, and in most transplant programmes, kidneys from those aged over 60 or 65 years will be classified as 'marginal' organs. Nevertheless, as discussed also in Chapter 14.2, survival of recipients of such kidneys even so remains better than wait-listed patients not transplanted at all. The problem of the elderly donor has extended with the increasing desire in many transplant programmes to use older living donors as well. Here, there is the additional worry of engendering renal failure in the donor from poorer compensatory responses following nephrectomy, thus creating a renoprival state. This has inhibited most programmes from undertaking this to any major extent; however, in Norway, elderly donors have been used more widely for greater than a decade (Opeltz 1998; Doyle *et al.* 2000). The level of renal function below which it may be considered 'safe' to take a kidney is not yet established, but most units would be reluctant to use older donors with a GFR of less than 60–70 ml/min. It is known that in younger donors, compensatory growth of the remaining kidney is highly variable, from no change to doubling of postnephrectomy function with a mean final figure of about 70–75 per cent of the original GFR; but also that this response is blunted in aged animals.

However, GFR measurement is not usually practicable in older and other 'marginal' cadaver donors, and histology has been suggested as a method capable of distinguishing good from less useful organs. Using the algorithm of Smith *et al.* (1989), a healthy person of 60 years should have on average 20 per cent of sclerosed glomeruli, a 70-year-old at least 25 per cent, a 75-year-old 27.5 per cent, and at 80 years the figure will approach 30 per cent. In some of the consensus statements from expert committees, it has been recommended that cadaver donor kidneys aged 60–75 years should not be used for single kidney transplants if they contain 20 per cent or more of sclerosed glomeruli. Thus, only a minority of kidneys over the age of even 60 years would be acceptable for a single transplant if these criteria were followed, halving the potential number of 60–75-year-old kidneys for transplantation. It has been recommended further that all kidneys from donors aged more than 75 years only be used for double transplants (see Morales *et al.* 1988), or discarded altogether if glomerulosclerosis is greater than 50 per cent. However, again using the formula just discussed, we would only expect to encounter 27.5–30 per cent sclerosis at this age. This approach of performing a double transplant from elderly or other 'marginal' donors seems promising, and is under active investigation at the moment in a number of centres (Andres *et al.* 2000; Lu *et al.* 2000).

Other methods of assessing the potential of such organs have been explored, such as the excretion of enzymes during *ex vivo* perfusion (Daemen *et al.* 1997). Phosphorus nuclear magnetic resonance for ATP/ADP levels seems promising, but difficult to apply to human rather than rodent kidneys.

Acknowledgements

We are deeply indebted to Dr Carlos Guido Musso, Dr Carlos Adolfo Felix Musso, and Mr Anibal Mateo Enz for their valuable contribution to the studies in the elderly-elderly, and to Dr Jesús Garrido and Mr David James Harvey for help in the preparation of the manuscript.

References

Abernethy, D. R. (1999). Aging effects on drug disposition and effect. *Geriatric Nephrology and Urology* **9**, 15–19.

Adachi, T., Kawamura, M., Owada, M., and Hiramori, K. (2001). Effect of age on renal functional and orthostatic vascular response in healthy men. *Clinical and Experimental Pharmacolology and Physiology* **28**, 877–880.

Abreu, P. F., Ramos, L. R., and Sesso, R. (1999). Abnormalities of renal function in the elderly. *Geriatric Nephrolology and Urology* **9**, 141–145.

Adler, S., Lindeman, R. D., Yiengst, M. J., Beard, E., and Shock, N. W. (1968). Effect of acute acid loading on urinary acid excretion by the aging human kidney. *Journal of Laboratory and Clinical Medicine* **72**, 278–289.

Agarwal, B. N. and Cabebe, F. G. (1980). Renal acidification in elderly subjects. *Nephron* **26**, 291–295.

Anderson, S., Meyer, T. W., and Brenner, B. M. Mechanisms of age-associated glomerular sclerosis. In *Renal Function and Disease in the Elderly* (ed. J. F. Macías-Núñez and J. S. Cameron), pp. 49–66. London: Butterworths, 1987.

Andres, A. *et al.* (2000). Double versus single renal allografts from aged donors. *Transplantation* **69**, 2060–2066.

Arnel, M. and Gollapudi, S. (2001). Functional decline in Aging and disease: a role for apoptosis. *Journal of the American Geriatrics Society* **49**, 1234–1240.

Baylis, C. and Corman, B. (1998). The aging kidney: insights from experimental studies. *Journal of the American Society of Nephrology* **9**, 699–709.

Benetos, A. *et al.* (2001). Telomere length as an indicator of biological aging: the gender effect and relation with pulse pressure and pulse wave velocity. *Hypertension* **37**, 381–385.

Bengelé, H. N., Mathias, R. S., and Alexander, E. A. (1981). Impaired natriuresis after volume expansion in the aged rat. *Renal Physiology* **4**, 22–29.

Bengelé, H. N., Mathias, R., Perkins, J. N., McNamara, E. R., and Alexander, E. A. (1983). Impaired renal and extrarenal adaption in old rats. *Kidney International* **23**, 684–690.

Biswas, K. and Mulkerrin, E. C. (1997). Potassium homoeostasis in the elderly. *Quarterly Journal of Medicine* **90**, 487–492.

Böhler, J., Glöer, D., Reetze-Bonorden, P., Keller, E., and Schollmeyer, P. J. (1993). Renal function reserve in elderly patients. *Clinical Nephrology* **39**, 145–150.

Brown, W. W., Davis, B. B., Spry, L. A., Wongsurawat, N., Malone, D., and Domoto, D. T. (1986). Aging and the kidney. *Archives of Internal Medicine* **146**, 1790–1796.

Burini, R., Da Silva, C. A., Ribeiro, M. A. C., and Campana, A. D. (1973). Concentracão de sodio e de potassio no soro e plasma de individuos normais. Influencia da idade, do sexo e do sistema de colheita do sangue sobre os resultados. *Revista de Hospitale Clinico da Facultad do Medicina de São Paulo* **28**, 9–14.

Butterfield, W. J. H., Keen, H., and Whichelow, M. (1967). Renal glucose threshold variations with age. *British Medical Journal* **4**, 505–507.

Ceruso, D., Squadrito, G., Quartarone, M., and Parisi, M. (1970). Comportamento della funzionalita renale e degli elttroliti ematici ed urinary dopo aldosterone in soggetti anziani. *Giornale di Gerontologia* **18**, 1–6.

Chien, S., Usami, S., and Simmons, R. L. (1966). Blood volume and age: repeated measurements on normal men. *Journal of Applied Physiology* **21**, 583–588.

Chutka, D. S., Evans, J. M., Fleming, K. C., and Mikkelson, K. G. (1995). Drug prescribing for elderly patients. *Mayo Clinic Proceedings* **70**, 685–693.

Claesson, S., Morrison, A., Wertheimer, A. I., and Berger, M. L. (1999). Compliance with prescribed drugs: challenges for the elderly population. *Pharmacy World Science* **21**, 256–259.

Cockroft, D. W. and Gault, M. N. (1976). Prediction of creatinine clearance from serum creatinine. *Nephron* **16**, 31–41.

Cohen, J. L. (1986). Pharmacokinetic changes in aging. *American Journal of Medicine* **80** (Suppl. 5A), 31–38.

Cohn, J. E. and Shock, N. W. (1949). Blood volume studies in middle aged and elderly males. *American Journal of Medical Sciences* **217**, 388–391.

Cox, J. R. and Orme, J. E. (1973). Body water, electrolytes and psychological test performance in elderly patients. *Gerontologica Clinica* **15**, 203–208.

Daemen, J. W. *et al.* (1997). Glutathione-S-transferase as predictor of functional outcome in transplantation of machine-preserved non-heart beating donor kidneys. *Transplantation* **63**, 83–93.

Danziger, R. S., Tobin, J. D., Becker, L. C., Lakatta, E. E., and Fleg, J. C. (1990). The age-associated decline in glomerular filtration rate in healthy normotensive volunteers. Lack of relationship to cardiovascular performance. *Journal of the American Geriatrics Society* **38**, 1127–1132.

Darmady, E. M., Offer, J., and Woodhouse, M. A. (1973). The parameters of the ageing kidney. *Journal of Pathology* **109**, 195–207.

Davidson, A. J., Talner, D. B., and Downs, M. (1969). A study of the angiographic appearances of the kidney in an aging normal population. *Radiology* **92**, 975–983.

Davies, D. F. and Shock, N. W. (1950). Age changes in glomerular filtration rate, effective renal plasma flow, and tubular excretory capacity in adult males. *Journal of Clinical Investigation* **29**, 490–507.

De Leon, W., García, A., and De Jesus, P. I. (1933). Normal weights of visceral organs in adult Filipinos. *Philippine Journal of Science* **52**, 111.

de Santo, N., Anastasio, P., Coppola, S., Barba, G., Jadanza, A., and Capasso, G. (1991). Age-related changes in renal reserve and renal tubular function in healthy humans. *Child Nephrology and Urology* **11**, 33–40.

Dontas, A. S., Marketos, S., and Papanayioutou, P. (1972). Mechanisms of renal tubular defects in old age. *Postgraduate Medical Journal* **48**, 295–303.

Doyle, S. E., Matas, A. J., Gillingham, K., and Rosenberg, M. E. (2000). Predicting clinical outcome in the elderly renal transplant recipient. *Kidney International* **57**, 2144–2150.

Duraković, Z. (1986). Creatinine clearance in the elderly: a comparison of direct measurement and calculation from serum creatinine. *Nephron* **44**, 66–69.

Edelman, I. S. and Leibman, J. (1959). Anatomy of body water and electrolytes. *American Journal of Medicine* **27**, 256–260.

Editorial (1984). Thirst and osmoregulation in the elderly. *Lancet* **ii**, 1017–1018.

Edmonds, C. J., Jasani, B. M., and Smith, T. (1975). Total body potassium and body fat estimation in relationship to height, sex, age, malnutrition and obesity. *Clinical Science and Molecular Medicine* **48**, 431–440.

Eiam-Ong, S. and Sabatini, S. (2002). Effects of aging and potassium depletion on renal collecting tubule K^+-controlling ATPases. *Nephrology* **7**, 87–91.

Epstein, F. H. and Prasad, P. (2000). Effect of furosemide on medullary oxygenation in younger and older subjects. *Kidney International* **57**, 2080–2083.

Epstein, M. (1996). Aging and the kidney. *Journal of the American Society of Nephrology* **7**, 1106–1122.

Epstein, M. and Hollenberg, N. H. (1976). Age as a determinant of renal sodium conservation in normal man. *Journal of Laboratory and Clinical Medicine* **87**, 411–417.

Epstein, M. and Hollenberg, N. H. (1979). Renal 'salt wasting' despite apparently normal renal, adrenal and central nervous system function. *Nephron* **24**, 121–126.

Evrin, P.-E. and Wibell, L. (1972). The serum levels and urinary excretion of β Cr-EDTA clearance as a measure of glomerular filtration rate. *Scandinavian Journal of Clinical and Laboratory Investigation* **41**, 611–616.

Ferris, D. and Menyah, D. K. (2001). Reducing the use of inappropriate medications in the hospitalized elderly. *American Journal of Health-System Pharmacology* **58**, 1588–1592.

Fliser, D., Zeir, M., Nowalk, R., and Ritz, E. (1993). Renal functional reserve in healthy elderly subjects. *Journal of the American Society of Nephrology* **3**, 1371.

Fliser, D., Franek, E., Joest, M., Block, S., Mutschler, E., and Ritz, E. (1997a). Renal function in the elderly: impact of hypertension and cardiac function. *Kidney International* **51**, 1196–1204.

Fliser, D., Franek, E., and Ritz, E. (1997b). Renal function in the elderly—is the dogma of an inexorable decline of renal function correct? *Nephrology, Dialysis, Transplantation* **12**, 1553–1555.

Fliser, D. and Ritz, E. (2001). Serum cystatin C concentration as a marker of renal dysfunction in the elderly. *American Journal of Kidney Diseases* **37**, 79–83.

Frassetto, L. A., Morris, R. C. Jr., and Sebastian, A. (1996). Effect of age on blood acid-base composition in adult humans: role of age-related renal functional decline. *American Journal of Physiology* **271**, 1114–1122.

Fuiano, G. *et al.* (2001). Renal hemodynamic response to maximal vasodilating stimulus in healthy older subjects. *Kidney International* **59**, 1052–1058.

Galinsky, D., Meller, Y., and Shany, S. The aging kidney and calcium-regulating hormones: vitamin D metabolites, parathyroid hormone and calcitonin. In *Renal Function and Disease in the Elderly* (ed. J. F. Macías-Nuñez and J. S. Cameron), pp. 121–142. Butterworths: London, 1987.

Granerus, G. and Aurell, M. (1981). Reference values for Cr-EDTA clearance as a measure of glomerular filtration rate. *Scandinavian Journal of Clinical and Laboratory Investigation* **41**, 611–616.

Grimley Evans, J. and Bond, J. (1997). The challenges of age research. *Age and Ageing* **26** (Suppl. 4), 43–46.

Goldberg, T. H., Martin, S., and Finkelstein, S. (1987). Difficulties in estimating glomerular filtration rate in the elderly. *Archives of Internal Medicine* **147**, 1430–1433.

Goldman, R. Modern ideas about the renal function in the elderly. In *Geriatrics for the Practitioner* (ed. A. N. J. Reinders Folmer and J. Shouten), pp. 157–166. Amsterdam: Excerpta Medica, 1981.

Hackbarth, H. and Harrison, D. E. (1982). Changes with age in renal function and morphology in C57BL/6, CBA/HT6, and B6CBAFI mice. *Journal of Gerontology* **37**, 540–547.

Helderman, J. H., Vestal, R. E., Rowe, J. W., Tobin, J. D., Andres, R., and Robertson, G. L. (1978). The response of arginine vasopressin to intravenous ethanol and hypertonic saline in man: the impact of aging. *Journal of Gerontology* **33**, 39–47.

Hippius, M. *et al.* (2001). Adverse drug reaction monitoring—digitoxin overdosage in the elderly. *International Journal of Clinical Pharmacology and Therapeutics* **39**, 336–343.

Hiraide, K. (1981). Alterations in electrolytes with aging. *Nihon University Journal of Medicine* **23**, 21–31.

Hollenberg, N. K., Adams, D. F., Solomon, H. S., Rashid, A., Abrams, H. L., and Merrill, J. P. (1974). Senescence and the renal vasculature in normal man. *Circulation Research* **34**, 309–316.

Holley, H. E., Hunt, J. C., Brown, A. L., Kincaid, O. W., and Sheps, S. G. (1964). Renal artery stenosis. A clinical pathological study of normotensive and hypertensive patients. *American Journal of Medicine* **37**, 14–22.

Hugonot, R., Dubos, G., and Mathes, G. (1978). Étude expérimentale des troubles de la soif du vieillard. *La Revue de Gériatrie* 4 September, 179–191.

Joaquin, A. M. and Gollapudi, S. (2001). Functional decline in aging and disease: a role for apoptosis. *Journal of the American Geriatric Society* **49**, 1234–1240.

Kampmann, J., Siersbaek-Nielsen, K., Kristensen, K., and Molholm-Hansen, J. (1974). Rapid evaluation of creatinine clearance. *Acta Medica Scandinavica* **196**, 517–520.

Kaplan, C., Pasternack, B., Shah, H., and Gallo, G. (1975). Age-related incidence of sclerotic glomeruli in human kidneys. *American Journal of Pathology* **80**, 227–234.

Kappel, N. and Olsen, S. (1980). Cortical interstitial tissue and sclerosed glomeruli in the normal human kidney, related to age and sex. *Virchows Archiv: Pathologie Histologie* **387**, 271–277.

Karlberg, B. E. and Tolagen, K. (1977). Relationships between blood pressure, age, plasma renin activity and electrolyte excretion in normotensive subjects. *Scandinavian Journal of Clinical and Laboratory Investigation* **37**, 521–528.

Keller, F. (1987). Kidney function and age (letter). *Nephrology, Dialysis, Transplantation* **2**, 382.

Kimmel, P. L., Lew, S. Q., and Bosch, J. P. (1996). Nutrition, ageing and GFR: is age-associated decline inevitable? *Nephrology, Dialysis, Transplantation* **11**, 85–87.

Kirkland, J. L., Lye, M., Levy, D. W., and Banerjee, A. K. (1983). Patterns of urine flow and electrolyte secretion in healthy elderly people. *British Medical Journal* **285**, 1665–1667.

Kleeman, C. R. Water metabolism. In *Clinical Disorders of Fluid and Electrolyte Balance* (ed. M. H. Maxwell and C. R. Kleeman), p. 697. New York: McGraw-Hill, 1972.

Kromhout, D., Broberg, U., Carlmark, B., Karlsson, S., Nissel, O., and Reizenstein, P. (1977). Potassium depletion and ageing. *Comprehensive Therapeutics* **3**, 32–37.

Laine, G., Goulle, J. P., Houlbreque, P., Gruchy, D., and Leblanc, J. (1977). Clairance de la créatinine. Valeurs de réference en fonction de l'age et du sexe. *Nouvelle Presse Médicale* **30**, 2690–2691.

Lakatta, E. G. (1987). Cardiac muscle changes in senescense. *Annual Review of Physiology* **49**, 519–531.

Larsson, M., Jagenburg, R., and Landahl, S. (1986). Renal function in an elderly population. *Scandinavian Journal of Clinical Laboratory Investigation* **46**, 593–598.

Lewis, W. H. and Alving, A. S. (1938). Changes with age in the renal function of adult men. Clearance of urea, amount of urea nitrogen in the blood, concentrating ability of kidneys. *American Journal of Physiology* **123**, 505–515.

Lindeman, R. D. (1990). Overview: renal physiology and pathophysiology of ageing. *American Journal of Kidney Diseases* **16**, 275–282.

Lindeman, R. D. (1991). Is a high protein intake harmful to the aging human kidney? *Geriatric Nephrology and Urology* **1**, 113–119.

Lindeman, R. D., Van Buren, H. C., and Raisz, L. G. (1960). Osmolar renal concentrating ability in healthy young men and hospitalized patients without renal disease. *New England Journal of Medicine* **262**, 1396–1409.

Lindeman, R. D., Tobin, J., and Shock, N. W. (1985). Longitudinal studies on the rate of decline in renal function with age. *Journal of the American Geriatrics Society* **33**, 278–285.

López-Novoa, J. M. and Rodríguez-Puyol, D. (1997). Mecanismos de envejecimiento celular. *Nefrología* **17** (3), 15–22.

Lu, A. D. *et al.* (2000). Outcome in recipients of dual transplants. *Transplantation* **69**, 281–285.

Lye, M. (1981). Distribution of body potassium in healthy elderly subjects. *Gerontology* **27**, 286.

Macías-Núñez, J. F. and Cameron, J. S. *Renal Function and Disease in the Elderly*. London: Butterworths, 1987.

Macías-Núñez, J. F. *et al.* (1978). Renal handling of sodium in old people: a functional study. *Age and Ageing* **7**, 178–181.

Macías-Núñez, J. F., García-Iglesias, C., Tabernero-Romo, J. M., Rodríguez-Commes, J. L., Corbacho-Becerra, L., and Sanchez-Tomero, J. A. (1980). Renal management of sodium under indomethacin and aldosterone in the elderly. *Age and Ageing* **9**, 165–172.

Macías-Núñez, J. F. *et al.* (1981). Estudio del filtrado glomerular en viejos sanos. *Revista Española de Geriatria y Gerontologia* **16**, 113–124.

Macías-Núñez, J. F. *et al.* (1983). Comportamiento del riñon del viejo en la sobrecarga de acidos. *Nefrología* **3**, 11–16.

Macías-Núñez, J. F., Bondía Román, A., and Rodriguez-Commes, J. L. Physiology and disorders of water balance and electrolytes in the elderly. In *Renal Function and Disease in the Elderly* (ed. J. F. Macías-Núñez and J. S. Cameron), pp. 67–93. London: Butterworths, 1987.

Macías-Núñez, J. F., López-Novoa, J. M., and Martínez Maldonado, M. (1996). Acute renal failure in the aged. *Seminars in Nephrology* **16**, 330–338.

McDonald, R. K., Solomon, D. H., and Shock, N. W. (1951). Aging as a factor in the hemodynamic changes induced by a standard pyrogen. *Journal of Clinical Investigation* **30**, 457–462.

McLachlan, M. Anatomic structural and vascular changes in the aging kidney. In *Renal Function and Disease in the Elderly* (ed. J. F. Macías-Núñez and J. S. Cameron), pp. 3–26. London: Butterworths, 1987.

McLachlan, M. S. F., Guthrie, J. C., Anderson, C. K., and Fulker, M. J. (1977). Vascular and glomerular changes in the ageing kidney. *Journal of Pathology* **121**, 65–77.

Melk, A. *et al.* (2000). Telomere shortening in kidneys with age. *Journal of the American Society of Nephrology* **11**, 444–453.

Meyer, B. R. (1989). Renal function in ageing. *Journal of the American Geriatrics Society* **37**, 791–800.

Miller, J. H., McDonald, R. K., and Shock, N. W. (1952). Age changes in the maximal rate of renal tubular reabsorption of glucose. *Journal of Gerontology* **7**, 196–200.

Miller, P. D., Krebs, R. A., Neal, B. J., and McIntyre, D. O. (1982). Hypodipsia in geriatric patients. *American Journal of Medicine* **73**, 354–356.

Morales, J. M. *et al.* (1998). Trasplante renal en pacientes de edad avanzada con un riñón de donante añoso. *Nefrología* **18** (Suppl. 5), 32–46.

Musso, C. G., Macías-Núñez, J. F., Musso, C. A. F., Algranati, L. S., and dos Ramos Farias, E. (2000). Fractional excretion of sodium in old people on low sodium diet. *The FASEB Journal* **14**, A659.

Musso, C. G., Maytin, S., Fainstein, I., Algranati, L. S., and dos Ramos Farias, E. (1999). Water metabolism in elderly with immobility syndrome. *XV International Congress of Nephrology*, Buenos Aires, (abstracts), p. 69.

Musso, C. G., Macías-Núñez, J. F., Fainstein I., Algranati, L. S., and dos Ramos Farias, E. (2000). Water metabolism in demented elderly. *The FASEB Journal* **14**, A658.

Myers, J., Morgan, T., Waga, S., and Manley, K. (1982). The effect of sodium intake on blood pressure related to the age of the patients. *Clinical and Experimental Pharmacology and Physiology* **9**, 287–289.

Neugarten, J., Gallo, G., Silbiger, S., and Kasiske, B. (1999). Glomerulosclerosis in aging humans is not influenced by gender. *American Journal of Kidney Diseases* **34**, 884–888.

Nicholl, S. R. *et al.* (1991). Assessment of creatinine clearance in healthy subjects over 65 years of age. *Nephron* **59**, 621–625.

Nyengaard, J. R. and Bendtsen, T. F. (1992). Glomerular number and size in relation to age, kidney weight, and body surface in normal man. *Anatomical Record* **232**, 194–201.

Opeltz, G. (1998). The influence of recipient age on kidney transplant outcome. *Nephrology* **2** (Suppl. 1), s211–s214.

Phillips, P. A. *et al.* (1984). Reduced thirst after water deprivation in healthy elderly men. *New England Journal of Medicine* **311**, 753–759.

Refoyo, A. and Macías-Núñez, J. F. (1991). The maintenance of plasma sodium in the healthy aged. *Geriatric Nephrology and Urology* **1**, 65–68.

Roberts, M. M. and Robinson, A. G. (1993). Hyponatremia in the elderly: diagnosis and management. *Geriatric Nephrology and Urology* **3**, 43–50.

Robertson, G. L. (1984). Abnormalities of thirst regulation. *Kidney International* **25**, 460–469.

Rodeheffer, R. J., Gerstenblith, G., Becker, L. C., Fleg, J. L., Wesifeldt, M. L., and Lakatta, E. G. (1984). Exercise cardiac output is maintained with advancing age in healthy human subjects: cardiac dilatation and increased stroke volume compensate for a diminished heart rate. *Circulation* **69**, 203–213.

Rodriguez-Puyol, D. (1998). The aging kidney. *Kidney International* **54**, 2247–2265.

Rowe, J. W., Shock, N. W., and De Fronzo, R. A. (1976a). The influence of age on the renal response to water deprivation in man. *Nephron* **17**, 270–278.

Rowe, J. W., Minaker, K. L., Sparrow, D., and Robertson, G. L. (1982). Age-related failure of volume–pressure-mediated vasopressin release. *Journal of Clinical Endocrinology and Metabolism* **54**, 661–664.

Scharf, S. and Christophidis, N. (1991). Pharmacokinetics and pharmacodynamics in the elderly. *Australian Journal of Hospital Pharmacy* **21**, 198–202.

Scharf, S. and Christophidis, N. (1993). Prescribing for the elderly: 1. Relevance of pharmacokinetics and pharmacodynamics. *Medical Journal of Australia* **158**, 395–402.

Schou, M., Thomson, K., and Vestergaard, P. (1986). The renal lithium clearance and its correlation with other biological variables: observation in a large group of physically healthy persons. *Clinical Nephrology* **25**, 207–211.

Schück, O. and Nádvorníkova, H. (1987). Short acidification test and its interpretation with respect to age. *Nephron* **46**, 215–216.

Seeling, M. S. and Preuss, H. G. (1994). Magnesium metabolism and perturbation in the elderly. *Geriatric Nephrology and Urology* **4**, 101–111.

Seymour, D. G., Henschke, P. J., Cape, R. D. T., and Campbell, A. J. (1980). Acute confusional states and dementia in the elderly: the role of dehydration/volume depletion, physical illness and age. *Age and Ageing* **9**, 137–406.

Shannon, R. P., Minaker, K. L., and Rowe, J. W. (1984). Aging and water balance in humans. *Seminars in Nephrology* **4**, 346–353.

Shock, N. W. and Yiengst, M. J. (1948). Experimental displacement of the acid–base equilibrium of the blood in aged males. *Federation Proceedings* **7**, 114–119.

Smith, S. M., Hoy, W. E., and Cobb, L. (1989). Low incidence of glomerulosclerosis in normal kidneys. *Archives of Pathology and Laboratory Medicine* **113**, 1253–1255.

Solomon, L. R. and Lye, M. (1990). Hypernatraemia in the elderly patient. *Gerontology* **36**, 171–179.

Solomon, L. R., Sangster, G., and Lye, M. (1992). Hyponatremia in the elderly patient. *Geriatric Nephrology and Urology* **2**, 63–74.

Sorensen, F. H. (1977). Quantitative studies of the renal corpuscle IV. *Acta Microbiologica et Pathologica Scandinavica* **85**, 356–365.

Sourander, L. The kidney. In *Geriatrics* (ed. D. Platt), pp. 202–221. Berlin: Springer, 1983.

Steffes, M. W., Barbosa, J., Bagsea, J. M., Matas, A. J., and Mauer, M. W. (1983). Quantitative glomerular morphology of the normal human kidney. *Laboratory Investigation* **49**, 82–86.

Swift, C. G. (1994). Pharmacokinetics and prescribing in the elderly. *Journal of Antimicrobial Chemotherapy* **34**, 25–32.

Takazakura, E., Sawabu, N., Handa, A., Takada, A., Shinada, A., and Takeuchi, J. (1972). Intrarenal vascular change with age and disease. *Kidney International* **2**, 224–230.

Takemoto, S. and Terasaki, P. I. (1988). Donor age and recipient age. *Clinical Transplantation* 345–356.

Tauchi, H., Tsuboi, K., and Okutani, J. (1971). Age changes in the human kidney of the different ages. *Gerontologia* **17**, 87–97.

Van den Noortgate, N., Janssens, W. H., Afschrift, M., and Lameire, N. H. (2001). Renal function in oldest-old on acute geriatric wards. *International Urology and Nephrology* **32**, 531–537.

Vestal, R. E. (1997). Aging and pharmacology. *Cancer* **80**, 1302–1310.

Wesson, L. G. Renal hemodynamics in physiological states. In *Physiology of the Human Kidney* (ed. L. G. Wesson), p. 96. New York: Grune & Stratton, 1969.

Wörum, I., Fulöp, T., Csongör, J., Foris, G., and Leóvey, A. (1984). Interrelation between body composition and endocrine system in healthy elderly people. *Mechanisms of Aging and Development* **28**, 315–324.

Yamada, T., Endo, T., Ito, K., Nagata, H., and Izumiyama, T. (1979). Age-related changes in endocrine and renal function in patients with essential hypertension. *Journal of the American Geriatrics Society* **27**, 280–292.

Zimmer, A. W., Calkins, E., Hadley, E., Ostfeld, A. M., Kaye, K. M., and Kaye, K. (1985). Conducting clinical research in geriatric populations. *Annals of Internal Medicine* **103**, 270–283.

General reading

Brown, W. W., Davis, B. B., Spry, L. A., Wongsurawat, N., Malone, D., and Domoto, D. T. (1986). Aging and the kidney. *Archives of Internal Medicine* **146**, 1790–1796.

Lindeman, R. D. (1990). Overview: renal physiology and pathophysiology of ageing. *American Journal of Kidney Diseases* **16**, 275–282.

Macías-Núñez, J. F. and Cameron, J. S., ed. *Renal Function and Disease in the Elderly*. London: Butterworths, 1987.

Meyer, B. R. (1991). Renal function in aging. *Journal of the American Geriatrics Society* **37**, 791–800.

Sarris, E. and Wilkinson, R. (1991). Aging in the kidney. *Journal of Nephrology* **2**, 67–74.

1.6 Imaging in nephrology

1.6.1 Imaging techniques

1.6.1.i Ultrasound

Jean-Michel Correas and Olivier Hélénon

Ultrasonography of the urinary tract has become the primary modality for the evaluation of genitourinary diseases, due to its availability, safety profile, low cost, and minimal invasiveness. It provides not only anatomical information, such as the presence of a kidney in the lumbar fossa or the dilatation of the urinary tract, but also functional information obtained from the Doppler study. The recent introduction of an ultrasound contrast agent (USCA) without renal toxicity improves the sensitivity of the Doppler evaluation and provides additional quantitative and functional information. However, the ultrasound examination remains operator dependent and its diagnostic capabilities can be limited by technical issues such as bowel gas interposition or attenuation of the ultrasound beam due to depth.

Principles of ultrasound imaging

Ultrasound imaging benefits from recent improvements in technology that lead to increased spatial resolution in B-mode imaging as well as increased sensitivity, frame rate, and resolution in the Doppler modalities.

Grey scale imaging

It still relies on the pulse-echo principle, where the ultrasound pulse emitted by the transducer travels in the tissues. A small amount of energy is backscattered to the probe at each interface where the acoustical impedance changes. This energy is maximized when the direction of the pulse is perpendicular to the surface of the scattering element (specular reflection). The angle of insonation requires continuous opti-mization to remain as close as possible to the specular reflection. This is why each organ or abnormality should be studied using multiple planes of view by moving the transducer. The backscattered echo is displayed by the grey scale of the ultrasound system after signal processing using non-linear compression of the signals. This compression is required due to the difference between the dynamic range of the ultrasound system (60–100 dB) and the dynamic range of the monitor (30 dB). The postprocessing exhibits a non-linear relationship between the echo amplitude and the displayed echoes to enhance the contrast between a lesion and the surrounding tissues, or between two different tissues within the same organ (such as cortex and medulla). The texture of the organ results from a stationary interference pattern (speckle). The identification of an organ or abnormality results from a relative difference in texture and echogenicity from the surrounding tissues.

The frequency range of the ultrasonic pulses varies from 2 to 14 MHz in clinical practice. The higher frequencies provide higher resolution but suffer from attenuation, and are chosen for superficial structures. Thus, the ultrasound image results from a compromise between resolution and penetration. The attenuation is compensated by a logarithmic amplification of the echoes, called time-gain compensation. Real-time ultrasound imaging is obtained by moving the scan line very fast to cover the entire imaging plane. Four different probes can be distinguished. In linear and curvilinear-array scanners, a large number of small transducers are arranged in a line or a curve. A small number of these elements are excited together and the beam is rapidly swept among the different groups of elements to create real-time imaging. Usually, linear probes are built with high-frequency transducers (7–15 MHz), while curvilinear arrays exhibit lower frequencies (2–7 MHz). Phased-array scanners are built with lesser number of transducers with lower frequencies. They are excited with a short delay (or phase) that increases from one side to the other. This allows steering and electronic focusing of the ultrasound beam. The change in the scan line can also be obtained by mechanical rotation of the element, such as in endovascular or some transrectal probes.

Recently, B-mode imaging has been improved with the development of digital signal processing, broadband transducers and increased bandwidth. The digital architecture of ultrasound systems improves the control of signal processing. Newer transducers offer an increased frequency width, which allows emission of a broadband pulse with a very rich frequency content, from 2 to 5 MHz for an abdominal probe of 3.5 MHz central frequency, for example. They allow better penetration and resolution, because higher frequencies are used for building the superficial plane, and simultaneously lower frequencies are selected for the deeper areas. Another improvement comes from the development of USCAs. The resonant properties of the tissues can be used to increase the relative difference between the structures of close backscatter. This imaging modality was called harmonic imaging at the beginning. More recently, the detection of the non-linear components of the signals has been improved with the introduction of multipulse techniques, called phase inversion. Two inverted pulses are transmitted for each transducer. The backscatter information is summed in the digital beamformer. Linear response from the tissues cancels while non-linear response is enhanced. Because the non-linear response of liquids strongly differs from that of tissues, the detection of cysts and dilatation of the pyelocaliceal system significantly improves. Compounding imaging is another improvement where the alteration of the ultrasound beam due to the subcutaneous fat is reduced. The pulse from each transducer can be stirred electronically, so that the target is seen from multiple angles from each crystal. The signal processing can combine compounding and non-linear imaging to maximize tissue information and reduce noise (Fig. 1).

Doppler imaging

The Doppler technique allows assessment of the haemodynamics of the entire renal vasculature (arteries and veins), from the main extrarenal vessels to the arcuate vessels. The interpretation of the colour and spectral information relies on the normal blood flow characteristics and the changes induced by stenosis, arteriovenous fistula, etc. The Doppler shift is the difference between the transmitted and received frequencies after hitting a moving target (red blood cells). The principle of all Doppler techniques is based upon the Doppler equation. The Doppler shift is proportional to the velocity of the target, the transmitted frequency, and the cosine of the insonation angle between the ultrasound beam and the direction of the vessel. This angle should be reduced as much as possible by optimal positioning of the probe. If the angle reaches 0, the cosine is equal to 1 and the Doppler shift is maximized. By coincidence, the range of ultrasound frequencies in clinical practice fits into the range of audible frequencies.

Continuous-wave Doppler is not appropriate for the Doppler examination of the urinary tract, because it does not allow spatial discrimination. All vessels encountered by the ultrasonic pulse will add some changes to the Doppler shift. In contrast, pulsed-wave Doppler allows spatial discrimination of the signals. Short bursts of ultrasound signals are transmitted. The depth of the Doppler window is determined by the length of time between each pulse. The longer the system waits, the deeper the gate is located. The size of the Doppler window is controlled by the length of time for which the detection gate remains open. The same transducer is usually used for both emission and reception of the pulses. The direction of the flow is detected by a demodulator using phase quadrature detection. To obtain adequate sampling of the signals, the pulse repetition frequency (PRF) should be at least twice the peak frequency of the Doppler signals recorded from the vessel. If not, aliasing phenomena occur and the spectral analysis shows a folding over of the signals that induces ambiguous flow information. The limit of correct Doppler signal sampling depends on the ultrasound frequency, the angle of insonation, and the depth. The position of the pulsed-wave Doppler window can be guided by the real-time anatomical grey scale imaging. This modality is called duplex Doppler, and is the basis for detection of vascular diseases (Fig. 2).

The Doppler signals reflect the haemodynamic information obtained from multiple scatterers located within the vessels. The information is displayed on the monitor of the ultrasound system as a curve, which shows the variation of the frequency and intensity of the signals (power spectrum) as a function of time. The instantaneous relative power for each frequency is calculated using fast Fourier transform. The flow is coded as positive if the scatterers are moving towards the probe, and negative if they are moving away.

Colour Doppler ultrasonography allows detection of the vascular information upon an entire area of the image, and not only at the level of a single Doppler window, such as pulse-wave Doppler, using the concept of a multigate system. A Doppler line with multiple small spectral Doppler windows is moved across the colour box. The flow information cannot be displayed with the same time–frequency curve as in pulsed-wave Doppler, as too many samples are taken almost simultaneously. That is why the average Doppler shift frequency is instantaneously calculated and superimposed with a colour map on the real-time B-mode image. To reach an acceptable frame rate, the calculation is speeded up using an autocorrelation technique. This processing compares the frequency components of the entire line of echoes from one pulse to the next, to reduce computer processing. Recently, the sensitivity, spatial resolution, and frame rate of colour Doppler imaging have been improved with the introduction of the

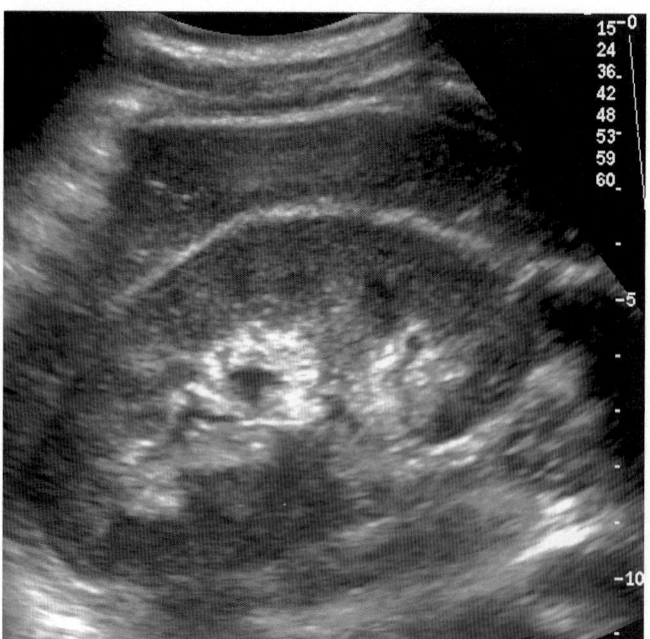

Fig. 1 Longitudinal view of a normal kidney studied with harmonic compounding imaging. Note the hypoechoic appearance of the pyramids.

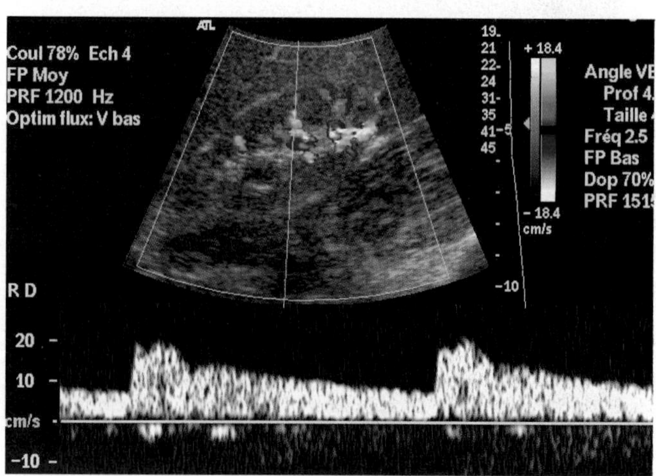

Fig. 2 Pulsed-wave Doppler analysis of the interlobar artery: normal spectrum.

digital architecture of ultrasound systems and the technology of transducers (Fig. 3). Newer signal processing such as cross-correlation techniques, tracking the movement of a target in the imaging plane, or broadband colour Doppler (dynamic flow) offers better resolution.

Power Doppler imaging allows detection of smaller vessels with low flow (Fig. 4). It relies on the coding of the power of the spectrum instead of the Doppler shift. Thus, the colour map usually exhibits a single colour scale, as the directional information of the flow is lost.

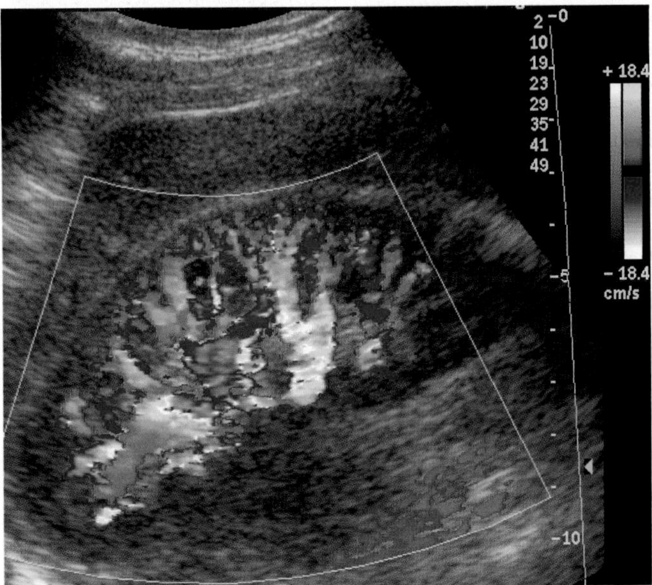

Fig. 3 Colour Doppler ultrasonography of the right kidney using a longitudinal view: note the filling of the distal cortex up to the capsule with the colour signals.

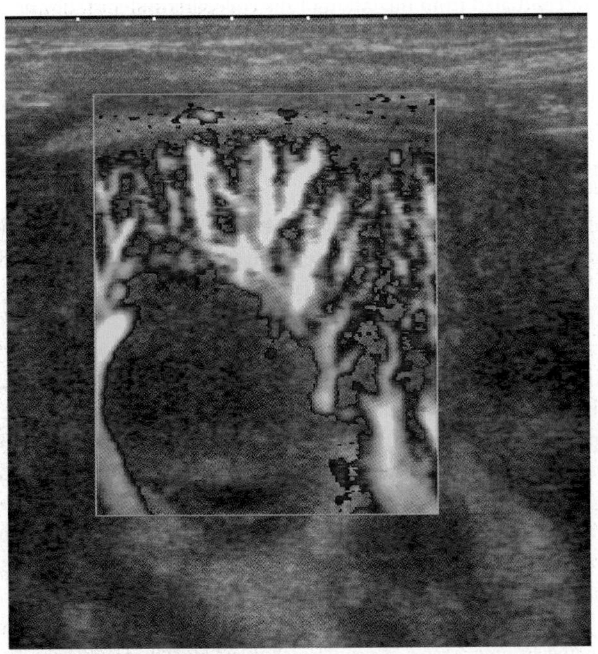

Fig. 4 Power Doppler imaging of a renal transplant at high frequency. Note the excellent resolution and sensitivity, with detection of the arcuate and interlobular arteries.

The signal is proportional to the amount of scatterers in the imaging plane. The persistence is increased in order to increase the signal-to-noise ratio. The main limitation of the power Doppler technique is the lack of haemodynamic information, such as flow direction, acceleration, or turbulence. Recently, some manufacturers have introduced a new power Doppler modality that codes for the flow direction.

The diagnosis of vascular diseases still relies on the spectral analysis obtained from the pulsed-wave Doppler that contains much more information about the haemodynamics of the vessel than the colour or power Doppler techniques. Colour Doppler is then used for the detection of the vascular segment with abnormal blood flow, where the pulsed-wave Doppler window will be moved in order to study the blood flow disturbances.

Doppler measurements

Pulsed-wave Doppler allows measurements of velocity after correction of the angle of insonation. This angle should remain at less than 60° to limit large errors in the measurements. Peak systolic velocity, mean velocity, and end-diastolic velocity can be calculated. When the downstream impedance is low, such as in the distal renal vascular bed, blood flow in diastole is quite high. When vascular impedance increases, the diastolic blood flow reduces. Two indices are mainly used to evaluate the impedance status, the resistive index (Pourcelot) and the pulsatility index. They exhibit little dependence on the angle of insonation. The resistive index is calculated as the ratio between the difference peak systolic velocity minus the end-diastolic velocity and the peak systolic velocity. The pulsatility index is calculated as the ratio between the difference peak systolic velocity minus the minimal diastolic velocity and the mean integrated velocity.

Ultrasound contrast agents

The concept of contrast enhancement is extending the usefulness of ultrasound imaging thanks to an improvement in USCA persistence and efficacy. The most recent USCAs are based on stabilized microbubbles. The persistence of the microbubbles have been dramatically increased using gases different from air and shells of various stiffness (Correas *et al.* 2001). The gas has been replaced by perfluorocarbon gases, which exhibit low solubility and low diffusibility in the plasma. Microbubble contrast agents exhibit an excellent safety profile with no renal toxicity. Their clinical potential has been further increased by the development of specific ultrasound sequences based on non-linear ultrasound imaging that exploit microbubble-specific interactions with the ultrasound beam. They improve the detection of the macro- and microvessels. Initially, they were developed to improve the Doppler examination in case of technical failure, due to attenuation of the ultrasound beam (Kim *et al.* 1999). With improvements in Doppler techniques, this application is slowly disappearing. The development of new imaging sequences that take advantage of the resonant properties of the microbubbles allows real-time visualization of the blood flow from large vessels to microcirculation. These sequences detect the non-linear properties either by selecting the frequency components (harmonic imaging) or by combining pulses (pulse inversion imaging, coherent contrast imaging). Pulse inversion imaging is a technique that relies on the emission of two inverted pulses by each transducer. When the two inverted pulses are summed in the digital beamformer, the linear response from the tissues mostly cancels. In the presence of resonating microbubbles, the sum of distorted pulses does not cancel.

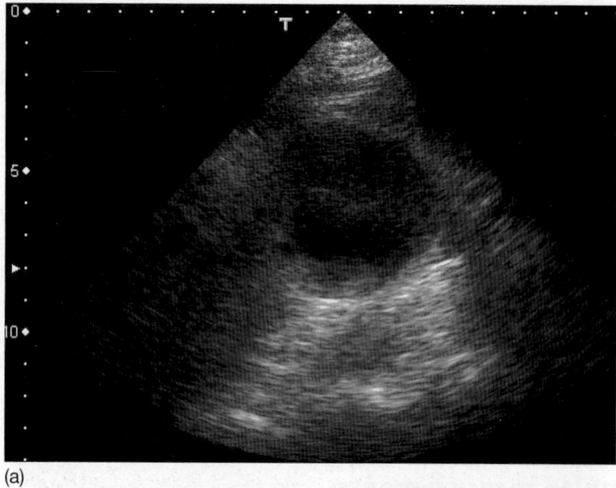

(a)

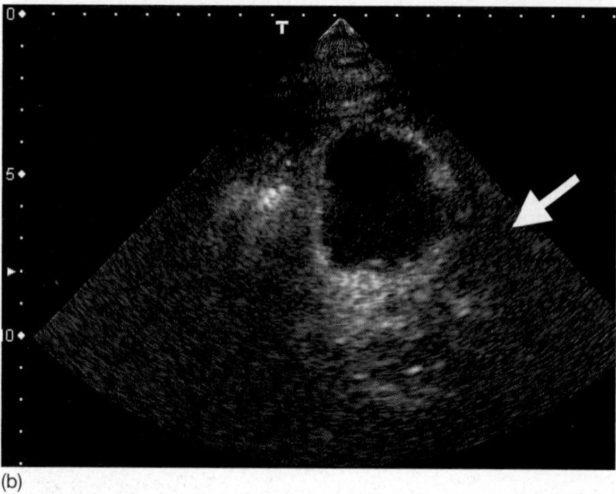

(b)

Fig. 5 Contrast-enhanced study of a cystic lesion: (a) At baseline, the deeper wall of the cyst is thickened. (b) After injection of an ultrasound contrast agent, the cyst is scanned at low mechanical index. The deeper wall strongly enhances the signal and an additional mural nodule is detected (arrow).

This approach can be developed at high acoustic pressures where most of the microbubbles can be destroyed, or at very low acoustic pressures preserving the integrity of the microbubbles (Fig. 5). Contrast-enhanced imaging allows quantification of the signal enhancement and provides functional information. Relative local blood flow and volume can be extracted. More studies are required to precisely define the impact of USCAs in urinary tract assessment.

Grey scale ultrasonography of the kidneys and the urinary tract

Technical considerations

Grey scale ultrasonography allows a non-invasive morphological evaluation of the urinary system. Whereas a contrast medium is usually not required, recently developed USCAs may improve the diagnostic performance in selected cases. No preparation is needed except for a full bladder that permits assessment of the bladder wall, the distal portions of the ureters, and the evaluation of postvoiding residual urine.

Capabilities and limitations

Kidneys

The number and location of the kidneys, their size and shape, and the status of the collecting system are accurately assessed. Each kidney is formed by approximately 11 lobes, with central medulla (pyramids) containing the tubules, surrounded by the cortex. The pyramids exhibit a triangular shape with a large base oriented towards the capsule and the apex oriented towards the sinus (Fig. 1). The renal cortex makes indentations between pyramids, called columns of Bertin. When they are enlarged, these columns of Bertin mimic a renal tumour. The normal echostructure and surrounding vascularity are helpful in diagnosing this anatomical variant (Fig. 6). The cortical echogenicity should be compared to that of the medulla, liver, and spleen. The sonographic corticomedullary differentiation of the normal renal parenchyma can be determined in most cases. It is increased in medical renal diseases. Ultrasonography can detect solid and cystic parenchymal masses that are usually responsible for a capsular budging, as most renal masses originate from the subcapsular cortex. One of the most relevant clinical benefits of ultrasonography is the increased early detection of renal cell carcinomas. Up to 83 per cent of asymptomatic renal tumours are incidentally detected using ultrasound (Fig. 7) (Siemer *et al.* 2000). Most benign cystic lesions, including simple cysts and minimally complicated cysts, are accurately identified with ultrasonography. More complex cystic masses and solid renal neoplasms cannot be accurately classified by ultrasound and require computed tomography (CT) or magnetic resonance imaging characterization (Fig. 5). On the other hand, ultrasonography may provide additional diagnostic information for differential diagnosis of some renal masses that remain equivocal at CT.

The centrally located sinus contains fatty tissues, segmental arteries and veins, lymphatics, and the collecting system. The sinus complex is highly echogenic and should be screened for solid or cystic mass (parapelvic cysts) identification, as well as a markedly hyperechoic renal stone producing acoustic shadowing. The parapelvic cysts should be differentiated from dilatation of the collecting system. They do not branch as the collecting system and usually displace the calyceal tree.

In addition to some diagnostic and therapeutic procedures that can benefit from ultrasound guidance, intraoperative ultrasound remains the only available tool that enables renal parenchymal sparing surgery.

Urinary tract

The normal collecting system is not seen except with high-resolution transducers in renal transplants or thin patients, or when the renal pelvis is extrarenal as a normal variant. Dilatation of the calyces usually indicates obstructive uropathy or a postobstructive low-pressure dilated urinary tract. Obstructive dilatation of the collecting system (Fig. 8) cannot be differentiated from non-obstructive dilatation in ultrasound (Webb 2000), except when the resistive index is increased by more than 10 per cent compared to the normal side (Platt *et al.* 1993). The normal ureters are not seen, except the hypoechoic mural portion of the distal ureter up to the meatus. Dilated ureters, however, can be seen and examined for the detection of an obstructive ureteral calculus at four levels: the proximal subpyelic lumbar portion, the presacral portion that crosses the iliac vessels anteriorly, and the distal pelvic segment posterior to the bladder and within the bladder wall (Fig. 9). The mid-portion of a dilated lumbar ureter is usually not seen. Non-lithiasic lesions and abnormalities of the urinary tract including urothelial neoplasms, blood clot, papillary necrosis, etc. are poorly assessed with ultrasound.

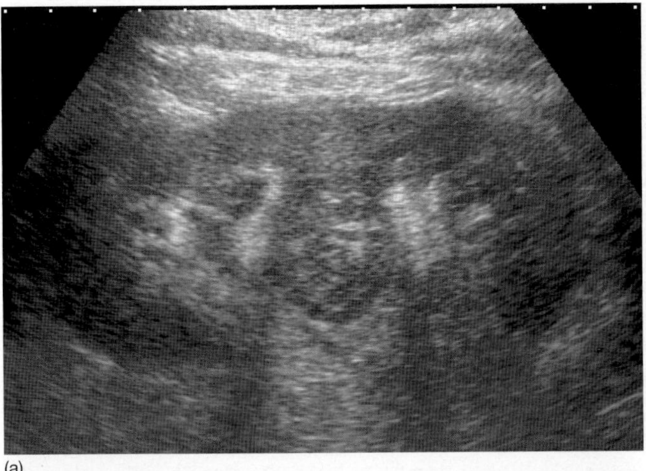

(a)

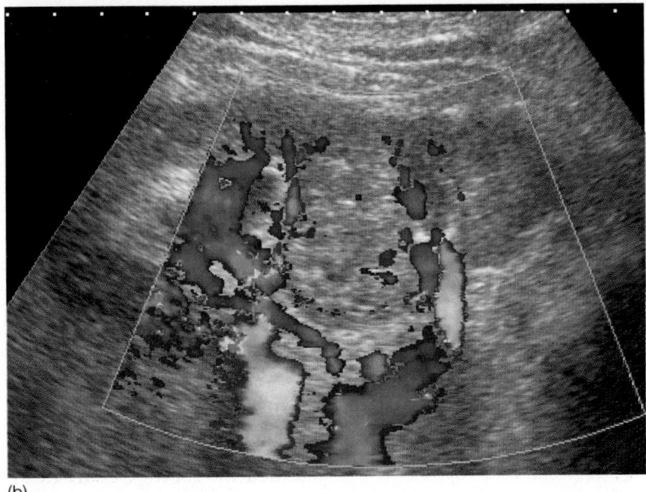

(b)

Fig. 6 Pseudotumour: hypertrophy of a column of Bertin in the middle of the left kidney, studied with B-mode (a) and colour Doppler ultrasonography (b).

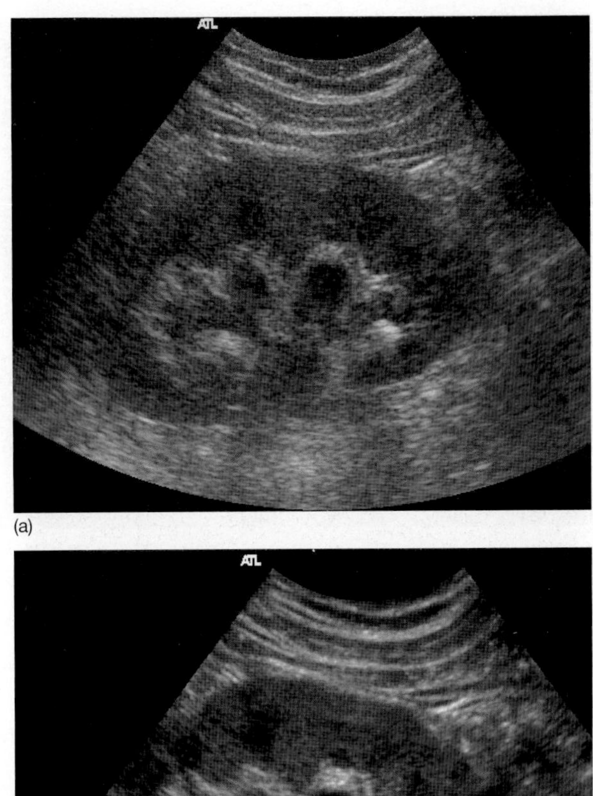

(a)

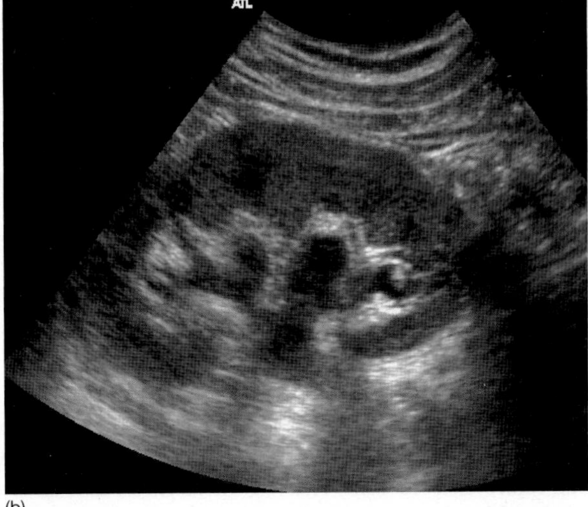

(b)

Fig. 8 Dilatation of the calyceal tree and the renal pelvis. Note that the dilatation is better seen with non-linear imaging (b) compared to conventional B-mode (a).

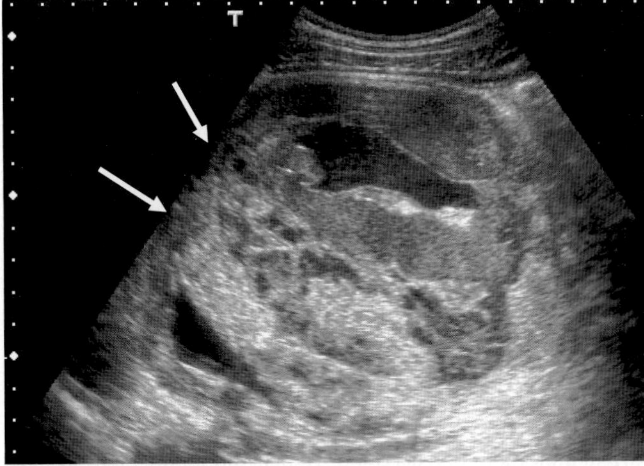

Fig. 7 Large renal tumour incidentally discovered (arrows).

Current indications of grey scale ultrasonography

Indications for using grey scale ultrasound include:

- detection and characterization of renal cysts;
- detection of solid renal masses;
- primary assessment of renal dysfunction;
- diagnosis of a pelvicalyceal filling defect due to a non-opaque calculus;
- screening patients for hydronephrosis;
- evaluation of perinephric fluid collections;
- screening acute pyelonephritis for renal abscess formation;
- screening patients for familial disorders such as polycystic kidney disease;
- screening renal transplant recipients for urological complications;

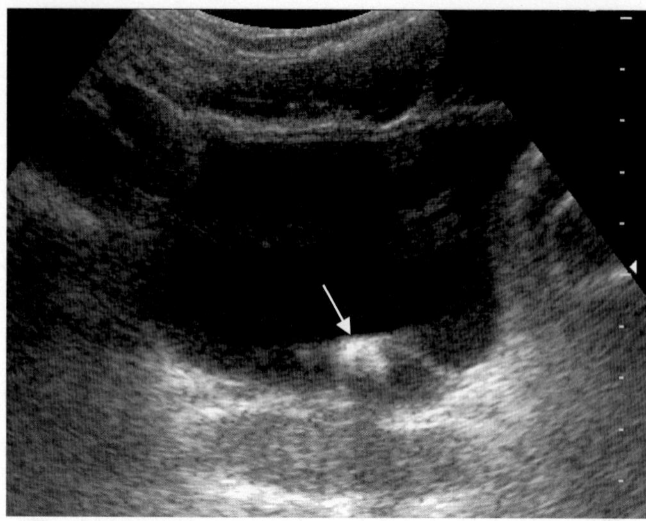

Fig. 9 Ureteral calculus in the bladder wall (arrow).

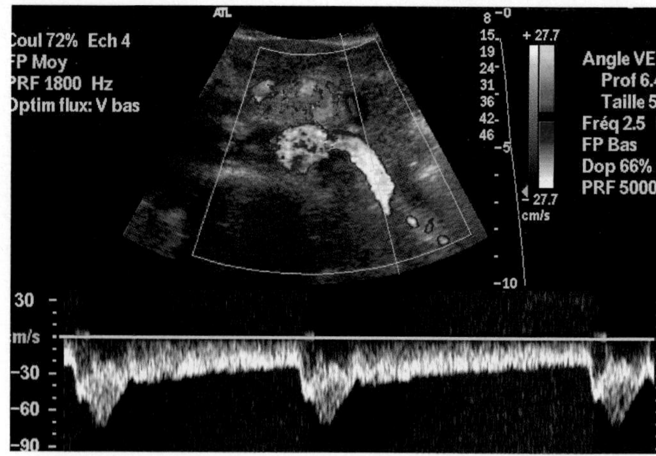

Fig. 10 Colour and spectral analysis of a normal left renal artery.

- screening fetal renal disorders (hydronephrosis, multicystic kidney, etc.);
- guiding biopsies and other percutaneous interventional procedures.

Doppler ultrasonography of the renal vasculature

Technical considerations

The combined Doppler examination of the renal vasculature, including duplex Doppler and colour Doppler ultrasonography, is an efficient but still controversial modality enabling the diagnosis of renal artery stenosis and other vascular disorders. By providing real-time visualization of the renal vascular tree, colour Doppler ultrasound facilitates the identification of the renal artery and allows a direct analysis of haemodynamic changes (Fig. 10). The diagnosis of renal artery stenosis requires duplex Doppler interrogation of intrarenal arteries and extrarenal portions of the renal arteries. Doppler ultrasound should screen the renal arteries for haemodynamic changes at the level of the stenosis, including flow acceleration and spectral broadening, and downstream intrarenal flow repercussion in cases of tight renal artery stenosis. Other vascular disorders can be depicted using colour Doppler and duplex Doppler ultrasonography interrogation obtained from the site of colour encoding alterations.

Capabilities and limitations

Colour Doppler ultrasonography enables investigation of all levels of the vascular supply to native kidneys except vessels in the superficial cortex. Normal blood flow, as defined on spectral analysis, can be depicted from the main renal artery to interlobar branches into the deep cortex. The main Doppler waveform parameters obtained from intrarenal arterial branches include: a normal systolic–diastolic modulation, the acceleration time of early systole, and the resistive index. The so-called tardus parvus waveform (loss of normal systolic–diastolic modulation), a prolonged acceleration time (>70 ms), and a marked decrease in resistive index compared to the opposite side may indicate a tight stenosis of the upstream main renal artery trunk. An increased resistive index (RI > 0.70) reflects a rise in intrarenal arterial resistance that can be seen in non-glomerular nephropathies (Platt *et al.* 1990).

A major limitation of Doppler ultrasound is the difficult and incomplete assessment of renal vessels due to anatomical factors relative to patient corpulence or bowel gas. A technically successful study and an accurate assessment of renal vessels require skilled hands and a good knowledge of the normal renal arterial blood supply. The presence of supernumerary arteries, as well as a well-developed collateral blood supply, can preserve normal downstream arterial flow in cases of tight stenosis. Moreover, arterial branches arising from a patent supernumerary artery could be sampled during Doppler interrogation resulting in normal waveforms in the case of a tight stenosis or even thrombosis involving the second main renal artery.

The diagnosis of primary renal vein thrombosis or tumour thrombus with colour Doppler ultrasonography is accurate, provided the examination is technically adequate (Platt *et al.* 1993). However, early intrarenal venous branch thromboses are usually missed either with colour Doppler ultrasonography or CT.

Among intrarenal vascular disorders, arteriovenous malformations and iatrogenic arteriovenous lesions, such as arteriovenous fistulas and arterial false aneurysms, are accurately detected by colour Doppler ultrasonography in most cases (Helenon *et al.* 1997). These iatrogenic lesions are usually detected after renal biopsy or following a percutaneous endourologic procedure. The lower sensitivity of colour Doppler ultrasonography in the diagnosis of renal infarction and cortical necrosis is due to the deep location of the native kidneys and the small size of some vascular defects (especially cortical necrosis). USCAs are very useful in this case. The infarcted area appears as a microbubble-free renal parenchyma, and thus does not enhance. Microaneurysms associated with renal vasculitis such as polyarteritis nodosa are not seen in colour Doppler ultrasonography.

Current indications of renal colour Doppler ultrasonography

Current indications of renal colour Doppler ultrasonography include:

- the screening of patients at risk of renovascular hypertension or renal failure for renal artery stenosis and thrombosis;

- the detection of renal artery aneurysms;
- the screening of patients for bland or tumour thrombus;
- the detection of renal peripheral infarction;
- the differentiation between glomerulonephritis from other tubulointerstitial and/or vascular medical renal diseases (responsible for elevated resistive index);
- the screening of patients for postbiopsy vascular complications;
- the screening of patients with macroscopic recurrent haematuria for a vascular cause (arteriovenous malformation).

Ultrasound of the prostate and male genital organs

Prostate

Ultrasound examination of the prostate is performed using a transrectal approach (intrarectal probe) (Fig. 11). The examination includes the assessment of the upper urinary tract, evaluation of the postvoiding residual urine, estimation of the prostatic volume, and screening for peripheral zone nodule. Colour Doppler ultrasound can depict focal hypervascular malignant lesions within the peripheral zone. Transrectal ultrasonography is also indicated in male infertility to detect obstructive causes that involve the ejaculatory ducts (lithiasis, intraprostatic cystic lesions) and seminal vesicle abnormalities (agenesis, cystic vesicle).

External male genital organs

Scrotum and other external male genital organs are studied using a high-frequency (7–12 MHz) linear probe that provides a high-resolution

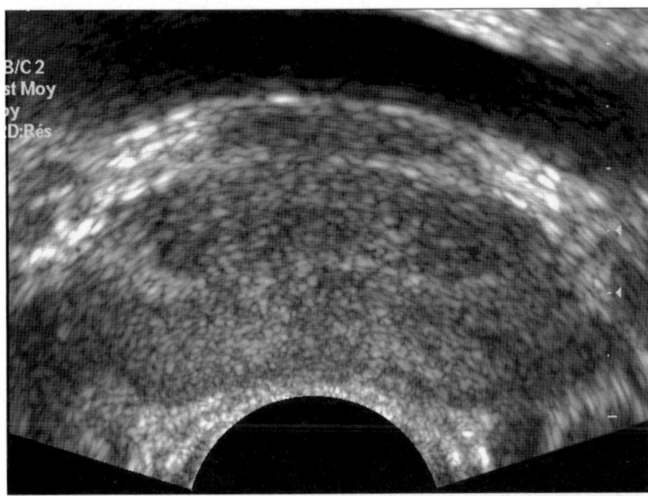

(a)

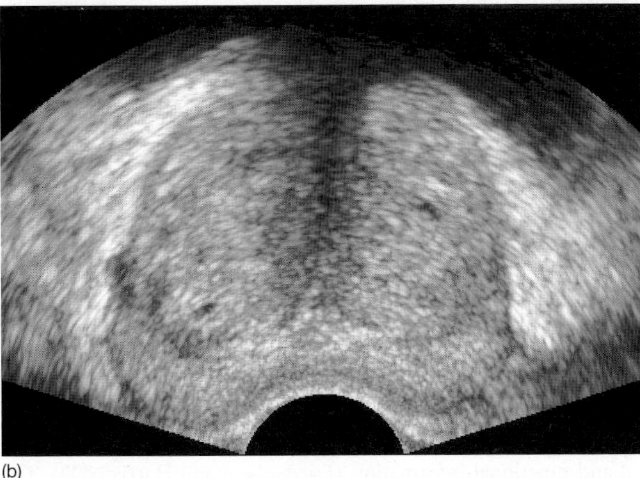

(b)

Fig. 11 Transrectal assessment of the prostate: normal feature (a) and benign hypertrophy (b).

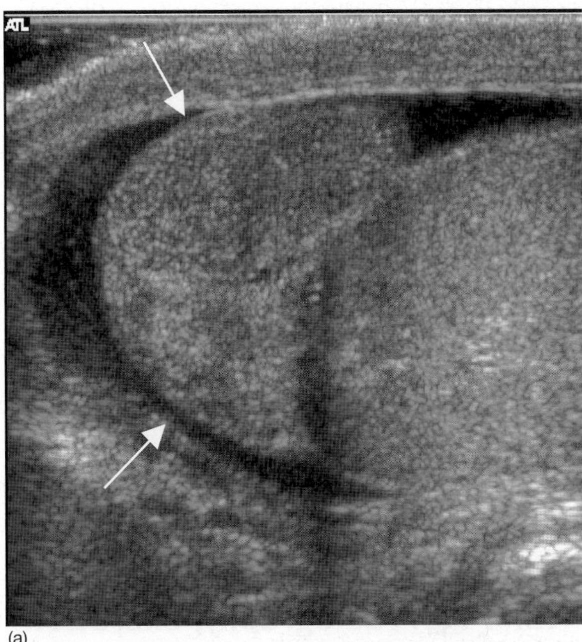

(a)

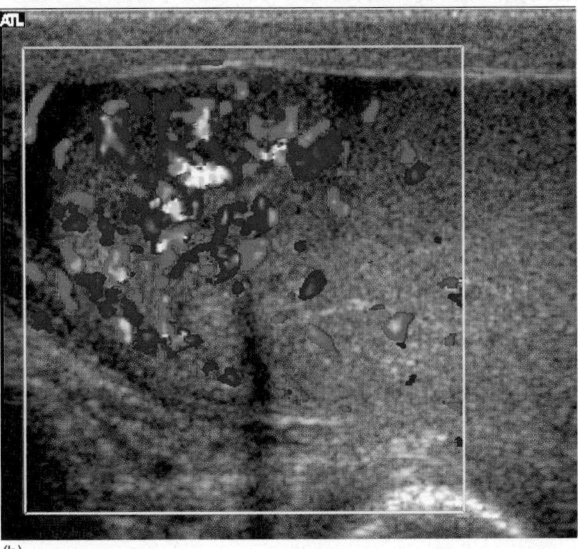

(b)

Fig. 12 Epididymitis: at the top of the testis, the head of the epididym is enlarged on B-mode (a) and the vascularity is strongly increased (b).

image of the testis, epididymis, and cavernous corpus. Urethra and periurethral tissues can also be assessed using retrograde saline infusion in selected cases. The colour Doppler assessment of the testis is accurate and provides diagnostic information that helps differentiate inflammatory disorders (hypervascular) from torsion or neoplasia (Fig. 12). Moreover, colour Doppler ultrasonography and spectral analysis are used in the diagnosis of male infertility due to spermatic venous reflux and male sexual dysfunction of arterial origin.

References

Correas, J. M., Bridal, L., Lesavre, A., Méjean, A., Claudon, M., and Hélénon, O. (2001). Ultrasound contrast agents: properties, principles of action, tolerance and artifacts. *European Radiology* **11**, 1316–1328.

Helenon, O., Melki, P., Correas, J. M., Boyer, J. C., and Moreau, J. F. (1997). Renovascular disease: Doppler ultrasound. *Seminars in Ultrasound, CT, and MR* **18**, 136–146.

Kim, A. Y., Kim, S. H., Kim, Y. J., and Lee, I. H. (1999). Contrast-enhanced power Doppler sonography for the differentiation of cystic renal lesions: preliminary study. *Journal of Ultrasound in Medicine* **18**, 581–588.

Platt, J. F., Rubin, J. M., Ellis, J. H., Di Pietro, M., and Sedman, A. B. (1990). Intrarenal arterial Doppler sonography in patients with nonobstructive renal disease: correlation of resistive index with biopsy findings. *AJR. American Journal of Roentgenology* **154**, 1223–1227.

Platt, J. F., Rubin, J. M., and Ellis, J. H. (1993) Acute renal obstruction: evaluation with intrarenal duplex Doppler and conventional US. *Radiology* **186**, 685–688.

Siemer, S. *et al.* (2000). Value of ultrasound in early diagnosis of renal cell carcinomas. *Der Urologe* **39**, 149–153.

Webb, J. A. W. (2000). Ultrasonography and doppler studies in the diagnosis of renal obstruction. *BJU International* **86** (Suppl. 1), 25–32.

1.6.1.ii Plain radiography, excretion radiography, and contrast radiography

Akira Kawashima and Andrew J. LeRoy

Introduction

Radiology is an integral component in the evaluation of the urinary tract. For decades, excretion radiography following intravenous administration of iodinated contrast media, which is also called intravenous urography (IVU), intravenous pyelography (IVP), and excretory urography (EXU), has been the primary imaging modality of the urinary tracts. In recent years, other imaging modalities such as ultrasonography, computed tomography (CT), and magnetic resonance imaging (MRI) are being used with increasing frequency to compensate for the limitations of IVU. Like excretion radiography, these cross-sectioned imaging examinations have their limitations. Plain radiography, contrast radiography, and excretion urography still remain important in the diagnosis of some urinary tract diseases (Hattery *et al.* 1988; Banner 2001; Dyer *et al.* 2001).

This section will outline basic uroradiological imaging with each subsection providing information on technique, indications, complications, and normal anatomical findings. Radiographic findings relevant to specific pathology, such as renal masses, will be presented in their respective sections and chapters.

Plain radiography

Plain radiography of the abdomen and pelvis is most often referred to as a KUB (kidneys, ureters, and bladder) film or an abdominal 'flat plate' (Fig. 1), and can provide important information about urinary calculi (Figs 2 and 3), calcifications, renal masses (Fig. 2), renal size and contour, bony changes, and bowel gas (Dyer *et al.* 1998; Barbaric and Pollack 2000). An anteroposterior (AP) projection radiograph of the abdomen in supine position may also be referred to as a scout (preliminary) film prior to intravenous (IV) or direct contrast injection for a conventional urogram. This scout radiograph helps establish appropriate radiographic exposure technique factors, evaluate the patient's positioning, and confirms that residual oral contrast material from previous studies has been eliminated from the gut. The indications for the examination and patient risk factors should be reviewed carefully. A menstrual history should be obtained in women of child-bearing age. Radiation exposure should always be limited appropriately. The presence of a fetal skeleton on the scout film justifies postponing the planned contrast study. A scout film is imperative prior to contrast studies because stones and calcifications can be obscured by contrast material in the urinary tract on subsequent films.

The appropriately positioned AP radiograph includes the area cephalad to both adrenals and extends caudal to 2 cm below the symphysis pubis. The kidneys are often suboptimally visualized by overlying bowel gas. Additional views in an oblique projection and plain nephrotomograms are helpful for further evaluation of calcifications or masses. A combination of plain radiographs and non-contrast coronal tomography is valuable in evaluating patients with known metabolic stone disease or in defining residual stone burden after surgical stone therapy.

Anatomical landmarks

Several abdominal and pelvic organs can be identified on plain films. Organs such as the liver, spleen, kidneys, and bladder can be outlined on the film based on the contrasting densities of the organs themselves compared to surrounding mesenteric or retroperitoneal fat. The outline of the kidneys is helpful both for assessing size and focal cortical scarring and for delineating intrarenal calcifications. The psoas muscle margins can usually be seen on the plain radiograph (Fig. 1), but is obscured by retroperitoneal fluid or mass.

Plain films of the abdomen and pelvis can demonstrate abnormalities of the bowel gas pattern (i.e. adynamic ileus, mechanical obstruction, faecal impaction) and also allow for evaluation of skeletal anomalies, such as sacral agenesis and spinal dysraphism.

Excretion radiography

Excretion radiography is frequently used as a non-invasive screening procedure for the entire urinary tract because it displays both anatomical and functional information (Friedenberg and Harris 2000). The current indications for excretion radiography include: (a) haematuria (macroscopic and microscopic); (b) suspected urothelial tumours or

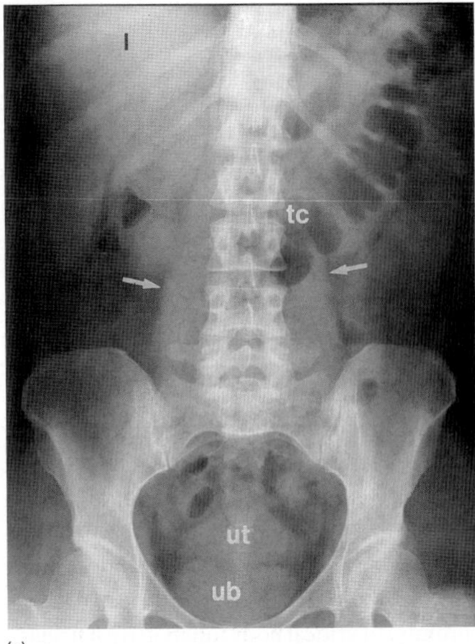

(a)

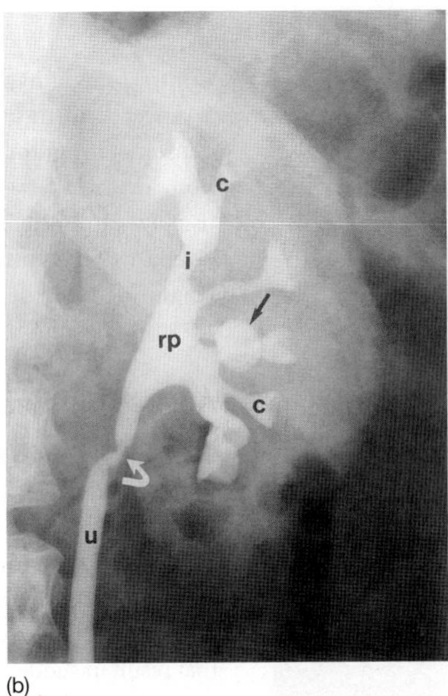

(b)

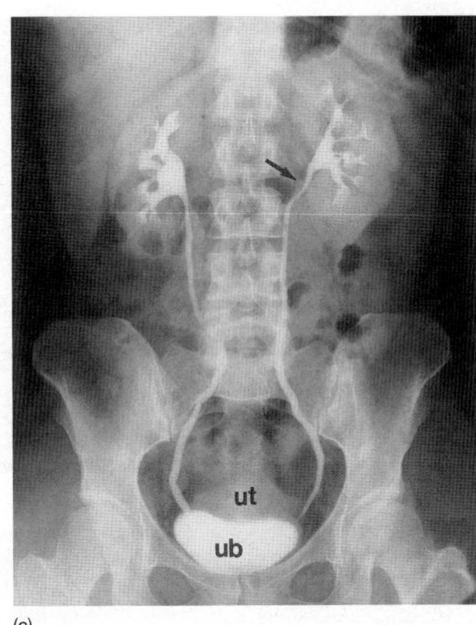

(c)

Fig. 1 Excretion radiography: (a) Plain radiograph of the abdomen and pelvis reveals normal contour of the kidneys and the medial margin of the psoas muscles (arrows). Liver (l), transverse colon (tc), urinary bladder (ub), and uterus (ut). (b) Magnified view of the left kidney with abdominal compression 8 min after IV contrast material administration. Calyx (c), infundibulum (i), renal pelvis (rp), proximal ureter (u). Calyx which projects posteriorly is seen *en face* (arrow). Normal fold of the ureter at the ureteropelvic junction (curved arrow). (c) Abdominal radiograph after release of ureteral compression reveals normal ureters and urinary bladder (ub). The left ureter at the ureteropelvic junction (arrow) is better distended and straight. Uterus (ut).

papillary necrosis; (c) surveillance protocol for patients with prior urothelial malignancy; (d) stone disease, often in conjunction with ultrasonography and CT; (e) complicated or unusual urinary tract infections (including tuberculosis); (f) preoperative evaluation for select endourological procedures; and (g) postoperative evaluation of urological surgical procedures.

Patient preparation

A thorough pre-examination bowel prep with a mild laxative (e.g. $1^1/_4$ ounces of extract of senna) the night before the procedure is desirable to cleanse the colon of stool, which may interfere with optimal visualization of the urinary tract. Withholding of fluid and solid food overnight is advantageous for optimal renal concentration and excretion of the contrast medium. An empty stomach also decreases the possibility of aspiration of solid food by a vomiting patient after IV contrast administration.

Filming procedure

A plain abdominal radiograph (KUB) prior to the administration of IV contrast media is essential. After the contrast medium is injected, abdominal compression is applied. Approximately 2–3 min after the contrast material has been administered, nephrotomograms (usually three) are obtained to visualize the renal parenchyma (nephrographic phase) (Hattery *et al.* 1988). Radiographs 8–10 min after the contrast injection demonstrate the calyces, pelves, and proximal ureters (pyelographic phase) (Fig. 1). The ureters are generally well visualized on the 10-min decompression radiograph. Films of the bladder (often including a postvoid film) conclude the examination.

Diuretic excretion radiography (modified excretion radiography)

This modification of excretion radiography is reserved for those patients suspected of having volume-dependent hydronephrosis in whom an initial (dehydrated) excretion radiography revealed no obstruction. With a brisk diuresis after frusemide injection (Lasix, 20 mg IV), a borderline ureteropelvic junction or ureteral narrowing may become inadequate to transport the increased urine volume and may result in hydronephrosis and reproduce the patient's symptoms.

Contrast media

Intravenous iodinated contrast material is excreted by glomerular filtration with little or no tubular excretion, with subsequent concentration in postglomerular tubules and collecting ducts and progressive opacification of the urinary tract. Urine concentrations are determined by the dose administered, the glomerular filtration rate (GFR), and the renal tubular function. As the urine is concentrated in the collecting ducts, the relative concentration of the contrast agent is enhanced 50–100-fold.

Traditional urographic contrast media consist of three atoms of iodine attached to a benzene ring (tri-iodinated benzoic acid derivatives) (Katzberg 1997). Older agents include the sodium or meglumine salts of diatrizoate (Renografin, Hypaque) and iothalamate (Conray), all of which are categorized as high-osmolar contrast media (HOCM) with a mean osmotic load of 1400–2400 mOsm/kg water, exceeding serum by a factor of 5–7.

The widely used newer non-ionic, low osmolar contrast agents such as iohexol (Omnipaque), iopamidol (Isovue), and ioversol (Optiray) offer

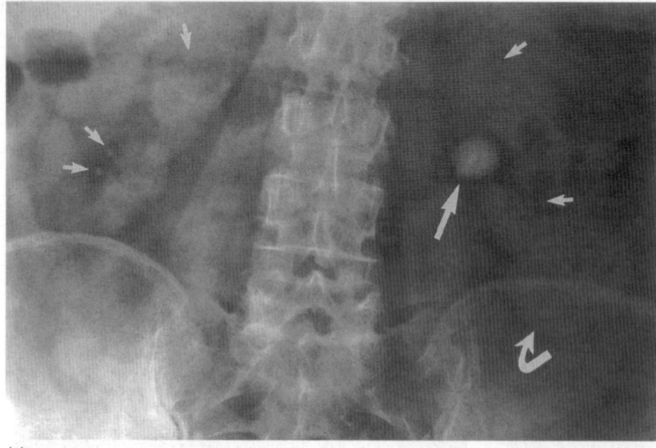

(a)

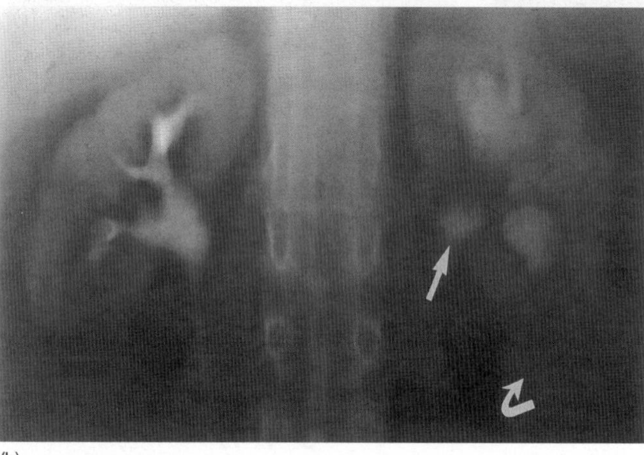

(b)

Fig. 2 Patient with renal stones and renal cell carcinoma: (a) Plain radiograph demonstrates bilateral renal calculi (short arrows) with the largest over the left renal hilum (long arrow). A round mass is projected over the lower pole of the left kidney (curved arrow). (b) Nephrotomogram after IV contrast administration demonstrates left hydronephrosis with pyelocaliectasis and delayed excretion caused by the large stone at the left renal pelvis near the ureteropelvic junction (straight arrow). The small bilateral renal calculi lie in calyces. The mass originates from the lower renal pole (curved arrow), which was shown to be an enhancing mass on CT (not shown) and proved to be a renal cell carcinoma at surgery.

a somewhat more comfortable, safer examination to patients who are sensitive to the older HOCM and produce fewer adverse effects, although the rare life-threatening reactions are not eliminated by the use of these low-osmolar contrast media (LOCM) (Palmer 1988; Katayama *et al.* 1990). LOCM has approximately a 50–100 per cent reduction in osmolarity with an equivalent iodine load, ranging from 411 to 796 mOsm/kg of water. Although the cost of LOCM has come down over the last 10 years, LOCM are still 3–4 times more expensive than HOCM in the United States. Because of this, some hospitals have adopted a limited use of LOCM in high-risk patients. The use of LOCM is preferred for patients with a significant history of allergy, including reactions to previously administered contrast media, any patient whose general condition appears fragile (e.g. cardiac compensation, advanced age or debility, electrolyte imbalance), and patients with renal functional impairment, blood dyscrasia, and risk of aspiration (Cohan *et al.* 1998).

Dosage

Contrast medium can be administered either as a bolus injection or as a slower drip infusion. The bolus injection allows for a rapid and dense nephrogram when films are obtained 2–3 min after the injection. In the average-sized adult, 60–100 ml of contrast medium is usually administered. Larger (>100 kg) and/or older patients with decreased GFRs often receive 100–150 ml of contrast to optimize the diagnostic value of their urographic examination.

Adverse effects

The majority of adverse effects with iodinated contrast media are mild or moderate and only observation, reassurance, and support are required. However, the more severe adverse effects often have a mild or moderate onset of symptoms or prodrome. Reactions to contrast agents usually occur within 20 min following IV injection. The severe contrast reactions most threatening to patients are those unanticipated events that result in sudden compromise of critical body functions, particularly systemic anaphylactoid reactions or profound cardiovascular collapse.

The aetiology of contrast medium reactions can be classified as anaphylactoid (idiosyncratic), non-anaphylactoid, and combined although the physiological mechanisms involved in these reactions are not fully understood. Anaphylactoid reactions, which mimic systemic allergic responses, usually occur unexpectedly and the specific reaction pathway is uncertain. Other reactions (non-anaphylactoid) related to osmotic, chemotoxic, direct organ toxicity, or vasomotor effects are more predictable and better understood.

Anaphylactoid (idiosyncratic) reactions are generally classified as (a) mild, (b) moderate, and (c) severe (Cohan *et al.* 1998). Minor side-effects, by definition, are not serious and for the most part do not require therapy. Nausea and vomiting are the most common adverse reactions encountered with HOCM. Other minor reactions include altered taste, warmth, headache, dizziness, shaking, nasal congestions, itching, pallor, flushing, chills, sweats, rash, hives (less than four), swelling, and anxiety. These symptoms are usually self-limited, but observation is required to confirm resolution and/or lack of progression. No treatment is necessary beyond comfort measures. Patient reassurance is usually helpful. Moderate reactions include tachycardia, brachycardia, hypertension, mild hypotension, dyspnoea, bronchospasm, wheezing, and pronounced cutaneous reaction such as extensive hives (four or more than four) or diffuse erythema. The observed clinical signs and symptoms of moderate reactions should be considered as indications for immediate treatment (Table 1). These situations require close, careful observation of possible progression into a life-threatening event. Patients with moderate symptoms such as systemic urticaria or facial oedema are treated with antihistamines and subcutaneous adrenaline. Severe types of reactions include laryngeal oedema, and/or profound hypotension and often require small doses of 1 : 10,000 dilution of adrenaline IV. Other severe types of reactions include convulsion, arrhythmias, unresponsiveness, and cardiopulmonary arrest. All severe reactions require prompt recognition and treatment by the radiologist and hospitalization is almost always required.

Approximately 5–12 per cent of patients demonstrate an allergic or histamine-type reaction to HOCM. In patients with a history of multiple allergies, especially with seafood sensitivity, the reaction rate increases to approximately 15 per cent (threefold), with the majority of these being mild. Yet, it is slightly higher in those who have a history

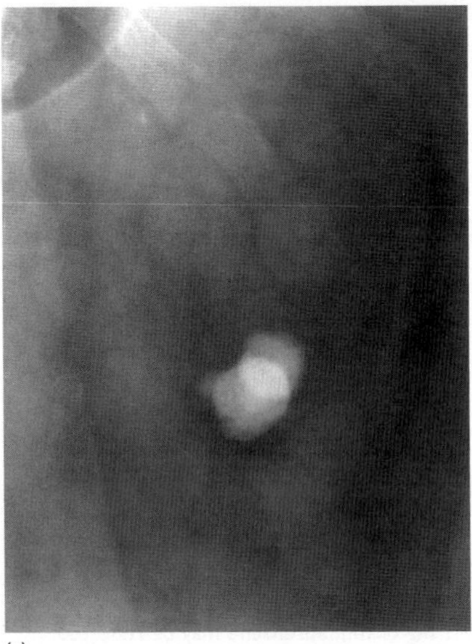
(a)

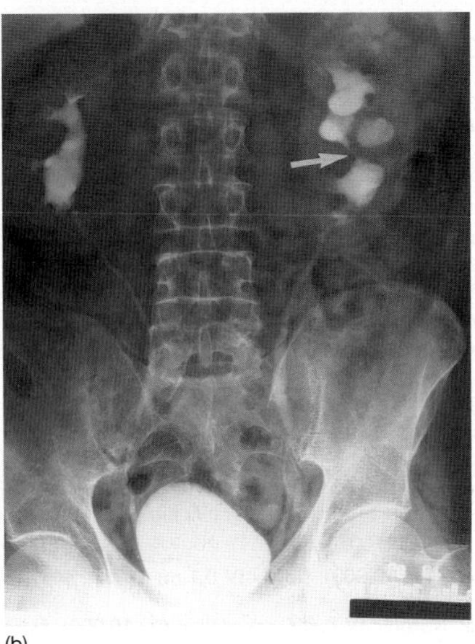
(b)

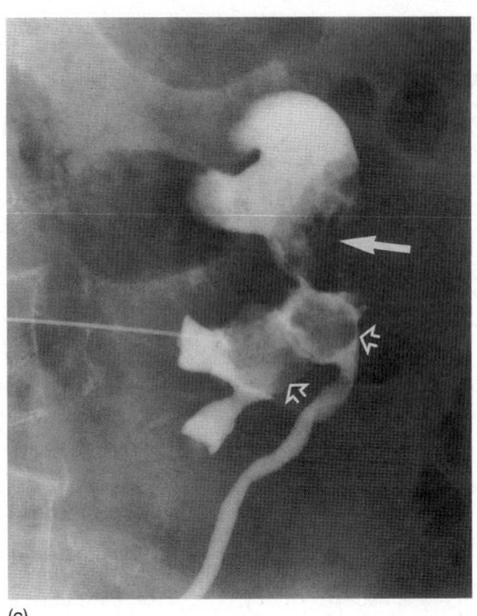
(c)

Fig. 3 Patient with renal stones and transitional cell carcinoma: (a) Magnified view of plain radiograph demonstrates two adjacent stones projected over the lower pole of the left kidney. (b) Excretory radiograph shows the left renal stones in the lower intrarenal collecting system. Note irregular narrowing of the left renal pelvis (arrow) with associated caliectasis. Kidneys are congenitally malrotated bilaterally. (c) Magnified view of antegrade pyelogram following a percutaneous needle puncture of a lower pole calyx shows a large filling defect in the mid- to upper-left renal pelvis with urothelial irregularity (arrow), characteristics of urothelial tumour. The two stones (open arrows) lie in the lower left collecting system.

of asthma or an allergic reaction to prior administration of contrast medium. Serious contrast reactions are rare and occur in 1 or 2 per 1000 examinations using HOCM. In a review of the literature, deaths range from 1 : 40,000 to 1 : 170,000 patients following IV administration of HOCM (Cohan *et al.* 1998).

LOCM is associated with a decreased occurrence of anaphylactoid reactions and with a decrease in the incidence of repeated anaphylactoid reactions in patients with a history of allergies. Serious contrast reactions to LOCM are rarer than HOCM and occur in 0.16 per 1000 examinations using LOCM. Currently, the incidence of fatal outcomes after LOCM has decreased to 0.9 per 100,000. This change likely reflects improvement in contrast media design (LOCM) and the increased use of LOCM for patients with risk factors, as well as the proper recognition and treatment of all contrast reactions.

Prophylactic corticosteroids are strongly recommended for 'at risk' patients who require contrast media (Table 2) (Lasser 1988; Greenberger and Patterson 1991). They should also receive LOCM. However, no regimen has eliminated repeat reactions completely. Pretesting is not predictive, may itself be dangerous, and is not recommended (Yamaguchi *et al.* 1991).

Contrast media may induce physiological changes (non-anaphylactoid reactions) due to either their hypertonicity or chemotoxicity. Many of the symptoms caused by hypertonicity are lessened with LOCMs. HOCM can cause increased cardiac output and decreased peripheral vascular resistance by expanding the intravascular space. Peripheral vasodilation can result in a sensation of warmth or burning and reflux tachycardia. Bradycardia has also been reported and thought to be due to direct vasovagal reaction. HOCM and, to a lesser degree, LOCM can inhibit aggregation of platelets and cause blocking thrombin generation, thereby prolonging partial thromboplastin, prothrombin, and thrombin time. These changes induce a diuresis and can result in the loss of electrolytes and contraction of the systemic volume. Rare cases of neurotoxicity have been reported related to contrast volumetric overdose with induction of seizures, although the exact dose at which this occurs is not known.

Contrast-media-induced acute renal failure

IV contrast media may aggravate pre-existing renal disease in a small percentage of patients with underlying azotemia by a process not yet understood. Aetiological factors that have been proposed include: (a) renal haemodynamic changes, (b) direct tubular toxicity, and (c) intratubular obstruction as a result of tubular cell injury (Katzberg 1997; Cohan *et al.* 1998). There is no standard definition for reporting contrast-media-induced nephrotoxicity. The definition of 'significant' changes varies considerably among studies. Acute contrast-material-induced nephrotoxicity has been defined as an increase in the baseline creatinine values of 20–50 per cent or an absolute increase from 0.5 to 1.0 mg/dl (Katzberg 1997). Most cases of contrast-media-induced nephrotoxicity are unrecognized because serum creatinine concentration is not systematically monitored. This nephrotoxicity is usually self-limited. Serum creatinine usually peaks within 3–5 days, and usually returns to baseline within 10–14 days (Katzberg 1997). Nephrotoxicity is extraordinarily unlikely when kidney function is normal. Patients with diabetic nephropathy whose creatinine is elevated appear to be the most vulnerable. Compared to HOCM, LOCM use reduces the risk of the development of contrast nephropathy (Barrett and Carlisle 1993). However, the reduced risk may be minimal.

Those patients at high risk for contrast-induced nephropathy are more susceptible when dehydrated and when exposed to increasing volumes of contrast agents. Therefore, in high-risk patients, adequate hydration (avoidance of dehydrating preparations) may be beneficial.

Table 1 Reactions to iodinated contrast material and treatment

Type of reactions	**Treatment**
Pruritus	If severe, diphenhydramine PO/IV 25–50 mg or chlorpheniramine 4 mg PO
Uriticaria	Contrast injection discontinued if not completed Minimal (few scattered lesions): observation If diffuse or symptomatic, diphenhydramine PO/IV 25–50 mg, if severe, adrenaline SQ (1 : 1000), 0.1–0.3 ml
Angioedema	Closely monitor the airway, O_2 by mask Isotonic IV fluids, adrenaline SQ (1 : 1000), 0.1–0.3 ml (0.1–0.3 mg) If severe or associated with hypotension or airway compromise, adrenaline IV (1 : 10,000), 0.1 mg (1 ml)
Diffuse erythema	O_2 by masks, isotonic IV fluid If hypotensive: adrenaline IV (1 : 10,000), 0.1 mg (1 ml) Hydrocortisone (Solu-Cortef) IV 200–300 mg
Bronchospasm	O_2 6–10 l/min by mask, isotonic IV fluids, β-agonist inhalers, metaproterenol (Alupent), and albuterol (Proventil) adrenaline SQ (1 : 1000), 0.1–0.3 ml If hypotensive, adrenaline (1 : 10,000), slowly IV 0.1 mg (1 ml)
Laryngeal oedema	O_2 6–10 l/min by mask, isotonic IV fluids, adernaline (1 : 10,000), slowly IV 0.1 mg (1 ml), adrenaline may be repeated as needed up to maximum of 1 mg
Pulmonary oedema	Elevate torso, O_2 6–10 l/min by mask, frusemide (lasix) 20–40 mg IV push (slowly) Transfer to intensive care unit or emergency department
Hypotension with bradycardia (vagal reaction)	Legs elevated 60° or more, or Trendelenburg position, O_2 by mask, isotonic Ringer's lactate or normal saline IV fluids, atropine 0.6–1.0 mg IV push slowly (up to a total dose of 0.04 mg/kg in adults, 2–3 mg)
Hypotension with tachycardia	Legs elevated 60° or more, or Trendelenburg position, O_2 6–10 l/min by mask, isotonic Ringer's lactate or normal saline IV fluids, if poorly responsive, adrenaline IV (1 : 10,000), 0.1 mg/1 mL, adrenaline may be repeated as needed up to maximum of 1 mg
Hypertensive crisis	O_2 6–10 l/min, maintain IV access, nitroglycerin 0.4 mg tablet sublingual (may repeat 3×) or topical 2 per cent nitroglycerin ointment, apply 1 in. strip, transfer to intensive care unit or emergency department
Angina pectoris	O_2 6–10 l/min by mask, IV fluids, nitroglycerin 0.4 mg tablet sublingual (may repeat 3×), transfer to intensive care unit or emergency department
Seizures/convulsions	O_2 6–10 l/min by mask, maintain IV access, consider diazepam (Valium) 5 mg or midazolam (Versed) 2.5 mg, refer to emergency room for further evaluation and work-up

Modified from Cohan *et al.* (1998).

Table 2 Premedication

Corticosteroid/antihistamine (Greenberger and Patterson 1991) Predonisone 50 mg po 13 h, 7 h, and 1 h prior to contrast exam Diphenhydramine (Benadryl) 50 mg po 1 h prior
Corticosteroid alone (Lasser and Berry 1991) Methylprednisolone (Medrol) 32 mg po 12 h and 2 h prior to contrast exam

Because treatment options are limited once oliguric renal failure has developed, most clinical effort has been aimed at prevention of contrast-induced acute renal failure. In addition to active hydration by IV isotonic saline solution, several studies have suggested that various pharmacological agents may be of benefit in preventing contrast-induced acute renal failure, including the adenosine receptor antagonist theophylline (Katholi *et al.* 1995; Pflueger *et al.* 2000), and the antioxidant acetylcysteine (Tepel *et al.* 2000).

In patients with underlying chronic renal failure who undergo regular dialysis, contrast media are readily cleared by dialysis because these are not protein-bound. Unless there is significant underlying cardiac dysfunction, or a very large volume of contrast media is used, there is no need for urgent dialysis. The use of LOCM is still suggested to limit intravascular fluid volume fluctuations and their cardiovascular effects.

Patients with multiple myeloma may occasionally experience acute renal failure following IV contrast administration. Dehydration of the patient is a predisposing factor, so fluid restriction, vomiting, or laxative prior to excretion radiography should be avoided in patients with myeloma.

In diabetic patients with normal renal function, taking the oral antihyperglycaemic agent metformin (glucophage), it is beneficial to stop the metformin for at least 48 h after administration of IV contrast material to minimize the risk of developing metformin-associated lactic acidosis.

Subcutaneous extravasation of contrast medium is not uncommon. Such extravasation may result in local pain, erythema, and swelling. These symptoms usually resolve with local therapy including both warm and cold compression and elevation of affected extremity. Extravasated LOCM is better tolerated than HOCM. Rarely, significant tissue necrosis and dermal sloughing can occur unpredictably with even very small amounts of extravasation (Cohan *et al.* 1996). An immediate surgical consultation is indicated when patients develop increased swelling or pain after 2–4 h, altered tissue perfusion, changes in sensation in the affected extremity, and skin ulceration.

The normal excretion urogram

The renal parenchyma is optimally assessed during the nephrographic phase of urography. The normal kidney may range from 9 to 13 cm in cephalocaudal dimension depending on sex and age. The left kidney is frequently larger that the right kidney by approximately 0.5 cm. The kidneys are sharply marginated and smooth in contour. Congenital fetal lobulation is a common normal variant, and can be differentiated from scars from prior renal infarction or inflammation by their smooth contour and regular spacing and relationship to normal calices. Renal parenchyma measures 3–3.5 cm in thickness in the polar regions and 2–2.5 cm in the interpolar regions. The number of calyces may vary considerably. Each calyx (minor calyx) is deeply cupped and surrounds one papilla. The peripheral portion of the calyx is called the fornix. A group of calyces, termed compound calices, drains two to four papillae and is frequently seen in the polar regions where the cortical columns are deficient or thin. Two or more infundibula (major calyces), each leading to single or multiple calices, arise separately from the pelvis. Conventionally, all branches from the renal pelvis, whether single or multiple, are termed infundibula. Normal infundibula are straight without bowing or displacement. The renal pelvis sometimes appears to be outside the confines of the kidneys, where it often has a distended appearance (the extrarenal pelvis).

The upper ureter usually begins as a smooth extension from the renal pelvis and descends lateral to the transverse processes of the upper lumbar vertebra. The middle third of the ureter is usually superimposed on the transverse processes of the lower lumbar vertebra. The ureter crosses anterior to the iliac vessels at a slightly higher position on the right than the left. The distal ureter courses posterolaterally and then anteromedially to enter the bladder. Peristalsis activity may change the size and shape of the calyces, pelvis, and ureter from film to film. When the bladder is progressively distended, it is smoothly marginated and appears roughly spherical. On a postvoid film, the mucosal pattern of the bladder is frequently identified.

CT urography

Cross-sectional imaging studies including ultrasound, CT, and MRI have been increasingly used to assess the renal parenchyma because it has been shown that with diminishing size of a renal mass, the sensitivity of EXU decreased dramatically. With the introduction of helical CT, CT urography has been increasingly used as a more definitive study for the evaluation of urinary tracts. The renal parenchyma is evaluated with CT scans before and after IV contrast administration, and then the collecting system is visualized by one of several methods, including conventional abdominal radiographs (Vrtiska *et al.* 2000), CT scanned projection radiographs (CT scout, scanogram) (Kawashima *et al.* 2001), or reformatted images generated from thin-section multidetector helical CT images obtained during the excretory phase of contrast enhancement (Chow and Sommer 2001; Caoili *et al.* 2002). This evolving technique has the potential to replace standard excretory radiography in the majority of patient evaluations.

Contrast radiography

Retrograde pyelography

Retrograde pyelography is the opacification of the ureter and pelvicaliceal system via the direct retrograde injection of contrast media at the time of cystoscopy (Fig. 4) (Imray *et al.* 2000). The examination may be done in a cystoscopic suite, or the ureter may be cannulated and the patient may be subsequently brought to the radiology department for the examination. The examination is best performed with fluoroscopy and appropriate spot and overhead films. When a urothelial lesion is suspected, subsequent endoscopy with brushing or biopsy of the lesion for a pathological diagnosis may be performed under fluoroscopic control.

Retrograde pyelography is performed to investigate lesions of the ureter and renal collecting system that cannot be adequately defined by EXU or to visualize the collecting systems and ureters when EXU is contraindicated (renal failure, severe prior contrast reaction). Retrograde pyelography is used to visualize the ureteral stump remaining after nephrectomy in a patient with haematuria or positive urinary cytology.

The procedure is performed using a sterile technique and is contraindicated in a patient with infected urine because of the risk of

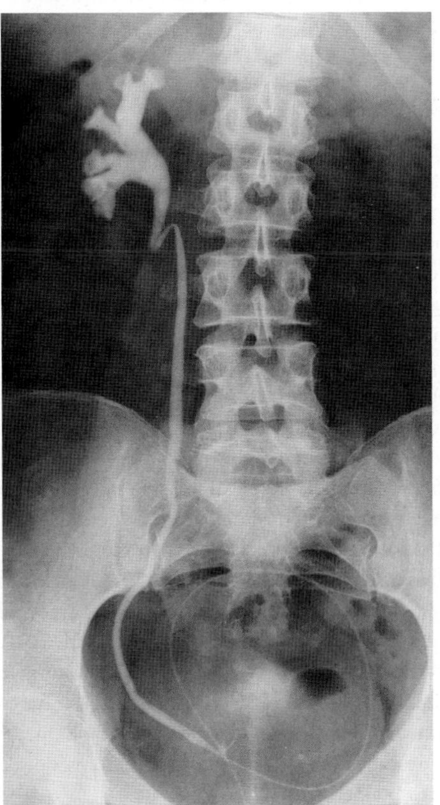

Fig. 4 Retrograde pyelogram reveals normal contrast filling of the right ureter and intrarenal collecting system.

introducing bacteria into the upper collecting system or blood stream. Retrograde pyelography cannot be performed when patients cannot or should not undergo cystoscopy (e.g. patients recovering from recent bladder or urethral surgery). The procedure may be impossible to complete in patients with a very large prostate preventing proper cannulation of the ureter, in patients with tortuous ureters, or following ureteral reimplantation.

Delayed films can be obtained after retrograde pyelography to evaluate the drainage of the collecting system. Delayed films are best obtained after the patient has been upright for a short period of time. Retrograde pyelography in the presence of significant obstruction can be potentially dangerous because of the risk of bacterial spread into the upper tract above the obstruction. If significant obstruction is identified during retrograde pyelography then ureteral stent placement should be considered.

Complications of retrograde pyelography include ureteral perforation, infection, and contrast reaction. The most common ureteral injury during retrograde pyelography is perforation, occurring during advancement of the catheter or guide wire. These injuries are usually managed with either observation or stent placement depending upon the extent of the injury. Introduction of infection is a risk and retrograde pyelography should be avoided in patients with infected urine. If the retrograde pyelography procedure must be performed, adequate antibiotic coverage is required, and if obstruction is present then stent placement must be considered. Up to 10–15 per cent of contrast media can be absorbed during retrograde pyelography. Therefore, caution is advised in patients with a known contrast allergy. Fluoroscopic monitoring of retrograde pyelography is helpful to avoid excess contrast volume injection, reducing the amount of extravasation from the distended upper collecting system.

Antegrade pyelography

Antegrade pyelography is performed to visualize the upper tract when excretion radiography is unsatisfactory and retrograde pyelography cannot be performed (e.g. ureteral diversion). This technique can delineate the site or nature of upper urinary tract obstruction if retrograde pyelography has failed or alternative imaging techniques (Ultrasonography, CT, MRI) are not definitive. Antegrade pyelography is indicated to ascertain whether a dilated collecting system is obstructed or not when azotaemia and/or oliguria occurs after renal transplantation. Pyelography is an essential component of upper urinary tract urodynamic testing (Whitaker test).

Antegrade pyelography is contraindicated in patients with an uncorrectable bleeding diathesis, diffuse skin infection over the puncture site, or anatomic anomalies that preclude safe renal puncture. A non-dilated collecting system is not a contraindication. Although it is technically challenging to percutaneously puncture a non-dilated collecting system, it can usually be accomplished successfully.

The renal pelvis is percutaneously punctured with a 21-gauge thin-walled needle from a posterior or posterolateral approach (Fig. 3). Renal localization is provided by means of contrast excreted after an IV injection or, in the event of a non-visualizing kidney, with ultrasound. The procedure is carried out under fluoroscopic control and spot films are obtained.

Among the complications of this procedure is inadvertent puncture of adjacent intra-abdominal structures. Although puncture of the renal vein, kidney parenchyma, liver, spleen, or colon is possible, few, if any, complications result because of the small size of the needle. Some contrast extravasation into the perinephric tissues usually occurs with any antegrade pyelogram. However, the transparenchymal puncture tract is very small and rapidly seals off after the needle has been removed if no collecting system obstruction is present. Comprehensive antegrade pyelography may be technically difficult and time consuming and, on rare occasions, may be unsuccessful if the collecting system is not dilated.

Cystography

Static cystography

Static cystography provides information on bladder volume, contour, position, and continuity. Static cystography is performed to assess suspected bladder rupture, to demonstrate bladder diverticula, delineate vesicoenteric fistulae, and to assess postoperative healing following open bladder or distal ureteral surgery.

Contraindications to passage of a Foley catheter may make attempts at cystography inadvisable, but there are no absolute contraindications to cystography itself. When a patient has sustained pelvic trauma, the integrity of the urethra must first be established before blindly inserting a urethral catheter. This often requires retrograde urethrography (RUG) before formal cystography to prevent further urethral injury during catheter placement. Complications of cystography are rare. Excessively forceful injection may result in bladder rupture or disruption of a fresh suture line, but these events are rare.

The technique of cystography is basic and an initial scout film is obtained prior to injection of contrast. Contrast enhanced imaging of the lower urinary tract provides valuable information on the function and anatomy of the bladder and urethra. A total of 300–400 ml of contrast material is instilled either in a retrograde fashion through a transurethral Foley catheter or in an antegrade manner through a suprapubic tube. A postdrainage film is obtained and is considered a mandatory part of a trauma cystogram because a small amount of contrast extravasation may be hidden posteriorly behind the opacified distended bladder.

The normal cystogram

The distended bladder is a smooth walled organ with either a round or an oval shape. The oval shaped bladder is often aligned vertically in the female and horizontally in the male. In the newborn, the bladder lies above the symphysis pubis and descends as the child grows. In the older child and adult the bladder base lies at or below the level of the symphysis pubis.

Voiding cystourethrography

Voiding cystourethrography (VCUG) provides anatomical information about the lower urinary tract during the physiological act of micturition. VCUG is performed to diagnose vesicoureteral reflux, to assess bladder emptying, and to evaluate the urethra for posterior urethral valves in the infant male, urethral stricture disease, and urethral diverticula, particularly in female patients. VCUG is useful in assessing certain types of voiding dysfunction (e.g. detrusor external sphincter dyssynergia, neuropathic bladder) and demonstrating reflux into an ectopic ureter which inserts into the urethra.

The bladder is filled with contrast material using a transurethral catheter as for a static cystogram. Once filled, the older child or adult patient is asked to void in the upright position. The procedure is monitored with videofluoroscopy and recorded with either spot films or videorecording. In male patients, the voiding films should be obtained with the pelvis in a 45° oblique position similar to RUG, so that the entire length of urethra is better demonstrated.

The normal voiding cystourethrogram

The bladder is smoothly marginated and roughly spherical in shape. Normally urine is held at the bladder neck. In male patients, the posterior urethra extends from the bladder neck to the external sphincter. The prostatic urethra is the widest section of the entire urethra in calibre during micturition. The verumontanum (urethral crest) is located on the posterior wall of the prostatic urethra. The membranous urethra is short (1 cm) and narrow. The anterior urethra is divided into the bulbous and penile portions. In female patients, the urethra averages 4 cm in length (Fig. 5).

Retrograde urethrography

RUG provides detailed visualization of the anterior urethra in the male. Unlike a voiding cystourethrogram, RUG incompletely visualizes the posterior urethral because of the resistance to retrograde flow provided by the external urethral sphincter. Complete evaluation of the entire urethra often requires both procedures, which may be performed at separate intervals. RUG is rarely indicated in female patients.

RUG is most frequently indicated to assess suspected or known urethral stricture disease, suspected urethral trauma, and to demonstrate urethral diverticula, fistulae, and neoplasms. Retrograde urethrograms should be performed in all patients with pelvic trauma prior to cystography in order to minimize further urethral injury.

Retrograde urethrograms are obtained during injection of water-soluble contrast material with the distal urethra occluded by a 12- to 14-F Foley catheter or Brodny clamp. The patient is placed in a 45° oblique position with the dependent hip acutely flexed and the penis draped over the thigh.

RUG with the use of a double balloon Trattner catheter is performed to assess the female urethra and to diagnose urethral diverticula (Older and Hertz 2000), which has recently been replaced by other imaging modalities such as MRI. Contrast material is directly injected into the urethra between the two balloons.

Manipulation of the urinary tract, however, including injection of contrast material under pressure as during a retrograde urethrogram should be performed in the absence of acute urethritis to minimize the risk of bacteraemia. Intravasation of contrast material into the corpus cavernosum and spongiosum may occur during the procedure. LOCM should be employed when patients are contrast sensitive.

The normal retrograde urethrogram

The male urethra consists of anterior and posterior segments (Fig. 6). On the lateral urethrogram, the verumontanum is indicated as an oval-filling defect in the posterior urethra. Below the verumontanum lies the external sphincter. On RUG, this portion of the urethra may not dilate and the proximal portion of the bulbar urethra appears to taper at this point. This finding should not be misinterpreted as urethral pathology. Another area of normal narrowing in the male urethra that may be confused for a pathological stricture occurs in the proximal urethra of children. On the lateral urethrogram, the junction of the smooth muscle of the proximal urethra with the striated muscle of the distal urethra may be represented by a shallow anterior indentation.

Loopography and pouchgraphy

After cystectomy, anastomoses of the ureters to an isolated intact segment (loop) of ileum, transverse colon, or a detubularized large or small bowel segment (pouch) is the most common method of establishing permanent urinary diversion (Spring and Deshon 2000; Banner 2001). The isolated but otherwise intact bowel loop serves as a simple conduit for urinary flow transporting urine outward towards the stoma in a continuous, rhythmic, isoperistaltic way. The detubularized pouch,

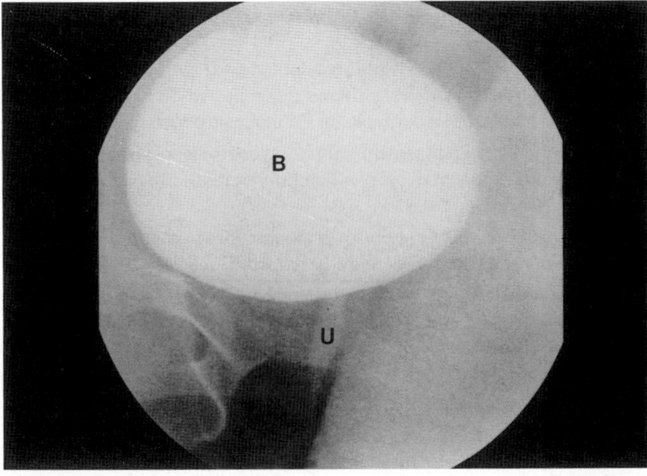

Fig. 5 Voiding cystourethrogram demonstrates normal bladder (B) and female urethra (U). No vesicoureteral reflux.

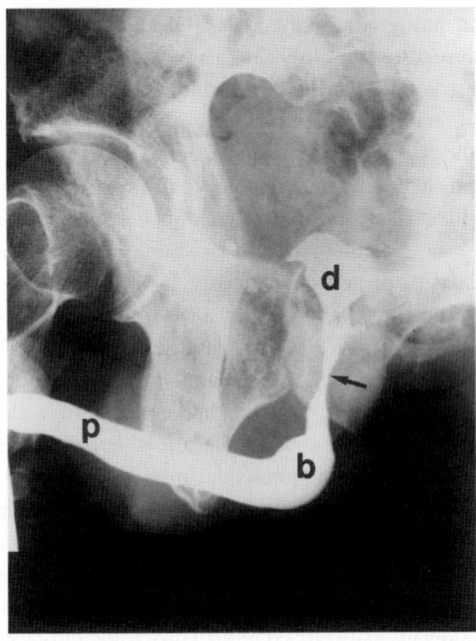

Fig. 6 Retrograde urethrogram in male patient. Anterior urethra consists of bulbous (b) and penile (p) segments. Posterior urethra consists of prostatic and membranous (arrow) segments. Prior transurethral resection defect at the prostatic urethra (d) and bladder neck.

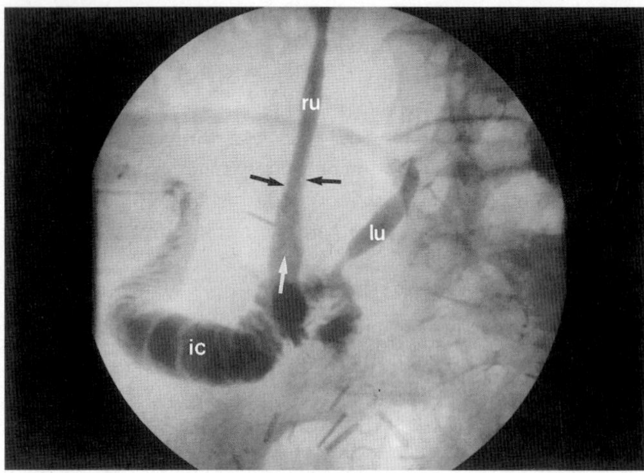

Fig. 7 Loopogram shows contrast filling of the ileal loop with reflux into the distal ureters bilaterally. The small nodular irregularity of the mucosa of the distal right ureter (arrows) was proven to be recurrent urothelial tumour by biopsy. Ileal loop (ic), right ureter (ru), and left ureter (lu).

on the other hand, lacks the contractivity to propel urine to the outside, thus becoming a reservoir (e.g. neobladder, continent diversion) rather than a conduit. Therefore, detubularized pouches are continent of urine and require intermittent catheterization for emptying. Radiographic examination of loops or pouches is referred to as loopography or pouchgraphy, respectively.

A loopogram is performed to visualize the upper urinary tracts by reflux of injected contrast media (Fig. 7). This procedure is utilized in postoperative patients with progressive renal failure and replaces transurethral retrograde pyelography in excluding ureteral obstruction. In such patients, the absence of reflux may indicate ureteral anastomotic obstruction. On the other hand, neobladder and continent diversion ureteral anastomoses are often of an antirefluxing nature. Therefore, the absence of reflux into the ureters on pouchgrams may not indicate urinary obstruction. Loopography or pouchgraphy is also performed to evaluate the bowel conduit or pouch for suspected intrinsic disease (e.g. filling defects, anastomotic or other leaks, loop stenosis), capacity, or peristaltic activity. Loopography is essential to delineate the anatomy of a urinary diversion and probable site of ureteral implantation prior to any planned endourological or interventional procedures on the diverted ureters.

Following a scout, the stoma of the ileal conduit is catheterized with a 14- or 20-F Foley catheter. Water-soluble contrast material is injected to fill the conduit. Fluoroscopic images are obtained with specific attention to the presence or absence of ureteral reflux. The catheter is then removed and the conduit and upper urinary tracts are evaluated for emptying. To assess a continent urinary pouch or reservoir, the stoma (for a cutaneous diversion) or urethra (for an orthotopic diversion, neobladder) is catheterized and a Foley catheter placed into the reservoir.

There are no absolute contraindications to the retrograde study of a urinary conduit or reservoir. Patients with current or previous urinary tract infections should receive prophylactic antibiotics because forced reflux of infected urine results in pyelonephritis.

References

Banner, M. P. Diagnostic uroradiology. In *Clinical Manual of Urology* (ed. P. Hanno, S. B. Malkowicz, and A. J. Wein), pp. 87–133. New York NY: McGraw-Hill, 2001.

Barbaric, Z. L. and Pollack, H. M. Abdominal plain radiography. In *Clinical Urography* Vol. 1 (ed. H. M. Pollack and B. L. McClennon), pp. 67–146. Philadelphia, PA: W.B. Saunders, 2000.

Barrett, B. J. and Carlisle, E. J. (1993). Metaanalysis of the relative nephrotoxicity of high- and low-osmolality iodinated contrast media. *Radiology* **188**, 171–178.

Caoili, E. M. *et al.* (2002). Urinary tract abnormalities: initial experience with multi-detector row CT urography. *Radiology* **222**, 353–360.

Chow, L. C. and Sommer, F. G. (2001). Multidetector CT urography with abdominal compression and three-dimensional reconstruction. *American Journal of Roentgenology* **177**, 849–855.

Cohan, R. H., Ellis, J. H., and Garner, W. L. (1996). Extravasation of radiographic contrast material: recognition, prevention, and treatment. *Radiology* **200**, 593–604.

Cohan, R. H., Matsumoto, J. S., and Quagliano, P. V. *Manual on Contrast Media.* Reston VA: American College of Radiology, 1998.

Dyer, R. B., Chen, M. Y., and Zagoria, R. J. (1998). Abnormal calcifications in the urinary tract. *Radiographics* **18**, 1405–1424.

Dyer, R. B., Chen, M. Y., and Zagoria, R. J. (2001). Intravenous urography: technique and interpretation. *Radiographics* **21**, 799–821; discussion 822–824.

Friedenberg, R. M. and Harris, R. D. Excretory urography. In *Clinical Urography* Vol. 1 (ed. H. M. Pollack and B. C. McClennon), pp. 147–281. Philadelphia, PA: W.B. Saunders, 2000.

Greenberger, P. A. and Patterson, R. (1991). The prevention of immediate generalized reactions to radiocontrast media in high-risk patients. *Journal of Allergy and Clinical Immunology* **87**, 867–872.

Hattery, R. R. *et al.* (1988). Intravenous urographic technique. *Radiology* **167**, 593–599.

Imray, T. J., Lieberman, R. P., and Pollack, H. M. Retrograde pyelography. In *Clinical Urography* Vol. 1 (ed. H. M. Pollack and B. L. McClennon), pp. 282–302. Philadelphia, PA: W.B. Saunders, 2000.

Katayama, H. *et al.* (1990). Adverse reactions to ionic and nonionic contrast media. A report from the Japanese Committee on the Safety of Contrast Media. *Radiology* **175**, 621–628.

Katholi, R. E. *et al.* (1995). Nephrotoxicity from contrast media: attenuation with theophylline. *Radiology* **195**, 17–22.

Katzberg, R. W. (1997). Urography into the 21st century: new contrast media, renal handling, imaging characteristics, and nephrotoxicity. *Radiology* **204**, 297–312.

Kawashima, A. *et al.* (2001). Improved CT scanned projection radiographs (SPRs) utilizing enhanced algorithms: can improved CT SPRs replace conventional film-screen radiographs for CT urography? *Radiology* **221** (P), 501.

Lasser, E. C. (1988). Pretreatment with corticosteroids to prevent reactions to i.v. contrast material: overview and implications. *American Journal of Roentgenology* **150**, 257–259.

Lasser, E. C. and Berry, C. C. (1991). Adverse reactions to contrast media. Ionic and nonionic media and steroids. *Investigative Radiology* **26**, 402–403.

Older, R. A. and Hertz, M. Cystourethrography. In *Clinical Urography* Vol. 1 (ed. H. M. Pollack and B. L. McClennon), pp. 303–355. Philadelphia, PA: W.B. Saunders, 2000.

Palmer, F. J. (1988). The RACR survey of intravenous contrast media reactions. Final report. *Australasian Radiology* **32**, 426–428.

Pflueger, A. *et al.* (2000). Role of adenosine in contrast media-induced acute renal failure in diabetes mellitus. *Mayo Clinic Proceedings* **75**, 1275–1283.

Spring, D. B. and Deshon, G. E., Jr. Radiology of vesical and supravesical urinary diversions and orthotopic bladder replacements. In *Clinical Urography* Vol. 1 (ed. H. M. Pollack and B. L. McClennon), pp. 357–377. Philadelphia, PA: W.B. Saunders, 2000.

Tepel, M. *et al.* (2000). Prevention of radiographic-contrast-agent-induced reductions in renal function by acetylcysteine. *New England Journal of Medicine* **343**, 180–184.

Vrtiska, T. J. *et al.* (2000). CT urography: description of a novel technique using a uniquely modified multidetector-row CT scanner. *Radiology* **217** (P), 225.

Yamaguchi, K. *et al.* (1991). Prediction of severe adverse reactions to ionic and nonionic contrast media in Japan: evaluation of pretesting. A report from the Japanese Committee on the Safety of Contrast Media. *Radiology* **178**, 363–367.

1.6.1.iii Percutaneous nephrostomy and ureteral stenting

François Cornud, M. Gouahdni, Y. Chrétien, and Olivier Hélénon

Percutaneous nephrostomy (PCN) represents the base upon which interventional uroradiology has developed. Since the early 1980s, it emerged that percutaneous access to the kidney could be performed by applying angiographic techniques familiar to most radiologists. As PCN indications increased, the procedure proved to be safe and it rapidly appeared that access to the ureter through the nephrostomy tract was possible, which permitted endoureteral manipulations and ureteric stenting.

Technique

Patient preparation (Richards and Jones 1993; Banner 1998a)

Haemostatic evaluation, antibiotics prior to and following decompression in patients with suspected urinary tract infection, monitoring of vital signs, electrocardiogram, and oxygen saturation during the procedure and postprocedural monitored observation are done under the supervision of an anaesthetist. We perform interventional procedures on patients under local anaesthesia assisted by an intravenous sedation. In selected cases, our anaesthetists elect to perform a general anaesthesia if prolonged endoureteral manipulations are planned, particularly if a combined antegrade–retrograde approach is necessary (Cornud *et al.* 1991a).

Patient position

Although the prone or prone oblique position is usually recommended (Richards and Jones 1993; Banner 1998a), we prefer to place the patient in an oblique supine position (with the ipsilateral flank elevated) to puncture the lumbar fossa. This permits to maintain a retrograde access to the bladder or to the cutaneous stomia when combined antegrade and retrograde endoureteral manipulations are planned (Cornud 1991a,b). Moreover, the oblique supine position is much more comfortable for the anaesthetist who keeps a safe and quick access to the airways of the patient should respiratory problems occur during the procedure. The skin of the lumbar fossa is scrubbed with povidone–iodine, and the patient and entire fluoroscopic table are draped in sterile fashion.

Puncture guidance

Sonography is of inestimable value in patients with hydronephrosis, particularly in pregnant women in whom the entire procedure can often be successfully accomplished with only real-time ultrasound (US) guidance (Banner 1998a). However, apart from this exception, most interventional radiologists (Richards and Jones 1993; Banner 1998a) use, once the collecting system has been punctured under US guidance, fluoroscopy for the remainder of the procedure, including the injection of contrast material. If additional endoureteral manipulations are anticipated, the collecting system can be repunctured under fluoroscopic guidance if the initial site of entry into the collecting system does not appear to be optimal for subsequent manipulations. In our experience, as in most groups, the initial puncture under fluoroscopic guidance is used for percutaneous stone management (LeRoy 1998), endopyelotomy (Lee 1998), percutaneous ablation of transitional cell carcinoma (Kellett 2000), or other circumstances in which entry into a particular calyx is desired (Banner 1998b). Fluoroscopic localization for stone management is particularly recommended for opaque calyceal calculi, which serve as a target for the nephrostomy needle. In this circumstance, we inject air to opacify the pelvicalyceal complex (Fig. 1). It avoids

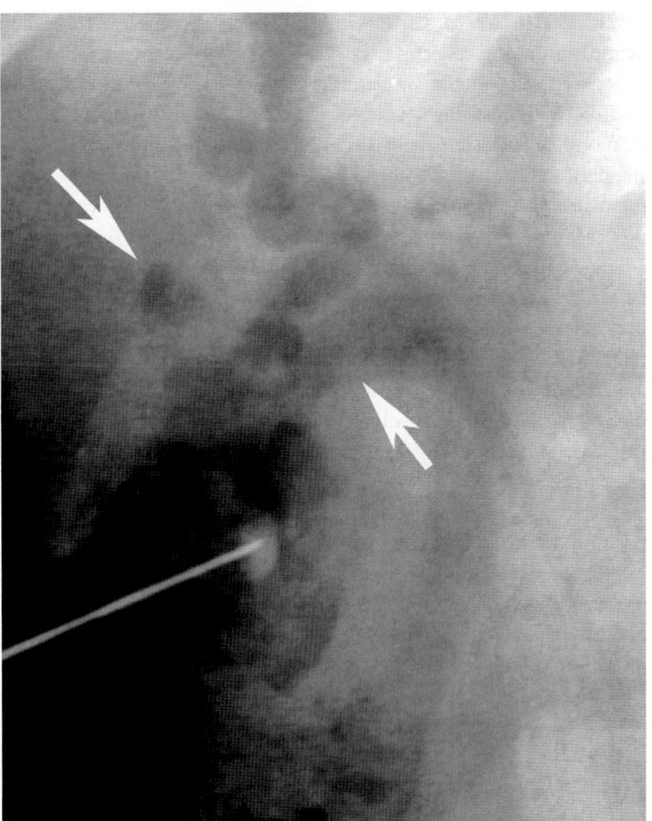

Fig. 1 Pyelography with injection of air. The lower pole calyx has been punctured under sonographic guidance with a lumbar puncture 20-gauge, 10-cm long needle and, after urine has been obtained, a few millilitres of air has been injected which provides an excellent delineation of the pelvicalyceal system (arrows). PCN and percutaneous nephrolithotomy were subsequently performed.

extravasation of contrast material, which can obscure fluoroscopic visualization of the stone. Transplanted kidneys are a particular situation (Banner 1998a). When obstruction of a renal transplant is questioned but not definitively established by means of ultrasonography, a thin-needle antegrade pyelogram is usually indicated. In this case, the contrast material is injected into the renal pelvis to assess the point of obstruction. If a PCN is then indicated, the definitive puncture is made into an anterolateral calyx, preferably a mid- or lower-pole calyx. Needle puncture into the upper pole of the allograft might inadvertently traverse the peritoneal cavity before entering the collecting system. If a PCN becomes necessary into a transplanted kidney that has been placed into the peritoneal cavity, a computerized tomography (CT) scan should be available to assess neighbouring structures that might be in the path of the needle and catheter. CT-guided needle puncture may be advisable under these circumstances.

Any PCN requires an optimal entry site that is, as often as possible, below the 12th rib, lateral to the paraspinal muscles, along the posterior axillary line so that the needle should traverse renal parenchyma along the relatively avascular posterolateral (the so-called Broedel's line) and enter a posteriorly oriented calyx before entering the collecting system. Such an approach will almost always avoid inadvertent puncture of the retroperitoneal colon. Ureteral stenting, as further discussed, may be facilitated by entering a mid- rather than a lower-pole calyx. The initial renal puncture is done with a 20-gauge lumbar puncture needle to opacify the kidney with contrast material or almost routinely now in our practice with air, which provides an excellent delineation of the collecting system (Fig. 1). This is then followed by fluoroscopically guided puncture of the calyx of choice with the 18-gauge nephrostomy needle (20-cm long, stainless steel trocar with diamond-tip stylet) that will accept a 0.038-in. guidewire over which a standard nephrostomy catheter can be passed. We favour the other popular alternative, which is to use a so-called introducer system. In this case, the collecting system is punctured from the flank with a 20-gauge 10- or 15-cm long needle, an 0.018-in. platinum-tip guidewire is inserted, and the needle exchanged for a 3–5 F coaxial catheter that allows, after the 3 F catheter and small wire are removed, the introduction of a 0.038-in. stiff Teflon Amplatz guidewire through the 5 F catheter left in place through the percutaneous tract. Renal puncture with an 18-gauge needle is thereby avoided, limiting the rate of vascular complications. Whatever the chosen needle, the nephrocutaneous track is then dilated with polyethylene fascial dilators and the nephrostomy catheter is passed over the guidewire. Although the final position of the pigtail nephrostomy catheter should be checked by injecting contrast, the collecting system should not be distended if the urine is infected, as pyelotubular or pyelovenous backflow may result in bacteraemia and urosepsis.

Indications (Banner 1998a)

Percutaneous nephrostomy has been used primarily to provide urinary drainage for relief of renal or ureteral obstruction. It is now widely used to provide access to the renal collecting system, ureter, or bladder for diagnostic or therapeutic procedures. These include ureteral stent placement, ureteral stricture dilation or incision, urinary stone removal, biopsy of urothelial lesions, retrieval of foreign bodies and fungus balls, bypass of ureteral injuries to dry ureteral fistulae, and nephroscopically directed surgical procedures, such as endopyelotomy (Lee 1998) or endoscopic resection of urothelial tumours (Kellett 2000).

Contraindications

The only absolute contraindication to PCN is a severe uncorrected bleeding disorder. Although the severe electrolyte imbalance that may accompany obstructive uropathy (i.e. hyperkalaemia) may be more rapidly corrected by utilizing haemodialysis prior to PCN, in practice, urinary decompression is usually the initial therapeutic procedure for such patients.

Complications (Rickards *et al.* 1993; Banner 1998a)

Complications of PCN can be vascular, infectious, or catheter-related.

Only occasionally, PCN-related bleeding requires transfusion or even embolization (Thomson and Walters 1993). Bleeding complications are minimized by correcting coagulation abnormalities, if possible, prior to PCN and by using small needles directed towards posterolateral calyces. If large blood clots form in the collecting system and impair catheter drainage, repeated gentle saline irrigation can ensure catheter patency until the thrombolytic effect of the urokinase in the patient's urine lyses the clots. Bleeding pseudoaneurysms and arteriovenous fistulae should be suspected when gross haematuria persists for several days, new intrapelvic clots develop, or the haematocrit drops significantly, renal arteriography is indicated, subsequently followed by embolization if necessary. A significant reduction in haematocrit should also raise the suspicion of a PCN-induced subcapsular or perinephric haematoma. Following PCN placement, subcapsular haematomas may be seen on CT in up to 13 per cent of patients with normal bleeding parameters; they are usually small and rarely require additional treatment.

Symptomatic infection occurs most often in patients with positive urine cultures, urinary obstruction, infection-related urinary calculi, and urostomies. In these high-risk patients, PCN often exacerbates existing infection that is minimized by administering appropriate antibiotics intravenously for 24 h (if possible) prior to PCN and by limiting intrarenal manipulations and contrast injections until obstruction is relieved and high concentrations of intraparenchymal antibiotics can be achieved.

Insertion of a PCN catheter can occasionally produce injury to organs adjacent to the kidney or along the path of the nephrostomy needle. An intercostal approach to the kidney is associated with a higher incidence of complications than in a subcostal one. Twenty-four intercostal nephrostomies may result in atelectasis, pleural effusion or pleural puncture, and subsequent pneumothorax, hydrothorax, or haemothorax. When employed, needle puncture should be made on expiration and as lateral as feasible to minimize the chances of pleural transgression. PCN catheters placed above the 12th rib can also irritate intercostal muscles. Injuries to various solid and hollow organs (liver, spleen, colon, duodenum, biliary tract) can rarely occur as a result of PCN placement. Nephrocolic fistula (LeRoy 1998), one of the more feared complications, may result from inadvertent needle perforation of the colon and subsequent dilation of the nephrostomy track for stone removal. Nephrocolic fistulae can usually be managed in non-operative, endourological fashion.

Percutaneous antegrade ureteral stenting

Technique for stent insertion

The insertion of a ureteral stent depends on the ability to negotiate a ureteral obstruction or bypass a ureteral leak. Ureteral obstructions can often be negotiated in antegrade (percutaneous) fashion, even if retrograde cystoscopic catheterization is not possible. Such situations are encountered in various cases such as a tumour obstructing a ureteral orifice, a distal ureteral angulation secondary to spread of prostatic or gynaecologic malignancy, or more generally tight ureteral stenoses. Approximately 90 per cent of obstructed or leaking ureters can be stented percutaneously. Failure of antegrade stenting can easily be bypassed by a combined retrograde and antegrade approach, which achieves a virtually 100 per cent success rate of stenting (de Baere *et al.* 1995; Watson *et al.* 2002). When the pelvic ureter is severed completely, re-entry into the bladder may be accomplished provided the distance to the bladder is short and there are no vascular or digestive interposed structures. The so-called ureteroneocystostomy can be performed with a transeptal needle (Lang 1988) or an electrode using electrocautery (Cornud *et al.* 1991b) to re-establish continuity in a completely occluded distal ureter (Fig. 2). In the special case of ureteral diversion to a bowel conduit or an enterocystoplasty, an obstructed ureter can be stented in either antegrade or retrograde fashion, once a guidewire and catheter have been percutaneously manipulated past the stricture, through the conduit, and out of the stoma. Prior to stenting, the stenosis is dilated with a high-pressure angioplasty balloon (Banner 1998b) or incised with a cutting balloon device (Cornud *et al.* 2000), which allows a 1-cm-deep incision of any ureteral or ureterodigestive stenosis. This cutting balloon is also one of the treatment options of primary or secondary ureteropyelic obstructions (Chandhoke *et al.* 1993), which can be treated either from an antegrade or retrograde approach.

Indications (Banner 1998c)

Percutaneous ureteral stenting developed as a logical consequence of PCN. When retrograde endoscopic placement of a ureteral stent is not feasible or possible, percutaneous ureteral stenting can provide urinary diversion to the bladder or a bowel conduit or reservoir without the need for an external collection device. Most patients find a ureteral stent more comfortable, convenient, and cosmetically acceptable than a nephrostomy catheter. Long-term stenting (months to years) is most frequently performed to bypass a malignant ureteral obstruction. If the stenosis is tight, we dilate with a high-pressure angioplasty balloon to ensure easy placement of the stent. Short-term stenting has a great importance in conjunction with non-operative treatment of renal and ureteral calculi. If retrograde endoscopically guided or fluoroscopically guided manipulations successfully displace mid- or upper-ureteral calculi into the kidney, ureteral stents ensure that the stones do not migrate back into the ureter prior to extracorporeal shock wave lithotripsy (ESWL) or percutaneous nephrolithotomy (PCNL). Ureteral stents facilitate localization of upper urinary tract calculi during ESWL. Following ESWL, stents allow for antegrade urinary drainage while stone fragments pass into the bladder. In patients with renal allografts (Banner 1998b), stents have an important role in the management of the

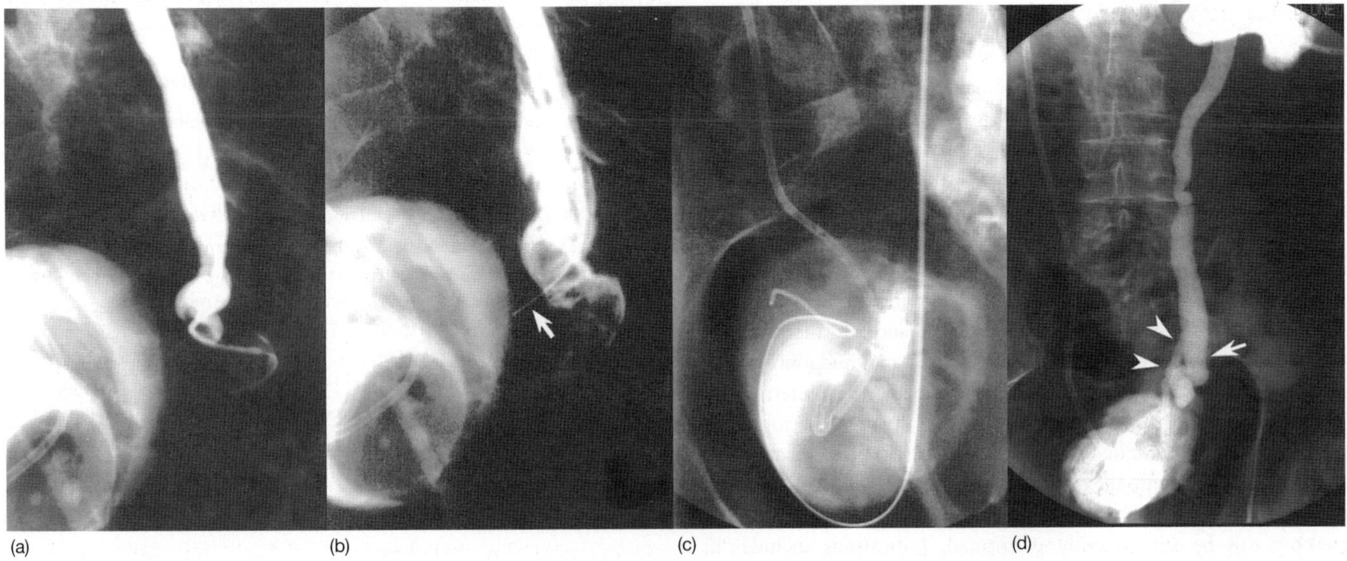

(a) (b) (c) (d)

Fig. 2 Ureteroneocystostomy in a case of impassable stenosis of the iliac portion of the left ureter. (a) Antegrade urogram shows total obstruction of the left pelvic ureter, related to a breast carcinoma. Passage of the stenosis with different kind of wires and catheters was only possible on a few centimetres. Contrast medium in the bladder has been retrogradely injected through a Foley catheter. (b) The ureteral wall has been perforated with a rigid end of an Amplatz guide wire and the bladder has been fully distended to reduce the distance between the ureter and the bladder wall. The catheter–guide-wire combination was oriented towards the bladder wall and cutting current was applied. (c) The bladder wall has been perforated and the preshaped catheter has been coiled into the bladder. (d) Antegrade pyelogram showing normal patency of the stent through the neotract (arrowheads) and filling of the distal portion of the ureter with contrast medium (arrow).

ureteral complications of renal transplantation, namely obstruction, dehiscence, fistula, or necrosis. Stents may obviate the need for further surgery or allow postponement of definitive surgical correction until renal function has been stabilized and immunosuppression has been reduced.

Complications of ureteral stents (Banner 1998c)

Complications associated with indwelling ureteral stents include encrustation, fragmentation, and stent migration. Stent encrustation is the natural history of all types of stents, although it varies with stent composition. Maintaining a high output of uninfected acid urine can minimize encrustation. If stents are left indwelling for longer than 6 months, they become a 'forgotten' indwelling ureteral stent, leading to an increased risk for loss of renal function. Stents placed in pregnant women with calculus ureteral obstruction are often impressively encrusted by the time of parturition if not periodically exchanged. Stents should be replaced at most every 6 months, and more often in patients who are prone to develop stent obstruction by mucus from a bowel conduit or reservoir. A rare complication of indwelling ureteral stents is the development of a fistula between the stented ureter and the iliac artery, most often observed in patients with pre-existing compromised ureteral vascularity due to prior pelvic surgery and irradiation. These patients develop often-impressive haematuria. Awareness of this rare, but life-threatening condition is crucial for prompt treatment and stoppage of bleeding can be successfully achieved with embolotherapy (Quillin *et al.* 1994) or iliac artery stenting with a metallic stent.

Transconduit retrograde ureteral stenting (Banner 1998c)

Drainage for an obstructed kidney whose ureter has been anastomosed to a bowel conduit has traditionally been provided by PCN, as conduit endoscopy does not provide consistent adequate visualization of the anastomosis for catheterization. However, fluoroscopically controlled transconduit retrograde catheterization of ureters that have been diverted to a bowel conduit can be done in patients with patent low-grade ureteroenteral anastomoses. The technique involves initial opacification of the urinary conduit and demonstration of ureteral reflux, advancement of a curved-tip angiographic catheter and hydrophilic wire through the urostomy stoma and into the proximal conduit adjacent to the ureteral anastomosis, manipulation of the catheter to approximate the expected ureteral orifice, and intermittent contrast injection through the catheter. When the ureter retrogradely fills, a straight hydrophilic-coated guidewire is reinserted through the catheter and passed into the distal ureter. The catheter is then advanced over the guidewire into the distal portion of the diverted ureter and stenting can be subsequently performed. Indications include, in patients with an ureterodigestive diversion, the need to provide renal drainage for partially obstructing ureteral or anastomotic strictures or renal calculi, insertion of ureteral catheters prior to ESWL, removal of ureteral calculi, brush biopsy of upper urinary tract, and retrograde exchange of ureteral stents (Drake and Cowan 2002). If the retrograde transconduit approach is not successful, a subsequent PCN can be performed.

References

Banner, M. P. Percutaneous nephrostomy. In *Radiologic Interventions. Uroradiology* (ed. M. P. Banner), pp. 3–27. Baltimore: Williams and Wilkins, 1998a.

Banner, M. P. Ureteral stricture management: balloon catheter dilation. In *Radiologic Interventions. Uroradiology* (ed. M. P. Banner), pp. 128–138. Baltimore: Williams and Wilkins, 1998b.

Banner, M. P. Antegrade and retrograde ureteral stenting. In *Radiologic Interventions. Uroradiology* (ed. M. P. Banner), pp. 96–127. Baltimore: Williams and Wilkins, 1998c.

Chandhoke, P. S. *et al.* (1993). Endopyelotomy and endoureterotomy with the acucise ureteral cutting balloon device: preliminary experience. *Journal of Endourology* **7** (1), 45–51.

Cornud, F. *et al.* (1991a). Long-term results of angioplasty balloon dilatation of stenosed ureterodigestive anastomoses. Effect of prolonged pattern with large caliber prosthesis. *Journal of Urology* **97** (1), 11–14.

Cornud, F. E. *et al.* (1991b). Impassable ureteral strictures: management with percutaneous ureteroneocystostomy. *Radiology* **180** (2), 451–454.

Cornud, F. *et al.* (2000). Percutaneous incision of stenotic uroenteric anastomoses with a cutting balloon catheter: long-term results. *Radiology* **214** (2), 358–362.

de Baere, T. *et al.* (1995). Combined percutaneous antegrade and cystoscopic retrograde approach in the treatment of distal ureteric fistulae. *Cardiovascular Interventional Radiology* **18** (6), 349–352.

Drake, M. J. and Cowan, N. C. (2002). Fluoroscopy guided retrograde ureteral stent insertion in patients with a ureteroileal urinary conduit: method and results. *Journal of Urology* **167** (5), 2049–2051.

Kellett, M. J. (2000). Interventional uroradiology: an update. *BJU International* **86** (Suppl. 1), 164–173.

Lang, E. K. (1988). Percutaneous ureterocystostomy and ureteroneocystostomy. *American Journal of Roentgenology* **150** (Suppl. 5), 1065–1068.

Lee, W. L. Percutaneous therapy for ureteropelvic junction obstruction. In *Radiologic Interventions. Uroradiology* (ed. M. P. Banner), pp. 59–67. Baltimore: Williams and Wilkins, 1998.

LeRoy, A. J. Percutaneous procedures for nephrolithiasis. In *Radiologic Interventions. Uroradiology* (ed. M. P. Banner), pp. 28–46. Baltimore: Williams and Wilkins, 1998.

Quillin, S. P., Darcy, M. D., and Picus, D. (1994). Angiographic evaluation and therapy of ureteroarterial fistulas. *AJR. American Journal of Roentgenology* **162** (4), 873–878.

Rickards, D. and Jones, S. Percutaneous nephrolithotomy. In *Practical Interventional Uroradiology* (ed. D. Rickards, S. Jones, K. R. Thompson, and M. D. Rifkin), pp. 35–44. London: Edward Arnold, 1993.

Rickards, D., Jones, S., and Kellett, M. J. Percutaneous nephrostomy. In *Practical Interventional Uroradiology* (ed. D. Rickards, S. Jones, K. R. Thompson, and M. D. Rifkin), pp. 23–34. London: Edward Arnold, 1993.

Thomson, K. R. and Walters, N. A. Therapeutic urogenital angiography. In *Practical Interventional Uroradiology* (ed. D. Rickards, S. Jones, K. R. Thompson, and M. D. Rifkin), pp. 97–108. London: Edward Arnold, 1993.

Watson, J. M., Dawkins, G. P., Whitfield, H. N., Philp, T., and Kellett, M. J. (2002). The rendezvous procedure to cross complicated ureteric strictures. *BJU International* **89** (3), 317–319.

1.6.1.iv Renal arteriography

Francis G. Joffre and Lisette El Hajj

During the last two decades, the use of arteriography has been challenged by new imaging techniques: renal ultrasonography and renal colour Doppler ultrasonography, helical computed tomography (HCT), and magnetic resonance angiography (MRA) (Richter *et al.* 1993; Rubin *et al.* 1994). Concomitantly, techniques of arterial catheterization and contrast media have improved, and digital techniques have greatly simplified the collection of images. Thus, arteriography is being used less, whereas endovascular interventional radiology has rapidly developed.

Renal arteriography technique

Opacification of the renal arteries can currently be obtained by intra-arterial injection of radiological contrast medium (CM).

Catheterization technique (Joffre 1998)

It is currently performed under local anaesthesia after simple premedication. Use of neuroleptanalgesia is rarely necessary except in the case of endovascular treatment. Percutaneous arterial puncture according to Seldinger's technique mostly concerns the femoral artery. Rarely, a transhumeral or transradial approach is used. The small diameter (4 F) of the catheters used reduces the haemorrhagic risk of the arterial puncture, allowing the investigation to be performed as a day case.

The first step is global aortography, generally in the front position (Fig. 1). It is essential to study well and precisely the renal arteries ostia where sites of atheromatous plaques are frequent. This may require additional injections in an oblique position particularly in presence of severe aortic atheromatous lesions. Aortography is also necessary to detect accessory renal arteries (20–30 per cent). Selective catheterization of one or several renal arteries may be needed to evaluate intrarenal vasculature if necessary.

Imaging technique

Since the past decade, digitalization, which assigns a numerical value to each point of the collected image of an X-ray intensifier, has replaced the classic photographic process (Hillman 1989). This digital processing has considerably improved the conditions of the angiography.

The advantages of digitalization are very important: (a) The dose of CM is reduced to 50 per cent lower than conventional doses. Abdominal aortography requires only 30 ml of low osmolality CM with an iodine concentration of 250 mg/100 ml. (b) Patient and operator exposure to irradiation is decreased due to shorter examination time. (c) Post-treatment of image is possible, suppressing the majority of poor-quality pictures in the case of obesity, presence of intestinal gas, or incomplete apnea. Real-time subtraction (removal of some superimpositions) and contrast enhancement are the main possibilities. (d) The digital image can be easily stored and transmitted by PACS (picture, archiving, and communication system).

For renal arteriography of a transplanted kidney (Irving and Khoury 1983), the approach is identical, the choice of the side depending on the type of arterial anastomosis (controlateral for terminoterminal anastomosis with hypogastric artery, ipsilateral for lateroterminal anastomosis with external iliac artery). The use of a balloon occluding catheter placed under the anastomosis allows to reduce the dose of CM used (Fig. 2).

Renal arteriography in patients with renal insufficiency (see also Chapters 1.6 and 9.7)

The association of renal artery stenosis and chronic renal failure is not rare in elderly patients in whom renal arteriography and endovascular treatment may be required (see Chapter 9.7).

Contrast media nephrotoxicity occurs in approximately 15 per cent of the patients with renal impairment following renal arteriography, and

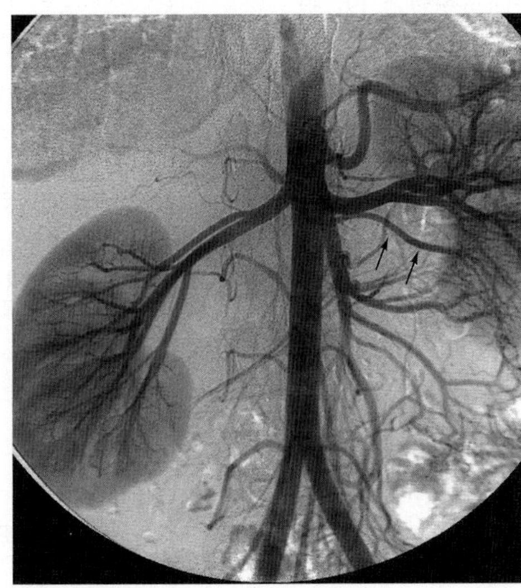

Fig. 1 Global aortography: normal aspect. Note the presence of an inferior polar renal artery (arrows).

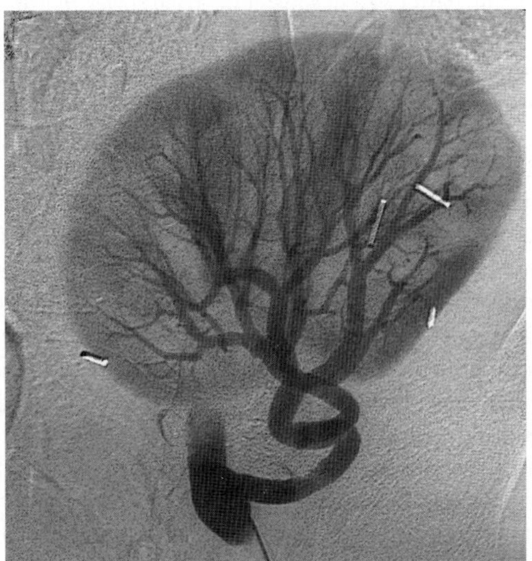

Fig. 2 Selective renal arteriography in a transplanted kidney. Good opacification of the normal renal vasculature by using a balloon occluding catheter placed in the left external iliac artery under the renal artery.

the risk of adverse effects rises to 31 per cent after renal angioplasty (percutaeous transluminal renal angioplasty, PTRA) (Spinosa *et al.* 1999). Prevention of CM nephrotoxicity should be implemented (see Chapter 1.6) as follows: (a) Identification of risk factors such as renal failure, diabetes mellitus, proteinuria, heart failure, other nephrotoxic drugs. (b) Use of low-osmolarity CM. (c) Substitution by CO_2 or gadolinium chelates (Hammer *et al.* 1999; Kan *et al.* 1999). The image quality is inferior but this is usually sufficient for diagnosis and endovascular treatment. However, replacement of CM with gadolinium remains controversial (Nyman *et al.* 2002). (d) Adequate intravenous (IV) administration of isotonic saline, during and after the procedure (Solomon *et al.* 1994), and/or antioxidant drug (acetylcysteine) (Tepel *et al.* 2000), and/or theophylline (Huber *et al.* 2002).

Complications

Local complications are currently extremely rare for an operator with good expertise. They are certainly lower than 1 for 1000 with the material used today, for an arteriography alone. These exceptional complications are represented by haematoma of the groin and cholesterol emboli due to endoaortic manipulation of the catheter. The main general complications are secondary to CM nephrotoxicity and can be largely prevented (Otal *et al.* 2000).

Normal arteriogram

Arteriographic investigation of the renal vasculature takes place in three successive phases (Joffre and Russ 1997): arterial, parenchymatous, and venous (Fig. 1). The arterial phase is very short, about 2 s, and allows evaluation of the renal pedicle and the intrarenal branches. Before they enter the hilum of the kidney, renal arteries give rise to extrarenal branches which can be seen by selective injection of CM. These include the inferior adrenal, the capsular, the pelvic, the superior ureteric arteries. These arteries supply the perirenal arterial circle and vascularize the most external zone of the renal cortex (cortex corticis) through the perforans arteries. Intrarenal vasculature is extremely variable from one side to the other and from one subject to another. The most typical scheme is the subdivision into one prepyelic branch and one retropyelic. Each of these arteries gives rise to segmentary branches which are divided into lobar branches and interlobar branches which pass through Bertin's columns and become arcuate arteries by curving at the bases of the pyramids of Malpighi. Branches of arcuate arteries are not visualized because they are masked by the parenchymatous opacification. All these branches are considered as terminal, without any anastomotic relation between them. Multiple renal arteries are found in about 20–30 per cent of cases, either two or more, and rarely, three renal arteries (Fig. 1). The parenchymal opacification (nephrography) is mainly cortically induced by the opacification of the glomerular capillaries. It starts 2 s after the CM injection. The cortex is well visualized as well as its internal radiated extension, which correspond to Bertin's columns and which define non-opacified pyramids of Malpighi (Fig. 1). The returning venous phase appears after 10 s. Opacification of the renal vein trunk is usually faint according to the injected dose (Fig. 1). Renal arteriography allows a precise display of the renal vasculature. However, it does not provide an axial view of the renal trunk such as angio-HCT or MRA (see Chapters 1.6.1.v and vi).

Indications

For the last decades, radiological investigation of renal arteries has been considerably modified (Khauli 1994). Today, colour Doppler, HCT, and/or MRA supply renal arteriography to screen and provide the main information necessary for the management of renal artery stenosis which is the main vascular pathology of the kidney. However, in this frequent situation, renal arteriography is necessary for guiding an endovascular treatment. Therefore, the remaining diagnostic indications for renal arteriography are limited and in the vast majority of patients this technique is combined with endovascular treatment.

Diagnostic arteriography

These indications are rare and restricted to complex vascular lesions for which the information provided by less invasive imaging techniques (HCT, MRA) is insufficient to determine the possibilities of endovascular or surgical treatment: complex dysplastic lesions of the renal artery trunk and branches, renal artery aneurysms, acute obstruction of renal artery and branches. In this last condition, arteriography allows us to determine the cause of occlusion (embolism, acute thrombosis secondary to stenosis, aortic dissection, spontaneous or traumatic dissection of renal artery). It also allows to assess the site and extension of the obstruction, thereby guiding the therapeutic choice (surgical or endovascular embolectomy, thrombectomy, *in situ* thrombolysis, endoprosthesis, etc.).

Some patients with gross haematuria in whom all investigations remain negative may benefit from renal arteriography. In these patients, arteriography is an essential diagnostic tool to identify vascular malformations, or congenital arteriovenous fistula (Fig. 3a and b). Renal arteriography is also indicated when a vascular intrarenal haemorrhagic lesion is suspected, occurring spontaneously, or associated with an iatrogenic trauma (e.g. bleeding angiomyolipoma or needle biopsy).

Renal arteriography may also be used as a diagnostic element when periarteritis nodosa is suspected. It must be performed before renal biopsy. It allows us to establish an almost definite diagnostic for revealing microaneurysms of variable size and number, which are frequently associated with stenosis or obstructive lesions of the intrarenal branches (Helenon *et al.* 1977).

Renal arteriography and endovascular treatment

Renal arteriography is mandatory for determining the indication, the therapeutic strategy, guiding the procedure, and evaluating the results of all endovascular treatment of renal artery diseases which are performed by selective and/or subselective catheterization of this artery. The indication must remain the result of close discussion between radiologists and the medicosurgical team. Advantages and risks of each method must be considered before any therapeutic decision (Mitty and Gribetz 1982).

Renal embolization (Lieberman *et al.* 1983; Beaujeux *et al.* 1995)

Renal embolization consists of introducing, by an appropriate catheter, various materials which intend to occlude the vascular lumen. The vascular obstruction must be, according to the clinical indication, proximal or as much distal as possible, localized or diffused and respecting as much as possible the healthy parenchyma. It can also be temporary or definitive. Different materials can be used according to the aim sought: resorbable particles, *in situ* injection of polymer paste, absolute alcohol, balloon release, and metallic spirals. Therapeutic drugs can also be associated with the injected fragments (chemoembolization of some malignant tumours). The indication for renal embolization can be grouped into three categories.

- Preoperative embolizations: the aim is to decrease the tumoural vascularization and thus to facilitate surgery by decreasing blood loss and making dissection easier. Agreement is far from complete concerning the real usefulness of this technique, which must be restricted only to voluminous and highly vascular tumours.
- Treatment of symptoms by embolization: it is most often palliative and aimed at treating a symptom, haematuria, pain, mostly in non-surgical tumoural pathology. However, the treatment of post-trauma (mainly postrenal biopsy) haematuria and/or perirenal haematoma by embolization represents a particularly efficient and attractive solution since selective catheterization allows us to preserve as much as possible the healthy parenchyma: it is particularly the case in haematuria caused by needle biopsy.
- Treatment of diseases by embolization: embolization can be proposed as a therapeutic method for definitive treatment of vascular malformation (Fig. 3a and b), some renal angiomyolipomas (Fig. 4a and b), and palliative treatment of some inoperable renal cell carcinomas. Unilateral or bilateral 'radiologic nephrectomy' can also be used in some cases of uncontrollable symptoms such as malignant hypertension, heavy proteinuria, untreatable ureteral fistula.

Embolization risks are moderate. Secondary manifestations related to renal infarction are constant and transitory, as for instance, lumbar

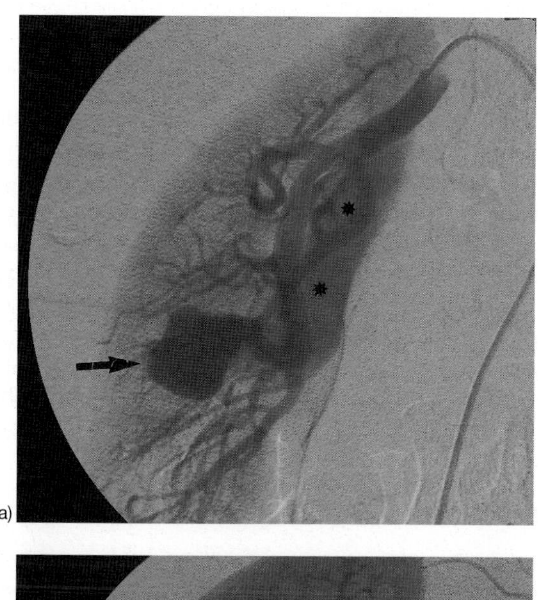

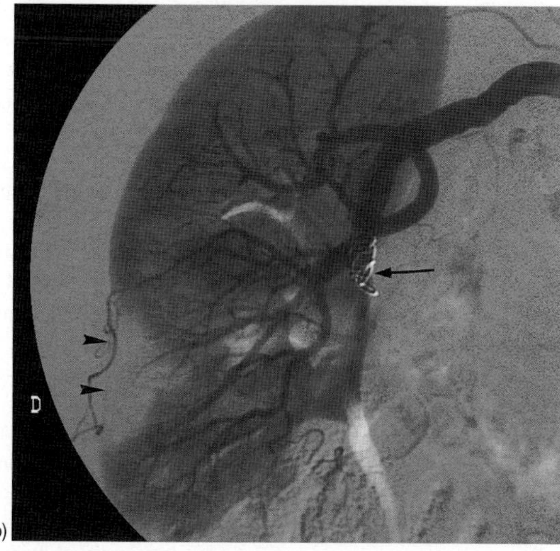

Fig. 3 Arteriovenous renal malformation. (a) Right renal arteriography in a patient with macroscopic haematuria. Opacification of an arteriovenous aneurysm of the lower pole (arrow) with early venous opacification (*). (b) Arteriographic control after embolization with coils of the feeding artery (arrow). Moderate ischaemic zone of the lower pole (arrowheads).

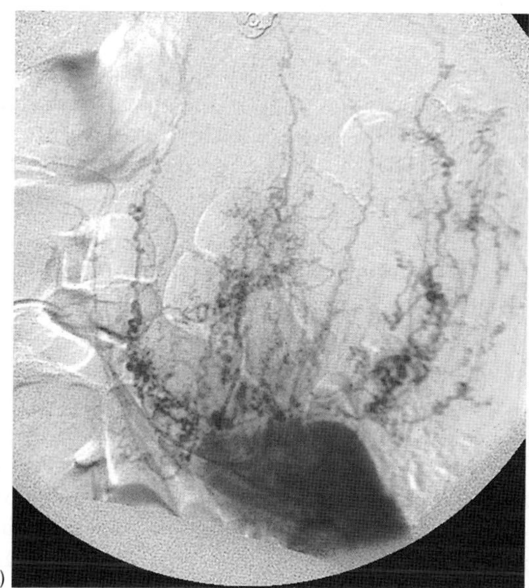

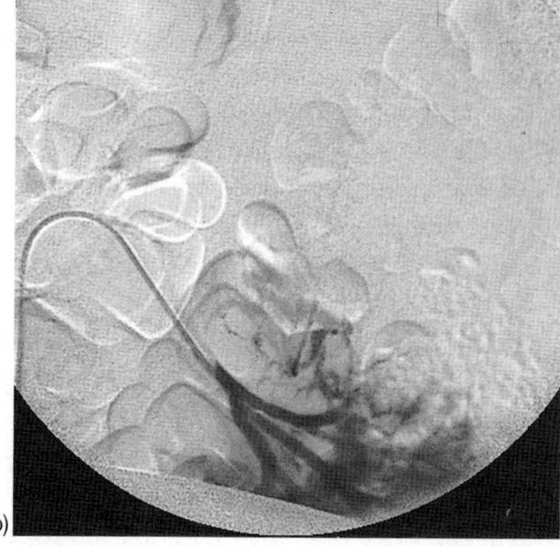

Fig. 4 Embolization of a huge renal angiomyolipoma with acute retroperitoneal haemorrhage in a pregnant woman: (a) selective left renal arteriography showing hypervascularization of the tumour; (b) control after embolization of particles: almost complete occlusion of the tumoural hypervascularization.

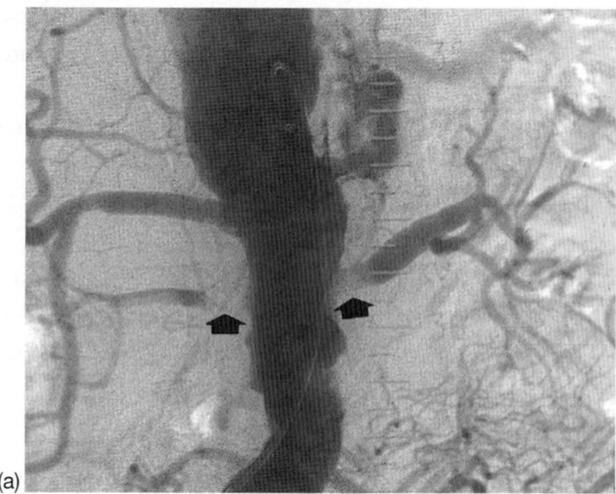

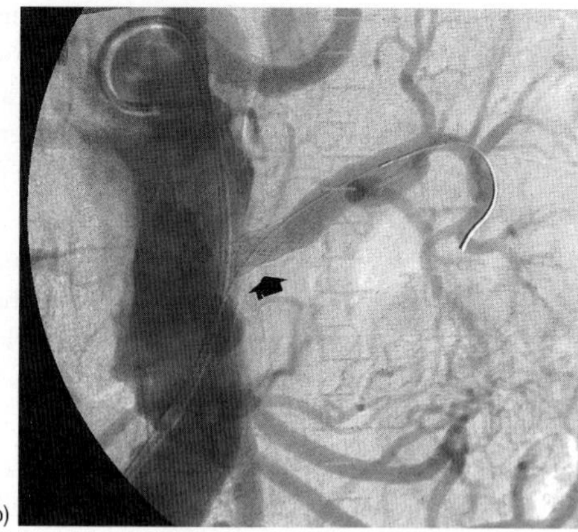

Fig. 5 Renal angioplasty. (a) Aortography for ischaemic nephropathy with severe hypertension, progressive renal insufficiency, and subacute pulmonary oedema: important aortic atheroma, occlusion of the right renal artery (arrow) with non-functioning and atrophic right kidney, ostial stenosis of the left renal artery (arrow). (b) Aortographic control after stenting of the left renal artery (arrow).

pain, sometimes fever, and leucocytosis. The migration of embolic fragments into the aortic lumen must be avoided by a careful radioscopic control during the injection. Since the possibility of an abscess which would occur within tumoural necrosis cannot be ruled out, antibiotic therapy is justified in some cases.

Percutaneous transluminal renal angioplasty

Since the first description in 1978 by Gruntzig, PTRA has been progressively considered as the initial therapeutic approach to renal artery stenosis (RAS) whenever possible. Due to the introduction of endoprostheses, the results are comparable to those of surgery with a lower morbidity and mortality (Hennequin *et al.* 1994). PTRA provides good, long-term anatomical results in approximately 85 per cent of patients. Immediate failures become exceptional with the use of stents. Major complications occur in less than 5 per cent and immediate surgery is required in less than 0.5 per cent of patients. Mid-term recurrences are observed in 15 per cent of the cases and are closely related to the quality of the immediate the result.

Clinical results are not always related to anatomic results and are totally different in atheromatous patients and in the case of fibromuscular dysplasia. In renovascular hypertension, a clinical benefit is obtained in approximately 50 per cent of all atheromatous stenoses and in 85 per cent of stenoses due to fibromuscular dysplasia. Results are worse in patients with renal insufficiency, many of them tend to be older, with extensive atheromatous lesions and probably nephroangiosclerosis. A clinical benefit is obtained in approximately 50 per cent of the cases.

Indications concern significant and symptomatic RAS in patients with two main categories of symptoms: (a) Patients with hypertension due to RAS (renovascular hypertension). In this situation, the aim of the treatment is to control the hypertension. (b) Patients with RAS, which is responsible for progressive renal insufficiency (ischaemic nephropathy). In the latter case, the indication mostly aims at preserving the renal vasculature (Fig. 5a and b).

Despite the good results in several categories of patients with such fibromuscular dysplasia, multiple points of controversy persist, particularly concerning the indications.

In terms of evidence-based medicine, the universally admitted indications of PTRA are the following: significant and accessible RAS with (a) uncontrolled hypertension with two medications, (b) progressive renal insufficiency, and (c) acute onset of cardiac insufficiency with recurrent pulmonary oedema. In all other situations, the benefit of PTRA has never been clearly demonstrated and indications must be largely discussed case by case (for clinical indications see also Chapter 9.7).

Therefore, a multidisciplinary discussion estimating risks and benefits is justified before the therapeutic decision (Sacks 2000).

References

Beaujeux, R. *et al.* (1995). Superselective endovascular treatment of renal vascular lesions. *Journal of Urology* **153**, 14–17.

Gruntzig, A. *et al.* (1978). Treatment of reno-vascular hypertension with percutaneous transluminal dilatation of renal artery stenosis. *Lancet* **i**, 801–802.

Hammer, F. D. *et al.* (1999). Gadolinium dimeglumine: an alternative contrast agent for digital substraction angiography. *European Radiology* **9**, 128–136.

Helenon, Ch. *et al.* (1977). Aspects de l'artériographie au cours de l'évolutivité des lésions de la péri-artérite noueuse. *Journal de Radiologie* **58**, 45–50.

Hennequin, L. M. *et al.* (1994). Renal artery stent placement: long-term results with the wallstent endoprosthesis. *Radiology* **191**, 713–719.

Hillman, B. J. (1989). Imaging advances in the diagnostic of reno-vascular hypertension. *AJR. American Journal of Roentgenology* **153**, 5–14.

Huber, W *et al.* (2002). Effects of theophylline on contrast material-induced nephropathy in patients with chronic renal insufficiency: controlled, randomized, double-blinded study. *Radiology* **223**, 772–779.

Irving, J. D. and Khoury, G. A. (1983). Digital substraction angiography in renal transplant recipients. *Cardiovascular Interventional Radiology* **6**, 224–230.

Joffre, F. Renal angiography. In *Oxford Textbook of Clinical Nephrology* 2nd edn. Vol. 1 (ed. A. M. Davison, J. S. Cameron, J. P. Grunfeld, D. N. S. Kerr, Z. E. Ritz, and C. G. Winearls), pp. 132–137. Oxford: Oxford University Press, 1998.

Joffre, F. and Russ, P. D. Anatomy and conventional imaging of the kidneys and upper urinary tract. In *Imaging of Abdominal and Pelvic Anatomy* Chapter 26 (ed. F. Weill and Manco-Johnson), pp. 250–278. New York: Churchill Livingstone, 1997.

Kan, J. H. *et al.* (1999). Carbon dioxide guided endovascular renal artery intervention: initial results. *Journal of Interventional Radiology* **14**, 29–35.

Khauli, R. B. (1994). Defining the role of renal angiography in the diagnosis of renal artery disease. *American Journal of Kidney Diseases* **24**, 679–684.

Lieberman, S. F. *et al.* (1983). Percutaneous vaso-occlusion for non malignant renal lesions. *Journal of Urology* **129**, 805–809.

Mitty, H. A. and Gribetz, M. E. (1982). The status of interventional uroradiology. *Journal of Urology* **127**, 2–9.

Morcos, S. K., Thomsen, H. S., Webb, J. A., and Esur (1999). Contrast-media safety committee. Contrast-media induced nephrotoxicity: a consensus report. *European Radiology* **9**, 1602–1613.

Nyman, U. *et al.* (2002). Are gadolinium-based contrast media really safer than iodinated media for digital substraction angiography in patients with azotemia. *Radiology* **223**, 311–318.

Otal, Ph. *et al.* (2000). Imagery and endovascular treatment of renal artery stenosis in the diabetic patient. *Diabetes and Metabolism* **26**, 97–102.

Richter, C. S. *et al.* (1993). Assessment of renal artery stenosis by contrast magnetic resonance angiography. *European Radiology* **3**, 493–498.

Rubin, G. D. *et al.* (1994). Spiral CT of renal artery stenosis: comparison of three dimensional rendering technique. *Radiology* **190**, 181–189.

Sacks, D., Rundback, J. H., and Martin, L. G. (2000). Renal angioplasty/stent placement and hypertension in the year 2000. *Journal of Vascular Interventional Radiology* **11**, 949–953.

Solomon, R. *et al.* (1994). Effects of saline, mannitol and furosemide on acute decrease in renal function induced by radio-contrasts agents. *New England Journal of Medicine* **331**, 1416–1420.

Spinosa, D. J. *et al.* (1999). Renal insufficiency: usefulness of gadolinium enhanced renal angiography for diagnosis and percutaneous treatment. *Radiology* **210**, 663–672.

Tepel, M. *et al.* (2000). Prevention of radiographic-contrast-agent-induced reductions in renal function by acetyl-cysteine. *New England Journal of Medicine* **20**, 180–184.

1.6.1.v CT scanning and helical CT

Bernard E. Van Beers and André Noël Dardenne

Introduction

Since the beginning of the 1990s, helical computed tomography (CT) has become the standard CT method to assess the abdomen and the urinary tract. It has replaced conventional, sequential CT for this purpose. Conventional CT is a method in which X-ray exposure and patient translation alternate. Organs are scanned slice by slice. In contrast, helical CT scanning is based on the continuous rotation of the X-ray tube when the patient is moved through the gantry. It allows scanning complete organs or anatomical regions during a single breath hold. The increased speed of helical CT scanning avoids misregistrations that occur in sequential scanning because of inconsistent levels of inspiration from scan to scan. The image quality of multiplanar and three-dimensional reformations is improved and studies of large volumes can be repeated during several phases after the injection of contrast agents (Kopka *et al.* 1997). Because helical CT scanning is now the routine CT method in the urinary tract, this chapter is mainly devoted to it. Helical CT has a major role in diagnostic imaging of the kidney and upper urinary tract. It helps to assess tumours, trauma, stones, as well as vascular and inflammatory lesions (Kawashima *et al.* 1997a; Liu *et al.* 2000; Harris *et al.* 2001). Because of its cross-sectional nature and increased sensitivity to small differences in contrast, helical CT has replaced conventional urography for these indications. The longitudinal or craniocaudal resolution of CT is limited so that evaluation of subtle lesions of the urothelium remains difficult (McNicholas *et al.* 1998). However, CT urography obtained with new-generation multislice helical CT scanners may challenge the role of conventional urography in the depiction of the urinary collecting system (Caoili *et al.* 2002).

Helical CT is more accurate than sonography for the evaluation of renal lesions (Zagoria 2000) and the detection of urolithiasis (Sheafor *et al.* 2000). Magnetic resonance imaging has some advantages over CT. Its greater contrast sensitivity may be useful in the detection of tumourous enhancement with contrast agents in equivocal cases. Contrast-enhanced magnetic resonance imaging also may be used for the characterization of renal lesions in patients with renal insufficiency. Still the availability, speed, and cost of helical CT favour its use for the assessment of focal renal lesions in most patients.

Techniques of helical CT

Multislice helical CT scanning

The volume coverage speed of helical CT can be substantially improved by new CT systems equipped with a multiple-row detector array as opposed to the single-row detector array used in single slice helical CT. These multislice CT scanners acquire several slices in a single rotation of the X-ray tube and detector assembly. Compared with single-slice helical CT, multislice helical CT provides a substantial improvement in speed with comparable diagnostic image quality. Larger volumes are thus scanned in a given time with multislice helical CT scanners than with single slice CT scanners.

Alternatively, the same volume can be scanned with thinner slices. Thin slices improve the spatial resolution in the longitudinal axis, the grading of vessel stenosis, and the characterization of small renal lesions (Brink *et al.* 1995; Bae *et al.* 2000). Lesion characterization is improved with thin-slice CT because partial volume averaging of the lesions with surrounding tissue is decreased. To avoid partial volume averaging, the section thickness should not be larger than half the diameter of the evaluated mass. With multislice helical CT, a section thickness of 1–3 mm is used routinely (Caoili *et al.* 2002).

Reconstruction techniques

Conventional CT is basically an anisotropic imaging modality. This means that the longitudinal resolution determined by the slice thickness (up to 10 mm in conventional scanning) and the reconstruction interval are worse than the in-plane or transverse resolution (<1 mm). Because of this poor longitudinal resolution, two-dimensional multiplanar reformations and three-dimensional reconstructions are rarely used with conventional CT. With helical CT, and particularly multislice helical CT, the longitudinal resolution is greatly improved for two reasons. First, large volumes can be scanned rapidly with thin slices during a single breath-holding interval. Second, from the volumetric acquisition, overlapping cross-sectional images can be reconstructed without increasing patient dose.

Because of the high longitudinal resolution of multislice helical CT, high-quality two-dimensional multiplanar reformations and three-dimensional reconstructions can be obtained routinely. This results in an important improvement and wide acceptance of CT angiography and CT urography (Caoili *et al.* 2002; Schreyer *et al.* 2002).

Two-dimensional reconstruction techniques include multiplanar reformations in the coronal or sagittal plane and curved planar reformations in any projection drawn by the operator. With multiplanar reformations, the urinary tract can be displayed in a format similar to that of an intravenous urogram or a conventional angiogram with the advantage that adjacent organs are depicted. Multiplanar reformations also reduce the load of transverse images. Curved reformations are useful to display the whole length of the renal arteries or ureters. However, the method is very 'operator dependent'. Inaccurate plane selection can falsely simulate vascular stenoses or exclude true stenoses. Methods of automatic selection of a plane passing through the centre of the vessel or perpendicular to its main axis have been developed.

Three-dimensional reconstruction techniques include surface rendering, maximum intensity projection, and volume rendering (Fig. 1) (Prokop *et al.* 1997). Volume rendering is the most complicated, but has the potential to be the most informative of the three reconstruction methods (Johnson *et al.* 1999).

The operator dependence of multiplanar reformations and three-dimensional reconstructions should be emphasized. Therefore, two-dimensional reformations and three-dimensional displays should be interpreted together with the transverse source images (Prokop *et al.* 1997).

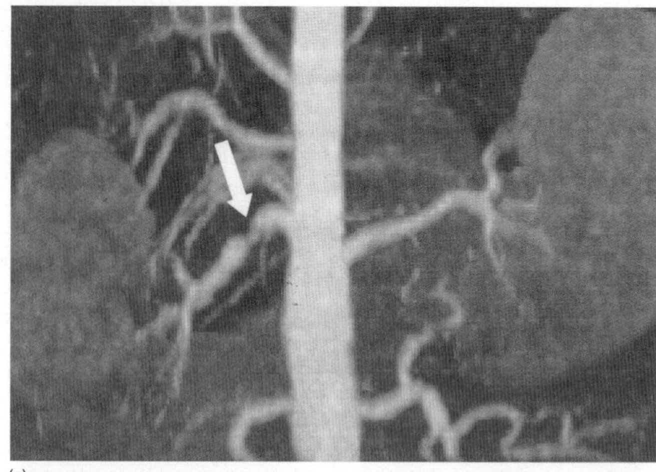

(a)

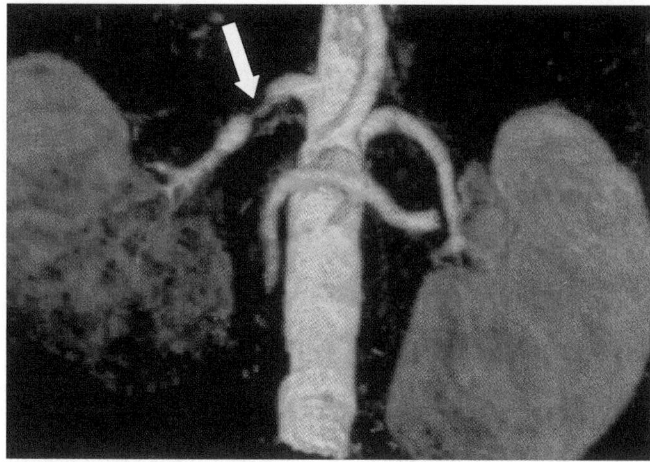

(b)

Fig. 1 Stenosis of left renal artery. Maximum intensity projection image (a) and volume rendered reconstruction (b) clearly show severe stenosis (arrow) of left renal artery with poststenotic dilatation.

Multiphasic scanning

With helical CT, scanning of the kidneys can be performed before contrast material administration and at defined phases after contrast material injection, including the corticomedullary, nephrographic, and excretory phases. Scanning before contrast material injection should always be performed to detect renal calcifications or urolithiasis and to characterize renal lesions. Indeed, baseline density measurements are necessary in renal lesions to determine if density enhancement is present after contrast material injection. In patients with acute flank pain, unenhanced CT is widely performed to detect ureteral calculi. In patients with flank pain but without visible stones on unenhanced CT, contrast-enhanced CT should be performed to rule out renal infarction, acute pyelonephritis, or a renal tumour.

After bolus injection (2.5–4 ml/s) of contrast material (80–150 ml), imaging of patients with renal lesions should be repeated during the corticomedullary, the nephrographic, and/or excretory phase. In the absence of precontrast CT examination, delayed CT (more than 15 min after contrast material injection) of incidentally discovered high-attenuating renal mass enables differentiation of high-density cysts from renal neoplasm by documentation of de-enhancement as a proof of vascularity and, hence, neoplasm (Macari and Bosniak 1999).

The corticomedullary phase is the first phase of renal signal enhancement. It usually occurs between 25 and 80 s after initiation of contrast injection. During this phase the contrast material is mainly located in the vessels and the lumina of the proximal cortical tubules. The highly enhanced cortex is clearly differentiated from the poorly enhanced and hypovascular medulla. Assessing the corticomedullary phase may cause significant errors. Small hypovascular tumours of the renal medulla or small hypervascular tumours of the cortex may be missed, and poorly or inhomogeneously enhanced medulla may be misdiagnosed as a renal mass. Nevertheless, imaging during the corticomedullary phase remains useful for several reasons. The vascularization of tumours and inflammatory lesions may be better appreciated during this phase than during later phases. Normal corticomedullary enhancement can be useful to differentiate normal variants such as prominent columns of Bertin from renal masses. Renal arterial and venous enhancement and the imaging of other organs such as the liver are optimal soon after injection. Imaging during the corticomedullary phase is thus useful to determine the extension of malignant renal tumours in the abdomen (Kopka *et al.* 1997).

The second phase, the nephrographic phase, includes the passage of contrast material through the tubules. It usually starts 85–100 s after contrast material injection. The renal parenchyma is homogeneous. The nephrographic phase is the best phase for the detection and the characterization of renal lesions (Fig. 2) (Kopka *et al.* 1997). During the third phase, the excretory phase, the contrast material enhances the collecting system. This phase starts within 3–5 min after contrast material injection. The nephrogram remains homogeneous, but its attenuation decreases as the plasma level of contrast material decreases. This phase is useful to show lesions of the urothelium (Caoili *et al.* 2002). Abdominal compression of the ureters may be used to improve the distension of the renal pelvis and the calices.

For CT angiography, signal enhancement should be high in the renal arteries and absent in the renal veins. Therefore, contrast agents are injected at high rates (3–5 ml/s) and imaging is initiated soon after the injection. The time to peak enhancement in the arteries depends on contrast material volume, injection rate, and patient's circulation time. Patients with cardiovascular diseases have wide variations in circulation time which can be assessed by the injection of a small test bolus before the actual scan or by methods of bolus triggering that automatically detect the arrival of the bolus in the aorta. Test bolus injection or bolus triggering is mainly useful to detect renal artery stenoses in patients with atheromatosis. These patients are typically old with a high prevalence of cardiovascular comorbidities and altered circulation time. In contrast, a fixed delay between contrast material injection and scanning initiation can be used for CT angiography in young renal donors.

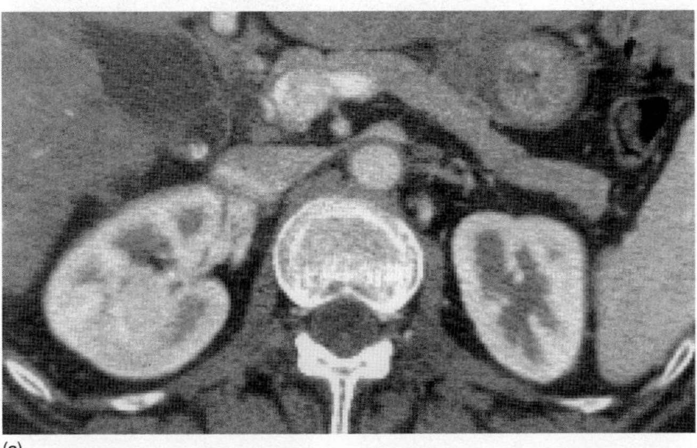

(a)

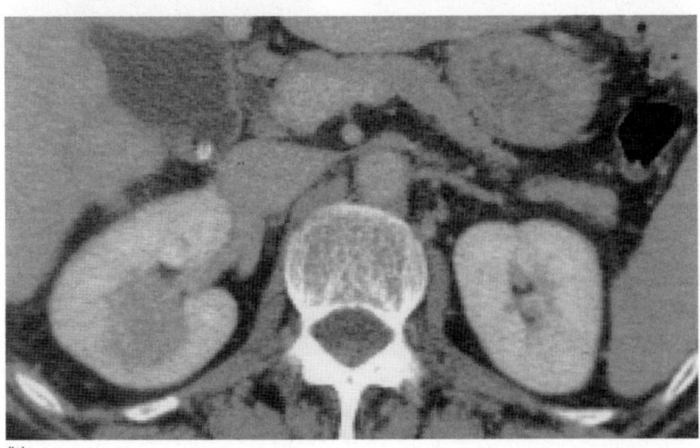

(b)

Fig. 2 Hypervascular renal cell carcinoma of the right kidney. Contrast between tumour and kidney is higher during the nephrographic phase (b) than during the corticomedullary phase (a) of renal enhancement.

Measurement of renal perfusion and function

Renal perfusion, glomerular filtration, and tubular function can be assessed with fast repeated CT scanning of the aorta and kidney during the transit of contrast material (Miles 1991; Tsushima *et al.* 1999; Krier *et al.* 2001). Two approaches have been used to measure renal perfusion with CT. The first is based on the fractionation of cardiac output (Miles 1991), and the second on the mean transit time equation (Krier *et al.* 2001). The glomerular filtration rate has mainly been calculated by a mathematical analysis designed to measure the permeability of the blood–brain barrier (Tsushima *et al.* 1999). Renal flow reserve can also be determined by repeated measurements of renal blood flow during a pharmacological challenge with short-acting vasodilators.

The measurement of renal perfusion and function with CT offers interesting perspectives for research and clinical applications. However, functional CT is not widely used. Limitations include the use of iodinated contrast agents in patients with compromised renal function and the radiation exposure due to repeated scanning of the same region of interest to construct time–density curves. Renal perfusion and glomerular filtration can also be measured with magnetic resonance imaging, without the risk inherent to contrast-enhanced CT.

Radiation dose

CT is a relatively high-dose technique that is more and more used. Indications for CT have widened and the technique is now extensively used in benign diseases and in young patients for whom radiation protection is paramount (Golding and Schrimpton 2002). Controversy exists about the carcinological potential of radiation exposure associated with CT. The relationship between these radiation exposures and biological risk for patients is determined by mathematical extrapolation derived from changes observed after exposure to much higher levels of radiation. Nevertheless, the risk associated with radiation exposure from CT cannot be considered negligible. The effective dose of an abdominal CT examination often reaches 10 mSv. It has been estimated that this dose increases the lifetime risk of fatal cancer by 1 in 2000 (Golding and Schrimpton 2002). Multislice CT will probably further increase the population dose from CT as a result of new applications and the easiness to perform extended examinations and multiphasic examinations.

A European Commission Working Party addresses the problem of radiation dose in CT and develops European guidelines for quality criteria, including reference dosimetry based on the practical dose quantities of weighted CT dose index ($CTDI_w$) and dose length product (DLP). Practically speaking, the potential benefit of CT has to be weighted against its biological cost and the exposure parameters should be adjusted to deliver the minimum dose (Golding and Schrimpton 2002). The length of patient scanned should be adapted to the clinical question. Radiation dose may be lowered by decreased tube current and/or increased pitch defined as the collimation divided by the table feed. However, these factors also determine image noise, low contrast resolution, image quality, and therefore clinical efficacy. A trade-off thus exists between image quality and exposure (Golding and Schrimpton 2002). Technical measures such as attenuation-based modulation of the tube current may significantly reduce the dose without sacrificing image quality.

Renal arteries

Helical CT angiography can be used to assess most lesions of the renal arteries. It has a reported sensitivity and specificity of at least 90 per cent for the detection of renal artery stenosis (Kaatee *et al.* 1997). It is more accurate than Doppler sonography and captopril scintigraphy for this purpose (Vasbinder *et al.* 2001). A meta-analysis shows that CT angiography and gadolinium-enhanced MR angiography have similar diagnostic performance (Vasbinder *et al.* 2001). A potential disadvantage of CT angiography is that, in contrast to MR angiography, large volumes of contrast material are needed for adequate opacification of the renal arteries. This increases the risk of inducing nephrotoxicity. Fibromuscular dysplasia can also be demonstrated with CT angiography. However, the demonstration of subtle or peripheral lesions with CT angiography remains limited.

Helical CT angiography is a good alternative to renal angiography and intravenous urography for living renal donor assessment (Rubin *et al.* 1995). Some small accessory arteries may be missed at CT angiography. However, the accuracy and predictive values of CT angiography in the detection of accessory arteries exceed 90 per cent. In addition, venous anatomy, incidental renal tumours or other renal lesions can be demonstrated with helical CT. Other benefits of helical CT over renal angiography are lower morbidity, improved donor convenience, and lower cost.

Helical CT angiography is also suitable to identify crossing vessels in kidneys with obstruction of the ureteropelvic junction (Fig. 3) (Rouviere *et al.* 1999). Congenital obstruction of the ureteropelvic junction is most likely caused by abnormal musculature. The role of crossing vessels in the pathogenesis of the obstruction as well as their influence on the results of endourological procedures remains controversial. Van Cangh *et al.* (1994) showed that crossing vessels have a significant negative influence on the outcome of endoureteropyelotomy. This provides a rationale for preoperative screening of crossing vessels.

Helical CT angiography can provide all the necessary information for surgical or endovascular repair of abdominal aortic aneurysms (Van Hoe *et al.* 1996). In particular, CT angiography is superior to conventional arteriography to show the proximal extent of the aortic aneurysm relative to the renal arteries. The higher speed and longitudinal coverage of multislice helical CT is useful to demonstrate associated iliofemoral artery disease.

Helical CT is also useful to demonstrate other diseases of the renal arteries and veins, including dissection, thrombosis, and aneurysms. Small and distal aneurysms, as observed in polyarteritis nodosa, may not always be detectable with CT angiography. Finally, CT angiography is helpful in the follow-up of postoperative patients, particularly those who have undergone renal transplantation, angioplasty, or stent placement (Hofmann *et al.* 1999).

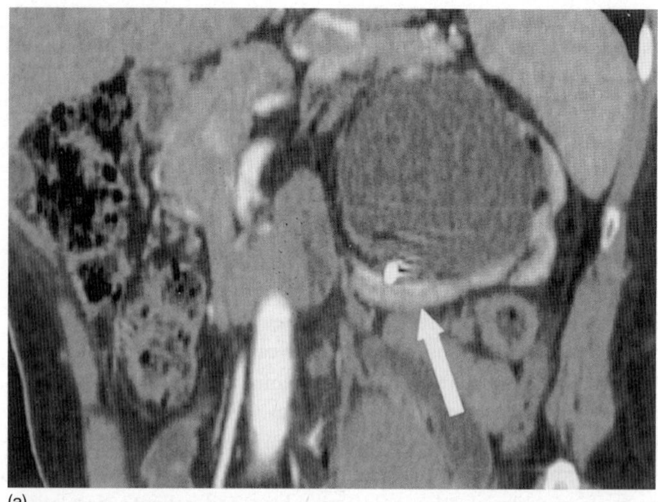

(a)

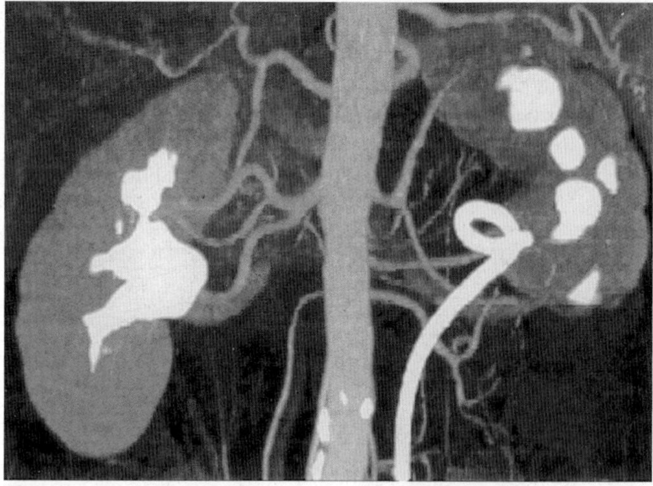

(b)

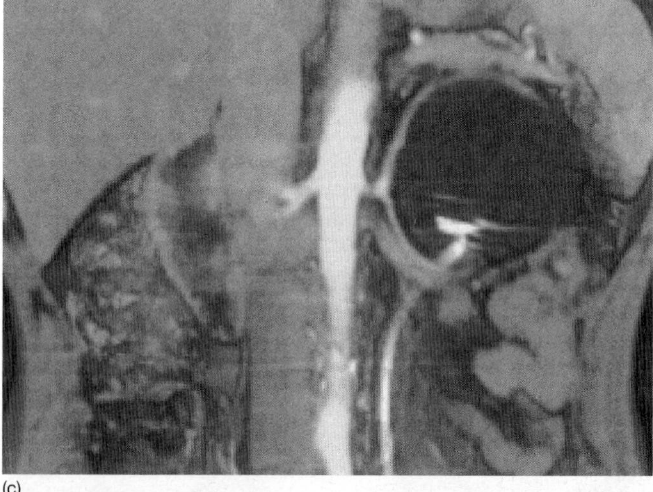

(c)

Fig. 3 Obstruction of left ureteropelvic junction. Coronal oblique reconstruction (a) shows renal artery and vein (arrow) crossing beneath dilated left renal pelvis, but the whole length of these vessels is not demonstrated. The maximum intensity projection image (b) better demonstrates the whole length of the left renal artery, but the less-enhanced left renal vein and unenhanced renal pelvis are not clearly seen. Volume rendered reconstruction (c) clearly shows a dilated pelvis and crossing artery and vein.

Renal masses

Cystic lesions

Most of the small, incidentally detected renal lesions are benign cysts. Simple cysts usually have typical imaging features at sonography and

CT when they are larger than 1 cm. With CT, the simple cyst has a smooth, thin wall, a water density content that is homogeneous throughout (0–20 HU), and no enhancement following IV administration of contrast material (Bosniak 1986). Partial volume averaging and beam hardening artefactually increases attenuation numbers in cysts and may mimic enhancement after contrast material administration (Bae *et al.* 2000). However, this pseudoenhancement of renal cysts after administration of contrast material is usually below 10 HU.

Despite this limitation, CT is superior to sonography for the detection and characterization of renal masses (Zagoria 2000). However, sonography rather than CT remains the most cost-effective method for the workup of a renal mass detected at urography, because most renal masses are benign cysts that are readily diagnosed at sonography (Einstein *et al.* 1995). Any mass detected initially on sonography or evaluated with sonography after detection with urography that does not meet the strict sonographic criteria for a simple cyst should be further evaluated with CT (Zagoria 2000). Cystic lesions can be further divided, using Bosniak's classification, into four categories (Bosniak 1986; Siegel *et al.* 1997). *Category I lesions* are uncomplicated simple cysts that have characteristic findings at imaging. *Category II lesions* are benign as well, but do not have all the characteristic imaging findings of simple renal cysts. The lesion may contain a few thin septations or calcifications or may be hyperdense. If hyperdense, these cysts have a diameter lower than 3 cm and exhibit homogeneous attenuation. A lot of haemorrhagic or infected cysts fall in this category. *Category III lesions* may show thick or irregular walls, septations, or calcifications. Some of these lesions correspond to complicated cysts or benign cystic tumours, but others correspond to malignant cystic tumours. These lesions are thus indeterminate and theoretically should be surgically explored and possibly removed. *Category IV lesions* are solid elements that enhance with contrast media. Bosniak's classification is useful for the assessment of renal cystic lesions (Fig. 4).

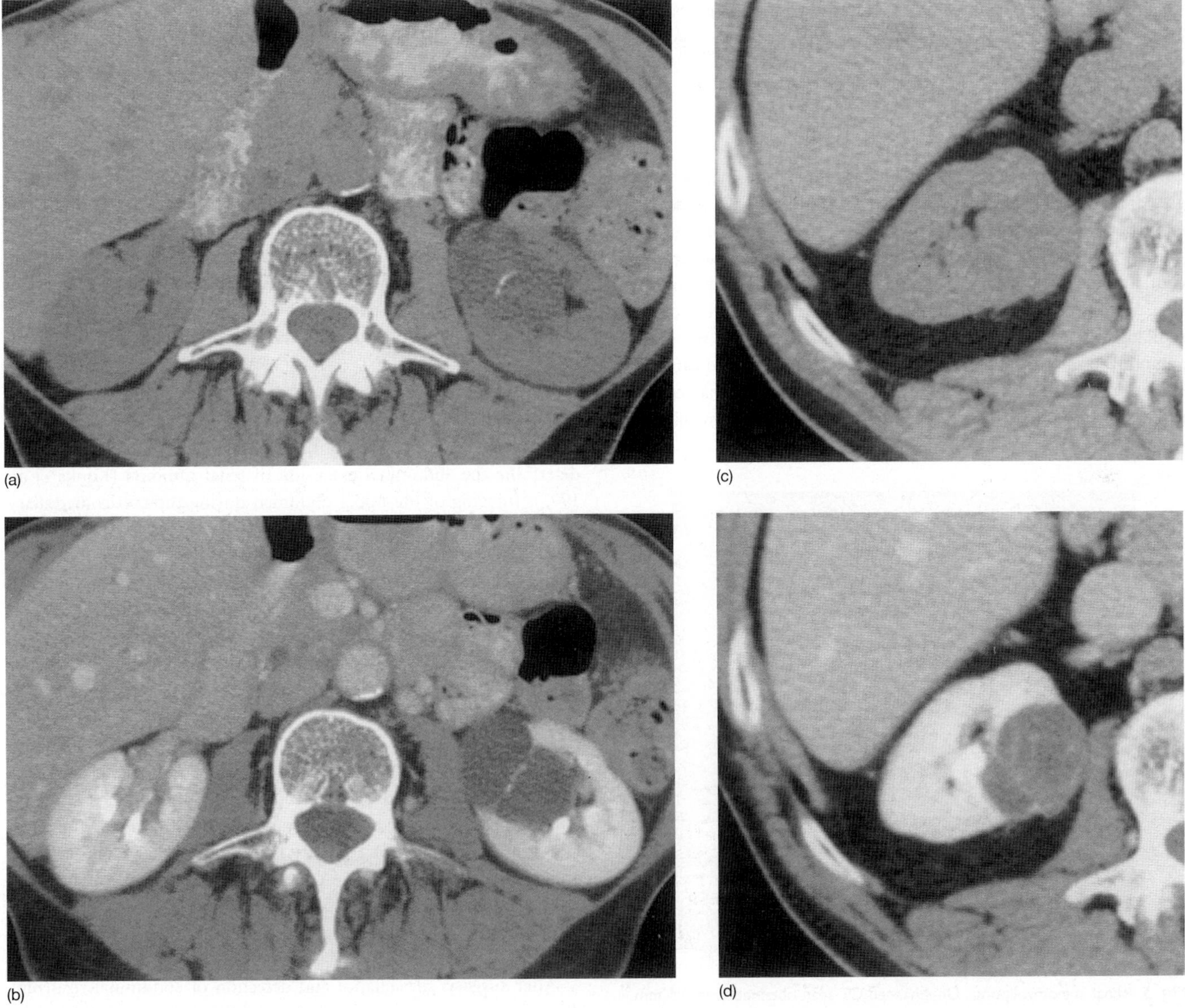

Fig. 4 Bosniak's classification of renal cystic lesions. CT scans before contrast material injection (a) and during the nephrographic phase (b) in a patient with category II lesion show left renal cyst containing fine, partially calcified septum. CT scans before contrast material injection (c) and during the nephrographic phase (d) in another patient with category IV lesion show cystic lesion containing solid, enhancing components in the right kidney.

However, some interobserver variation in the distinction between category II and III lesions may affect the choice between surgical and conservative management (Siegel *et al.* 1997).

Helical CT is valuable in the detection of tumours in patients with cystic diseases. This is especially relevant in patients with von Hippel–Lindau disease in whom renal cell carcinomas are frequent and often multifocal (see Chapter 16.6). Screening of renal tumours and nephron-sparing surgery are of value in patients with von Hippel–Lindau disease (Chauveau *et al.* 1996). In contrast, screening in patients who are on dialysis and have acquired cystic kidney disease remains controversial because the yield of renal tumours is relatively low (Choyke 2000).

Helical CT is useful in other cystic diseases. Thin-section CT demonstrates medullary cysts in patients with nephronophthisis cystic renal medulla complex (Elzouki *et al.* 1996). In patients with autosomal dominant polycystic kidney disease, CT shows the most frequent complications, including cyst haemorrhage or infection and obstructive urinary calculi (Gupta *et al.* 2000). Helical CT allows one to distinguish localized cystic disease from autosomal dominant polycystic kidney disease and cystic tumours including cystic nephroma (Slywotzky and Bosniak 2001).

Solid masses

On unenhanced CT scans, attenuation of solid renal masses will be greater than 20 HU or less than −10 HU. In addition, solid masses will enhance after contrast material injection. The detection of regions of interest of less than −10 HU in a renal mass indicates that the lesion contains fat and is diagnostic of angiomyolipoma in nearly every case (Fig. 5) (Bosniak *et al.* 1988). Very few renal cell carcinomas contain radiologically detectable fat. In contrast, approximately 5 per cent of angiomyolipomas contain no demonstrable fat on CT and cannot be characterized with imaging. Helical CT is more sensitive than conventional CT in showing fatty components in small angiomyolipomas using small and overlapping sections (Silverman *et al.* 1996). It is important to diagnose angiomyolipomas with CT. Indeed, angiomyolipomas smaller than 4 cm should not be treated because the bleeding risk is low. Whereas most angiomyolipomas can be characterized with CT, other solid tumours often do not have characteristic features and are indistinguishable from renal cell carcinoma.

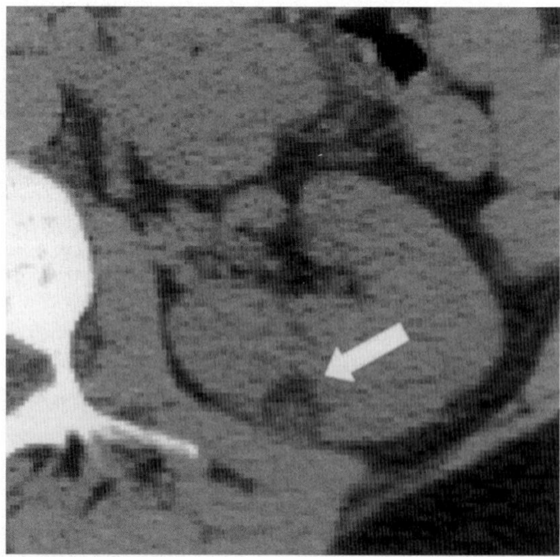

Fig. 5 Renal angiomyolipoma. Unenhanced CT scan obtained with 2.5-mm collimation reveals low-density, fatty component (arrow) in a small left renal tumour. Unenhanced, thin slices of the kidneys should be obtained to demonstrate tiny fat components in tumours.

Renal cell carcinoma is the most common primary malignancy of the kidney. This tumour accounts for 2 per cent of all cancers. In recent years, the widespread application of CT and sonography for other indications has led to increased detection of renal cell carcinoma as an incidental finding. At present, 25–50 per cent of renal cell carcinomas are diagnosed after the incidental detection of a renal mass as compared with 10 per cent or less before the use of cross-sectional imaging (Zagoria 2000). Tumours found incidentally are typically smaller than those that produce symptoms and are more likely to be resected for cure, leading to improved prognosis. However, several biases may play a role in this apparent improved survival (Black and Welch 1997). Epidemiological data have shown that the rapid incidence of renal cell cancer in the United States between 1975 and 1995 is only partly explained by the increased detection of presymptomatic tumours with imaging. A real increase is suggested by the upward trend in incidence for more advanced tumours and by a corresponding increase in kidney cancer mortality during that period (Chow *et al.* 1999).

The growth rate of small incidentally discovered renal tumours is variable. Tumours that are destined to grow and possibly metastasize do so early and most small tumours grow at a low rate or not at all (Bosniak *et al.* 1995). The standard therapy for small, incidentally discovered renal cell carcinoma remains surgical excision before the tumour metastasizes, but watchful waiting may be an appropriate alternative, especially in patients who are elderly or those who have an increased risk of perioperative mortality and morbidity.

Tumour extension

Computed tomography is the imaging method most often used to determine the abdominal extension of renal tumours (Kopka *et al.* 1997). Imaging of the upper abdomen during the corticomedullary phase of enhancement is important to detect liver metastases and tumour invasion of the renal vein. Helical CT is accurate in the assessment of macroscopic renal vein involvement in patients with renal cell carcinoma (Fig. 6). The same holds true for macroscopic adrenal involvement (Gill *et al.* 1994). Therefore, adrenal sparing nephrectomy may be considered when the adrenal gland appears normal at CT. Helical CT remains limited to determine early perinephric tumour spread, invasion of adjacent organs, and metastasis to normal-sized lymph nodes (Zagoria 2000; Sheth *et al.* 2001).

Nephron sparing surgery is increasingly performed in select patients with localized renal cell carcinoma. This treatment is effective, providing long-term control with preservation of renal function. However, nephron sparing surgery is technically challenging. Three-dimensional reconstructions of the CT data are useful to show the arterial and venous anatomy of the kidney and to delineate the precise relationship between the tumour and the surface of the kidney, the collecting system and the renal vessels (Fig. 7) (Sheth *et al.* 2001).

After surgery, surveillance and detection of abdominal recurrent disease can be performed with helical CT (Scatarige *et al.* 2001). The need to perform surveillance CT in patients with T1 tumours of less than 4 cm remains questionable (Levy *et al.* 1998).

Non-tumourous focal lesions

Inflammatory masses such as renal and perirenal abscesses can be detected with CT (Kawashima *et al.* 1997a). An abscess appears as a well-defined mass with a necrotic centre and a thick, irregular wall (Fig. 8). Signs of uncomplicated acute pyelonephritis include striated, wedge-shaped, or rounded renal areas of decreased contrast enhancement, renal enlargement, perinephric stranding, and wall thickening of the calices, pelvis, and ureter. The use of CT is not routinely indicated in uncomplicated renal infection. CT may be performed in patients whose clinical diagnosis is unclear, patients who fail to respond to conventional treatment, and high-risk patients.

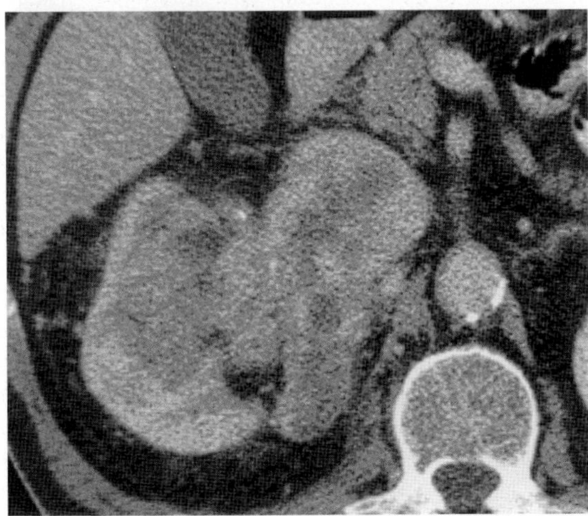

Fig. 6 Advanced renal tumour. Transverse contrast-enhanced CT scan shows large renal tumour with heterogeneous thrombus within the renal vein and inferior vena cava.

CT is currently the most useful imaging modality to diagnose xanthogranulomatous pyelonephritis. The typical CT findings in diffuse xanthogranulomatous pyelonephritis include an enlarged, nonfunctioning kidney, a central calculus, and multiple rounded hypoattenuating masses with peripheral enhancing rims, typically arranged in a hydronephrotic pattern. These hypodense masses correspond to dilated calices or inflammatory tissue. The perirenal and pararenal spaces are commonly involved (Kawashima *et al.* 1997a). A focal form of xanthogranulomatous pyelonephritis may mimic a renal tumour at CT.

In renal infarction, the CT findings include wedge-shaped areas without contrast enhancement, high-attenuation cortical rim peripheral to the lesions, and perinephric stranding (Fig. 9). The cortical rim sign is seen in about 50 per cent of cases with renal infarction and is thought to be due to an intact renal collateral circulation. The cortical rim sign can be seen in other conditions, including renal vein thrombosis and acute tubular necrosis.

Renal trauma

Helical CT is the imaging modality of choice in the evaluation of blunt abdominal injury (Harris *et al.* 2001). Volume scanning can be performed rapidly and requires less patient collaboration than conventional CT scanning (Schreyer *et al.* 2002). Helical CT helps in evaluation of the severity of parenchymal injury, including parenchymal devascularization due to vessel injury, and demonstrates lesions of the vascular pedicle and the upper urinary tract. In blunt abdominal trauma, helical CT is often performed for screening of the entire abdomen and the kidneys are visualized during the corticomedullary phase. Imaging of the upper urinary tract during the excretory phase should be performed to show contrast extravasation caused by injury of the renal collecting system and ureteropelvic junction (Kawashima *et al.* 1997b). Integration of the imaging findings with clinical

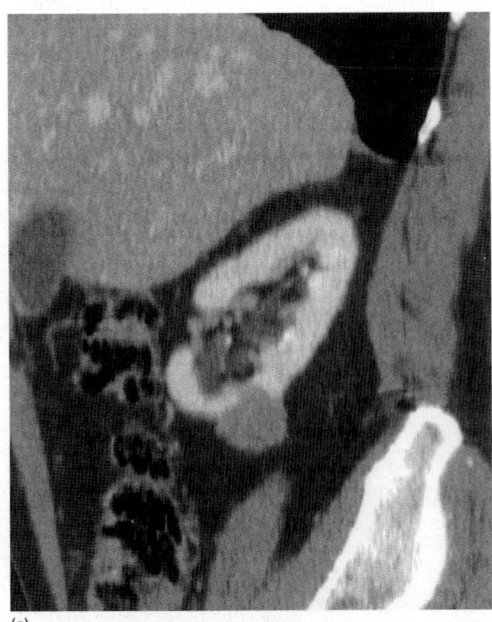

(a)

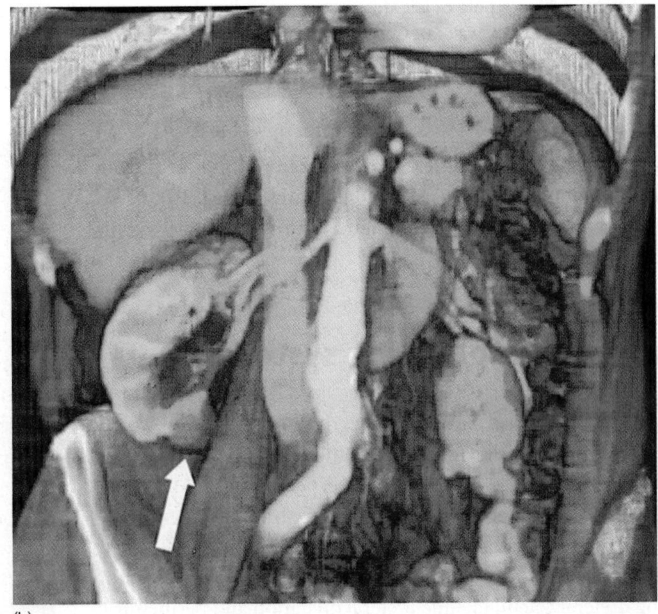

(b)

Fig. 7 Small renal cell carcinoma. Sagittal reconstruction (a) shows a small, peripheral tumour. Volume rendered reconstruction (b) shows that the tumour does not extend into the renal hilum.

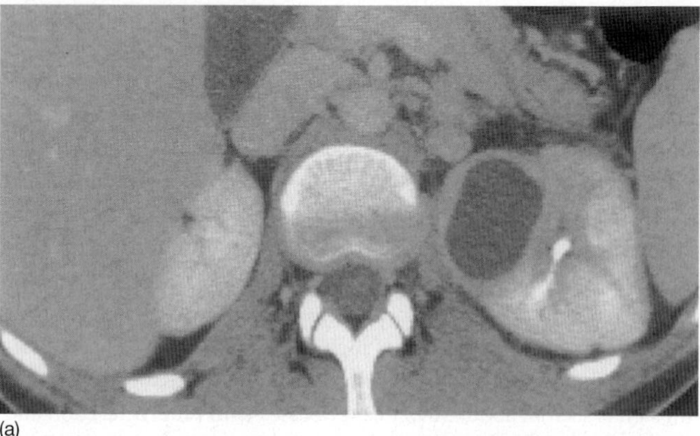

(a)

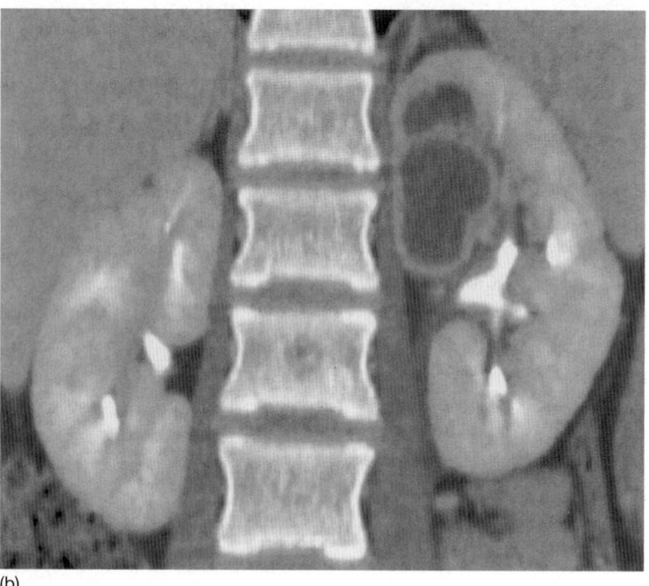

(b)

Fig. 8 Renal abscess. Upper pole of left kidney contains well-defined mass with necrotic centre and thick wall (a). Coronal reconstruction shows lack of communication between abscess and calices (b).

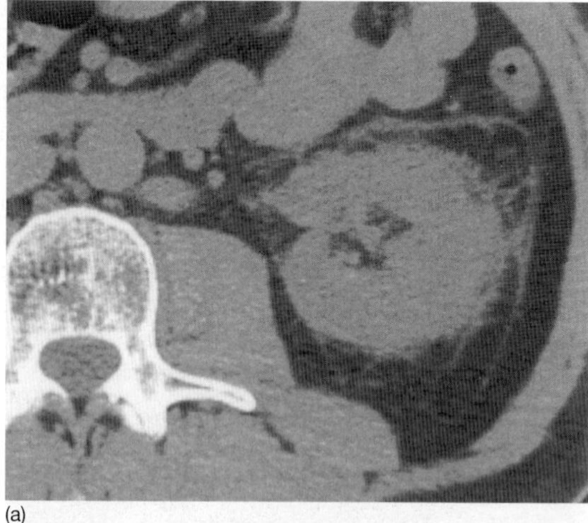

(a)

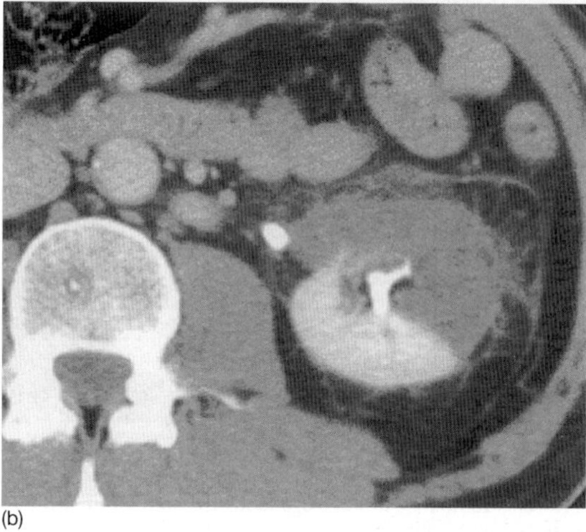

(b)

Fig. 9 Renal infarct. Unenhanced CT scan (a) in a patient with acute left flank pain shows perinephric stranding. After IV injection of contrast material, absence of contrast enhancement in anterior part of kidney is demonstrated (b).

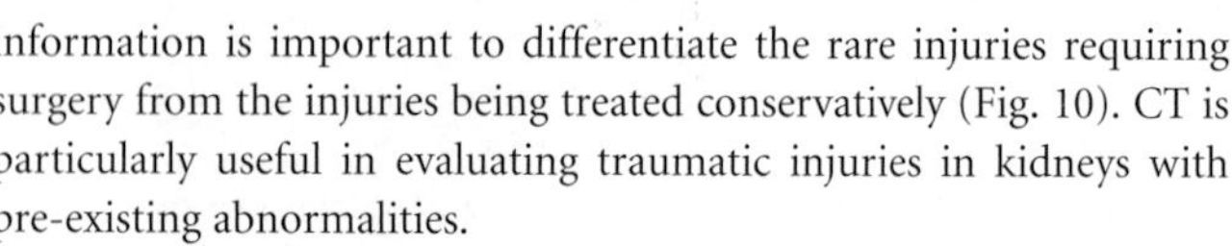

information is important to differentiate the rare injuries requiring surgery from the injuries being treated conservatively (Fig. 10). CT is particularly useful in evaluating traumatic injuries in kidneys with pre-existing abnormalities.

Lesions in the collecting system

Urinary calculi

Helical CT has become the reference method for the diagnosis of urolithiasis (Fig. 11) (Liu *et al.* 2000; Van Beers *et al.* 2001). Almost all urinary calculi are clearly seen within the urinary tract as high-density structures. Only calculi caused by indinavir sulfate intake have lower, soft-tissue density and may be undetected at CT. Accessory signs of obstructing ureteral calculi include ureteral dilatation and perinephric stranding. However, these signs may be absent in long-standing calculous obstruction and may be observed in other lesions such as acute pyelonephritis, renal infarction, and neoplasms (Kawashima *et al.* 1997a,b). Sometimes, ureteral calculi may be difficult to distinguish

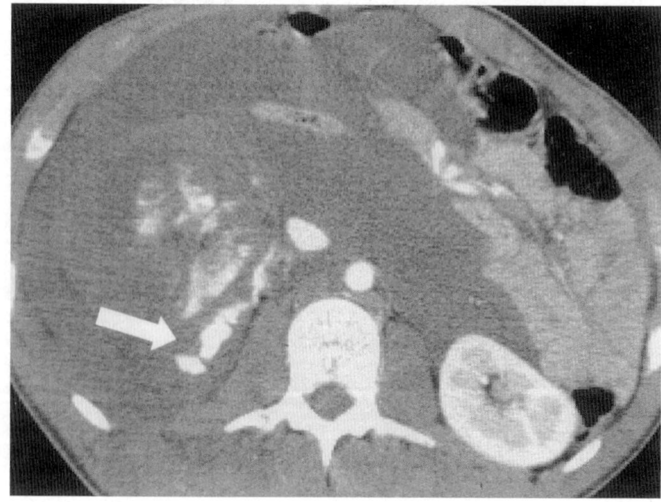

Fig. 10 Renal trauma. CT scan during early phase after injection of contrast material shows shattered right kidney, huge retroperitoneal haematoma, and active haemorrhage (arrow) from right renal pedicle.

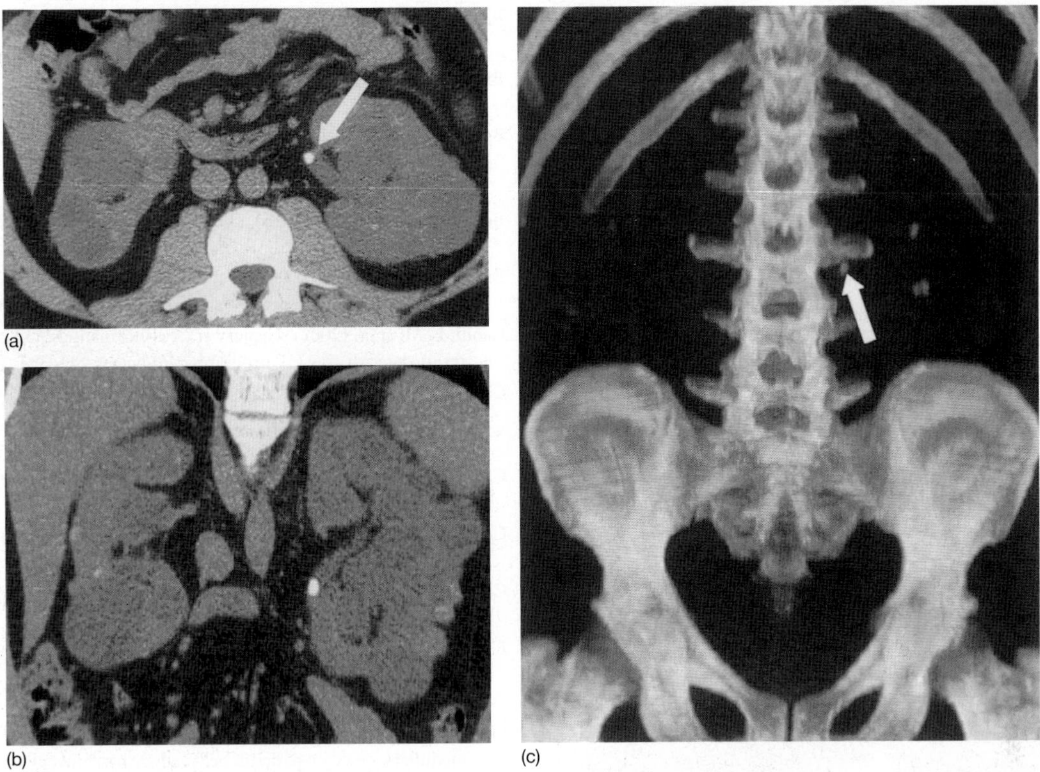

Fig. 11 Ureteral stone in a patient with cystic disease of kidneys. Transverse CT scan (a) and coronal–oblique reconstruction (b) show calculus (arrow) in the proximal part of the left ureter of a patient with multiple renal cysts. Maximum intensity projection image (c) shows ureteral (arrow) and left renal calculi in a format similar to the conventional radiograph.

from extraurinary calcifications, especially when the ureter is not dilated. In these cases, contrast-enhanced CT during the excretory phase is useful to confirm the diagnosis.

Helical CT is superior to abdominal radiography, intravenous urography, and sonography for the detection of renal and ureteral calculi (Sheafor *et al.* 2000). Furthermore, unenhanced helical CT may show extraurinary causes of acute flank pain. However, the radiation dose delivered by unenhanced helical CT of the urinary tract is around 3.5–6.5 mSv. This dose is higher than that of urography, even if low-dose protocols are used for CT (Liu *et al.* 2000). Because of this biological cost, the universal use of CT in patients with suspected renal colic remains limited. Selective use of CT in patients in whom abdominal radiography and sonography fail to show the cause of symptoms has been proposed, especially in Europe (Catalano *et al.* 2002).

Abnormalities of the collecting system

Experience with CT in the evaluation of abnormalities of the collecting system, such as renal tubular ectasia, tubular necrosis, caliceal diverticulum, and urothelial tumour remains limited (McNicholas *et al.* 1998; Caoili *et al.* 2002). The feasibility of showing these lesions with multislice helical CT has been demonstrated, but additional studies comparing CT urography with conventional urography should be performed. CT urography with scanning during multiple phases before and after injection of contrast material has the advantage to combine in one examination the morphological information about the renal vessels, the renal parenchyma, and the urinary collecting system. CT urography may challenge conventional urography and sonography in the evaluation of patients with haematuria (Fig. 12). The high dose of CT urography remains a limitation. The effective dose lies between 35 and 55 mSv, when scanning of the urinary tract is performed during four phases (Caoili *et al.* 2002). An alternative to excretory CT is to remove the patient from the CT scanner before the excretory phase and to obtain conventional radiography of the contrast-filled ureters in a general radiography room. However, cross-sectional imaging of the contrast-filled urinary tract is not obtained (McNicholas *et al.* 1998).

Conventional CT is limited to assess the local stage of transitional cell tumours. It remains to be determined if helical CT can improve this tumour staging. Finally, CT is useful to show the extent of various periureteral lesions that cause urinary obstruction.

Conclusions

Helical CT has become the standard CT technology to assess the urinary tract. Volume scanning of the kidneys and urinary collecting system can be performed at different phases before and after the injection of contrast material. Thin slices can be reconstructed at arbitrarily determined intervals and two-dimensional multiplanar reformations and three-dimensional reconstructions can be obtained. Important applications of helical CT are in the assessment of renal arterial diseases, the detection, characterization, and staging of renal tumours, the evaluation of renal trauma, and the detection of urinary calculi. For these applications, helical CT is more accurate than conventional

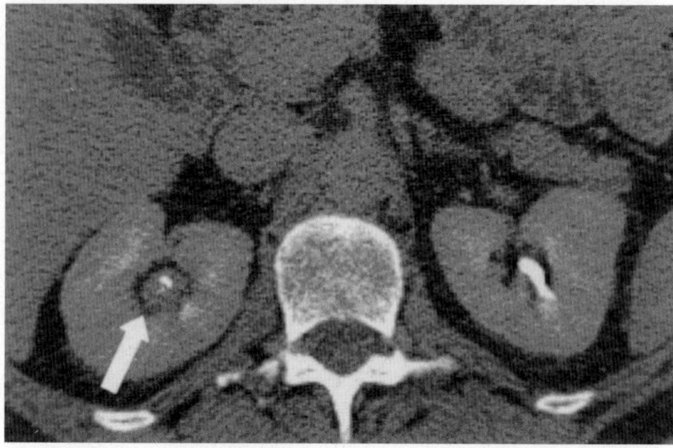

(a)

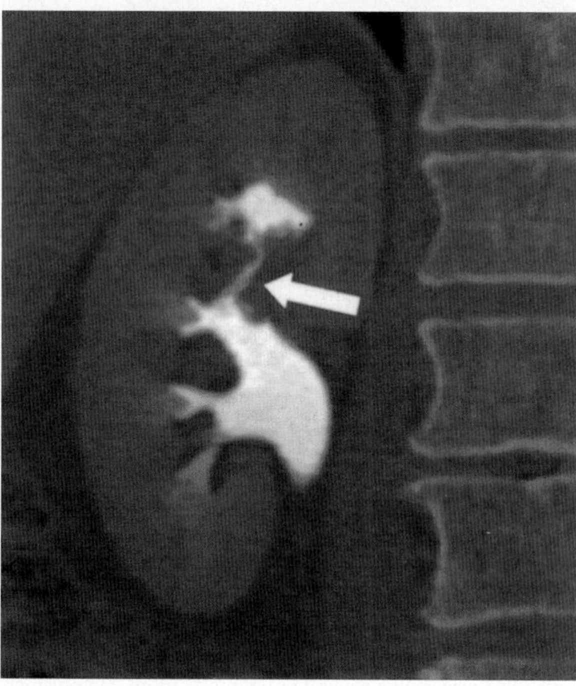

(b)

Fig. 12 Transitional cell carcinoma of upper calyx in a patient with haematuria. Transverse CT scan obtained with 1-mm collimation reveals mural thickening (arrow) of upper right calyx (a). Coronal reconstruction shows irregular stenosis (arrow) of upper calyx (b).

urography and sonography. In addition, CT urography may become an alternative to urography to assess lesions of the urinary collecting system. The cost-effectiveness of helical CT should be assessed further. These cost-effectiveness studies should take into account the biological cost of CT due to its relatively high radiation burden. This is especially relevant in young patients with benign disease, such as urinary calculi.

References

Bae, K. T. *et al.* (2000). Renal cysts: is attenuation artifactually increased on contrast-enhanced CT images? *Radiology* **216**, 792–796.

Black, W. C. and Welch, H. G. (1997). Screening for disease. *AJR. American Journal of Roentgenology* **168**, 3–11.

Bosniak, M. A. (1986). The current radiological approach to renal cysts. *Radiology* **158**, 1–10.

Bosniak, M. A. *et al.* (1988). CT diagnosis of renal angiomyolipoma: the importance of detecting small amounts of fat. *American Journal of Roentgenology* **151**, 497–501.

Bosniak, M. A. *et al.* (1995). Small renal parenchymal neoplasms: further observations on growth. *Radiology* **197**, 589–597.

Brink, J. A. *et al.* (1995). Technical optimization of spiral CT for depiction of renal artery stenosis: *in vitro* analysis. *Radiology* **194**, 157–163.

Caoili, E. M. *et al.* (2002). Urinary tract abnormalities: initial experience with multi-detector row CT urography. *Radiology* **222**, 353–360.

Catalano, O. *et al.* (2002). Suspected ureteral colic: primary helical CT versus selective helical CT after unenhanced radiography and sonography. *AJR. American Journal of Roentgenology* **178**, 379–387.

Chauveau, D. *et al.* (1996). Renal involvement in von Hippel–Lindau disease. *Kidney International* **50**, 944–951.

Chow, W. H. *et al.* (1999). Rising incidence of renal cell cancer in the United States. *Journal of the American Medical Association* **281**, 1628–1631.

Choyke, P. L. (2000). Acquired cytic kidney disease. *European Radiology* **10**, 1716–1721.

Einstein, D. M. *et al.* (1995). Evaluation of renal masses detected by excretory urography: cost-effectiveness of sonography versus CT. *American Journal of Roentgenology* **164**, 371–375.

Elzouki, A. Y. *et al.* (1996). Thin-section computed tomography scans detect medullary cysts in patients believed to have juvenile nephronophthisis. *American Journal of Kidney Disease* **27**, 216–219.

Gill, I. S. *et al.* (1994). Adrenal involvement from renal cell carcinoma: predictive value of computerized tomography. *Journal of Urology* **152**, 1082–1085.

Golding, S. J. and Schrimpton, P. C. (2002). Radiation dose in CT: are we meeting the challenge? *British Journal of Radiology* **75**, 1–4.

Gupta, S. *et al.* (2000). CT in the evaluation of complicated autosomal dominant polycystic kidney disease. *Acta Radiologica* **41**, 280–287.

Harris, A. C. *et al.* (2001). CT findings in blunt renal trauma. *Radiographics* **21**, S201–S214.

Hofmann, L. V. *et al.* (1999). Three-dimensional helical CT angiography in renal transplant recipients: a new problem-solving tool. *American Journal of Roentgenology* **173**, 1085–1089.

Johnson, P. T. *et al.* (1999). Renal artery stenosis: CT angiography-comparison of real-time volume-rendering and maximum intensity projection algorithms. *Radiology* **211**, 337–343.

Kaatee, R. *et al.* (1997). Renal artery stenosis: detection and quantification with spiral CT angiography versus optimized digital subtraction angiography. *Radiology* **205**, 121–127.

Kawashima, A. *et al.* (1997a). CT of renal inflammatory disease. *Radiographics* **17**, 851–866.

Kawashima, A. *et al.* (1997b). Ureteropelvic junction injuries secondary to blunt abdominal trauma. *Radiology* **205**, 487–492.

Kopka, L. *et al.* (1997). Dual-phase helical CT of the kidney: value of the corticomedullary and nephrographic phase for evaluation of renal lesions and preoperative staging of renal cell carcinoma. *American Journal of Roentgenology* **169**, 1573–1578.

Krier, J. D. *et al.* (2001). Noninvasive measurement of concurrent single-kidney perfusion, glomerular filtration, and tubular function. *American Journal of Physiology Renal Physiology* **281**, F630–F638.

Levy, D. A. *et al.* (1998). Stage specific guidelines for surveillance after radical nephrectomy for local renal cell carcinoma. *Journal of Urology* **159**, 1163–1167.

Liu, W. *et al.* (2000). Low-dose nonenhanced helical CT of renal colic: assessment of ureteric stone detection and measurement of effective dose equivalent. *Radiology* **215**, 51–54.

Macari, M. and Bosniak, M. A. (1999). Delayed CT to evaluate renal masses incidentally discovered at contrast-enhanced CT: demonstration of vascularity with deenhancement. *Radiology* **213**, 674–680.

McNicholas, M. M. *et al.* (1998). Excretory phase CT urography for opacification of the urinary collecting system. *American Journal of Roentgenology* **170**, 1261–1267.

Miles, K. A. (1991). Measurement of tissue perfusion by dynamic computed tomography. *British Journal of Radiology* **64**, 409–412.

Prokop, M. *et al.* (1997). Use of maximum intensity projections in CT angiography: a basic review. *Radiographics* **17**, 433–451.

Rouviere, O. *et al.* (1999). Ureteropelvic junction obstruction: use of helical CT for preoperative assessment. Comparison with intra-arterial angiography. *Radiology* **213**, 668–673.

Rubin, G. D. *et al.* (1995). Assessment of living renal donors with spiral CT. *Radiology* **195**, 457–462.

Scatarige, J. C. *et al.* (2001). Patterns of recurrence in renal cell carcinoma: manifestations on helical CT. *American Journal of Roentgenology* **177**, 653–658.

Schreyer, H. H., Uggowitzer, M. M., and Ruppert-Kohlmayer, A. (2002). Helical CT of the urinary organs. *European Radiology* **12**, 575–591.

Sheafor, D. H. *et al.* (2000). Nonenhanced helical CT and US in the emergency evaluation of patients with renal colic: prospective comparison. *Radiology* **217**, 792–797.

Sheth, S. *et al.* (2001). Current concepts in the diagnosis and management of renal cell carcinoma: role of multidetector CT and three-dimensional CT. *Radiographics* **21**, S237–S254.

Siegel, C. L. *et al.* (1997). CT of cystic renal masses: analysis of diagnostic performance and interobserver variation. *American Journal of Roentgenology* **169**, 813–818.

Silverman, S. G. *et al.* (1996). Small (< or = 3 cm) hyperechoic renal masses: comparison of helical and conventional CT for diagnosing angiomyolipoma. *American Journal of Roentgenology* **167**, 877–881.

Slywotzky, C. M. and Bosniak, M. A. (2001). Localized cystic disease of the kidney. *AJR. American Journal of Roentgenology* **176**, 843–849.

Tsushima, Y. *et al.* (1999). Use of contrast-enhanced computed tomography to measure clearance per unit renal volume. A novel measurement of renal function and fractional vascular volume. *American Journal of Kidney Disease* **33**, 754–760.

Van Beers, B. E. *et al.* (2001). Value of multislice helical CT scans and maximum-intensity-projection images to improve detection of ureteral stones at abdominal radiography. *American Journal of Roentgenology* **177**, 1117–1121.

Van Cangh, P. J. *et al.* (1994). Long-term results and late recurrence after endoureteropyelotomy: a critical analysis of prognostic factors. *Journal of Urology* **151**, 934–937.

Van Hoe, L. *et al.* (1996). Supra- and juxtarenal aneurysms of the abdominal aorta: preoperative assessment with thin-section spiral CT. *Radiology* **198**, 443–448.

Vasbinder, G. B. *et al.* (2001). Diagnostic tests for renal artery stenosis in patients suspected of having renovascular hypertension: a meta-analysis. *Annals of Internal Medicine* **135**, 401–411.

Zagoria, R. J. (2000). Imaging of small renal masses: a medical success story. *American Journal of Roentgenology* **175**, 945–955.

1.6.1.vi Magnetic resonance imaging

Akira Kawashima and Bernard F. King, Jr.

Introduction

Since its introduction in the mid-1980s, magnetic resonance (MR) imaging has emerged as a powerful imaging tool for the evaluation of patients with genitourinary disease. MR imaging of the kidneys and retroperitoneum is a useful alternative to computed tomography (CT) in patients in whom the use of iodinated contrast media is contraindicated or in patients at risk for radiation exposure. MR imaging has its distinct advantages over existing imaging approaches (Kressel *et al.* 2000; Banner 2001). Unlike CT, MR imaging has the capability to generate direct multiplanar (coronal, sagittal, and oblique) images without reformation. Many individual tissue properties of the MR signal, such as MR-proton density, relaxation rates (*T*1 and *T*2), flow, chemical shift, diffusion, and perfusion, contribute to soft tissue contrast. MR imaging demonstrates excellent contrast detail in normal tissues (e.g. kidneys, uterus, and prostate) and lesions frequently appear more conspicuous. MR imaging can provide specific information (e.g. blood flow, static fluid, and fat suppression). Fat suppression techniques may be useful in improving depiction of pathology when the kidneys are bright (i.e. when *T*2-weighted or gadolinium enhanced *T*1-weighted images). MR techniques are remarkably sensitive to blood flow and are useful in assessing renal and pelvic blood vessels. Blood-vessel MR imaging is known as MR angiography (MRA). MR contrast agents do not have nephrotoxicity in the small doses that are used and are safe to use in patients with impaired renal function.

Fast MR imaging as a result of the increased efficiency of MR imaging data acquisition has significantly decreased imaging times, making breath hold imaging practical. Breath hold acquisition techniques eliminate respiratory motion and allow for a substantial improvement in clinical MR imaging of the abdomen. Continued technological improvements are making MR acquisition times comparable with or superior to those for CT (Keogan and Edelman 2001).

Contraindications to an MR imaging examination are few but may be important. Patients with pacemakers, ferromagnetic intracranial aneurysm clips, cochlear implants, metallic ocular foreign bodies, and certain older heart valve prostheses cannot be safely imaged (Shellock and Kanal 1996; Sawyer-Glover and Shellock 2000). Open magnets, sedation, or general anaesthesia may be necessary in examining patients with claustrophobia or paediatric patients. Large, obese patients may not be able to be imaged because of limitations in the diameter of the gantry opening or the weight limits of the examining table. There has been no indication that use of clinical MR examination with or without MR contrast agents during pregnancy has produced deleterious effects. MR imaging can be considered during pregnancy only if the benefit of the procedure outweighs the benefits of alternative non-ionizing diagnostic imaging studies.

Principles

The complicated physics of MR is beyond the scope of this chapter. A simplified model can explain the phenomenon of imaging (Dunnick *et al.* 2001). Protons within the patient can be thought of as small spinning bar magnets. Hydrogen has an odd number of particles in the nucleus with a single proton. When a patient is placed in a large magnetic field, the hydrogen protons within the body align, and this alignment leads to the formation of a net magnetic vector within the patient. By applying radiofrequency (RF) pulses (excitation) to the patient, this vector can be made to deflect away from the main direction of the magnetic field. When the RF pulse is turned off, the protons will 'relax' back to the direction of the magnetic field. As they return to the direction of the main magnetic field, they resonate and release a small amount of specific RF energy. An antenna (coils) lying outside the patient in the magnet will have a current induced within the antenna by this resonant RF energy. This energy originates from the tissues and its magnitude is related to the intensity of the pixel in the MR image. When this information is digitized and processed, cross-sectional anatomical images of slices of the body are provided.

Pulse sequences

Superior soft tissue contrast resolution is one of the key advantages of MR imaging over CT. Unlike CT, MR imaging contrast arises from a complex relationship of many different factors including proton density, magnetic relaxation (*T*1 and *T*2 relaxation times) constants, magnetic susceptibility, and flow. It is possible to 'weight' the relative contribution to image contrast of all these factors in a single image to create images with different tissue contrast (i.e. *T*1-weighted, *T*2-weighted, proton density weighted, etc.). The main approach to MR tissue characterization is to rescan the patient with different pulse sequence parameters (*T*1-weighted and *T*2-weighted images). Most of the tissues can be differentiated by significant differences in their characteristic *T*1 and *T*2 relaxation times. The return to the equilibrium state after the excitation pulse ceases is called magnetic relaxation, which involves two exponential time constants (*T*1 and *T*2 relaxation times). *T*1 and *T*2 relaxation times are features of the three-dimensional (3D) molecular environment that surrounds each proton in the tissue imaged (Table 1). The *T*1 relaxation time, otherwise known as the spin lattice relaxation time, is a measure of a proton's ability to exchange energy with its surrounding chemical matrix, and is a measure of how quickly a tissue can become magnetized. The *T*2 relaxation time, termed the spin–spin or transverse relaxation time, conveys how quickly a given tissue loses its magnetization.

*T*1-weighted imaging

An image in which the contrast is primarily due to the differences of *T*1 relaxation values in the tissues is produced by a relatively short time of recovery [time of repetition (TR) of 250–600 ms] and a relatively short time of echo [time of echo (TE) of 10–20 ms] on spin echo pulse sequences. On *T*1-weighted spin echo MR imaging, tissues with short relaxation times appear bright. *T*1-weighted images are a good way to assess the morphology and anatomy of organs because of a relatively stronger signal intensity (Fig. 1a). Breath-hold *T*1-weighted images can be obtained with spoiled gradient echo (SPGR) pulse sequences, which can improve image quality by reducing motion.

Table 1 Relative *T*1 and *T*2 values for tissues and body fluid in the genitourinary system

	T2\T1	***T*1-weighted image**			
		Absent (markedly low SI)	**Long *T*1 (low SI)**	**Intermediate *T*1 (intermediate SI)**	**Short *T*1 (high SI)**
*T*2-weighted image	Long *T*2 (markedly high SI)		Urine, simple cysts, oedema, inflammation, neoplasm	Proteinaceous fluid (complicated cysts, abscess)	Subacute haemorrhage (extracellular methemoglobin)
	Long *T*2 (high SI)		High free water tissue (kidneys, testes, peripheral gland of prostate, seminal vesicle, penis)		Subacute haemorrhage (extracellular methemoglobin)
	Intermediate *T*2		High bound water tissue (adrenal, central gland of prostate, muscle)		Fat (adipose tissue, fatty bone marrow)
	Short *T*2 (low SI)				Gadolinium contrast agent
	Absent (markedly low SI)	Air, gas, calculi, compact bone, haemosiderin, ion deposition, highly concentrated gadolinium contrast			

SI, signal intensity.

Modified from Mitchell *et al.* (1987).

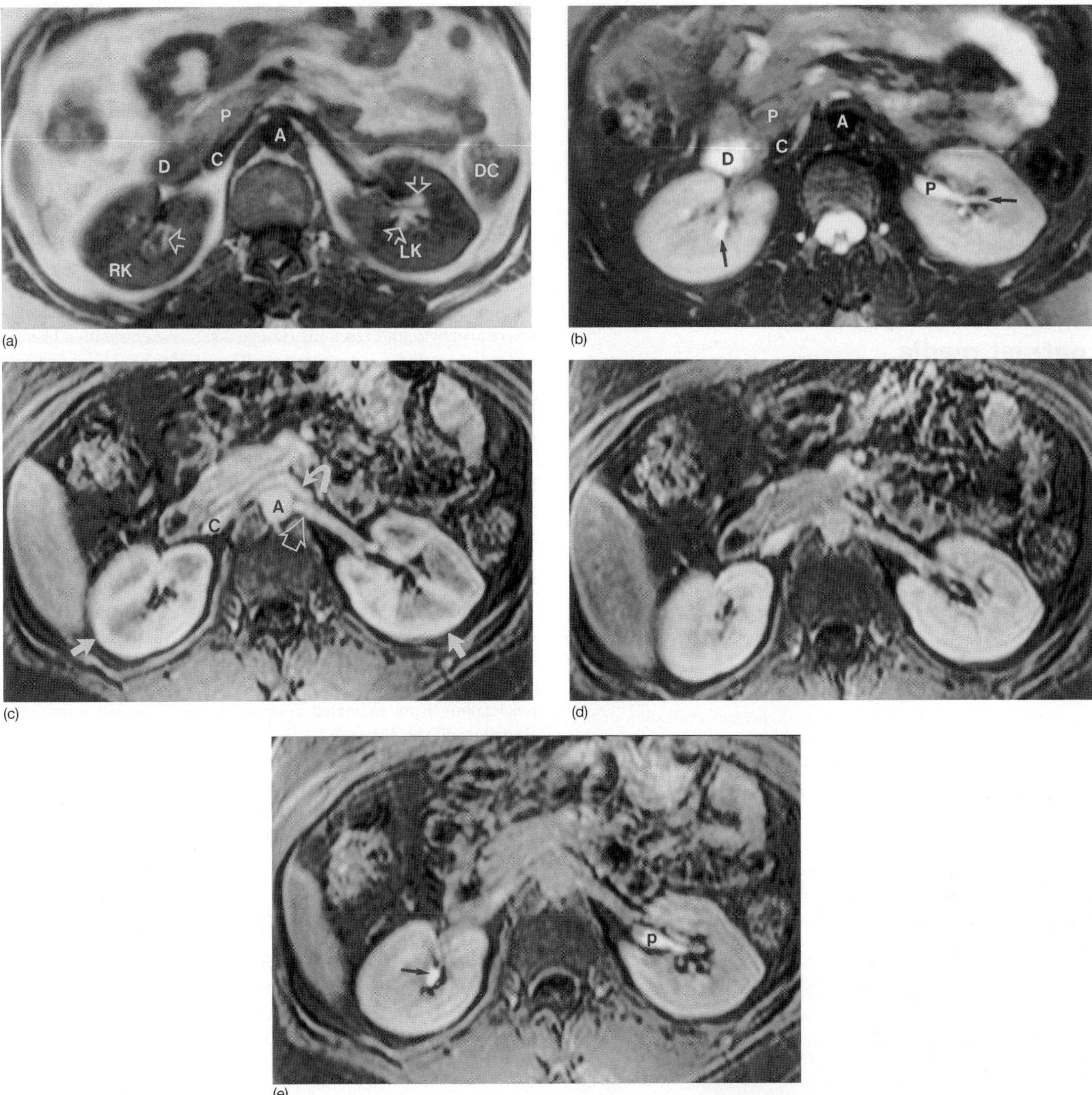

Fig. 1 Normal kidneys. (a) Axial *T*1-weighted spin echo image obtained at the level of the mid-kidneys reveals that kidneys of intermediate signal intensity are surrounded by retroperitoneal fat, which appears bright. The renal sinus appears bright because of fat. A, abdominal aorta; C, inferior vena cava; D, duodenum; P, pancreatic head; and DC, descending colon. (b) The kidneys appear hyperintense on *T*2-weighted fast spin echo image with fat suppression. The retroperitoneal fat signal intensities are suppressed. Urine in the renal collecting systems (arrows, calices and P, left renal pelvis) appears markedly bright similar to cerebrospinal fluid and fluid in the bowel loops. A, abdominal aorta; C, inferior vena cava; D, duodenum; and P, pancreatic head.
(c) Breath-hold dynamic enhanced *T*1-weighted spoiled gradient echo (SPGR) image with fat suppression 40 s after starting IV administration of gadolinium contrast demonstrates increased enhancement of the cortices (straight arrows) with the corticomedullary interface representing the cortical nephrographic phase. Open arrow, proximal left main renal artery; curved arrow, proximal left main renal vein; A, abdominal aorta; and C, inferior vena cava.
(d) Dynamic enhanced *T*1-weighted SPGR image with fat suppression 70 s after gadolinium injection demonstrates homogeneous renal enhancement during the nephrographic phase. (e) Delayed enhanced *T*1-weighted image with fat suppression demonstrates excreted contrast material in the intrarenal collecting systems bilaterally, representing the pyelographic phase.

*T*2-weighted imaging

A long TR (2000–4000 ms), long TE (60–120 ms) spin echo pulse sequence produces a *T*2-weighted image. On *T*2-weighted pulse sequences, tissues with long relaxation times (e.g. kidney) appear brighter (Fig. 1b). Pathological conditions such as tumours, inflammation, or trauma will have long relaxation times because of oedema and will appear bright on *T*2-weighted images. Static fluid such as urine appears markedly bright on *T*2-weighted images due to its very long relaxation time.

Gadolinium magnetic resonance contrast media

Intravascular MR contrast agents are used to help provide additional image contrast during MR imaging (Figs 1c–e and 2). Gadolinium is a lanthanide metal with a K-shell configuration of unpaired electrons, which results in its paramagnetic character. Gadolinium in the free state is toxic. However, when bound to chelates, gadolinium is safe for human use. Gadolinium chelates, following intravenous (IV) injection, are virtually eliminated by the kidneys via glomerular filtration. Four gadolinium chelates currently approved clinically in the United States include gadopentetate dimeglumine (Magnevist), gadoteridol (ProHance), gadodiamide (Omniscan), and gadoversetamide (OptiMARK). Gadolinium shortens *T*1 relaxation. Therefore, *T*1-weighted pulse sequences are used after IV administration of gadopentetate chelates (0.1–0.2 mmol/kg). Dynamic enhanced imaging, using *T*1-weighted breath-hold SPGR sequences, permits evaluation of the enhancement properties of parenchymal tissue or masses.

Adverse reactions to gadolinium are encountered with a much lower frequency than is observed after administration of iodinated contrast media. The frequency of all adverse events after IV injection of gadolinium chelates causing hives (urticaria) is found in less than 1 per cent of patients (Runge 2000). Although most adverse events resulting from administration of iodinated contrast media occur within 30 min of administration, reactions to gadopentetate dimeglumine injection can develop more than 1 h after the gadolinium is injected. In a series of 21,000 patients reviewed in 1996, moderate to severe anaphylactoid reactions occurred with a frequency of 0.04 per cent (Murphy *et al.* 1996). Two (0.01 per cent) of these patients developed severe anaphylactoid reactions, which were considered life-threatening. Fatal reactions to gadolinium chelates are very rare, but have been reported (Jordan and Mintz 1995). MR contrast agents currently approved for clinical use appear to have the same incidence of severe anaphylactoid reactions (Runge 2000). Patients with a history of reactions to iodinated contrast media seemed to be at increased risk (~2.0–3.7 times compared to those without allergies) (Niendorf *et al.* 1991; Cohan *et al.* 1998) and are more than twice as likely to have an adverse reaction to gadolinium (6.3 per cent of 857 patients). Treatment of moderate to severe adverse reactions to gadolinium-based contrast media is similar to that of moderate or severe reactions to iodinated contrast media. Personnel must be trained and equipment readily available for management and/or resuscitation of patients receiving IV administration of gadolinium chelate for MR imaging.

Gadolinium chelates, in the small doses used clinically, are not nephrotoxic (Runge 2000). Contrast-enhanced MR imaging has often been performed in lieu of contrast-enhanced CT in patients with pre-existing azotaemia (who are at increased risk of developing worsening renal failure from iodinated contrast media). The MR agents are cleared readily by dialysis.

Other MR contrast agents utilize other elements such as manganese (mangafodipir, Teslascan) or iron oxide (ferumoxides, Ferridex). These non-gadolinium contrast agents are primarily used for liver imaging and appear to have little use for imaging of the kidneys.

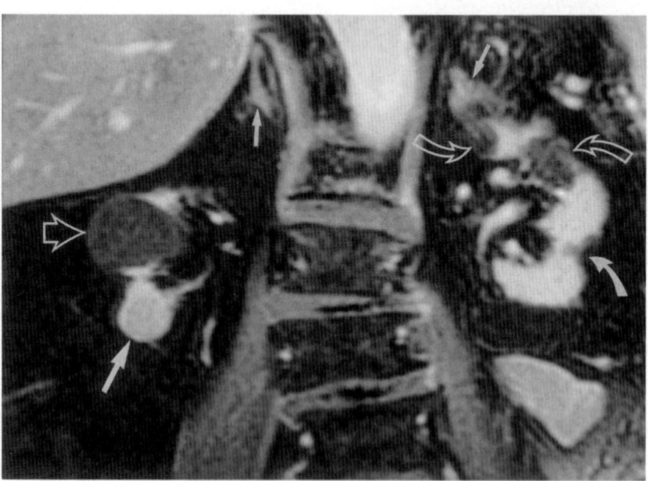

Fig. 2 Renal cell carcinoma in a 72-year-old man with renal failure. Enhanced *T*1-weighted SPGR image with fat suppression in the coronal plane reveals a small solid mass in the lower pole of the atrophic right kidney (long straight arrow), which is enhanced compared to unenhanced *T*1-weighted images (not shown), characteristic of a tumour. Simple cyst in the right kidney (straight open arrow) and two small cysts in the left kidney (curved open arrows). Focal cortical scarring of the lower left kidney (curved solid arrow). Normal adrenal glands (short arrows).

Magnetic resonance angiography

MRA is increasingly used to assess arterial and venous diseases. Earlier MRA techniques utilized flow related motion sensitive techniques for non-invasive vascular imaging. These flow related (or 'bright blood') MR angiographic techniques are divided into those affecting signal amplitude [time-of-flight (TOF) MRA] and those based on phase shift effects of flowing blood [phase-contrast (PC) imaging]. The TOF gradient echo technique is the most basic of the 'bright blood' MR angiographic techniques. The increased signal results from the wash-in of previously fully relaxed spins between RF excitations. The TOF technique is useful in assessing renal vein and in diagnosing thrombosis in the renal vein and inferior vena cava (IVC) (Kallman *et al.* 1992; Roubidoux *et al.* 1992). With the PC MR technique, the flow direction and velocity information are encoded in the phase shift of moving protons and can be displayed with relative degrees of brightness on MRA. PC MR requires specification of the range of velocities to be encoded [velocity encoding value (VENC)]. These 'bright blood' MRA techniques, however, have been limited by various technical challenges including dephasing and motion artefacts. MRA of the renal arteries has now moved from the 'bright blood' pulse sequences to breath-hold, contrast-enhanced, *T*1-weighted 3D volumetric data

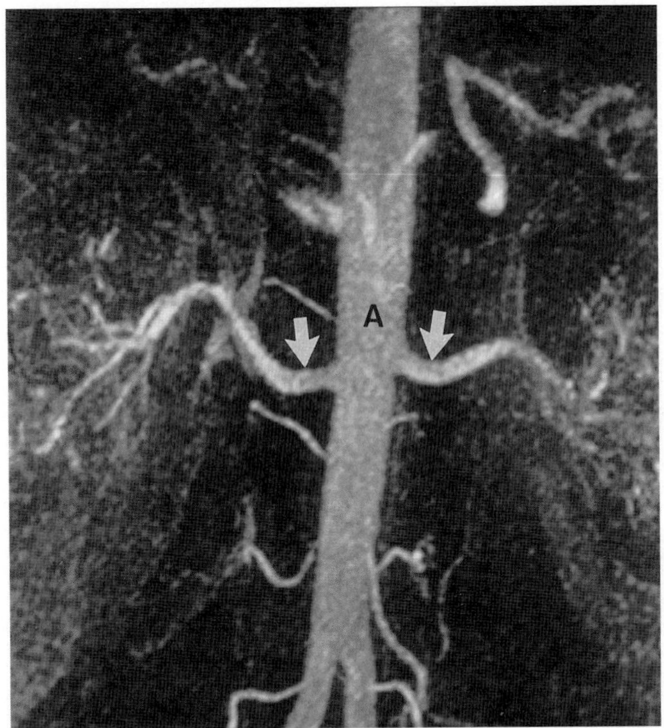

Fig. 3 High-spatial-resolution gadolinium-enhanced 3D MR angiogram reveals normal single main renal arteries bilaterally.

acquisitions. Contrast-enhanced 3D MRA relies on the significant $T1$-shortening effects of the infused paramagnetic contrast material in the blood vessel (Prince *et al.* 1995). The 3D gadolinium-enhanced MRA technique produces a contrast arteriogram without risks of iodinated contrast or ionizing radiation.

MRA is a time-efficient and safe test when compared with conventional catheter directed arteriography. Optimal MRA of the renal arteries utilizes a phased array torso coil and a smaller field-of-view (FOV) (26–30 cm) (Figs 3 and 4). This 'high-spatial-resolution' MRA of the renal arteries has proven to be highly sensitive and specific for renal artery disease, including fibromuscular dysplasia (FMD) (Fain *et al.* 2001). In addition to smaller FOVs (26–30 cm), MRA of the renal arteries is enhanced with pulse sequences utilizing a centric view read-out of the *k*-space to capture the arterial phase of the bolus following gadolinium administration. This centric read-out of the *k*-space can significantly reduce the overlapping venous signal. Finally, an accurate bolus tracking method (i.e. MR fluoroscopy) is vital to assure maximizing contrast-enhanced signal in the aorta and renal arteries (Riederer *et al.* 2000). Large FOV (40 cm) 3D MRA with a second injection can assess aortoiliac arteries (Fain *et al.* 2001). The visibility of the intrarenal vessels is still limited when compared to conventional angiography. Although false-negative studies are rare on MRA, slight overestimation of the degree of renal stenosis can occur and may lead to a false-positive diagnosis. To some extent this tendency to overestimate stenoses can be compensated for by performing PC MRA (Marcos and Choyke 2000; Schoenberg *et al.* 2002). As with conventional angiography, MRA is still only an anatomical test, which provides little information about the functional significance of a stenosis. It is highly accurate in determining the number of renal arteries,

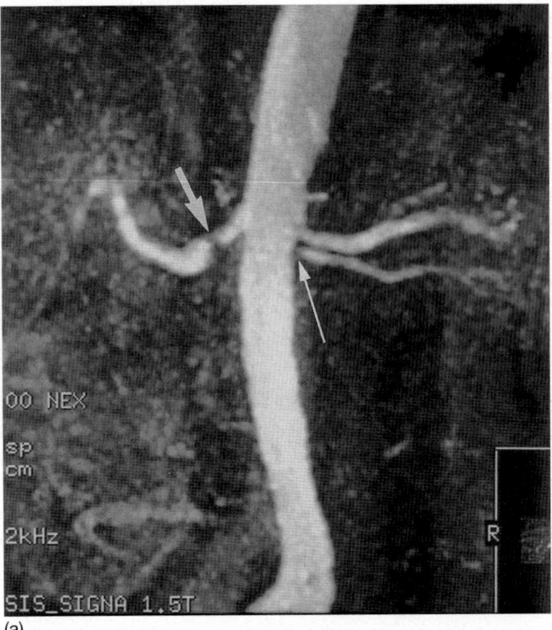

(a)

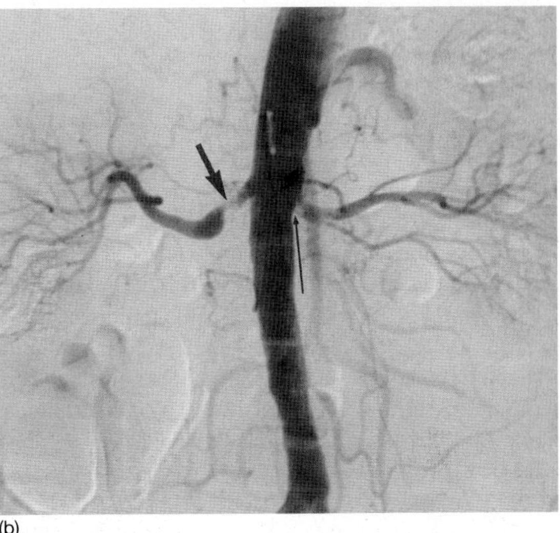

(b)

Fig. 4 Bilateral renal artery stenoses. (a) High-spatial-resolution enhanced 3D MR angiogram demonstrates a high grade stenosis of the single right main renal artery (short arrow) and focal stenosis of the accessory left renal artery (long arrow). The left main renal artery is negative for stenosis. (b) Digital subtraction catheter directed aortogram corresponds to the MR angiographic findings of bilateral renal artery stenoses indicated with short and long arrows.

the size of the kidneys, and the presence of any anatomical variants. MR imaging can be combined with a functional test similar in concept to captopril nuclear renography. This test, termed MR renography together with MRA may be helpful to determine functional significance in the work-up of renovascular hypertension (Lee *et al.* 2001).

Magnetic resonance urography

MR urography is another potential application of MR imaging (Nolte-Ernsting *et al.* 2001). Several different approaches are available.

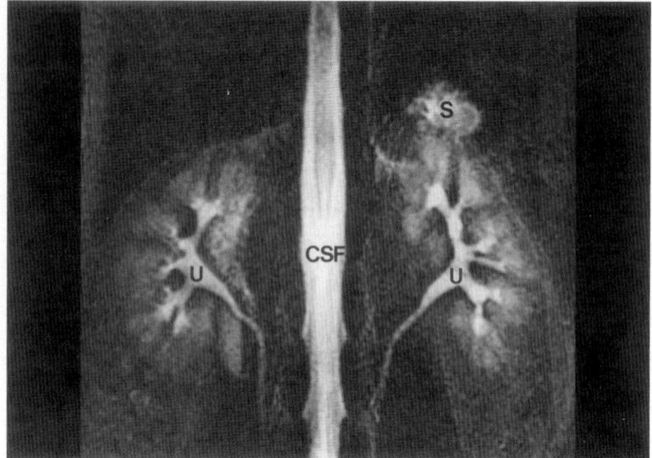

Fig. 5 Coronal MR urogram utilizing heavily *T*2-weighted SSFSE sequence during breath holding. Urine (U) in the intrarenal collecting systems and proximal renal pelvis appears markedly bright similar to the cerebrospinal fluid (CSF) and fluid in the gastric fundus (S).

The most common technique utilizes a fast heavily *T*2-weighted sequence acquired in a single breath-hold. These are usually half-Fourier transformation fast spin echo sequences [single shot fast spin echo (SSFSE) General Electronic Medical Systems or half-Fourier single-shot turbo spin-echo (HASTE) Siemens Medical Systems] (Fig. 5). These static-fluid MR urography techniques provide excellent rendering of the urinary tract, particularly dilated urinary tract. Another popular method is gadolinium-enhanced excretory MR urography (Nolte-Ernsting *et al.* 1998). This technique utilizes a pulse sequence that is very similar to gadolinium-enhanced MR angiographic pulse sequences. However, gadolinium-enhanced MR urography is obtained 5–10 min after gadolinium administration. This technique is further improved with a simultaneous dose of furosemide (5–10 mg) and is particularly useful in assessing non-obstructed urinary tracts.

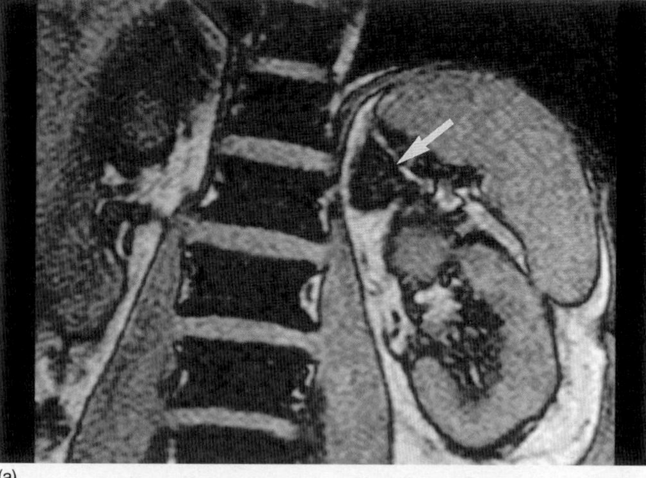
(a)

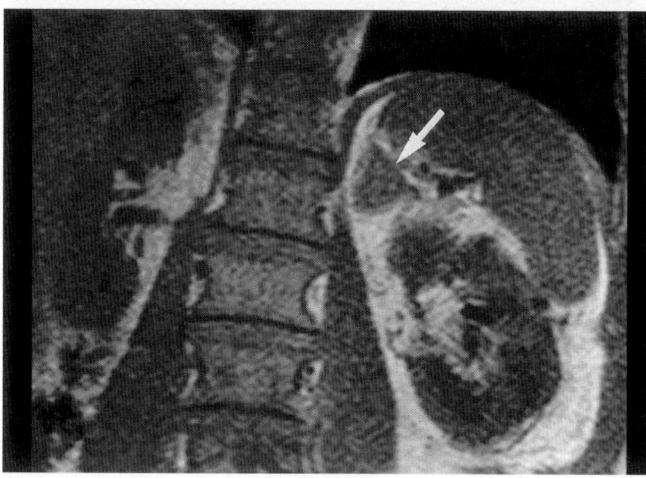
(b)

Fig. 6 Adrenocortical adenoma. (a,b) Left suprarenal mass (arrow) appears significantly dark on coronal out-of-phase *T*1-weighted SPGR image (a) compared to that on the in-phase image (b), characteristic of benign adrenocortical adenoma with abundant intracellular lipids.

Interpretations and indications

Adrenal gland and retroperitoneum

Normal adrenal glands appear in inverted V or Y configuration. Most of the normal adrenal glands are well outlined by the retroperitoneal fat on axial *T*1-weighted images; this may be augmented by thin sectioning or coronal or sagittal views. The gland appears hypointense to the liver and about isointense to the muscle. *T*2-weighted images are unnecessary if the adrenal glands appear normal on high-quality *T*1-weighted images; differentiation of the adrenal cortex from the medulla is generally not possible on routine MR images.

Out-of-phase and in-phase chemical shift gradient echo pulse sequences can differentiate benign adrenocortical adenomas from metastases (Mitchell *et al.* 1992). Benign adrenal adenomas naturally contain a moderate amount of intracellular lipid, whereas metastases do not. Out-of-phase MR images result in a cancellation of signal in lipid-rich benign adenomas because the intracellular lipid and water oppose each other and cancel the resultant signal within the pixel (Fig. 6). The extremely high signal intensity of pheochromocytomas on *T*2-weighted images is very helpful in diagnosing these lesions. Unfortunately, not all pheochromocytomas have these imaging characteristics (Varghese *et al.* 1997; Krebs and Wagner 1998).

With multiplanar capabilities, MR imaging is valuable in determining the origin of large abdominal masses whose sites of origin are not always obvious with other modalities. Such lesions often arise in the adrenal gland. In retroperitoneal fibrosis, MR imaging and CT are useful in demonstrating the extent of involvement but neither of these techniques can be used to differentiate benign from malignant masses (Amis 1990).

Kidney

On *T*1-weighted images, the renal cortex is isointense or slightly higher in signal intensity than the medulla with the corticomedullary differentiation, depending on the patient's age and hydration status. On *T*2-weighted images, the cortex is isointense or slightly hypointense compared to the medulla.

The most common uses of MR in the evaluation of the kidneys include MRA of the renal arteries, MR imaging of indeterminate renal masses shown on other imaging studies (Balci *et al.* 1999), and staging of known renal malignancies (Choyke *et al.* 1997; Pretorius *et al.* 1999). MR evaluation of indeterminate renal masses should begin with axial *T*1-weighted images (with and without fat saturation) and axial fast spin-echo *T*2-weighted images. These images allow for proper identification of the mass as well as provide vital tissue characterization with regard to potential fat content or haemorrhagic components. The most vital portion of an MR examination of an indeterminate renal mass is a dynamic gadolinium-enhanced *T*1-weighted SPGR pulse sequence. This is performed coronally in a single breath-hold utilizing 2D-SPGR sequence (Fig. 1c–e). The coronal or axial 2D-SPGR sequence is acquired before gadolinium administration, at 40 s (the cortical nephrographic phase), at 70 s (the early homogeneous nephrographic phase), and at 120 s (the late homogeneous nephrographic phase) after gadolinium administration. Excreted contrast medium starts to appear in the collecting system (the pyelographic phase) 3 min following IV contrast injection. The goal is to identify any vascular enhancement of the mass in question, which would indicate a tumour. Subtraction of the precontrast acquisition from the 120-s acquisition appears to be the most sensitive technique to detect vascular enhancement of the renal mass. MR imaging is the most accurate method for detecting renal vein and IVC tumour thrombi in patients with renal cell carcinoma compared to ultrasonography and enhanced CT (Kallman *et al.* 1992). MR imaging is also useful in determining whether the filling defects in the renal vein and IVC is due to a thrombus or a tumour (Aslam Sohaib *et al.* 2002). Gadolinium-enhanced MRA and MR venography in addition to cross-sectional and 3D display can also provide presurgical 'road mapping' prior to surgery. This can be especially helpful in nephron sparing surgery.

MRA depicts renal arterial and venous lesions with exquisite detail and is also becoming a primary imaging study in patients with suspected renal aneurysms, arteriovenous communications, and renal vein occlusion (Prince *et al.* 1997).

Newer techniques are now available and can be used to make a rough assessment of the overall and split renal functions, and renal blood flow.

Ureter

The intrarenal collecting system is generally not well visualized on routine imaging unless dilated. The renal pelvis, particularly extrarenal type pelvis, appears dark on *T*1-weighted images and markedly bright on *T*2-weighted images, characteristics of a fluid filled structure. The renal pelvis and ureter can be identified on *T*1-weighted images by the surrounding retroperitoneal fat. The normal ureteral wall is not well visualized. MR urography utilizing breath-hold heavily *T*2-weighted SSFSE or HASTE sequence is helpful in depicting a dilated upper urinary tract and in identifying the level of urinary obstruction.

Bladder

The bladder wall is well demarcated by perivesical fat but is often indistinguishable from the low-intensity urine on *T*1-weighted images. On *T*2-weighted images, the low-intensity bladder wall is well outlined by high-intensity urine.

With its multiplanar capability and various pulse sequences that allow for fast dynamic enhanced imaging, MR imaging has the potential to become the imaging modality of choice in staging bladder cancer (Barentsz *et al.* 1999; MacVicar 2000). With MR imaging, all the observations previously possible with CT are not only possible, but in addition, it has the advantage of being better able to differentiate between superficial and deep muscle invasion of the bladder wall and to assess invasion of the perivesical fat. MR can detect enlarged adenopathy.

MR imaging is also useful for the evaluation of patients with stress urinary incontinence. Pelvic floor laxity and abnormalities of the supporting fascia can be demonstrated in incontinent women by fast sagittal and coronal MR imaging obtained at rest and at maximal pelvic floor strain (Fielding *et al.* 1998; Pannu *et al.* 2000). Fast MR sequences (SSFSE and HASTE) of the pelvic floor can be utilized to obtain these images during active straining which allows for the detection and delineation of cystoceles, rectoceles, enteroceles, and uterine prolapse.

Prostate and seminal vesicles

The prostate is well outlined by the fat plane and is homogeneous in signal intensity on *T*1-weighted MR images. The glandular prostate is subdivided into the peripheral gland and the central gland (Coakley and Hricak 2000). The peripheral gland includes the peripheral zone and the most posterior and cephalad portion of the central zone. On *T*2-weighted images, the peripheral gland appears as a high-signal-intensity area in the posterior and posterolateral aspect of the gland surrounding the intermediate to low-intensity central gland. The central gland and the non-glandular elements of the prostate, consisting of the prostatic urethra and anterior fibromuscular stroma, have the same signal characteristics. In young men, the peripheral gland generally constitutes 70 per cent of the glandular tissues and is very bright on *T*2-weighted images. In older men, the central gland is mainly composed of the enlarged transitional zone from benign prostatic hyperplasia, and becomes heterogeneous on *T*2-weighted images. Prostatic cancer typically appears as areas of decreased signal in the peripheral gland on *T*2-weighted images. Unfortunately, prostatitis and postbiopsy fibrosis can have a similar appearance.

The use of an external multicoil array and/or an endorectal surface coil improves resolution and contrast in imaging the prostate. MR imaging of the male pelvis is primarily used to stage prostate cancer. Endorectal-coil MR imaging can assess gross extracapsular extension of the tumour and involvement of the seminal vesicle, preventing unnecessary surgery. Body-coil MR imaging can detect pelvic lymphadenopathy.

Proton MR spectroscopy of the prostate is able to depict cellular metabolites. The region of prostate cancer is identifiable based on reduced citrate and elevated choline. Recent technical developments with 3D MR spectroscopic imaging combined with MR imaging can improve tumour localization and volume measurement compared with those with MR imaging alone (Kurhanewicz *et al.* 1996; Scheidler *et al.* 1999; Coakley *et al.* 2002).

The seminal vesicles appear as symmetrically paired ovoid cystic structures. MR imaging is valuable for the evaluation of patients with ejaculatory dysfunction (e.g. haematospermia, painful ejaculation) and useful in detecting stones, mass, and obstruction of the seminal tract and prostate.

Urethra

High-resolution MR imaging with phased-array pelvic and endorectal coils has dramatically enhanced the ability to visualize abnormalities of the female urethra and periurethral tissues (Siegelman *et al.* 1997; Ryu and Kim 2001). MR imaging is accurate in diagnosing diverticula of the female urethra. The male urethra is rarely visualized on routine images unless a transurethral Foley catheter is inserted. MR imaging is useful in staging carcinoma of the male and female urethra.

References

Amis, E. S., Jr. (1990). Retroperitoneal fibrosis. *Urologic Radiology* **12**, 135–137.

Aslam Sohaib, S. A. *et al.* (2002). Assessment of tumor invasion of the vena caval wall in renal cell carcinoma cases by magnetic resonance imaging. *Journal of Urology* **167**, 1271–1275.

Balci, N. C. *et al.* (1999). Complex renal cysts: findings on MR imaging. *American Journal of Roentgenology* **172**, 1495–1500.

Banner, M. P. Diagnostic uroradiology. In *Clinical Manual of Urology* (ed. P. Hanno, S. B. Malkowicz, and A. J. Wein), pp. 87–133. New York, NY: McGraw-Hill, 2001.

Barentsz, J. O. *et al.* (1999). Fast dynamic gadolinium-enhanced MR imaging of urinary bladder and prostate cancer. *Journal of Magnetic Resonance Imaging* **10**, 295–304.

Choyke, P. L. *et al.* (1997). Renal cancer: preoperative evaluation with dual-phase three-dimensional MR angiography. *Radiology* **205**, 767–771.

Coakley, F. V. and Hricak, H. (2000). Radiologic anatomy of the prostate gland: a clinical approach. *Radiologic Clinics of North America* **38**, 15–30.

Coakley, F. V. *et al.* (2002). Prostate cancer tumor volume: measurement with endorectal MR and MR spectroscopic imaging. *Radiology* **223**, 91–97.

Cohan, R. H., Matsumoto, J. S., and Quagliano, P. V. *Manual on Contrast Media*. Reston VA: American College of Radiology, 1998.

Dunnick, N. R. *et al.* Diagnostic techniques. In *Textbook of Uroradiology* (ed. N. R. Dunnick, C. M. Sandler, J. H. Newhouse, and E. S. Amis, Jr.), pp. 49–72. Philadelphia, PA: Lippincott Williams & Wilkins, 2001.

Fain, S. B. *et al.* (2001). High-spatial-resolution contrast-enhanced MR angiography of the renal arteries: a prospective comparison with digital subtraction angiography. *Radiology* **218**, 481–490.

Fielding, J. R. *et al.* (1998). MR imaging of pelvic floor continence mechanisms in the supine and sitting positions. *American Journal of Roentgenology* **171**, 1607–1610.

Jordan, R. M. and Mintz, R. D. (1995). Fatal reaction to gadopentetate dimeglumine. *American Journal of Roentgenology* **164**, 743–744.

Kallman, D. A. *et al.* (1992). Renal vein and inferior vena cava tumor thrombus in renal cell carcinoma: CT, US, MRI and venacavography. *Journal of Computer Assisted Tomography* **16**, 240–247.

Keogan, M. T. and Edelman, R. R. (2001). Technologic advances in abdominal MR imaging. *Radiology* **220**, 310–320.

Krebs, T. L. and Wagner, B. J. (1998). MR imaging of the adrenal gland: radiologic–pathologic correlation. *Radiographics* **18**, 1425–1440.

Kressel, H. Y. *et al.* Magnetic resonance imaging. In *Clinical Urography* Vol. 1 (ed. H. M. Pollack and B. L. McClennan), pp. 525–554. Philadelphia, PA: W.B. Saunders, 2000.

Kurhanewicz, J. *et al.* (1996). Three-dimensional H-1 MR spectroscopic imaging of the in situ human prostate with high (0.24–0.7 cm^3) spatial resolution. *Radiology* **198**, 795–805.

Lee, V. S. *et al.* (2001). MR renography with low-dose gadopentetate dimeglumine: feasibility. *Radiology* **221**, 371–379.

MacVicar, A. D. (2000). Bladder cancer staging. *BJU International* **86** (Suppl. 1), 111–122.

Marcos, H. B. and Choyke, P. L. (2000). Magnetic resonance angiography of the kidney. *Seminars in Nephrology* **20**, 450–455.

Mitchell, D. G. *et al.* (1987). The biophysical basis of tissue contrast in extracranial MR imaging. *American Journal of Roentgenology* **149**, 831–837.

Mitchell, D. G. *et al.* (1992). Benign adrenocortical masses: diagnosis with chemical shift MR imaging. *Radiology* **185**, 345–351.

Murphy, K. J., Brunberg, J. A., and Cohan, R. H. (1996). Adverse reactions to gadolinium contrast media: a review of 36 cases. *American Journal of Roentgenology* **167**, 847–849.

Niendorf, H. P. *et al.* (1991). Safety of gadolinium-DTPA: extended clinical experience. *Magnetic Resonance in Medicine* **22**, 222–228 (discussion 229–232).

Nolte-Ernsting, C. C. *et al.* (1998). Gadolinium-enhanced excretory MR urography after low-dose diuretic injection: comparison with conventional excretory urography. *Radiology* **209**, 147–157.

Nolte-Ernsting, C. C., Adam, G. B., and Gunther, R. W. (2001). MR urography: examination techniques and clinical applications. *European Radiology* **11**, 355–372.

Pannu, H. K. *et al.* (2000). Dynamic MR imaging of pelvic organ prolapse: spectrum of abnormalities. *Radiographics* **20**, 1567–1582.

Pretorius, E. S. *et al.* (1999). Renal neoplasms amenable to partial nephrectomy: MR imaging. *Radiology* **212**, 28–34.

Prince, M. R. *et al.* (1995). Breath-hold gadolinium-enhanced MR angiography of the abdominal aorta and its major branches. *Radiology* **197**, 785–792.

Prince, M. R. *et al.* (1997). Hemodynamically significant atherosclerotic renal artery stenosis: MR angiographic features. *Radiology* **205**, 128–136.

Riederer, S. J. *et al.* (2000). Three-dimensional contrast-enhanced MR angiography with real-time fluoroscopic triggering: design specifications and technical reliability in 330 patient studies. *Radiology* **215**, 584–593.

Roubidoux, M. A. *et al.* (1992). Renal carcinoma: detection of venous extension with gradient-echo MR imaging. *Radiology* **182**, 269–272.

Runge, V. M. (2000). Safety of approved MR contrast media for intravenous injection. *Journal of Magnetic Resonance Imaging* **12**, 205–213.

Ryu, J. and Kim, B. (2001). MR imaging of the male and female urethra. *Radiographics* **21**, 1169–1185.

Sawyer-Glover, A. M. and Shellock, F. G. (2000). Pre-MRI procedure screening: recommendations and safety considerations for biomedical implants and devices. *Journal of Magnetic Resonance Imaging* **12**, 92–106.

Scheidler, J. *et al.* (1999). Prostate cancer: localization with three-dimensional proton MR spectroscopic imaging—clinicopathologic study. *Radiology* **213**, 473–480.

Schoenberg, S. O. *et al.* (2002). Morphologic and functional magnetic resonance imaging of renal artery stenosis: a multireader tricenter study. *Journal of the American Society of Nephrology* **13**, 158–169.

Shellock, F. G. and Kanal, E. *Magnetic Resonance: Bioeffects, Safety, and Patient Management*. Philadelphia, PA: Lippincott-Raven, 1996.

Siegelman, E. S. *et al.* (1997). Multicoil MR imaging of symptomatic female urethral and periurethral disease. *Radiographics* **17**, 349–365.

Varghese, J. C. *et al.* (1997). MR differentiation of phaeochromocytoma from other adrenal lesions based on qualitative analysis of T2 relaxation times. *Clinical Radiology* **52**, 603–606.

1.6.1.vii Isotope scanning

John M.H. De Klerk, Henk Stevens, Hein A. Koomans, and Jaap J. Beutler

Introduction

The application of nuclear medicine techniques for diseases of the kidneys is more varied than for most other organs. Functional studies measure renal plasma flow, glomerular filtration rate (GFR), renal transit time, and bladder kinetics. Imaging studies can visualize various components of the kidney.

Radionuclides have been applied extensively to clearance methodology including continuous infusion, single infusion, and simplified single injection techniques. In routine practise, however, single-injection clearance methods, which are relatively simple and provide sufficient accuracy to meet clinical demands, are usually adequate. Importantly, the results are highly reproducible when measurements are carefully performed and have lower standard error than creatinine clearance. In addition radionuclide techniques offer the possibility to assess clearance by individual kidneys.

After the introduction of gamma camera-based techniques during the 1960's, renal imaging became available and greatly expanded the potential areas in which renal radiopharmaceuticals could be applied. Imaging procedures involve the renal cortex, medulla, collecting system, bladder, penis, and testis.

Renal radiopharmaceuticals

The radiopharmaceuticals available for assessing renal function and anatomy are grouped into three categories depending on their most important excretory function: those excreted by glomerular filtration, those excreted by tubular excretion, and those retained in the renal tubules for long periods (Table 1).

Glomerular filtration

Inulin clearance remains the gold standard to measure GFR, but it is expensive, time consuming, and requires a steady-state plasma concentration and accurate and timed urine collection (Blaufox 1996).

Table 1 An overview of renal radiopharmaceuticals

Renal handling	Radiopharmaceutical	Imaging	Clinical use
Glomerular filtration	^{51}Cr-EDTA	No	GFR
	^{99m}Tc-DTPA	Yes	GFR
Tubular secretion	^{123}I/^{131}I-OIH	Yes	ERPF
	^{99m}Tc-MAG3	Yes	ERPF
	^{99m}Tc-EC	Yes	ERPF
Tubular retention	^{99m}Tc-DMSA	Yes	Cortical imaging
	^{99m}Tc-GH	Yes	Cortical imaging

The radionuclide of choice to assess GFR is ^{51}Cr-EDTA because its clearance is considered to be closest to that of inulin. However, the clearance of technetium-99m-diethylenetriamine pentaacetic acid (^{99m}Tc-DTPA), which is also excreted by glomerular filtration, correlates well with that of ^{51}Cr-EDTA, since recent DTPA formulations have minimized the serum protein binding of the tracer that was responsible for its lower plasma clearance rate with respect to EDTA. ^{99m}Tc-DTPA gives plasma clearance values very similar to inulin and with a similar transit time through a similar distribution volume. ^{99m}Tc-DTPA can also be used for gamma camera imaging, in contrast to ^{51}Cr-EDTA (Gunasekera and Peters 1996). ^{99m}Tc-DTPA is the least expensive renal radiopharmaceutical and provides a low radiation dose to patients. A small fraction may be bound to protein, but this is not a problem for routine measurement of GFR. The extraction fraction (percentage of the agent extracted with each pass through the kidney) of ^{99m}Tc-DTPA is approximately 20 per cent; for this reason, in patients with impaired renal function, this radiopharmaceutical is not useful for imaging studies. In such cases, agents with higher extraction efficiencies such as ^{99m}Tc-mercaptoacetyltriglycine (MAG3) and iodine-131 or iodine-123 *ortho*-iodohippurate (OIH or hippuran) are more appropriate.

Tubular secretion

p-Aminohippuric acid (PAH) is the gold standard for the measurement of tubular cell function and its clearance is a measurement of effective renal plasma flow (ERPF). However, it is not well suited for routine studies. The clinical need for a compound that can easily measure ERPF and renal tubular cell function led to the development of ^{131}I-OIH and ^{123}I-OIH. These compounds are cleared primarily by secretion in the proximal tubules, and only for a small fraction by glomerular filtration. Its clearance rate is approximately 500–600 ml/min in subjects with normal kidney function and is an indication of ERPF. Extraction of ^{131}I-OIH requires delivery of the compound to the kidney (renal plasma flow) and extraction from the plasma (proximal tubules). Injury to the proximal tubules may depress the clearance of these radiopharmaceuticals, even though renal plasma flow is not decreased. The measured ERPF is proportional to true renal plasma flow in normal subjects, but the ERPF may decrease disproportionately to the renal plasma flow in disorders such as renal artery stenosis, ischaemia, and partial thrombosis of the renal vein. The main disadvantages of ^{131}I-OIH are the suboptimal imaging characteristics of ^{131}I. ^{123}I-OIH has better imaging qualities, but ^{123}I is more expensive and less available.

^{99m}Tc-MAG3 is highly protein bound and is also cleared mainly by the proximal tubules. It was introduced by Fritzberg *et al.* (1986). Its extraction fraction is 40–50 per cent, more than twice that of ^{99m}Tc-DTPA. Because of its higher extraction fraction, ^{99m}Tc-MAG3 can provide better scintigraphic images than ^{99m}Tc-DTPA, particularly in patients with impaired renal function. Although the clearance of ^{99m}Tc-MAG3 is only 50–60 per cent of ^{131}I-OIH, the former is more protein bound and tends to remain in the intravascular compartment. Furthermore, unlike ^{131}I-OIH, ^{99m}Tc-MAG3 does not enter the red cells to a significant degree. For these reasons, a greater proportion of ^{99m}Tc-MAG3 remains in the plasma, and the increased plasma concentration compensates for the lower extraction fraction, so that ^{99m}Tc-MAG3 is excreted from the body at essentially the same rate as ^{131}I-OIH. Because of the similar rates of excretion, the renogram curves are almost identical. The clearance of ^{99m}Tc-MAG3 is highly correlated with the clearance of ^{131}I-OIH, and therefore can be used as an independent indicator of ERPF and renal function. During constant infusion, the MAG3/OIH clearance ratio is 0.47 ± 0.06 in normal subjects (Prenen 1991).

Since ^{99m}Tc-MAG3 is more protein bound than ^{131}I-OIH or ^{99m}Tc-DTPA, blood pools in the liver are more prominent in the early images, particularly in patients with impaired renal function. Furthermore, approximately 0.5 per cent of the injected dose of ^{99m}Tc-MAG3 accumulates in the gallbladder within 30–60 min of injection. Gallbladder activity can become more prominent in patients with impaired renal function. The gallbladder is not a problem on early images, but in rare instances it can simulate pelvic or caliceal activity on delayed images. If this question arises, it can be resolved by a lateral view.

^{99m}Tc-L,L and D,D-ethylenedicysteine (EC) are both excellent radiopharmaceuticals for renal studies. Evaluation of ^{99m}Tc-EC in animals, healthy humans, and patients with various renal disorders revealed that the renal clearance of ^{99m}Tc-EC is higher than that of ^{99m}Tc-MAG3, and that it more closely approaches that of OIH (Moran 1999).

Tubular retention

^{99m}Tc-dimercaptosuccinic acid (DMSA) is an excellent cortical imaging agent and is used when high-resolution anatomic scintigraphic images are required. It concentrates largely in the renal cortex and to a lesser degree in the liver. Its body retention is considerably longer than that of DTPA because of its strong binding to plasma proteins. This high protein binding may also account for its liver uptake. At 2 h postinjection, approximately 50 per cent of the injected dose is retained in the kidneys, leading to a very high kidney-to-liver ratio of 35 : 1. At this point, there is no visualization of the urinary collecting system, and thus the optimum time for imaging. At this time-point the cortex-to-medullary ratio of DMSA has been reported to be 22 : 1 and the glomerular-to-interstitial ratio to be 1 : 27 (Hosokawa *et al.* 1978). Autoradiographic studies reveal that most of the DMSA activity is concentrated in the cytoplasm of proximal tubular cells and less in the microsomes or nuclei. Minor activity is found in distal tubules or loops of Henle (Willis *et al.* 1977; Hosokawa *et al.* 1978). After this time-point of 2 h, kidney uptake of DMSA slows down until 6 h, when a plateau is reached. In patients with poor renal function, late images are better than early scintigrams because of the improved kidney-to-background ratio (Taylor 1982).

^{99m}Tc-glucoheptonate (GH) (glucose mono-carboxyl acid), is both filtered by the glomerulus and bound by the tubules. About 50 per cent of the injected dose is protein bound, and therefore glomerular filtration is partial. Early imaging allows assessment of perfusion, excretion, and transit through the collecting system. At 2 h, approximately 10 per cent is bound to renal tubules, significantly less than with DMSA. In subjects with normal renal function, most of the injected dose is rapidly excreted; however, 10–15 per cent of the injected dose remains bound to the renal tubules, and at 2–4 h late static scintigrams of the renal parenchyma can be obtained after the collecting system activity has been cleared (Taylor and Nally 1995).

Renal clearance measurement

Renal radiopharmaceuticals have been used extensively for renal clearance studies with continuous infusion, single injection, simplified single injection, and *in vivo* camera techniques. From a single injection of a renal radiopharmaceutical, bi-exponential fitting of the radioactivity derived from multiple blood samples over time is generally approved as an accurate method to quantify renal function for clinical use. Procedures using urinary excretion, which require the continuous infusion of radiopharmaceuticals and timed urine collection, remain the prime methods for research purposes but not for clinical use. The growing need for simplification has led to the replacement of multicompartmental models requiring multiple blood samples by single compartment models that need only two to three blood samples, or even only one blood sample (Blaufox *et al.* 1996). This one or two blood sample method is an alternative to the multiple blood sample method using iodohippurate, ^{99m}Tc-DTPA or ^{51}Cr-EDTA, and ^{99m}Tc-MAG3. In many situations, a single blood sample, or at most two, suffices to provide a reasonably accurate estimate of renal function. Renal uptake calculated by gamma camera renography is a good indicator for separate as well as global kidney function. Algorithms to quantify renal function from renograms have been developed for several renal radiopharmaceuticals. These techniques are easy and non-invasive, but less accurate than the blood sampling method. For these gamma-camera-based methods, there is at present consensus only on the determination of relative clearance (Prigent *et al.* 1999). Nonetheless, these methods are attractive in clinical practice, particularly for use in children, because blood sampling and counting are avoided and the results are immediately available from the computers (Itoh *et al.* 1996). The camera-based methods may play an important role in serial monitoring of renal function. The intraobserver reproducibility in calculating relative renal function has a coefficient of variation of 2–4 per cent (Moonen *et al.* 1994). An UK audit and analysis of quantitative parameters obtained from gamma camera renography stressed that one shoud be very prudent with the diagnosis of improved or deteriorated renal function based on whole kidney mean transit times obtained from different hospitals (Houston *et al.* 2001). However, relative function has comparatively good consistency between hosptitals.

The committee of radionuclides in nephrourology recommends to use the full disappearance curve or a continuous infusion with urine collection for the most reliable estimation of renal clearance. It should be noted that plasma clearances are indirect and subject to variation in non-renal disappearance. In comparison, urinary clearances have the advantage of being direct, but subject to problems with urine collection.

In clinical practice, the single-sample technique is adequate in a patient with a GFR greater than or equal to 30 ml/min. When GFR less than 30 ml/min, or in situations where there may be a third space (patients with ascites and oedema or any other abnormal fluid accumulation), indirect clearance techniques are not reliable and urine collection should be used.

For GFR measurement, the recommended agent is ^{99m}Tc-DTPA, which requires standardization since protein binding varies among products from different manufacturers, or ^{51}Cr-EDTA, which may provide more accurate values for GFR, but cannot be used for imaging. The method described by Watson (1992), which is based on the Groth 4-h methodology, is recommended by the international consensus committee (Blaufox *et al.* 1996). Two accurate simplified methods have been proposed for clinical routine in children. The 'slope–intercept method' is based on the determination of only the late exponential by means of at least two blood samples around 2 and 4 h postinjection. The accuracy of the slope–intercept method compared with the multiple blood sampling for clearance values is as low as 10 ml/min. Late blood samples have been advocated in the case of renal failure (renal clearance <10–15 ml/min). The second method, the 'distribution-volume' method, is based on a single blood sample at 2 h. This method is valid for children of any age and the results are identical to those of the slope–intercept method. However, this approach is not valid in patients with poor renal function (GFR < 30 ml/min/1.73 m^2) (Piepsz *et al.* 2001).

The Tauxe method (Tauxe *et al.* 1982) is recommended for measuring the ERPF. The optimum time for a single sample is at 44 min, but the use of a time in the range 39–49 min will yield acceptable results. ERPF values can be achieved by using ^{123}I, ^{131}I-, or ^{125}I-OIH.

^{99m}Tc-MAG3 can also be used to assess ERPF. Bubeck approach (Bubeck *et al.* 1993) or the Russell equations (Russel *et al.* 1995) can be applied. Russel's approach uses two samples that may provide some additional accuracy under certain circumstances, but in most cases a single sample will provide sufficient information.

Clinical applications

Renal failure

Nuclear medicine plays no part in the immediate assessment of apparent acute renal failure, when the emphasis should be on the rapid recognition of reversible factors and identification of life-threatening disorders. The diagnostic role of renographic imaging is limited to (a) differentiation between acute renal failure due to acute tubulus necrosis or to acute glomerular disease, (b) acute loss of perfusion of (parts) of the kidney(s), or (c) acute interstitial nephritis. More often, nuclear techniques are used to assess prognosis (Table 2).

Diagnosis

1. ^{131}I-Hippuran uptake capacity in the first 2 min after injection divided by the injected dose (HUC2), measured by the gamma camera, can differentiate between acute renal failure caused by acute tubular necrosis (ATN) or acute glomerular disease. When HUC2 exceeds 3, ATN is the most likely diagnosis (Abels-Fransen *et al.* 1983).
2. Acute loss of unilateral renal perfusion is usually caused by *renal arterial embolism* or *aortic dissection*. More rare causes are acute thrombosis as a final event in the progression of renal artery stenosis or as a complication of renal artery dissection due to fibromuscular dysplasia or trauma. In all these cases, there is absence of perfusion in the acute phase, but within 24–48 h a collateral circulation is present which may give the appearance of a satisfactory blood pool. In cortical necrosis following obstetric catastrophe, the same pattern of blood pooling from collaterals can be found and differentiates from cortical necrosis from ATN which has a much better prognosis. Renal vein thrombosis produces a swollen patchy kidney, with poor perfusion on renal scintigraphy. However, this diagnosis can better be established by computed tomography (CT) or magnetic resonance (MR) scanning.
3. Acute interstitial nephritis most commonly occurs as a hypersensitivity reaction to a variety of drugs, in association with a variety of infections or inflammatory diseases such as sarcoidosis. In most cases, the diagnosis is clear from the clinical picture or renal biopsy, but in the absence of renal histology, nuclear techniques may be helpful to differentiate between other forms of renal failure. Gallium-67 scintigraphy may be used, showing marked bilateral uptake.

Prognosis

Progressive accumulation of OIH or ^{99m}Tc-MAG3 is a good prognostic feature in ATN. In diseases associated with extreme reduction in perfusion, such as haemolytic–uraemic syndrome or in systemic sclerosis, failure of ^{99m}Tc-MAG3 uptake is a poor prognostic feature (Hilson 1998). The typical ^{99m}Tc-MAG3 images in ATN show a relatively well preserved renal perfusion phase followed by progressive uptake of the radiopharmaceutical in the parenchyma and no excretion. This pattern probably results from intratubular obstruction or preserved tubular cell with reduced tubular cell secretion (Blaustein *et al.* 2002).

Table 2 Scintigraphic patterns in nephrological disorders

Disease	Radiopharmaceutical	Scintigraphic pattern	Clinical role
Acute tubular necrosis	^{131}I/^{123}I-OIH	Progressive uptake, no excretion	Prognosis; differentiation from acute glomerular disease
	^{99m}Tc-MAG3	Progressive uptake, no excretion	Prognosis
Renovascular (occlusion)	^{99m}Tc-MAG3	No selective uptake	Diagnosis and prognosis
	^{99m}Tc-DTPA	No perfusion	Diagnosis and prognosis
Rhabdomyolysis	^{99m}Tc-HDP	Muscle and renal uptake	Diagnosis
Acute interstitial nephritis	Gallium-67	Marked bilateral uptake	Diagnosis and therapy response
Haemolytic–uraemic syndrome	^{99m}Tc-DTPA ^{131}I/^{123}I-OIH ^{99m}Tc-MAG3	Marked reduction of perfusion	Prognosis
Acute glomerulonephritis	^{99m}Tc-DTPA ^{99m}Tc-MAG3	Reduced perfusion	Little/no role
Systemic sclerosis	^{99m}Tc-MAG3	Failure of uptake	Prognosis

Miscellaneous

In rhabdomyolysis, renal scintigraphy has little to offer. ^{99m}Tc-DTPA may show severe impairment of perfusion, and there may be some uptake of ^{99m}Tc-MAG3, which improves with recovery. A ^{99m}Tc-HDP bone scintigram can show tracer uptake by the affected muscles together with marked uptake of the tracer in the renal parenchyma.

Obstruction

Diuresis renography is based on the washout rate of the radiopharmaceutical from the upper urinary collecting system (Fig. 1). The method has proved useful in both the diagnosis of obstruction and the serial follow-up of split urinary tract drainage. There is still a great variation in the technique and interpretation of the test between different centres. Conventional diuresis renography involves an intravenous injection with a radiopharmaceutical, in combination with a diuretic (frusemide) being administered intravenously either 15 min before (F − 15), simultaneous (F0), at 10 min (F + 10), or 20 min (F + 20) after administration of the radiopharmaceutical (O'Reilly *et al.* 1996; Adeyoju *et al.* 2001; Boubaker *et al.* 2001). There is no evidence to suggest that any of these timings is superior, although the F − 15 technique is preferred for patients with severe hydronephrosis (Adeyoju *et al.* 2001). Of course, if there is difficult venous access, a single injection is recommended. The general comments on hydration for patient preparation for renographic studies apply particularly to patients scheduled for diuresis renography. It is imperative that the patient is well hydrated with good urine output (Gordon *et al.* 2001).

Patients found to have hydroureteronephrosis by ultrasonography are candidates for diuresis renography in order to determine whether obstruction is present (Figs 2 and 3). Causes of dilatation include vesicoureteric reflux, previous obstruction (posterior urethral valves), congenital malformations (prune belly syndrome, megacalyces/megaureter), non-compliant bladder, and urinary tract obstruction (congenital stenosis, tumour, lithiasis). Most of these causes can be diagnosed by intravenous urography, ultrasonography, CT, MR scanning, or endoscopy. Renography plays a small part in the determination of the aetiology, but it is helpful to assess the indication and the effect of intervention. A good response on frusemide indicates the absence of obstruction and no need for intervention. If surgery is considered, ^{99m}Tc-DMSA is used to assess the amount of vital parenchyma and to predict functional recovery after surgical relief of obstructed kidneys in children (Thompson and Gough 2001). Preoperative DMSA scintigraphy avoids the need for prolonged nephrostomy. Primary nephrectomy was often done to avoid this.

Renal infection

The role of renography in diagnosis and follow-up of urinary tract infection in adults is limited. The classification of the urinary tract infection as lower versus upper remains controversial in paediatrics, mainly due to the lack of classic symptoms. In addition, laboratory tests of blood and urine have shown poor sensitivity and specificity for this task. Renal cortical scintigraphy with DMSA is the investigation of choice to establish acute pyelonephritis (APN) in children. It shows areas with no uptake in the the renal cortex. A recent prospective study showed that as many as 9 per cent of patients with APN would have been missed on the basis of equivocal or negative urine cultures (Levtchenko *et al.* 2001). In children with urinary tract infection, there

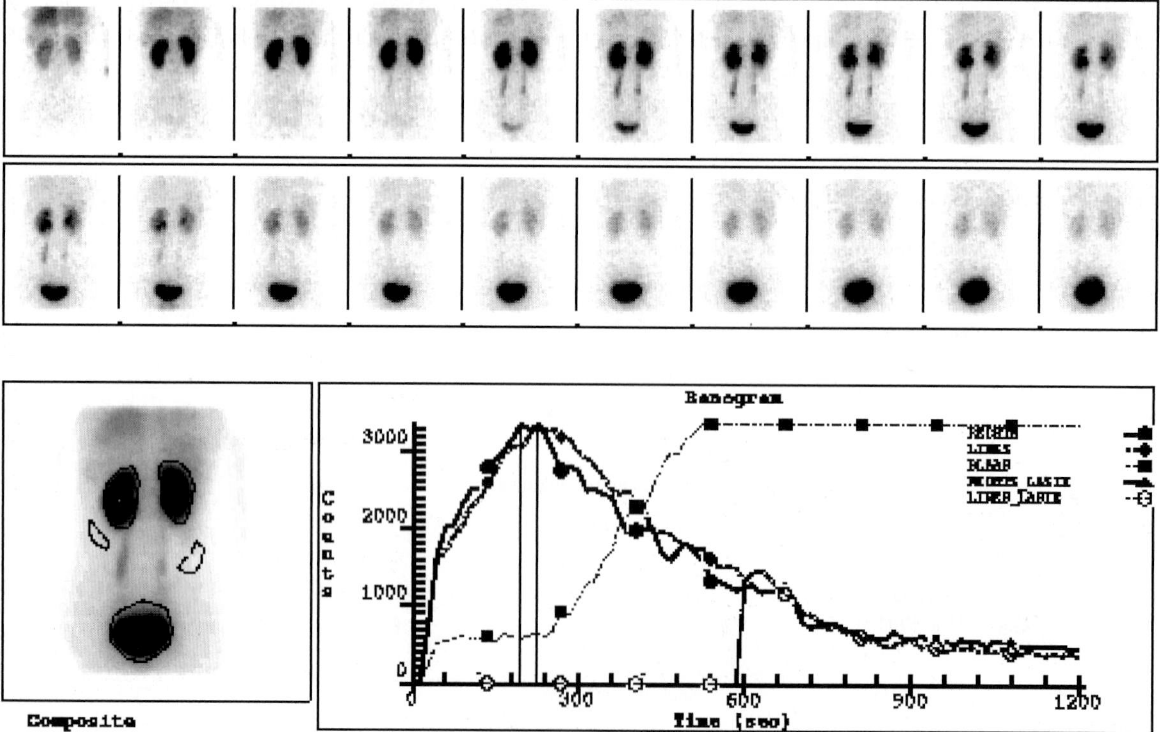

Fig. 1 A normal ^{99m}Tc-MAG3 renogram, showing good bilateral uptake and excretion of the radiopharmaceutical. Images in the upper rows are 1-min frames (total study: 20 min).

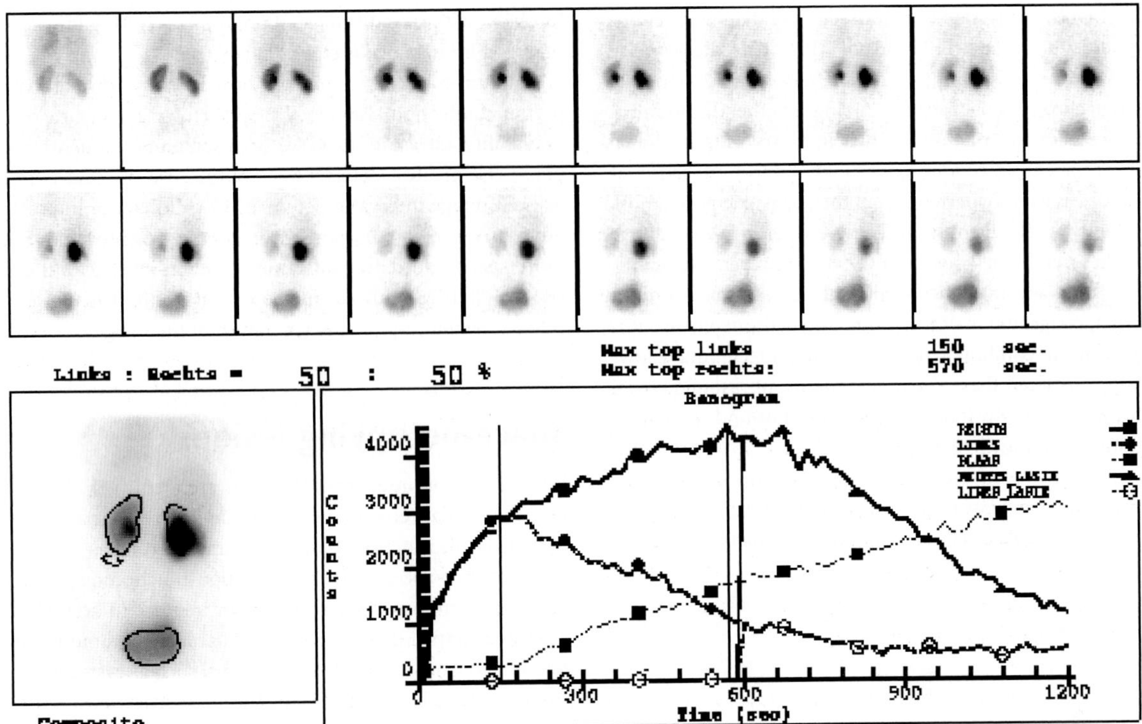

Fig. 2 F + 10 frusemide renogram showing a good response on frusemide (administered intravenously in the 10th minute) indicating no obstruction of the right kidney.

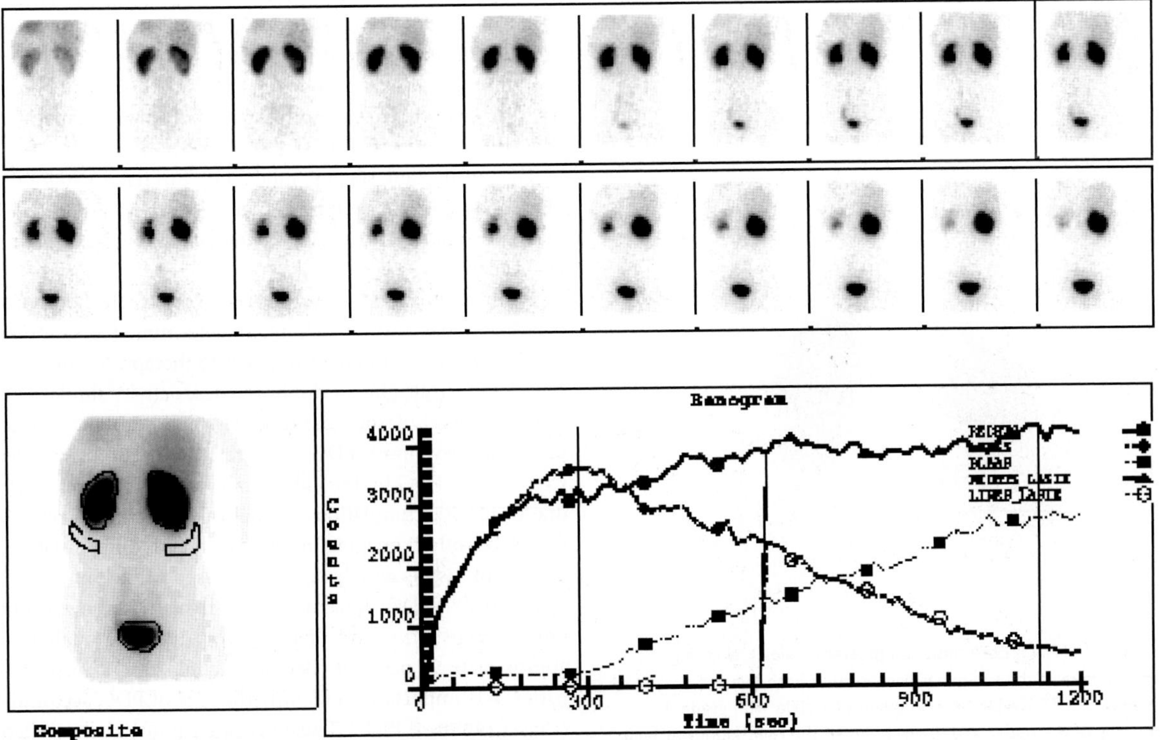

Fig. 3 Renogram (F + 10) showing no response on frusemide indicating obstruction of the right kidney.

is evidence that DMSA scintigraphy is more sensitive than intravenous urography or ultrasound to detect lesions of APN or its late sequelae (Piepsz 2002). DMSA scintigraphy is indeed a very reliable technique in the diagnosis of chronic renal cortical scarring, whether due to infections or to sterile vesicoureteric reflux (Rossleigh 2001) (Fig. 4). Renal scarring from recurrent infection remains an important cause of end-stage renal disease and hypertension in the paediatric population. DMSA scintigraphy is useful to monitor the efficiency of preventive treatments of these children (Rossleigh 1998). However, the scintigraphic picture is not specific, since similar pictures can be found in renal abscess, cyst, congenital malformations, and hydronephrosis. It is therefore mandatory to combine scintigraphy with a technique allowing differentiation between these situations, that is, ultrasound. Focal defects on DMSA scintigraphy in the absence of ultrasound abnormalities are suggestive of parenchymal infection (Piepsz 2002). Presently, DMSA imaging is considered the gold standard for the diagnosis of APN in children. However, Sfakianakis *et al.* found in retrospective and prospective studies that MAG3-F0 scintigraphy is as sensitive as DMSA

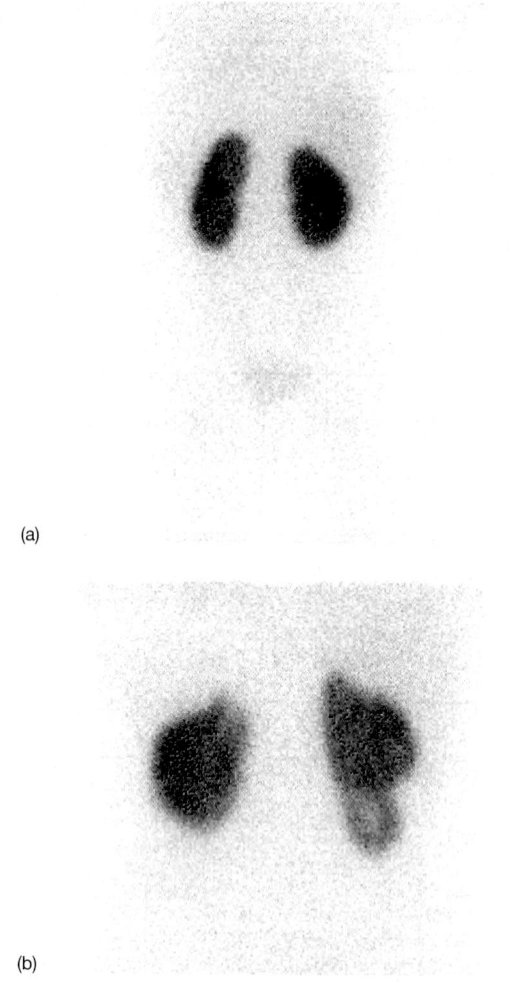

Fig. 4 (a) Normal ^{99m}Tc-DMSA scintigram (posterior view), showing a homogeneous uptake of the radiopharmaceutical in both kidneys. (b) Posterior view of a ^{99m}Tc-DMSA scintigram of a child with grade 4 reflux nephropathy of the upper and lower poles of the right kidney as well as the upper pole of the left kidney, showing lack of uptake in this region as late sequela of former infections.

for APN, with the advantage of providing results within 25 min rather than 2–3 h (Sfakianakis *et al.* 2000).

Gallium-67 (^{67}Ga) citrate can be used for the detection of renal and perirenal infection (Patel *et al.* 1980). However, because of their ready availability, ultrasound and CT are used more frequently for this purpose. The greatest deterrent to routine use of ^{67}Ga is probably the delayed image interval of 24–48 h. In children, an important issue is the relatively high radiation burden to the growing child. Perhaps even more specific to detect infection are ^{111}In-labelled white blood cells (Rossleigh 1998). An advantage of this method is the lack of bowel activity, facilitating the interpretation of the images.

Space-occupying lesions

When space-occupying renal lesions are identified, those comprising non-functional renal tissue should be differentiated from those with demonstrable function. Photopenic areas (i.e. areas without uptake of the radiopharmaceutical) caused by non-functioning parenchyma may represent tumours, cysts, abscesses, or infarcts. Infarcts usually appear as wedge-shaped defects. Solid lesions, such as tumours, may be differentiated from fluid-filled collections, such as cysts and abscesses, by sonography, CT, or MRI. A functioning, space occupying mass may represent a pseudotumour. Causes include hypertrophic columns of Bertin, focal regenerating nodules, fetal lobulation, dromedary kidney, and distortion of normal renal architecture by ectopic renal arteries (Harbert *et al.* 1996).

Hypertrophic Bertin's columns and unusual renal shape occasionally mimic intrarenal masses on IVP and ultrasound. These lesions concentrate renal radiopharmaceuticals and can so be differentiated from truly pathological lesions such as renal cell carcinoma and other solid masses. Normal uptake of the radiopharmaceutical in a renal mass essentially rules out malignancy. On the other hand, an area of absent uptake indicates the need for further imaging studies. Exceptions are rare tumours such as oncocytoma and mesoblastic nephroma, which have been reported to concentrate renal radiopharmaceuticals (Hartman *et al.* 1981; Lautin *et al.* 1981).

Diagnostic and staging modalities for renal carcinoma include ultrasonography, urography, CT, arteriography, and MRI. No specific radiopharmaceuticals, which accumulate in renal cell carcinoma only, are available.

Positron emission tomography (PET) using F-18-fluorodeoxyglucose (^{18}F-FDG) has proved helpful in determining diagnosis and prognosis of tumours and their response to therapy. Normal renal tubular cells demonstrate glucose-6-phosphatase activity similar to that in the heart. However, despite the relatively high hexokinase concentration in the kidney, most FDG is excreted without being metabolized. Excretion of FDG by the kidney can lead to interpretation problems due to FDG accumulation in renal calyces. When a renal tumour is found by other imaging modalities, good differentiation between malignant tissue and benign tissue is possible by quantifying the uptake of ^{18}F-FDG; since malignant tissue will show a much higher uptake. Sensitivity and specifity for detecting malignant lesions approximate 90 per cent (Belhocine *et al.* 2001). Correlation of PET with CT is important to identify the area of FDG accumulation precisely. Combined PET/CT scanners are commercially available.

Whole-body PET is useful to identify sites of metastatic lesions in patients with renal cell carcinoma. FDG-PET can be used to follow the response to chemotherapy or immunotherapy, a decrease in metabolic activity indicating favourable response. In addition to diagnosis of malignancies, nuclear medicine has a potential role in treatment of renal cell carcinoma using radiolabelled monoclonal antibodies (Mab). Trials with Mab G250 labelled to the therapeutic radionuclide ^{131}I are ongoing. The Mab G250 is reactive with the antigen G250, which is expressed on the cell surface of nearly all renal cell carcinomas. To optimize radioimmunotherapy, newer techniques such as multiple step (pretargeting) approaches are being developed. In this so-called 'pretargeting' approach, the antitumour antibody and the therapeutic radionuclide are administered separately (Boerman *et al.* 1999; Divgi *et al.* 2001).

Finally, when partial nephrectomy is considered or performed, preoperative and postoperative renal scintigraphy may contribute to the assessment and follow-up of the function of the remnant kidney.

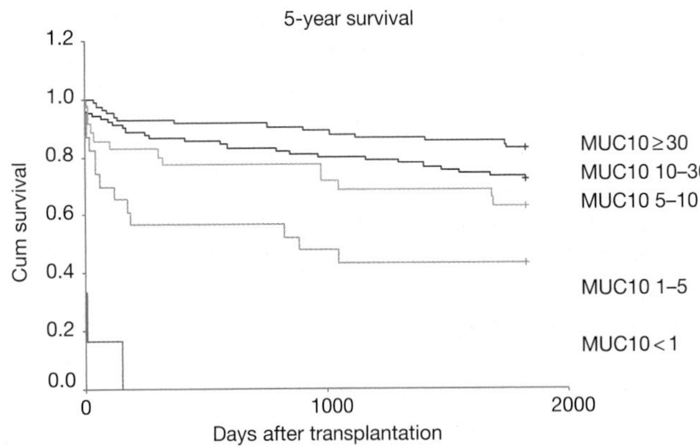

Fig. 5 Survival of the renal transplants within the five different groups of MUC10, 83, 72, 63, 43 and 0 per cent, respectively. Differences are significant, $p < 0.001$ (Kaplan–Meier survival analysis).

Trauma

During the evaluation by radiological imaging in patients with renal trauma, scintigraphy can provide additional information on specific issues. First, early phase renography can establish whether or not blood flow through one of the renal arteries or its branches has been interrupted. Second, parenchymal scintigraphy can determine the renal function when suspected contusion or haematoma is diagnosed by other imaging modalities. Finally, renal scintigraphy can be used to detect urine extravasation. All three issues can be easily studied by Tc-MAG3 scintigraphy. Immediate first pass extravasation indicates a vascular lesion, whereas late (>4 min) extravasation indicates a lesion in the drainage system. Leaks in the vicinity of the kidney may sometimes be confused with parenchymal uptake or radioactivity in the ureter. It is therefore necessary to see whether a consistent focus remains after washout of activity from the kidney and urinary. Extravasation in the pelvic region can be another source of confusion, because it may be difficult to discern bladder activity from adjacent extravasated urine. A comparison of pre- and postvoiding images usually facilitates the distinction. Alternatively, single photon emission computer tomography (SPECT) can be helpful for localization using three-dimensional imaging.

Transplantation renography

With the help of renography it is possible to quantify and visualize renal perfusion, and to visualize the urinary outflow tract. Transplant renography provides qualitative information about different surgical complications, for example, arterial stenosis, venous and arterial thrombosis, infarction, bleeding, and urinary obstruction or leakage and can be used to assess renal function.

Different tracers may be used for transplantation renography (^{131}I-OH Hippuran, ^{99m}Tc-MAG3, and ^{99m}Tc-DTPA). ^{99m}Tc-MAG3 is now mostly used for renal transplantation scintigraphy. Transplant renography is performed in a dynamic phase after bolus injection of ^{99m}Tc-MAG3. Various quantitative parameters from dynamic renal scintigraphy have been derived to facilitate the detection and follow-up of renal graft pathology. These quantitative parameters can be divided into parameters assessing renal graft perfusion and parameters evaluating parenchymal function. Perfusion parameters are mainly based on the first-pass technique, which measures the rate of appearance of the activity in the kidney graft or the ratio of the integral of activity under the transplanted kidney and arterial curves like the Hilson's perfusion index (PI), Kirchner's K/A ratio and renal transit time (El Maghraby 1998). These perfusion parameters may help to differentiate between early graft pathology due to acute rejection and to tubular, because the latter is accompanied by a better perfusion. However, routine application of the perfusion parameters in transplant renography has been limited mainly due to the lack of diagnostic power and to a large interobserver variability in calculating these parameters. The parenchymal function can be measured by registration of the total tracer uptake at a certain time point taken after the perfusion phase. Several studies have shown that the parenchymal function short after transplantation has a prognostic value for later function (Russel *et al.* 2000; Stevens *et al.* 2001). A study in 256 patients who underwent renal transplantation in our hospital showed that the MUC10 (uptake capacity of ^{99m}Tc-MAG3 during the first 10 min) measured within 48 h after transplantation is prognostic for the 5-year renal transplant survival (Fig. 5) (Stevens *et al.* 2001).

Finally, the study of perfusion and uptake of ^{99m}Tc-MAG3 or ^{99m}Tc-DMSA can used to establish arterial and venous thrombosis and renal infarction. Furthermore, the excretory pattern of ^{99m}Tc-MAG3 can be helpful in discriminating postrenal obstruction from other causes of renal failure and to detect urine leakage.

Renal-artery stenosis

In nuclear medicine, angiotensin-converting enzyme (ACE) inhibition renography is the test of choice to detect patients with renal artery stenosis (Prigent 1993; Taylor *et al.* 1996). The brief and quickly acting ACE inhibitor captopril is commonly used for this purpose. In patients with a haemodynamically significant stenosis this causes a fall in GFR, which can be viewed by renography.

Unfortunately, captopril renography can produce false-positive results, especially in populations in which the prevalence of renal artery stenosis is low. Therefore, its use should be restricted to patients with a high suspicion on renal artery, that is, hypertensive populations with a prevalence of renal artery stenosis greater than 10–20 per cent.

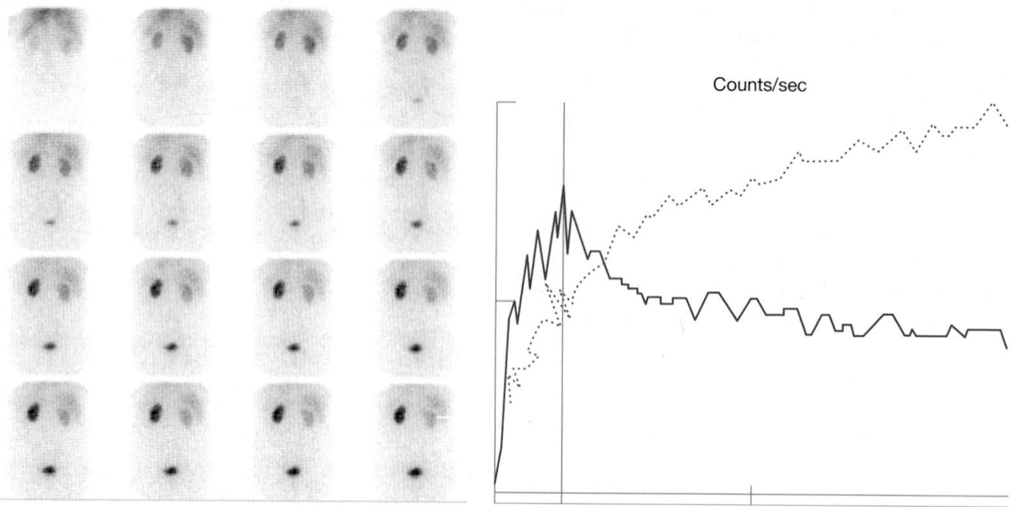

Fig. 6 Renogram and curve of a patient suffering from left-sided renal-artery stenosis (dotted line left kidney).

As a radiopharmaceutical, ^{99m}Tc-MAG3, ^{99m}Tc-DTPA, or ^{131}I-OH Hippuran can be used. Nowadays, mostly ^{99m}Tc-MAG3 is used, because of superior imaging possibilities. Renography is performed in a dynamic phase after bolus injection of ^{99m}Tc-MAG3 and prior oral administration of captopril. Captopril renography can be used as such, or can be compared with a renography without captopril. Captopril renography has a sensitivity and specificity that range between 57 and 100 per cent and 41 and 100 per cent, respectively (Prigent 1993; Vasbinder *et al.* 2001). Comparing captopril renography with a baseline renography increases the specificity, but is slightly at cost of the sensitivity. There are no differences in diagnostic accuracy between the different tracers. Comparable results are obtained in patients with mild renal failure and in patients with bilateral stenosis (Fommei *et al.* 1991). In contrast to the high sensitivity of captopril renography to detect patients with bilateral disease, the sensitivity of this modality to identify both stenotic kidneys is low. In almost all cases, only the most affected kidney shows an abnormal pattern (van de Ven *et al.* 2000).

Differences in the reported accuracy may be attributed to a number of factors, including variation in criteria for a positive test as well as in criteria for a significant stenosis on the arterial angiogram and interobserver variation (Krijnen *et al.* 2002).

In our Institute, captopril renography is used as such. The curves are scored with respect to time to maximal activity (T_{max}), downslope or excretory phase, and the fractional uptake of the kidneys. The renogram (Fig. 6) is considered to indicate probable renal-artery stenosis if the relative uptake of one of the kidneys is less than 40 per cent, or if the T_{max} in one or both kidneys is greater than 6 min. The sensitivity and specificity to detect renal artery stenosis is around 90 per cent (van der Ven 2000).

In patients with advanced renal failure, the specificity of captopril renography may be low. To improve this, the administration of furosemide to accelerate tracer wash out, and comparison with a theoretical 'expected curve' have been advocated. Using these methods, the sensitivity and specificity, are 79–96 per cent and 95 per cent, respectively (Erbslöh-Moller *et al.* 1991; Rocatello and Picciotto 1997).

To standardize captopril renography, consensus guidelines have been developed (Taylor *et al.* 1998). According to the consensus, the renograms can be graded into three groups: low probability, intermediate probability, and high probability. Low probability ($<$10 per cent) includes normal findings on captopril renography or abnormal findings that improve after ACE inhibition. Intermediate probability (sensitivity $>$ 90 per cent, specificity 50–70 per cent) have abnormal baseline findings, but the renogram stays unchanged after ACE inhibition. High probability ($>$90 per cent) is associated with marked changes of the renogram curve after ACE inhibition, including reduction in relative uptake and prolongation of the renal and parenchymal transit time, increase in the 20 min/peak ratio and prolongation of T_{max} (Taylor *et al.* 1996, 1998). Bilateral abnormal but identical curves are probably due to intrinsic parenchymal disease rather than to renal artery stenosis (Balink *et al.* 2001).

Aspirin can be used as an alternative for captopril. The rationale for this idea is the increased dependency of the circulation of poststenotic kidney on prostaglandins. Aspirin, which inhibits prostaglandin synthesis, causes preglomerular vasoconstriction, with the double effect of decreasing renal blood flow and glomerular capillary pressure and therefore the GFR. In a recent comparative study, aspirin renography was accurate for the identification of renal artery stenosis, but the results were not better than captopril renography (van der Ven *et al.* 2000).

References

Abels-Fransen, G. J. *et al.* (1983). The predictive value of hippuran uptake in acute renal failure. *Proceedings of the European Dialysis Transplantion Association* **20**, 641–645.

Adeyoju, A. A. B. *et al.* (2001). The choice of timing for diurectic renography: the F + 0 method. *BJU International* **88**, 1–5.

Balink, H. *et al.* (2001). Captopril renography and the relevance of abnormal but bilateral identical curves in the diagnosis of renal artery stenosis. *Nuclear Medicine Communications* **22**, 971–974.

Belhocine, T. Z. *et al.* Positron emission tomography imaging. Genitourinary carcinoma. In *Nuclear Oncology Diagnosis and Therapy* (ed. I. Khalkali, J. C. Maublant, and S. J. Goldsmith), pp. 403–416. Philadelphia, PA: Lippincott Williams & Wilkins, 2001.

Blaufox, M. D. *et al.* (1996). Report of the radionuclides in nephrourology committee on renal clearance. *Journal of Nuclear Medicine* **37**, 1883–1890.

Blaustein, D. A. *et al.* (2002). The role of technetium-99m-MAG3 renal imaging in the diagnosis of acute tubular necrosis of native kidneys. *Clinical Nuclear Medicine* **27**, 165–168.

Boerman, O. C. *et al.* (1999). Pretargeting of renal cell carcinoma: improved tumor targeting with a bivalent chelate. *Cancer Research* **59**, 4400–4405.

Boubaker, A. *et al.* (2001). F + 0 renography in neonates and infants younger than 6 months: an accurate method to diagnose severe obstructive uropathy. *Journal of Nuclear Medicine* **42**, 1780–1788.

Bubeck, B. *et al.* (1993). Renal clearance determination with one blood sample: improved accuracy and universal applicability by a new calculation principle. *Seminars in Nuclear Medicine* **23**, 73–86.

Divgi, C. R. *et al.* Renal carcinoma: monoclonal antibody therapy. In *Nuclear Oncology Diagnosis and Therapy* (ed. I. Khalkhali, J. C. Maublant, and S. J. Goldsmith), pp. 417–422. Philadelphia, PA: Lippincott Williams & Wilkins, 2001.

El Maghraby, T. A. *et al.* (1998). Renographic indices for evaluation of changes in graft function. *European Journal of Nuclear Medicine* **25** (11), 1575–1586.

Erbslöh-Möller, B. *et al.* (1991). Furosemide–^{131}I-hippuran renography after angiotensin-converting enzyme inhibition for the diagnosis of renovascular hypertension. *American Journal of Medicine* **90**, 23–29.

Fommei, E. *et al.* (1991). European Captopril Radionuclide Multicentre Study. Preliminary results. *American Journal of Hypertension* **4**, 690S–697S.

Fritzberg, A. R. *et al.* (1986). Synthesis and biological evaluation of Tc-99m-MAG3 as a hippuran replacement. *Journal of Nuclear Medicine* **27**, 111–116.

Gordon, I. *et al.* (2001). Guidelines for standard and diuretic renography in children. *European Journal of Nuclear Medicine* **28**, BP21–BP30.

Gunasekera, R. D., Allison, D. J., and Peters, A. M. (1996). Glomerular filtration rate in relation to extracellular fluid volume: similarity between Tc-99m-DTPA and inulin. *European Journal of Nuclear Medicine* **23**, 49–54.

Harbert, J. C., Andrich, M. P., and Peller, P. J. The genitourinary system. In *Nuclear Medicine Diagnosis and Therapy* (ed. J. C. Harbert, W. C. Eckelman, and R.D. Neumann), pp. 713–743. New York: Thieme Medical Publishers, Inc, 1996.

Hartman, D. S. *et al.* (1981). Mesoblastic nephroma. *American Journal of Radiology* **136**, 69–74.

Hilson, A. T. W. Renal failure. In *Nuclear Medicine in Clinical Diagnosis and Treatment* (ed. I. C. P Murray and P. J. Ell), pp. 339–347. Edinburg: Churchill Livingstone, 1998.

Hosokawa, S., Kawamura, J., and Yoshida, O. (1978). Basic studies on the intrarenal localization of renal scanning agent Tc-99m DMSA. *Acta Urologica Japan* **24**, 61–65.

Houston, A. S. *et al.* (2001). UK audit and analysis of quantitative parameters obtained from gamma camera renography. *Nuclear Medicine Communications* **22**, 559–566.

Itoh, K. *et al.* (1996). Quantification of renal function with a count-based gamma camera method using technetium-99m-MAG3 in children. *Journal of Nuclear Medicine* **37**, 71–75.

Krijnen, P. *et al.* (2002). Interobserver agreement on captopril renography for assessing renal vascular disease. *Journal of Nuclear Medicine* **43**, 330–337.

Lautin, E. M. *et al.* (1981). Radionuclide imaging and computer tomography in renal oncocytoma. *Radiology* **138**, 185–190.

Levtchenko, E. N. *et al.* (2001). Role of Tc-99m-DMSA scintigraphy in the diagnosis of culture negative pyelonephritis. *Pediatric Nephrology* **16**, 505–506.

Moonen, M. *et al.* (1994). Determination of split renal function from gamma camera renography: a study of three methods. *Nuclear Medicine Communications* **15**, 704–711.

Moran, J. K. (1999). Technetium-99m-EC and other potential new agents in renal nuclear medicine. *Seminars in Nuclear Medicine* **29**, 91–101.

O'Reilly, P. H. *et al.* (1996). Consensus on diuresis renography for investigating the dilated upper urinary tract. *Journal of Nuclear Medicine* **37**, 1872–1876.

Patel, R. *et al.* (1980). Gallium-67 scan: aid to diagnosis and treatment of renal and perirenal infections. *Urology* **16**, 225–228.

Piepsz, A. (2002). Cortical scintigraphy and urinary tract infection in children. *Nephrology, Dialysis, Transplantation* **17**, 560–562.

Piepsz, A. *et al.* (2001). Guidelines for glomerular filtration rate determination in children. *European Journal of Nuclear Medicine* **28**, BP31–BP36.

Prenen, J. A. C. *et al.* (1991). Technetium-99m-MAG3 versus iodine-123-OIH: renal clearance and distribution volume as measured by a constant infusion technique. *Journal of Nuclear Medicine* **32**, 2057–2060.

Prigent, A. (1993). The diagnosis of renovascular hypertension: the role of captopril renal scintigraphy and related issues. *European Journal of Nuclear Medicine* **20**, 625–644.

Prigent, A. *et al.* (1999). Consensus report on quality control of quantitative measurements of renal function obtained from the renogram: international consensus committee from the scientific committee of radionuclides in nephrourology. *Seminars in Nuclear Medicine* **29**, 146–159.

Roccatello, D. and Picciotto, G. (1997). Captopril-enhanced scintigraphy using the method of the expected renogram: improved detection of patients with renin-dependent hypertension due to functionally significant renal artery stenosis. *Nephrology, Dialysis, Transplantation* **12**, 2081–2086.

Rossleigh, M. A. Renal infection. In *Nuclear Medicine in Clinical Diagnosis and Treatment* (ed. I. C. P Murray and P. J. Ell), pp. 265–275. Edinburgh: Churchill Livingstone, 1998.

Rossleigh, M. A. (2001). Renal cortical scintigraphy and diuresis renography in infants and children. *Journal of Nuclear Medicine* **42**, 91–95.

Russel, C. D. *et al.* (1995). A single injection, two-sample method for measuring renal technetium-99m-MAG3 clearance in both children and adults. *Nuclear Medicine and Biology* **22**, 55–60.

Russell, C. D. *et al.* (2000). Prediction of renal transplant survival from early postoperative radioisotope studies. *Journal of Nuclear Medicine*, **41** (8), 1332–1336.

Sfakianakis, G. N. *et al.* (2002). Diuretic MAG3 scintigraphy (F0) in acute pyelonephritis: regional parenchymal dysfunction and comparison with DMSA. *Journal of Nuclear Medicine* **41**, 1955–1963.

Stevens, H. *et al.* (2001). Quantitative renography 48 hours after renal transplantation predicts long term survival. *European Journal of Nuclear Medicine* **28**, 1677–1681.

Tauxe, W. H. *et al.* (1982). New formulas for the calculation of effective renal plasma flow. *European Journal of Nuclear Medicine* **7**, 51–54.

Taylor, A., Jr. (1982). Quantification of renal function with static imaging agents. *Seminars in Nuclear Medicine* **4**, 330–334.

Taylor, A., Jr. and Nally, J. V. (1995). Clinical applications of renal scintigraphy. *American Journal of Radiology* **164**, 31–41.

Taylor, A. *et al.* (1996). Consensus report on ACE inhibitor renography for detecting renovascular hypertension. *Journal of Nuclear Medicine* **11**, 1876–1882.

Taylor, A. *et al.* (1998). Procedure guideline for diagnosis of renovascular hypertension. *Journal of Nuclear Medicine* **39**, 1297–1302.

Thompson, A. and Gough, D. C. S. (2001). The use of renal scintigraphy in assessing the potential for recovery in the obstructed renal tract in children. *BJU International* **87**, 853–856.

Vasbinder, G. B. C. *et al.* (2001). Diagnostic tests for renal artery stenosis in patients suspected of having renovascular hypertension: a meta-analysis. *Annals of Internal Medicine* **135** (6), 401–411.

van der Ven, P. J. G. *et al.* (2000). Aspirn renography and Captopril renography in the diagnosis of renal artery stenosis. *Journal of Nuclear Medicine* **41**, 1337–1342.

Watson, W. S. (1992). A simple method of estimating filtration rate. *European Journal of Nuclear Medicine* **19**, 827.

Willis, K. W. *et al.* (1977). Renal localization of Tc-99m-stannous glucoheptonate and Tc-99m-stannous dimercaptosuccinate in the rat by frozen section autoradiography. *Radiation Research* **69**, 475–488.

1.6.2 Imaging strategies in clinical nephrology

1.6.2.i Haematuria, infection, acute renal failure, and obstruction

Sven Dorph

Introduction

This chapter deals with strategies for imaging of the kidneys and urinary tract in various typical clinical situations in nephrology. It is important to realize that only main guidelines can be given, since the approach may depend on the individual patient, on the equipment available, and on particular local radiological experience and expertise.

Ultrasound, computed tomography (CT), magnetic resonance (MR), and nuclear medicine, which have appeared stepwise during the past 30 years, have all reached a high degree of technical refinement and diagnostic potential. They have gradually broadened the scope of nephrological imaging and radically changed imaging strategy in many clinical situations. One obvious result of this development is the far more limited use of intravenous urography, which was formerly the cornerstone in all diagnostic work-up of the kidneys and urinary tract. Typically, the number of urograms has been reduced by a factor of five in most radiological departments all over the world. However, urography still has an important, although more limited role to play.

A. Investigation of haematuria

Haematuria can be gross or microscopic and can originate from any site of the urinary tract. While gross haematuria should always lead to a thorough diagnostic work-up (Grossfield and Carroll 1998), microscopic haematuria is often found incidentally and the handling of this situation remains an issue.

Haematuria can be (a) symptomatic and (b) asymptomatic.

(a) Haematuria associated with other symptoms from the urinary tract is typically of urological origin. However, also a number of nephrological diseases may present with haematuria and other urinary tract symptoms, for instance, acute pyelonephritis, sloughed papillae in papillary necrosis, and urinary tract tuberculosis with complicating local obstruction. In such cases, the cause of the haematuria may be so obvious that the work-up can be simplified with these diagnoses in mind and occasionally there is no need for imaging at all (acute uncomplicated pyelonephritis).

(b) Haematuria with no accompanying urinary tract symptoms can have both urological and nephrological origin. It has numerous causes including renal and urothelial malignancies. Therefore, imaging is most often required, even when the haematuria is only microscopic.

Imaging

Urography, direct pyelography, ultrasound, CT, and MR are all useful to evaluate the urinary tract in patients with haematuria. There are no data that compare the value of each of these modalities as initial examination. Consequently, evidence-based guidelines cannot be given (Grossfield *et al.* 2001). Since MR is less generally available, more time consuming, and expensive than the other modalities it is not used as an initial study. Among the other three modalities intravenous urography is currently the initial study of choice for most radiologists if kidney function is normal or at least near normal.

Some important reasons are listed in Table 1. The disadvantages of urography are listed in Table 2.

The most important disadvantage is the fact that about 30 per cent of renal masses smaller than 3 cm are not detected with the urogram alone (Amendola *et al.* 1988) and even larger tumours can be overlooked if they do not deform renal contour or displace the calyces. This is true even with meticulous urographic techniques (abdominal compression, tomography, oblique projections). Also, when the urogram raises suspicion of a mass it is rarely sufficiently characterized. Consequently, a normal urogram or a urogram suggesting a mass should be followed by one of the three other modalities, all of which are superior in this respect. CT and MR have the highest sensitivity for both detection and characterization of solid renal masses (Amendola *et al.* 1988; Choyke *et al.* 1997), CT being most widely used for the above mentioned reasons. But, ultrasound is so good in distinguishing the many simple cysts from ambiguous cysts and solid tumours that it is considered the most cost-effective modality to follow the urogram (Einstein *et al.* 1995) (Fig. 1). However, ultrasound is less reliable than CT to detect and characterize small, ambiguous cysts and solid tumours (Jamis-Dow *et al.* 1996). Therefore, CT must follow ultrasound to exclude a parenchymal malignancy and to characterize a tumour already found. CT is also the single best modality to detect and evaluate stones and renal and perirenal infections and their complications.

Intravenous urography is the best imaging modality to detect urothelial tumours in the pelvicalyceal system and ureters (Fig. 2). Direct pyelography is often used to verify the diagnosis (Fig. 3). High sensitivity rates with CT have also been reported (Buckley *et al.* 1996), but its efficacy compared with urography remains to be demonstrated.

Bladder tumours are often detected by all the imaging modalities, but only cystoscopy can exclude a bladder malignancy.

Table 1 Advantages of urography as initial study in asymptomatic haematuria

Standardized and easily available
Relatively inexpensive
Excellent overview of entire tract
Most detailed visualization of pelvicalyceal system (with adjacent parenchyma) and ureters
Easy and most rewarding to communicate to the clinician

Table 2 Diasadvantages of urography

Requires kidney function
Insensitive in small renal masses
Cannot distinguish cyst from solid tumour
Only indirectly visualizes processes neighbouring the kidney and urinary tract

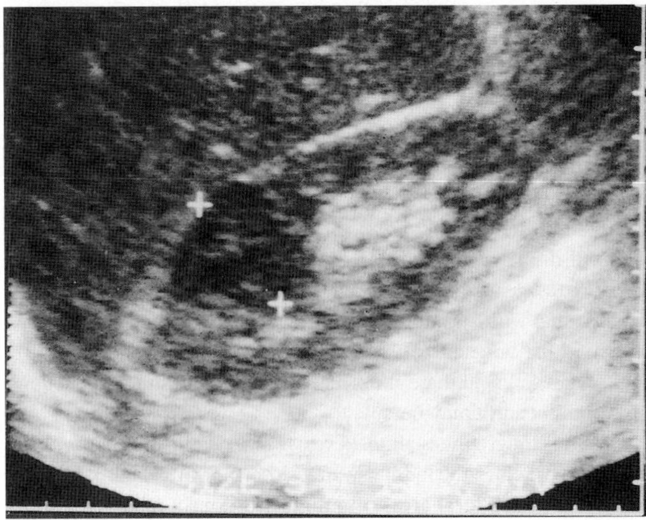

Fig. 1 Small, round, slightly hypoechogenic mass in upper anterior aspect of right kidney: renal cell carcinoma. CT is needed for verification and staging. Courtesy of Hans Henrik Holm, MD, Herlev, Denmark.

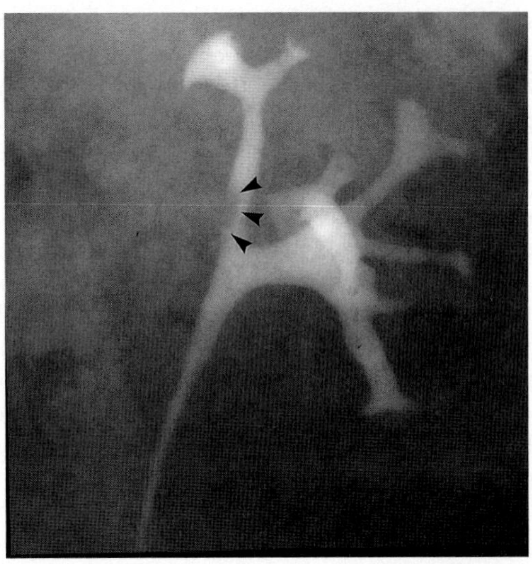

Fig. 3 When a small papilloma is suspected on the urogram, retrograde pyelography is often helpful to verify or exclude. Tiny papilloma (arrow heads) in upper calyx major of left kidney.

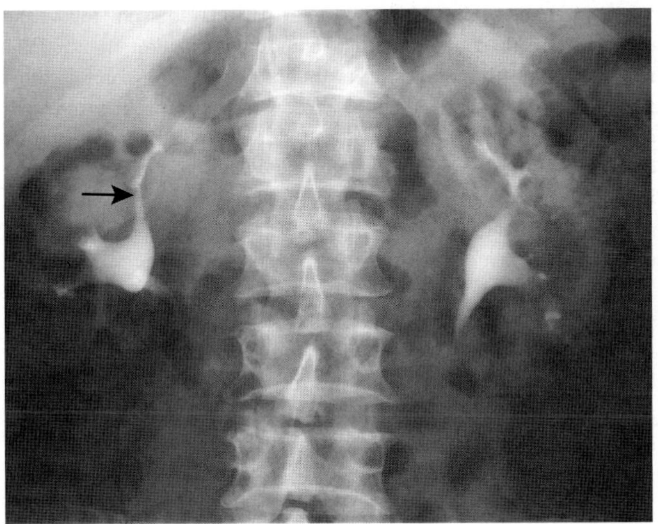

Fig. 2 Urography is best to detect small urothelial tumours in the pelvicalyceal system and ureter. The tiny filling defect (arrow) in the upper right calyx major was a papilloma.

There are radiologists who advocate the use of CT as the initial imaging study in haematuria because of its high efficacy in detecting and characterizing a wide range of underlying pathology.

The development of spiral CT from single detector to multidetector row volumetric aquisition technique has had a significant recent impact on imaging of the urinary tract, since it is now possible to combine the sensitivity and specificity of CT for stones and small parenchymal masses with those of urography for urothelial abnormalities into one single examination. The term CT-urography has been widely adopted and covers a variety of techniques where CT is either combined with urographic elements or directly replaces urograms in the form of planar reformatted images (Newhouse *et al.* 2001; Hertz 2002).

Also MR-techniques have been introduced to detect and characterize disease in the kidneys and urinary tract (MR-urography) (Kawashima *et al.* 2003).

Although there has still not been much research on the cost-effectiveness of CT and MR urography compared with conventional radiologic techniques in haematuria and other urologic symptoms, CT-urography is now being increasingly used and is expected gradually to replace the urogram in many clinical situations. MR-urography is already serving as an alternative imaging to urography and CT-urography in pregnant women, children and in patients with contraindication to iodinated contrast media.

In patients with renal insufficiency and other risk factors preventing the use of intravenous contrast media, a combination of scout films and ultrasound of the kidneys and bladder is a good alternative. It gives valuable information on the kidney disease if it is not known and detects both renal masses, stones, and obstruction with reasonable safety and often demonstrates a bladder tumour. CT with no contrast can provide a safer exclusion of stone disease, and cystoscopy, possibly combined with retrograde pyelography, can exclude urothelial malignancy when needed.

B. Investigation of urinary tract infection and reflux

Urinary tract infection (see Section 7)

Pathology and complications

In acute pyelonephritis, the bacteria spread through the papillary ducts and cause an acute tubulointerstitial inflammation along the course of the medullary rays. It may involve the full thickness of the whole kidney, sometimes one or more lobes or only part of a lobe with sharp demarcation between inflamed and normal parenchyma. The affected tissue gets hyperaemic and swollen and microabscesses may form. When only part of a kidney is affected, it is termed acute focal pyelonephritis. Many other terms, inspired by the subtle changes made visible by CT (lobar nephronia, segmental bacterial nephritis, etc.) are not used any more (Talner *et al.* 1994).

When microabscesses coalesce they may form an abscess, which will gradually be surrounded by a fibrous wall against the surrounding normal tissue. If the wall is incomplete or the abscess superficial, a breakthrough may result in a perirenal abscess. When the inflammation is primarily located in the urothelium and there is concurrent obstruction, the process is termed pyonephrosis. A pyonephrosis may also result in a perinephric abscess via pyelosinous extravasation.

Emphysematous pyelonephritis is the most severe form of acute pyelonephritis with bacterial gas formation in the pelvicalyceal system, in the renal interstitium, and in the subcapsular or perirenal space. It is seen in patients with deficient host response, most commonly due to diabetes mellitus. The mortality is high.

Imaging

Imaging is unnecessary in uncomplicated acute pyelonephritis in adult patients. It is indicated when there is poor response to treatment, frequent attacks, diabetes mellitus, immunosuppression, signs and symptoms of obstruction, history of stones, vesicoureteric reflux (VUR), or functional or neurogenic disturbance of micturition.

The following modalities are used: ultrasound, intravenous urography, CT scanning, dimercaptosuccinic acid (DMSA) scintigraphy, MR scanning, direct pyelography, and/or voiding cystourethrography.

Uncomplicated acute pyelonephritis

Although imaging is generally not indicated in uncomplicated acute pyelonephritis it may occasionally be used, particularly when there is severe loin pain mimicking acute ureteric obstruction. The chance of detecting radiological abnormalities in uncomplicated acute pyelonephritis depends on how early after onset of symptoms the examination is performed. Global or focal swelling, decreased density of contrast medium, striations in the nephrogram, delayed excretion, and calyceal compression are characteristic but unspecific urographic signs, which can be expected to be present or at least partly present in about 50 per cent of patients within the first 24 h (Kanel *et al.* 1988). Ultrasound is not very useful either. It can show kidney swelling and may show decreased echogenicity in affected portions of the kidney or increased echogenicity in the case of haemorrhage. Power Doppler increases the sensitivity slightly by showing decreased vascularity in the same areas (Sakaraya *et al.* 1998). CT with its higher contrast resolution and axial display will disclose more subtle nephrographic abnormalities such as generalized or focal, wedge shaped areas of decreased density often with striations after intravenous contrast and increased density in the same areas on delayed scans (Dalla Palma *et al.* 1997) (Fig. 4). However, all these abnormalities will diminish rapidly following successful antibiotic therapy.

DMSA scintigraphy is almost exclusively used in children in order to disclose whether the kidney is affected or not. It is highly sensitive by demonstrating focal areas of diminished uptake. The same information can be obtained from MR but scintigraphy is more practical in children (Lonergan 1998). In adult patients, interest is mainly focused on complications such as stone or abscess or obstruction for which urography, ultrasound, and CT are more useful.

Complicated pyelonephritis

When an acute pyelonephritis in adult patients does not follow the expected benign course or when clinical information indicates an increased risk of harmful effect of the infection and/or complications (vide supra), imaging is indicated. Intravenous urography has traditionally been the primary imaging modality in complicated pyelonephritis and it is still widely used as the initial study, not in order to study the inflammatory process in the kidney but to discover the underlying abnormality predisposing to infection. It is particularly useful to demonstrate congenital anomalies of almost any kind, for instance, medullary sponge kidney, where the dilated collecting ducts and the characteristic calcifications are diagnostic (see Chapter 17.5). Urography is also well suited to diagnose and localize obstruction, to visualize scarring of the kidney, and to diagnose papillary necrosis (Fig. 5). Radiopaque stones are precisely located to the tract and any obstructive effect demonstrated. Emphysematous pyelonephritis can be diagnosed readily on the

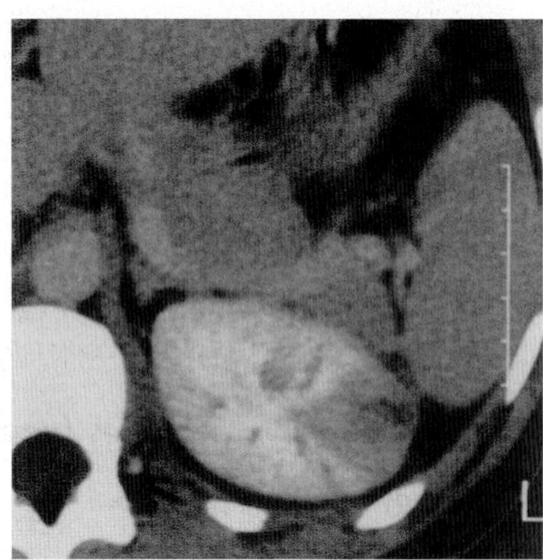

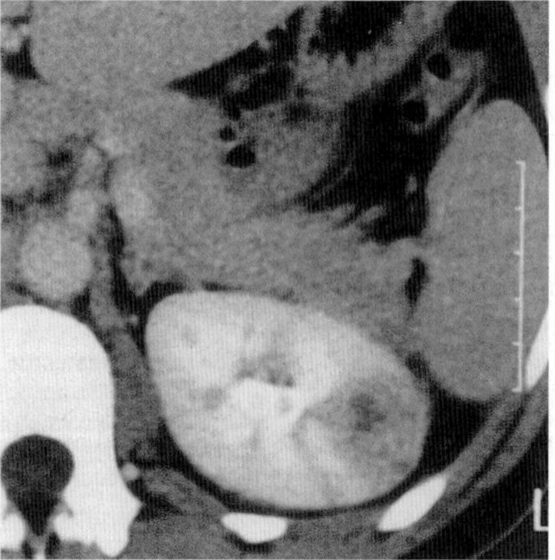

Fig. 4 Postcontrast CT of acute focal pyelonephritis. Nephrographic defect in wedge shaped area of kidney with central small area of liquefaction, which may be the beginning of an abscess. Courtesy of L. Dalla Palma, MD, Trieste, Italy.

scout films of the urogram as well as on non-enhanced CT by the demonstration of gas in the pelvicalyceal system, kidney, or perirenal space [Fig. 6(a) and (b)]. The urographic signs of renal or perirenal abscess and pyonephrosis are usually too inconsistent to be useful.

Ultrasound combined with scout films is also recommended as initial study in complicated pyelonephritis (Webb 1997). Ultrasound is a rapid and easy method to exclude obstruction, larger calculi, and renal and perirenal abscess. However, in the acute phase, it may be difficult to distinguish abscess from acute pyelonephritis, when there is no clear-cut fluid containing process. Serial studies may be of help as well as ultrasound-guided needle aspiration. Pyonephrosis can often be suspected by ultrasound when there is a combination of hydronephrosis and low-level echoes within the collecting system.

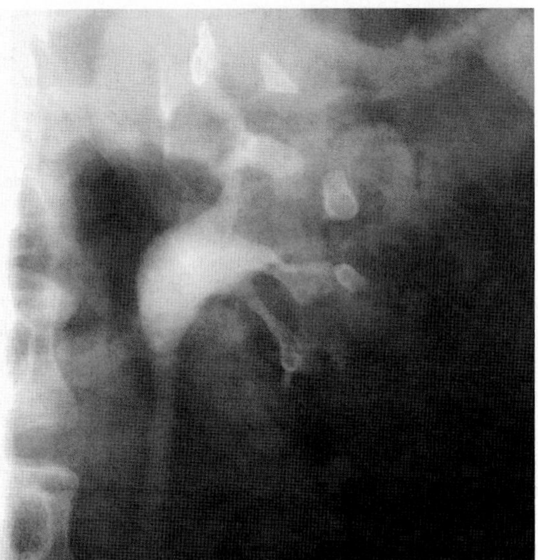

Fig. 5 Urogram demonstrating papillary necrosis. Sloughed papillae presenting as filling defects surrounded by contrast medium.

CT before and after intravenous contrast is currently the imaging study of choice to look for complications to the infection. It is more sensitive than ultrasound to visualize subtle parenchymal abnormality and to detect both renal and perirenal abscess (Fig. 7).

Therefore, if ultrasound is normal in patients with systemic infection, which could originate from the urinary tract, or in patients who simply fail to respond to antibiotic treatment, CT is indicated. CT is also helpful to identify stones containing little or no calcium.

There are radiologists and clinicians who prefer CT as the initial study in acute complicated pyelonephritis despite the increased costs. It is generally recommended in diabetics and other patients with decreased immunological response early after the onset of symptoms.

MR can readily demonstrate inflammatory lesions in the kidney but the technique should probably be reserved to special problem-solving, particularly for patients who cannot be given an iodinated contrast medium. Generally, it plays no significant role in the routine evaluation of pyelonephritis or its complications.

Direct pyelography may occasionally be indicated in obstruction, which cannot otherwise be sufficiently visualized. It must be remembered that it is an invasive procedure, which can cause spread of inflammation especially via pyelosinous reflux. In acute pyelonephritis, it should only be done under antibiotic cover. It may be retrograde or preferably antegrade, especially when nephrostomy is expected.

Voiding cystourethrography is used to demonstrate VUR in children. In adult patients it is only rarely indicated.

Genitourinary tuberculosis (see Chapter 7.3)

The kidneys are infected by a haematogenous spread, most often from the lungs. It is a bilateral infection, but the involvement is often very asymmetrical, so that the least affected side may look normal on imaging. Lower tract involvement is the result of spread from the kidneys. Kidney calcifications are frequent (50 per cent). Other characteristic features are scar formation and strictures resulting in hydrocalyx or hydronephrosis and cavitations in the parenchyma with breakthrough to the calyces. Obstruction caused by strictures can occur in any part

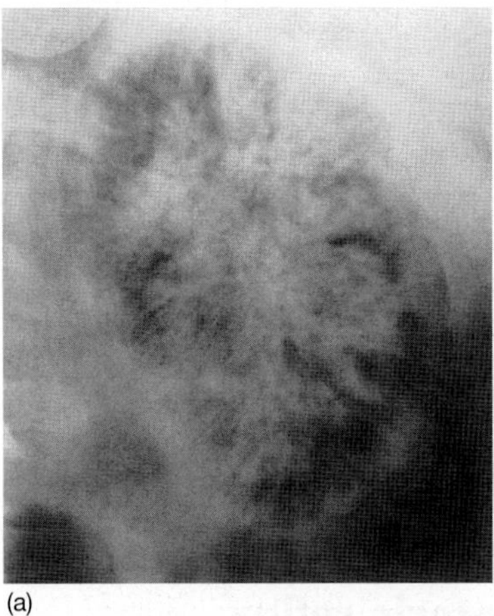

(a)

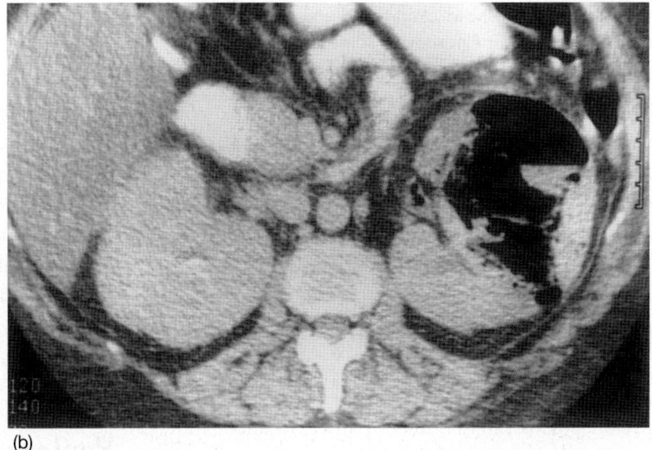

(b)

Fig. 6 Emphysematous pyelonephritis. (a) Plain radiograph of left kidney. Streaks of gas in renal interstitium radiating from the centre to the periphery. Thin rim of subcapsular gas also present, but no visible gas in the pelvicalyceal system. (b) CT showing extensive gas in anterolateral aspect of left kidney with fluid level, subcapsular abscess. From Talner, L. B. Imaging in acute renal infection. In *Syllabus for RSNA Categorical Course in Genitourinary Radiology*, 1994, pp. 39–48. With permission.

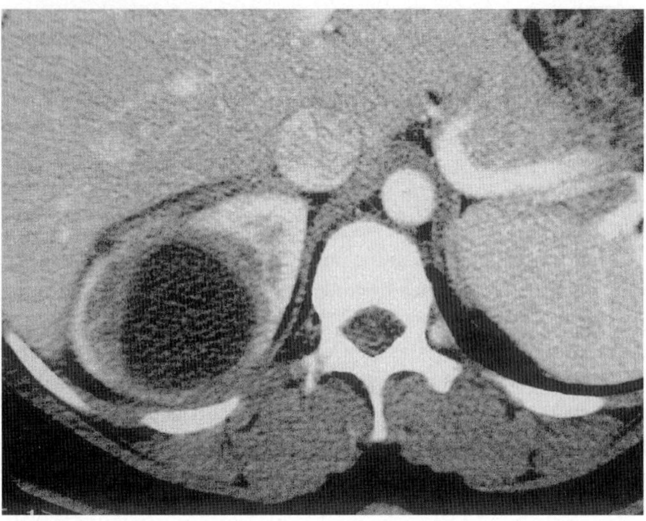

Fig. 7 Contrast enhanced CT of renal abscess. A 26-year-old woman with 3 weeks of right flank pain and recent fever. *E. coli* in blood and urine. About 60 cm^3 pus drained percutaneously. Courtesy of Lee Talner, MD, Seattle, WA.

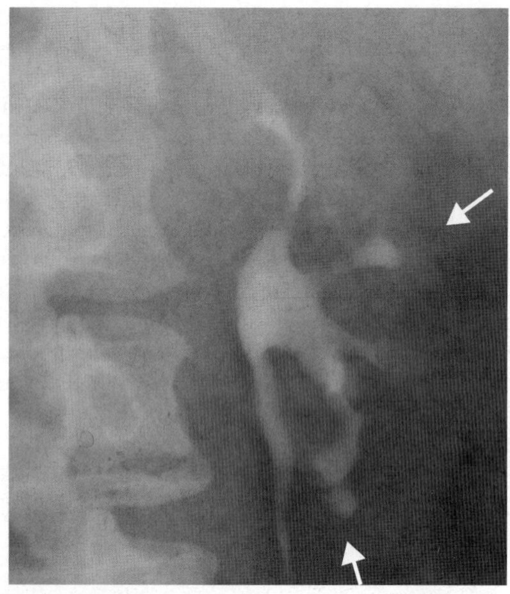

Fig. 9 Focal parenchymal atrophy associated with blunting of a middle and a lower pole calyx (arrows).

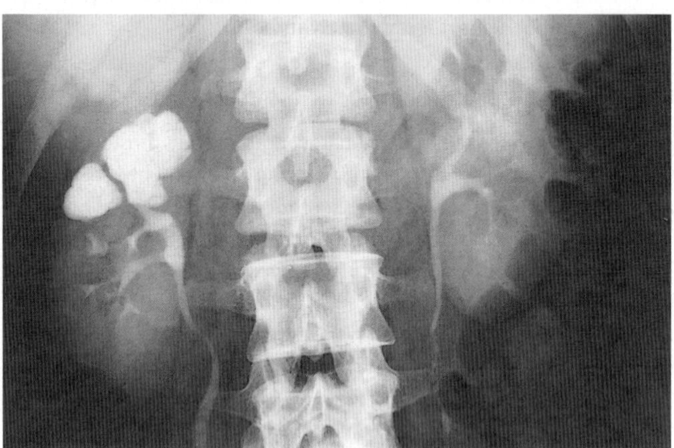

Fig. 8 Renal tuberculosis. Urogram shows cavitation of the upper calyx caused by infundibular stenosis. Scout film showed some stone material in the calyx.

of the urinary tract and can result in 'autonephrectomy'. When the kidneys are functioning, intravenous urography is best to demonstrate the damage (Fig. 8), but ultrasound and CT may also be useful.

Late complications of urinary tract infection

Uncomplicated pyelonephritis rarely results in any permanent morphological or functional damage of the kidney. In complicated pyelonephritis, on the other hand, whatever the cause may be, there is always risk of permanent damage either in the form of globar atrophy or focal scarring with calyceal clubbing, particularly characteristic of reflux nephropathy (see Chapter 17.2).

Intravenous urography, ultrasound, and CT can all demonstrate permanent parenchymal reduction following complicated pyelonephritis. Urography is best to visualize the calyceal abnormalities in focal scarring (Kenney 1990) (Fig. 9).

Necrotizing papillitis: Diabetics with small arterial disease of the kidneys are at risk of necrotizing papillitis as a relatively early complication to acute pyelonephritis. Sloughed papillae may cause superimposed obstruction. Intravenous urography and/or retrograde pyelography are best to demonstrate the papillary necrosis (Fig. 5).

Xanthogranulomatous pyelonephritis is a specific reaction of the kidney parenchyma to chronic infection (see Chapters 7.2 and 18.1). It mainly occurs in obstructed kidneys. There is almost invariably renal calculi, often of the staghorn type. On intravenous urography there is usually no excretion in the affected kidney. Ultrasound typically shows a central irregular mass with a calculus and dilated calyces. CT is best to demonstrate the entire process (Fig. 10) (Parker and Clark 1989).

Pyeloureteritis cystica presents as multiple, fluid-filled cysts in the lining of the pelvis and/or ureter, and sometimes the bladder. It is a special reaction of the urothelium to chronic infection. It never causes obstruction. Urography is the only non-invasive imaging study that reliably demonstrates the small cysts as filling defects (Fig. 11). When disseminated, the diagnosis is clear, but when localized they can mimic small papillomas (Menendez *et al.* 1997).

Long-standing urinary tract infection can furthermore result in squamous metaplasia, leucoplakia, cholesteatoma, and malakoplakia in the lining of the urinary tract. Diagnoses are rarely suggested based on radiological findings in these conditions.

Vesicoureteric reflux (see Chapter 17.2)

Micturitioncystourethrography (MCU) is the first study to diagnose VUR. No preparation is needed except that the child should not be

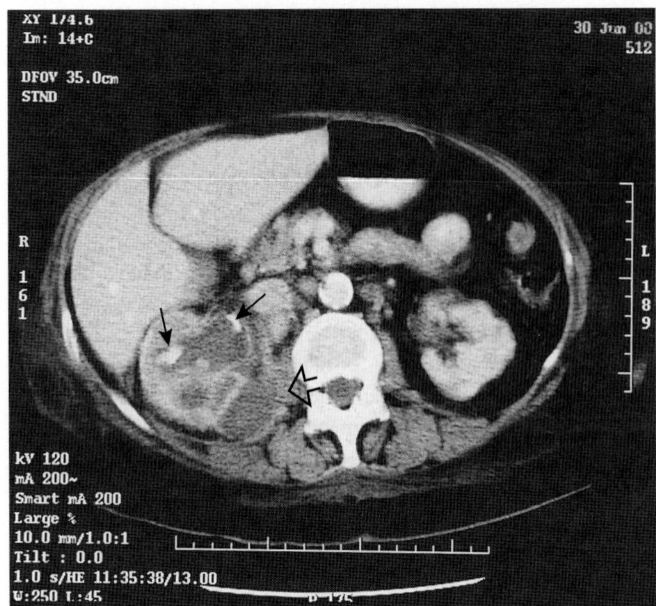

Fig. 10 Xanthogranulomatous pyelonephritis in right kidney in a male patient with *Proteus mirabilis* infection. Enhanced CT shows two calculi (black arrows), gross hydronephrosis, and extension of the inflammatory process to the perinephric space (open arrow). The kidney was non-functioning.

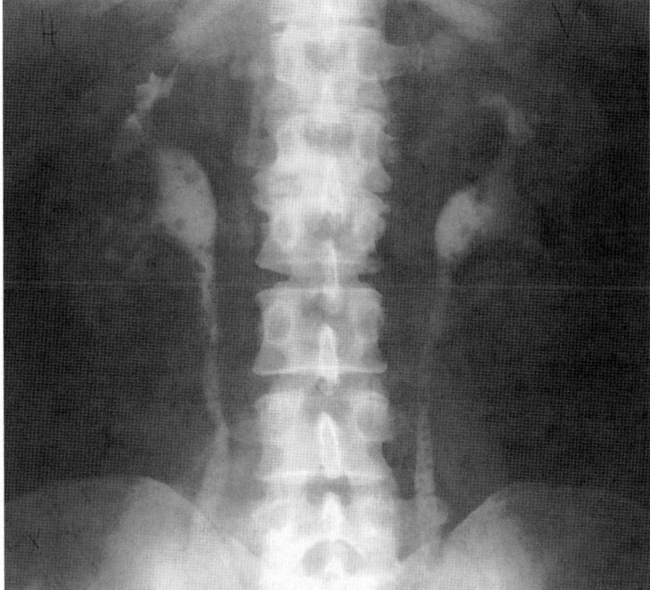

Fig. 11 Pyeloureteritis cystica. Urogram showing bilaterally multiple filling defects in the lining of the pelvicalyceal system and ureters.

too overloaded with fluid since a high urinary flow may suppress reflux. A small catheter is placed in the bladder, which is then slowly (drip-infusion) filled with dilute (30 per cent) radiopaque contrast medium under gravity control. Reflux is looked for by intermittent fluoroscopy during filling and when the bladder is full. Older children are then asked to void after removal of the catheter, while in babies and infants, spontaneous voiding due to bladder filling is waited for. Voiding is videotaped to look for reflux, bladder emptying, and bladder and urethral abnormalities. VUR is classified into five grades according to an international classification from 1981. MCU in adults is performed similarly.

The advantage of MCU is that it offers a very detailed anatomic study of the lower tract including the posterior urethra in male infants (posterior urethral valve). Direct isotope cystography is performed like MCU except that an isotope, technetium-99m pertechnetate, is instilled in the bladder and the reflux is recorded in the gamma camera. The advantage of this technique is that the radiation dose is significantly less compared with MCU. However, the anatomical details are poor. It is, therefore, not recommended as a first study in boys, but can be used in girls when bladder outlet obstruction is not expected.

Indirect isotope cystography is performed by intravenous injection of the isotope which is excreted in the urine. After 20–30 min the isotope reaches the bladder and the isotope concentration in the renal pelvis and ureter decreases. Reflux can then be indentified as refilling of these structures with full bladder and/or during voiding. The advantage is the physiological filling of the bladder without need for catheterization (Peters *et al.* 1990). The disadvantage is a significantly higher percentage of false-negative studies compared with the direct methods. It is used in children older than 3 years for follow-up.

The chronic changes or scars in the kidney, best demonstrated by intravenous urography, are described in Chapter 17.2. Exact information on the degree of functional damage is obtained by a combination of glomerular filtration rate (GFR) and static renography. Renography provides very useful information on the relative function of the kidneys. It is best performed with ^{99m}Tc-dimercaptosuccinic acid (^{99}Tc-DMSA). It is reabsorbed in the proximal tubules and images functional renal parenchyma. GFR and a renogram provide a baseline for future investigations and treatment decisions.

C. Acute renal failure and obstruction

Acute renal failure (see Section 10)

Imaging

There are two crucial questions that should be answered immediately in patients with renal failure:

1. What is the size of the kidneys?
2. Is there evidence of urinary obstruction?

Small kidneys indicate chronic renal failure that so far may have been clinically silent. Normal sized or enlarged kidneys, on the other hand, tell us that the disease is probably acute or of recent onset.

Obstruction leading to renal failure is almost invariably bilateral. However, in patients with chronic renal insufficiency, even a slight and unilateral obstruction may result in acute renal failure. It is, therefore, important to look for even the slightest sign of obstruction when the kidneys are small.

Ultrasound is the best available imaging modality to determine kidney size and screen for obstruction (Webb 1994). It is rapid, cheap, easily available, harmless, and does not require kidney function. It readily provides kidney size and shape and will reveal most cases of chronic obstruction, since this will be associated with dilated calyces and pelvis. In acute obstruction, ultrasound may fail, when there is no or only very slight dilatation (see below). Ultrasound promptly identifies patients with adult polycystic kidney disease and depicts the presence of renal calculi, which may cause or accompany renal failure.

When acute renal failure is due to necrotizing or proliferative disorders of the glomerulus, ultrasound will show bilaterally large, smooth kidneys with a homogeneous pattern of normal to increased echogenicity in the absence of hydronephrosis. These findings indicate a renal parenchymal disease, but provide no clue to its specific nature. There seems to be some correlation between increased cortical echogenicity and the level of renal failure (Hricak *et al.* 1982), but in clinical practice changes in echogenicity are based on the subjective impression of the examiner. Decreased cortical echogenicity may be seen in renal lymphoma, acute pyelonephritis, and renal vein thrombosis, while medullary sponge kidneys, medullary nephrocalcinosis, and renal tubular acidosis will present with increased medullary echogenicity.

Normal sized kidneys with normal parenchyma should raise suspicion of prerenal causes of renal failure or acute nephrotoxicity.

Intravenous urography is no longer used in patients with severe renal insufficiency. This is due to the fact that ultrasound can provide the same or even better information and to the concern over the use of water-soluble contrast media in these patients who are susceptible to further decrease in kidney function (Tubin *et al.* 1998). However, scout films should still be taken to detect renal calculi.

CT is indicated when ultrasound is inconclusive. It is highly sensitive to demonstrate small calcifications, and parenchymal stones, which are non-opaque on scout films because of low calcium content, are often visible. CT can detect hydronephrosis even without the use of an intravenous contrast medium, and the course of a dilated ureter can often be followed on the cross-sectional images directly to the point of obstruction, when it is located above the bladder. Also, the nature of the obstruction can be identified or at least suspected in quite a few cases.

CT also provides renal size and the amount of remaining renal parenchyma, although this is not a reliable indicator of potential renal function in the case of obstruction. Only a decompression can reveal the reversibility of renal insufficiency.

Angiography has an extremely limited role in renal failure. Acute occlusion of the renal arteries is detected by echo-Doppler. Some systemic diseases associated with renal failure may present multiple microaneurysms in the renal arterial bed, which can only be demonstrated by angiography (polyarteritis nodosa).

Antegrade and retrograde pyelography are useful when non-invasive imaging fails to identify obstruction located to the ureter as the cause of renal failure.

MR can readily demonstrate kidney anatomy and diagnose obstruction in renal failure but it is not used much since ultrasound and CT are cheaper and more readily available. Loss of corticomedullary distinction was initially reported to be a characteristic feature in some forms of medical renal disease (Fig. 12). However, the finding has been shown to be too unspecific to be of much practical use.

Acute obstruction of the upper urinary tract

Acute obstruction of the ureter will result in prompt increase in the hydrostatic pressure proximal to the obstruction, provided the kidney filtrates. The level of pressure will depend on the degree and duration of the obstruction, the escape of urine due to backflow, the capacity of the upper urinary tract proximal to the obstruction, and the condition of the kidney. The higher and more acute the pressure increase, the greater the chance of forniceal rupture with escape of urine to the renal sinus (pyelosinus backflow) and retroperitoneal spaces from where it is usually absorbed through veins and lymph channels (pyelovenous and pyelolymphatic backflow). This is a mechanism that will protect the kidney from damaging effects of very high pressure. However, it is also a potential source of spread of inflammation from infected urine.

The rise in pressure is short lived with a gradual subsequent decline due to backflow, to the compliance of the pelvicalyceal system and ureter with gradual dilatation, and reduced renal blood flow and filtration rate. Chronic obstruction will often eventually have normal or subnormal pressure (Talner *et al.* 2000).

Aetiology

A calculus lodged in the ureter is by far the most common course of acute obstruction. Less common are sloughed papillae, blood clots, and accidental ureteric ligation. Bladder tamponade from severe bleeding can cause acute bilateral ureteric obstruction.

Imaging

Intravenous urography has for many years been the cornerstone for imaging of acute ureteric obstruction. It is readily available, relatively inexpensive and safe, and allows visualization of the entire urinary tract. It is highly accurate in demonstrating acute obstruction even in the acute setting. Since there may be only minimal dilation in the early phase of acute ureteric obstruction, interest is also focused on subtle asymmetry in contrast opacification of the collecting system and the kidney parenchyma (Table 3). In many cases the stone can be suspected on the scout film and its intraluminal location proved on late films when the contrast filled ureter can be traced to the stone. In such cases the diagnosis is established, but also when there is no stone visible, the subtle signs in Table 3 are often sufficient to establish the diagnosis of acute ureteric obstruction or a recently passed ureteric stone (Fig. 13).

In case of forniceal rupture, which occasionally occurs when the urographic contrast medium induces an osmotic load, contrast medium dissects in the renal sinus tissue and often to the perirenal and periureteral space in a characteristic pattern (Fig. 14).

Ultrasound is highly sensitive in demonstrating moderate to severe dilation of the pelvicalyceal system and a combination of scout films and ultrasound has been proposed as primary imaging in acute ureteric colic (Dalla Palma *et al.* 1993). However, this degree of dilatation is rarely encountered in these patients and it is difficult to distinguish, by ultrasonography, between a normal extrarenal pelvis and mild dilatation due to acute obstruction. Direct visualization of the obstructing calculus is often possible, when it is located at the ureteropelvic and ureterovesical junction, while the rest of the ureter is only rarely visible, even when it is dilated. Doppler sonography to

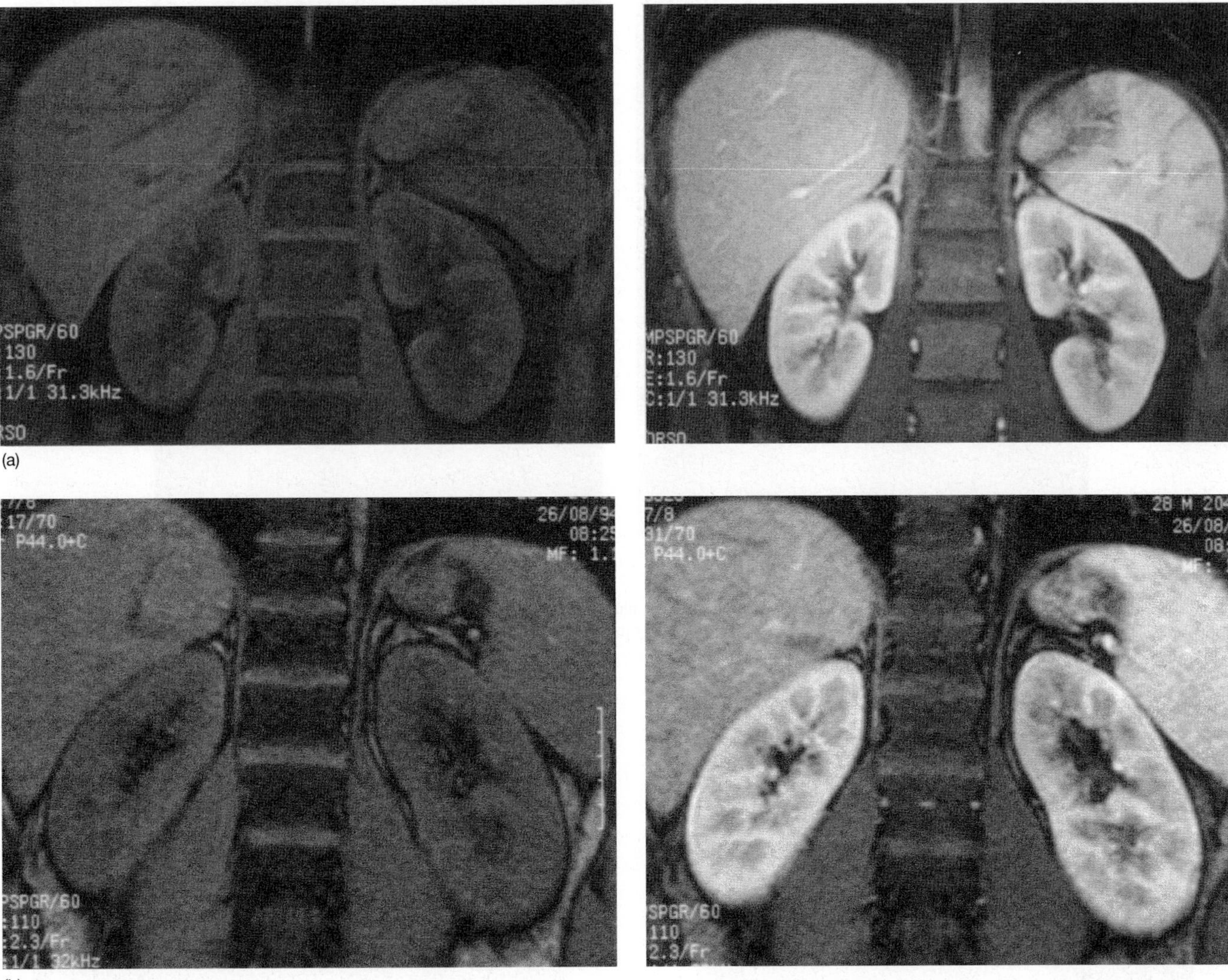

Fig. 12 (a) A dynamic, gadolinium enhanced gradient echo MR sequence before and immediately after injection of the contrast agent in a patient with normal kidneys. Distinct corticomedullary demarcation both before and after contrast. (b) Same sequence in a patient with nephrotic syndrome and acute renal failure. A corticomedullary distinction is not possible on the precontrast images and the demarcation is blurred on the postcontrast images. Courtesy of Gabriel Kristin, MD, Rotterdam, The Netherlands.

Table 3 Urographic signs of acute ureteric obstruction

Modest renal enlargement
Increasingly dense nephrogram
Delayed calyceal opacification
Minimal or moderate dilatation of collecting system and ureter proximal to obstruction
Spontaneous pyelosinous reflux

evaluate ureteral jets in the bladder (Burge *et al.* 1991) and measurements of resistive index, which should increase in response to acute obstruction (Rodgers *et al.* 1992), have been advocated, but their value has not been finally established.

In 1995, unenhanced spiral CT from the upper kidney poles to the bladder base was introduced as alternative imaging in patients with acute ureteric colic (Smith *et al.* 1995). It has been shown to be extremely useful and has been accepted all over the world. Sensitivity and specificity rates for diagnosis of acute ureteric obstruction are reported to be higher than for urography. The method is easy, fast, and relatively inexpensive and precludes the use of contrast material. It is highly sensitive for stone detection both in the kidneys and the ureter and the mildly dilated urinary tract can often be traced to the obstructing stone. Global swelling of the kidney and particularly perinephric oedema are signs of an acute obstruction affecting the kidney, confirming the diagnosis with high accuracy (Fig. 15). Quite a few causes of abdominal pain other than ureteric stone can also be diagnosed or suspected by this technique. Unenhanced spiral or multislice CT have gradually taken over the role of urography as primary imaging in patients with acute ureteric colic (Dobbins *et al.* 1998).

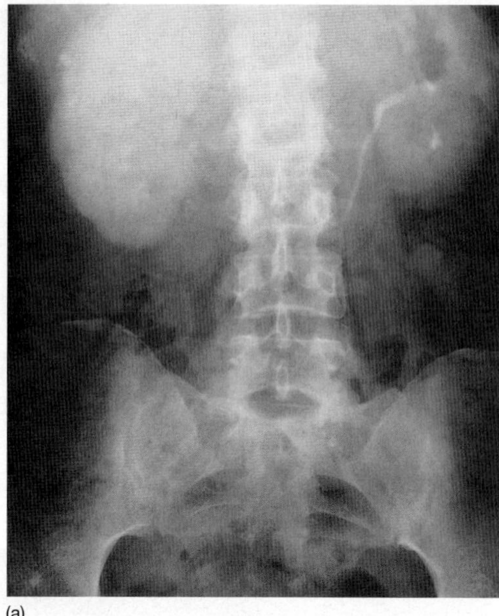
(a)

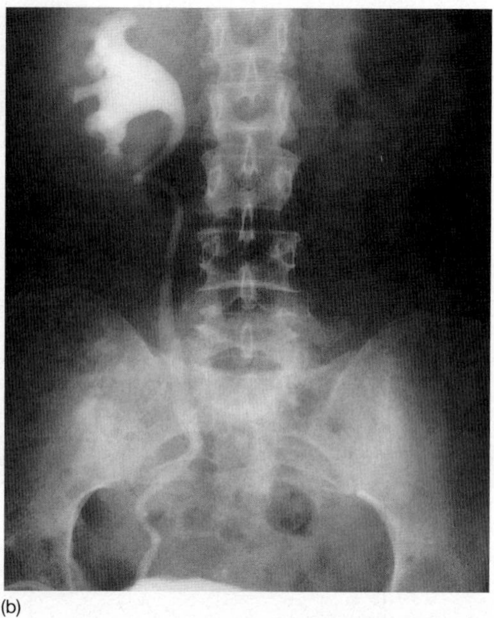
(b)

Fig. 13 Urogram in acute right distal ureteric obstruction. (a) Thirty-minute film. Delayed excretion in a slightly globular right kidney with a dense nephrogram. The ureteric stone showed to be localized at the uretero-vesical junction. (b) Three-hour film. Mild hydronephrosis and ureteric dilatation to the obstructing stone hidden by bladder contrast.

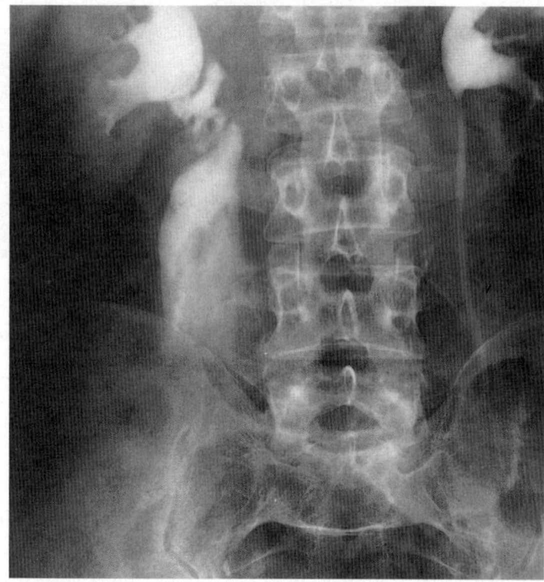

Fig. 14 Acute obstruction can result in rupture of the fornix of calyces (pyelosinous backflow) and extravasation of contrast can extend to the periureteral tissue.

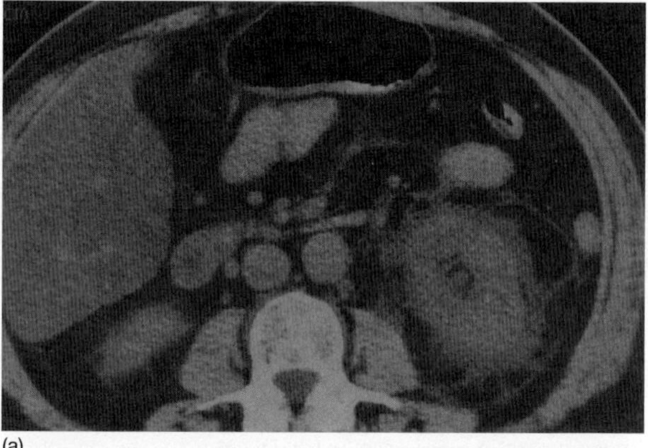
(a)

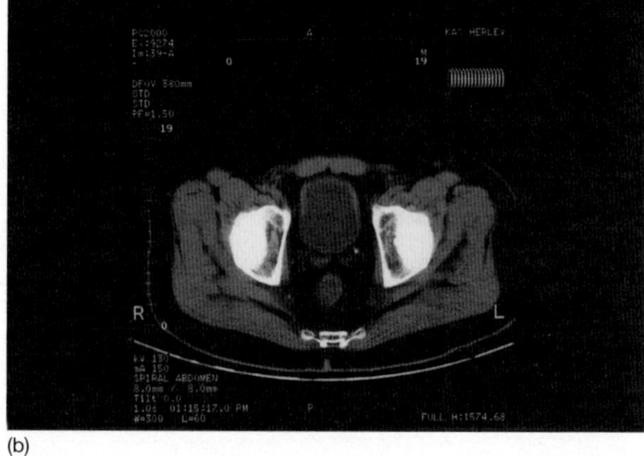

(b)

Fig. 15 (a) and (b) Spiral non-enhanced CT of acute left ureteric obstruction. Global swelling of kidney, perirenal stranding, and a stone in the distal ureter. During recent years, CT has become the study of choice in acute ureteric colic.

MR in acute obstruction has not been investigated much. While direct visualization of stones is not possible, pyeloureteric distension may be visualized and since gadolinium contrast is excreted like iodinized media, the same parenchymal and excretory changes should be expected as with urography. However, so far MR has not found a significant place in the clinical diagnosis of acute ureteric obstruction.

Radionuclide studies are not helpful to establish a diagnosis of acute obstruction but are useful to evaluate the relative function of the kidneys during later follow-up.

References

Amendola, M. *et al.* (1988). Small renal cell carcinomas: resolving a diagnostic dilemma. *Radiology* **166**, 637–641.

Buckley, J. A. *et al.* (1996). Transitional cell carcinoma of the renal pelvis: a retrospective look at CT staging with pathologic correlation. *Radiology* **201**, 194–198.

Burge, H. J. *et al.* (1991). Ureteral jets in healthy subjects and in patients with unilateral ureteral calculi: comparison with colour Doppler US. *Radiology* **180**, 437–442.

Choyke, P. L. (1997). Renal cancer: preoperative evaluation with dual phase three-dimensional MR imaging. *Radiology* **205**, 767–771.

Dalla Palma, L. *et al.* (1993). Ultrasonography and plain film versus urography in ureteric colic. *Clinical Radiology* **47**, 333–336.

Dalla Palma, L., Pozzi-Mucelli, R. S., and Pozzimucelli, F. (1997). Delayed CT in acute renal infection. *Seminars in Ultrasound, CT and MR* **18**, 122–128.

Dobbins, J. *et al.* (1998). Unenhanced helical computed tomography for suspected urinary tract stones: current state of the art. *Emergency Radiology* **5**, 97–102.

Einstein, D. M. *et al.* (1995). Evaluation of renal masses detected by excretory urography: cost effectiveness of sonography versus CT. *American Journal of Roentgenology* **164**, 371–375.

Grossfield, G. D. and Carroll, P. R. (1998). Evaluation of asymptomatic microscopic hematuria. *Urologic Clinics of North America* **25**, 661–676.

Grossfield, G. D. *et al.* (2001). Evaluation of asymptomatic microscopic hematuria in adults: The American Urological Association best practice policy recommendations. Part II. Patient evaluation, cytology, voided markers, imaging, cystoscopy, nephrology evaluation, and follow-up. *Urology* **57**, 604–610.

Hertz, B. R. (2002). The current status of CT urography. *Critical Reviews in Computed Tomography* **43**, 219–241.

Hricak, H. *et al.* (1982). Renal parenchymal disease: sonographic–histologic correlation. *Radiology* **144**, 141–147.

Jamis-Dow, C. A. *et al.* (1996). Small (<3 cm) renal masses: detection with CT versus US and pathologic correlation. *Radiology* **198**, 785–788.

Kanel, K. T. *et al.* (1988). Intravenous pyelogram in acute pyelonephritis. *Archives of Internal Medicine* **148**, 2144–2148.

Kawashima, A. *et al.* (2003). CT urography and MR urography. *Radiologic Clinics of North America* **43**, 945–961.

Kenney, P. J. (1990). Imaging of chronic renal infections. *American Journal of Roentgenology* **155**, 485–494.

Lonergan, G. J. (1998). Childhood pyelonephritis: comparison of gadolinium enhanced MR imaging and renal cortical scintigraphy for diagnosis. *Radiology* **207**, 377–384.

Menendez, B. *et al.* (1997). Cystic pyeloureteritis: review of 34 cases. Radiology aspects and differential diagnosis. *Urology* **50**, 31–37.

Newhouse, J. H. *et al.* Radiologic investigation of patients with hematuria. In *ACR Appropriateness Criteria (VA)*, pp. 1–5. American College of Radiology, 2001.

Parker, M. D. and Clark, R. L. (1989). Evolving concepts in the diagnosis of xanthogranulomatous pyelonephritis. *Urologic Radiology* **11**, 7–15.

Peters, A. M., Morony, S., and Gordow, I. (1990). Indirect radionuclide cystography demonstrates reflux under physiological conditions. *Clinical Radiology* **41**, 44–47.

Rodgers, P. M., Bates, J. A., and Irving, H. C. (1992). Intrarenal Doppler ultrasound studies in normal and acutely obstructed kidneys. *British Journal of Radiology* **65**, 207–212.

Sakaraya, M. E. *et al.* (1998). The role of power Doppler ultrasonography in the diagnosis of acute pyelonephritis. *British Journal of Urology* **81**, 360–363.

Smith, R. D. *et al.* (1995). Acute flank pain: comparison of non-contrast-enhanced CT and intravenous urography. *Radiology* **194**, 789–794.

Talner, L. B. *et al.* (1994). Acute pyelonephritis: can we agree on terminology? *Radiology* **192**, 297–305.

Talner, L. B., O'Reilly, P. H., and Roy, C. Urinary tract obstruction. In *Clinical Urography* 2nd edn. (ed. H. M. Pollack and B. L. McClennan), pp. 1846–1966. Philadelphia: W.B. Saunders, 2000.

Tubin, M. E., Murphy, M. E., and Tessler, F. N. (1998). Current concepts in contrast media-induced nephropathy. *American Journal of Roentgenology* **171**, 933–939.

Webb, J. A. W. (1997). The role of imaging in adult urinary tract infection. *European Radiology* **7**, 837–843.

Webb, J. A. W. (1994). The role of ultrasonography in the diagnosis of intrinsic renal disease. *Clinical Radiology* **49**, 589–591.

1.6.2.ii Hypertension and suspected renovascular disease

Jean-Michel Correas and Olivier Hélénon

Introduction

The diagnoses of renovascular diseases (RVDs) include a wide variety of occlusive and non-occlusive vascular disorders that can be classified with respect to their anatomical location. Pedicular arteriovenous disorders include renal artery stenosis (RAS), occlusion and aneurysm, and renal vein (RV) thrombosis, while peripheral intrarenal vascular disorders include arteriovenous malformation, iatrogenic arteriovenous fistula and false aneurysm, and parenchymal ischaemic disorders. Four non-invasive imaging techniques are currently available in the diagnosis of RVD: colour Doppler ultrasonography (CDUS), computed tomography angiography (CTA), magnetic resonance angiography (MRA), and renal scintigraphy. Digital intra-arterial subtraction angiography remains the gold standard and allows transluminal therapeutic applications. However, it remains an invasive procedure that requires the administration of iodinated contrast agents, with their potential nephrotoxicity. The use of angiography should be optimized as a single step diagnostic–therapeutic procedure following a non-invasive diagnostic strategy applied in a selected patient population.

Technical considerations

Ultrasound imaging

Colour Doppler ultrasound is a non-invasive and inexpensive modality the main limitation of which is the accessibility of the renal arteries to the ultrasound beam. Ultrasound benefits from recent and major technical improvements, resulting in a strong increase in colour and spectral Doppler sensitivity. New modalities, such as power Doppler and dynamic flow, can help in the detection of renal vessels. Moreover, the ultrasonic signals can be enhanced by intravenous (IV) injection of microbubble ultrasound contrast agents (Claudon *et al.* 2000). These agents are capable of passing through the lung capillaries after a peripheral IV injection and can recirculate for a few minutes.

Their tolerance is excellent with no allergic reactions or renal toxicity reported until now. Specific ultrasound sequences have been developed to take advantage of the resonant properties of the microbubbles. The increase in the backscattered signals allows a reduction in the number of technically inadequate examinations.

Computed tomography

The computed tomography (CT) performance for the assessment of RVD has changed with the recent introduction of multidetector row helical technology (see Chapter 1.6.1.v). The main limitations of CTA are the administration of iodinated contrast agents with their potential nephrotoxicity and the risk of allergic reactions, the presence of large arterial wall calcifications that reduces the ability to detect and quantify stenosis, the impossibility of assessing intraparenchymal vessels, and the exposure to radiation increased by the number of scans.

Magnetic resonance imaging

Since 1990, magnetic resonance imaging (MRI) technology has evolved rapidly with the introduction of phased array probes and high field systems with fast commuting gradients. Using this fat-suppressed *T*1-weighted sequence, the lumen of the abdominal vessels become hyperintense following a bolus of gadolinium contrast medium (0.1–0.2 mmol/kg). The acquisition can be easily repeated during arterial, venous, and various delayed phases. The detection of renal arteries and the diagnosis of RAS rely on the analysis of both native and reconstructed multiplanar views using maximal intensity projections (MIPs). The examination includes the assessment of the renal parenchyma with *T*2-weighted spin echo sequence and *T*1-weighted spin or gradient echo sequences before and after administration of the gadolinium contrast medium. Dynamic contrast-enhanced sequences are performed with breath-hold two-dimensional (2D) spoiled gradient echo sequences. The main limitations of MRI and MRA are the usual MRI contraindications (see Chapter 1.6.1.vi).

Renovascular hypertension

The diagnosis of renovascular hypertension (RVH) includes three steps: (a) the diagnosis of the anatomic arterial lesion, (b) the detection of haemodynamically significant RAS, and (c) the functional evaluation of RAS. Imaging modalities are mostly involved in the first two steps. Functional imaging relies on angiotensin-converting enzyme (ACE) inhibitor sensitized tests. RAS is the main cause of RVH, caused by atherosclerosis or fibromuscular dysplasia.

Doppler ultrasound diagnosis of RAS

Grey-scale imaging of renal artery (RA) can reveal focal narrowing and beady features in fibromuscular dysplasia and thickening/calcification of the arterial wall in atherosclerotic lesions. CDUS is helpful to guide pulsed Doppler interrogation of the main and accessory RA and their branches and, especially, at the level of flow disturbances detected by colour coding alterations. CDUS allows grading of RAS (Table 1). In haemodynamically significant RA stenosis (≥50 per cent in diameter), CDUS characteristics include (Kliewer *et al.* 1993; Hélénon *et al.* 1995): intrastenostic acceleration with high systolic peak velocity (>150 cm/s), renal-to-aortic ratio of peak systolic velocity above 3.5, poststenotic turbulent flow, and for tight stenosis over 75 per cent downstream intrarenal repercussions responsible for slowed Doppler waveforms with loss of systolic–diastolic modulation known as the tardus–parvus pattern (Fig. 1). The lack of tardus–parvus effect distally to critical stenosis is attributed to the compliance of the arterial walls and the presence of well-developed collateral blood supply that may compensate for the pressure drop. In such cases, distal Doppler waveforms may exhibit a decrease in resistive index (RI) with an increased side difference (>10 per cent), a prolonged acceleration time (>70 m s) with loss of the early systolic peak and a decreased acceleration (<3 m/s^2) (Kliewer *et al.* 1993; Schwerk *et al.* 1994; Hélénon *et al.* 1995). However, because of high inter- and intraoperator variability, such subtle quantitative criteria are of low diagnostic value. Intrarenal arterial flow repercussions are almost constant in severe RAS and, thus, help to diagnose indirectly most of the severe RAS when the interrogation of extrarenal RA failed. ACE inhibitors may sensitize CDUS demonstration of downstream intrarenal repercussion of RAS (Schwerk *et al.* 1994; Oliva *et al.* 1998).

In non-significant (<50 per cent) RAS, CDUS can demonstrate a mild acceleration at the site of the stenosis without additional abnormality. The diagnosis of a slight RA narrowing relies on the detection of grey-scale features. The detection of these RA lesions should

Table 1 RAS grading using colour Doppler ultrasound

Angiography	**Spectral analysis**			
Stenosis Ø (%)	**Intrastenotic**	**Poststenotic**	**Intrarenal**	
<50	Acceleration	Normal	Normal	1
50–75	Acceleration	Turbulence	Normal	1
>75	Acceleration	Turbulence	Tardus–parvus	3
>75 compensated	Acceleration	Turbulence	Accel. time ↑ Δ RI ↑	2
>95 preocclusive	No signal	Slowed flow	Tardus–parvus	3
100	No signal	No signal	Tardus–parvus	3
100	No signal	No signal	No signal	

Intrarenal Doppler pattern

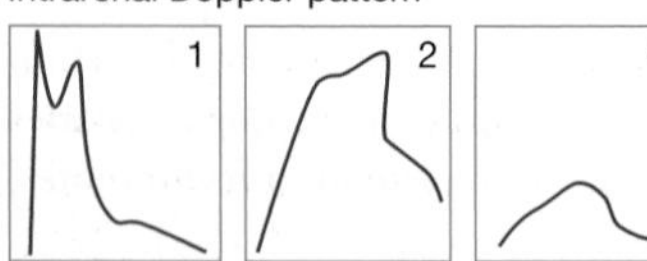

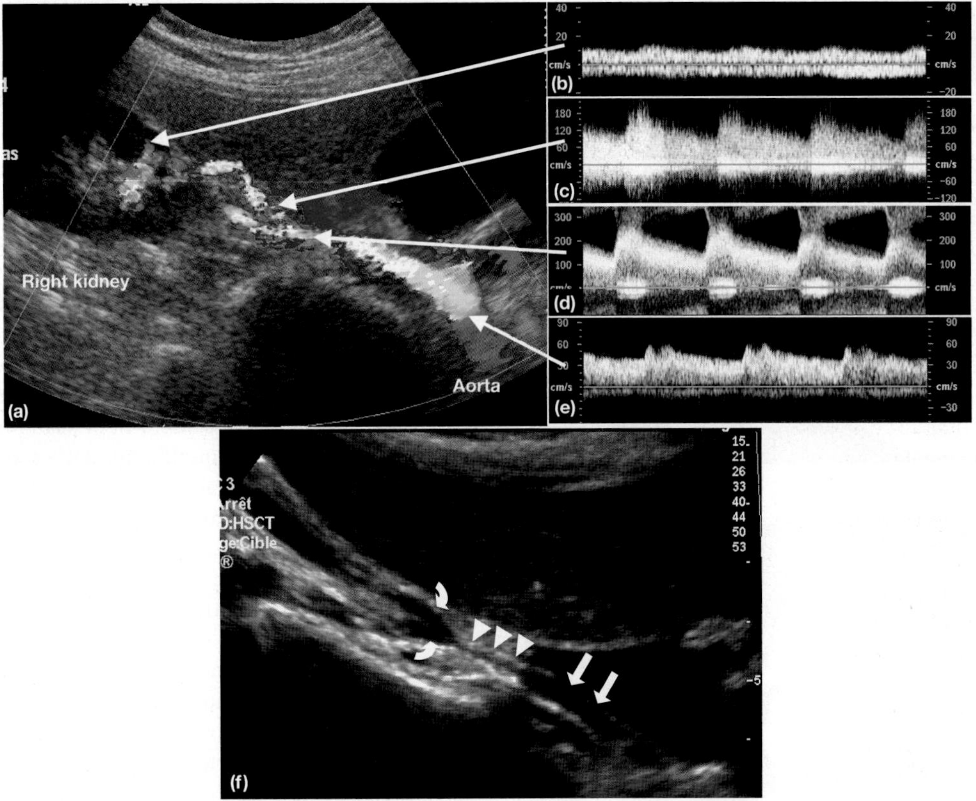

Fig. 1 Colour Doppler ultrasonography in a 38-year-old woman with suspicion of renovascular hypertension. (a) Axial transhepatic study displaying the overall course of the right renal artery, from the aorta (right) to the kidney (left). (b) Spectral Doppler analysis from an interlobar artery, showing the tardus–parvus pattern. (c) Spectral Doppler analysis obtained from the distal main renal artery, showing strong turbulence (reversed flow and poorly defined envelope). (d) Spectral Doppler analysis obtained at the level of the stenosis, showing acceleration above 3.0 m/s. (e) Spectral Doppler analysis from the initial segment of the main RA, showing normal blood flow. (f) Non-linear compounding imaging detects the normal retrocava main RA (straight arrow), the dysplastic segment at the end of the RA, and the normal pattern of the main segmental branches of the RA. These recordings along the RA are typical for a haemodynamically significant renal artery over 75 per cent in diameter in case of fibromuscular dysplasia.

prompt follow-up with CDUS whereas angiography is not mandatory until haemodynamical alterations occur. Depending upon the diagnostic criteria, the sensitivity and specificity of CDUS for RAS detection range from 87 to 98 per cent and 91 to 99 per cent, respectively (Hélénon *et al.* 1995; Miralles *et al.* 1996).

CTA diagnosis of RAS

CTA allows appropriate analysis of the aorta (detecting calcified plaques and aneurysms) and the extrarenal vessels (main and accessory arteries and veins). Large calcified plaques can over- or underestimate the degree of stenosis. The MIP algorithm usually overestimates the degree of stenosis, particularly in case of eccentric calcifications. In fibromuscular dysplasia, CTA findings include string-of-pearls pattern and aneurysms. However, the detection and grading of fibromuscular stenosis remain difficult and usually require additional study with CDUS or angiography.

Contrast-enhanced CT can also detect morphological changes of the stenotic kidney, with reduction in size and delayed nephrography. The detection rate of accessory renal arteries is 96 per cent (Kim *et al.* 1998) (Fig. 2). The overall sensitivity and specificity of CTA in the detection of RAS over 50 per cent in diameter range from 90 to 96 per cent and 94 to 97 per cent respectively (Kaate *et al.* 1997; Kim *et al.* 1998). When the main RA alone is considered, the sensitivity and specificity increase to 100 and 97 per cent, respectively (Kim *et al.* 1998).

MRA diagnosis of RAS

MRA also allows evaluation of both the aorta and extrarenal vessels. RAS MR findings are almost the same as CTA. If the resolution of MR images remains inferior to that of CT images, MR is less artefacted by calcified arterial wall plaques. MRA can under- or overestimate the degree of main RAS (respectively in 14 and 21 per cent of the cases) (Gilfeather *et al.* 1999) (Fig. 3). The detection of accessory RA is higher for MRA than for CDUS (De Cobelli *et al.* 2000). The sensitivity and specificity of MRA for the detection of significant RAS are 95–100 and 90–93 per cent, respectively, for 3D spoiled gradient echo sequences (Gilfeather *et al.* 1999; De Cobelli *et al.* 2000).

Diagnosis of RA occlusion

Chronic RA occlusion is the ultimate stage of an atherosclerotic RAS. It is an uncommon cause of RVH which may be associated with accelerated renal failure. CDUS findings include both severe intrarenal velocimetric abnormalities (tardus–parvus pattern or absent Doppler

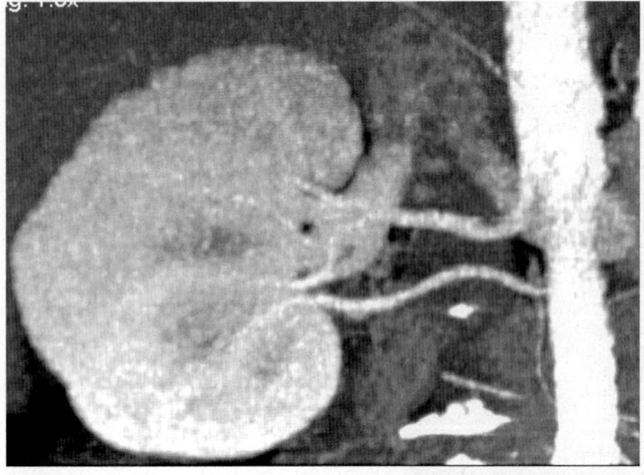

(a)

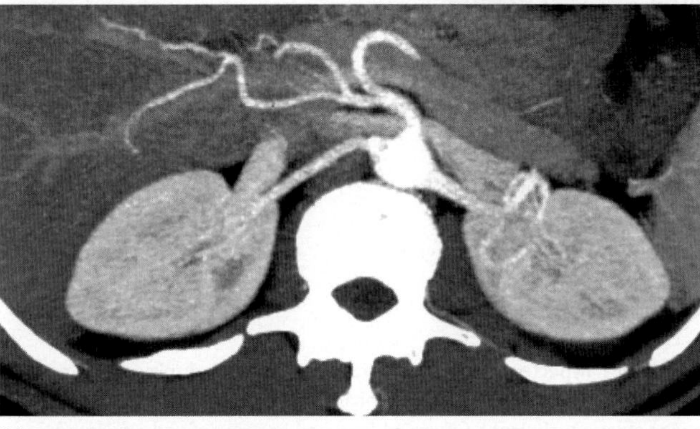

(b)

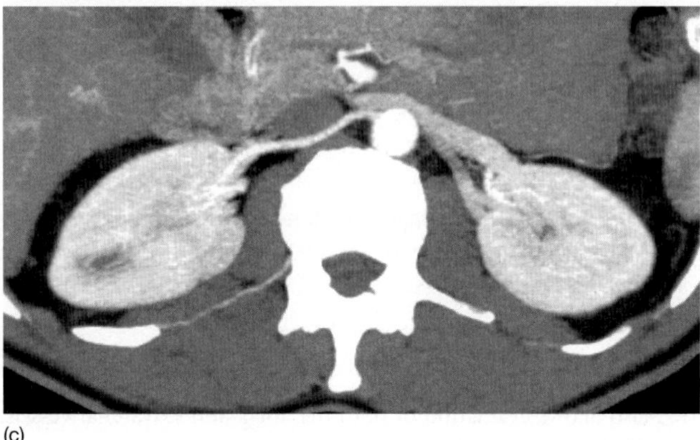

(c)

Fig. 2 CTA reconstruction in MIP in the coronal (a) and axial planes (b) and (c). (a) Coronal oblique reformat confirms the presence of two renal arteries, the main one rising from the usual anterior-lateral wall of the aorta, the accessory one rising 2 cm below. (b) and (c) Axial MIP reformat on the main (b) and accessory (c) RA, ruling out the diagnosis of RAS.

signal) and direct visualization of the mute RA, which is the only way to differentiate RA occlusion from tight RAS associated with severe downstream repercussions. The presence of flow within intrarenal arteries (tardus–parvus waveforms) is due to the development of collateral blood supply. The lack of intrarenal arterial flow could result from limited sensitivity of CDUS to reduced flow.

At MRA and CTA, the initial segment of the RA is not opacified during both arterial and delayed scanning. The diagnosis can be difficult because these two techniques overestimate the degree of stenosis. On MRA, the lack of signals is usual in severe RAS.

Strategy (see also Chapter 9.7)

The role of screening is to detect a RAS that can benefit from revascularization by means of a non-invasive tool (Fig. 4). CDUS is a useful and efficient first step imaging modality, provided that an experienced operator is available, particularly in patients with impaired renal function that precludes the use of iodinated contrast agents (Hélénon *et al.* 1995; Ozbek *et al.* 1995). Technological improvements combined with ultrasound contrast agents have reduced the rate of technical failure to less than 5 per cent for the assessment of main RA. MRA is indicated in patients with technically insufficient CDUS and high risk of RAS, or when angiography is contraindicated (renal failure, severe allergy to iodinated contrast medium). In practice, the use of MRA has three limitations: patient tolerance, low availability, and high cost. With the absence of contraindication to iodinated contrast medium, CTA is an alternative to CDUS and MRA, with a higher availability and a lower cost than MRI, particularly when the examination is technically inadequate or when no experienced operator is available. The role of ACE inhibitor scintigraphy remains controversial (Oliva *et al.* 1998). Today, it is the best test to diagnose functional RAS when the relationship between stenosis and hypertension remains clinically doubtful and/or when indication to treat the stenosis is unclear. A similar approach using an ACE inhibitor is under development with CDUS and MRI (Grenier *et al.* 1996).

RA aneurysm

Causes of RA aneurysm include atherosclerosis, fibrodysplasia, neurofibromatosis, or Ehlers–Danlos syndrome. They are classified as saccular, fusiform, dissecting, and intrarenal types. They usually arise from a renal arterial branch or distally from the main RA. CDUS demonstrates an echo-lucent mass filled with colour Doppler signal. Spectral analysis shows a turbulent flow with a reverse component within the aneurysm but without the to-and-fro pattern.

In CT, suggestive circumlinear calcifications can be detected at the baseline. Contrast-enhanced CT at the arterial phase demonstrates the flowing lumen. Multiple plane reconstruction is helpful to demonstrate the precise origin and relationship before surgical repair (Kawashima *et al.* 2000). Small aneurysms of the cortical arterial bed accompanying polyarteritis nodosa cannot be detected. MRA can also detect main RA aneurysms and is not artefacted by the wall calcifications. However, today MRI techniques suffer from insufficient resolution to analyse the precise relationship of the aneurysm to the main RA and its branches.

The RA false aneurysm is an iatrogenic complication of surgical and percutaneous renal procedures. The flowing cavity arises from the injured artery without venous drainage. Ultrasound shows a hypoechoic round-shaped mass located within the renal parenchyma that is filled with colour signal on CDUS. Spectral analysis obtained at the level of the communicating channel demonstrates a typical to-and-fro sign which reflects both systolic feeding arterial flow and diastolic draining arterial flow. At CTA, the false aneurysm appears as a contrast filling pouch.

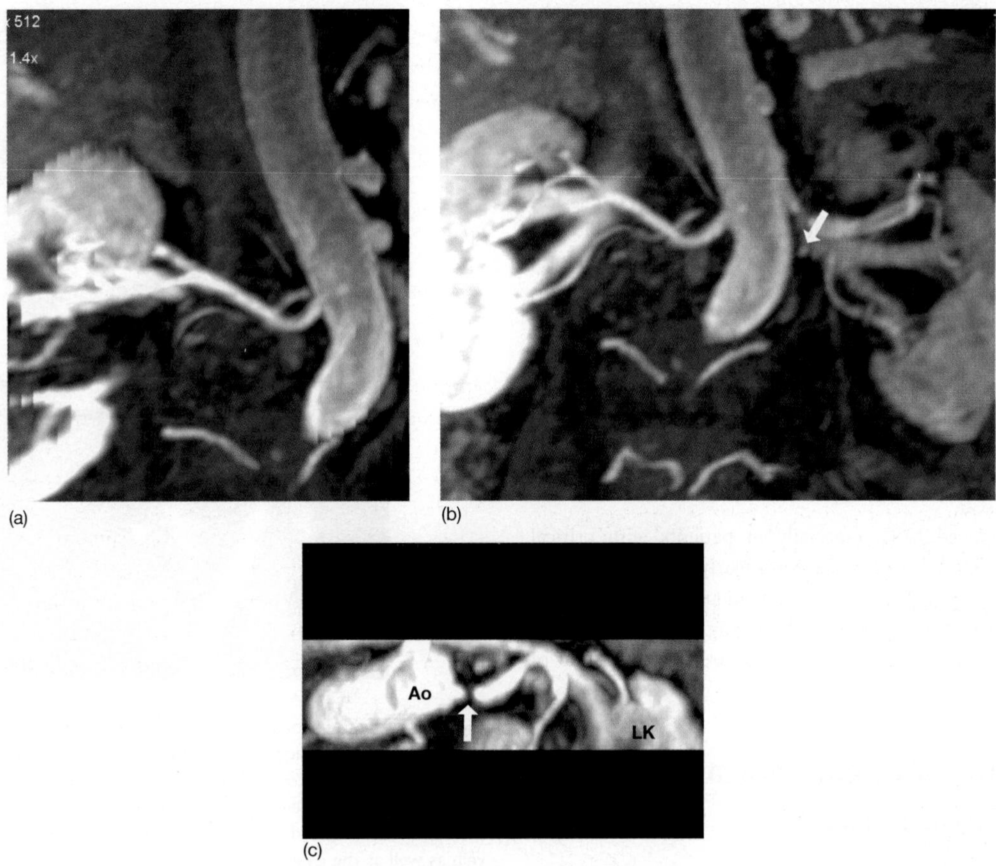

Fig. 3 MRA with MIP reconstructions in coronal (a) and (b) and axial plane (c). (a) Normal aspect of the right RA. (b) Significant RAS on the left side, with postostium disappearance of the signals (arrow). (c) Axial reformat on the left RAS (Ao: aorta, LK: left kidney, arrow showing the RAS).

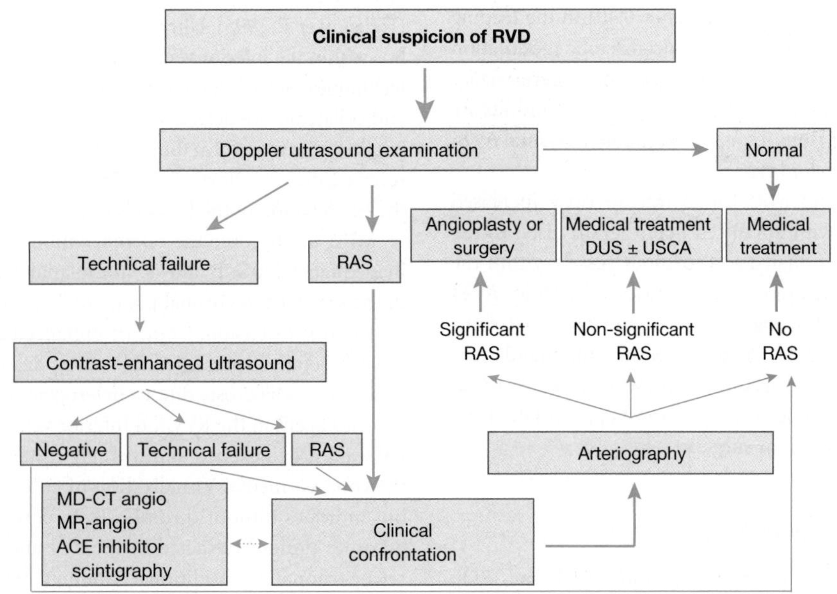

Fig. 4 Diagnostic algorithm in suspected renovascular disease.

Renal peripheral infarction

Renal infarction is mostly due to the embolism mechanism in patients with cardiovascular diseases and RA spontaneous dissection. At CDUS, segmental infarcts appear as hypoechoic areas with complete loss of Doppler signals. Although CDUS is a valuable method in the detection of renal allograft necrosis (Hélénon *et al.* 1992), it is less accurate for the diagnosis of perfusion defects in native kidneys because of their deep location. Ultrasound contrast agents are helpful in improving the performance of CDUS in case of technical problems and/or a small infarct size.

Contrast-enhanced CT easily demonstrates the presence of renal infarction, as a wedge-shaped non-enhancing area typically associated with a subcapsular enhanced rim of cortex. The size of parenchymal loss depends on both the distribution of the occluded artery and the collateral circulation. The infarcted parenchyma starts to shrink and will leave a cortical scar.

Gadolinium-enhanced MRI, especially in patients with critical renal failure, is also a modality of choice particularly when early accurate diagnosis is clinically required. The infarcted area exhibits a slight increase in signal intensity in $T2$-weighted imaging and is hypointense in $T1$-weighted imaging. Postcontrast findings are similar to that of CT features.

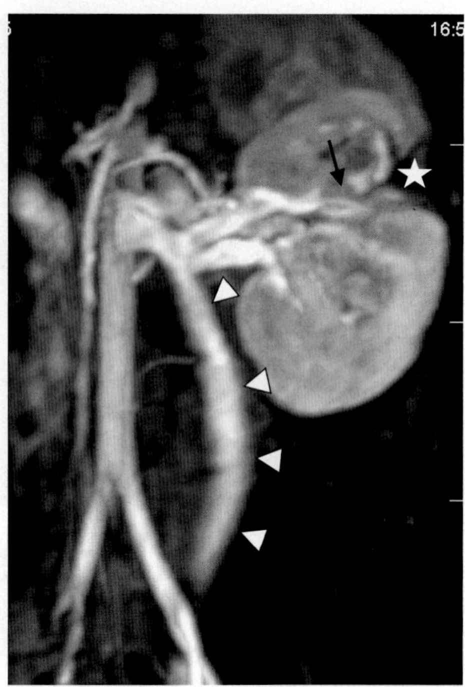

Fig. 5 MRA with coronal MIP reconstructions, in a 46-year-old woman with severe hypertension starting after surgery for a small renal cell carcinoma (tumourectomy). The defect corresponding to the ablation of the renal tumour is well seen (star). A large vein rises from the deep side of the tumourectomy bed at the junction with the sinus (arrow). The left renal vein as well as the ovarian vein, are enlarged in which flow is inverted (arrow heads). These are typical features of a postsurgical AV fistula. The diagnosis was confirmed by angiography.

Posttraumatic and congenital arteriovenous disorders

Arteriovenous (AV) fistulas result in most cases from a vascular injury (trauma, surgery, biopsy, nephrostomy, and nephrolithotomy for calculus extraction). Congenital AV malformation (AVM) is a rare and usually asymptomatic disease. CDUS appears to be the only non-invasive modality enabling the detection of postbiopsy AV fistulas. Such lesions produce local tissue vibration from flow turbulence detected on CDUS by a perivascular artefact (Hélénon *et al.* 1995; Ozbek *et al.* 1995). Typically, spectral analysis shows accelerated and highly turbulent flow at the site of the AV shunt, increased flow velocities with marked decrease of RI measurements (<0.40) in the feeding artery and increased flow velocities with systolic–diastolic modulation in the draining vein. Congenital AVM also generate a perivascular artefact at the site of the AV shunt at CDUS. Large vascular conduits are also detected within the renal sinus in cases of pseudoaneurysmal AVM whereas they are not in the cirsoid type.

Contrast-enhanced CT and MRI can detect an early increased venous drainage associated with a reduced nephrogram distal to the AV fistula (Fig. 5). A focus of dilated and tortuous vessels within the deep parenchyma can be demonstrated in cases of cirsoid AVM whereas a large aneurysmal flowing conduit within the renal sinus is associated with saccular AVM. Angiography is still mandatory, especially when colour Doppler suggests the presence of an AVM, to establish the final diagnosis and determine the most appropriate treatment (transcatheter embolization or surgery).

Renal vein thrombosis

Thrombosis in medical disease (such as nephrotic syndrome, SLE, hypercoagulopathy, dehydration) should be distinguished from tumour thrombosis (in renal cell carcinoma, transitional cell carcinoma, or adrenal carcinoma). CDUS appears to be particularly useful in the diagnosis of RV thrombosis since it provides in most cases an accurate non-invasive assessment of the RVs in patients with impaired renal function. The diagnosis of RV thrombosis requires identification of the enlarged and echogenic vein with no flow or peripheral flow with CDUS (Hélénon *et al.* 1995). Ultrasound also evaluates the extent of the thrombus within the inferior vena cava, particularly using non-linear imaging techniques. Segmental and interlobar vein blood flow can be inverted, and collaterals are detected in the retroperitoneum. Spectral analysis of renal arteries is useful at the early stage showing increased RI values (with reversed diastolic flow). Contrast-enhanced ultrasound is useful when the examination of the RVs fails due to poor anatomical conditions.

MRA has become the reference modality in cases with technically inadequate CDUS. It allows multiplanar reconstructions, particularly in the sagittal and coronal planes to improve the evaluation of the RV thrombosis extension. Contrast-enhanced CT is also useful when the renal function is preserved. However, delayed acquisition is required to avoid misdiagnosis due to heterogeneous mixing of the iodinated contrast agent in the RVs and inferior vena cava. At the early stage, the RV walls are thickened and strongly enhanced after administration of the contrast media. Visualization of enhancement within the thrombus indicates tumour thrombosis. In chronic RV thrombosis, the RV becomes thinner retracted to the clot and collaterals are seen in the retroperitoneum. Additional findings include enlargement of the kidney, oedema in the renal sinus and perirenal space, and coarse striations of the nephrogram.

References

Claudon, M., Plouin, P. F., Baxter, G. M., Rohban, T., and Maniez-Devos, D. (2000). Renal arteries in patients at risk of renal arterial stenosis: multicenter evaluation of the echo-enhancer SH U 508A at color and spectral Doppler US. *Radiology* **214**, 739–746.

De Cobelli, F., Venturini, M., Vanzulli, A., Sironi, S., Salvioni, M., Angeli, E., Scifo, P., Garancini, M. P., Quartagno, R., Bianchi, G., and Del Maschio, A. (2000). Renal arterial stenosis: prospective comparison of color Doppler US and breath-hold, three-dimensional, dynamic, gadolinium-enhanced MR angiography. *Radiology* **214**, 373–380.

Gilfeather, M., Yoon, H. C., Siegelman, E. S., Axel, L., Stolpen, A. H., Shlansky-Goldberg, R. D., Baum, R. A., Soulen, M. C., and Schnall, M. D. (1999). Renal artery stenosis: evaluation with conventional angiography versus gadolinium-enhanced MR angiography. *Radiology* **210**, 367–372.

Grenier, N., Trillaud, H., Combe, C., Douws, C., Jeandot, J., and Gosse, Ph. (1996). Diagnosis of renovascular hypertension with captopril-sensitized dynamic MR of the kidney: feasability and comparison with scintigraphy. *American Journal of Roentgenology* **166**, 835–843.

Hélénon, O. *et al.* (1992). Gd-Dota-enhanced MR imaging and color Doppler US of renal allograft necrosis. *Radiographics* **12**, 21–33.

Hélénon, O. *et al.* (1995). Color Doppler US of renovascular disease in native kidneys. *Radiographics* **15**, 833–854.

Kaate, R., Beek, F. J., de Lange, E. E., van Leeuwen, M. S., Smits, H. F., van der Ven, P. J., Beutler, J. J., and Mali, W. P. (1997). Renal artery stenosis: detection and quantification with spiral CT angiography versus optimized digital subtraction angiography. *Radiology* **205**, 121–127.

Kawashima, A., Sandler, C. M., Ernst, R. D., Tamm, E. P., Goldman, S. M., and Fishman, E. K. (2000). CT evaluation of renovascular disease. *Radiographics* **20**, 1321–1340.

Kim, T. S. *et al.* (1998). Renal artery evaluation: comparison of spiral CT angiography to intra-arterial DSA. *Journal of Vascular Interventional Radiology* **9**, 553–559.

Kliewer, M. A. *et al.* (1993). Renal artery stenosis: analysis of Doppler waveform parameters and tardus–parvus pattern. *Radiology* **189**, 779–787.

Miralles, M., Cairols, M., Cotillas, J., Gimenez, A., and Santiso, A. (1996). Value of Doppler parameters in the diagnosis of renal artery stenosis. *Journal of Vascular Surgery* **23**, 428–435.

Oliva, V. L., Soulez, G., Lesage, D., Nicolet, V., Roy, M. C., Courteau, M., Froment, D., Rene, P. C., Therasse, E., and Carignan, L. (1998). Detection of renal artery stenosis with Doppler sonography before and after administration of captopril: value of early systolic rise. *American Journal of Roentgenology* **170**, 169–175.

Ozbek, S. S., Memis, A., Killi, R., Karaca, E., Kabasakal, C., and Mir, S. (1995). Image-directed and color Doppler ultrasonography in the diagnosis of postbiopsy fistulas of native kidneys. *Journal of Clinical Ultrasound* **23**, 239–242.

Schwerk, W. B., Restrepo, I. K., Stellwaag, M., and Klose, K. J. and Schade-Brittinger C. (1994) Renal artery stenosis: grading with image-directed Doppler US evaluation of renal resistive index. *Radiology* **190**, 785–790.

1.6.2.iii Renal biopsy—procedure and complications

Claudio Ponticelli

The aim of the biopsy procedure is to provide a sample of kidney tissue of good quality and size to allow a correct histological interpretation while not causing severe complications to the patient.

Percutaneous needle core biopsy is, by far, the most frequently used technique. Open renal biopsy or transjugular renal biopsy have been proposed for few selected cases in which percutaneous biopsy is contraindicated.

Procedure

Percutaneous renal biopsy

The choice of the technique and the needle is important. Until a few years ago, percutaneous renal biopsy was performed by using hand-driven disposable trucut needles of 14 gauge. A significant advance has come in the shape of automated biopsy guns. Cutting needles are similar to the trucut but advancement of the needle is obtained by triggering the spring-loaded mechanisms. Automated devices have several advantages, including easier training of the operator, less chance of crush artefact of the core, less time for which the needle remains in the kidney, and less risk of laceration in the tissue.

A number of different needle sizes are available for percutaneous kidney biopsy. The most commonly used gauges range from 14 to 18. Larger needles may obtain renal samples of sufficient size but may expose the patient to a higher risk of complications, while thinner needles may have the opposite advantages and drawbacks.

Few studies have compared standard 14-gauge needles with spring-loaded, smaller-diameter needles. A greater number of glomeruli per core was observed in the 14-gauge cores than in the 18-gauge cores (Doyle *et al.* 1994), but the rates of adequate biopsies were similar (Riehl *et al.* 1994) or even higher (Cozens *et al.* 1992) with the automated smaller needles. A prospective randomized trial of three different sizes of core-cutting needles for renal transplant biopsy using a semiautomated gun showed that the larger needle provided more tissue and glomeruli but were associated with more pain (Nicholson *et al.* 2000). Many nephrologists are now using 16-gauge needles as a compromise between the need of a sufficient size of tissue and the need of clinical safety. Adequate quantity of tissue for diagnosis may be obtained with this needle size in 98.9 per cent of biopsies either in native or in transplanted kidneys (Chan *et al.* 2000).

The biopsy of a native kidney is done with the patient in a prone position upon a firmly rolled sheet compressing the upper abdomen and lower ribs and fixing the kidney. The lower pole of the kidney is chosen for biopsy as it is furthest away from the renal pelvis and large renal vessels and it falls in a natural anatomical triangle where the kidney is almost subcutaneous. The biopsy is generally performed on the left kidney to reduce the risk of inadvertently passing the needle through a major renal artery or vein.

The lower pole is usually localized by ultrasonography. Ultrasound can be exploited to perform the biopsy under continuous real-time guidance, either by a needle guide attached to the probe or by free

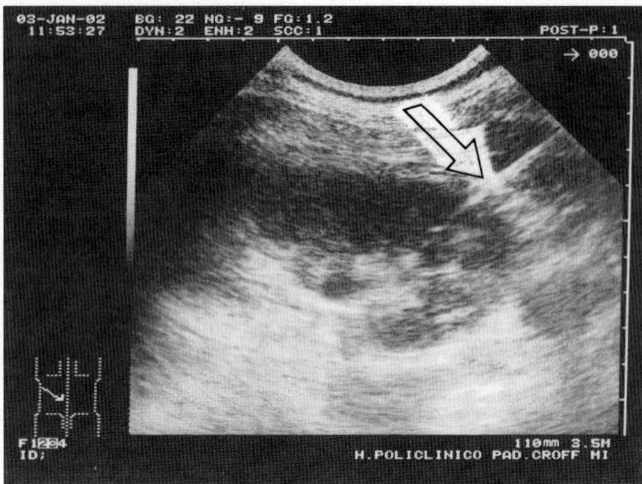

Fig. 1 Biopsy needle entering the lower pole of the kidney (real-time ultrasound).

hand introduction of the needle, which is continuously visualized by the transducer (Fig. 1). A few centres now use real-time computed tomography rather than ultrasonography as a guide for biopsy.

After local anaesthesia, a small incision is made through the skin. The biopsy needle, either mounted on a biopsy gun or driven by hand, is advanced to the renal capsule under ultrasound control in order to avoid the calyceal system and large vessels. The patient is invited to breathe deeply in order to follow the movements of the kidney through the movements of the needle. Then, the patient is asked to hold the breath so that the kidney remains firm. The gun is then fired and the needle withdrawn. After biopsy has been done, the specimen is checked under a dissection microscope or stereo lens to ascertain if there is cortical tissue. Two specimens containing cortical tissue are generally required to obtain adequate material for light, immunofluorescence, and electron microscopy.

For transplanted kidneys the technique is the same. However, the patient is in a supine position. The area chosen for biopsy should be away from the hilum. Real-time ultrasound scanning is necessary not only to localize and orient the position of the transplanted kidney but also to exclude the possible presence of intestinal loops which can rarely be placed on top of the graft.

Open renal biopsy

When it is considered that percutaneous biopsy involves an undue risk, an open surgical renal biopsy can be considered. This technique allows accurate haemostasis and can provide an adequate specimen of the renal cortex. The use of a needle is advisable to avoid crushing artefacts. Laparascopic retroperitoneal biopsy has also been used in difficult cases (Gupta *et al.* 2000; Jackman and Bishoff 2000).

Unfortunately, as patients selected for open biopsy are at risk, severe haemorrhagic complications are not unusual even with open renal biopsy.

Transjugular renal biopsy

A novel technique of renal biopsy through the internal jugular vein has been proposed for patients with bleeding disorders or other contraindications to renal biopsy (Mal *et al.* 1992). The technique appears to be safe and effective in patients with advanced liver disease as well (Sam *et al.* 2001). In a large comparative study it was found that the use of transjugular biopsy provided diagnostic yield and safety similar to those of percutaneous renal biopsy (Cluzel *et al.* 2000).

Renal biopsy in childhood

Renal biopsy may be a difficult procedure in children. In the past, general anaesthesia and open renal biopsy were largely used. Today, however, intravenous sedation and percutaneous renal biopsy represent the preferred procedure for most children. Intravenous administration of benzodiazepine, midazolam, ketamine, or Pethco (pethidine, chlorpromazine, and promethazine) can provide effective deep sedation in childhood, without the need of ventilation or intubation. Ultrasound-guided biopsy with automated devices can give a greater yield of diagnostic tissue and reduce the risk of severe complications when compared with non-automated methods (Feneberg *et al.* 1998; Simckes *et al.* 2000). Microinvasive 18-gauge, automated, spring-loaded disposable needles are generally used in infants. After the procedure, the site of biopsy is compressed for several minutes.

In children with morbid obesity, solitary kidney, anticoagulation, multiple bilateral renal cysts or other relative or absolute contraindications to a percutaneous procedure, laparoscopic renal biopsy proved to be a safe and effective technique (Gimenez *et al.* 1998).

Pre- and postoperative care

Preparation for biopsy

Ultrasonography is necessary before biopsy to know the size and the localization of the kidneys, as well as the possible presence of morphological abnormalities, cysts, or neoplasms.

In hypertensive patients, blood pressure should be lowered to normal values by adequate therapy. Aspirin and non-steroidal anti-inflammatory drugs should be stopped at least 4–5 days before biopsy to avoid their influence on platelet function. Coagulation disorders should be excluded by determining the blood platelet count, the partial thromboplastin time, and the prothrombin time. However, the most reliable haemostatic test in renal patients is the bleeding time, which reflects the platelet plug formation at the transect ends of blood vessels and is an indirect indicator of the platelet function. Normal values range between 3 and 7 min. Bleeding time is generally prolonged in uraemia. A transient shortening of bleeding time can be obtained by the infusion of desmopressin (DDAVP), which increases factor-VIII coagulant activity in uraemic patients (Mannucci *et al.* 1983). Infusion over 30 min of 0.3 μg/kg body weight diluted in 50 ml of physiological saline may normalize the bleeding time for 4–8 h in most uraemic patients.

Postoperative care

Following the biopsy of a native kidney, the patient must remain in the prone position upon a rolled sheet or pillow, for at least 1 h to improve compressive haemostasis. Following the biopsy of a transplanted kidney, firm pressure is applied to the needle entry site for 5 min. In our institution patients are instructed to remain under bed rest for 24 h. Blood pressure, pulse rate, and urine samples are monitored frequently. Even in apparently uncomplicated cases we check haematocrit and ultrasonography the day after biopsy.

Complications

Renal biopsy is an invasive procedure which may expose the patient to the risks of several complications particularly in patients with renal failure. In a review of 20 series including 14,492 percutaneous renal biopsies, Parrish (1992) found that 0.3 per cent of the procedures were followed by surgery and death related to the biopsy was observed in 0.12 per cent. The need for surgery or death were not reported in more recent series (Fraser and Fairley 1995; Hergesell *et al.* 1998), but the impression is that the rate of minor complications has not been reduced by the use of automated biopsy guns and real-time ultrasonography. About 90 per cent of complications can be identified within 24 h from the procedure. Shorter periods of observation may miss an early diagnosis in a consistent number of cases (Whittier and Korbet 2004).

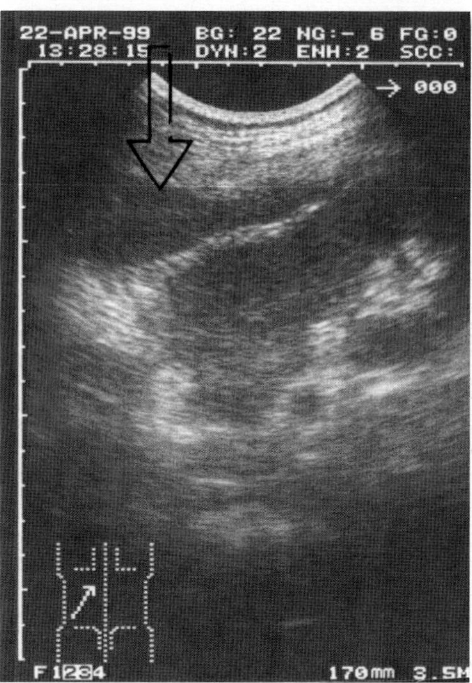

Fig. 2 Postbiopsy perirenal haematoma (ultrasound).

Haematuria

Transient microscopic haematuria virtually occurs in all patients. In recent reports, gross haematuria has been reported to range between 2 and 5 per cent (Fraser *et al.* 1995; Hergesell *et al.* 1998; Tang *et al.* 2002). Bleeding frequently stops within a few hours but it may be severe and prolonged. Macroscopic haematuria may be associated with clots, colicky pain, urinary obstruction, and in the most severe cases with haemorrhagic shock. Puncture of the renal calyceal system, large vessel damage, aneurysms, and arteriovenous fistulas are the main causes.

Strict bed rest is recommended in patients with gross haematuria. High urine flow rates may help to prevent urinary obstruction by clots. Angiography and the embolization of the bleeding artery are needed in prolonged, severe haemorrhage.

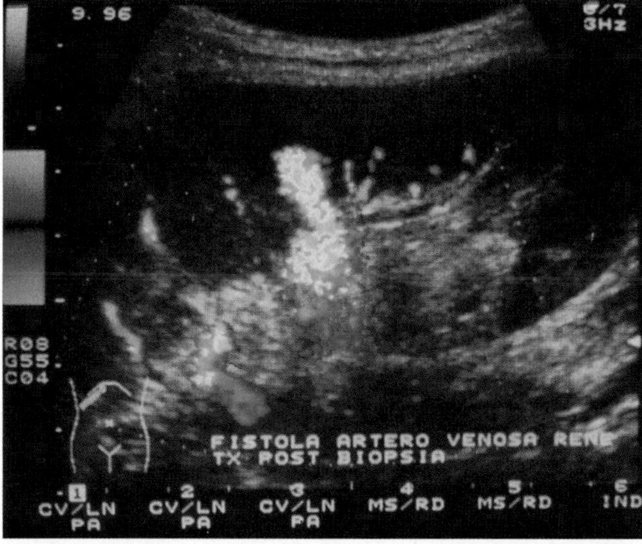

Fig. 3 Huge postbiopsy arteriovenous fistula at echocolour Doppler.

Perirenal haemorrhage

The incidence of clinically significant haematomas ranges between 2 and 3 per cent (Mendelssohn and Cole 1995; Hergesell *et al.* 1998). Perirenal bleeding usually occurs immediately after biopsy, but can be delayed for some days or even weeks. Loin tenderness and consistent decrease in haematocrit occur in patients with large perirenal haematomas. Computerized tomography and/or ultrasonography can be helpful in supporting the diagnosis, localizing the haematoma, and following its outcome (Fig. 2). Severe anaemia, impairment of renal function due to compressive ischaemia, and perinephric abscesses are the most severe complications of haematomas. In most cases bed rest is sufficient, but in more severe cases surgical evacuation of the haematoma and local compressive haemostasis or repair of capsular lacerations are needed.

Arteriovenous fistulas

This complication can occur in 10–15 per cent of patients examined by angiography or colour Doppler (Fig. 3). However, in most patients an arteriovenous fistula is asymptomatic and heals spontaneously within some months. Other patients present persistent haematuria, hypertension, or high-output cardiac failure. A non-invasive diagnosis of arteriovenous fistula can be reached by colour Doppler sonography. In severe cases the occlusion of the fistula can be obtained by arterial embolization.

Aneurysms

The formation of arteriolar aneurysms is a rare complication of renal biopsy. The involvement of arcuate arteries may be responsible for arterial hypertension and/or gross haematuria.

Other complications

Inadvertent puncture of the spleen, pancreas, liver, intestine as well as laceration of renal, mesenteric, and subcostal arteries have been reported as exceptional complications in the past. Today, with the use of ultrasonography it is almost impossible for such complications to occur with an experienced operator.

Rare cases of oligoanuria may occur as a result of posthaemorrhagic hypotension or of the compression by a perirenal haematoma.

References

Chan, R., Common, A. A., and Marcuzzi, D. (2000). Ultrasound-guided renal biopsy: experience using an automated core biopsy system. *Canadian Association of Radiologists Journal* **51**, 107–113.

Cluzel, P. *et al.* (2000). Transjugular versus percutaneous renal biopsy for the diagnosis of parenchymal diseases: comparison of sampling effectiveness and complications. *Radiology* **215**, 689–693.

Cozens, N. J. A., Muchison, J. T., Allan, P. L., and Winney, R. J. (1992). Conventional 15 G needle technique for renal biopsy compared with ultrasound-guided spring-loaded 18 G needle biopsy. *British Journal of Radiology* **65**, 594–597.

Doyle, A. J., Gregory, M. C., and Terreros, D. A. (1994). Percutaneous native renal biopsy: comparison of a 1.2 mm spring-driven system with a traditional 2-mm hand-driven system. *American Journal of Kidney Diseases* **23**, 498–503.

Feneberg, R. *et al.* (1998). Percutaneous renal biopsy in children: a 27-year experience. *Nephron* **79**, 438–446.

Fraser, I. R. and Fairley, K. F. (1995). Renal biopsy as an outpatient procedure. *American Journal of Kidney Diseases* **25**, 876–878.

Gimenez, L. F. *et al.* (1998). Laparoscopic renal biopsy. *Kidney International* **54**, 525–529.

Gupta, M. *et al.* (2000). Laparoscopic-assisted renal biopsy: an alternative to open approach. *American Journal of Kidney Diseases* **36**, 636–639.

Hergesell, O. *et al.* (1998). Safety of ultrasound-guided percutaneous renal biopsy—retrospective analysis of 1090 consecutive cases. *Nephrology, Dialysis, Transplantation* **13**, 975–977.

Jackman, S. V. and Bishoff, J. T. (2000). Laparoscopic retroperitoneal renal biopsy. *Journal of Endourology* **14**, 833–838.

Mal, F. *et al.* (1992). The diagnostic yield of transjugular renal biopsy. Experience in 200 cases. *Kidney International* **41**, 445–449.

Mannucci, P. M. *et al.* (1983). Deamino-8-D-arginine vasopressin shortens the bleeding time in uremia. *New England Journal of Medicine* **308**, 8–12.

Mendelssohn, D. C. and Cole, E. H. (1995). Outcome of percutaneous kidney biopsy, including those of solitary native kidneys. *American Journal of Kidney Diseases* **26**, 580–585.

Nicholson, M. L. *et al.* (2000). A prospective randomized trial of three different sizes of core-cutting needle for renal transplant biopsy. *Kidney International* **58**, 390–395.

Parrish, A. E. (1992). Complications of percutaneous renal biopsy: a review of 37 years experience. *Clinical Nephrology* **38**, 135–141.

Riehl, J. *et al.* (1994). Percutaneous renal biopsy: comparison of manual and automated puncture techniques with native and transplanted kidney. *Nephrology, Dialysis, Transplantation* **9**, 1568–1574.

Sam, R. *et al.* (2001). Transjugular renal biopsy in patients with liver disease. *American Journal of Kidney Diseases* **37**, 1304–1307.

Simckes, A. M., Blowey, D. L., Gyves, K. M., and Alon, U. S. (2000). Success and safety of same-day kidney biopsy in children and adolescents. *Pediatric Nephrology* **14**, 946–952.

Tang, S. *et al.* (2002). Free-hand, ultrasound guided percutaneous renal biopsy: experience from a single operator. *European Journal of Radiology* **41**, 65–69.

Whittier, W. L. and Korbet, S. (2004). Timing of complications in percutaneous renal biopsy. *Journal of the American Society of Nephrology* **15**, 142–147.

1.6.2.iv Renal masses

Olivier Hélénon, Jean-Michel Correas, and Arnaud Méjean

Computed tomography (CT) is the gold standard for detecting and characterizing renal masses and staging renal cell carcinoma (RCC). Ultrasonography plays a key role in screening renal masses. With the exception of typical renal cysts, most renal masses remain indeterminate by ultrasonography. However, ultrasonography may provide additional diagnostic information over CT in selected cases among renal masses that remain equivocal at CT. Moreover, ultrasonography is the only available intraoperative tool that may help remove a small tumour during renal parenchymal sparing surgery. Magnetic resonance imaging (MRI) also helps in characterizing indeterminate masses in selected cases and is deemed to be a substitute gold standard in patients with severe contraindication to iodinated contrast agents especially those with significant renal failure or at risk of contrast medium nephrotoxicity.

Detection of renal masses

Although, renal CT using a dedicated protocol, is the gold standard, most renal masses are incidentally detected on abdominal ultrasonography or CT. One of the most relevant clinical benefits of ultrasonography is the increased early detection of RCCs. Up to 83 per cent of asymptomatical renal tumours are incidentally detected at ultrasonography (Siemer *et al.* 2000). At initial screening, the tumour is significantly smaller (5.5 cm) and at a lower local tumour stage than those depicted in symptomatic patients (7.8 cm) (Siemer *et al.* 2000).

Characterization of renal masses

Renal masses include three categories with respect to the size and the gross architecture of the lesion: indeterminate very small masses, cystic, and solid renal masses.

Indeterminate very small masses

Very small lesions of less than 10 mm in diameter usually remain unclassified because of the partial volume effect that prevents accurate CT attenuation measurement (Fig. 1). With the exception of patients at risk of renal tumours such as familial-hereditary renal tumour disease (von Hippel–Lindau, familial tubulopapillary RCC) and patients with history of removed RCC, such lesions in the general population are likely to be microcysts and do not require further workup.

If better characterization is needed, MRI may help demonstrate the fluid content of very small cysts (bright signal intensity on $T2$-weighted image) because of a higher contrast resolution compared to CT.

Cystic renal masses

Characterization of cystic masses relies on Bosniak's classification, which consists of four categories (Table 1) (Bosniak 1986): benign (category I) and minimally complicated cysts (II) (Figs 1 and 2); indeterminate cystic masses (III) including cystic tumours (Fig. 3) and complex cysts; cystic RCCs (IV) (Fig. 4). Category III often poses difficult diagnostic problems with cystic neoplasms, whereas categories II and IV are without doubt benign minimally complicated cysts and cystic/necrotic RCCs, respectively.

Category III complex cysts result mostly from intracystic haemorrhage or infection which can exhibit thick peripheral wall, irregularity, septations, and calcifications with or without peripheral postcontrast enhancement. High attenuation values within a cystic mass suggest haemorrhage within a benign cyst when the mass is of rather small size (<3 cm) with extension beyond the renal outline by at least a fourth of its circumference (in order that the lack of wall thickening can be confidently verified); with CT numbers higher than 50 HU, homogeneous, sharply marginated, either on pre- or postcontrast scans with no change after contrast enhancement (lack of enhancement) (Fig. 5).

Small RCCs with spontaneous high attenuation values (due to previous intratumoural haemorrhage or iron deposits) and small hypovascularized tumours (mostly tubulopapillary RCCs) with undetectable or only subtle postcontrast tumour tissue enhancement are rare conditions that can mimic a hyperdense complex cyst. Such pitfalls should be avoided using a strict CT scanning technique and making certain that the lesion meets all the above mentioned diagnostic criteria of hyperattenuating benign cysts.

A spontaneously isodense (>20, <50 HU) avascular (with no obvious postcontrast enhancement) mass should be viewed as a possible small hypovascularized tumour especially when the CT scanning technique is inadequate, and should prompt ultrasonographic examination or CT repeat examination. In ultrasonography, hyperdense cysts are typically anechoic in about 30–50 per cent of the cases. When ultrasonography or a technically appropriate CT scan are not conclusive, MRI may be indicated to demonstrate a homogeneous bright signal or fluid-iron level pattern within the lesion in both *T*1- and *T*2-weighted images. Such a typical pattern is encountered in about 50 per cent of haemorrhagic cysts. MRI can also be useful in

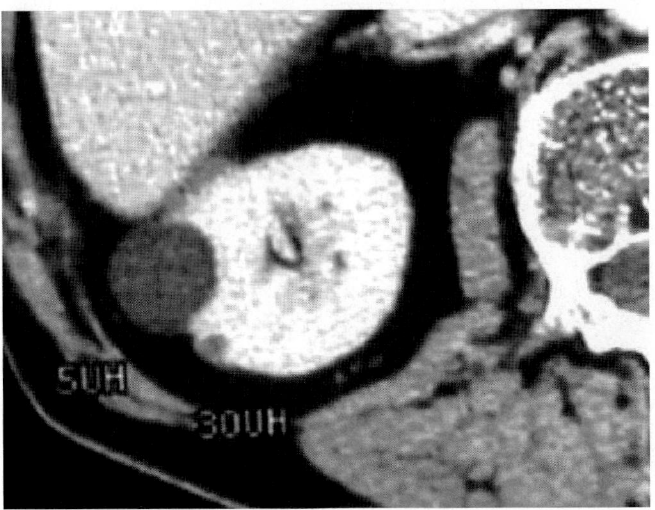

Fig. 1 Contrast-enhanced CT shows typical cortical cyst (type I according to Bosniak classification) with water attenuation values (5 HU) and indeterminate very small mass that exhibit equivocal CT attenuation measurements (30 HU).

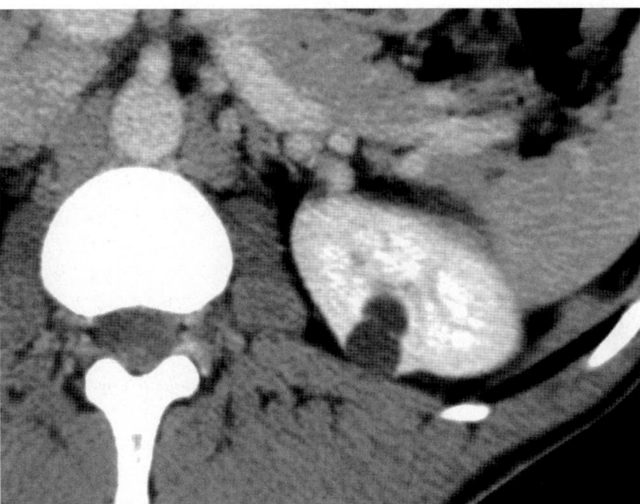

Fig. 2 Contrast-enhanced CT shows minimally complicated cortical cyst (type II according to Bosniak classification) containing a fine and smooth septum.

Table 1 CT-based classification of cystic renal masses (Bosniak 1986)

Category	Precontrast CT	Postcontrast CT	Diagnosis
I	Water attenuation (−10 to +20 HU) Homogeneous and sharp margins No wall, no septa, no calcification	No enhancement Homogeneous and sharp	Simple benign cyst
II	Water or high (50–100 HU) internal attenuation values (hyperdense cyst) Homogeneous and sharp margins One or two fine (<1 mm), smooth septa Delicate calcification	No enhancement Homogeneous and sharp	Mildly complicated cyst (haemorrhage, infection)
III	Inhomogeneous fluid (20–50 HU) Thick irregular calcification(s) Uniform wall thickening More numerous or thicker septa	Wall/septa enhancement	Complex benign cyst Multilocular cystic nephroma Cystic RCC Multilocular cystic RCC
IV	Inhomogeneous fluid content Thick irregular wall or septa Irregular margins, mural nodule	Solid enhancing tissue	Cystic/necrotic RCC Multilocular cystic RCC

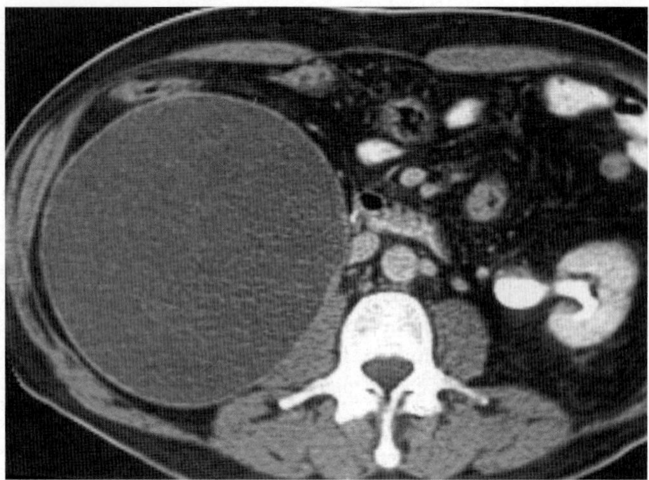

Fig. 3 Atypical cystic RCC. Post-contrast CT scan shows indeterminate type III right renal mass according to Bosniak classification with thick regular wall.

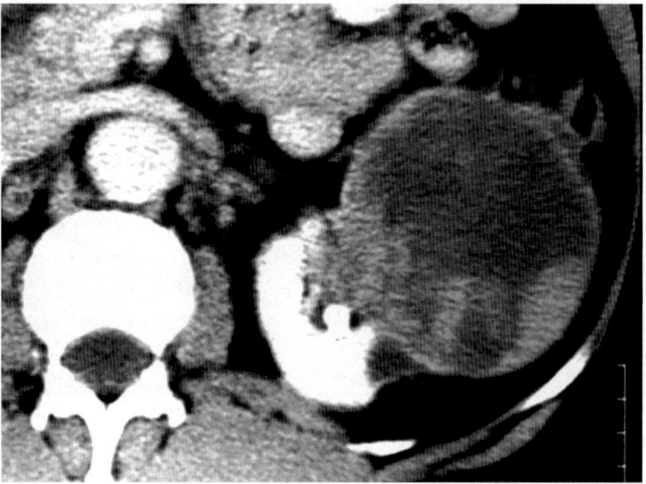

Fig. 4 Typical cystic RCC. Post-contrast CT scan shows type IV cystic renal mass with thick irregular wall and mural nodules consistent with a pseudocystic necrotic carcinoma.

demonstrating a minimal postcontrast enhancement in solid tumours with poor vascularity (tubulopapillary RCC) or within the wall of cystic RCCs (Tello *et al.* 2000).

Solid renal masses

The goals of imaging in characterizing solid renal tumours are: (a) to differentiate renal tumours from normal variants or pseudotumours that may mimic a neoplasm; (b) to differentiate benign from malignant renal tumours, especially angiomyolipoma (AML) from non-fatty renal tumours that should be removed. CT enables an accurate diagnosis of typical large necrotic RCCs and benign AMLs containing macroscopic fat tissue. Other tumours that do not exhibit typical CT features are indeterminate solid renal masses including atypical renal primary and secondary neoplasms and unusual inflammatory renal masses that can mimic renal neoplasm.

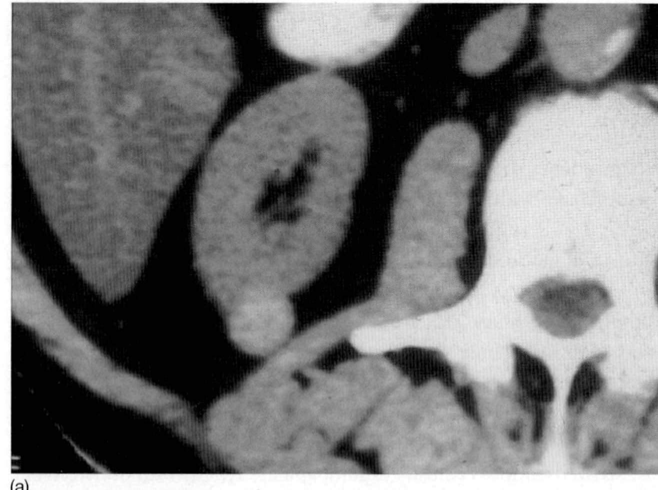

(a)

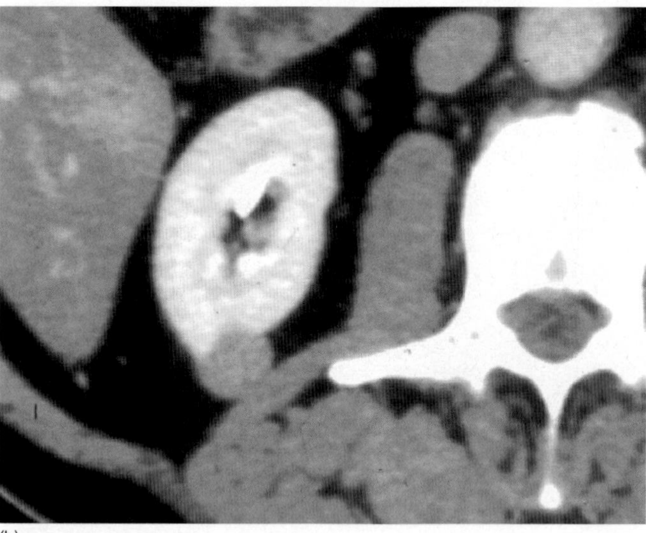

(b)

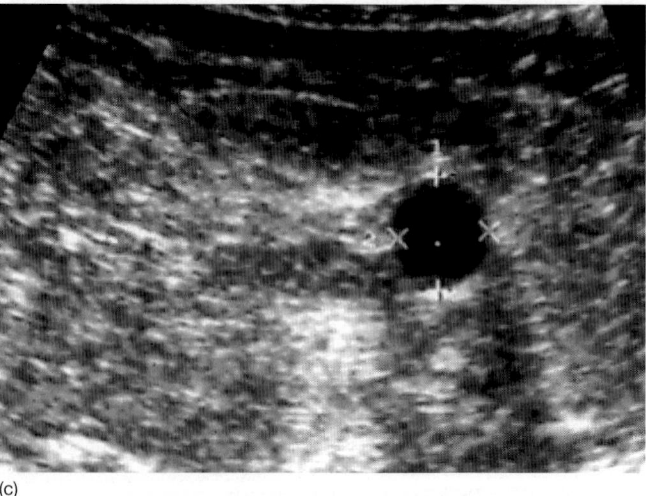

(c)

Fig. 5 Typical hyperattenuating renal cyst. Pre- (a) and post-contrast (b) CT scans show a small hyperattenuating (70 HU) homogeneous and sharp renal mass with no change after contrast enhancement. (c) Ultrasonography shows a typical anechoic appearance of the cyst.

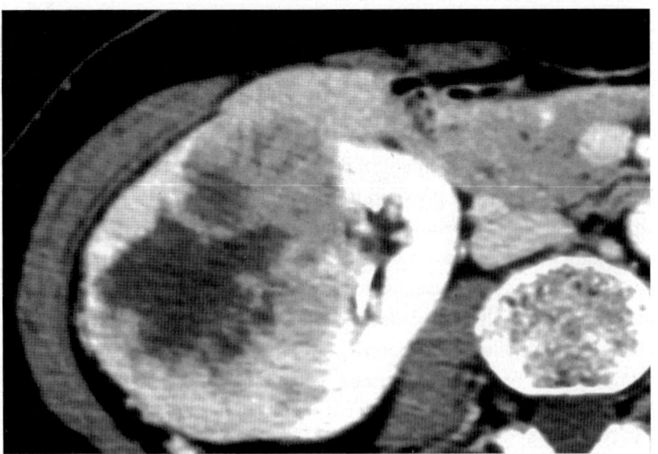

Fig. 6 Typical RCC of the right kidney. Contrast-enhanced CT shows a large heterogeneous renal tumour with intratumoural necrotic areas.

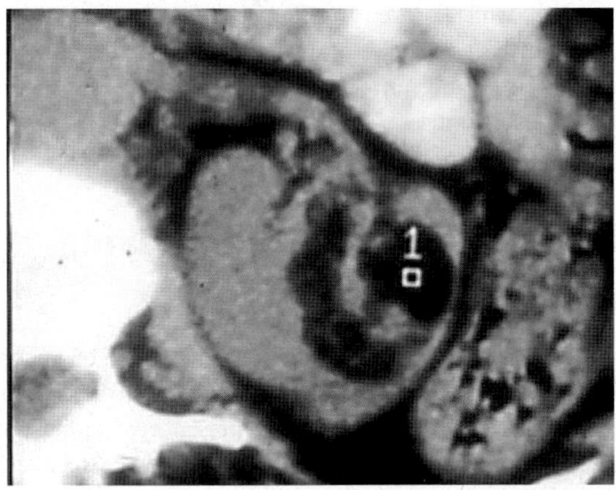

Fig. 7 Typical angiomyolipoma of the left kidney. Pre-contrast CT scan shows obvious fat attenuation values (−65 HU) within the lesion.

Typical large renal cell carcinoma

Large RCCs, typically, show a heterogeneous pattern due to intratumoural necrotic areas with early and marked tumour tissue enhancement on postcontrast scans, sometimes associated with scattered calcifications (Fig. 6). Although this finding does not contribute to a definitive diagnosis, it is highly suggestive of RCC and should lead to enlarged nephrectomy. On the other hand, the association between a large renal tumour and a finding that suggests a venous tumour invasion also strongly suggests malignancy and likely an RCC irrespective of the appearance of the lesion.

Typical angiomyolipoma

AML is the only benign tumour of the kidney that can be almost specifically diagnosed by imaging. The diagnosis relies on the detection of intratumoural fat which is characteristic of AML.

Presence of intratumoural areas of fat density (<−20 HU) on CT, which may require thin (≤5 mm) sections, is the key diagnostic feature of AML (Fig. 7). A varying amount of soft tissue is also visible and relates to the degree of enhancement of the lesion following administration of IV contrast. Ultrasonography typically shows a well defined, hyperechoic lesion. Although a markedly hyperechoic (isoechoic to renal sinus) lesion is highly suggestive of AML, it is not specific (about 30 per cent of small RCCs appear as a hyperechoic mass) and therefore requires CT confirmation. Contrary to earlier reports, echogenicity of AML does not seem to correlate with the amount of intratumoural fat (Hélénon *et al.* 1997). In a patient presenting with a renal mass, the evidence of a fat component within the lesion helps to rule out an RCC and avoid surgery in most cases. However, isolated observations do report the presence of fat in various types of renal neoplasms including Wilm's tumours, oncocytomas, liposarcomas, large RCCs invading perirenal fat, large RCCs with lipid-producing necrosis, and RCCs containing areas of osseous metaplasia (Hélénon *et al.* 1997).

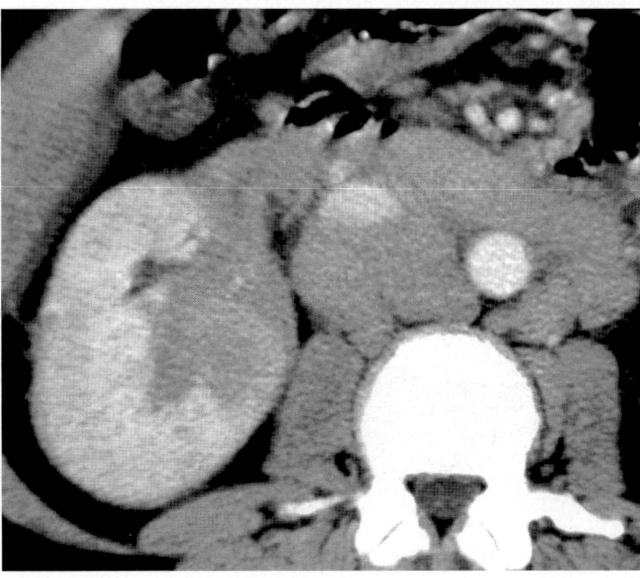

Fig. 8 Renal lymphoma of the right kidney. Post-contrast CT scan shows infiltrative renal mass associated with retroperitoneal lymph nodes involvement.

Indeterminate solid renal masses

The clinical history and some CT findings may help suggest the histopathological nature of an indeterminate solid mass in cases of large oncocytomas that may exhibit a stellate central scare; tubulopapillary RCCs with hypovascular behaviour, chronic or acute inflammatory lesions (focal acute pyelonephritis, chronic abscesses and xanthogranulomatous pyelonephritis), renal lymphoma, metastases, and multiple hereditary renal neoplasms (von Hippel–Lindau disease).

The current indications of fine needle ultrasonography- or CT-guided biopsies are multiple and/or bilateral tumours or infiltrative renal tumours associated with extrarenal manifestations that suggest renal metastases or lymphoma (Fig. 8).

Staging of renal cell carcinoma

Although CT remains the first choice modality to assess the local extension of RCC and lymph node involvement, MR can be used in

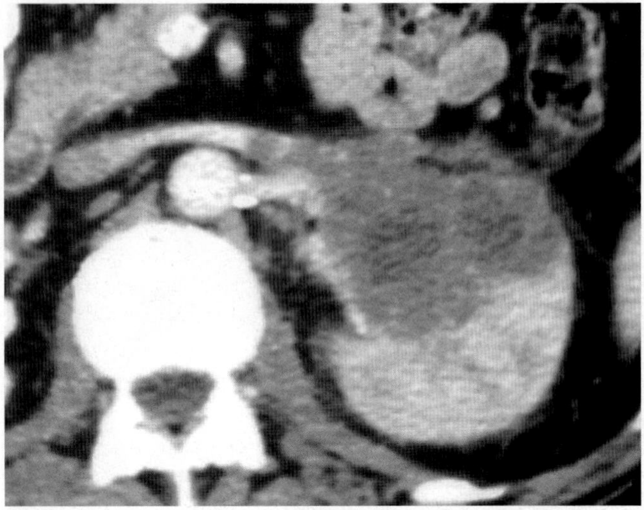

Fig. 9 Infiltrative RCC with left renal vein invasion. Contrast-enhanced CT scan shows an infiltrative tumour of the left kidney with tumour thrombus extension involving the proximal portion of the renal vein.

cases of a severe contraindication to iodinated contrast IV injection as previously mentioned. On the other hand, MRI is reported to be the most accurate modality for assessing venous tumour thrombus extension (Goldfarb *et al.* 1990). In clinical practice, CT and Doppler sonography are often combined primarily to assess the venous involvement of an RCC (Fig. 9). MRI is the modality of choice when CT and sonographic findings are inconclusive, particularly regarding the thrombus extent within the inferior vena cava. The second role of MR in this field consists in assessing neighbouring organ involvement when CT is equivocal, usually in cases in which a large tumour arising from the upper pole of the kidney extends towards the medial aspect of the spleen or the inferior aspect of the right lobe of the liver.

References

Bosniak, M. A. (1986). The current radiological approach to renal cyst. *Radiology* **158**, 1–10.

Goldfarb, D. A. *et al.* (1990). Magnetic resonance imaging for assessment of vena caval tumor thrombi: a comparative study with venacavography and computerized tomography scanning. *Journal of Urology* **144**, 1100–1104.

Hélénon, O. *et al.* (1997). Unusual fat-containing tumors of the kidney: a diagnostic dilemma. *Radiographics* **17**, 129–144.

Siemer, S. *et al.* (2000). Value of ultrasound in early diagnosis of renal cell carcinomas. *Urologe* **39**, 149–153.

Tello, R., Davidson, B. D., O'Malley, M., Fenlon, H., Thomson, K. R., Witte, D. J., and Harewood, L. (2000). MR imaging of renal masses interpreted on CT to be suspicious. *American Journal of Roentgenology* **174**, 1017–1022.

1.6.2.v Living donor workup

Claudio Ponticelli and Marco Cappelletti

The continuous improvement of the results of renal transplantation has allowed to extend the possibilities of transplantation to patients with advanced age or comorbid conditions, and this has further widened the discrepancy between a longer and longer waiting list and the limited possibility of offering a cadaveric kidney. On the other hand, in spite of the improved results with cadaveric renal transplants living donor transplantation still allows a superior graft survival, especially in the long-term, and has been recommended whenever possible by the European Best Practice Guidelines for Renal Transplantation (Berthoux *et al.* 2000). The data of the United Network for Organ Sharing (Gjertson and Cecka 2000) showed that the 10-year graft survival probability was 39 per cent for cadaveric kidneys, 50 per cent for kidneys from parents, 55 per cent for kidneys from spouses, 56 per cent for kidneys from siblings, and 69 per cent for kidneys from identical siblings. A further advantage of living donation is the possibility of realizing a preemptive transplantation, which proved to offer better results than transplants performed in dialysis patients (Mange *et al.* 2001). As a consequence, the use of related and unrelated living donors has progressively increased in most countries.

Evaluation of the potential living kidney donor

The workup of a potential living kidney donor should be as complete as possible: (a) to ensure that the donor is healthy with minimal risks from nephrectomy; (b) to exclude the presence of kidney disease; (c) to exclude the risk of transmitting disease to the recipient; and (d) to ascertain the separate function of the two kidneys and the absence of anatomical abnormalities which might threaten the success of transplantation.

The need for a thorough clinical work-up is further stressed by the fact that about 40 per cent of potential donors are excluded on immunological or clinical grounds (Saunders *et al.* 2000).

Medical evaluation (see also Section 13)

Several steps may be suggested to obtain a complete medical evaluation of the donor (Table 1).

1. Blood ABO compatibility between donor and recipients is usually the first analysis. Most transplant units tend to discard donors who are ABO incompatible with recipients although successful outcome may be obtained with transplants from ABO incompatible living donors (Ishida *et al.* 2000). The medical history must be carefully studied. Drug addicts and patients with cancer, hypertension, renal diseases, diabetes mellitus, or other systemic diseases with potential renal involvement usually preclude the donation (Table 2). Physical examination should uncover any potential cause of exclusion, such as hypertension without a good control of cardiovascular disease, pulmonary insufficiency, chronic infection, or malignancy.

Table 1 Main steps and non-invasive procedures for evaluation of potential living donors

(A)	ABO blood typing Medical history Physical examination
(B)	Chemistry: serum creatinine, urea, sodium, potassium, calcium, phosphorus, total protein albumin, glucose, cholesterol, triglycerides, liver enzymes, bilirubin Creatinine clearance (iothalamate when possible) Haematology: complete blood count Urine: urinalysis (with measurement of microalbuminuria) urine culture Hepatitis virus: HbsAg, HCV HIV
(C)	Electrocardiogram (optional echocardiography or cardiac scintigraphy) Chest radiograph (optional pulmonary function tests) Cytomegalovirus, Epstein–Barr herpes simplex, varicella-zoster, antibodies titres In females pregnancy tests, gynaecological examination when older than 40 years. In males, prostatic specific antigen when older than 50 years HLA typing Cross-match

Table 2 Exclusion criteria for living donation

Cardiovascular disease
Diabetes mellitus
Uncontrolled hypertension
Proteinuria > 300 mg/day
Creatinine clearance < 70 ml/min
Kidney stones
Multiple cysts
Sickle trait
Transmittable infections (including HIV, HBV, and HCV)
Malignancy
Pregnancy

2. As a second step, the donor's blood chemistry should be checked and urinalysis should be carried out to rule out the presence of renal diseases, liver diseases, or diabetes.
3. As a third step, the cardiorespiratory function should be evaluated, it should be assessed whether the donor is a carrier of potentially transmittable viruses, and the presence of malignancy should be excluded. The HLA histocompatibility between donor and recipient is usually checked. If a choice exists between several live donors with similar clinical characteristics, priority should be given to the donor with the lower number of HLA mismatches. However, good results can be obtained even when there is no compatibility at all, as in the case of spouses (Gjertson and Cecka 2000). Whether or not the recipient has preformed anti-HLA antibodies, a cross-match between the serum of the recipient and the lymphocytes of the donor is mandatory. A positive cross-match against T cells is a formal contraindication to transplant the kidney of particular donor to a particular recipient, the risk of hyperacute rejection being extremely elevated. More controversy exists about the prognostic significance of cross-match positivity against B cells, which is done by the flow cytometry technique. Large surveys reported that positive cross-match against B cells is associated with a poorer outcome of the graft (4–6 per cent) (Cho and Cecka 2001). However, a recent study showed that 77 per cent of B-cell cross-match positivity is not related to HLA antibodies and does not affect graft survival. In a minority of patients B-cell cross-match is associated with lower early but not long-term graft survival (Le Bas-Bernadet *et al.* 2003). Thus a positive B-cell cross-match does not necessarily contraindicate kidney transplantation.

The prognostic significance of positive cross-match with historical sera but negative with current sera has been debated. Some investigators reported a decreased graft survival both in sensitized (Speiser and Jeannet 1995) and in nonsensitized patients with a positive historical cross-match (Karpinski *et al.* 2002). Other studies showed that if antibodies are disappeared and only naive cytotoxic T cells are present a successful transplant may be feasible (van Kampen *et al.* 2002).

Imaging techniques

Imaging techniques are of paramount importance for the evaluation of the potential living donor. It is obviously necessary to ascertain the presence of two kidneys, to evaluate the separate function for each of them, to exclude renal abnormalities or malignancy, which preclude transplantation, and to assess the number and the state of the major renal vessels.

Renal ultrasonography is usually the first and simplest imaging investigation. It may show whether the kidneys are normal or whether there are abnormalities such as stones, hydronephrosis, a small kidney, etc. When possible, ultrasonography should be associated with echo colour Doppler which can show artery stenosis, arteriovenous fistula, aneurysms, or other abnormalities.

Renal sequential scintigraphy provides information about the separate function of the two kidneys and can show a possible hypoperfusion of one kidney.

In the past, many centres used intravenous pyelography to evaluate the urinary tract. Today this investigation is considered to be optional as other imaging techniques can offer a more complete evaluation.

The greatest hurdle for the potential donor to be accepted in the evaluation process has been the aortogram which can define the renal artery anatomy (Fig. 1). This invasive procedure carries a 1.4 per cent rate of complications (Egglin *et al.* 1995) such as contrast reaction, puncture site bleeding, groin haematoma, arterial dissection, or, thrombosis (Table 3). The use of spiral computed tomography (CT) or magnetic resonance angiography have simplified the procedure of defining donor vascular anatomy (Lerner *et al.* 1999). An advantage of these techniques is the administration by vein, thus avoiding most of the potential complications of intra-arterial puncture. Another important advantage is the possibility of knowing not only the number, the location, and the branching pattern of the renal arteries but also the number, the location, and the branching pattern of renal veins, adrenal veins, and gonadal veins (Halpern *et al.* 1999). Only small amounts of radiocontrasts are needed for spiral CT (Fig. 2). Delayed films can give

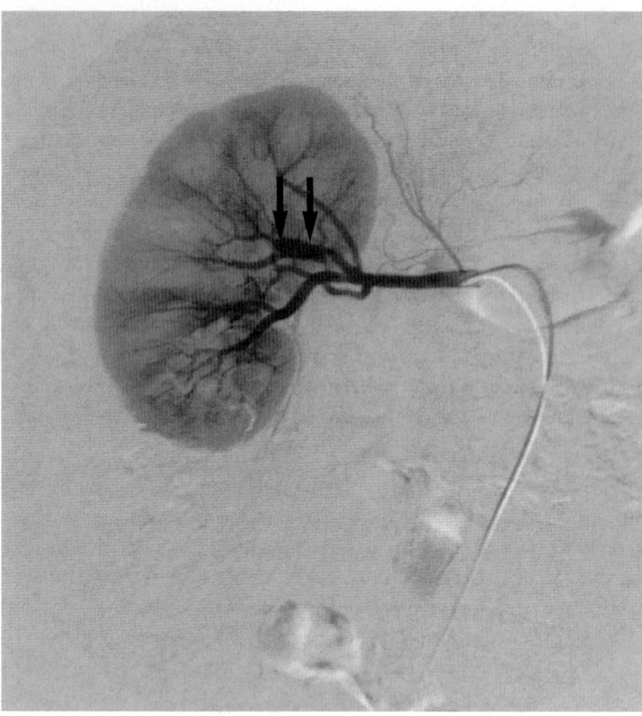

Fig. 1 Renal angiography in a potential donor. An intrarenal aneurysm was discovered. The kidney donation was ruled out and the aneurysm was successfully treated with a stent.

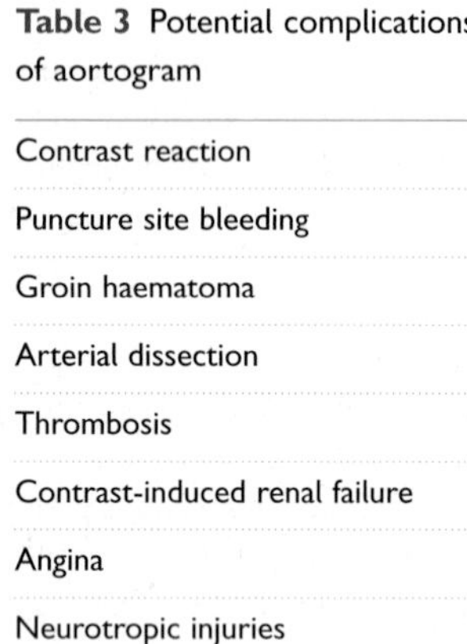

Table 3 Potential complications of aortogram

Contrast reaction
Puncture site bleeding
Groin haematoma
Arterial dissection
Thrombosis
Contrast-induced renal failure
Angina
Neurotropic injuries

details of the excretory apparatus, thus making the intravenous pyelography unnecessary (Herts 1999). CT angiography needs a 5-min study which is a further advantage over the multiexam sequence. Magnetic resonance angiography is a safe technique because the administered contrast agent, gadolinium, is free of renal toxicity and has a low incidence of allergic reactions. Moreover, this technique eliminates the exposure to ionizing radiation. Disadvantages of these techniques are the low availability and the cost. However, use of CT angiography, plus conventional therapy instead of excretory urography and conventional arteriography can result in a 35–50 per cent reduction in cost of imaging studies in potential renal donors (Cochran *et al.* 1997).

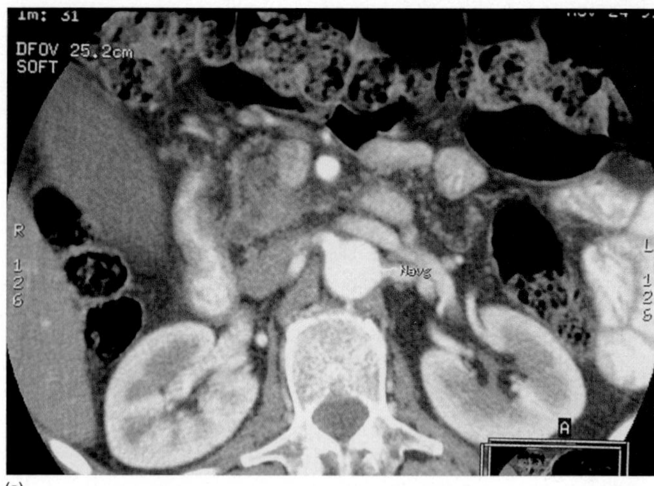

(a)

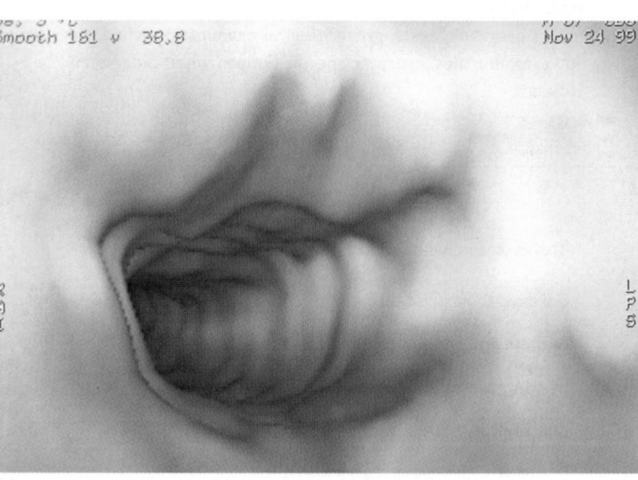

(b)

Fig. 2 (a) CT section of the origin of renal arteries. The axial image is unable to follow the renal arteries completely. (b) The curvilinear reconstruction based on the processing of the axial images allows to visualize the renal arteries completely.

References

Berthoux, F. *et al.* (2000). European best practice guidelines for renal transplantation (part 1). *Nephrology, Dialysis, Transplantation* **15** (Suppl. 7), 1–85.

Cho, Y. W. and Cecka, J. M. Crossmatch tests—an analysis of UNOS data from 1991–2000. In *Clinical Transplants* (ed. J. M. Cecka and P. I.), pp. 237–246. UCLA, Los Angeles, 2001.

Cochran, S. T. *et al.* (1997). Helical CT angiography for examination of living renal donors. *American Journal of Radiology* **168**, 1569–1573.

Egglin, T. K. *et al.* (1995). Complications of peripheral arteriography: a new system to identify patients at increased risk. *Journal of Vascular Surgery* **22**, 787–794.

Gjertson, D. W. and Cecka, J. M. (2000). Living unrelated donor kidney transplantation. *Kidney International* **58**, 491–499.

Halpern, E. J. *et al.* (1999). US, CT, and MR evaluation of accessory renal arteries and proximal renal arterial branches. *Academy of Radiology* **6**, 299–304.

Herts, B. R. (1999). Triphasis helical CT of the kidneys: contribution of vascular phase scanning in patients before urologic surgery. *American Journal of Radiology* **173**, 1273–1277.

Ishida, H. *et al.* (2000). Anti-AB titer changes in patients with ABO incompatibility after living related kidney transplantations. *Transplantation* **70**, 681–685.

Karpinski, M. *et al.* (2002). Flow cytometry crossmatching in primary renal transplants with a negative anti-human globulin enhanced cytotoxic crossmatch. *Journal of the American Society of Nephrology* **12**, 2807–2814.

Le Bas-Bernadet, S. *et al.* (2003). Identification of antibodies involved in B-cell cross-match in renal transplantation. *Transplantation* **75**, 477–482.

Lerner, L. B., Henriques, H. F., and Harris, R. D. (1999). Interactive 3-dimensional computerized tomography reconstruction in evaluation of the living renal donor. *Journal of Urology* **161**, 403–407.

Mange, K., Jaffe, M. M., and Feldman, H. I. (2001). Effect of the use or nonuse of long-term dialysis on the subsequent survival of renal transplants from living donors. *New England Journal of Medicine* **344**, 726–731.

Saunders, R. N. *et al.* (2000). Workload generated by a living donor programme for renal transplantation. *Nephrology, Dialysis, Transplantation* **15**, 1667–1672.

Speiser, D. E. and Jeannet, M. (1995). Renal transplantation to sensitised patients: decreased survival probability associated with a positive historical crossmatch. *Transplant Immunology* **3**, 330–334.

Van Kampen, C. A. *et al.* (2002). Primed CTLs specific for HLA class I may still be present in sensitized patients when anti-HLA antibodies have disappeared: relevance for donor selection. *Transplantation* **73**, 1286–1290.

1.6.2.vi Transplant dysfunction

Olivier Hélénon, Jean-Michel Correas, Arnaud Méjean, and Emmanuel Morelon

Introduction

The main role of imaging is to detect vascular and urological complications that do not require biopsy and can lead to reconstructive surgery or percutaneous management. The first step imaging modality of choice in most cases is colour Doppler ultrasonography (CDUS). The following discussion will focus on the diagnosis of vascular damages including causes of early and delayed postoperative renal failure and postbiopsy vascular injuries.

Diagnosis of early postoperative renal failure

Acute tubular necrosis

This is the most common cause for early postoperative anuria that typically occurs immediately after graft revascularization. The major diagnostic problem at that stage is excluding other causes for early anuria and especially acute vascular occlusion. CDUS typically shows a normal parenchymal vascular supply with a high resistive arterial flow (resistive index > 0.80) and normal systolic peak.

A small number of acute tubular necrosis (ATN) (13 per cent) is associated with a reversed flow during diastole, which reflects very severe ischaemia of the graft. In some rare cases, intrarenal arterial spectra are very similar to those obtained in acute venous occlusion or diffuse cortical necrosis (see below). Unlike such vascular complications, which usually lead to the transplant loss, severe ATN is associated with a patent renal vein and preserved normal cortical vascular supply on colour Doppler imaging.

Acute thrombosis of the renal artery

This rare complication usually occurs very early after transplantation and leads to massive infarction. Typically, CDUS shows a total lack of intrarenal vascular flow (Grenier *et al.* 1991; Hélénon *et al.* 1992). However, in some rare cases passive reflux of blood from the iliac vein can be responsible for a preserved intrarenal to-and-fro venous flow (Hélénon *et al.* 1992).

Incomplete occlusion of the renal artery

Incomplete twisting or severe anastomotic malformation can be responsible for a tight stenosis and immediate postoperative anuria. Such a condition should be suspected when poor vascularity is shown within the graft with a marked decrease of arterial velocities and a loss of normal systolic–diastolic modulation as shown by pulsed Doppler interrogation of intrarenal arteries (see below, Fig. 4b).

Acute thrombosis of the renal vein

It is a rare complication in adults, which results in renal parenchymal venous infarction because of the absence of venous collateral pathways in the graft.

Spectral analysis from intrarenal arteries typically exhibits a narrowed systolic peak followed by a plateau-like reversed diastolic flow (Fig. 1a) associated with a total lack of intrarenal and pedicular venous signals (Reuther *et al.* 1989; Hélénon *et al.* 1992). Consequently, contrast-enhanced magnetic resonance imaging (MRI) or computed tomography (CT) scan should be performed in order to confirm the diagnosis of complete venous thrombosis associated with renal cortical infarction (Fig. 1b).

Segmental infarction due to proximal vascular damage

Occlusion of a renal arterial branch or a polar artery with separate anastomosis is the more frequent early vascular complication. Such vascular damage produces limited infarction, which can result in sudden and unexplained reduction in renal function early after transplantation. An increase in serum lactic dehydrogenase (LDH) may strongly suggest the diagnosis, which relies on the demonstration of a focal lack of colour flow and pulsed Doppler signal at CDUS (Hélénon *et al.* 1992). Small superficial infarcts may result in false negatives since normal vascularity of the superficial cortex is not assessed by conventional CDUS. Overall sensitivity and specificity of CDUS for the detection of renal allograft necrosis are 76 and 95 per cent, respectively (Hélénon *et al.* 1994). The use of ultrasound contrast agents (IV administration of microbubbles) increases the sensitivity of sonography in the detection of small defects and helps differentiate hypoperfused areas from true infarcts (Correas *et al.* 1999).

Contrast-enhanced MRI provides accurate, non-invasive and non-nephrotoxic evaluation (compared to iodinated contrast-enhanced CT) of perfusion defects (Fig. 2). The overall sensitivity and specificity of contrast-enhanced MRI in the diagnosis of renal allograft necrosis are 96 and 100 per cent, respectively (Hélénon *et al.* 1994).

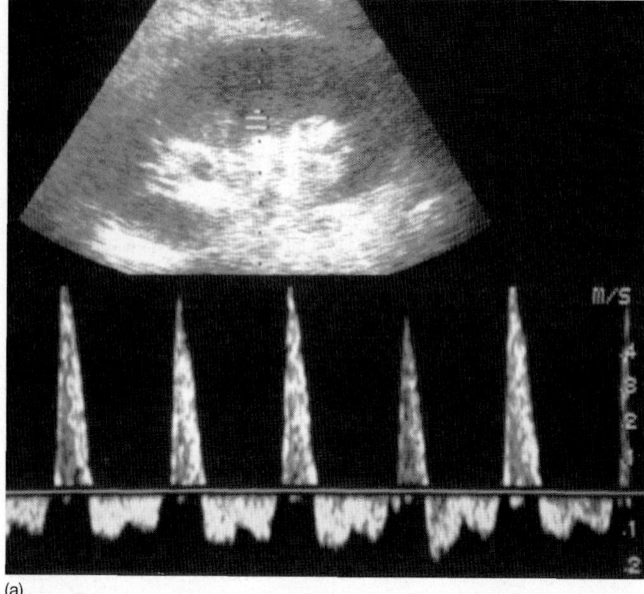

(a)

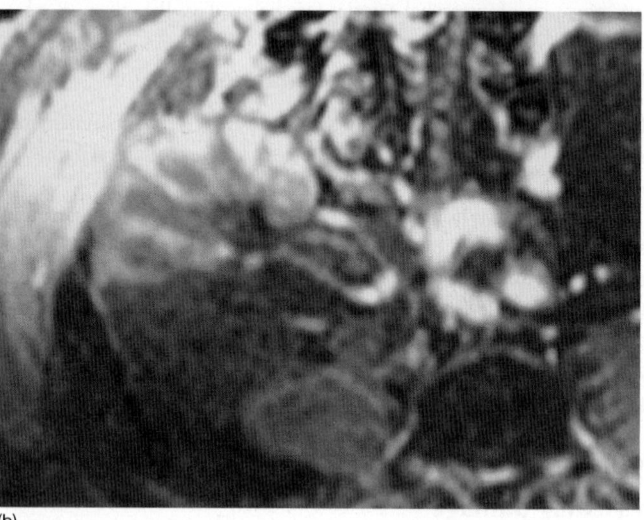

(b)

Fig. 1 Acute renal vein thrombosis. Spectral analysis obtained from segmental renal arteries shows plateau-like reversed diastolic flow (a) associated with total lack of venous signal (not shown). Contrast-enhanced MRI (b) confirms occlusion of the renal vein with diffuse infarction of the renal parenchyma.

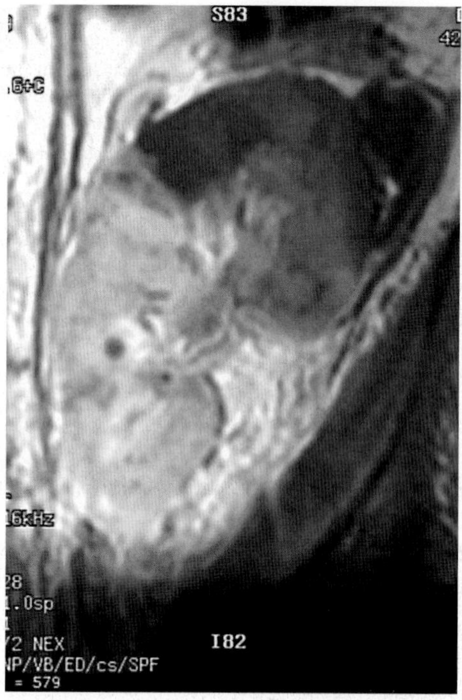

Fig. 2 Segmental renal infarction. Contrast-enhanced MRI (coronal view) shows a large area of cortex without contrast-enhancement involving the upper pole of the kidney.

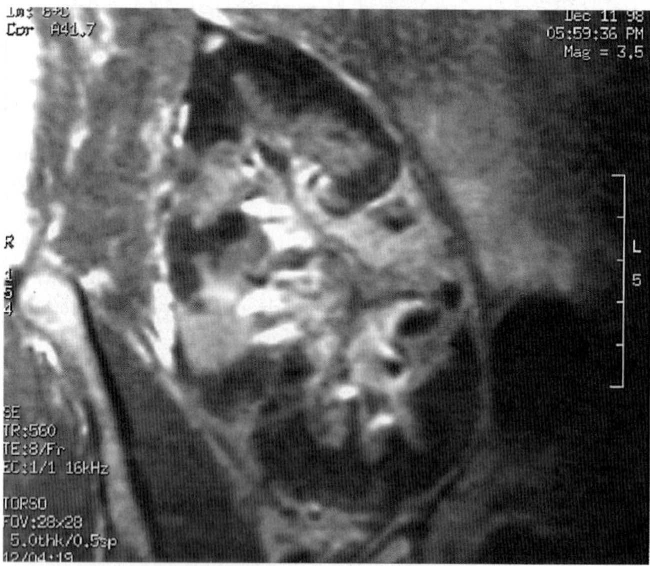

Fig. 3 Accelerated rejection with diffuse cortical necrosis. Postcontrast MRI (coronal view) shows multiple and diffuse cortical defects.

Distal vascular damage due to accelerated acute rejection

Accelerated acute rejection leads to destruction of the graft usually within the first 10 days after surgery. Typically, severe ischaemia of the cortex is responsible for highly increased resistive indices (RIs) with reversed flow in diastole and subsequently diffused cortical necrosis which lead to nephrectomy. Contrast-enhanced MRI provides an accurate evaluation of cortical necrosis (Fig. 3) except in cases of small superficial patches. It should be performed to confirm the diagnosis and to assess more precisely the extent of necrosis in order to help the physician in the management of such a complication (transplant nephrectomy versus prolonged immunosuppressive treatment with imaging follow-up of the cortical vascularity).

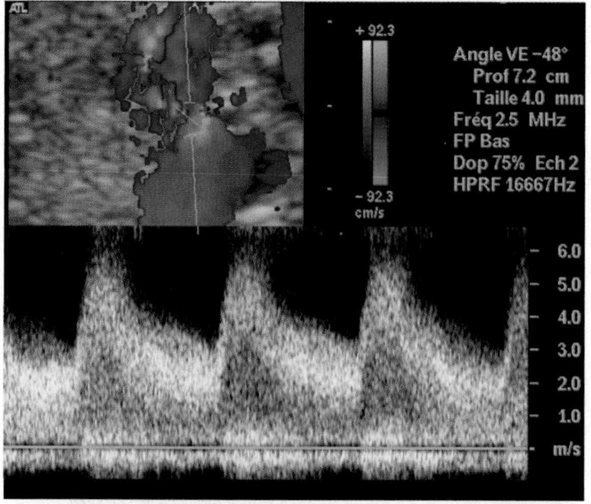

(a)

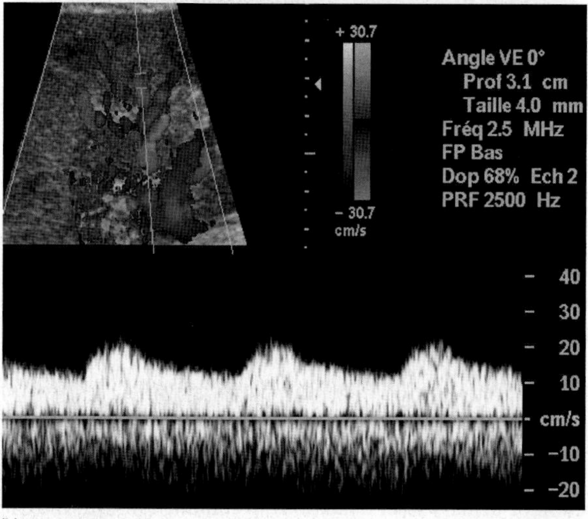

(b)

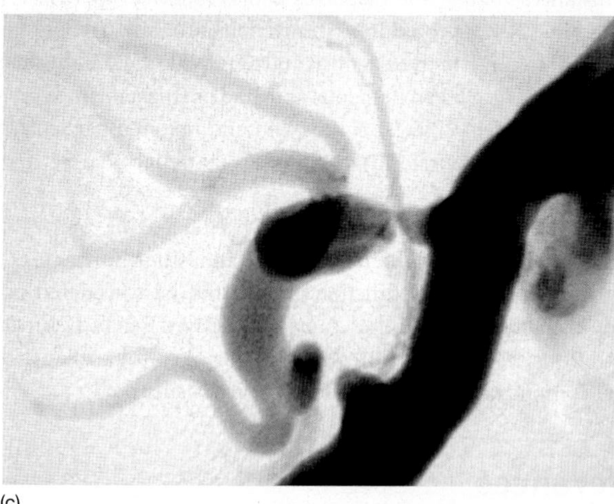

(c)

Fig. 4 Severe stenosis of the renal transplant artery. Spectral analysis obtained from the renal artery shows a marked acceleration (up to 500 cm/s) and spectral broadening due to turbulence (a). Intrarenal arterial spectrum (b) shows slowed arterial flow with loss of systolic–diastolic modulation related to the downstream repercussion of a tight (>75%) stenosis. Angiogram obtained before transluminal angioplasty (c).

Diagnosis of a delayed renal failure

Causes of episodes of renal failure during the first months following renal transplantation that do not occur immediately after surgery can be divided into two clinical categories: non-immunological causes including urinary tract complications, vascular complications, drug nephrotoxicity, and immunological causes (see Section 13).

Imaging provides no specific criteria for rejection (Kelcz *et al.* 1990; Meyer *et al.* 1990). Thus, the main role of CDUS and other imaging modalities is to screen for urinary tract and vascular complications and particularly renal artery stenosis at that stage. On the other hand, when the diagnosis of rejection is established, CDUS with assessment of RIs appears to be a useful tool in the follow-up of the treatment efficacy.

Renal artery stenosis

Renal artery (RA) stenosis is the most frequent vascular complication causing prolonged renal failure during the first months following surgery. Although RA stenosis occurs in a high percentage of transplant recipients, only a small number of cases of severe stenosis are associated with significant renal failure and/or renovascular hypertension. The stenosis involves more frequently the proximal segment of the main RA and the perianastomotic portion. Stenoses that are located on the distal portion of the main RA or on an RA branch are not rare (approximately 25 per cent among all transplant artery stenoses).

The same criteria that are applied in native kidneys are used to diagnose transplant artery stenosis. They include (Grenier *et al.* 1991; Brown *et al.* 2000): intrastenotic acceleration and poststenotic turbulent flow and/or parvus–tardus waveforms obtained from intrarenal arteries in cases of tight (≥80 per cent) stenoses (Fig. 4). The sensitivity and specificity of CDUS for the detection of main RA stenosis have been evaluated at between 90–95 and 95–100 per cent, respectively. Intra-arterial angiography is indicated in the preoperative assessment of the arterial tree. MR angiography or spiral CT scan have provided interesting results but may be insufficient in the preoperative assessment of the arterial tree because of the poor visibility of distal branches. MR angiography using bolus injection of a gadolinium complex provides the best diagnostic performance without contrast-induced nephrotoxicity (Ferreiros *et al.* 1999).

Postbiopsy vascular complications

Postbiopsy arteriovenous fistula

The presence of an arteriovenous (AV) shunt produces local tissue vibration that results in the so-called perivascular artefact on colour flow image (Fig. 5) (Grenier *et al.* 1991; Brown *et al.* 2000). Typically, spectral analysis shows accelerated and highly turbulent flow at the site of the AV shunt, increased systolic–diastolic flow velocities with marked decrease of RI measurements (0.35–0.45) in the feeding artery, and increased flow velocities with systolic–diastolic modulation in the draining vein.

Most cases recover spontaneously (spontaneous AV shunt occlusion) and do not require further imaging except CDUS follow-up. The presence of an AV fistula (AVF) should contraindicate renal biopsy without colour Doppler guidance. Less than 5 per cent of AVFs require a specific treatment. Intra-arterial angiography with transluminal selective embolization is indicated when AVF is responsible for a severe haematuria. Some rare cases associated with impairment of graft

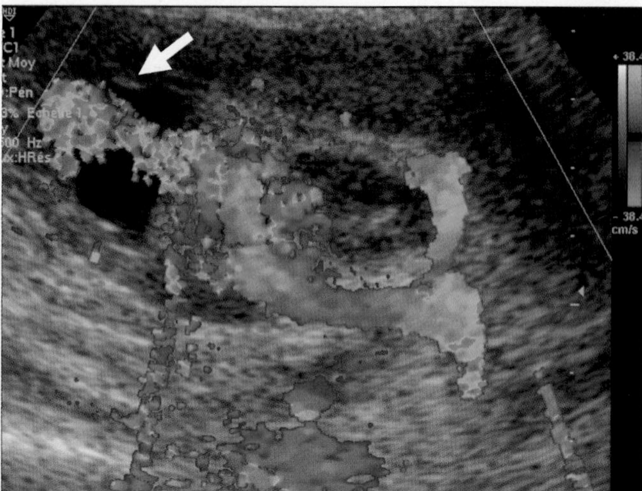

Fig. 5 Postbiopsy AVF. CDUS shows intrarenal perivascular artefact at the level of the arteriovenous shunt (arrow).

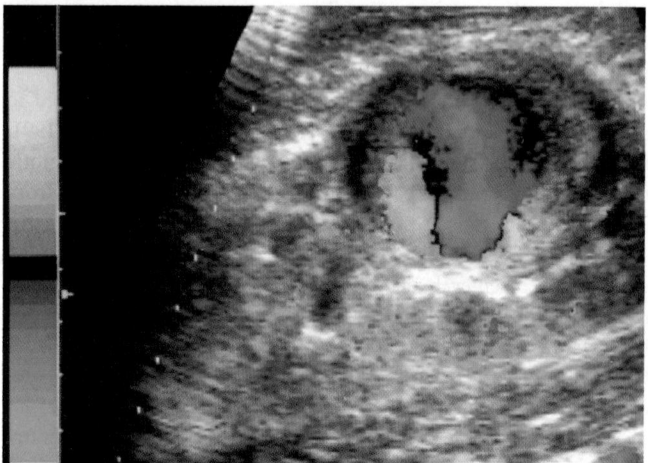

Fig. 6 Postbiopsy false aneurysm. CDUS shows a pseudocystic cortical mass filled with colour flow signal with arterial systolic–diastolic modulation.

function due to a steal effect relative to a high volume flow through the AV shunt can also benefit from selective endovascular occlusion.

Renal artery false-aneurysm

RA false-aneurysm (FA) is a rare but serious iatrogenic complication occurring in less than 1 per cent of renal biopsies. Rare cases are associated with the presence of an AVF. The flowing cavity arises from the injured artery without venous drainage. Ultrasound shows a hypoechoic round shaped mass filled with colour signal on the CD image (Fig. 6). Spectral analysis obtained at the level of the communicating channel demonstrates a typical finding known as the to-and-fro sign, which reflects both systolic feeding arterial flow and diastolic draining arterial flow. Large (>2 cm) and/or subcapsular FAs need to be treated using endovascular occlusion of the injured vessel in order to avoid bleeding.

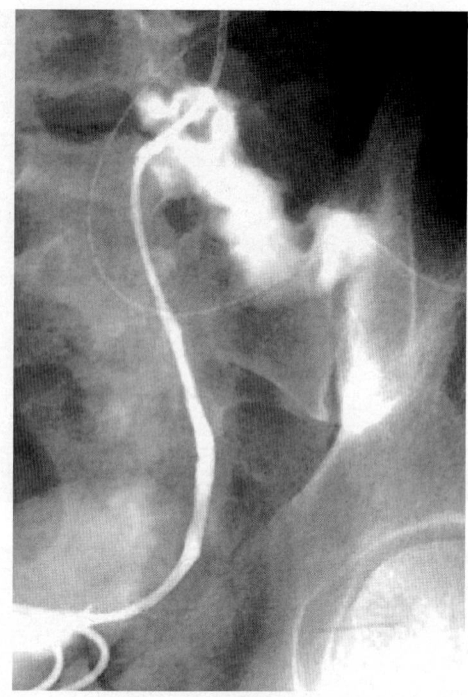

Fig. 7 Ureteral leak after renal transplantation with pyeloureteric anastomosis. Pyelogram after retrograde stent placement.

Urological complications

They include early postoperative complications and delayed urinary tract disorders. Perirenal haematoma or abscess formation, lymphocele, ureteral anastomotic leakage, or early stenosis may occur during the first week after transplantation. Ultrasound findings (perirenal fluid collection or urinary tract dilatation) in conjunction with the clinical circumstances suggest the diagnosis and is followed up with CT or conventional X-ray procedures (intravenous urogram, pyelogram, or cystogram) to confirm the diagnosis and to provide accurate evaluation of the lesion (Fig. 7). Percutaneous antegrade management of ureteral damages is efficient (Bhagat *et al.* 1998) and required particularly in patients with vesicoureteric anastomosis that precludes retrograde stent insertion.

Urinary tract disorders such as acute pyelonephritis, ureteral anastomotic stenosis, vesicoureteric reflux, and stone formation may lead to delayed renal dysfunction and should be considered in the differential diagnosis of other causes of delayed renal dysfunction. Conventional X-ray procedures and CT play key roles in such urological complications which are often clinically silent.

References

Bhagat, V. J. *et al.* (1998). Ureteral obstructions and leaks after renal transplantation: outcome of percutaneous antegrade ureteral stent placement in 44 patients. *Radiology* **209**, 159–167.

Brown, E. D. *et al.* (2000). Complications of renal transplantation: evaluation with US and radionuclide imaging. *Radiographics* **20**, 607–622.16.

Correas, J. M., Hélénon, O., and Moreau, J. F. (1999). Contrast-enhanced ultrasonography of native and transplanted kidney diseases. *European Radiology* **9** (Suppl. 3), S394–S400.

Ferreiros, J. *et al.* (1999). Using gadolinium-enhanced three-dimensional MR angiography to assess arterial inflow stenosis after kidney transplantation. *American Journal of Roentgenology* **172**, 751–757.

Grenier, N. *et al.* (1991). Detection of vascular complications in renal allografts with color Doppler flow imaging. *Radiology* **178**, 217–223.

Hélénon, O. *et al.* (1992). Gd-DOTA enhanced MR imaging and color Doppler US characteristics of infarction in transplanted kidneys. *Radiographics* **12**, 21–33.

Hélénon, O. *et al.* (1994). Renal allograft necrosis: value of color Doppler ultrasound and Gd-DOTA-enhanced MR imaging. *Transplantation Proceedings* **26**, 300.

Kelcz, F., Pozniak, M. A., Pirsch, J. D., and Oberly, T. D. (1990). Pyramidal appearance and resistive index: insensitive and nonspecific sonographic indicators of renal transplant rejection. *AJR. American Journal of Roentgenology* **155**, 531–535.

Meyer, M., Paushter, D., and Steinmuller, D. R. (1990). The use of duplex Doppler ultrasonography to evaluate renal allograft dysfunction. *Transplantation* **50**, 974–978.

Reuther, G., Wangura, D., and Baner, H. (1991). Acute renal vein thrombosis in renal allograft: detection with duplex Doppler US. *Radiology* **170**, 557–558.

1.7 Renal biopsy: indications for and interpretation

Claudio Ponticelli, Michael J. Mihatsch, and Enrico Imbasciati

The introduction of renal biopsy in clinical practice has represented one of the most important advances in the field of clinical nephrology. Renal biopsy has contributed greatly to a rational classification of intrinsic renal diseases and, therefore, to a better knowledge of the pathogenetic mechanisms involved. In spite of the flood of new and less invasive tests, renal biopsy is still an irreplaceable tool in assessing diagnosis and prognosis and guiding the treatment of many renal diseases. It is being more frequently used, especially with the advancement of new biopsy guns and real-time ultrasound guidance.

Indications for renal biopsy

The value of renal biopsy for management of patients with renal disease has been a subject of great debate. Theoretically, biopsy should be considered whenever clinical and laboratory data are not sufficient to define the nature of the disease, to assess the outcome, and to optimize the treatment. However, the indication in individual patients requires an accurate balance of risk–benefit ratio. This can be assessed from an evaluation of information that we can expect, from a knowledge of the clinical features, and from knowledge of renal morphology. Few studies have examined this issue prospectively or retrospectively (Paone and Meyer 1981; Turner *et al.* 1986; Cohen *et al.* 1989; Richards *et al.* 1994). These studies show that renal biopsy was relevant in defining diagnosis in 44–63 per cent, outcome in 32–57 per cent, and treatment in 31–42 per cent of the patients investigated. Differences were largely dependent on the clinical setting. Patients with adult nephrotic syndrome, acute or rapidly progressive renal failure, were those who most often benefited from biopsy, since the information obtained significantly influenced treatment decisions. On the contrary, biopsy rarely altered management of patients with microscopic haematuria or isolated proteinuria.

Idiopathic nephrotic syndrome (see also Chapters 3.3 and 3.4)

In the absence of a systemic disease, it is likely that a nephrotic syndrome is caused either by a minimal change disease, or a focal segmental glomerulosclerosis or a membranous nephropathy. Until recently, it was uniformly agreed that renal biopsy was an essential procedure in patients with idiopathic nephrotic syndrome, not only in terms of diagnosis but also in selecting treatment. However, some clinicians restrict their use of renal biopsy in this condition. Paediatricians, for example, think that most nephrotic children up to the age of 8 years should first receive an 8-week course of high-dose prednisone before considering renal biopsy (Brodehl 1991). In fact, childhood lipoid nephrosis is by far the most common cause of the nephrotic syndrome and usually responds with a complete remission of proteinuria within a few days or some weeks of corticosteroid therapy. These clinicians would reserve renal biopsy for steroid-resistant patients or for children with clinical and laboratory features (such as hypertension, renal insufficiency, multiorgan involvement, haematuria, unselective proteinuria) which suggest an underlying renal disease other than minimal change nephropathy.

A similar approach cannot be applied to adults with an idiopathic nephrotic syndrome. There is, in fact, evidence that no more than 60 per cent of adults with minimal change nephrotic syndrome are in complete remission after an 8-week course of prednisone but more than 80 per cent are without proteinuria after 16 weeks of treatment (Nolasco *et al.* 1986). Even more striking, the experience of Korbet *et al.* (1988) shows that only 32 per cent of patients older than 40 years achieved a complete remission within 8 weeks of corticosteroids, but that 77 per cent had responded by 16 weeks of treatment and 94 per cent became free of proteinuria with more prolonged therapy. Using the short-term approach a large number of late-responding patients would be considered as steroid-resistant and would not be treated further. As for focal glomerulosclerosis, a number of studies (Pei *et al.* 1987; Banfi *et al.* 1991; Rydel *et al.* 1995; Cattran *et al.* 1999; Ponticelli *et al.* 1999) have reported that 40–60 per cent of patients with focal glomerulosclerosis and nephrotic syndrome can respond with a complete remission of proteinuria, when treated with aggressive and prolonged corticosteroid therapy, cytotoxic agents, or cyclosporin. Without biopsy these patients would not receive potentially beneficial treatment.

Disappointing results would also be obtained with the administration of a short course of prednisone in patients with membranous nephropathy (see Chapter 3.7). An English multicentre trial has shown that an 8-week course of alternate-day prednisone does not interfere with the natural course of membranous nephropathy (Cameron *et al.* 1990), which is contrary to results reported by the American Collaborative Study Group (Collaborative Study of the Adult Idiopathic Nephrotic Syndrome 1979). On the other hand, other controlled trials in idiopathic membranous nephropathy showed that a 6-month course with methylprednisolone alone or, even better, with methylprednisolone and chlorambucil (Ponticelli *et al.* 1992) or methylprednisolone and cyclophosphamide (Ponticelli *et al.* 1998) favours remission of the nephrotic syndrome and protects renal function in the long-term (Ponticelli *et al.* 1995). Without renal biopsy, patients with membranous nephropathy would receive a useless short-term course of prednisone while being excluded from a potentially helpful treatment. The value of renal biopsy in the idiopathic nephrotic syndrome is further stressed by prospective studies showing that about 50 per cent of clinically predicted diagnoses and prognoses changed after renal biopsy (Paone and Meyer 1981; Turner *et al.* 1986; Cohen *et al.* 1989; Richards *et al.* 1994). Moreover, in some cases biopsy can show that what appears clinically to be an idiopathic nephrotic syndrome is actually secondary to a systemic disease such as amyloidosis, myeloma, or lupus.

We conclude that since there is no way other than renal biopsy of diagnosing the underlying disease correctly in patients with idiopathic nephrotic syndrome, and since data are emerging to suggest a role for treatment in several instances, most adults should undergo renal biopsy in order to better assess their diagnosis and prognosis and to decide on possible treatment, which today may be tailored using the results of biopsy.

Acute renal failure (see also Section 10)

Prerenal oligoanuria and urinary tract obstruction can be easily diagnosed without renal biopsy. The most frequent cause of acute renal failure is tubular necrosis. In most cases, the diagnosis of acute tubular necrosis is made correctly on clinical grounds. In these cases biopsy adds little to prognosis and nothing to the choice of therapy. Thus, in anuric patients, renal biopsy should be reserved for doubtful cases in order to detect causes other than acute tubular necrosis, which may benefit from specific treatment (Fuiano *et al.* 2000). Biopsy may also be useful in those patients who fail to regain renal function after four or more weeks (Table 1).

Rapidly progressive renal failure

In patients with rapid deterioration of renal function when an acute inflammatory process involving glomeruli, small vessels, or interstitium is suspected, renal biopsy is generally needed. In these instances, the clinical diagnosis may be difficult and incomplete. Presenting features of these conditions may be an unexplained renal function impairment, with normal kidney size. In this clinical setting, renal biopsy despite a high risk of complication is the determining factor in identifying potentially treatable patients.

In some cases a diagnosis can be made on clinical grounds and be confirmed serologically. These cases include postinfectious glomerulonephritis, mixed cryoglobulinaemia, and Goodpasture's syndrome. Even in these instances, however, renal biopsy may be of help in evaluating the possible reversibility of the lesions and in deciding therapy. In other instances, a wide spectrum of primary or systemic diseases with different histological features may be revealed by renal biopsy. The prognosis and therapeutical approach are clearly different in each of these settings. Interstitial nephritis is a histological diagnosis which can be found in a number of patients with unexplained renal function deterioration. Fever, rash, and eosinophilia are present only in a minority of the cases. False results with eosinophiluria are frequent. Some vasculitides may be difficult to recognize, although the detection of antibodies to components of neutrophil cytoplasm (anti-neutrophil anticytoplasmic antibodies, ANCA) has allowed an easier and earlier diagnosis. Renal biopsy is extremely useful to confirm diagnosis in doubtful cases, in assessing the prognosis for patients with renal failure, and in deciding whether or not it is helpful to treat the patient aggressively. Multiple myeloma may present with an acute renal failure with no symptoms of the underlying disease (Border and Cohen 1980) and the same may occur for primary amyloidosis (Zawada *et al.* 1987). Thus, in most cases of progressive or unexplained acute renal failure renal biopsy can provide useful and irreplaceable information.

Table 1 Indications for renal biopsy in acute renal failure

Gradual onset of acute renal failure
No obvious cause of acute renal failure
Heavy proteinuria
Significant haematuria
Clinical evidence or history of systemic disease
Prolonged oliguria

Microscopic haematuria

There is no rule for the indications for renal biopsy in patients with isolated haematuria with or without asymptomatic proteinuria. In patients with isolated microscopic haematuria an accurate study of the urine sediment by phase-contrast microscopy is recommended. A prevalence of monomorphic erythrocytes may indicate a postglomerular source of bleeding. A detailed history of prescribed and 'over the counter' medications (phenacetin/paracetamol) and urological work-up should be considered in these cases, particularly in adults over 50 years of age, for whom haematuria may be the only sign of an underlying cancer. The presence of 75–80 per cent of dysmorphic erythrocytes and/or more than 4–5 per cent of acanthocytes strongly suggests an underlying glomerular disease. These patients are generally affected by one of three disorders: IgA nephritis, hereditary nephritis, or thin basement membrane disease. Only renal biopsy can allow a firm diagnosis in these cases, but the indication is optional, since there are no therapeutic measures available. In clinical practice, we prefer to follow-up the patients and to postpone biopsy until proteinuria, hypertension, or renal function deterioration develop. However, we perform renal biopsy in patients who, for joining insurance companies or for whatever other reason, want a definite diagnosis and information about the long-term prognosis or, for eugenic reasons, in women of childbearing age to detect the presence of Alport's syndrome or other hereditary diseases.

Isolated non-nephrotic proteinuria

There is no agreement on the indications for renal biopsy in patients with proteinuria less than 1–2 g per day, normal renal function, and mild urine sediment abnormalities. Some of these patients have orthostatic proteinuria, others have an underlying nephrosclerosis or a reflux nephropathy causing a secondary focal glomerulosclerosis. In these cases, renal biopsy is of little help. However, biopsy should be considered if the clinical setting is compatible with a primary glomerular disease. There is evidence that a proteinuria more than 1 g per day is associated with a poor long-term prognosis in patients with IgA nephritis (D'Amico *et al.* 1986). Randomized controlled trials showed that a course with corticosteroids (Pozzi *et al.* 1999, 2004) or with fish-oil (Donadio *et al.* 1999) may protect renal function in these patients. Thus, renal biopsy is important in taking therapeutic decisions in these instances. Other patients may have a primary focal and segmental glomerulosclerosis or an idiopathic membranous nephropathy. As treatment with steroids or immunosuppressive agents are generally not indicated in this setting, some nephrologists prefer to postpone biopsy until proteinuria or serum creatinine increase. Others, however, are inclined to perform biopsy in order to have a definite diagnosis and to exclude systemic diseases which may initially manifest with an isolated renal involvement, as in some cases of sarcoidosis, systemic lupus erythematosus, amyloidosis etc.

Chronic renal insufficiency

Chronic renal failure represents a contraindication to renal biopsy. However, for patients with moderate renal insufficiency and a normal-sized kidney, a kidney biopsy may be indicated to recognize the type of renal disease and the potential reversibility of histological lesions. In several cases of membranous nephropathy (Torres *et al.* 2002), lupus nephritis (Moroni *et al.* 1999), and IgA nephritis (Ballardie and Roberts 2002) with renal dysfunction a trial with corticosteroids and cytotoxins proved to be of benefit.

Diabetic nephropathy

The appearance of proteinuria or renal dysfunction in a patient with long-lasting diabetes associated with retinopathy or neuropathy is very likely to be due to diabetic glomerulosclerosis. In these patients renal biopsy is rarely indicated (Olsen and Mogensen 1996). However, non-diabetic renal disease may develop in diabetic patients. Moreover, a multitude of glomerulopathies may be associated with diabetic nephropathy, including membranous nephropathy (Silva *et al.* 1983), minimal change nephropathy (Parving *et al.* 1992), acute glomerulonephritis (Monga *et al.* 1989), anti-GBM nephritis (Ahuja *et al.* 1998), and IgA nephritis (Mak *et al.* 2001). These events are particularly frequent in type II diabetes mellitus (Richards *et al.* 1992). Thus, proteinuric non-insulin-dependent diabetic patients without retinopathy may require renal biopsy.

Lupus nephritis

There are few doubts that clinical and biological data are generally sufficient for diagnosing lupus nephritis. However, renal biopsy is the only tool that permits the correct classification of lupus nephritis. For this purpose, biopsy should be evaluated by light microscopy, immunofluorescence, and preferably electron microscopy. A patient with haematuria, proteinuria, and normal or subnormal renal function may have any class of underlying glomerular lesions and unpredictable severity of histological lesions. This may imply a different prognosis and different therapeutic approaches. Moreover, there are instances in which the diagnosis can be difficult. A few patients may present initially with renal disease and only exhibit systemic and biological manifestations of lupus later in their course. This is relatively frequent for patients with an underlying membranous nephritis. In some cases, the biological markers of lupus may be absent for years and the differential diagnosis from idiopathic and lupus membranous nephritis can be established only by biopsy, which may show mesangial immune deposits, occasional subendothelial deposits, a full house immunofluorescence pattern typical of lupus, or endothelial tubuloreticular inclusions. A different situation is represented by those patients who have no clinical evidence of renal involvement despite underlying glomerular lesions at biopsy. Usually, this silent nephritis is characterized by mesangial or mild focal proliferative lesions but, exceptionally, it may be associated with diffuse proliferative glomerulonephritis.

It has been well documented that glomerular pathology is a reliable indicator of prognosis in lupus nephritis. A good correlation between the WHO classification and its most recent classification (Weening *et al.* 2004) and the short-term renal outcome has been found. Of the five classes devised in the WHO classification patients with minimal changes (class I), pure mesangial lesions (class II), or focal proliferation limited to few glomeruli (class III) were found to have little probability of progression although transformations to more severe forms have been observed. More controversial was the prognosis for membranous nephritis (class V), which was usually considered to be an indolent disease although a review of the literature reported that about 37 per cent either died or developed renal failure (Donadio 1992). There was consensus that patients with extended focal proliferation and those with diffuse proliferative glomerulonephritis (class IV) had the worst prognosis, but with marked variability in the clinical course. Because of this, efforts have been made to better define the histological features associated with a poor renal prognosis in patients with lupus nephritis. The original WHO classification was expanded by adding several subclasses which took into account the extension of active and sclerosing lesions (Churg *et al.* 1995). In particular, membranous nephritis was further subdivided according to the presence of mesangial (Vb), focal (Vc), or diffuse (Vd) proliferation. Patients with a membranous pattern associated with signs of glomerular inflammation in more than 50 per cent of the glomeruli or with diffuse proliferation (Vd) have been found to have a poorer prognosis than class IV patients (Najafi *et al.* 2001). A further contribution was made by the introduction of activity and chronicity indices, which summed the semiquantitative scores of certain histological features, including vascular and tubulointerstitial lesions, not considered in the WHO classification. Austin *et al.* (1983) reported that the index of activity (including lesions such as fibrinoid necrosis, cell proliferation, interstitial inflammation etc.) and the index of chronicity (including irreversible lesions such as glomerular sclerosis, interstitial fibrosis etc.) could help in predicting the risk of renal failure and in orientating the therapy. Others, however, raised objections about the reproducibility of the standard indices of activity and chronicity and did not find a good correlation between these indices and renal outcome (Schwartz *et al.* 1993; Wernick *et al.* 1993). More recently, the classification of lupus glomerulonephritis has been revised again. The original scheme of the WHO classification has been maintained, but the classes and subclasses have been unequivocally defined, by incorporating selective refinements of activity and chronicity criteria (Weening *et al.* 2004).

Whether, and when, renal biopsy should be repeated in lupus patients is still far from being established. Excellent results can be obtained by intensive clinical monitoring, which allows prompt and vigorous treatment of renal flares, characterized either by an increase in plasma creatinine, or by an increase in urinary protein excretion (Moroni *et al.* 1996). However, only repeat biopsy allows to document transformation from one histological class to another and to establish the long-term prognosis. A good correlation between clinical signs and histology is usually found in patients with clinical improvement. Stable histological features are usually seen in patients with persistent nephrotic syndrome. Conversely, the histological picture in patients with impaired renal function is unpredictable (Moroni *et al.* 1999). In these particular patients who are those at higher risk of irreversible uraemia, repeat renal biopsy is not only fully justified, but is almost mandatory in order to evaluate whether or not the patient may benefit from further treatment.

Renal transplantation (see also Chapters 13.3.3 and 13.3.4)

There are a number of possible indications for core renal biopsy of a transplanted kidney. In the early post-transplant period, renal biopsy can show whether oligoanuria is caused by acute tubular necrosis or by irreversible lesions, for example, infarction, and hyperacute, accelerated rejection. Graft biopsy has also been largely used to differentiate acute rejection from drug toxicity, infections, or other causes of allograft dysfunction.

In a later period, transplant biopsy may help in diagnosing whether a slow deterioration of renal function is caused by chronic rejection, by calcineurin-inhibitor toxicity, by recurrent disease, by a polyoma virus infection, or by a *de novo* glomerulonephritis.

Acute rejection

Renal biopsy is helpful not only for a correct diagnosis but also for assessing the prognosis and for establishing treatment of an acute rejection.

The Banff working classification (Racusen *et al.* 1999) proposed to categorize acute rejection into three grades (Table 2). More recently, this categorization has been revisited by adding some diagnostic criteria for humoral rejection. These include the presence of C4d deposits in peritubular capillaries, circulating donor-specific antibodies, and either neutrophils in the peritubular capillaries and glomeruli, or intimal fibrosis or acute tubular injury (Racusen *et al.* 2003). If renal biopsy remains a valid tool for a correct diagnosis, it must be pointed out that there are several limits to this technique. For example, interstitial inflammation and tubulitis (Fig. 1) are typical features of acute rejection. However, mononuclear inflammatory infiltrates can occur in stable allografts, which maintain normal function without any adjunctive therapy (Meehan *et al.* 1999). Even tubulitis is non-specific in itself as it may occur in acute tubular necrosis, drug-induced toxicity, and even in grafts with normal function. Moreover, there is a large interobserver variability in interpreting the grade of tubulitis (Furness and Taub 2001).

Only intimal arteritis (Fig. 2) can be considered to be specific for acute rejection and also grading the severity of rejection rests mainly on the type and severity of arterial lesions. This implies that graft biopsies without representative arteries are often inadequate.

Protocol biopsies performed every few weeks or months showed an unexpectedly high incidence of histological signs of mild rejection in patients with stable graft function (Rush *et al.* 1998; Nickerson *et al.* 1999). The significance of these 'subclinical rejections' is still undetermined, however, because of the poor specificity of tubulitis and interstitial inflammation, the poor reproducibility of results between different observers, and the risk that overimmunosuppression may overcome the potential advantage of detecting a mild rejection.

Table 2 Categorization of acute rejection according to Banff classification (Racusen *et al.* 1999)

Banff
Grade I
Interstitial inflammation >25% of parenchyma
(a) Tubulitis (>4 mononuclear cells/tubular cross-section)
(b) Tubulitis (>10 mononuclear cells/tubular cross-section)
Grade II
(a) Significant interstitial inflammation and/or mild to moderate arteritis
(b) Moderate to severe intimal arteritis comprising >25% of the luminal area
Grade III
Transmural arteritis and/or arterial fibrinoid change and necrosis of smooth cells with accompanying inflammation

Calcineurin-inhibitor toxicity

Both cyclosporin and tacrolimus may exert a similar nephrotoxicity, which may include acute graft function deterioration, haemolytic–uraemic syndrome, and chronic renal toxicity.

In the milder forms of acute nephrotoxicity the morphologic changes mainly affect proximal tubules, which show isometric vacuolization, giant mitocondria, and microcalcifications. More severe toxicity is associated with the development of an arteriolopathy characterized either by focal myocyte necrosis in the media of small arteries or by nodular hyalinosis (Mihatsch *et al.* 1983a).

The most severe form of acute toxicity is represented by the haemolytic–uraemic syndrome, which is characterized histologically by the typical features of thrombotic microangiopathy with mucinoid intimal thickening, severe luminal restriction of the small arterial vessels, and glomerular thrombosis (Mihatsch *et al.* 1995). Several cases of salvage of kidney allografts have been reported after the discontinuance of the offending drug (Young *et al.* 1996).

The main problem with the use of calcineurin inhibitors is represented by the development of a chronic progressive nephropathy. This is usually heralded by the appearance of arteriolopathy, which may

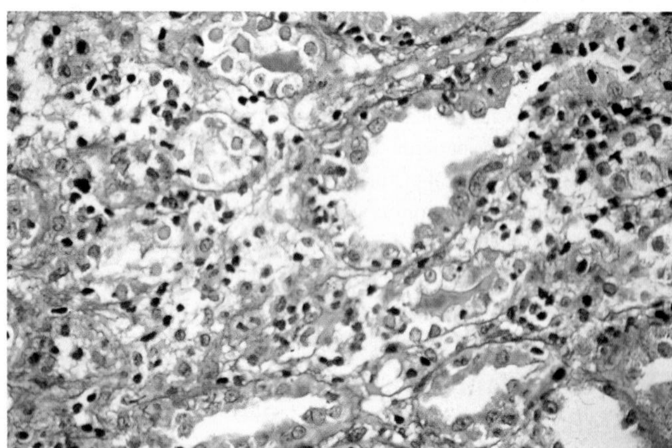

Fig. 1 Interstitial cellular rejection with tubulitis.

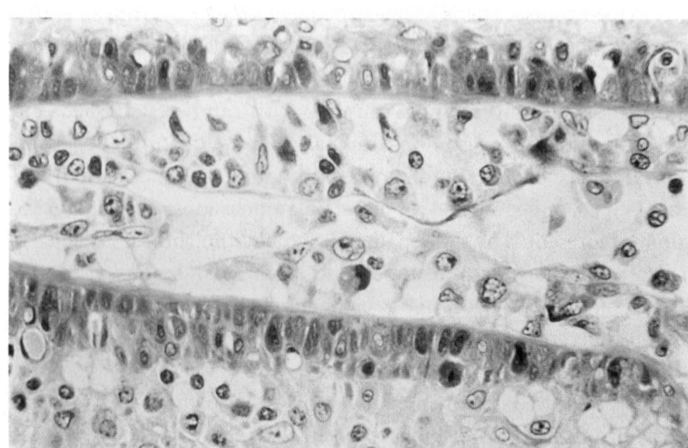

Fig. 2 Infiltrative and proliferative endoarteritis.

progress to vascular occlusion with consequent interstitial fibrosis and glomerular obsolescence (Nankivell *et al.* 2003).

Chronic allograft nephropathy

This term encompasses all the cases of slowly progressive graft dysfunction not caused by well identifiable factors. Both alloantigen-dependent and -independent mechanisms may concur in the development of chronic allograft nephropathy, although there is an indirect participation of immunological factors also in cases triggered by alloantigen-independent mechanisms (Ponticelli 2000).

Histologically, the main lesions consist of fibrous intimal thickening of arterial vessels associated with glomerular and tubulointerstitial changes. Not only are the arterioles affected, as in the case of calcineurin-inhibitor toxicity, but intimal fibrosis is also present in the interlobular arteries and even in the main renal artery (Mihatsch *et al.* 1995). Initially, there are proliferative changes of the intimal and smooth muscle cells, followed by progressive vascular sclerosis, and obliteration (Colvin 1996). The glomeruli may show an increase in mesangial cell and matrix, thickening and duplication of glomerular basement membrane, with scarring and adhesion (Habib and Broyer 1993). The peritubular capillaries may show thickening and multilayering of the basement membrane (Monga *et al.* 1992). Progression of scarring may be monitored by means of a protocol biopsy (Serón *et al.* 2002; Nankivell *et al.* 2003).

Polyoma virus nephritis

Polyoma BK virus infection may be reactivated by an intensive immunosuppression mostly with tacrolimus and mycophenolate mofetil and may lead to a progressive interstitial nephritis with graft loss in a significant number of cases (Fig. 3). Its incidence is about 5–6 per cent (Ramos *et al.* 2002). The diagnosis is based on a combination of viral intranuclear inclusion bodies in epithelial cells (tubular and glomerular parietal cells), epithelial cell necrosis, and accompanying interstitial nephritis at graft biopsy, urine cytology showing typical decoy cells, and viral load in plasma (Nickeleit *et al.* 2003). In patients treated with tacrolimus and mycophenolate mofetil, routine immunochemistry for the detection of SV 40 large T-antigen is recommended in the evaluation of biopsies to make the diagnosis as early as possible.

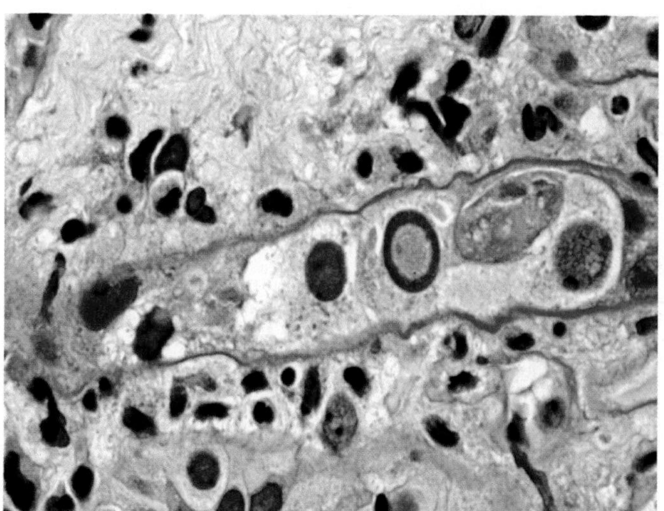

Fig. 3 Polyoma BK virus nephritis. Typical cytopathic changes of tubular epithelial cells with inclusions and extensive necrosis.

Contraindications

Renal mass

The presence of polycystic kidney disease is a formal contraindication to renal biopsy. Large cysts and renal neoplasms are not an absolute contraindication, if they can be well localized. Renal biopsy under the guidance of ultrasonography or an open surgical biopsy should be done in these cases.

Solitary kidney

This condition is generally considered as a contraindication to percutaneous renal biopsy. An exception is the transplanted kidney, which is commonly biopsied both because it is easy to puncture, being almost subcutaneous, and because compressive haemostasis can be carried out. However, technical advances, such as real-time ultrasound guidance and automated biopsy guns, have improved the safety profile of biopsy a native solitary kidney. Good results have been obtained in selected cases both in adults (Mendelssohn and Cole 1995) and in children (Greenbuaum *et al.* 2000). Open biopsy is an alternative option in patients with a solitary kidney.

Chronic renal failure

Patients with decreased renal function have a high rate of complications. Moreover, useful information cannot be obtained from the biopsy of small, contracted kidneys. For these reasons, renal biopsy should be considered only in patients with almost normal-sized kidneys after careful control of hypertension and correction of coagulation disorders.

Urinary infection

The presence of an active, untreated infection of the upper urinary tract is considered a contraindication to renal biopsy, in view of the potential communication between the collecting system and a possible perirenal haematoma, with consequent catastrophic infection of the haematoma.

Hypertension

The risk of complications after biopsy is directly related to the degree of elevation of blood pressure. Although normalization of blood pressure with antihypertensive agents may reduce the risks of renal biopsy, nevertheless, the transection of sclerotic vessels is more likely to produce severe haemorrhage. Uncontrolled hypertension should be considered as a high-risk factor for complications.

Coagulation disorders

Haemorrhagic diathesis is a formal contraindication to renal biopsy. Many patients with renal dysfunction present a prolongation of the skin bleeding time associated with normal results on coagulation tests. The risk of haemorrhagic complications after biopsy is high in patients with very prolonged bleeding time. However, in many cases preoperative infusion of desmopressin (0.3 μmol/kg over 30 min) can achieve normal values of the bleeding time for some hours and allow renal biopsy.

Miscellaneous

Renal artery aneurysm, marked calcified atherosclerosis, perinephric abscess, and horseshoe kidney are generally considered as contraindications to percutaneous renal biopsy. However, in particular cases an open biopsy may be considered if the clinical situation warrants the risk.

In pregnancy, renal biopsy before 30 weeks of gestation is not associated with significant complications (Chen *et al.* 2001). However, in the pre- or postpartum period it is often complicated by perirenal haematomas (Kuller *et al.* 2001). Thus, biopsy should be considered only if it may offer the opportunity to make a diagnosis other than severe pre-eclampsia in a patient remote from term.

Patients with AL amyloidosis may have a factor X deficiency due to binding of this factor to the amyloid tissue deposit (Choufani *et al.* 2001). Moreover, vascular amyloid deposits may impair vascular occlusion and vasoconstriction after transection of vascular structures by biopsy. In view of the increased risk of haemorrhage, patients with amyloidosis should be assessed carefully to rule out possible haemostatic defects.

Biopsy specimen processing

Since biopsies of native kidneys are usually done only once per lifetime, no doubt should remain about the diagnosis of the renal disease.

To allow optimal evaluation of a renal biopsy, sufficient cortical tissue should be available for light microscopy, immunofluorescence, and electron microscopy although in most cases the diagnosis can already be achieved with a combination of light microscopy and immunofluorescence. Among 5000 biopsies, we found immunohistology essential for the definite diagnoses in 21 per cent. Electronmicroscopy is helpful in unclear cases or essential in each 8 per cent of biopsies.

For electron microscopy, it is advisable to take two cores. Two or three small pieces of cortical tissue are cut from one of the two specimens and put in the fixative solution as quickly as possible. The light microscopy specimen is laid on a strip of heavy filter paper and plunged into the fixative. The tissue cylinder chosen for immunohistology is placed on a block-holder previously covered by a supporting substance and is immersed in isopentane precooled by liquid nitrogen. If only one specimen is available, the fragment for immunohistology can be obtained by cutting the cylinder of tissue longitudinally. However, this manoeuvre can produce massive crushing artefacts. Preferably, immunohistology can be performed in formalin-fixed and paraffin-embedded tissue (Bolton and Mesnard 1982; Fogazzi *et al.* 1989).

The choice and the optimization of the methods used for tissue processing in the three techniques are of paramount importance in obtaining maximum information. The reader can find detailed descriptions of these techniques elsewhere (Zollinger and Mihatsch 1978). Here, we summarize the guidelines for optimal tissue processing.

Light microscopy

Fixation in neutral, phosphate-buffered 4 per cent formalin is recommended for routine examination. Good results can also be obtained with fixation in Dubosq–Brazil; however, specimens processed with this fixative cannot be used for immunohistology. Alcoholic dehydration and embedding in paraffin or paraplast is commonly used to process renal biopsies. Numbered slides are then obtained from the paraffin block by cutting serial 2 μm sections. A regular thickness is important for semiquantitative or morphometric examination. To obtain thinner (0.5–1 μm) sections, methyl methacrylate has been proposed as the embedding medium (Striker *et al.* 1978). However, this technique is time consuming, limits the selection of stains, does not allow immunohistology, and thus cannot be recommended for routine use. Sections should be stained routinely with haematoxylin–eosin, periodic acid–Schiff reagent, silver methenamine, Masson trichrome stain, or acid fuchsin orange G (AFOG) stain (Zollinger and Mihatsch 1978). If amyloidosis is suspected, sections should be stained with Congo red and examined under polarized light.

Immunohistology

Immunohistological techniques are usually performed in renal biopsies in order to recognize and characterize deposits of immunoglobulin and complement factors. Immunofluorescence is more commonly used, but immunoperoxidase is also applied since it offers advantages with stability of the stain and with the use of light microscopy for examination. Various immune sera are available commercially for both techniques: anti-IgG, -IgA, -IgM, -C3, -C4, -C1q, -fibrin(ogen). Anti-light-chain sera should be used routinely. Additional antisera, such as those specific for other complement components, for coagulation factors, for viral or amyloid antigens, may be useful in selected cases.

The intensity of staining of the individual sera is semiquantitatively scored. In order to obtain reproducible data, standardization of the techniques is necessary. Artefacts should be avoided. Poorly preserved specimens during the snap-freezing procedure, thick sections, and non-specific fixation of the sera or of the free-labelling material are the most common causes of misinterpretation. Immunohistology is generally performed on cryostat sections from frozen specimens. Formalin-fixed and paraffin-embedded specimens can be used by applying conjugated antisera to sections previously treated by proteolytic digestion with trypsin or pronase. This method is more complex and time consuming than that on frozen sections. It gives comparable results for immunoglobulins, fibrin, and light-chain detection, but is less sensitive for complement factors (Bolton and Mesnard 1982; Fogazzi *et al.* 1989). The background staining is often higher especially for IgG but overall the morphology is much better and special equipment is not necessary.

Electron microscopy

Ultrastructural studies are expensive and time consuming. In some centres, therefore, small tissue specimens are routinely embedded in resin, but are examined by electron microscopy only when diagnosis has not been obtained by light and immunofluorescence microscopy.

Standard processing for electron microscopy includes fixation in glutaraldehyde, postfixation in osmium, embedding in epon, and preparation of semithin sections and ultrathin sections, which are stained by uranyl acetate and lead citrate. Silver impregnation of ultrathin sections is an additional staining procedure, seldom used, for evaluation of basement membrane abnormalities. Immunoelectron microscopy can be applied to routine biopsy material. The method gives reproducible results in different forms of glomerulonephritis and allows the routine biopsy material to be used for studying subcellular mechanisms in immune complex deposition and removal (Ihling *et al.* 1994). Scanning electron microscopy and histochemistry on electron microscopy are further possible applications of this technique, which, however, requires special preparation of the specimens.

General guidelines for renal biopsy evaluation

Evaluation of the biopsy specimen by different techniques is included in a stepwise diagnostic process, where clinical and laboratory data are integrated and correlated with morphological findings (Table 3).

The first step in a renal biopsy analysis is low-power evaluation of the light microscopy slides. This allows assessment of the proportion of cortical and medullary tissue and detection of rough abnormalities such as infarcted areas or large scars. The adequacy of the specimen is evaluated from the number of glomeruli observed, although this criterion is not absolute, but depends on the underlying disease and on the purpose of the study. When the lesion is confined to the glomeruli and is diffuse, even a single glomerulus may be sufficient for diagnosis. Clearly, however, other associated interstitial and vascular changes or the degree of glomerular obsolescence cannot be assessed. When the lesion is focally distributed the representativeness of the specimen is directly proportional to the number of glomeruli. The accuracy of biopsy evaluation in these conditions can be assessed quantitatively, considering the actual number of abnormal glomeruli and the size of the specimen (Corwin *et al.* 1988). In general, for the evaluation of glomerular lesions a biopsy should contain at least five glomeruli. For tubulointerstitial lesions a biopsy size of 6–10 glomeruli is necessary (Oberholzer *et al.* 1983). In order to improve the accuracy of histological evaluation, it can be useful to cut a large number of sections and also to study semithin sections.

The second step consists of an analytical examination of features of glomeruli, tubules, interstitium, and vessels by light microscopy. For each of these structures several histological parameters must be considered (Table 4). Careful examination at high-power magnification, especially of sections stained by silver methenamine and trichrome techniques, is needed for identifying the lesions.

The third step consists of the interpretation of immunohistology and electron microscopy findings. Immunohistological findings should be evaluated by considering for each antiserum the site of fixation on different structures, the extension and the distribution of positively stained material, the intensity of the staining, and the morphological characteristics of deposits. These findings are very important in diagnosis, especially in glomerular diseases. For each histological type of glomerular disease, a well-defined immunohistological pattern can be identified on the basis of the antigen composition, conformation, and allocation of deposits on glomerular structures (Fig. 4). In addition, some diseases, such as IgA mesangial deposits nephropathy, antibasement membrane glomerulonephritis, and subtypes of crescentic glomerulonephritis, cannot be correctly classified without immunohistology.

Table 3 Stepwise evaluation of renal biopsy

Evaluation of clinical and laboratory data
Study at low-power magnification (adequacy and preliminary examination)
Analytical study of light microscopy features (glomeruli, tubules, interstitium, vessels)
Presumptive diagnosis and correlation with clinical data Evaluation of immunohistological and electron microscopy findings
Confirmation of diagnosis, or: Revision of light microscopy and clinical data
Final diagnosis, stating of lesions, and evaluation of prognosis indices

Many peculiar abnormalities may be recognized only by electron microscopy (Table 5). Ultrastructural studies are essential for the diagnosis of thin-basement-membrane nephropathy, Alport's syndrome, and other hereditary diseases, in the initial phase of diabetic nephropathy, in dense-deposit disease, in cryoglobulinaemic nephropathy, in some cases of amyloidosis, in type 3 collagen glomerulopathy (Imbasciati *et al.* 1991) and in the so-called fibrillary glomerulopathies (Korbet *et al.* 1994). In glomerular disease an ultrastructural study provides detailed information about glomerular basement membrane changes, the characteristics of the deposits, and of some cellular abnormalities. These findings may allow recognition of morphological subtypes of membranous nephropathy, membranoproliferative glomerulonephritis, and lupus nephropathy. Finally, some findings related to dissolution of the deposits or accumulation of basement membrane-like material may give pointers to the duration of the pathological phenomena.

The final step is a comprehensive evaluation of histological, clinical, and laboratory findings. Discrepancies between clinical and pathological data should stimulate both a critical revision of biopsy data or further laboratory investigations. Renal biopsy is not only irreplaceable in the recognition of a well-defined pathological entity to insert the patient in a nosological framework, but may also provide

Table 4 Items for analytical evaluation of light microscopy

Glomeruli	Mononuclear cells in vasa recta
Number of glomeruli	Tubules
Number of obsolescent glomeruli	Epithelial cell (proximal)
Size and shape of glomerular tuft	Swelling or flattering
Bowman's capsule	Vacuolization (size of vacuoles)
Bowman's space	Brush border loss
Capsular adhesion	Inclusion (hyaline, crystals)
Crescents (number, size, and type)	Foamy transformation
Leucocytes in capillary loops	Nuclear changes
Mesangial cell proliferation	Mitoses
Mesangial matrix increase	Necrosis
Capillary lumen patency	Tubular lumen
Deposits	Size and patency
Basement membrane features	Casts (type and size)
Segmental sclerosis	Cells (erythrocytes, leucocytes, epithelial) and cell debris
Glomerular capillary necrosis	Crystals
Glomerular capillary thrombosis	Basement membrane
Juxtaglomerular apparatus	Interstitium
Vessels	Oedema
Arteries/arterioles	Leucocyte infiltration
Intimal fibrosis	Granuloma formation
Intimal proliferation	Red blood cell extravasation
Mucoid transformation (onion-skin)	Fibrosis
Elastic reduplication	Foam cells
Hyaline or fibrinoid deposits	Lymph casts
Medial hypertrophy	Crystals or calcified aggregates
Necrosis	
Thrombosis	
Leucocyte infiltration	
Peritubular capillaries and venules	
Congestion	
Leucocyte infiltration	

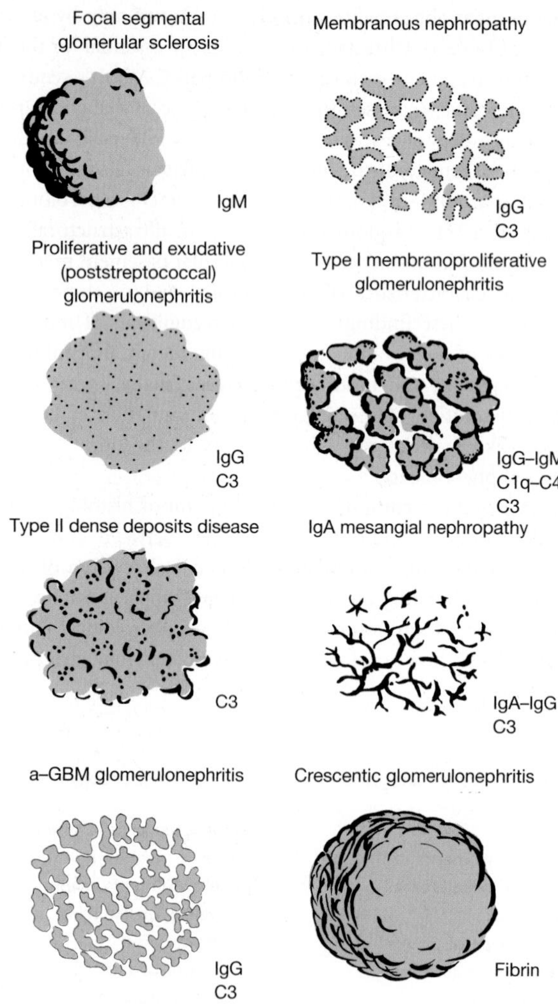

Fig. 4 Characteristic immunohistological patterns of the different types of primary glomerulonephritis.

information on the activity or chronicity of the lesions, as well as on staging or subclassification of pathological patterns. It is seldom that the inadequacy of the biopsy specimen, the presence of extensive sclerosing lesions, the presence of an unclassifiable pattern, or the superimposition of two different pathological processes preclude a firm classification. However, even when the final morphological diagnosis remains uncertain, renal biopsy may suggest a diagnostic hypothesis.

Analytical approach to biopsy findings

Identification of some basic morphological changes plays a key role in renal biopsy interpretation. This type of analysis may be schematic and is not always applicable. However, it represents an effort to establish a correlation between morphological changes and pathogenetic mechanisms underlying renal lesions. These changes may be isolated or may coexist with other lesions. They will be described briefly, considering light and electron microscopy together.

Glomerular lesions

Glomerular changes can be divided into three categories (Fig. 5): (a) changes of cellular components; (b) changes resulting from deposition of immune material; and (c) changes of extracellular components.

Changes of cellular components include intracapillary (endothelial or mesangial) proliferation, infiltration of capillary loops (by polymorphonuclear and/or mononuclear cells), extracapillary or crescentic proliferation. The use of monoclonal antibodies may be helpful in characterizing the cells causing hypercellularity, for example, monocytes, and lymphocytes (Hooke *et al.* 1987; Castiglione *et al.* 1988). Detailed evaluation of podocytes sometimes gives the clue for a definite diagnosis. Fabry's disease is characterized by a massive accumulation of myelin figures or massive vasuolization or protein storage of podocytes may indicate segmental hyalinosis sclerosis in deeper sections of the glomerulus.

Table 5 Electron microscopy findings relevant for diagnosis

Electron microscopy findings	Disease
Glomerular cell	
Foot process effacement of podocytes	Minimal change nephropathy
Microtubular inclusions (virus-like structures)	Lupus nephritis
Cytoplasmic inclusions of storage material	Lecithin–cholesterol acyltransferase deficit disease—Fabry's disease
Mesangial cell interposition	Membranoproliferative glomerulonephritis
Leucocytes (polymorphonuclear, lymphocytes, and monocytes) and platelets in capillary loops	Acute glomerulonephritis, lupus nephritis Cryoglobulinaemia
Extracellular glomerular structures	
Mesangial matrix increase and interposition	Glomerulonephritis
Lamina densa abnormalities (thickening, thinning, splitting, reticulation)	Alport syndrome
Lamina rara interna widening	Haemolytic–uraemic syndrome, scleroderma, transplant glomerulopathy
Basement membrane new formation	Glomerulonephritis
Collagen deposition	Nail patella syndrome
Fibrin in loops	Collagen type 4, haemolytic–uraemic syndrome
Dense deposits allocation (subepithelial, subendothelial, mesangial, intramembranous) and characterization (size and shape, osmiophilia, structure)	Glomerulonephritis
Microfibrils (amyloid and non-amyloid)	Amyloidosis–fibrillosis

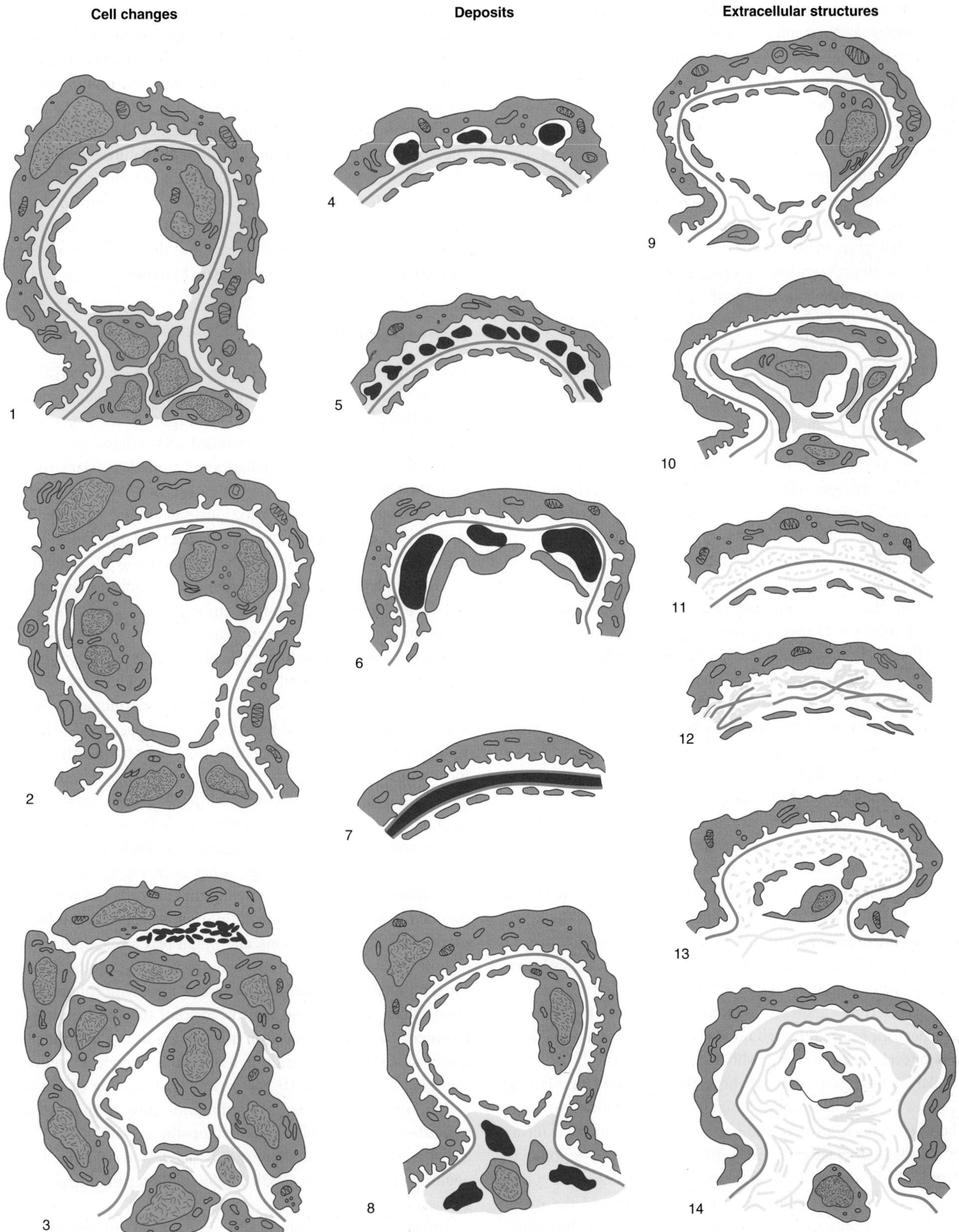

Fig. 5 Schematic representation of glomerular changes classified according to the structure involved (cell deposits and extracellular structures). (1) Mesangial cell proliferation; (2) leucocyte infiltration; (3) extracapillary proliferation with crescent formation; (4) subepithelial deposits (hump-like); (5) subepithelial deposits (membranous nephropathy); (6) subendothelial deposits (membranoproliferative glomerulonephritis type I); (7) intramembranous dense deposits (membranoproliferative glomerulonephritis type II); (8) mesangial deposits; (9) mesangial matrix increase; (10) mesangial interposition; (11) new formation of basement membrane; (12) lamina densa reticulation (Alport's syndrome); (13) lamina rara internal widening with fine granular material (haemolytic–uraemic syndrome, systemic sclerosis, malignant hypertension); (14) glomerular sclerosis with capillary lumen obliteration.

Glomerular deposits can be identified in mesangial, subendothelial, intramembranous, and subepithelial positions. Two types of the last deposits can be distinguished: (a) those typical of postinfections (post-streptococcal) glomerulonephritis, termed humps, which are scattered, globular, or elongated and lean on the lamina rara externa; and (b) those typical of membranous nephropathy, which are in contact with the lamina densa.

A great variety of changes can be identified in extracellular structures. These changes may be the consequence of immune injury, haemodynamic abnormalities, biochemical abnormalities in diabetes, direct endothelial injury in haemolytic uraemic syndrome, or hereditary abnormalities in Alport's syndrome. A reciprocal effect between cellular and extracellular changes of the glomerular structure exists, and it has been demonstrated that platelets, mononuclear cells, and mesangial cells may produce factors that promote mesangial proliferation, basement membrane and matrix formation, and eventually sclerosis.

Tubular lesions

Since renal biopsy is seldom performed in patients with acute tubular necrosis, tubular changes reflecting acute injury are rarely encountered in biopsies as isolated findings. Conversely, tubular cell swelling, vacuolation, and necrosis are frequently found in association with acute and severe glomerulonephritis, interstitial nephritis, vasculitis, graft rejection, and drug toxicity. Severe acute tubular lesions consisting of protein and/or necrotic cell cast may also be observed in patients with minimal change nephrotic syndrome complicated by acute renal failure (Imbasciati *et al.* 1981). A peculiar type of cast composed of dense and fractured material surrounded by multinucleated giant cells may be seen in patients with multiple myeloma and renal dysfunction. Erythrocyte casts may be seen in some cases of acute renal failure in patients with IgA nephropathy (Praga *et al.* 1985) or other types of glomerulonephritis characterized by macroscopic haematuria and tubular lesions (Fogazzi *et al.* 1995).

Tubular lesions may assume particular relevance in renal transplantation. Acute tubular necrosis is relatively frequent in cadaveric renal transplantation. Tubulitis (i.e. the tubular infiltration by lymphocytes) is considered to be a reliable marker of acute rejection (Solez *et al.* 1993). When acute rejection occurs early in the post-transplant period, tubular lesions may reflect both immunological and ischaemic insults. The use of cyclosporin in transplantation has introduced another cause of tubular damage. Some tubular lesions (i.e. isometric vacuolization, giant mitochondria, and calcification of individual necrotic cells), although non-specific, have been considered suggestive of cyclosporin toxicity (Mihatsch *et al.* 1983).

A tubular change observed in patients with chronic and long-lasting renal diseases is tubular atrophy. A significant correlation has been found between tubular atrophy and impairment of glomerular filtration rate (Mackensen-Haen *et al.* 1981). Two patterns of this lesion may be observed. The first is always accompanied by a thinning of the tubular basement membrane characterized by a reduction of the outer diametre. Epithelial cells are decreased in size and show a clear cytoplasm and loss of brush border. In the second pattern, the outer diameter may be unchanged or even increased, although the epithelium is flattened and dedifferentiated. The lumen may be widened and may contain hyaline casts. The tubular basement membrane is usually thickened. Tubular atrophy develops in a variety of renal disorders associated with glomerular obsolescence and interstitial fibrosis. Inflammatory destruction of parts of the nephron, narrowing of the major blood vessels, or obliteration of peritubular capillaries with consequences of reduced blood supply to tubular cells are probably the cause of tubular atrophy. Large areas of atrophic tubules with basement membrane thinning is typically seen in case of narrowing of larger extra- or intrarenal arteries. Tubular destruction may play a key role in the loss of renal function in chronic renal failure. Some studies have shown that tubular obliteration may lead to a tubular glomeruli, which are unaltered glomeruli deprived of their connection to the proximal tubule. This process may be the main reason for deterioration of renal function in tubulointerstitial disease, but there is some evidence that it can also occur in glomerular diseases (Marcussen 1992).

Interstitial tissue

Diffuse interstitial infiltration of leucocytes is characteristic of drug-induced interstitial nephritis. Inflammatory cells, mainly mononuclear and scattered eosinophils and polymorphs, or even granulomas, fill interstitial spaces, which are expanded and oedematous. Cells tend to accumulate in peritubular capillaries and around vascular structures, and even infiltrate into the tubules. Other causes of acute interstitial nephritis are bacterial and viral infections, sarcoidosis, systemic lupus erythematosus, and other immune-mediated renal diseases. In many cases, the cause of interstitial nephritis remains unknown (Cameron 1988).

Acute interstitial rejection is another condition characterized by diffuse interstitial infiltration by mononuclear cells. These cells may fill peritubular capillaries and penetrate into the tubules, leading to so-called tubulitis, which is a typical sign of acute rejection.

Mononuclear cells infiltrating interstitial spaces may be seen, independently of nephron loss, in primary glomerulonephritis, in lupus nephritis, and in essential mixed cryoglobulinaemia (D'Amico 1988). Mild to severe focal interstitial inflammation is frequently found. Small foci of interstitial infiltration are generally localized near obsolescent glomeruli and atrophic tubules. In lupus nephritis, interstitial inflammation has been found to correlate with the activity of glomerular lesions and to have prognostic significance (Park *et al.* 1986).

According to these findings, it has been suggested that interstitial infiltration may be an active reaction that parallels glomerular injury. It may be mediated by mechanisms in some aspects independent of those producing glomerular lesions, and might play a role in the progression of glomerular diseases. Pyelonephritis gives rise to another type of interstitial inflammation mainly characterized by polymorphonuclear leucocytes, which infiltrate and destroy adjacent tubules, tubular cells, and basement membranes. Electron microscopy, usually not the method of choice to study the interstitium, has recently became attractive in renal transplants. In peritubular capillaries, multilayering of the basement membranes was described as a lesion indicating chronic rejection and correlated with transplant glomerulopathy (Hvala *et al.* 2001). This lesion is, however, entirely unspecific as it is also found in analgesic nephropathy (Mihatsch 1983b), following interstitial nephritis and in glomerulonephritis.

Interstitial fibrosis may be a consequence of inflammation, tubular obstruction, glomerular obsolescence, and ischaemia. Interstitial fibrosis, usually in association with tubular atrophy, is an obvious parameter of chronicity in any type of renal disease, and may be predictive of the outcome in membranous nephropathy (Wehrmann *et al.* 1989), lupus nephritis (Austin *et al.* 1983), and in IgA nephropathy (D'Amico *et al.* 1986).

Vascular lesions

Arteriolar changes are the main characteristic of several diseases, such as hypertension, diabetes mellitus progressive systemic sclerosis, thrombotic thrombocytopenic purpura, haemolytic–uraemic syndrome, micropolyarteritis. Vascular lesions may also appear in chronic renal diseases as a consequence of arterial hypertension, immune deposits, and/or adaptative changes of intrarenal haemodynamics. A peculiar form of vascular damage can be seen in patients treated with cyclosporin. The lesion, which is similar to that observed in haemolytic uraemic syndrome, has been described in kidneys of patients treated with cyclosporin for organ transplantation (Mihatsch *et al.* 1983) or autoimmune disease (Mihatsch *et al.* 1988).

Arterial and arteriolar lesions are commonly grouped into a few main categories (Fig. 6), although the criteria for differential diagnosis among pathological groups are not clearly established. It is useful to recognize some basic changes, which alone or in combination may contribute to the lesion. They include endothelial swelling or necrosis, proliferation of myofibroblasts, new basement membrane formation, accumulation of immune granular or filamentous material (mucoid transformation) (Hsu and Churg 1980), reduplication of the elastic membranes, fibrinoid necrosis of the vascular wall, and leucocyte infiltration and thrombotic

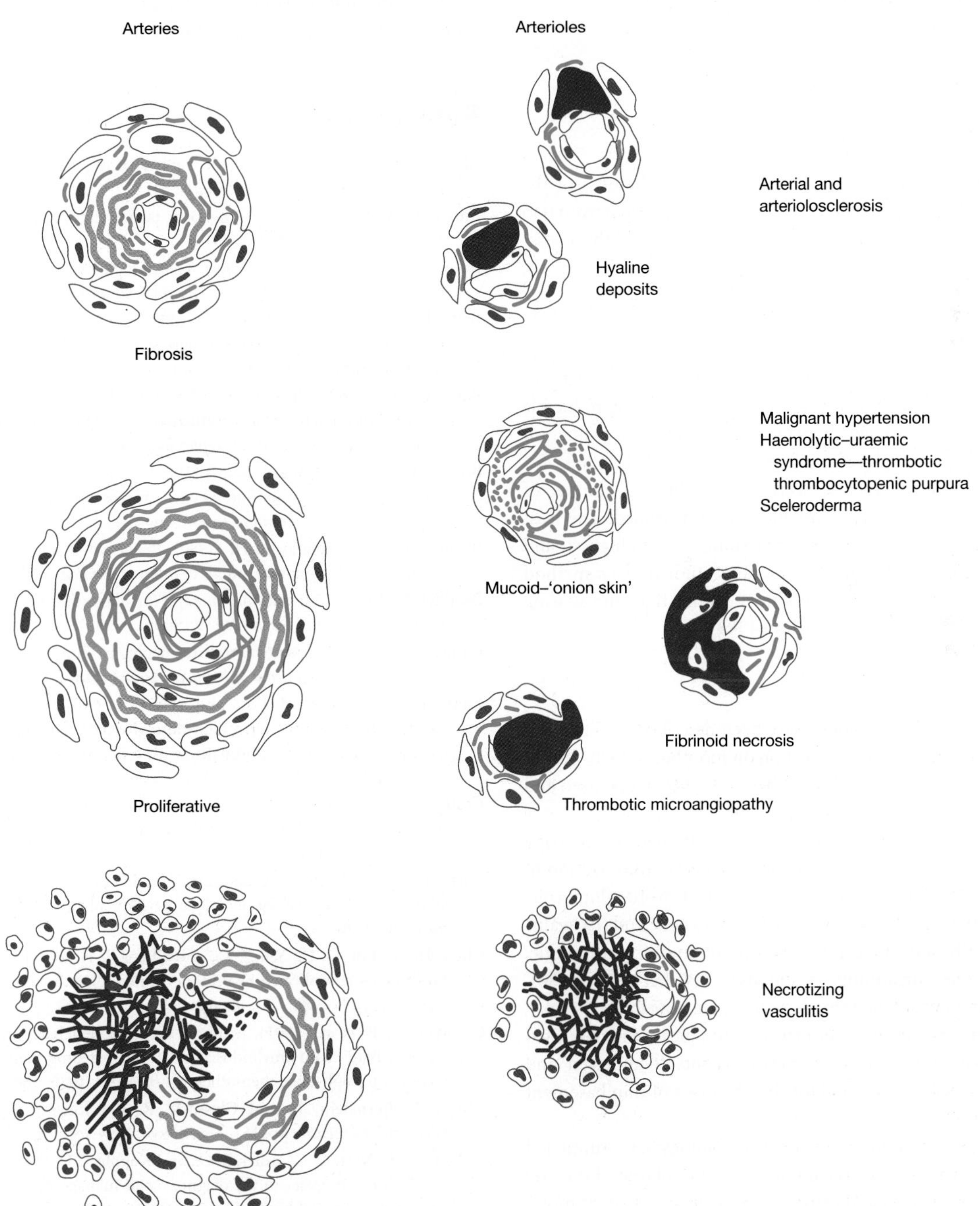

Fig. 6 Schematic representation of the main pathological patterns of vascular diseases involving the kidney.

obliteration of the lumen. Unfortunately, the pathogenesis of the diseases that involve renal microvasculature is largely unknown. Endothelial injury produced by different aetiological factors may initiate a variety of pathological events within the vessel wall and the lumen: within the vessel wall accumulation of fine fibrillar material on the subendothelial side, overproduction of basement membrane, insudation of proteinaceous material, necrosis and/or proliferation of myofibroblasts; in the vascular lumen endothelial damage promotes platelet aggregation, fibrin deposition, and thrombosis. Considering that endothelial injury is the common event of different disorders, it seems reasonable to group within the same histopathological pattern haemolytic–uraemic syndrome, thrombotic thrombocytopenic purpura, malignant nephrosclerosis, and progressive systemic sclerosis and radiation nephropathy.

Semiquantitative evaluation and morphometry

The degree of severity and the distribution (in focal lesions) of the different morphological parameters can be arbitrarily scored from 0 to 3 or 4+. Relatively objective criteria can be established for the assessment of some lesions, such as tubular atrophy or interstitial fibrosis, where the percentage of tissue area covered by this change may be evaluated approximately. Obsolescent glomeruli, glomeruli focally involved by proliferative or sclerosing lesions, crescents, and glomerulocapsular adhesions can be evaluated numerically. Semiquantitative evaluation of renal biopsy has been demonstrated to be a reproducible method (Pirani *et al.* 1964), which increases the accuracy of evaluation of the biopsy and provides useful information in predicting the outcome and in making therapeutic decisions. If a limited number of cases are studied, the ranking technique is recommended. The least severe lesion is ranked 1, the most severe lesion is ranked highest, and this may correspond to the number of cases studied. This method allows a better correlation with laboratory values than the scoring system from 0 to 3+ (Solez and Whelton 1983).

Morphometry

Different morphometric techniques have been described for light and electron microscopy. For basic information on morphometry the reader is referred to standard monographs (Weibel 1979, 1980; Gundersen and Osterby 1982).

The prerequisites for morphometric analysis by light microscopy are: (a) absolute standardized preparation of material from fixation to embedding; (b) sufficient sample size (at least 6–10 glomeruli) (Oberholzer *et al.* 1983); (c) uniform section thickness; and (d) evaluation of identically stained sections. The point-counting technique, which is very time consuming, is still used (Weibel 1979, 1980). Alternatively, different semiautomatic systems are available.

In electron microscopy, morphometric techniques are mainly used for basement membrane thickness measurements (Gundersen and Osterby 1982), which are essential for the diagnosis of thin basement membrane disease.

The advent of new techniques of molecular biology have stimulated studies on the mechanisms of renal injury at molecular level directly on renal tissue. Production and expression of a great variety of molecules have been investigated in experimental animals by new techniques such as reverse transcription polymerase chain reaction or *in situ* hybridization. There is a great interest in applying these methods even in human renal biopsies to better understand the role of inflammatory mediators and other factors that regulate production of extracellular matrix components (Schena and Gesualdo 1994). Glomerular mRNA levels of molecules relevant for podocyte function may be helpful for establishing diagnosis and predict prognosis in some proteinuric diseases. Schmid *et al.* 2003 found that the expression ratio of podocyn to synaptopodin, the two genes with the most disparate expression, allowed a robust separation between focal segmental glomerulosclerosis and minimal change disease and expression markers were able to predict steroid responsiveness in these cases. The same group of investigators, using small microarrays dedicated to genes involved in cell-cell contact, matrix turnover, and inflammation found a strong correlation between gene expression data and progression of renal disease (Henger *et al.* 2004).

References

Ahuja, T. S. *et al.* (1998). Diabetic nephropathy with anti-GBM nephritis. *American Journal of Kidney Diseases* **31**, 127–130.

Austin, H. A., III *et al.* (1983). Prognostic factors in lupus nephritis. *American Journal of Medicine* **75**, 382–391.

Baker, R. J. and Pusey, C. D. (2004). The changing of acute tubulointerstitial nephritis. *Nephrology, Dialysis, Transplantation* **19**, 8–10.

Ballardie, F. W. and Roberts, I. S. D. (2002). Controlled prospective trial of prednisolone and cytotoxic in progressive IgA nephropathy. *Journal of the American Society of Nephrology* **13**, 142–148.

Banfi, G. *et al.* (1991). The impact of prolonged immunosuppression on the outcome of idiopathic focal segmental glomerulosclerosis with nephrotic syndrome in adults. *Clinical Nephrology* **36**, 53–59.

Bolton, W. K. and Mesnard, R. M. (1982). New technique of kidney tissue processing for immunofluorescence microscopy. Formol sucrose/gum sucrose/paraffin. *Laboratory Investigation* **47**, 206–213.

Border, W. A. and Cohen, A. H. (1980). Renal biopsy diagnosis in clinically silent multiple myeloma. *Annals of Internal Medicine* **93**, 43–46.

Brodhel, J. (1991). Conventional therapy for idiopathic nephrotic syndrome in children. *Clinical Nephrology* **9** (Suppl. 1), 8–15.

Cameron, J. S. (1988). Allergic interstitial nephritis: clinical features and pathogenesis. *Quarterly Journal of Medicine* **66**, 97–116.

Cameron, J. S., Healey, M. J. R., and Adu, D. (1990). The Medical Research Council Trial of short-term high-dose alternate day prednisone in idiopathic membranous nephropathy with a nephrotic syndrome in adults. *Quarterly Journal of Medicine* **74**, 133–156.

Castiglione, A., Bucci, A., D'Amico, G., and Atkins, R. C. (1988). The relationship of infiltrating renal leukocytes to disease activity in lupus and cryoglobulinaemic glomerulonephritis. *American Journal of Nephrology* **50**, 14–23.

Cattran, D. C. *et al.* (1999). A randomized trial of cyclosporine in patients with steroid-resistant focal segmental glomerulonephritis. *Kidney International* **56**, 2220–2226.

Chen, H. H., Lin, H. C., Yeh, J. C., and Chen, C. P. (2001). Renal biopsy in pregnancies complicated by undertermined renal disease. *Acta Obstetrica Gynecologica Scandinavica* **80**, 888–893.

Choufani, E. B. *et al.* (2001). Acquired factor X deficiency in patients with amyloid light chain amyloidosis: incidence, bleeding manifestations, and response to high-dose chemotherapy. *Blood* **97**, 1885–1887.

Churg, J., Bernstein, J., and Glassock, R. J. *Classification and Atlas of Glomerular Diseases*, pp. 151–156. Tokyo, New York: Igaku-Shoin, 1995.

Cohen, A. H., Nast, C. C., Adler, S. G., and Kopple, J. D. (1989). Clinical utility of kidney biopsies in the diagnosis and management of renal disease. *American Journal of Nephrology* **9**, 309–315.

Collaborative Study of the Adult Idiopathic Nephrotic Syndrome (1979). A controlled study of short-term prednisone treatment in adults with membranous nephropathy. *New England Journal of Medicine* **301**, 1301–1306.

Colvin, R. B. (1996). The renal allograft biopsy. *Kidney International* **50**, 1069–1082.

Corwin, H. L., Schwartz, M. N., and Lewis, E. J. (1988). The importance of sample size in the interpretation of the renal biopsy. *American Journal of Nephrology* **8**, 85–89.

D'Amico, G. (1988). Role of interstitial infiltration in glomerular disease. *Nephrology, Dialysis, Transplantation* **3**, 596–600.

D'Amico, G. *et al.* (1986). Prognostic indicators in idiopathic IgA mesangial nephropathy. *Quarterly Journal of Medicine* **59**, 363–378.

Donadio, J. V., Jr. (1992). Treatment of membranous nephropathy in systemic lupus erythematosus. *Nephrology, Dialysis, Transplantation* **7** (Suppl. 1), 97–104.

Donadio, J. V. *et al.* (1999). The long-term outcome of patients with IgA nephropathy treated with fish oil in a controlled trial. *Journal of the American Society of Nephrology* **10**, 1772–1777.

Fogazzi, G. B., Bajetta, M. T., Banfi, G., and Mihatsch, M. (1989). Comparison of immunofluorescent findings in kidney after snap-freezing and formalin fixation. *Pathology Research and Practice* **185**, 225–230.

Fogazzi, G. B., Imbasciati, E., Moroni, G., Scalia, A., Mihatsch, M. J., and Ponticelli, C. (1995). Reversible acute renal failure from gross hematuria due to glomerulonephritis: not only in IgA nephropathy and not associated with intratubular obstruction. *Nephrology, Dialysis, Transplantation* **10**, 624–629.

Fuiano, G. *et al.* (2000). Current indications for renal biopsy: a questionnaire-based survey. *American Journal of Kidney Diseases* **35**, 448–457.

Furness, P. N. and Taub, N. (2001). International variation in the interpretation of renal transplant biopsies. Report of the CERTPAP Project. *Kidney International* **60**, 1998–2012.

Greenbaum, L. A. *et al.* (2000). Pediatric biopsy of a single native kidney. *Pediatric Nephrology* **15**, 66–69.

Gundersen, H. J. G. and Osterby, R. (1982). Optimizing sampling efficiency of stereological studies in biology: or do more less well! *Journal of Microscopy* **121**, 65–73.

Habib, R. and Broyer, M. (1993). Clinical significance of allograft nephropathy. *Kidney International* **44** (Suppl. 43), S95–S98.

Henger, A. *et al.* (2004). Gene expression fingerprints in human tubulointerstitial inflammation and fibrosis as prognostic markers of disease progression. *Kidney International* **65**, 904–917.

Hooke, D. H., Gee, D. C., and Atkins, R. C. (1987). Leukocyte analysis using monoclonal antibodies in human glomerulonephritis. *Kidney International* **31**, 964–972.

Hsu, H. C. and Churg, J. (1980). The ultrastructure of mucoid 'onionskin' intimal lesions in malignant nephrosclerosis. *American Journal of Pathology* **99**, 67–80.

Hvala, A. *et al.* (2001). Interstitial capillary in normal and in transplanted kidneys: an ultrastructural study. *Ultrastructural Pathology* **25**, 295–299.

Ihling, Ch. *et al.* (1994). Immunoelectron microscopy of different forms of glomerulonephritis in routine biopsy material. *Pathological Research Practice* **190**, 417–422.

Imbasciati, E. *et al.* (1981). Acute renal failure in idiopathic nephrotic syndrome. *Nephron* **28**, 186–191.

Imbasciati, E. *et al.* (1991). Collagen type III glomerulopathy: a new idiopathic glomerular disease. *American Journal of Nephrology* **11**, 422–429.

Korbet, S. M., Schwartz, M. M., and Lewis, E. J. (1988). Minimal-change glomerulopathy of adulthood. *American Journal of Nephrology* **8**, 291–297.

Korbet, S. M., Schwartz, M. M., and Lewis, E. J. (1994). The fibrillary glomerulopathies. *American Journal of Kidney Diseases* **23**, 751–765.

Kuller, J., D'Andrea, N. A., and Mc Mahon, M. J. (2001). Renal biopsy and pregnancy. *American Journal of Obstetrics and Gynecology* **184**, 1093–1096.

Mackensen-Haen, S., Bader, R., Grund, K. E., and Bohle, A. (1981). Correlation between renal cortical interstitial fibrosis, atrophy of the proximal tubules and impairment of the glomerular filtration rate. *Clinical Nephrology* **15**, 167–171.

Mak, S. K. *et al.* (2001). Prospective study on renal outcome of IgA nephropathy superimposed on diabetic glomerulosclerosis in type 2 diabetic patients. *Nephrology, Dialysis, Transplantation* **16**, 1183–1188.

Marcussen, N. (1992). Atubular glomeruli and the structural basis for chronic renal failure. *Laboratory Investigation* **66**, 265–284.

Meehan, S. M. *et al.* (1999). The relationship of untreated borderline infiltrates by the Banff criteria to acute rejection in renal allograft biopsies. *Journal of the American Society of Nephrology* **10**, 1806–1814.

Mendelssohn, D. C. and Cole, E. H. (1995). Outcomes of percutaneous kidney biopsy, including those of solitary native kidneys. *American Journal of Kidney Diseases* **26**, 580–585.

Mihatsch, M. J. *et al.* (1983a). Morphological findings in kidney transplants after treatment with cyclosporine. *Transplantation Proceedings* **15**, 2821–2836.

Mihatsch, M. J. *et al.* (1983b). Capillary sclerosis of the urinary tract and analgesic nephropathy. *Clinical Nephrology* **20**, 285–301.

Mihatsch, M. J. *et al.* (1988). Cyclosporin associated nephropathy in patients with autoimmune diseases. *Klinische Wochenschrift* **66**, 43–47.

Mihatsch, M. J., Ryffel, B., and Gudat, F. (1995). The differential diagnosis between rejection and cyclosporine toxicity. *Kidney International* **48** (Suppl. 52), S63–S69.

Monga, G. *et al.* (1989). Pattern of double glomerulopathies: a clinicopathologic study of superimposed glomerulonephritis on diabetic glomerulosclerosis. *Modern Pathology* **2**, 407–414.

Monga, G. *et al.* (1992). Intertubular capillary changes in kidney allografts: a morphologic investigation on 61 renal specimens. *Modern Pathology* **5**, 125–130.

Moroni, G. *et al.* (1996). Nephritic flares are predictors of bad long-term outcome in lupus nephritis. *Kidney International* **50**, 2047–2053.

Moroni, G. *et al.* (1999). Clinical and prognostic value of serial renal biopsies in lupus nephritis. *American Journal of Kidney Diseases* **34**, 530–539.

Najafi, C. C. *et al.* (2001). Significance of histologic patterns of glomerular injury upon long-term prognosis in severe lupus glomerulonephritis. *Kidney International* **59**, 2156–2163.

Nankivell, B. J. *et al.* (2003). The natural history of chronic allograft nephropathy. *New England Journal of Medicine* **349**, 2288–2290.

Nickerson, P. *et al.* (1999). Efect of increasing baseline immunosuppression on the prevalence of clinical and subclinical rejection: a pilot study. *Journal of the American Society of Nephrology* **10**, 1801–1805.

Nickeleit, V., Singh, H. K., and Mihatsch, M. J. (2003). Polyomavirus nephropathy: morphology, pathophysiology, and clinical management. *Current Opinions in Nephrology and Hypertension* **12**, 599–605.

Nolasco, F., Cameron, J. S., Heywood, E. F., Hicks, J., Ogg, C., and Williams, D. G. (1986). Adult-onset minimal change nephrotic syndrome: a long-term follow-up. *Kidney International* **29**, 1215–1223.

Oberholzer, M., Torhorst, J., and Mihatsch, M. J. (1983). Minimum sample size of kidney biopsies for semiquantitative and quantitative evaluation. *Nephron* **34**, 192–195.

Olsen, S. and Mogensen, C. E. (1996). How often is NIDDM complicated with non-diabetic renal disease? An analysis of renal biopsy and the literature. *Diabetologia* **39**, 1638–1645.

Paone, D. B. and Meyer, L. R. E. (1981). The effect of biopsy on therapy in renal disease. *Archives of Internal Medicine* **141**, 1039–1041.

Park, M. H., D'Agati, V., Appel, G. B., and Pirani, C. L. (1986). Tubulointerstitial disease in lupus nephritis: relationship to immune deposits, interstitial inflammation, glomerular changes, renal function and prognosis. *Nephron* **44**, 309–319.

Parving, H. H. *et al.* (1992). Prevalence and causes of albuminuria in non-insulin-dependent diabetic patients. *Kidney International* **41**, 758–762.

Pei, Y., Cattran, D., Delmore, T., Katz, A., Lang, A., and Rance, P. (1987). Evidence suggesting undertreatment in adults with idiopathic focal segmental glomerulosclerosis. Regional Glomerulonephritis Registry Study. *American Journal of Medicine* **82**, 938–944.

Pirani, C. L., Pollack, V. E., and Schwartz, F. D. (1964). The reproducibility of semiquantitative analyses of renal histology. *Nephron* **1**, 230–246.

Ponticelli, C. *et al.* (1992). Methylprednisolone and chlorambucil as compared with methylprednisolone alone for the treatment of idiopathic membranous nephropathy. *New England Journal of Medicine* **327**, 599–603.

Ponticelli, C. *et al.* (1995). A 10-year follow-up of a randomized study with methylprednisolone and chlorambucil in membranous nephropathy. *Kidney International* **48**, 1600–1604.

Ponticelli, C. *et al.* (1998). A randomized study comparing methylprednisolone plus chlorambucil versus methylprednisolone plus cyclophosphamide in idiopathic membranous nephropathy. *Journal of the American Society of Nephrology* **9**, 444–450.

Ponticelli, C. *et al.* (1999). Can prolonged treatment improve the prognosis in adults with focal segmental glomerulosclerosis? *American Journal of Kidney Diseases* **34**, 618–625.

Ponticelli, C. (2000). Progression of renal damage in chronic rejection. *Kidney International* **57** (Suppl. 75), S62–S70.

Pozzi, C. *et al.* (1999). Corticosteroids in IgA nephropathy: a randomized controlled trial. *Lancet* **355**, 883–887.

Pozzi, C. *et al.* (2003). Corticosteroid effectiveness in IgA nephropathy: long-term results of a randomized, controlled trial. *Journal of the American Society of Nephrology* **15**, 157–163.

Praga, M. *et al.* (1985). Acute worsening of renal function during episodes of macroscopic haematuria in IgA nephropathy. *Kidney International* **28**, 69–74.

Racusen, L. C. *et al.* (1999). The Banff 97 working classification of renal allograft pathology. *Kidney International* **55**, 713–723.

Racusen, L. C. *et al.* (2003). Antibody-mediated rejection criteria—an addition to the Banff 97 classification of renal allograft rejection. *American Journal of Transplantation* **3**, 708–714.

Ramos, E. *et al.* (2003). Clinical course of polyoma virus nephropathy in 67 renal transplant patients. *Journal of the American Society of Nephrology* **13**, 2145–2151.

Richards, N. T. *et al.* (1992). Increased prevalence of renal biopsy findings other than diabetic glomerulopathy in type II diabetes mellitus. *Nephrology, Dialysis, Transplantation* **7**, 397–399.

Richards, N. T. *et al.* (1994). Knowledge of renal biopsy alters patient management in over 40 per cent of cases. *Nephrology, Dialysis, Transplantation* **9**, 1255–1259.

Rydel, J. J., Korbet, S. M., Borok, R. Z., and Schwartz, M. M. (1995). Focal and segmental glomerular sclerosis in adults: presentation, course and response to therapy. *American Journal of Kidney Diseases* **25**, 534–542.

Rush, D. *et al.* (1998). Beneficial effects of treatment of early subclinical rejection: a randomized study. *Journal of the American Society of Nephrology* **9**, 2129–2134.

Schena, F. P. and Gesualdo, L. (1994). Renal biopsy—beyond histology and immunofluorescence. *Nephrology, Dialysis, Transplantation* **9**, 1541–1544.

Schmid, H. et al. (2003). Gene expression profiles of podocyte-associated molecules as diagnostic markers in acquired proteinuric diseases. *Journal of American Society of Nephrology* **14**, 2958–2966.

Schwartz, M. N. *et al.* (1993). Irreproducibility of the activity and chronicity indices limits their utility in the management of lupus nephritis. *American Journal of Kidney Diseases* **21**, 374–377.

Silva, F., Pace, E. H., Burns, D. K., and Krous, H. (1983). The spectrum of diabetic nephropathy and membranous glomerulopathy: report of two patients and review of the literature. *Diabetic Nephropathy* **2**, 28–32.

Serón, D. *et al.* (2002). Reliability of chronic allograft nephropathy diagnosis in sequential protocol biopsies. *Kidney International* **61**, 727–733.

Solez, K. and Whelton, A. *Acute Renal Failure: Correlations Between Morphology and Function.* New York: Dekker, 1983.

Solez, K. *et al.* (1993). International standardization of criteria for the histologic diagnosis of renal allograft rejection: the Banff working classification of kidney transplant pathology. *Kidney International* **44**, 411–422.

Striker, G. E., Quadracci, L. J., and Cutler, R. E. *Use and Interpretation of Renal Biopsy.* Philadelphia: Saunders, 1978.

Torres, A. *et al.* (2002). Conservative versus immunosuppressive treatment of patients with idiopathic membranous nephropathy. *Kidney International* **61**, 219–227.

Turner, M. W., Hutchinson, T. A., Barre, P. E., Prichard, S., and Jothy, S. (1986). A prospective study on the impact of the renal biopsy in clinical management. *Clinical Nephrology* **26**, 217–221.

Weening, J. J. *et al.* (2004). The classification of glomerulonephritis in systemic lupus erythematosus revised. *Journal of the American Society of Nephrology* **15**, 241–250.

Wehrmann, M. *et al.* (1989). Long-term prognosis of chronic idiopathic membranous glomerulonephritis. *Clinical Nephrology* **31**, 67–76.

Weibel, E. R. *Stereological Methods. Vol. I. Practical Methods for Biological Morphometry.* London: Academic Press, 1979.

Weibel, E. R. *Stereological Methods. Vol. II. Theoretical Foundations.* London: Academic Press, 1980.

Wernick, R. M. *et al.* (1993). Reliability of histologic scoring for lupus nephritis: a community-based evaluation. *Annals of Internal Medicine* **119**, 805–811.

Young, B. A., Barsch, C. L., Alpers, C. E., and Davis, C. L. (1996). Cyclosporine-associated thrombotic microangiopathy/hemolytic uremic syndrome following kidney and kidney–pancreas transplantation. *American Journal of Kidney Diseases* **28**, 561–571.

Zawada, E. T., Jensen, R., Hicks, D., Putnam, W., and Ramirez, D. (1987). Nephrotic syndrome and renal failure in an elderly man. *American Journal of Nephrology* **7**, 482–489.

Zollinger, H. U. and Mihatsch, J. M. *Renal Pathology in Biopsy.* Berlin: Springer-Verlag, 1978.

1.8 Immunological investigation of the patient with renal disease

Jo H.M. Berden and Jack F.M. Wetzels

Introduction

The kidney is an important target of immune-mediated injury. Our understanding of the pathogenesis of immunological diseases has been greatly facilitated by detailed studies of the time course of changes in kidney morphology in various animal models. A well-known example is the renal injury that occurs after injecting bovine serum albumin (BSA)–anti-BSA complexes in rabbits, a model of serum sickness, and a prototypical example of an immune complex disease. It is now well established that many primary glomerular diseases are immune-mediated (Ambrus and Sridhar 1997). Furthermore, the kidney may be the target in various infectious diseases, auto-immune disorders, and systemic vasculitides (Ledford 1997).

Renal injury may be evoked by humoral (antibody) or cellular immune responses. Three mechanisms can be defined. The kidney may be the target of antibodies that are directed against kidney specific antigens, exciting a type II immunological reaction. Anti-glomerular basement membrane (anti-GBM) disease is the best-known example, caused by antibodies directed against collagen IV, an intrinsic component of the GBM. More often, the kidney is involved in a type III immunological reaction caused by the deposition of immune complexes. These immune complexes may either be formed in the circulation or *in situ*, by the binding of an antibody to an antigen planted in the glomerular capillary wall. Size, charge, and composition of the immune complexes determine their final localization, for example, subendothelial deposits in the initial stage of poststreptococcal glomerulonephritis and subepithelial deposits in membranous glomerulopathy. The most common systemic disease with immune complex mediated renal injury is systemic lupus erythematosus (SLE). The kidney is also frequently involved in vasculitis. In this latter condition injury is probably also mediated by cellular responses. Although various autoantibodies may be present in the circulation of patients with systemic vasculitis, there is no evidence of antibody or complement deposition in the kidneys.

Assays directed at the evaluation of the immune response and particularly at the recognition of (auto)-antibodies have proved to be valuable tools in establishing a diagnosis and/or monitoring of disease activity in patients with renal diseases. An alphabetical overview of various immunological markers and associated renal diseases is given in Table 1.

Laboratory techniques

Although an in-depth discussion of the various laboratory assays is beyond the scope of this chapter, we will briefly address the most important techniques. For the practicing clinician, it is important to realize that test results are dependent on the techniques used and to be aware of pitfalls.

Electrophoresis

This is a simple technique, where a mixture of proteins is applied to an agar gel and subsequently separated by applying a charge over the gel. Protein electrophoresis of serum shows the typical pattern with separation of albumin, $\alpha1$, $\alpha2$, β, and γ globulins. More specific assays are based on the principle that antigens and antibodies form precipitates. Examples are immunoelectrophoresis or immunofixation, where proteins are separated by charge and precipitated by antibodies that diffuse into the gel. If specific antibody–antigen reactions occur these are visible as precipitation lines in the gel. In immunonephelometry the antigens and antibodies form insoluble complexes in solution that are detected by light scatter.

Indirect immunofluorescence

With this technique, antibodies directed at tissue antigens can be visualized. Tissue slides (varying from kidney to specific cell lines) are exposed to serum. Antibodies directed to antigens that are expressed in the tissue/cells will bind. These antibodies are visualized by adding a fluorescent secondary antibody directed at human immunoglobulins. The fluorescent pattern and the tissue type provide clues with respect to the antigens involved. Anti-GBM antibodies will cause linear immunofluorescence (IF) in the glomeruli on normal kidney sections and antinuclear antibodies will react with the nucleus of cell lines. The indirect IF technique is subject to several pitfalls: the specificity of the antigens is unclear, and most laboratories use only anti-IgG antibodies as secondary antibodies, which will not detect immunoglobulin A (IgA) or IgM class antibodies.

Enzyme-linked immunoabsorbent assay

In direct enzyme-linked immunoabsorbent assay (ELISA), antigens are coated on a plate. Antibodies will bind, and can be visualized with a ligand, usually a secondary antibody labelled with an enzyme. The enzyme converts a colourless substrate into a chromogen, which can be measured. In the ELISA assay, the sensitivity and specificity are determined by the nature and conformational shape of the coated antigens, the sort of ligand, and the epitope specificity of the antibody. The specificity and sensitivity of an ELISA can be increased by an indirect technique, the so-called antigen capture ELISA. In this technique, plates are coated with specific antibodies, which bind the antigen under investigation.

Table 1 Overview of immunological markers in renal diseases

Immunological marker		Associated systemic or renal disease
Screening assays		
ANA	+	SLE; autoimmune diseases
ANCA	+	M. Wegener; microscopic polyangiitis; renal limited vasculitis; Churg–Strauss syndrome
Antibody specificity		
Cardiolipin	+	Antiphospholipid syndrome
Centromere	+	Cutaneous sclerosis
C1q	+	SLE nephritis
DNAse B	+	Poststreptococcal glomerulonephritis
DsDNA	+	SLE
ENA	+	MCTD; M. Sjögren; scleroderma; SLE
α fodrin	+	M. Sjögren
GBM	+	Anti-GBM disease; Goodpasture's syndrome
Histone	+	Drug-induced SLE; SLE
MPO	+	See ANCA
Nucleosome	+	SLE nephritis
Phospholipid	+	See anticardiolipin/lupus anticoagulant
Proteinase 3	+	See ANCA
RNP	+	Mixed connective tissue disease
SS-A (Ro)	+	SLE; M. Sjögren
SS-B (La)	+	M. Sjögren
Streptolysin O (ASO)	+	Poststreptococcal glomerulonephritis
Topoisomerase I	+	Systemic scleroderma
Complement		
C1q	D	SLE (80%; ♂>♀)
CH50	↓/D	See C3/C4
C2	D	SLE (25%; ♂>♀); IgA nephropathy, HSP, MPGN type I
C3	↓	SLE, type I MPGN, DDD, postinfectious glomerulonephritis
	D	SLE (seldom)
C4	↓	SLE, cryoglobulinaemia
	D	SLE (75%)
Factor H	↓	HUS
	D	HUS; DDD
C3 nephritic factor	+	DDD; partial lipodystrophy
C5–C9	D	SLE (seldom)
Miscellaneous		
Cryoglobulins	+	Cryoglobulinaemia; SLE; M. Sjögren; lymphoma; HCV
IgA	↑	IgA nephropathy
	D	SLE
Lupus anticoagulant	+	Antiphospholipid syndrome; SLE
Paraproteins	+	Amyloidosis, MIDD, cast-nephropathy
vWF protease activity	↓	TTP

Abbreviations: ANA, antinuclear antibodies; ANCA, antineutrophil cytoplasmic antibodies; ENA, extractable nuclear antigens; GBM, glomerular basement membrane; MPO, myeloperoxidase; PR3, proteinase 3; ASO, antistreptolysin O; MIDD, monoclonal immunoglobulin deposition disease; DDD, dense deposit disease; HSP, Henoch–Schönlein purpura; MCTD, mixed connective tissue disease; HCV, hepatitis C virus; HUS, haemolytic uraemic syndrome; TTP, thrombotic thrombocytopaenic purpura; MPGN, membranoproliferative glomerulonephritis; D, deficiency; +, presence; ↓, decrease; ↑, increase.

This technique ensures to a greater extent that the antigen remains in its native conformation. Subsequently, antibodies reactive with the captured antigen can be detected.

Immunoblotting techniques

This technique is used to further characterize the antigen specificity of an antibody. The protein mixture is separated depending on size or change by gel chromatography and the molecules are then transferred to a nitrocellulose membrane. These blots are incubated with serum samples. After binding, antibodies are visualized by enzyme labelled secondary antibodies. The blotted proteins are identified in a marker lane by labelled antibodies of known specificity, which allows the determination of antibody specificities in the sample under investigation by comparison.

Immunoglobulins

Immunoglobulin A

IgA comprises 15–20 per cent of all immunoglobulins. In serum, most IgA is present in its monomeric form (MW 160 kDa). Two classes of IgA are recognized, IgA1 (80 per cent) and IgA2 (20 per cent). Plasma concentrations of IgA may be increased in up to 50 per cent of patients with IgA nephropathy (D'Amico 1988). However, normal values do not exclude the presence of IgA nephropathy, and elevated levels of IgA can be found in patients with hepatitis, liver cirrhosis, and Sjögren's disease. Thus, the sensitivity and specificity of measurement of serum IgA levels for the diagnosis of IgA nephropathy are rather low. Recent studies have documented abnormal glycosylation of IgA in patients with IgA nephropathy. These alterations in the IgA molecule, with a reduction of galactosyl and sialic acid residues, may be important in the pathogenesis. Abnormally glycosylated IgA demonstrates increased binding to lectin and is less effectively cleared by the sialoglycoprotein receptor. The importance of altered glycosylation is supported by the finding that this altered form of IgA is preferentially present in the mesangial IgA deposits of patients with IgA nephropathy (Allen *et al.* 2001). Although at present the biochemical characterization of IgA is purely a research tool, such measurements may provide a better clue for the diagnosis of IgA nephropathy in the future. Some investigators have observed high levels of IgA antigliadin antibodies in patients with IgA nephropathy.

IgA deficiency is the most common form of immunoglobulin deficiency, occurring in 1 out of 800 persons. IgA deficiency is associated with an increased incidence of systemic autoimmune diseases including SLE.

Paraproteins

Paraproteins are monoclonal immunoglobulins, synthesized and excreted by an abnormal clone of B lymphocytes. Paraproteins can consist of the intact immunoglobulin or contain only one part of the immunoglobulin molecule, either the heavy chain (G, A, M, D, or E) or the light chain (κ or λ). The light chains are also known as Bence Jones proteins.

Paraproteins can be recognized as a single band on serum or urine protein electrophoresis. The identity of the paraprotein must be confirmed by immunoelectrophoresis or immunofixation. A normal pattern of protein electrophoresis does not exclude the presence of a small amount of paraprotein. Also, the paraprotein may be masked in the β-globulin band.

Various renal diseases can be associated with a monoclonal gammopathy (see Chapter 4.2.1). In amyloidosis predominantly λ light chains are found, whereas κ light chains predominate in the monoclonal immunoglobulin deposition diseases (MIDD) and in patients with the Fanconi syndrome. In 15–30 per cent of patients with amyloidosis or MIDD, no monoclonal paraprotein is found in serum or urine. In contrast, light chains are present in the majority of patients with cast nephropathy, in fact, in the vast majority of these patients, the light chains account for more than 70 per cent of total urinary protein.

The detection of a monoclonal immunoglobulin on routine electrophoresis is common, especially in older persons. In fact, a paraprotein (at concentrations up to 30 g/l) is found in 2 per cent of persons over 50 years and older. These patients are usually classified as patients with a monoclonal gammopathy of undetermined significance (MGUS). Recent studies have clarified the prognosis. Although these patients are at some risk for the development of plasma cell related disorders (at a rate of 1 per cent per year), the likelihood for developing renal disease is low. Amyloidosis was seen in less than 1 per cent of patients after a follow-up of 15 years (Kyle *et al.* 2002).

The presence of Bence Jones proteins must be ascertained in patients with multiple myeloma, as well as in patients with acute or subacute renal failure. Although large concentrations of urinary light chains are pathogenic, smaller concentrations (<150 mg/l) are detected in up to one-third of patients with so-called MGUS. Urine dip sticks do not detect light chains, therefore, in patients under suspicion urine must be screened by biochemical techniques.

There is recent evidence that the paraproteins that deposit in the kidney have structural abnormalities. Identification of such biochemical abnormalities is not yet possible as routine investigation.

Cryoglobulins

Cryoglobulins are immunoglobulins or combinations thereof that precipitate in the cold and resolve upon rewarming to 37°C (Dammacco *et al.* 2001). Cryoglobulins are potent activators of the classical complement pathway, a likely mechanism to explain the vasculitis that occurs in medium- and small-sized vessels. Renal involvement is seen in up to 25 per cent of patients, typically with a MPGN type I like picture.

Cryoglobulins are classified based on their immunochemical composition (see Chapter 4.6) and can be associated with a variety of underlying diseases. In recent years, a high association between cryoglobulinaemia and hepatitis C virus (HCV) infection has become evident. In Mediterranean countries, almost 100 per cent of patients with cryoglobulinaemia are HCV positive, in other studies percentages have varied from 40 to 80 per cent. The association between HCV and cryoglobulins has been strengthened by the finding that the concentration of HCV RNA is 10–1000-fold higher in the cryoprecipitate than in the serum. For anti-HCV antibodies, the ratio is only 1 : 1.

For the detection of cryoglobulins in the serum, meticulous precautions at the time of blood collection must be taken. Blood must be drawn in a warm tube and kept at 37°C during clotting. The serum is then placed in a refrigerator for 1–3 days. The cryoprecipitate can be seen as a white precipitate in the bottom of the tube. After washing with warm saline to remove passively trapped proteins, the sample is stored at 4°C after centrifugation at 1400*g*. The resulting precipitate is quantitated as the cryocrit. Subsequently, the nature of the cryoglobulins must be investigated by immunochemical techniques such as immunofixation.

Modern techniques allow quantitation of minor amounts of cryoprecipitates. Values as low as 80 mg/l can be found in normal persons. Clinical features of cryoglobulinaemia are most often observed in patients with type II cryoglobulins, at concentrations generally exceeding 1 g/l.

The serum of patients with cryoglobulinaemia usually contains rheumatoid factor activity, resulting from the presence of an IgM with anti-IgG specificity. Serum complement C4 levels are usually very low, whereas C3 levels may be normal or low.

If no serum cryoglobulins are detected in a patient with cold insensitivity, purpura, livedo reticularis, and/or recurrent skin ulcera, a diagnosis of cryofibrinogenaemia must be considered (Blain *et al.* 2000).

Complement

The complement system is a group of tightly controlled plasma proteins, which after activation can evoke very potent biological effects. The activation pathways of the complement system, its most important components and regulatory proteins, and the biological effects are depicted in Fig. 1.

The complement system can be activated in three different ways, the classical pathway, the alternative pathway, and the recently discovered mannose binding lectin (MBL) pathway. All three pathways lead to the generation of an enzymatically active C3 convertase, which cleaves the central component C3 into C3a and C3b. C3b converts the C3 convertase to a C5 convertase, which cleaves C5 to C5a and C5b, the initiator of the formation of the C5b–C9 complex, the so-called membrane attack complex. To prevent continuous activation of the complement system regulatory (inhibitory) proteins are present such as factors H and I.

Individual components of the complement system can be measured by immunochemical methods. C3, C4, and factor B are most frequently measured, and allow to differentiate between alternative (low C3, normal C4) and classical (low C3 and low C4) pathway activation. The CH50 activity assay is a functional assay that measures the overall activity of the complement system after activation of the classical pathway. Absent or very low CH50 activity indicates a congenital deficiency of complement components such as C1q, C2, or C4. Use of the CH50 activity assay allows the detection of a special form of functional C1q deficiency, caused by a point mutation resulting in normal levels of non-functional C1q. Factor H levels can also be measured by immunochemical techniques. However, for factor H also functional deficiencies caused by gene mutations have been described that are not reflected by decreased protein levels. In patients with factor H deficiency decreased C3 levels may be found as a result of continuous unopposed alternative pathway activation. However, in many patients with (functional) factor H deficiency C3 levels are normal.

The complement system is frequently involved in renal diseases, mostly through activation of the classical pathway. In Table 2, we provide an overview of complement abnormalities in various renal diseases. It is important to realize that complement activation is not always reflected by decreased levels of C3 or C4. Sometimes, the increased

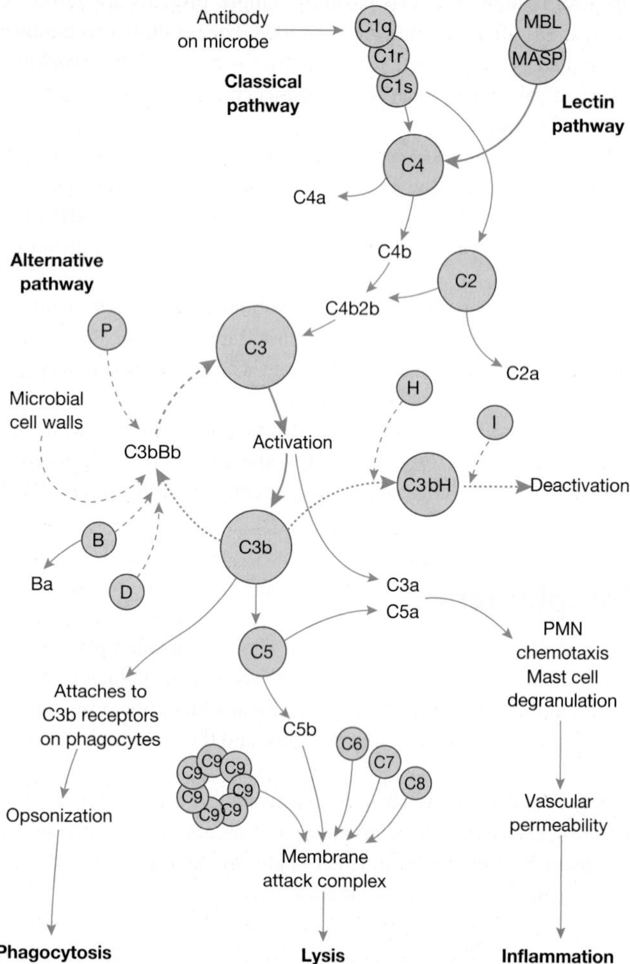

Fig. 1 Overview of the complement system. C4 is activated either by the classical pathway or by the lectin pathway. The classical pathway is activated by binding of C1q to antigen–antibody complexes. This activates C1r and C1s which cleave C4. The lectin pathway is activated if the mannan binding lectin (MBL) binds to mannose groups on bacteria. This activates the serine proteases MASP 1 and 2 (MBL associated serine protease). MBL and MASP are homologous to C1q, C1r, and C1s. Next, C2 can bind to C4b and then becomes susceptible to cleavage by C1s. After cleavage the classical C3 convertase (C4b2b) is formed, which cleaves C3 into C3b and C3a. The formation of C3b can also result from alternative pathway activation. Spontaneous C3 activation occurs spontaneously at a low level. If this activated C3b binds to factor B, the complex becomes susceptible to cleavage by factor D. This results in the formation of the alternative pathway C3 convertase C3bBb. However, factor H has a higher affinity for C3b than factor B. If factor H binds to C3b, the complex is cleaved by factor I resulting in inactivated C3b. Certain microbial surfaces favour the association between C3b and factor B and, therefore, activate the alternative pathway. Self surfaces promote the binding of factor H to C3b, thereby inhibiting alternative pathway activation. Generation of C3b is a central feature of complement activation, because of the biological functions associated with C3b formation namely opsonization/phagocytosis and proinflammatory responses via C3a and C5a. In addition, it forms the initial event in the formation of the so-called membrane attack complex C5b–C9 which drills holes in bacteria and cells. (Adapted from Playfair, J.H.L. and Lydyard, P.M. *Medical Immunology for Students*. Churchill and Livingstone, 1995, p. 8.)

Table 2 Complement levels in various renal diseases

	C4	C3	Factor B	
Poststreptococcal GN	N(-↓)	↓↓	N?	Only in acute phase
Lupus nephritis	↓↓	↓↓	N	Proportionally decreased
MPGN Type I	N-↓	↓	N	
MPGN Type II (DDD)	N	↓↓	↓	Due to presence of C3NeF
GN associated with chronic infections	↓	↓	N	
Cryoglobulinaemic GN	↓-↓↓	N or ↓	N	
ANCA-associated GN	N	N	N	
Anti-GBM disease	N	N	N	

Abbreviations: GN, glomerulonephritis; MPGN, membranoproliferative glomerulonephritis; DDD, dense deposit disease; C3NeF, C3 nephritic factor.

production of complement components, as a result of an acute phase response, outweighs the increased breakdown. Alternatively, activation of C3 may go unrecognized since antibodies are used that recognize an epitope that is present on intact C3 as well as on C3i. Some investigators, therefore, have claimed that measurements of complement breakdown products such as C3d are more specific indicators of complement activation. However, proof for this claim is limited. Alternatively, decreased levels of complement do not always reflect immunological injury. Temporary decreases of complement C3 and/or C4 can be found in various conditions such as atheroembolic disease, HUS/TTP, sepsis, pancreatitis, severe burns, use of contrast agents or inulin, cuprophan haemodialysis, cardiopulmonary bypass, haemolytic crisis in malaria, and porphyria (Hebert *et al.* 1991).

Congenital or acquired deficiencies of complement components deserve special consideration. There are well known associations between complement deficiencies and the development of various renal diseases (Table 1). Deficiencies of C1q, C2, and C4 are frequently associated with SLE. Deficiencies of factor H have been associated with familial and sporadic cases of the haemolytic–uraemic syndrome (HUS) and dense deposit disease (DDD).

C3 nephritic factor is an autoantibody that is associated with DDD. This autoantibody prevents the deactivation of C3b by factor H, either by binding to C3b or to factor H. Some patients with DDD and C3 nephritic factor have a typical appearance with partial lipodystrophy and the absence of fat tissue in the face and upper part of the body. The pathogenesis has been recently clarified: the adipocytes in the upper part of the body produce a protein called adipsin, which is identical to factor D. In the presence of C3 nephritic factor complement will be activated and mediate lysis of the adipocytes.

Antinuclear antibodies

Antinuclear antibodies (ANA) are directed against nuclear constituents, either nucleic acids or nucleoproteins. ANA can be detected in an indirect IF test by applying serum to fixed cell lines. Most commonly used are HeLa cells. A positive ANA on indirect IF can be found in up to 10 per cent of aged healthy persons. In most of these cases antibody specificities are undetermined and the finding is of no significance. Various defined specificities of ANA can be recognized (Table 1). The nuclear staining pattern can already provide an indication for the specificity of the ANA (see Fig. 2). A homogeneous or peripheral rim pattern is mainly caused by antibodies against the nucleosome or its components double stranded DNA (dsDNA) or histones. A speckled pattern is caused by antibodies against nucleoproteins like Sm, RNP, SS-A (Ro), or SS-B (La). A nucleolar staining is suggestive of anti-topo-isomerase I or anti-centromere antibodies.

The antibody specificities can be more precisely determined by additional testing. Specificity for dsDNA can be determined qualitatively by an indirect IF assay on *Crithidia luciliae*, a flagellate which contains a kinetoplast with pure dsDNA. For quantitative testing, the Farr assay is used, a modified RIA that specifically detects high avidity antibodies. The specificity for other defined nucleoproteins can be documented by an immunodiffusion technique using purified nuclear antigens (ENA) or an immunoblotting technique using an extract of nuclear and/or cytoplasmic antigens. Well-known specificities include antihistone, anti-Sm, anti-RNP, anti-SS-A, anti-SS-B, and antitopoisomerase I.

Both anti-dsDNA and anti-Sm antibodies are almost pathognomonic for SLE. Both specificities are included in the ACR criteria for SLE. Various other ANA are also frequently found in patients with SLE and correlate with specific disease associations (see Chapter 4.7).

Anti-C1q antibodies

The popularity of the use of assays for measurement of circulating immune complexes in the 1970s using C1q as a substrate revealed the presence of autoantibodies to C1q in many disease conditions (Siegert *et al.* 1999). These antibodies can be measured by using immobilized C1q either in ELISA or a RIA. To prevent binding of immune complexes or dsDNA to C1q these tests are performed at an increased ionic strength, mostly 0.3 M NaCl. These anti-C1q antibodies are frequently found in patients with lupus nephritis (30–60 per cent) but also in patients with MCTD, PAN (±30 per cent), cryoglobulinaemia, and MPGN (60–80 per cent). However, anti-C1q antibodies are also

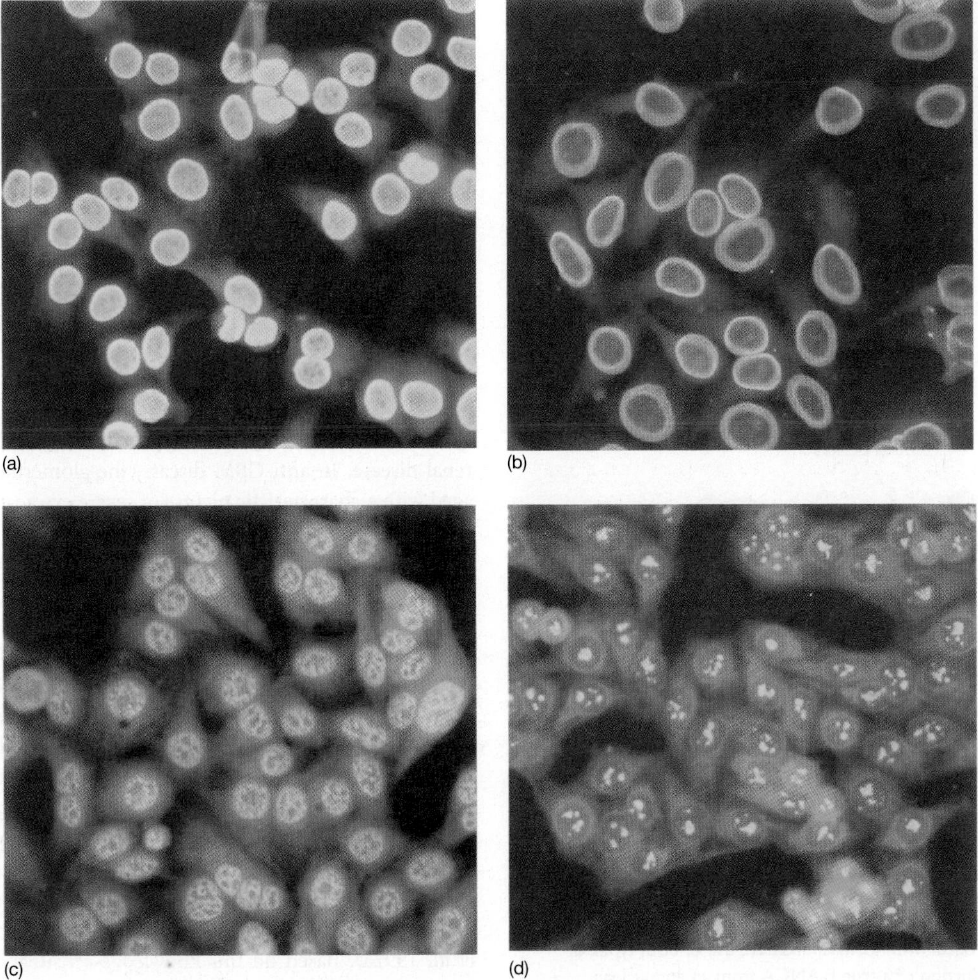

Fig. 2 The four common patterns of antinuclear staining. Homogeneous (a), peripheral (b), speckled (c), and nucleolar (d). (Reproduced with permission from Dieppe, P.A., Bacon, P.A., Bamji, A.N., and Watt, I. *Slide Atlas of Rheumatology*, Vol. 9 SLE. London: Gower, 1984, p. 9.6.)

present in healthy controls (5 per cent), the prevalence increasing with age (>70 years, 18 per cent positive).

Antineutrophil cytoplasmic antibodies

The discovery of antineutrophil cytoplasmic antibodies (ANCA) has been a major breakthrough in the differential diagnosis of vasculitis and rapidly progressive glomerulonephritis (RPGN). ANCA are directed against proteins that are predominantly present in the azurophilic granules of neutrophils. The screening assay for ANCA is indirect IF on ethanol fixed neutrophils. Under these conditions, three different patterns can be seen: cytoplasmic ANCA (C-ANCA), perinuclear ANCA (P-ANCA), or atypical ANCA (Fig. 3).

The difference in staining pattern between C-ANCA and P-ANCA is due to a fixation artefact. Ethanol fixation disrupts the lysosomal membrane and as a result the lysosomal proteins will leak into the cytoplasm. Cationic proteins (targeted by P-ANCA) will be attracted to the negatively charged nuclear membrane giving rise to the perinuclear staining pattern, whereas anionic or neutral proteins will be more evenly distributed in the cytoplasm (C-ANCA). On formalin-fixed neutrophils there are no differences, and only a C-ANCA staining pattern is seen.

P-ANCA must be differentiated from ANA that also give a perinuclear staining pattern. The effects of fixation can provide a clue. Whereas P-ANCA staining will change in a C-ANCA pattern on formalin fixed neutrophils, the perinuclear staining of ANA will remain unchanged. Furthermore, ANA staining can be observed when using other cells or tissues, whereas P-ANCA antibodies are neutrophil specific.

Most C-ANCA are directed against a 29 kDa protein called proteinase 3 (PR3). P-ANCA are most frequently directed against myeloperoxidase (MPO), although other antigenic targets may occur such as elastase, lactoferrin, lysosyme, cathepsin G, and bactericidal/permeability-increasing protein (BPI). The specificities of atypical ANCA are currently unknown (Savige *et al.* 2000).

The specificity of ANCA should be tested by ELISA assays for PR3 and MPO, which are widely available. These commercial assays only detect IgG class antibodies. Although there is concordance between C-ANCA staining and anti-PR3 positivity in ELISA and between P-ANCA staining and anti-MPO positivity, results are not always congruent, dependent on the assay used (Wang *et al.* 1997). Of C-ANCA positive sera, 44–84 per cent were positive in a PR3 ELISA, whereas P-ANCA positivity was confirmed by anti-MPO ELISA in 25–75 per cent of cases (Wang *et al.* 1997). In the latter study, only 35 per cent of P-ANCA positive sera proved MPO-ANCA positive in capture ELISA, immunoblot, and inhibition assays, indicating the common existence of other specificities. Up to 5 per cent of patients with vasculitis are negative in IIF but positive by a MPO or PR3 specific ELISA (Savige *et al.* 2000).

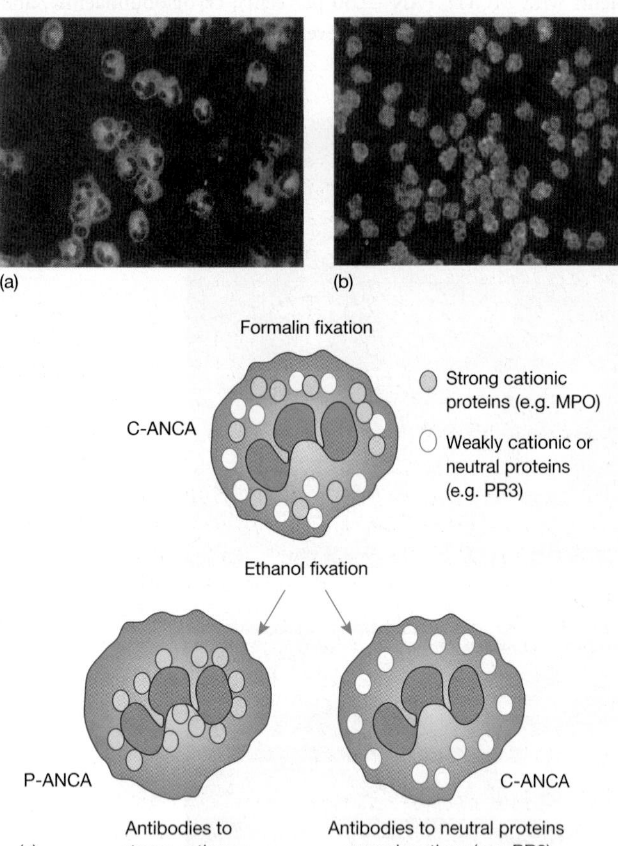

Fig. 3 Antinuclear cytoplasmic antibodies (ANCA). (a) and (b), indirect immunofluorescence techniques using ethanol-fixed neutrophils demonstrate perinuclear (p) (a) and cytoplasmic (c) (b) staining patterns, (c). The use of crosslinking fixatives (e.g. formalin) during the preparation of the neutrophil substrate leads to alterations in granule membranes, allowing positively charged constituents to migrate to the negatively charged nuclear membrane. Because this does not occur with formalin fixation, use of both types of fixation allows the distinction of a true P-ANCA from an antinuclear antibody (ANA). With formalin-fixed neutrophils, antibodies that would cause P-ANCA patterns (on ethanol-fixed cells) will display diffuse granular cytoplasmic staining, whereas nuclear staining would indicate the presence of an ANA. Abbreviations: MPO, myeloperoxidase; PR3, proteinase 3.

Anti-GBM antibodies

Anti-GBM disease is the prototypical example of antibody mediated renal disease. In anti-GBM disease, the glomerulus is severely damaged with a characteristic picture of severe extracapillary proliferation with capillary wall necrosis. Patients present with the clinical picture of a RPGN. In some patients, especially in smokers, the lungs may be involved too (classical Goodpasture's syndrome = pulmonary renal syndrome).

A renal biopsy in patients with anti-GBM disease discloses a typical picture on IF, with linear IF of Ig along the glomerular capillary wall. In most cases the causative antibody is of the IgG class; however, patients with IgA and IgM class anti-GBM antibodies have been described.

The presence in the serum of antibodies against the GBM was formerly studied by an indirect IF procedure using normal kidney tissue as substrate. This technique proved negative in up to 40 per cent of patients with anti-GBM glomerulonephritis. The anti-GBM antibodies are directed against a conformational epitope on the so-called non-collagenous (NC1) domain of the collagen IV $\alpha 3$ chain (Hellmark *et al.* 1997a). Based on this knowledge sensitive and specific ELISA assays have been developed using recombinant protein for the quantitative measurement of anti-GBM antibodies. These antibodies can be detected in high titres in almost every patient with anti-GBM disease. The specificity of the assay is very high, although low titres can be observed in other unrelated conditions. Of note, both IIF and ELISA regularly only detect IgG antibodies. Thus the rare patient with IgA or IgM anti-GBM antibodies may remain unrecognized.

In approximately 30 per cent of patients with anti-GBM antibodies ANCA antibodies can be found, in two-thirds with anti-MPO specificity. The co-occurrence of ANCA and anti-GBM antibodies is mostly associated with a more favourable course of the disease and in these patients treatment is more efficacious. The epitope of the anti-GBM antibodies in this subset of patients is not different (Hellmark *et al.* 1997b).

Anti-GBM antibodies can also be formed in patients with Alport's disease after renal transplantation (Brainwood *et al.* 1998; Kalluri *et al.* 2000). Alport's disease is caused by mutations in genes encoding for the $\alpha3$, $\alpha4$, or $\alpha5$ chains of collagen IV. These patients do not express these collagen chains in their native forms in their kidneys. After renal transplantation, some patients may develop a sometimes aggressive form of anti-GBM disease, causing renal failure. Recent studies have indicated that anti-GBM antibodies can be detected in almost all patients, linear deposits of IgG along the glomerular capillary wall are seen in 20–50 per cent of patients, whereas only a minority develop manifest anti-GBM disease. Several studies have addressed the potential epitopes of these antibodies. Although results are equivocal, many patients have antibodies that are directed against the NC1 domain of collagen $\alpha5$. These antibodies may not be detected by commercial anti-GBM ELISA assays that use the specific NC1 $\alpha3$ antigen as substrate.

Antiphospholipid antibodies

Antiphospholipid (PL) antibodies are associated with the recently defined antiphospholipid syndrome (APS), which is characterized by (recurrent) arterial and/or venous thromboses, and recurrent miscarriages (Levine *et al.* 2002). The kidney is often involved, with vascular lesions and variable thrombotic microangiopathy (TMA) (Nochy *et al.* 1999). The APS syndrome can be primary (without systemic autoimmunity) or secondary in patients with autoimmune diseases such as SLE (Daugas *et al.* 2002).

The first recognized anti-PL antibodies were the lupus anticoagulant (LAC) and the anticardiolipin (aCL) antibodies. The latter antibody is responsible for the false positive Venereal Disease Research Laboratory (VDRL) test that is often found in patients with SLE.

The LAC is defined as a serum factor that prolongs PL-dependent coagulation tests in platelet-poor plasma. Examples are the activated partial thromboplastin time, the kaolin clotting time or diluted Russell's viper venom clotting time (DRVVT). Tests are considered positive if the coagulation defect cannot be corrected by the addition of normal plasma, but becomes normal after addition of excess anionic phospholipids or freeze–thawed thrombocytes. There is large heterogeneity in the methods used to detect LAC activity (Jacobson *et al.* 2001). By only using the standard APTT test, with a cut-off value of 67 s, 47 per cent of LAC positive samples will be missed (Jacobson *et al.* 2001).

DRVVT is considered as the most sensitive test. The presence of LAC must be ascertained by using at least two independent tests. However, one should realize that the accuracy and reproducibility of the test procedures are low.

aCL antibodies are directed against cardiolipin, and can be detected in ELISA. Although some aCL antibodies have LAC activity, the results are not always overlapping. When searching for anti-PL antibodies, both tests are thus necessary. Recently, it has been demonstrated that anti-PL antibodies may be directed at various plasma proteins that have affinity for anionic phospholipids. In fact, aCL antibodies recognize a conformational epitope formed between CL and $\beta2$-glycoprotein I ($\beta2$GPI). Therefore, $\beta2$GPI is an essential co-factor in these assays. Additional specificities have included proteins such as prothrombin, protein C, protein S, and annexin V. Of note, these proteins are only recognized in the assays if bound to anionic surfaces. In ELISA, antigens must therefore be coated specifically on γ-irradiated polystyrene plates.

Although the association between the presence of anti-PL antibodies and thrombosis is now well recognized, the pathogenicity of the antibodies is unclear. aCL antibodies may be detectable in 2–4 per cent of healthy controls. The incidence is higher (15 per cent) in patients with rheumatoid arthritis or SLE (Merkel *et al.* 1996). Other specificities are also found with high frequency in patients with SLE. Nojima *et al.* (2001) reported a 21–56 per cent prevalence of antibodies to $\beta2$GPI, prothrombin, protein C, protein S, and annexin V in patients with SLE. Patients with positive LAC had significantly more frequent antibodies against protrombin and $\beta2$GPI, with no difference in the other antibody specificities.

The association between LAC and aCL antibodies and the APS is well established (Levine *et al.* 2002). In general LAC activity is more specific whereas aCL antibodies show higher sensitivity. It can be expected that our understanding of the APS and the role of the anti-PL antibodies in various clinical manifestations will improve with the development of more specific and better standardized assays. In a recent study, there was an association between antibodies against $\beta2$GPI and protrombin and arterial thrombosis, between antibodies against protein S and venous thrombosis, and between antiannexin V and fetal loss (Nojima *et al.* 2001). These results need to be confirmed in prospective studies.

Although the definition of the APS requires the documented presence of anti-PL antibodies (either LAC or aCL antibodies), several studies have presented patients with a clear clinical APS that were negative for LAC and aCL antibodies. In some patients, IgA aCL or antibodies exclusively directed against $\beta2$GPI were found (Lockshin *et al.* 2000).

Patients with an established APS need lifelong intensive oral anticoagulation. For the monitoring of the intensity of oral anticoagulation, the International Normalized Ratio (INR) is used aiming at an INR between 3.0 and 3.5. It should be realized that monitoring of the INR may be difficult in patients with LAC since some available tests may be influenced. In the presence of LAC values of INR may be falsely elevated, and the level of anticoagulation may be overestimated (Moll *et al.* 1997).

Antimicrobial responses

The kidney can be damaged in the course of many infectious diseases (see Chapter 3.12). A detailed discussion of these diseases and their diagnosis is beyond the scope of this chapter. We will briefly discuss poststreptococcal glomerulonephritis, hepatitis B, and hepatitis C.

Antibodies against streptococcal antigens

Poststreptococcal glomerulonephritis was once regarded as the best example of an immune-complex mediated glomerular disease, caused by entrapment in the glomerular capillary wall of complexes that consist of streptococcal antigens and antistreptococcal antibodies. More recently, cross reactive recognition of intrinsic glomerular antigens by the antistreptococcal antibodies has been put forward as an alternative explanation.

The identification of a prior streptococcal infection is based on the assessment of the production of antibodies directed against streptococcal antigens. Well-known examples are antibodies directed against streptolysin O (ASO). Using a single determination of the antibody titre, a pre-existent infection may be missed in up to 30–50 per cent of patients. Therefore, detection of a significant rise in antibody titre is probably more valuable. Still, many patients do not produce ASO antibodies, in particular, patients with a streptococcal skin infection. The detection of antibodies directed at other streptococcal antigens may be more sensitive and specific for the diagnosis of poststreptococcal infection. Examples are antibodies against deoxyribonuclease B (DNAse B), streptokinase, hyaluronidase, zymogen, GAPDH, and NAD+ glycolase. In a recent study in children with acute poststreptococcal glomerulonephritis, the sensitivity of ASO, anti-DNAse, and antizymogen titres was studied (Parra *et al.* 1998). When compared to controls, ROC curves showed superiority of antizymogen greater than anti-DNAse B greater than ASO. Sensitivity and specificity was 42 and 84 per cent for ASO, 73 and 89 per cent for anti-DNAse B, and 87 and 85 per cent for antizymogen. Of note, increased titres of ASO and to a lesser degree for the other antibodies were frequently observed in patients with upper respiratory tract infections or impetigo who did not experience a glomerulonephritis. Thus, the above-mentioned specificity of the assays does not hold if patients with infections are included without evidence of renal involvement.

Hepatitis C

Hepatitis C is held responsible for various renal diseases such as MPGN type I, membranous nephropathy, and cryoglobulinaemic glomerulonephritis (Lauer and Walker 2001). The detection of hepatitis C is based on the detection of antibodies against hepatitis C antigens. An enzyme immunoassay is used for screening. This test is very sensitive when used in a low-risk population (99 per cent). However, false positive results are common; therefore, positive results should always be confirmed by a recombinant immunoblot assay. False negative results may occur in patients with renal failure, patients using immunosuppression, and patients with cryoglobulinaemia. In patients with high suspicion for hepatitis C, HCV RNA can be detected by rt PCR, a very sensitive method that allows detection of virus as early as 2 weeks after infection. Since viral RNA is unstable, blood samples must be processed within 3 h. In patients with cryoglobulinaemia, viral RNA is mainly present in the cryoprecipitate, and special attention must be given that the blood is drawn at 37°C.

Hepatitis B

Various serological markers can be used to evaluate a hepatitis B infection, for example, HBsAg, HBe antigen and anti-HBs, and anti-HBc and anti-HBe antibodies. The test results provide an indication of the time sequence and the infectiosity of the hepatitis B infection (Wallach 2000). Some immunosuppressed patients (including patients on haemodialysis) may not develop antibodies upon exposure to the viral antigen. If suspicion is high, HBV DNA can be detected by sensitive PCR techniques. This technique provides a diagnosis and an indication of the viral load. The absence of the HBs-antigen in general argues for non-infectiosity; however, this is not the case if organs are used for transplantation. In HbsAg negative patients with antibodies against HBc, viral DNA is present in the liver and to a lesser extent in the kidney. Therefore, there is a risk of HBV transmission particularly if the organ is transplanted in a non-vaccinated recipient. In case of kidney transplantation the risks are much lower than that after liver transplantation (Delmonico and Syndman 1998).

Immunological studies in patients with specific renal syndromes: guidelines

Few studies have specifically assessed the value of testing specific immunological markers in establishing a diagnosis or monitoring disease activity in patients with renal diseases. We will briefly discuss the data that are most relevant for various clinical renal syndromes and several specific disease entities.

Nephrotic syndrome

Recent studies have argued against the routine testing of patients with proteinuria or a nephrotic syndrome (Howard *et al.* 1990; Chew *et al.* 1999). Measurement of ANA, rheumatoid factor, C3, C4, CH50, HbsAg, VDRL, cryoglobulins, and serum and urine electrophoresis did not improve diagnostic accuracy. Therefore, in almost all cases a renal biopsy is needed to establish a diagnosis. Based on the renal biopsy results (and sometimes on clinical grounds), additional serological tests can be performed that can strengthen the diagnosis and sometimes are helpful during follow-up.

Rapidly progressive glomerulonephritis/ acute nephritic syndrome

In patients with RPGN, glomerular damage occurs often very rapidly and is irreversible if treatment is postponed. Therefore, rapid diagnosis and early treatment is urgently needed. Serological markers can be very helpful in establishing a diagnosis in these patients. It is important to stress that a meticulous examination of the urinary sediment for the presence of dysmorphic erythrocytes and/or erythrocyte casts remains the most important diagnostic tool to differentiate between RPGN and other causes of acute renal failure.

The presence of high titres of anti-GBM antibodies in patients with RPGN is virtually pathognomonic for anti-GBM disease. By using the widely available, specific, and sensitive ELISA, a diagnosis can be made within a day. Although most centres still prefer to perform a renal biopsy, such an approach can be questioned. In patients with anti-GBM antibodies, a search for the presence of ANCA is warranted. Clinicians should be aware of the possibility that cases of anti-GBM disease are seldom caused by non-IgG antibodies that will not be detected in the standard assays.

Regular assessment of the anti-GBM antibody titres during follow-up may guide treatment. In general, antibodies will disappear within 12–16 weeks after start of treatment, and at that time point immunosuppressive treatment can be rapidly tapered and stopped. Renal transplantation in a patient with anti-GBM disease should be postponed until no anti-GBM antibodies are detected anymore for at least 3 months.

The finding of ANCA has a high predictive value in patients with RPGN. In fact, some authors have argued that in patients with extrarenal symptoms that fit with a multisystemic vasculitis, and who present with acute renal failure, the detection of ANCA is sufficient for the diagnosis and a renal biopsy may be omitted.

Data on the sensitivity and the specificity of ANCA for the diagnosis of systemic or renal limited vasculitis are given in Table 3 (Hagen *et al.* 1998). The diagnostic accuracy is best if ANCA are analysed by both IIF and ELISA techniques. In a recent meta-analysis, combined testing for C-ANCA/αPR3 and P-ANCA/αMPO showed a sensitivity of 85.5 per cent and a specificity of 98.6 per cent for the diagnosis of small vessel vasculitis (Choi 2001). One should realize that the high positive and negative predictive values in this and other studies only hold for patients with a (rapidly) deteriorating renal function, in whom the prevalence of systemic vasculitis is high. A recent analysis of Falk *et al.* (2000) clearly illustrates that predictability is much lower in patients with moderate renal failure (Table 4). In such patients, a renal biopsy is always needed to establish a diagnosis.

Table 3 Sensitivity and specificity of ANCA using combined IIF and ELISA in systemic vasculitis

	Sensitivity (%)	Specificity (%)
M. Wegener (*n* = 97)	73	98
Microscopic polyangiitis (*n* = 44)	67	98
Idiopathic RPGN (*n* = 12)	82	98

Adapted from Hagen *et al.* (1998). Numbers in parentheses represent number of patients in the study cohort. Specificity data are based on 184 disease controls.

Table 4 Estimated positive (PPV) and negative (NPV) predictive values of ANCA for pauci-immune crescentic glomerulonephritis

Clinical picture	PPV (%)	NPV (%)
RPGN	98	80
Nephritic syndrome and		
Screatinine > 270 μmol/l (A)	92	80
Screatinine 135–270 μmol/l (B)	77	98
Screatinine < 135 μmol/l (C)	47	99

Adapted from Falk *et al.* (2000). Data are for adult patients with observed prevalences of pauci-immune crescentic glomerulonephritis 47% for RPGN, 21% for A, 7% for B, and 2% for C.

Evaluation of ANCA activity is also of particular value in the follow-up of patients. In 50–60 per cent of patients, titres fluctuate parallel to disease activity. A favourable response to immunosuppressive treatment is found in 83 per cent of patients accompanied by a negative ANCA test after a median of 12 weeks (Jayne *et al.* 1995). The predictive value of a rise in ANCA titre (if measured monthly) for a clinical relapse has a sensitivity of 57 per cent and a specificity of 45 per cent. The specificity becomes even 72 per cent if transient increases after conversion from cyclophosphamide to azathioprine and rises at the moment of relapse are excluded. Similar results were found in a recent prospective study. The predictive value for a relapse of a rise in C-ANCA titre in IF was 57 per cent and 71 per cent if assessed in an PR3-ELISA (Boomsma *et al.* 2000). However, one should realize that disease quiescence is possible with persistently positive ANCA titres, and that relapses can occur while the ANCA test remains negative.

In patients with RPGN, who are anti-GBM and ANCA negative, additional serological tests may be done based on clinical symptoms or biopsy results (Fig. 4). The same holds true for patients with a nephritic syndrome and/or chronic renal failure. In these patients, abnormalities in serum complement levels, the presence of autoantibodies, or the detection of cryoglobulins or paraproteins are not enough sensitive or specific to establish a diagnosis; however, a positive finding may be helpful in confirming a diagnosis or may be used to guide treatment. Abnormalities in complement levels in renal diseases are given in Table 2. For most diagnoses there is no evidence that serial measurements of complement can be used to monitor disease activity.

Systemic lupus erythematosus

Laboratory tests are pivotal in establishing the diagnosis and may be helpful in monitoring the renal disease activity in patients with SLE. The ANA test is a valuable screening test with high sensitivity but low specificity. If positive, additional tests must be done to establish antibody specificities. The presence of anti-dsDNA and anti-Sm antibodies establishes a diagnosis of SLE with 85 per cent sensitivity and 93 per cent specificity. Antinucleosome antibodies (Bruns *et al.* 2000) and antibodies to C1q (Siegert *et al.* 1999) may be better predictors of renal involvement in SLE; however, prospective data are limited. Complement levels are not helpful in the diagnosis of SLE, but persistently low CH50

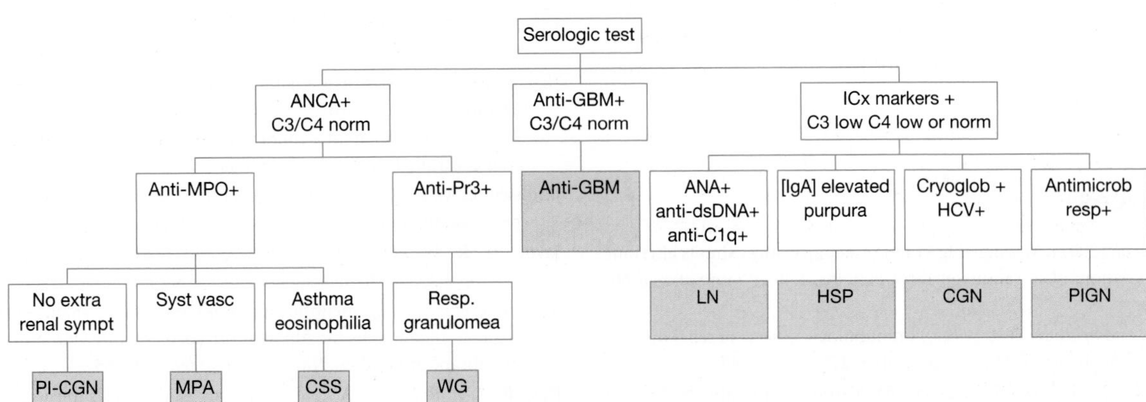

Fig. 4 Diagnostic approach of the patient with a rapidly progressive glomerulonephritis. Abbreviations: PI-CGN, pauci-immune crescentic GN; MPA, microscopic polyangiitis; CSS, Churg–Strauss syndrome; WG, Wegener's granulomatosis; anti-GBM, anti-GBM nephritis; LN, lupus nephritis; HSP, Henoch–Schönlein purpura; CGN, cryoglobulinaemic GN; PIGN, postinfectious GN; IC, immune-complex; [IgA], serum IgA concentration; HCV, hepatitis C virus.

values raises the possibility of a deficiency of one of the early complement factors.

Antinuclear antibody titres are valuable in monitoring SLE nephritis disease activity during follow-up. If anti-dsDNA is measured monthly by the Farr assay, onset or flares of lupus nephritis will be accompanied by increases of anti-dsDNA titres in more than 90 per cent of patients (ter Borg *et al.* 1990). Measurement of anti-C1q antibodies might even be more accurate in predicting renal relapses (Moroni *et al.* 2001). The likelihood of renal involvement in SLE patients who are negative for anti-C1q or anti-dsDNA antibodies is very low (specificity between 92 and 100 per cent) (Trendelenburg *et al.* 1999; Moroni *et al.* 2001). Unfortunately, the anti-C1q assay is not available for routine use.

Whether measurement of complement is valuable for monitoring disease activity is still unclear. Monitoring of C4 is not useful, although recently a low C4 value (<110 mg/l) at the moment of renal remission was identified as a risk factor for a flare (Illei *et al.* 2002). Measurement of C3 seems somewhat more valuable, with sensitivities ranging from 20 to 95 per cent and specificities between 74 and 94 per cent (Esdaile *et al.* 1996). Thus, in many patients with renal disease activity normal C3 levels are found, whereas decreased C3 levels may be present in patients without renal disease activity.

Thrombotic microangiopathy

TMA is a descriptive diagnosis and associated with various clinical syndromes (see Chapter). In the recent decade much progress has been made in defining the pathogenesis of these disorders (Ruggenenti *et al.* 2001). Abnormalities of factor H favour a diagnosis of the HUS whereas the presence of antiphospholipid antibodies is characteristic of APS.

Recently, evidence has emerged that thrombotic thrombocytopenic purpura (TTP) is related to abnormalities in the activity of serum von Willebrand factor (vWF) protease. This protease is a zinc metalloprotease called ADAMTS13, encoded by a gene on chromosome 9q34. This protease rapidly degrades large vWF multimers that are formed in the endothelial cells. A decreased activity of the protease results in the persistence of large vWF multimers in the circulation. These large multimers cause endothelial damage and promote thrombosis. Familial forms of TTP have been associated with a deficiency of this vWF protease. In several families, mutations in the ADAMTS13 gene have been found (Levy *et al.* 2001). The acquired form of TTP has been associated with a functional loss of vWF protease activity due to circulating antibodies. In patients with HUS, no persistent abnormalities in vWF protease activity have been detected (Furlan *et al.* 1998).

References

Allen, A. C. *et al.* (2001). Mesangial IgA1 in IgA nephropathy exhibits aberrant *O*-glycosylation: observations in three patients. *Kidney International* **60**, 969–973.

Ambrus, J. L. and Sridhar, N. R. (1997). Immunologic aspects of renal disease. *Journal of the American Medical Association* **278**, 1938–1945.

Blain, H. *et al.* (2000). Cryofibrinogenaemia: a study of 49 patients. *Clinical Experimental Immunology* **120**, 253–260.

Boomsma, M. M. *et al.* (2000). Prediction of relapses in Wegener's granulomatosis by measurement of antineutrophil cytoplasmic antibody levels. *Arthritis and Rheumatism* **43**, 2025–2033.

ter Borg, E. J. *et al.* (1990). Measurement of increases in anti-double-stranded DNA antibody levels as a predictor of disease exacerbation in systemic lupus erythematosus. *Arthritis and Rheumatism* **33**, 634–643.

Brainwood, D. *et al.* (1998). Targets of alloantibodies in Alport anti-glomerular basement membrane disease after renal transplantation. *Kidney International* **53**, 762–766.

Bruns, A. *et al.* (2000). Nucleosomes are major T and B cell autoantigens in systemic lupus erythematosus. *Arthritis and Rheumatism* **43**, 2307–2315.

Chew, S. T. H. *et al.* (1999). Role of urine and serum protein electrophoresis in evaluation of nephrotic-range proteinuria. *American Journal of Kidney Diseases* **34**, 135–139.

Choi, H. K. *et al.* (2001). Diagnostic performance of antineutrophil cytoplasmic antibody tests for idiopathic vasculitides: metaanalysis with a focus on antimyeloperoxidase antibodies. *Journal of Rheumatology* **28**, 1584–1590.

D'Amico, G. (1988). Clinical features and natural history in adults with IgA nephropathy. *American Journal of Kidney Diseases* **12**, 353–357.

Dammaco, F. *et al.* (2001). The cryoglobulins: an overview. *European Journal of Clinical Investigation* **31**, 628–638.

Daugas, E. *et al.* (2002). Antiphospholipid syndrome nephropathy in systemic lupus erythematosus. *Journal of the American Society of Nephrology* **13**, 42–52.

Delmonico, F. L. and Snydman, D. R. (1998). Organ donor screening for infectious diseases. *Transplantation* **65**, 603–610.

Esdaile, J. M. *et al.* (1996). Routine immunologic tests in systemic lupus erythematosus: is there a need for more studies? *Journal of Rheumatology* **23**, 1891–1896.

Falk, R. J. *et al.* (2000). ANCA glomerulonephritis and vasculitis: A Chapel Hill perspective. *Seminars in Nephrology* **20**, 233–243.

Furlan, M. *et al.* (1998). Von Willebrand factor-cleaving protease in thrombotic thrombocytopenic purpura and the hemolytic–uremic syndrome. *New England Journal of Medicine* **339**, 1578–1584.

Hagen, E. C. *et al.* (1998). Diagnostic value of standardized assays for antineutrophil cytoplasmic antibodies in idiopathic systemic vasculitis. *Kidney International* **53**, 743–753.

Hebert, L. A., Cosio, F. G., and Neff, J. C. (1991). Diagnostic significance of hypocomplementemia. *Kidney International* **39**, 811–821.

Hellmark, T., Segelmark, M., and Wieslander J. (1997a). Anti-GBM antibodies in Goodpasture syndrome; anatomy of an epitope. *Nephrology, Dialysis, Transplantation* **12**, 646–648.

Hellmark, T. *et al.* (1997b). Comparison of anti-GBM antibodies in sera with or without ANCA. *Journal of the American Society of Nephrology* **8**, 376–385.

Hoffmann, G. S. and Specks, U. (1998). Antineutrophil cytoplasmic antibodies. *Arthritis and Rheumatism* **41**, 1521–1537.

Howard, A. D. *et al.* (1990). Routine serologic tests in the differential diagnosis of the adult nephrotic syndrome. *American Journal of Kidney Diseases* **15**, 24–30.

Illei, G. G. *et al.* (2002). Renal flares are common in patients with severe proliferative lupus nephritis treated with pulse immunosuppressive therapy: long-term follow-up of a cohort of 145 patients participating in randomized controlled studies. *Arthritis and Rheumatism* **46**, 995–1002.

Jacobsen, E. M. *et al.* (2001). The evaluation of clotting times in the laboratory detection of lupus anticoagulants. *Thrombosis Research* **104**, 275–282.

Jayne, D. R. W. *et al.* (1995). ANCA and predicting relapse in systemic vasculitis. *Quarterly Journal of Medicine* **88**, 127–133.

Kalluri, R. *et al.* (2000). Identification of $\alpha3$, $\alpha4$, and $\alpha5$ chains of type IV collagen as alloantigens for Alport posttransplant anti-glomerular basement membrane antibodies. *Transplantation* **69**, 679–683.

Kyle, R. A. *et al.* (2002). A long-term study of prognosis in monoclonal gammopathy of undetermined significance. *New England Journal of Medicine* **346**, 564–569.

Lauer, G. M. and Walker, B. D. (2001). Hepatitis C virus infection. *New England Journal of Medicine* **345**, 41–52.

Ledford, D. K. (1997). Immunologic aspects of vasculitis and cardiovascular disease. *Journal of the American Medical Association* **278**, 1962–1971.

Levine, J. S., Branch, D. W., and Rauch, J. (2002). The antiphospholipid syndrome. *New England Journal of Medicine* **346**, 752–763.

Levy, G. C. *et al.* (2001). Mutations in a member of the ADAMTS gene family cause thrombotic thrombocytopenic purpura. *Nature* **413**, 488–494.

Lockshin, M. D., Sammaritano, L. R., and Schwartzman, S. (2000). Validation of the Sapporo criteria for antiphospholipid syndrome. *Arthritis and Rheumatism* **43**, 440–443.

Merkel, P. A. *et al.* (1996). The prevalence and clinical associations of anticardiolipin antibodies in a large inception cohort of patients with connective tissue diseases. *American Journal of Medicine* **101**, 576–583.

Moll, S. and Ortel, T. L. (1997). Monitoring warfarin therapy in patients with lupus anticoagulants. *Annals of Internal Medicine* **127**, 177–185.

Moroni, G. *et al.* (2001). Anti-C1q antibodies may help in diagnosing a renal flare in lupus nephritis. *American Journal of Kidney Diseases* **37**, 490–498.

Nochy, D. *et al.* (1999). The intrarenal vascular lesions associated with primary antiphospholipid syndrome. *Journal of the American Society of Nephrology* **10**, 507–518.

Nojima, J. *et al.* (2001). Association between the prevalence of antibodies to β_2-glycoprotein I, prothrombin, protein C, protein S, and annexin V in patients with systemic lupus erythematosus and thrombotic and thrombocytopenic complications. *Clinical Chemistry* **47**, 1008–1015.

Parra, G. *et al.* (1998). Antibody to streptococcal zymogen in the serum of patients with acute glomerulonephritis: a multicentric study. *Kidney International* **54**, 509–517.

Ruggenenti, P., Noris, M., and Remuzzi, G. (2001). Thrombotic microangiopathy, hemolytic uremic syndrome, and thrombotic thrombocytopenic purpura. *Kidney International* **60**, 831–846.

Savige, J. *et al.* (2000). Antineutrophil cytoplasmic antibodies and associated diseases: A review of the clinical and laboratory features. *Kidney International* **57**, 846–862.

Siegert, C. E. *et al.* (1999). Autoantibodies against C1q: view on clinical relevance and pathogenic role. *Clinical Experimental Immunology* **116**, 4–8.

Trendelenburg, M. *et al.* (1999). Lack of occurrence of severe lupus nephritis among anti-C1q autoantibody negative patients. *Arthritis and Rheumatism* **42**, 187–188.

Wallach, J. *Interpretation of Diagnostic Tests*. Philadelphia: Lippincott, Williams & Wilkins, 2000.

Wang, G. *et al.* (1997). Comparison of eight commercial kits for quantitation of antineutrophil cytoplasmic antibodies (ANCA). *Journal of Immunological Methods* **208**, 203–211.

1.9 The epidemiology of renal disease

Paul J. Roderick and Terry Feest

Introduction

Overview of epidemiological methods

The impact of epidemiological approaches on the understanding of chronic kidney disease was initially limited, but in the last decade there has been considerable increase in interest in this field (Whelton 1996; Elseviers and de Broe 2001). This largely stems from the recognition of the need for primary and secondary preventive strategies to reduce the health care burden of treating endstage renal failure (ESRF), which has grown inexorably in most developed countries. This chapter reviews some of the insights gained from such work in adults. It starts by considering epidemiological methods and the difficulties faced in applying them to chronic kidney disease (CKD).

Epidemiology is the study of the patterns of disease. The descriptive epidemiology of CKD investigates its frequency over time, place, and types of people. Measures of disease frequency are incidence rates ('new cases arising in a defined population in a given time period') and prevalence ('all cases with disease present in a defined population at a given point in time or over a period of time', so-called point and period prevalence, respectively). Analyses of patterns of incidence may generate hypotheses about the underlying causes of CKD, and prevalence data provide information on the current and likely future burden for health services for managing CKD.

Analytical epidemiology is concerned with elucidating the underlying causes of CKD in order to identify strategies for prevention, both in the population and individual patient. Clinical epidemiology covers the science of diagnosis, therapy, and prognosis of patients with CKD and is not the focus of this chapter.

Analytical epidemiological studies are observational and aim to determine the association between putative exposures (or 'risk factors') and CKD (Rothman 2002). A risk factor is an exposure or attribute of a person (or patient) which is associated with the occurrence of a disease. Such factors can be protective as well as associated with increased risk and they may be causal or non-causal. Non-causal factors may be markers of the disease itself or factors which are associated with causal factors (i.e. they are said to be confounded). Causal factors are the key targets for interventions.

There are established criteria for assessing whether a risk factor is causal. The most important is temporality, namely the cause must come before the effect. Other criteria include the strength of the increased risk, a dose–response relationship (i.e. increasing risk with increasing exposure), consistency in more than one well designed study, reversibility (i.e. disease occurrence is reduced after the risk factor is reduced), and biological plausibility. None except temporality is absolute (Rothman 2002).

There are four main methods of observational study: case–control, cohort, cross-sectional, and ecological. There are advantages and disadvantages of each of these four methods. Cohort studies start with a group of people free of disease, ascertain the distribution of the risk factor (and potential confounding factors) at baseline, and then follow them up prospectively over time to see whether these factors are associated with the incidence of disease. The risk measure is the ratio of incidence rates of the exposed and non-exposed groups expressed as a relative risk. Retrospective cohort studies utilize previously collected data on risk factors and identify outcomes contemporaneously. It is an efficient method where such data exist, such as in occupational settings, or using baseline data from previous cohort studies (Dubach *et al.* 1991; Calvert *et al.* 1997; Klag *et al.* 1997). Cohort studies provide the strongest evidence of causation because it is possible to establish temporality, but they need to be large for less frequent outcomes, and loss to follow-up may bias results.

The case–control design is efficient for rare diseases such as severe CKD as it starts with diseased individuals, ideally new incident cases, and assembles a comparative group of non-diseased controls. The frequency of the risk factor (and confounders) is ascertained retrospectively and compared between the two groups; the measure of association is the odds ratio which approximates to the relative risk (Nuyts *et al.* 1995; Perneger *et al.* 1999). Case–control studies have considerable potential for biases in the selection of cases and controls (i.e. selection should not be affected by the risk factor of interest, which can occur for example in taking hospital controls who may not be representative of the population's level of the risk factor under study), and in ascertaining risk factor information (e.g. the retrospective recall of previous exposures may differ between cases with disease and controls).

In cross-sectional studies disease status and risk factor information are collected at the same time, so such studies are unable to establish temporality and they study prevalent cases who may differ in the risk factor pattern from new cases (e.g. if the risk factor affects prognosis). Finally, in ecological studies risk factors and disease outcomes are correlated at a population level (Whittle *et al.* 1991). Whilst useful for generating hypotheses, such studies have less value for inferring causes because of confounding (the so-called 'ecological fallacy').

Challenges of studying chronic kidney disease using the epidemiological method

CKD poses some particular challenges for these epidemiological methods (Young 1997):

(1) More severe renal disease, especially ESRF, is a relatively rare event, which makes prospective cohort studies difficult unless they are very

large. The natural history from exposure to occurrence of disease may take many years requiring a long duration of follow-up which may be unfeasible.

(2) The early stages of CKD are not easily detectable clinically as the disease is often asymptomatic until a significant decline in function occurs, and even then symptoms are usually non-specific. Moreover, the sensitivity of routinely used markers of CKD such as serum creatinine is poor, so by the time such tests show abnormality, significant renal function has been lost, making study of the initiation of early renal damage difficult. In addition studies based on tests taken on patients who have presented to health care may be unrepresentative of CKD in the population.

(3) The natural history of CKD is complex, often with multiple risk factors operating, both at the stage of initiation of renal damage, and in its progression to severe CKD or ESRF. The timing and duration of exposures and their impact may vary during the natural history.

(4) The process of diagnostic classification tends to focus on one 'underlying cause', and may miss the importance of other contributing factors. Although CKD can arise as a complication of specific underlying diseases (assigned as the 'cause'), even in such cases it is often multifactorial.

(5) Precise diagnostic criteria for underlying 'causes' of CKD are not well established and vary in their interpretation and application between studies and Renal Registries. It is not possible to apply the gold standard diagnostic method of renal biopsy in community studies of CKD not least because of the associated hazards. Even in studies of cases starting renal replacement therapy (RRT), up to 40 per cent of cases requiring RRT are referred late, within months of requiring RRT. A high proportion of cases starting RRT have renal disease of unknown aetiology, as they present with bilateral small shrunken kidneys and no relevant prior history, and biopsy is contraindicated.

(6) If the diagnosis of CKD is associated with the putative exposure one can falsely derive an association, for example if exposed people are more actively tested or given the diagnosis based on the exposure. One example is the diagnosis of hypertensive nephropathy, especially in Blacks (Fernandes *et al.* 2000).

(7) Recall and measurement of prior exposures in case–control studies at the appropriate time in the natural history at which they might have affected renal function is problematic given the long and complex natural history. This particularly applies to occupational, drug, and environmental exposures (Fored *et al.* 2001).

(8) For any putative risk factor there is the need to consider confounders (i.e. alternative explanations) and factors along the causal pathway. For example, occupational exposures may be confounded by socioeconomic determinants, which in turn may act through access to health care; familial associations with CKD may be due to associations with underlying diseases such as diabetes.

(9) A potential complication for determining causal pathways is the phenomenon of 'reverse causation' whereby the disease itself alters risk factors. This mostly affects prognostic studies of advanced CKD; examples include the occurrence of low blood pressure (secondary to heart failure) and low serum cholesterol (secondary to malnutrition) as complications of advanced CKD. U-shaped and other non-linear relationships have been found between these variables and CKD outcomes in dialysis populations (Zager *et al.* 1998; Lowrie and Lew 2003; Miskulin 2003).

(10) A similar problem arises when studying cases under clinical care where the treatment of symptoms or disease manifestations will alter the relationship between risk factors and disease occurrence for example use of only certain types of analgesics in cases with CKD altering associations of drugs with CKD, and the use of antihypertensive agents to control blood pressure. This has been termed 'confounding by indication'.

(11) Many studies have used Registries of RRT to capture cases with ESRF accepted for RRT. There are powerful selection factors in acceptance for treatment, which may be associated with important risk factors/confounders such as age, gender, social status, and comorbidity. Such selection factors will also apply to a lesser extent to studying cases of CKD under nephrological care.

There are two widely used measures in Registry RRT studies: acceptance and prevalence rates.

Acceptance (or take-on) rates of RRT are 'new' cases started on RRT per year per million of a defined population. These rates are influenced not only by the underlying incidence of ESRF in the population, but also by levels of detection, referral and acceptance onto RRT, and the definition of a new case. Definitions vary; in the United States Renal Data System (USRDS) a new case is not included until after 90 days of starting RRT; this excludes patients with established ESRF who die in the first 90 days, and underestimates incidence and the workload for health care providers. However, ascertaining patients at day 0 is difficult. Some patients requiring haemodialysis may have acute renal failure; if those that die early are included as ESRF this may inflate estimates as some of these cases may have recovered renal function and not needed long-term RRT. Such differences in definition need to be borne in mind when comparing acceptance rates. Ideally acceptance rates should be standardized for age and gender to take into account demographic differences between populations or between time periods.

Prevalence rates, also called 'stock' rates, are measures of the total number of patients on RRT at any time (usually at the year end, i.e. point prevalence) in a defined population. They indicate the health care burden and costs of an RRT programme.

Measurement of renal function in epidemiological studies

Although the most valid measure of renal function is the glomerular filtration rate (GFR), methods to directly measure this are impractical for epidemiological studies (see Chapter 1.3). Whilst there are formulae to estimate GFR (Cockcroft and Gault 1976; Levey 1999), most studies of CKD have used serum creatinine (SCr). This is insensitive to early renal impairment, as it does not increase to outside the normal range until the GFR declines by 50 per cent (Duncan *et al.* 2001). In one study 15 per cent of outpatients having SCr measured had a normal SCr (<130) but abnormal estimated GFR, this proportion rising with age (Duncan *et al.* 2001). There has been a search for other markers. Cystatin C seems the most promising, studies suggesting that it may be more sensitive than SCr, especially in detecting early renal damage (Laterza *et al.* 2002), although it has not yet been used in epidemiological studies and is rarely used yet in clinical practice.

Definition of chronic kidney disease

There has been no agreed terminology, until recently, for less severe CKD (Hsu and Chertow 2000). The US National Kidney Foundation has now defined CKD to include conditions that affect the kidney with the potential to cause either progressive loss of kidney function, or complications arising from decreased function (National Kidney Foundation 2002). CKD is defined as:

Kidney damage of not less than 3 months as defined by structural or functional abnormalities of the kidney, with or without decreased GFR, manifest by either pathological abnormalities or markers of kidney damage in blood or urine or imaging; or decreased function GFR of less than 60 ml/min/1.73 m^2 for not less than 3 months with or without evidence of kidney damage.

CKD is divided into stages (Table 1).

ESRF is the irreversible deterioration of renal function to a degree that is incompatible with life without RRT, either by dialysis or transplantation. It is the end result of progressive CKD. In practice, ESRF is usually taken as a GFR of less than 15 ml/min. SCr above 500 μmol/l is a rough guide to ESRF.

The other important marker of renal damage is proteinuria which can be detected by semiquantitative dipstick, or from random or timed urine specimens for albumin to creatinine ratios and albumin quantification, respectively.

Table 1 Stages of chronic kidney disease

Stage	Description	GFR (ml/min/1.73 m^2)	Presence of raised BP/abnormal laboratory tests/symptoms
1	Kidney damage with normal or increased GFR	≥90	
2	Kidney damage with mild GFR fall	60–89	Bp/lab+/−
3	Moderate GFR fall	30–59	Bp/lab+sym+/−
4	Severe GFR fall	15–29	BP/lab++sym+
5	Endstage kidney failure	<15 or dialysis	BP/lab+++ sym++

Descriptive epidemiology of adult chronic kidney disease

Incidence and prevalence studies

Most epidemiological data are from the developed world. The incidence and prevalence of CKD in the population has been investigated using SCr results measured as part of urea and electrolyte tests by chemical pathology laboratories (Table 2). Early studies used urea but it was too inaccurate a measure (Pendreigh *et al.* 1972). As SCr is a specific although insensitive marker, such studies will underestimate CKD rates. Moreover, they will be biased by factors associated with requiring a blood test, which may be because of an acute illness, for chronic disease management, for routine testing before elective surgery, for insurance purposes, or for private health screening. They exclude many people with CKD who are asymptomatic and who have not had urea and electrolyte tests; amongst these are high-risk groups such as diabetics who have not had regular blood tests as part of active surveillance (Kissmeyer *et al.* 1999). However, such population-based studies of 'detected' CKD are more likely to be representative than nephrology clinic studies where even greater selection factors apply (Jungers *et al.* 1996). The most robust information comes from testing random samples of the population as part of health surveys (Jones *et al.* 1998a). In all studies, use of a single cut-off level may be misleading given the variation in SCr by age, gender, size, and ethnicity. The CKD rates will vary depending on the distribution of these characteristics in the population studied.

There are few incidence studies and they have been undertaken in areas with small ethnic minority populations. The pyramidal relationship of less severe CKD to ESRF is striking.

The prevalence of untreated ESRF is very similar to the incidence because of poor survival. There have been prevalence studies on less severe CKD although differences in the study design, cut-off chosen, and population and age group studied, leads to variation in the rates (Table 3). The variable definition of prevalence means some studies might include acute renal failure cases. Prevalence is highest in population surveys, and whilst severe CKD is not common, rates of mild CKD are high and appear to be greater in the United States than elsewhere.

The prevalence of albuminuria has been described in the US population using the NHANES III. Overall 1 per cent had macroalbuminuria, this proportion was greater the worse the renal function, rising from 0.7 per cent in those with an estimated GFR > 60 ml/min to 3.3 per cent in those between 30 and 60 ml/min and to 26 per cent if GFR was less than 30 ml/min (Garg *et al.* 2002).

Table 2 Incidence of chronic kidney disease in population studies

Study	Year	Location	Definition of CKD[a]	Annual rate pmp
Pasternak *et al.* (1985)	1973–1976	Finland	>230 >500	317 119
Drey (2000)	1992–1994	Southampton, UK	>150 μmol/l	1700
Khan *et al.* (1994)	1 year 1989/1990	Grampian, UK	>300 μmol/l >500 μmol/l	450 132
Feest *et al.* (1990)	2 years 1986–1987	Devon, North West England, UK	>500 μmol/l	148

[a] Persistent elevation over 6 months.

Table 3 Prevalence studies of chronic kidney disease

Study	Year	Place	Design	Pop. group or age cut-off	Creatinine cut-offs, μmol/l	Prevalence (%)
Pasternack *et al.* (1985)	1976	Finland	Opportunistic	Adult	>230 >500	0.067 0.012
Culleton *et al.* (1999)	1977–1983	United States	Cohort baseline	Mean 54	Male 136–235 Female 120–265	8.7 8.0
Iseki *et al.* (1997)	1983	Japan	Screening	>18	Male > 177 Female > 146 (equivalent to estimated GFR< 30 ml/min)	0.37
Jones *et al.* (1998a)	1988–1994	United States	Survey	>17	Male > 141 Female > 124	3.3 2.7
Garg *et al.* (2002)	1988–1994	United States	Survey	>20	Male > 177 Female > 146	1.09
Coresh *et al.* (2003)	1988–1994	United States	Survey	>20	K/DOQI stages 3 (GFR 30–59) 4 (GFR 15–29)	 4.3 0.2
Nissenson *et al.* (2001)	1994–1997	United States	Opportunistic	Adults	>168	1.1
Gregory *et al.* (1990)	1986/1987	United Kingdom	Survey	18–64	Male > 120 Female > 120 All > 150 All > 190	9 1 0.32 0.27
Finch *et al.* (1998)	1995/1995	United Kingdom	Survey	65+	Male > 169 Female > 136	2.5 2.5
Wannamethee *et al.* (1997)	1978–1980	United Kingdom	Cohort baseline	Men 45–59	>150	3.5
John *et al.* (personal communication 2002)	2000/2001	United Kingdom	Opportunistic	Adults > 16	Male > 180 Female > 135 >300	0.55 0.04
Magnason *et al.* (2002)	1967–1991	Iceland	Survey	30–79	>150	0.22

There have been no direct studies of the geographical variation in CKD incidence or prevalence. Likewise it has been difficult to establish time trends, as there are no routine data on CKD incidence or prevalence. The only data are based on RRT rates (reviewed below). Ad hoc studies have been one off using different methodologies, case definitions, and populations. Even data from repeated US NHANES surveys are hard to compare. The prevalence of SCr > 168 μmol/l in NHANES II (conducted in 1976–80) was 0.42 per cent for ages 12–74; NHANES III had different age cut-offs; for all ages the prevalence was 0.55 per cent in males and 0.25 per cent in females. It is, therefore, difficult to conclude from these data whether or not there is a time trend (Strauss *et al.* 1993; Jones *et al.* 1998a). There were no time trends in the prevalence data in Iceland (Magnason *et al.* 2002).

Renal replacement therapy acceptance rate patterns

RRT has been a great success story since the introduction of dialysis in the 1960s. All developed countries have seen a steady increase in acceptance rates. The main growth has been increases in rates of acceptance in over 65-year-olds, especially in the last decade. This is most likely due to changing ascertainment, referral, and acceptance onto RRT, rather than any major increase in the incidence of CKD/ESRF, although population ageing and trends in the incidence of Type 2 diabetes will have contributed.

As an example, in the United Kingdom the number and rate of patients accepted onto RRT has steadily increased over the last two decades, from 20 pmp in 1982 to 96 pmp in 1998. The types of patients being treated have changed dramatically. In the late 1970s RRT was restricted almost exclusively to those under 65, and patients with diabetic ESRF were rarely treated. Twenty years later nearly half of the cases being treated were over 65, and diabetic ESRF was the most common single cause of ESRF amongst those accepted (Fig. 1).

Internationally, there is still substantial variation in the most recent acceptance rates. The United States of America has the highest acceptance rate, closely followed by Japan (Table 4). In Europe the highest rate is seen in Germany (175 pmp in 2000). In Eastern Europe RRT programmes are developing fast although generally they are still smaller than in Western Europe (Rutkowski 2000). Overall prevalence of RRT worldwide was 240 pmp in 2001, whilst it was highest in North America (1400 pmp), Japan (1830 pmp), and Europe (490 pmp), followed by Latin America (310 pmp) and the Middle East (150 pmp) (Moeller *et al.* 2002). An important question is 'why have acceptance rates increased so much?' The factors contributing to the increase can be summarized as follows (van Dijk *et al.* 2001):

- Greater referral/acceptance;
- Increased incidence of ESRF due to demographic change (i.e. ageing);
- True increased incidence of ESRF due to change in underlying risk: this can be due to the increased incidence of underlying disease and/or reduction in competing risk such as cardiovascular mortality.

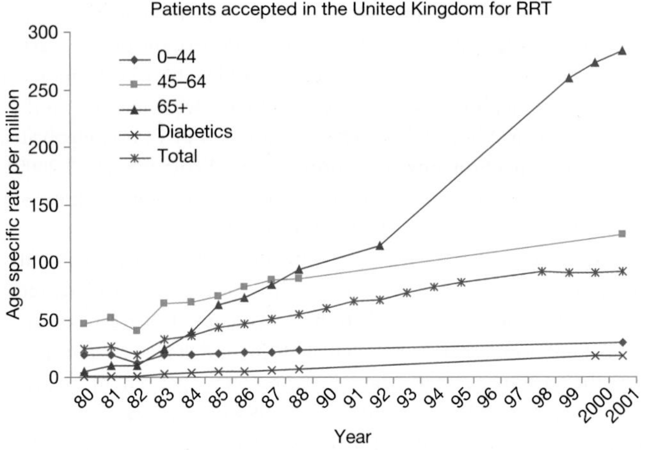

Fig. 1 Trends in acceptance rates for RRT in England (1981–2001).

Some of the increase in acceptance rates can be ascribed to greater awareness of ESRF, a lower threshold for referral of older sicker patients with ESRF to nephrologists, and a greater acceptance by nephrologists of such patients. This has partly been due to technical advances in dialysis therapy allowing for safe and long-term care of such patients. Studies of physicians' and nephrologists' attitudes over the last decade demonstrate this liberalization of attitudes (Challah *et al.* 1984; Parry 1996; McKenzie *et al.* 1998).

Mortality data as an indication of incidence of endstage renal failure

Mortality data from renal disease have been used as a proxy for incidence, but suffer from problems of under ascertainment and inaccuracy (Goldacre 1993; Perneger *et al.* 1993). Moreover, International Classification of Disease coding does not reliably distinguish between

Table 4 Patterns of RRT in different countries

Country	Year	Incident median age (years)	Incident rate (pmp)	Incident (%) DM	DM ESRF incident rate (pmp)	Prevalence (pmp)
Australia	2000	61	91	22	20	605
Austria	2000	64	129	33	43	714
Belgium-Dutch	2000	69	144	20	30	806
Canada	2000		143	32	46	609
Czech Rep	1998		136	37	50	563
Greece	2000	67	154	26	39	798
Japan	2000		253	37	94	1630
Norway	2000	65	89	15	13	577
Poland	1998		66	18	12	252
Spain Catalonia	2000	67	145	20	29	993
Spain	2000		132	18	23	848
Sweden	2000		125	25	31	712
Netherlands	2000	62	94	16	15	624
New Zealand	2000	58	107	36	39	610
Basque	2000	65	117	14	17	777
Germany	2000	66	175	36	63	870
Croatia	2000	62	106	28	30	620
United States	2000	64	333	43	142	1309
United Kingdom	2000	64	95	18	17	554

Sources: ANZData (2000), Canadian Organ Replacement Register (2000), USRDS (2000), Ansell *et al.* (2003), and ERA-EDTA.

acute and chronic forms of kidney disease. Temporal trends in deaths may reflect diagnostic patterns rather than true changes. Age standardized mortality rates from genitourinary diseases, which includes death from renal failure, declined consistently in England and Wales in the twentieth century (Roderick and Webster 1997). A similar trend was found in the United States of America in 1960–1986 (Hansen and Susser 1971). However, in the United States of America age specific trends increased during 1979–90, especially from mortality from diabetic nephropathy (Eberhardt *et al.* 1995).

Cause of chronic kidney disease and endstage renal failure

There are problems in classifying 'causes' of CKD and ESRF. Current classification systems were developed to classify ESRF cases accepted onto RRT. The three main Registry groups USRDS, ANZ, and EDTA have some variation in the coding systems used but they can be grouped (Maisonneuve *et al.* 2000):

Arteriopathic (i.e. renovascular disease, hypertensive disease);

Diabetic ESRF;

Glomerulonephritis;

Infective/obstructive (includes chronic pyelonephritis or reflux nephropathy, benign prostatic hypertrophy, neurogenic bladder, renal stones disease);

Congenital/familial/hereditary (e.g. adult polycystic kidney disease (PKD), Alport's syndrome, cystinosis, oxalosis);

Toxic (e.g. drug induced such as analgesic nephropathy, other toxic agents);

Neoplasms (e.g. kidney tumours);

Systemic (e.g. myeloma, systemic lupus erythematosus (SLE), amyloid, Henoch–Schönlein purpura, scleroderma, haemolytic uraemic syndrome);

Miscellaneous (e.g. Balkan nephropathy);

Uncertain.

Establishing such types of renal disease may be useful for individuals in informing prognosis and use of specific treatments, indicating risk of recurrence after transplantation, and in counselling families with hereditary conditions. In aggregate, cause data can indicate changing patterns and the public health importance of particular conditions. Routinely presented Registry cause data are limited as epidemiological measures, as they will be determined by referral/acceptance policies and population demography as well as by underlying disease patterns, and many patients have 'uncertain cause'. Moreover, the classification system imposes limitations, as the basis for ascribing cause is heterogeneous and not mutually exclusive (e.g. based on presumed nephrotoxin for analgesic nephropathy, presence of systemic illness for SLE, histology for glomerulonephritis (GN), morphology (PKD), and may confuse probable cause from consequence (hypertensive nephropathy).

Presenting a single cause does not cover the multifactorial nature of many cases of CKD. Whilst some cases of CKD are due to specific underlying diseases (such as PKD) many cases have no known cause, and even where there is an underlying condition or disease there may be several contributing factors. For example, for diabetic nephropathy occupational or environmental exposures, undiagnosed renovascular disease, cardiovascular risk factors such as smoking, obesity, drug use (e.g. NSAIDs), and bladder flow obstruction (due to autonomic neuropathy) may contribute to the initiation and progression of renal damage and each might be considered as the potential cause (Young 1997). Conversely diabetes may contribute to other causes of CKD by such mechanisms. Choosing a single cause can, therefore, be misleading.

Comparing studies is difficult because of varying definitions and diagnostic criteria, and the reliance on clinical judgement. For example, the degree to which biopsy is undertaken, and thereby histological evidence used to support the diagnosis of glomerulonephritis, varies. Fernandes showed that there is a specific problem of over-diagnosis of hypertensive nephropathy in Blacks in the United Kingdom, and of primary GN in Whites, whereas the diagnoses of PKD, pyelonephritis, and diabetic nephropathy were more robust (Fernandes *et al.* 2000). There was also evidence of over ascription of hypertensive disease in Blacks in the United States (Perneger *et al.* 1995a).

The cause of CKD is even more difficult to determine from population studies, as many cases do not have investigation, particularly renal biopsy. In a population-based study in Scotland 46 per cent of cases were of unknown cause, interstitial nephritis and diabetic nephropathy were the most frequent specific causes, and only 4 per cent had definite GN (Khan *et al.* 1994). In a study of patients with CKD who were under nephrologists' care the breakdown was different (Landray *et al.* 2001), with a much higher proportion having GN though even here 23 per cent were classified as an 'uncertain' cause (Table 5).

In the developed world, as the overall incidence of ESRF has increased, the contribution to the total of each individual cause has changed. Thus, whilst the incidence of GN may not have fallen, the percentage of patients with this, and many other primary renal diseases, is falling, as other causes, particularly systemic diseases such as diabetes, become more common. For example, in Canada GN fell from 20 to under 15 per cent between 1992 and 2000, and there were also small falls in pyelonephritis and PKD. In contrast diabetic ESRF rose from 24 to 32 per cent and there were smaller percentage rises in reno-vascular and hypertensive renal disease (Canadian Organ Replacement Register 2000) (Table 6). Trends in several European countries are shown in Fig. 2. As these proportional changes are in the context of rising acceptance rates, in absolute terms they are even greater. Patterns vary by age; in particular uncertain cause and renovascular disease are more common in the elderly. Thus, as more and

Table 5 Causes of CKD in patients under nephrologist care

	Per cent
Primary glomerulonephritis	21
Vascular disease	14
Diabetic nephropathy	8
Secondary GN	5
Pyelonephritis	9
Familial/congenital	10
Interstitial nephritis	5
Uncertain	23

Adapted from Landray *et al.* 2001.

Table 6 Acceptance rates and proportions by primary renal disease in four developed countries

	Australia	Canada	Canada	UK	USA
Year	2001	1992	2000	2001	1997–2000
Annual acceptance rate pmp and proportion (in brackets)					
Glomerulo nephritis[a]	21 (22%)	19 (20%)	20 (14%)	11 (12%)	28 (12%)
Hypertension	15 (15%)	10 (10%)	19 (13%)	5 (5%)	87 (23%)
Analgesic	5 (5%)		—	—	0.7 (0.2%)
Reflux	4 (4%)		—	—	2 (0.6%)
'Pyelo'[b]	—	7 (7%)	6 (4%)	10 (10%)	—
Diabetes	24 (25%)	24 (25%)	46 (32%)	18 (19%)	146 (44%)
Uncertain[c]	12 (12%)	14 (15%)	17 (12%)	19 (20%)	13 (4%)
PCKD	6 (6%)	6 (6%)	6 (4%)	7 (7%)	7 (2%)
Renovascular disease	Not recorded	7 (7%)	13 (9%)	10 (10%)	10 (3%)
Total	97	96	143	95	337 (in 2000)

[a] Proven by biopsy.

[b] Pyelonephritis (including both prostatic hypertrophy and chronic PN from childhood reflux nephropathy).

[c] Includes ascription of GN not biopsied.

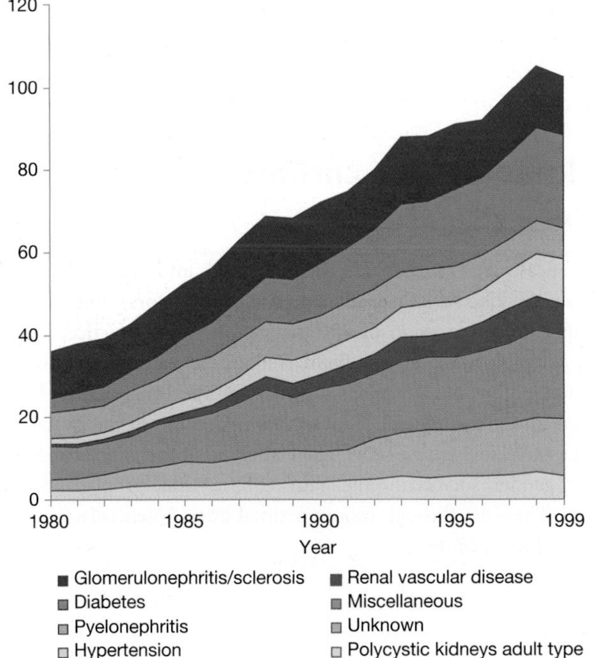

Fig. 2 Trends in causes of RRT in Europe (1980–1999).

more old patients are accepted for treatment, the changing patterns reflect the different age distributions of causes of ESRF.

Trends in RRT rates may be more informative of the underlying epidemiology in young people if it is assumed that all young cases are referred and accepted onto RRT. This approach has shown changes in patterns of specific underlying causes, such as the decline in analgesic nephropathy in Australia (Stewart *et al.* 1994).

In all Registries, data on the type of diabetes are unreliable. There is particularly large inter-country variation in diabetic ESRF rates. Whilst this can be partly explained by variation in ascription (i.e. to what extent the presence of proteinuria, other microvascular disease, or biopsy changes are required for the diagnosis), it is also due to patterns of diabetes especially Type 2, the effectiveness of preventive health measures, and referral patterns for diabetics with renal disease.

Population studies of the incidence of glomerulonephritis

Epidemiological studies of GN have been based on analysis of data from specific biopsy registers. However, there are several selection factors that will determine the pattern of GN identified. The likelihood of referral and indications for biopsy will vary between renal units and clinicians, and by the mode of clinical presentation (e.g. nephrotic syndrome, intermittent haematuria), which in turn varies by GN type. These patterns will vary by studies due to differences in country, time period, age distribution, and the inclusion or not of secondary GN, and classification schemes used for certain subtypes of GN (e.g. antiglomerular basement membrane, Wegener's, PAN vasculitis), and the known special interests of the centre concerned. The indications for biopsy in the elderly differ from younger groups with a lower proportion of the elderly having biopsy for urinary abnormalities (Davison and Johnston 1996).

Some studies have no defined denominator and so are not able to generate rates (Frimat *et al.* 1996). Results from some population

Table 7 Population studies of biopsy proven glomerulonephritis

Study	Year	Country	Rate pmp	Inclusive type GN	Types GN rate pmp		Male (%)	Age pattern
Schena (1997)	1993	Italy	Biopsy proven GN 34	1°, 2°	IgA Membranous GN FSGS Lupus MesP Vasculitis	8.4 4.9 2.5 2.6 1.6 1.6	65	
Briganti *et al.* (2001)	1995–1997	Victoria, Australia	All biopsy 215 proven GN 125	1°, 2° DM excl	IgA FSGS Vasculitis Lupus Membranous nephropathy	43 21 17 15 13	55	IgA commonest in <65 year olds, vasculitis commonest in >65 year olds
Heaf *et al.* (1999)	1985–1997	Denmark	Biopsy proven GN 39	1°, 2°	MesP Minimal change FSGS Cresentic Membranous GN	11 7 6 5 5	59	
Simon *et al.* (1994)	1976–1990	One region, France	Biopsy proven GN 82	1°	IgA Membranous nephropathy FSGS[a] Nephrosis	27 14 8 10	66	IgA 3–4 × commoner 20–59 versus elderly, membranous GN reverse
Rivera *et al.* (2002)	1994–1999	Spain	All biopsy 48	1°, 2°	IgA FSGS Lupus Minimal change	8 6 6 5	66 in adults	Vasculitis, membranous nephropathy > in over 65 s

[a] Excluding FSGS with nephrotic syndrome—these included in nephrosis.

studies are shown in Table 7. All are from developed countries. IgA is the most common form of primary GN where biopsy for haematuria has been commonly performed (Heaf *et al.* 1999). All types of GN are more common in males except for lupus. Age distribution varies by subtype; peak ages in both sexes were 25–34 for lupus, 55–64 for focal segmental glomerulosclerosis (FSGS) and membranous GN, 65–74 for vasculitis, and for IgA nephropathy 25–34 for females and 55–64 for males. Rarer causes of GN are minimal change (in adults), thrombotic microangiopathy, mesangiocapillary GN, postinfectious GN, anti-GBM antibody disease, and cryoglobulinaemia.

One study was able to ascertain incidence over time in one French region (Simon *et al.* 1994). There was a fall in the rate of GN in the period 1976–1990 attributed to a steady decline in mesangiocapillary GN poststreptococcal infection. IgA rates were steady suggesting an immunogenetic rather than environmental or infectious aetiology. In contrast, there was no change in biopsy proven GN in 1985–1997 in Denmark (Heaf *et al.* 1999).

The pattern of GN by clinical indication for biopsy is described in Schena's Italian study (Schena 1997). The most common indications and related GN type were nephrotic syndrome (27 per cent of biopsies) where membranous GN predominated, nephritis (5 per cent biopsies) where it was FSGS and IgA nephropathy, urinary abnormalities (40 per cent biopsies) including recurrent macroscopic haematuria where it was IgA nephropathy, and 'chronic renal impairment' (19 per cent biopsies) where it was IgA, membranous, and FSGS nephropathy.

Risk factors for chronic kidney disease

Theoretically risk factors can be separated into those factors that increase the risk of kidney damage *per se* (initiators) and those that promote the progression of CRD (promoters). In practice, it is not always possible to distinguish them as many factors do both. Moreover, in practice all would be targets for intervention. Initiators can be subdivided into proximal and distal factors in relation to the causal pathway. Distal factors are the more 'fixed' attributes (or characteristics) such as age, gender, socioeconomic status (SES), ethnic group, and family history. These act through more proximal often potentially modifiable factors which include:

Diabetes

Hypertension

Cardiovascular disease

Smoking, alcohol, obesity, dyslipidaemia, low birth weight

Occupational exposure to nephrotoxins, for example silica, hydrocarbon

Environmental exposure to nephrotoxins, for example lead, cadmium

Nephrotoxic drugs, for example analgesics

Congenital dysplasia/reflux nephropathy

Bladder outflow obstruction

Some glomerulonephritides

Autoimmune disease

Infection, for example HIV, hepatitis C

Neoplasia, for example myeloma.

This section focuses on the fixed sociodemographic factors associated with CKD. Many of the underlying conditions and risk factors associated with CKD are covered in separate chapters. The incidence of CKD could be reduced by interventions to prevent such conditions or factors (e.g. by population change in obesity and exercise to reduce the incidence of Type 2 diabetes) or prevention of the consequences (e.g. tight blood pressure and glucose control in diabetics).

Age

All incidence and prevalence studies have found that CKD is predominantly a disease of the elderly, with incidence rates rising steeply with age. In Feest's incidence study, ESRF annual rates were 58, 160, 282, 503, and 588 pmp in the age groups 20–49, 50–59, 60–69, 70–79, and 80+, respectively (Feest *et al.* 1990). Similarly in Khan's study the rate in the age group 50–69 was 159 pmp rising to 472 pmp in the 70–79 age group (Khan *et al.* 1994).

For less advanced CKD in the United States NHANES III study the prevalence of SCr over 126 μmol/l was 9.7 per cent in men of all ages, but 32.3 per cent in men over 70; corresponding figures in females were 1.8 and 9.3 per cent, respectively (Jones *et al.* 1998). Using SCr cut-offs equivalent to a GFR of less than 30 ml/min/1.73 m^2 Garg *et al.* (2002) showed prevalence of 0.17 per cent in 20–39 year olds, 0.40 per cent in 40–59 year olds and 2.22 per cent in 60–79-year-olds. Other population studies have also shown the age effect in SCr (Culleton *et al.* 1999; Caresh *et al.* 2001).

Nephrons start to decline in number during the third decade of life. As creatinine clearance declines, the ageing subject loses muscle mass and produces less creatinine. Thus, plasma creatinine may remain stable, hiding the progressive loss of renal function. In elderly people with low muscle mass and poor nutrition SCr may be a misleading guide to renal function. Calculations of creatinine clearance from serum creatinine, such as the Cockroft and Gault equation are unreliable in very old people and accurate urine collections are difficult: when available radioisotope techniques to measure creatinine clearance are better (Friedman *et al.* 1989).

On balance, in many people serum creatinine increases with age despite the loss of muscle mass (Stewart *et al.* 1994; Jones *et al.* 1998). By the age of 80 the creatinine clearance may be between 40 and 75 mls/min and the plasma creatinine as high as 140 μmol/l without overt renal disease (Kampmann *et al.* 1974). Epstein reviewed renal changes in the kidney with age (Epstein 1996). Longitudinal studies have shown that whilst there is some decline in reserve and a reduced ability to respond to challenges, these are not of clinical significance unless there is an acute challenge (e.g. drug) or superimposed pathological process such as vascular disease or hypertension which are increasingly common with age (Lindeman *et al.* 1985).

Gender

There is a male excess of CKD in most studies. In Nissenson's prevalence study in the United States, males had an overall prevalence of 1.6 per cent and females 0.8 per cent, this twofold ratio was maintained at all levels of SCr (Nissenson *et al.* 2001). The NHANES III study showed a substantial male excess, with mean values of 116 mmol/l in men and 96 mmol/l in women (Jones *et al.* 1998). Part of the excess is due to using the same cut-offs; a better comparison is to take gender specific cut-offs to allow for the lower muscle mass in women, but even so there is still a male excess (Table 8).

Registry data on RRT generally confirm the male excess. Whilst this could be due to gender inequity in referral/acceptance, there is increasing evidence of a sex difference in the incidence of most types of CKD, and of progression in all types of CKD (Silbiger and Neugarten 1995; Zeier *et al.* 1998). For example, there is an excess of immune-mediated primary glomerular disease such as membranous nephropathy in men (Mallick *et al.* 1987; Rosen *et al.* 1994) (Table 6). In some cases there is an interaction between race and gender—diabetic nephropathy is more common in African-American women than men, whilst the converse occurs in White women. Silbiger reviewed the effect of gender on progression and concluded that progression rates are faster in men independent of blood pressure and lipids (Silbiger and Newgarten 1995). Various mechanisms have been proposed. Data on gender differences in kidney anatomy and function are unclear. The female advantage is lost postmenopause suggesting a protective role for sex hormones, which are thought to act through a variety of mechanisms including mesangial cell function, cytokine production and release, and by vasoactive agents, although the exact mechanisms for gender differences remain to be elucidated.

Ethnicity

It has been recognized since the 1980s that Black populations in the United States have higher rates of treated ESRF than White populations, with particularly high rates of hypertensive and diabetic ESRF (Hiatt and Friedman 1982; Rostand *et al.* 1982). Age- and gender-adjusted rate ratios for all ESRF of 3.5–3.7 were found in the decade upto 1988, age-adjusted rates of hypertension were 6.2, diabetes 3.7, and glomerulonephritis 2.5 (Feldman *et al.* 1992).

This excess risk has also been demonstrated in many other indigenous or migrant minority populations including native Americans (Stahn *et al.* 1993; Robbins *et al.* 1996), Hispanics in the United States (Chiapilla and Feldman 1995; Pugh 1996), people of West African or Caribbean origin in the United Kingdom (Roderich *et al.* 1996), Indo-Asians in the United Kingdom (Higgins *et al.* 1995; Lightstone *et al.* 1995; Roderich *et al.* 1996), and Aborigines in Australia (Hay 2000), and Canada (Dyck and Jan 1998). A selection of such studies is shown in Table 9, based on acceptances for RRT.

The USRDS (2000b) data showed that age-adjusted rates of treated ESRF were increased 3.9-fold in Blacks, and 2.8-fold in native Americans compared to Whites, and 1.8-fold in Hispanics compared to non-Hispanics (USRDS 2000b). There were particularly high rates

Table 8 Prevalence (%) of raised serum creatinine in NHANES III 1988–1994

	>126 μmol/l	>143 μmol/l	>168 μmol/l
Males	9.7	2.5	0.55
Females	1.8	0.7	0.25

Table 9 Relative risks of being accepted for RRT in ethnic minorities

Ethnic group	Country	Period	Increased risk versus Whites (all CKD)	Increased risk versus Whites (DM ESRF)
Blacks (Klag *et al.* 1997)	United States	1973–1990	3.2 (age adjusted)	5.2
Native Americans (Stahn *et al.* 1993)	United States	1982–1988	2.8	5.8
Black (Roderick *et al.* 1996)	United Kingdom	1991/1992	3.7 (age adjusted)	6.5
Indo-Asians/Blacks (Higgins *et al.* 1995)	United Kingdom (Coventry)	1994/1995	4.5	
Indo-Asians (Roderick *et al.* 1996)	United Kingdom	1991/1992	4.2 (age adjusted)	5.8
Hispanics (Pugh *et al.* 1988)	United States	1978–1984	3	6
Aborigines (Spencer *et al.* 1998)	Australia Northern Territories	1993–1996	21 (age adjusted)	
Aborigines (Cass *et al.* 1999)	Australia New South Wales	1987–1998	1.4	2.5
Aborigines (Dyck and Jan 1998)	Canada	1981–1990	2.6 for non-diabetic ESRF	

of hypertensive and diabetic ESRF in Blacks (6.0- and 4.1-fold compared to Whites) and high rates of diabetic ESRF amongst native Americans (5.1-fold). UK data on ethnic minorities not only confirm the excess incidence of diabetic and hypertensive ESRF, but also show a high proportion of Indo-Asians with unknown cause presenting with small kidneys, and interstitial nephritis (Lightstone *et al.* 1995; Ball *et al.* 1997, 2001).

Population survey data using the US NHANES III confirm higher prevalence of raised creatinine levels in ethnic minority groups in the United States (Jones *et al.* 1998b). Long-term follow-up of the MRFIT study found an over threefold greater incidence of ESRF in African-American men compared to White men, which was partly reduced after controlling for income (Klag *et al.* 1997).

A common feature in these ethnic minorities is an early age of onset, high rate of diabetic ESRF and in some a female excess. The reasons are multifactorial, reflecting a complex mix of genetic and environmental influences. While there is a common pattern there is variation even within the same ethnic group (e.g. between different native American tribes, and amongst aboriginals from different parts of Australia) (Cass *et al.* 2001). Possible explanations for the high risks include a greater propensity to underlying conditions such as Type 2 diabetes and hypertension, socioeconomic circumstances which may amongst other effects influence access to health care, and an increased susceptibility to the effects of hypertension or diabetes. These are considered below.

Higher rates of diabetes

These populations have high rates of Type 2 diabetes associated with central obesity, insulin resistance, hyperlipidaemia, and hypertension. This is most marked in Pima Indians who have the highest rates of Type 2 diabetes in the world with virtually all ESRF being diabetic, but it is also true of other groups (Nelson *et al.* 1993). People of Indo-Asian origin living in the United Kingdom have a higher prevalence and mortality from Type 2 diabetes (Raleigh 1997). An important factor is a change in lifestyle to a Western pattern of food intake and exercise, which in some groups arose after migration. One theory is that ethnic minorities have a genotype geared to lay down fat in times of starvation ('thrifty genotype') but which predisposes to Type 2 diabetes in times of relative plenty (Neel *et al.* 1998). Another hypothesis is that it is due to a 'thrifty phenotype' arising from intrauterine starvation and consequent low birth weight, which transmits an intergenerational rather than genetic predisposition (Barker *et al.* 1989; Cruickshank *et al.* 2001). Paradoxically improvements in healthcare have reduced perinatal mortality and may have led to survival of a higher proportion of low birth weight babies, which is one reason cited for the high rates in Aborigines (Hay *et al.* 1998).

Higher rates of hypertension

This has been studied most in US Blacks and UK African and Afro-Caribbean populations. The latter have higher mortality from cerebrovascular and hypertensive disease (Raligh *et al.* 1996) and a higher prevalence of hypertension than Whites in the United Kingdom (Raleigh 1997). US Blacks have a higher prevalence of hypertension in NHANES studies (Jones *et al.* 1998). Mclellan *et al.* (1987) and Whittle *et al.* (1991) showed higher rates of hypertension and severe hypertension in Blacks compared to Whites. The MDRD trial baseline data showed that Black race was significantly and independently associated with hypertension (Buckalen *et al.* 1996). Such hypertension in Blacks is more salt sensitive than Whites (Jones and Agodoa 1993). The excess incidence in the national MRFIT cohort was reduced after control for systolic blood pressure (Klag *et al.* 1997).

Socioeconomic factors

Ethnic minority groups in developed countries tend to have socioeconomic disadvantages. The impact may be lifelong affecting each stage of childhood development, and adult life. Factors include greater exposure to childhood infection, exposure to occupational and environmental toxins, the impact of deleterious behaviours such as smoking and heavy alcohol consumption, and reduced access to timely preventive health care (e.g. for detection and management of BP) (Hoy, 2000). The risk of ESRF in Blacks was reduced after control for income and benefit receipt (Young *et al.* 1994; Perneger *et al.* 1995b; Klag *et al.* 1997).

Greater susceptibility to develop endstage renal failure

Whilst it is clear that all the factors above apply, studies which have adjusted for these have suggested that there is a greater susceptibility to develop renal damage in ethnic minorities. Brancati showed that the increased rate of diabetic ESRF in US Blacks was present even after adjusting for the prevalence of diabetes, hypertension, SES (education), and access to regular health care, suggesting an increased susceptibility to develop nephropathy (Braneati *et al.* 1992). Similar findings apply to Mexican Hispanics (Feldman 1992). McLellan *et al.* (1987) showed that the excess risk of hypertensive ESRF in Blacks could not be explained solely by higher rates of moderate or severe hypertension or poorer control: adjustment for age, sex, and hypertension still left a sevenfold excess risk. Whittle *et al.* (1991), using population health surveys as well as RRT data, showed that hypertensive ESRF was still increased 4.5-fold after adjustment for hypertension prevalence and severity, age, diagnosis, and education. The Hypertension Detection and Follow-Up study found that Blacks had higher levels of SCr, at similar levels of BP, than Whites (Shulman 1989). Blacks with hypertension are more likely to develop renal insufficiency than Whites (Feldman 1992), and microalbuminuria (Summerson *et al.* 1995; Grossfeld *et al.* 2001). However, in the prospective cohort study ARIC, Blacks who were diabetic had a threefold faster decline in renal function than Whites, but 80 per cent of the difference was due to modifiable factors such as socioeconomic factors, suboptimal glucose and blood pressure control, and smoking (Kropp *et al.* 1999).

Genetic influences are suggested by the strong familial relationships found in US Blacks (Freedman *et al.* 1993). There may be interethnic differences in renal responses to explain this (Smith *et al.* 1991), such as in the regulation of salt water and renal haemodynamics (Frohlich *et al.* 1983), the renin angiotensin system (Dunn and Janner 1974), and volume loading (Feldman *et al.* 1992). Low birth weight which is more prevalent in Blacks, may be associated with lower nephron numbers, thereby increasing susceptibility to develop nephropathy (Lopes and Port 1995; Konji *et al.* 1996).

Indo-Asians with Type 2 diabetes are more likely to develop microalbuminuria (Allawi *et al.* 1988), which is not explained by poorer BP or glucose control, or high triglyceride levels (Mather *et al.* 1998), and have a higher incidence of proteinuria (Koppiker *et al.* 1998; Earle *et al.* 2001). Small studies in nephrology and diabetic clinic populations have showed either no difference in the rate of decline between Whites and Indo-Asians with diabetic nephropathy or greater decline in Indo Asians (Koppiker *et al.* 1998; Earle *et al.* 2001).

A few studies illustrate the complexity of factors influencing CKD. In the Aborigines of the Northern Territories of Australia there has been an epidemic in the last 40 years of CKD together with hypertension, diabetes, and cardiovascular disease (Hoy 2000). Community studies of renal function (including the albumin/creatinine ratio) have shown this pattern to be multifactorial with influences of lower birth weight, childhood infection, diabetes, hyperlipidaemia, obesity, hypertension, and insulin resistance. This reflects rapid social change accompanied by social disadvantage (Spencer *et al.* 1998; Cass *et al.* 1999). The excess CKD is much less in Aboriginals in New South Wales, which may reflect better socioeconomic circumstances and access to health care in this more affluent area of Australia (Cass *et al.* 1999).

The effects of a generalized improvement in health care are not always beneficial in all areas. Nelson showed that in Pima Indians over the period 1955–1994 diabetic nephropathy in Type 2 diabetics increased despite better control of blood pressure and blood glucose, suggesting other powerful environmental or behavioural factors affecting risk (Nelson *et al.* 1998). This may in part reflect that by reducing deaths to competing factors such as cardiovascular disease, the population lived longer and then developed nephropathy (Table 8).

Socioeconomic status

There is strong evidence that the incidence of CKD and ESRF is positively associated with lower SES (Perneger *et al.* 1995c). The incidence rates of detected SCr concentration over 150 μmol/l in Southampton were highest in the most deprived areas (Drey 2000). Ecological studies in the United Kingdom, the United States, and Australia of RRT acceptances have shown associations with poorer areas. Such studies have the problem of ecological confounding (i.e. the alternative explanation such as the effects of ethnic minority populations) but they do raise the possibility of a true association (Roderick *et al.* 1999; Cass *et al.* 2001b). For example, modelling studies of acceptances onto RRT in England by area deprivation show positive associations with deprivation (Boyle *et al.* 1996; Roderick *et al.* 1999), although area deprivation was not found to be a factor associated with acceptance onto RRT in Scotland (Khaw *et al.* 1993; Metealfe *et al.* 1999). In the study of Whittles *et al.* (1991), lower level of education and low income of areas were independently associated with hypertensive RRT acceptance rates in the United States; Perneger *et al.* (1995b) found area income levels to be inversely associated with all RRT acceptance rates, and Brancati *et al.* (1992) showed that diabetic ESRF RRT acceptance rates were associated with income and education levels too in a similar design. A case–control study in Sweden of ESRF cases found that low SES was associated with an increased risk of ESRF; this was not explained by smoking, body mass index (BMI), alcohol, or analgesic consumption (Fored *et al.* 2003).

The socioeconomic disparity cannot be attributed to differential access to RRT services as one would hypothesize this would be inversely related to SES. More likely are social and environmental determinants such as increased exposure to nephrotoxins, higher incidence of diseases leading to CKD, behaviours such as smoking, and poorer access to preventive health care. There is evidence of socioeconomic gradients in underlying causes of CKD such as Type 2 diabetes and hypertension (Perneger *et al.* 1995a). Bakir and Dunea (2001) outline the factors contributing to higher incidence of CKD in US inner city areas—a complex interaction in poor largely ethnic minority communities with inadequate blood pressure detection and control, high levels of drug abuse and HIV infection.

As discussed above SES explains in part the excess risk of CKD in ethnic minority groups. The MRFIT follow-up study showed that the incidence of ESRF is associated with SES at baseline, and that this partly explains excess risk in Blacks (Klag *et al.* 1997).

Family history/genetic susceptibility

There is increasing interest in the inherited susceptibility to ESRF. This has been stimulated by the findings of familial clustering of risk, which has been found in all ethnic groups and for all types of CKD (Freedman and Satko 2000). For example, in a study of incident dialysis patients in the United States 20 per cent had a family history of ESRF (Freedman *et al.* 1997).

Several case–control studies have investigated aggregation in ESRF cases (Ferguson *et al.* 1988; Steenland *et al.* 1990; Spray *et al.* 1995; O'Dea *et al.* 1998; Rei *et al.* 1998; Freedman 1999). O'Dea *et al.* (1998) compared renal outcomes in relatives of index ESRF cases in Canada, in a largely White population with the spouses of index cases as a control group (i.e. to control for shared environmental exposure). They only looked at non-Mendelian disease and found a threefold higher frequency of renal failure in relatives than in spousal controls. This risk was particularly high for hypertensive renal failure, diabetic nephropathy, and interstitial nephritis (pyelonephritis). Similar findings were found in another study in White populations by Spray *et al.* (1995).

The risk associated with family history is even higher in Blacks (Freedman 1999). Freedman found in a diabetic ESRF case–control study an eightfold increased risk in Blacks, which was not explained by hypertensive or diabetes control, suggesting familial clustering (Freedman 1999). Bergman found that nearly half of the family members of index cases with hypertensive ESRF had evidence of renal disease; a quarter had ESRF, and 65 per cent had one first degree relative with nephropathy or ESRF (Bergman *et al.* 1996). Lei *et al.* (1998) showed that the risk of ESRF was increased in a dose–response manner (i.e. depending on the number of relatives affected), and it persisted after controlling for the presence of diabetes and hypertension, and was present if renal disease was defined as ESRF or less severe kidney disease. Jurkovitz *et al.* (2002) showed that screening family members of index cases with ESRF gave a high yield of previously undetected CKD.

Such studies suggest a shared genetic risk for CKD, although the alternatives include shared environment in childhood or early adulthood as well as greater predisposition to diabetes and hypertension. Using ESRF as the outcome may underestimate associations, especially where there is variable penetrance of any genetic factor. The search is now on for genetic markers. Many candidate genes have been reported to be associated with increased risk of nephropathy e.g. the ACEI/FD polymorphism is associated with Type 2 diabetic nephropathy (Freedman and Satko 2000). Most of these studies to date have been undertaken in the United States. There is a need to investigate this issue in other populations and ethnic minority groups at high risk of CKD.

Conclusion

Despite advances in the understanding of the epidemiology of CKD more research is needed on the patterns of CKD over time and between places, and on identifying the contributions of modifiable risk factors in initiating and hastening progression of CKD in order to improve the scope for preventing CKD.

References

Allawi, J., Rao, P. V., Gilbert, R., Scotti, G., Jarrett, R. J., and Keen, H. (1988). Microalbuminuria in non-insulin-dependent diabetes: its prevalence in Indian compared with Europid patients. *British Medical Journal* **296**, 462–464.

Ansell, D., Feest, T., and Byrne, C. UK Renal Registry Report 2002 (Fifth annual). Bristol: UK Renal Registry, 2003.

ANZ Data (Australian and New Zealand Dialysis and Transplant Registry) (2000). Report, 2000.

Bakir, A. A. and Dunea, G. (2001). Renal disease in the inner city. *Seminar on Nephrology* **21**, 334–345.

Ball, S., Cook, T., Hulme, B., Palmer, A., and Taube, D. (1997). The diagnosis and racial origin of 394 patients undergoing renal biopsy: an association between Indian race and interstitial nephritis. *Nephrology, Dialysis, Transplantation* **12**, 71–77.

Ball, S. *et al.* (2001). Why is there so much end-stage renal failure of undetermined cause in UK Indo-Asians? *Quarterly Journal of Medicine* **94**, 187–193.

Barker, D. J. P., Osmond, C., Golding, J., Kuh, D., and Wadsworth, M. E. J. (1989). Growth *in utero*, blood pressure in childhood and adult life, and mortality from cardiovascular disease. *British Medical Journal* **298**, 564–567.

Bergman, S., Key, B. O., Kirk, K. A., Warnock, D. G., and Rostant, S. G. (1996). Kidney disease in the first-degree relatives of African–Americans with hypertensive end-stage renal disease. *American Journal of Kidney Diseases* **27**, 341–346.

Boyle, P. J., Kudlac, H., and Williams, A. J. (1996). Geographical variation in the referral of patients with chronic end stage renal failure for renal replacement therapy. *Quarterly Journal of Medicine* **89**, 151–157.

Brancati, F. L., Whittle, J. C., Whelton, P. K., Seidler, A. J., and Klag, M. J. (1992). The excess incidence of diabetic end-stage renal disease among blacks. *Journal of the American Medical Association* **268**, 3079–3084.

Briganti, E. M. *et al.* (2001). The incidence of biopsy-proven glomerulonephritis in Australia. *Nephrology, Dialysis, Transplantation* **16**, 1364–1367.

Buckalew, V. M., Berg, R. L., Wang, S. R., Porush, J. G., Rauch, S., and Schulman, G. (1996). Prevalence of hypertension in 1795 subjects with chronic renal disease: the modification of diet in renal disease study baseline cohort. Modification of Diet in Renal Disease Study Group. *American Journal of Kidney Diseases* **28**(6), 811–821.

Calvert, G. M., Steenland, K., and Palu, S. (1997). End stage renal disease among silica exposed gold miners. A new method for assessing incidence among epidemiologic cohorts. *Journal of the American Medical Association* **277** (15), 1219–1223.

Canadian Organ Replacement Register 2000 Report. www.cihi.ca, 2000.

Cass, A., Gillin, A. G., and Horvath, J. S. (1999). End-stage renal disease in aboriginals in New South Wales: a very different picture to the Northern Territory. *The Medical Journal of Australia* **171**, 407–410.

Cass, A., Cunningham, J., Wang, Z., and Hoy, W. (2001a). Regional variation in the incidence of end-stage renal disease in indigenous Australians. *The Medical Journal of Australia* **175**, 24–27.

Cass, A., Cunningham, J., Wang, Z., and Hoy, W. (2001b). Social disadvantage and variation in the incidence of end-stage renal disease in Australian capital cities. *Australian and New Zealand Journal of Public Health* **25**, 322–326.

Challah, S., Wing, A. J., Bauer, R., Morris, R. W., and Schroeder, S. A. (1984). Negative selection of patients for dialysis and transplantation in the United Kingdom. *British Medical Journal* **288**, 1119–1122.

Chiapella, A. P. and Feldman, H. I. (1995). Renal failure among male Hispanics in the United States. *American Journal of Public Health* **85**, 1001–1004.

Cockcroft, D. W. and Gault, M. H. (1976). Prediction of creatinine clearance from serum creatinine. *Nephron* **16**, 31–41.

Coresh, J. *et al.* (2001). Prevalence of high blood pressure and elevated serum creatinine level in the United States: findings from the third National Health and Nutrition Examination Survey (1988–1994). *Archives of Internal Medicine* **161**, 1207–1216.

Coresh, J., Astor, B. C., Greene, T., Eknoyan, G., and Levey, A. S. (2003). Prevalence of chronic kidney disease and decreased kidney function in the adult US population: third National Health and Nutrition Examination Survey. *American Journal of Kidney Diseases* **41**, 1–12.

Cruickshank, J. K., Mbanya, J. C., Wilks, R., Balkau, B., McFarlane-Anderson, N., and Forrester, T. (2001). Sick genes, sick individuals or sick populations with chronic disease? The emergence of diabetes and high blood pressure in African-origin populations. *International Journal of Epidemiology* **30**, 111–117.

Culleton, B. F. *et al.* (1999). Prevalence and correlates of elevated serum creatinine levels: the Framingham Heart Study. *Archives of Internal Medicine* **159**, 1785–1790.

Davison, A. M. and Johnston, P. A. (1996). Glomerulonephritis in the elderly. *Nephrology, Dialysis, Transplantation* **11** (Suppl. 9), 34–37.

Drey, N., Roderick, P., Mullee, M., and Rogerson, M. (2003). A population-based study of the incidence and outcomes of diagnosed chronic kidney disease. *American Journal of Kidney Diseases* **42**, 677–684.

Dubach, E. C., Rosner, B., and Sturmer, T. (1991). An epidemiologic study of abuse of analgesic drugs. Effects of phenacetin and salicylate on mortality and cardiovascular morbidity (1968 to 1987). *New England Journal of Medicine* **324**, 155–160.

Duncan, L., Heathcote, J., Djurdjev, O., and Levin, A. (2001). Screening for renal disease using serum creatinine: who are we missing? *Nephrology, Dialysis, Transplantation* **16**, 1042–1046.

Dunn, M. J. and Tanner, R. L. (1974). Low-renin hypertension. *Kidney International* **5**, 317–325.

Dyck, R. F. and Tan, L. (1998). Non-diabetic end-stage renal disease among Saskatchewan aboriginal people. *Clinical and Investigative Medicine* **21**, 33–38.

Earle, K. K., Porter, K. A., Ostberg, J., and Yudkin, J. S. (2001). Variation in the progression of diabetic nephropathy according to racial origin. *Nephrology, Dialysis, Transplantation* **16**, 286–290.

Eberhardt, M. S., Wagener, D. K., Herman, W. H., Tomlinson-Marshall, L. A., and Hawthorne, V. M. (1995). Trends in renal disease morbidity and mortality in the United States, 1979 to 1990. *American Journal of Kidney Diseases* **26**, 308–320.

Elseviers, M. M. and de Broe, M. E. (2001). What can nephrologists learn from epidemiology? *Journal of Nephrology* **14** (2), 88–92.

Epstein, M. (1996). Aging and the kidney. *Journal of the American Society of Nephrology* **7** (8), 1106–1122.

European Renal Association/European Dialysis and Transplantation Association Registry (ERA-EDTA). www.era-edta.org.

Feest, T. G. *et al.* (1990). Incidence of advanced chronic renal failure and the need for end stage renal replacement therapy. *British Medical Journal* **301**, 897–900.

Feldman, H. I., Klag, M. J., Chiapella, A. P., and Whelton, P. K. (1992). End-stage renal disease in US minority groups. *American Journal of Kidney Diseases* **19**, 397–410.

Ferguson, R., Grim, C. E., and Opgenorth, T. J. (1988). A familial risk of chronic renal failure among Blacks on dialysis? *Journal of Clinical Epidemiology* **41** (12), 1189–1196.

Fernandes, P. F., Ellis, P. A., Roderick, P. J., Cairns, H. S., Hicks, J. A., and Cameron, J. S. (2000). Causes of end-stage renal failure in Black patients starting renal replacement therapy. *American Journal of Kidney Diseases* **36**, 301–309.

Finch, S. *et al. National Diet and Nutrition Survey People Aged 65 Years and Over*. London: Her Majesty's Stationery Office, 1998.

Fored, C. M., Ejerblad, E., Lindblad, P., Fryzek, J. P., Dickman, P. W., and Signorello, L. B. (2001). Acetaminophen, aspirin, and chronic renal failure. *New England Journal of Medicine* **345**, 1801–1808.

Fored, C. M. *et al.* (2003). Socioeconomic status and chronic renal failure: a population based case control study in Sweden. *Nephrology, Dialysis, Transplantation* **18**, 82–88.

Freedman, B. I. (1999). Familial aggregation of end-stage renal failure: aetiological implications. *Nephrology, Dialysis, Transplantation* **14** (2), 295–297.

Freedman, B. I. and Satko, S. G. (2000). Genes and renal disease. *Current Opinion in Nephrology and Hypertension* **9**, 273–277.

Freedman, B. I., Spray, B. J., Tuttle, A. B., Vardaman, M., and Buckalew, V., Jr. (1993). The familial risk of end-stage renal disease in African Americans. *American Journal of Kidney Diseases* **21**, 387–393.

Freedman, B. I., Tuttle, A. B., and Spray, B. J. (1995). Familial predisposition to nephropathy in African–Americans with non-insulin-dependent diabetes mellitus. *American Journal of Kidney Diseases* **25**, 710–713.

Freedman, B. I., Soucie, J. M., and McClellan, W. M. (1997). Family history of end-stage renal disease among incident dialysis patients. *Journal of the American Society of Nephrology* **8**, 1942–1945.

Friedmann, J. R., Norman, D. C., and Yoshikawa, T. T. (1989). Correction of estimated renal function parameters versus 24 hour creatinine clearance in ambulatory elderly. *Journal of American Geriatric Society* **37**, 145–147.

Frimat, L., Hestin, D., Aymard, B., Mayeux, D., Renoult, E., and Kessler, M. (1996). IgA nephropathy in patients over 50 years of age: a multicentre, prospective study. *Nephrology, Dialysis, Transplantation* **11**, 1043–1047.

Frohlich, E. D., Messerli, F. H., and Dunn, F. G. Comparison of renal hemodynamics in Black and White patients with essential hypertension. In *The Kidney in Essential Hypertension* (ed. F. H. Messerli). Boston: Nijhoff, 1983.

Garg, A. X., Kiberd, B. A., Clark, W. F., Haynes, R. B., and Clase, C. M. (2002). Albuminuria and renal insufficiency prevalence guides population screening: results from the NHANES III. *Kidney International* **61**, 2161–2175.

Goldacre, M. J. (1993). Cause-specific mortality: understanding uncertain tips of the disease iceberg. *Journal of Epidemiology and Community Health* **47**, 491–496.

Gregory, J., Foster, K., Tyler, H., and Wiseman, M. *The Dietary and Nutritional Survey of British Adults*. London: Her Majesty's Stationery Office, 1990.

Grossfeld, G. D. *et al.* (2001). Asymptomatic microscopic hematuria in adults: summary of the AUA best practice policy recommendations. *American Family Physician* **63**, 1145–1154.

Hansen, H. and Susser, M. (1971). Historic trends in deaths from chronic kidney disease in the United States and Britain. *American Journal of Epidemiology* **93**, 413–424.

Heaf, J., Lokkegaard, H., and Larsen, S. (1999). The epidemiology and prognosis of glomerulonephritis in Denmark 1985–1997. *Nephrology, Dialysis, Transplantation* **14**, 1889–1897.

Hiatt, R. A. and Friedman, D. G. (1982). Characteristics of patients referred for treatment of end stage renal disease in a defined population. *American Journal of Public Health* **72** (8), 829–833.

Higgins, R. M., Edmunds, M. E., and Dukes, D. C. (1995). End-stage renal failure in Indo-Asians. *Quarterly Journal of Medicine* **88**, 523–524.

Hoy, W. (2000). Renal disease in Australian aborigines. *Nephrology, Dialysis, Transplantation* **15**, 1293–1297.

Hoy, W. E. *et al.* (1998). Low birthweight and renal disease in Australian aborigines. *Lancet* **352**, 1826–1827.

Hsu, C. Y. and Chertow, G. M. (2000). Chronic renal confusion: insufficiency, failure, dysfunction, or disease. *American Journal of Kidney Diseases* **36**, 415–418.

Iseki, K., Ikemiya, Y., and Fukiyama, K. (1997). Risk factors of end-stage renal disease and serum creatinine in a community-based mass screening. *Kidney International* **51**, 850–854.

Jones, C. A. and Agodoa, L. (1993). Kidney disease and hypertension in Blacks: scope of the problem. *American Journal of Kidney Diseases* **21** (Suppl. 1), 6–9.

Jones, C. A. *et al.* (1998a). Serum creatinine levels in the US population: third National Health and Nutrition Examination Survey. *American Journal of Kidney Diseases* **32**, 992–999.

Jones, C. A. *et al.* (1998b). Serum creatinine levels in the US population: third National Health and Nutrition Examination Survey. *American Journal of Kidney Diseases* **32** (6), 992–999.

Jungers, P. *et al.* (1996). Age and gender-related incidence of chronic renal failure in a French urban area: a prospective epidemiologic study. *Nephrology, Dialysis, Transplantation* **11**, 1542–1546.

Jurkovitz, C., Franch, H., Shoham, D., Bellenger, J., and McClellan, W. (2002). Family members of patients treated for ESRD gave higher rates of undetected kidney disease. *American Journal of Kidney Diseases* **40**, 1173–1178.

Kampmann, J., Siersbaek-Nielsen, K., Kristensen, M., and Molholm Hansen, J. (1974). Rapid evaluation of creatinine clearance. *Acta Medica Scandinavica* **196**, 517–520.

Khan, I. H., Cheng, J., Catto, G. R., Edward, N., and MacLeod, A. M. (1993). Social deprivation indices of patients on renal replacement therapy (RRT) in Grampian. *Scottish Medical Journal* **38**, 139–141.

Khan, I. H., Catto, N. E., and MacLeod, A. M. (1994). Chronic renal failure: factors influencing nephrology referral. *Quarterly Journal of Medicine* **87**, 559–564.

Kissmeyer, L., Kong, C., Cohen, J., Unwin, R. J., Woolfson, R. G., and Neild, G. H. (1999). Community nephrology: audit of screening for renal insufficiency in a high risk population. *Nephrology, Dialysis, Transplantation* **14**, 2150–2155.

Klag, M. J., Whelton, P. K., Randall, B. L., Neaton, J. D., Brancati, F. L., and Stamler, J. (1997). End-stage renal disease in African-American and White men. 16-year MRFIT findings. *Journal of the American Medical Association* **277** (16), 1293–1298.

Konje, J. C., Bell, S. C., Morton, J. J., de Chazal, R., and Taylor, D. J. (1996). Human fetal kidney morphometry during gestation and the relationship between weight, kidney morphometry and plasma active renin concentration at birth. *Clinical Science* **91**, 169–175.

Koppiker, N., Feehally, J., Raymond, N., Abrams, K. R., and Burden, A. C. (1998). Rate of decline in renal function in Indo-Asians and Whites with diabetic nephropathy. *Diabetic Medicine* **15**, 60–65.

Krop, J. S. *et al.* (1999). A community-based study of explanatory factors for the excess risk for early renal function decline in Blacks vs Whites with diabetes: the atherosclerosis risk in communities study. *Archives of Internal Medicine* **159**, 1777–1783.

Landray, M. J. *et al.* (2001). Epidemiological evaluation of known and suspected cardiovascular risk factors in chronic renal impairment. *American Journal of Kidney Diseases* **38**, 537–546.

Laterza, O. F., Price, C. P., and Scott, M. G. (2002). Cystatin C: an improved estimator of glomerular filtration rate? *Clinical Chemistry* **48**, 699–707.

Lei, H. H., Perneger, T. V., Klag, M. J., Whelton, P. K., and Coresh, J. (1998). Familial aggregation of renal disease in a population-based case–control study. *Journal of the American Society of Nephrology* **9**, 1270–1276.

Levey, A. S., Bosch, J. P., Lewis, J. B., Greene, T., Rogers, N., and Roth, D. (1999). A more accurate method to estimate glomerular filtration rate from serum creatinine: a new prediction equation. Modification of Diet in Renal Disease Study Group. *Annals of Internal Medicine* **130** (6), 461–470.

Lightstone, L., Rees, A. J., Tomson, C., Walls, J., Winearls, C. G., and Feehally, J. (1995). High incidence of end-stage renal disease in Indo-Asians in the UK. *Quarterly Journal of Medicine* **88**, 191–195.

Lindeman, R. D., Tobin, J., and Schock, N. W. (1985). Longitudinal studies on the rate of decline in renal function with age. *Journal of the American Geriatric Society*, **33**, 278–285.

Lopes, A. A. and Port, F. K. (1995). The low birth weight hypothesis as a plausible explanation for the Black/White differences in hypertension, non-insulin-dependent diabetes, and end-stage renal disease. *American Journal of Kidney Diseases* **25**, 350–356.

Lowrie, E. G. and Lew, N. L. (2003). Death risk in haemodialysis patients: the predictive value of commonly measured variables and an evaluation of death rate differences between facilities. *American Journal of Kidney Diseases* **15**, 458–482.

Magnason, R. L., Indridason, O. S., Sigvaldason, H., Sigfusson, N., and Palsson, R. (2002). Prevalence and progression of CRF in Iceland: a population based study. *American Journal of Kidney Diseases* **40**, 955–963.

Maisonneuve, P. *et al.* (2000). Distribution of primary renal diseases leading to end stage renal failure in the United States, Europe, and Australia/New Zealand: results from an international comparative study. *American Journal of Kidney Diseases* **35** (1), 157–165.

Mallick, N. P., Short, C. D., and Hunter, A. H. (1987). How far since Ellis? The Manchester Study of Glomerular Disease. *Nephron* **46**, 113–124.

Mather, T. H., Chaturvedi, N., and Kehely, A. M. (1998). Comparison of prevalence and risk factors for microalbuminuria in South Asians and Europeans with type 2 diabetes mellitus. *Diabetic Medicine* **15**, 672–677.

McClellan, W., Tuttle, E., and Issa, A. (1987). Racial differences in the incidence of hypertensive end-stage renal disease (ESRD) are not entirely explained by differences in the prevalence of hypertension. *American Journal of Kidney Diseases* **12**, 285–290.

McKenzie, J. K., Moss, A. H., Feest, R. G., Stocking, C. B., and Siegler, M. (1998). Dialysis decision making in Canada, the United Kingdom and the United States. *American Journal of Kidney Diseases* **31** (1), 12–18.

Metcalfe, W., MacLeod, A. M., Bennett, D., Simpson, K., and Khan, I. H. (1999). Equity of renal replacement therapy utilization: a prospective population-based study. *Quarterly Journal of Medicine* **92**, 637–642.

Miskulin, D. C. *et al.* (2003). Comorbidity and its change predict survival in incident dialysis patients. *American Journal of Kidney Diseases* **41**, 149–161.

Moeller, S., Gioberge, S., and Brown, G. (2002). ESRD patients in 2001: global overview of patients, treatment modalities and development trends. *Nephrology, Dialysis, Transplantation* **17**, 2071–2076.

National Kidney Foundation (2002). K/DOQI clinical practice guidelines for chronic kidney disease: evaluation, classification and stratification. *American Journal of Kidney Diseases* **39** (Suppl. 1), Part 4, S46–S64.

Neel, J. V., Weder, A. B., and Julius, S. (1998). Type II diabetes, essential hypertension, and obesity as 'syndromes of impaired genetic homeostasis': the 'thrifty genotype' hypothesis enters the 21st century. *Perspectives in Biology and Medicine* **42** (44), 74.

Nelson, R. G., Knowler, W. C., Pettitt, D. J., Saad, M. F., and Bennett, P. H. (1993). Diabetic kidney disease in Pima Indians. *Diabetes Care* **16**, 335–341.

Nelson, R. G., Morgenstern, H., and Bennett, P. H. (1998). An epidemic of proteinuria in Pima Indians with type 2 diabetes mellitus. *Kidney International* **54**, 2081–2088.

Nissenson, A. R., Pereira, B. J., Collins, A. J., and Steinberg, E. P. (2001). Prevalence and characteristics of individuals with chronic kidney disease in a large health maintenance organization. *American Journal of Kidney Diseases* **37**, 1177–1183.

Nuyts, G. D. *et al.* (1995). New occupational risk factors for chronic renal failure. *Lancet* **346**, 7–11.

O'Dea, D. F., Mourphy, S. W., Hefferton, D., and Parfrey, P. S. (1998). Higher risk for renal failure in first degree relatives of White patients with end stage renal disease: a population based study. *American Journal of Kidney Diseases* **32**, 794–801.

Parry, R. G., Crowe, A., Stevens, J. M., Mason, J. C., and Roderick, P. (1996). Referral of elderly patients with severe renal failure: questionnaire survey of physicians. *British Medical Journal* **131**, 466.

Pasternack, A., Kasanen, A., Sourander, L., and Kaarsalo, E. (1985). Prevalence and incidence of moderate and severe chronic renal failure in south-western Finland, 1973–1976. *Acta Medica Scandinavica* **218**, 173–180.

Pendreigh, D. M. *et al.* (1972). Survey of chronic renal failure in Scotland. *Lancet* **1**, 304–307.

Perneger, T. V., Klag, M. J., and Whelton, P. K. (1993). Cause of death in patients with end-stage renal disease: death certificates vs registry reports. *American Journal of Public Health* **83** (12), 1735–1738.

Perneger, T. V., Whelton, P. K., Klag, M. J., and Rossiter, K. A. (1995a). Diagnosis of hypertensive end-stage renal disease: effect of patient's race. *American Journal of Epidemiology* **141**, 10–15.

Perneger, T. V., Whelton, P. K., and Flag, M. J. (1995b). Race and end stage renal disease socioeconomic status and access to health care as mediating factors. *Archives of Internal Medicine* **155**, 1201–1208.

Perneger, T. V., Klag, M. J., and Whelton, P. K. (1995c). Race and socio-economic status in hypertension and renal disease. *Current Opinion in Nephrology and Hypertension* **4**, 235–239.

Perneger, T. V., Whelton, P. K., Puddey, I. B., and Klag, M. J. (1999). Risk of end-stage renal disease associated with alcohol consumption. *American Journal of Epidemiology* **150**, 1275–1281.

Pugh, J. A. (1996). Diabetic nephropathy and end-stage renal disease in Mexican Americans. *Blood Purification* **14**, 286–292.

Pugh, J. A., Stevens, P., Eiflet, C. W., and Zapata, M. (1988). Excess incidence of treatment of end-stage renal disease in Mexican Americans. *American Journal of Epidemiology* **127**, 135–144.

Raleigh, V. S. (1997). Diabetes and hypertension in Britain's ethnic minorities: implications for the future of renal services. *British Medical Journal* **314**, 209–213.

Raleigh, V. S., Kiri, V., and Balarajan, R. (1996). Variations in mortality from diabetes mellitus, hypertension and renal disease in England and Wales by country of birth. *Health Trends* **28**, 122–127.

Rivera, F., Lopez-Gomez, J. M., and Perez-Garcia, R. (2002). Frequency of renal pathology in Spain 1994–1999. *Nephrology, Dialysis, Transplantation* **17**, 1594–1602.

Robbins, D. C. *et al.* (1996). Regional differences in albuminuria among American Indians: an epidemic of renal disease. *Kidney International* **49**, 557–563.

Roderick, P. J., Raleigh, V. S., Hallam, L., and Mallick, N. P. (1996). The need and demand for renal replacement therapy in ethnic minorities in England. *Journal of Epidemiology and Community Health* **50**, 334–339.

Roderick, P. and Webster, P. Renal Diseases. In *Health of Adult Brain: 1841–1994* (ed. J. Charlton and M. Murphy), pp. 1–17. London: National Statistics Office, 1997.

Roderick, P., Clements, S., Stone, N., Martin, D., and Diamond, I. (1999). What determines geographical variation in rates of acceptance onto renal replacement therapy in England. *Journal of Health Service Research Policy* **4**, 139–146.

Rosen, S., Tornroth, T., and Bernard, D. B. In *Membranous Glomerulonephritis* (ed. C. Craig Tisher and Barry M. Brenner), pp. 258–293. Philadelphia, PA: J.B. Lippincott Co, 1994.

Rostand, S. G., Kirk, K. A., Rutsky, E. A., and Pate, B. A. (1982). Racial differences in the incidence of treatment for end-stage renal disease. *New England Journal of Medicine* **306**, 1276–1279.

Rothman, K. J. *Epidemiology. An Introduction.* New York: Oxford University Press, 2002.

Rutkowski, B. (2000). Changing pattern of end-stage renal disease in central and eastern Europe. *Nephrology Dialysis Transplantation* **15**, 156–160.

Schena, F. P. (1997). Survey of the Italian Registry of renal biopsies. Frequency of the renal diseases for 7 consecutive years. The Italian Group of Renal Immunopathology. *Nephrology, Dialysis, Transplantation* **12**, 418–426.

Shulman, N. B. (1989). Prognostic value of serum creatinine and effect of treatment of hypertension on renal function in 8683 patients. *Hypertension* **13** (Suppl.), 180–193.

Silbiger, S. R. and Neugarten, J. (1995). The impact of gender on the progression of chronic renal disease. *American Journal of Kidney Diseases* **25**, 515–533.

Simon, P. *et al.* (1994). Epidemiology of primary glomerular diseases in a French region. Variations according to period and age. *Kidney International* **46**, 1192–1198.

Smith, S. R., Svetkey, L. P., and Derben, P. (1991). Racial differences in the incidence and progression of renal diseases. *Kidney International* **40**, 815–822.

Spencer, J. L., Silva, D. T., Snelling, P., and Hoy, W. E. (1998). An epidemic of renal failure among Australian Aboriginals. *The Medical Journal of Australia* **168**, 537–541.

Spray, B. J., Atassi, N. G., Tuttle, A. B., and Freedman, B. I. (1995). Familial risk, age at onset, and cause of end-stage renal disease in White Americans. *Journal of the American Society of Nephrology* **5**, 1806–1810.

Stahn, R. M., Gohdes, D., and Valway, S. E. (1993). Diabetes and its complications among selected tribes in North Dakota, South Dakota, and Nebraska. *Diabetes Care* **16**, 244–247.

Steenland, N. K., Thun, M. J., Ferguson, C. W., and Port, F. K. (1990). Occupational and other exposures associated with male end-stage renal diseasse: a case/control study. *American Journal of Public Health* **80** (2), 153–159.

Stewart, J. H., McCredie, M., Disney, A. P., and Mathew, T. H. (1994). Trends in incidence of end stage renal failure in Australia, 1972–1991. *Nephrology, Dialysis, Transplantation* **9**, 1377–1382.

Strauss, M. J., Port, F. K., Somen, C., and Wolfe, R. A. (1993). An estimate of the size of the US predialysis population with renal insufficiency and anemia. *American Journal of Kidney Diseases* **21**, 264–269.

Summerson, J. H., Bell, R. A., and Konen, J. C. (1995). Racial differences in the prevalence of microalbuminuria in hypertension. *American Journal of Kidney Diseases* **26**, 577–579.

US Renal Data System. USRDS 2000 Report. www.usrds.org, 2000a.

USRDS 2000 Annual Data Report. 12, 177–182. Bethesda, MD: National Institutes of Health, 2000.

van Dijk, P. C. *et al.* (2001). Renal replacement therapy in Europe: the results of a collaborative effort by the ERA-EDTA registry and six national or regional registries. *Nephrology, Dialysis, Transplantation* **16**, 1120–1129.

Wannamethee, S. G., Shaper, A. G., and Perry, I. J. (1997). Serum creatinine concentration and risk of cardiovascular disease. A possible marker for increased risk of stroke. *Stroke* **28**, 557–563.

Whelton, P. K. (1996). Challenges and evolving contributions of epidemiology in nephrology and hypertension. *Current Opinion in Nephrology and Hypertension* **5** (3), 203–204.

Whittle, J. C., Whelton, P. K., Seidler, A. J., and Klag, M. J. (1991). Does racial variation in risk factors explain Black–White differences in the incidence of hypertensive end-stage renal disease? *Archives of Internal Medicine* **151**, 1359–1364.

Young, E. W. (1997). An improved understanding of the causes of end-stage renal disease. *Seminar on Nephrology* **17** (3), 170–175.

Young, E. W., Mauger, E. A., Jiang, K. H., Port, F. K., and Wolfe, R. A. (1994). Socioeconomic status and end stage renal disease in the United States. *Kidney International* **45**, 907–911.

Zager, P. G. *et al.* (1998). *U* curve association of blood pressure and mortality in haemodialysis patients. *Kidney International* **54**, 561–569.

Zeier, M., Gafter, U., and Ritz, E. (1998). Renal function and renal disease in males or females—vive la petite difference. *Nephrology, Dialysis, Transplantation* **13**, 2195–2198.

2

The patient with fluid, electrolyte, and divalent ion disorders

2.1 Hypo–hypernatraemia: disorders of water balance

Nicolaos E. Madias and Horacio J. Adrogué

Disturbances in the serum sodium concentration, known as hyponatraemia and hypernatraemia, are the most common electrolyte disorders encountered in clinical practice. The resultant morbidity varies widely: hyponatraemia and hypernatraemia can be largely inconsequential but at times they can claim the patient's life. Although diagnosis and management can be straightforward, quite often they prove challenging even to experienced physicians. The complexity underlying these disorders is highlighted by the fact that dysnatraemias are frequently hospital-acquired—essentially iatrogenic. Further, some of their most dreaded consequences result not from the disorders themselves, but rather from inappropriate management. Optimal treatment of abnormalities in serum sodium concentration demands considerable pathophysiological insight, sound clinical judgement, and, when the dysnatraemia is severe, frequent monitoring of the patient's clinical status and laboratory parameters.

Serum tonicity and, thus, serum sodium concentration are tightly adjusted by the normally exquisite regulation of water homeostasis. Water intake and renal water excretion are adjusted through the control of thirst and the release of vasopressin (antidiuretic hormone, ADH). Therefore, hyponatraemia and hypernatraemia primarily reflect disruptions of water homeostasis. In this chapter, we first review principles of water homeostasis and then summarize the pathophysiological and clinical aspects of hyponatraemia and hypernatraemia.

Principles of water homeostasis

Body fluid tonicity and osmolality

Tonicity defines the forces that determine the net flux of water between two solutions separated by a membrane permeable to water but impermeable to certain solutes contained in the solutions. In such a system, water flows from the more dilute to the more concentrated solution (as defined by the concentration of those solutes that are constrained in their movement across the cell membrane). Osmolality, a physical property of solutions, refers to the forces generated by solutes that reduce the random movement of water molecules; such forces depend only on the concentration, not the nature, of all particles in the solution. Because some of the solutes that are regularly or frequently present in body fluids, most notably urea and ethanol, permeate cell membranes as freely as water, these solutes contribute to osmolality but have no impact on tonicity. This distinction is made by the term effective osmolality that is synonymous to tonicity.

Serum osmolality can be thoroughly assessed by three closely related variables: measured osmolality, calculated osmolality, and tonicity or effective osmolality. Serum osmolality, a property dependent on total solute concentration (i.e. all particles in solution), is measured with an osmometer. This instrument evaluates changes in other physical properties of particles in solution, such as the freezing point or the water vapour pressure of the solution, which are then 'translated' into osmolality. The value obtained, the measured serum osmolality, fails to differentiate between total solute and those solutes that translocate water from one compartment to another across cell membranes.

Calculated serum osmolality is obtained from the measured concentrations of sodium, glucose, and urea, the three major low-molecular-weight solutes contained in serum, as follows:

$$\begin{aligned}&\text{Serum osmolality, mOsm/kg } H_2O\\&\quad = [Na^+, \text{mmol/l}] \times 2 + [\text{glucose, mg/dl}]/18\\&\qquad + [\text{BUN, mg/dl}]/2.8 \qquad (1)\end{aligned}$$

where BUN refers to blood urea nitrogen, a commonly measured substitute of urea itself. The multiplier 2 overestimates the osmotic force created by sodium and its accompanying anions, as the activity (dissociation factor) of the sodium salts is approximately 1.86 in extracellular fluid (ECF) (due to ion interactions in a relatively concentrated solution). The dissociation factor would be precisely 2 in ideal solutions with maximal dilution and absence of substantial ion interactions. However, using 2 instead of 1.86 in Eq. (1) compensates for the osmotic contribution of other low-molecular-weight serum constituents (i.e. potassium, calcium, and magnesium and their accompanying anions) present at low concentrations. The concentration of glucose and urea (non-ionic solutes) expressed in mmol/l corresponds to their contribution to osmolality in mOsm/kg H_2O. When reported in mg/dl, a usual practice in many countries, glucose must be divided by 18 (molecular weight of glucose is 180) and BUN by 2.8 (28 being the contribution of nitrogen to the molecular weight of urea, which is 60) to convert mg/dl to mmol/l. On account of their large molecular weight, serum proteins make a meagre contribution to serum osmolality that is essentially ignored. Taking the average normal values for the three solutes included in Eq. (1), that is, 140 mmol/l for sodium, 90 mg/dl for glucose, and 15 mg/dl for BUN, one can derive a calculated osmolality of 290 mOsm/kg H_2O, a value virtually identical to the average normal serum osmolality measured with an osmometer. Barring laboratory error, the finding of an 'osmolar gap', defined as measured serum osmolality exceeding calculated serum osmolality by at least 10 mOsm/kg H_2O, must reflect either the presence in serum of additional low-molecular-weight solute(s) at substantial concentration(s) (e.g. ethanol, methanol, ethylene glycol, mannitol) or a substantial decrease in serum water content coupled with measurement of serum sodium concentration by flame photometry or an indirect electrode technique involving dilution of the sample (i.e. pseudohyponatraemia).

Serum tonicity or effective osmolality is calculated by adding the osmolar contribution of sodium and its accompanying anions to that of glucose, as follows:

$$\text{Serum tonicity (effective osmolality), mOsm/kg } H_2O = [Na^+, \text{mmol/l}] \times 2 + [\text{glucose, mg/dl}]/18 \quad (2)$$

Mannitol, an additional, albeit uncommon, solute that is compartmentalized in the ECF, contributes to serum effective osmolality. In contrast, urea crosses cell membranes freely, and, therefore, makes no contribution to serum effective osmolality. The normal range for effective osmolality is 275–290 mOsm/kg H_2O with an average value of 285 mOsm/kg H_2O. Corresponding values for serum osmolality are 280–295 mOsm/kg H_2O (normal range) with an average value of 290 mOsm/kg H_2O.

Water balance

Maintenance of water balance (homeostasis) requires identical levels of water intake and water losses. The daily obligatory (i.e. minimal) extrarenal water loss amounts to approximately 500 ml of water—the difference between water losses from the skin and lungs (dubbed insensible losses) of about 1000 ml and water production by oxidative metabolism of about 500 ml. A small amount of water is lost in the stool. In turn, the daily obligatory renal water loss depends on urinary solute excretion. Increases in solute excretion reduce the maximal urine osmolality, that is, that achieved in the presence of maximal levels of ADH, thereby increasing the daily obligatory renal water loss (Fig. 1). Daily ingestion of 70 g of protein and 10 g of sodium chloride, a usual diet in many countries, generates approximately 700 mOsm of solute that must be excreted by the kidney to strike daily solute balance. Considering a maximal urine concentration during antidiuresis of approximately 900 mOsm/kg H_2O when urine solute excretion is at 700 mOsm/day, the obligatory daily urine volume would be of the order of 800 ml. For this level of solute load, a minimum of 1300 ml (i.e. 800 + 500) of water must be ingested daily to replace the renal and extrarenal (insensible) fluid losses. Water homeostasis and body fluid tonicity would then remain normal. However, water intake can be substantially larger than the minimal amount; in such a case, a corresponding increase in renal fluid loss ensures water balance and normal body fluid tonicity. Taken to the extreme, at a maximal urine dilution of about 50 mOsm/kg H_2O, daily excretion of 14 l of urine can be attained for the same level of solute excretion (700/50) thereby accomodating up to 14.5 l of water intake (balancing renal and extrarenal losses) without risking a decrease in body fluid tonicity.

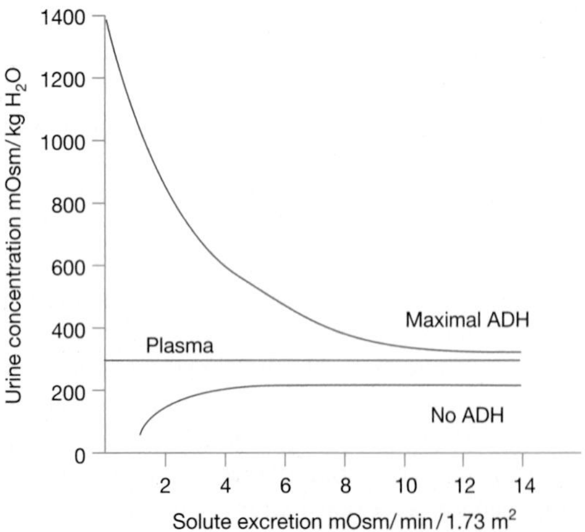

Fig. 1 Effect of solute excretion on maximal and minimal urine osmolality [maximal level of antidiuretic hormone (ADH) or absence of ADH, respectively]. [Modified from de Wardener H.E. and del Greco F. (1955). *Clinical Science* **14**, 715.]

The typical water intake of humans exceeds the minimum requirement for maintaining water balance and is largely determined by social and cultural influences. Thus, normal adults usually ingest approximately 1.5–2.5 l of water per day; the corresponding urine volume is of the order of 1–2 l per day assuming the usual, low rate of insensible losses. However, when exercise, hot weather, or high fever stimulates sweating and pulmonary ventilation, extrarenal water losses increase markedly, occasionally exceeding 5 l/day. The ensuing increase in serum tonicity stimulates thirst and vasopressin release; in turn, increase in water intake coupled with renal water conservation restores water balance and normal serum tonicity.

Role of thirst

Thirst plays a critical role in water balance as demonstrated by the fact that sustained hypertonicity and hypernatraemia occur only when thirst or access to water is impaired. Hypertonicity is the most potent stimulus for thirst. The level at which the sensation of thirst arises, the tonicity threshold for thirst, is reached with a 2–3 per cent increase in serum tonicity (i.e. to an average level of 290 mOsm/kg H_2O), a value that is normally about 5 mOsm/kg H_2O higher than that which stimulates vasopressin release. Some investigators, however, have reported similar tonicity thresholds for thirst and vasopressin release (Thompson *et al.* 1991). The tonicity sensors are neurons residing in the anterior hypothalamus close to the supraoptic nuclei. The same sensors might control both thirst and vasopressin release, but the existence of two different sensors has not been excluded. Activation or inhibition of these sensing cells appears to result from changes in cell volume triggered by tonicity-induced water shifts.

The ECF volume provides an additional control mechanism of thirst mediated by low-pressure baroreceptors located in the cardiac atria, whose discharge is transmitted to the brain via the vagus nerve. Hypovolaemia also stimulates the renin–angiotensin system, angiotensin II reaching the hypothalamus where it exerts a potent dipsogenic effect (Mann *et al.* 1987). Other factors also affect thirst, including a dry mouth and social influences.

Several factors mediate cessation of thirst or water satiety, such as the central tonicity sensors, oropharyngeal mechanoreceptors stimulated by swallowing large volumes of fluid, and distension of the stomach.

Role of vasopressin and the kidney

Arginine vasopressin, the human form of ADH, is a nine-amino acid peptide consisting of a six-amino acid ring with a three-amino acid side chain. Vasopressin is synthesized as a large prohormone in the cells of the supraoptic and paraventricular nuclei of the hypothalamus and transported in secretory granules to the neural lobe (neurohypophysis or posterior pituitary). In the secretory granule, the prohormone is cleaved and enzymatically processed into vasopressin, neurophysin, and the vasopressin-binding glycopeptide. Vasopressin is stored in secretory granules within the nerve terminals in the neurohypophysis, bound to its neurophysin. Depolarization of the nerve terminals, caused by activation of cation channels, releases the bound peptides, vasopressin and neurophysin, into the circulation, where vasopressin dissociates from the other peptide, becoming an active hormone (Oliet and Bourque 1993). Vasopressin is degraded in the liver and kidney, its half-life in the circulation being only 15–20 min.

Control of vasopressin secretion

ADH secretion is stimulated by hypertonicity and decreased ECF volume or arterial blood pressure (Fig. 2) (Robertson 1987). Released vasopressin leads to water retention by the kidney that in turn corrects hypertonicity and normalizes ECF volume and blood pressure. Conversely, hypotonicity decreases ADH release promoting water diuresis, negative fluid balance, and restoration of normal tonicity. A large water load lowers serum tonicity, shuts off ADH release and promotes excretion of more than 80 per cent of the ingested water within 4 h; about 90–120 min elapse before maximal diuresis appears, an interval required for absorption of water and degradation of circulating ADH. Volume expansion, on the other hand, has little effect on vasopressin release.

Tonicity

Only effective osmoles trigger vasopressin release. Thus, administration of hypertonic saline or mannitol increases serum tonicity, which in turn promotes water exit from the tonicity sensing cells; the resulting decrease in osmoreceptor cell volume elicits their activation. Conversely, urea, an ineffective osmole, crosses cell membranes freely and therefore fails to change serum tonicity or cell volume. At a serum tonicity less than 280 mOsm/kg H_2O, circulating vasopressin is undetectable under normal conditions (Fig. 2). The osmoreceptor cells are sensitive to changes in serum tonicity as small as 1 per cent, this exquisite response fostering the remarkable stability of serum tonicity. In fact, despite wide variations in water intake, serum tonicity normally does not fluctuate by more than 1–2 per cent. The tonicity threshold for ADH secretion ranges from 280 to 290 mOsm/kg H_2O, a variation due, in part, to the modulating influence of changes in ECF volume and blood pressure. At a tonicity of about 290 mOsm/kg H_2O the released vasopressin reaches serum levels that cause maximal antidiuresis in normal subjects. However, vasopressin levels progressively increase at higher levels of serum tonicity (Fig. 2).

Because serum sodium and its accompanying anions largely determine ECF tonicity (Eq. 2), serum sodium concentration is essentially the primary stimulus to vasopressin release. Glucose, the other potentially major extracellular solute, behaves as an effective osmole promoting ADH release only in states of insulin deficiency, such as uncontrolled diabetes mellitus (DM). In normal subjects, however, the hyperglycaemia-induced insulin release promotes glucose entry into the osmoreceptor cells thereby rendering glucose an ineffective osmole.

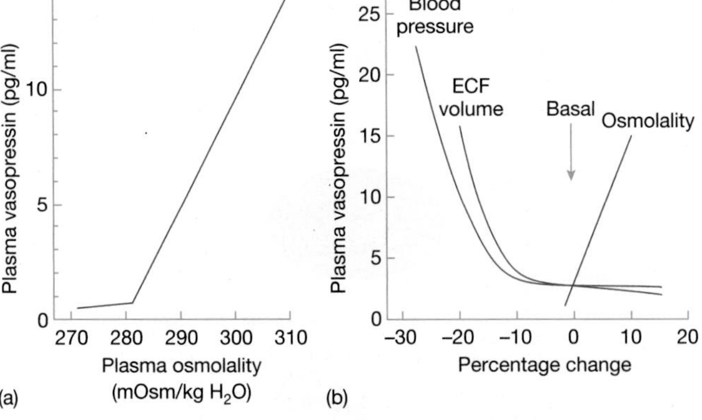

Fig. 2 Relationship between plasma vasopressin and osmolality (a) and plasma vasopressin and percentage change in blood pressure, ECF volume, and osmolality (b). A 5 per cent increase in serum osmolality is sufficient to change plasma vasopressin from undetectable levels to levels effecting maximal urine concentration. On the other hand, ECF volume or blood pressure must be reduced by 10–15 per cent to trigger vasopressin release. (Modified from Gennari 1998; Robertson 1992.)

ECF volume and blood pressure

The discharge rate from parasympathetic afferent nerves in the carotid sinus baroreceptors modifies vasomotor-centre activity in the medulla and, in turn, release of vasopressin produced in the paraventricular nuclei (Abramow *et al.* 1987). In contrast, the supraoptic nuclei participate only in tonicity-induced changes in ADH secretion. Thus, increased discharge from these afferent nerves in states of decreased effective circulating volume (e.g. vomiting, cirrhosis, heart failure) increases vasopressin release. Low-pressure receptors located in the left atrium have no significant role in ADH secretion in humans (only in the control of thirst) unless systemic blood pressure has also decreased (Bie *et al.* 1986). A 10 per cent reduction in ECF volume is required to stimulate ADH release; greater degrees of hypovolaemia cause an exponential increase in plasma vasopressin, yielding concentrations that far exceed those attained in response to hypertonicity (Fig. 2) (Baylis 1987). Blood pressure reductions lower than 10 mm Hg have little effect on vasopressin secretion, but more severe hypotension is a potent stimulus to ADH release.

Whereas hypovolaemia, a nonosmotic stimulus to ADH release, potentiates the ADH response to hypertonicity, it can also override the inhibitory effect on ADH secretion normally exerted by hypotonicity (Fig. 2). The latter concept finds important clinical application in the hyponatraemias associated with states of decreased effective circulating volume.

Other factors

Additional factors or conditions alter ADH secretion, most notably nausea, pain, surgery, pregnancy, and several drugs. Nausea is probably the strongest known stimulus to ADH release, as it can increase vasopressin up to 500-fold by mechanisms that remain undetermined. Pain, especially following surgery, triggers ADH release, which, together with a large intake of water or hypotonic fluids, promotes water retention and dilutional hyponatraemia.

Pregnancy is associated with a decrease in serum sodium of about 5 mmol/l because of a downward resetting of the osmoregulatory threshold for both vasopressin release and thirst (Lindheimer *et al.* 1989). Multiple factors, conditions, and drugs listed in Table 1 stimulate or inhibit vasopressin release; compounds are also listed that potentiate the renal effects of ADH or cause water retention by undefined mechanisms.

Effects of vasopressin

Vasopressin acts through its interaction with three types of receptors coupled to G proteins (Bichet *et al.* 1988; Sugimoto *et al.* 1994). The V1a receptor mediates pressor and proliferative effects in vascular

Table 1 Factors, conditions, and drugs that alter renal water excretion by changing the level or renal action of vasopressin (ADH)

Stimulation of ADH release	Inhibition of ADH release	Drugs that potentiate renal action of ADH	Drugs that cause water retention by unknown mechanism
Hypertonicity	Hypotonicity	Chlorpropamide	Haloperidol
Volume contraction	Volume expansion	Cyclophosphamide	Fluphenazine
Hypotension	Hypertension	Non-steroidal anti-inflammatory drugs	Amitriptyline
Nausea/emesis	Hormones/drugs	Acetaminophen	Thioridazine
Hypoglycaemia	Opioids (κ and agonists)		Fluoxetine
Severe heart failure	Sympathetic amines (β agonists)		Sertraline
Severe liver failure	Ethanol		Ecstasy
Hypothyroidism			
Adrenal insufficiency			
Hormones/drugs			
Angiotensin II			
Sympathetic amines (α1 agonists)			
Histamine			
Bradykinin			
Opioids (μ agonists)			
Nicotine			
Antipsychotics/ antidepressants			
Ifosfamide			
Chlorpropamide			
Carbamazepine			
Narcotics			
Vincristine			
Clofibrate			

smooth muscle cells as well as stimulation of coagulation through the release of procoagulant factors (factor VIII and von Willebrand's factor) from vascular endothelium and increased platelet aggregation. The V1b receptor, limited to anterior pituitary cells, facilitates the release of adrenocorticotropic hormone (ACTH). The V2 receptor, present in the basolateral membrane of the principal cells of cortical and medullary collecting tubules, mediates the ADH-induced stimulation of water permeability thereby permitting osmotic equilibration with the renal interstitium (Fig. 3) (Agre 2000). Vasopressin interaction with this receptor activates adenylate cyclase and generates the second messenger, cyclic AMP, which then initiates a sequence of events that leads to the exocytotic insertion of cytosolic water channels (aquaporin-2) into the apical membrane of the principal cells of the collecting tubule (Fig. 3) (Deen *et al.* 1994; Sasaki *et al.* 1994). These water channels permit water movement into the cells down a favourable osmotic gradient; water then rapidly exits across the basolateral membrane (via the constitutive water channel, aquaporin-3) to the systemic circulation. When the vasopressin effect dissipates, the water channels are removed from the apical membrane by endocytosis and returned to the cytoplasm (Harris *et al.* 1991). Vasopressin also stimulates the renal production of prostaglandin E_2 and prostacyclin within several renal structures, including the glomerular mesangium, thick ascending limb, collecting tubules, and medullary interstitium (Bonvalet *et al.* 1987). These prostaglandins reduce both the antidiuretic and vascular actions of ADH, thereby preventing an excessive antidiuretic response and possibly maintaining renal perfusion (Yared *et al.* 1985; Hebert *et al.* 1990). Further, vasopressin stimulates sodium reabsorption in the thick ascending limb of the loop of Henle in some species, but it is unclear whether this action occurs in humans.

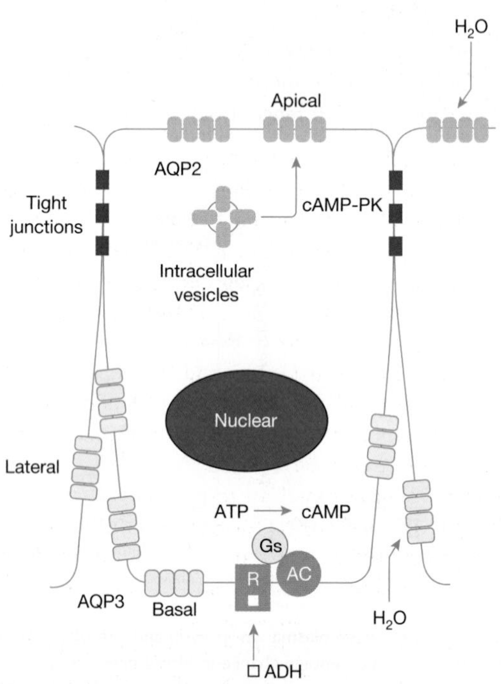

Fig. 3 Diagram of vasopressin effects on the collecting duct principal cell indicating water channel (aquaporin-2, AQP2) insertion in the apical membrane. The basolateral membrane contains a different constitutive water channel (aquaporin-3, AQP3). (Modified from Agre 2000.)

The kidney and water excretion

Regulation of water balance largely rests with the kidney's ability to excrete urine with an osmolality that varies from a minimum of 50 mOsm/kg H_2O to a maximum of 900–1400 mOsm/kg H_2O (Fig. 1). This wide range of urine osmolality reflects adjustments in collecting duct water permeability from a low value in the absence of vasopressin (production of dilute urine, water diuresis) to a high value in the presence of vasopressin (production of concentrated urine, antidiuresis).

The ability of the kidney to produce maximal urine dilution in states of water excess depends on three crucial steps, including: (a) adequate delivery of filtered fluid to the collecting tubule thereby ensuring sufficiently high flow rates that prevent the equilibration of collecting duct urine with the hypertonic renal interstitium; at low flow rates, osmotic equilibration can occur even in the absence of vasopressin thereby producing concentrated urine; adequacy of distal delivery requires a normal glomerular filtration rate and normal (not increased) proximal fluid reabsorption; (b) active sodium chloride transport without water in the thick ascending limb of the loop of Henle (impermeable to water), which reduces the osmolality of fluid entering the distal tubule to 50–100 mOsm/kg H_2O; and (c) absence of vasopressin, thereby maintaining the intrinsically low water permeability of the collecting duct.

On the other hand, the capacity of the kidney to produce maximal urine concentration and thus minimize water loss in states of water depletion requires the following critical steps: (a) active sodium chloride transport without water in the thick ascending limb of the loop of Henle (impermeable to water) thereby producing dilution of the tubular fluid and concentration of the renal interstitium; (b) enhancement of the effect of step (a) by the entry of sodium chloride into the descending limb of the loop of Henle (hairpin configuration) and the exit of water from this segment (through water channels known as aquaporin-1) thereby raising progressively the osmolality both of the luminal fluid of the descending limb of the loop of Henle and the renal interstitium from the corticomedullary junction to the inner medulla (Chou *et al.* 1999); this process is known as countercurrent multiplication mechanism (Sands and Kokko 1996); (c) maintenance of the corticomedullary osmotic gradient by the vasa recta (hairpin configuration similar to that of the loops of Henle and in direct juxtaposition with them) that reach osmotic equilibrium with the interstitium, as they are permeable to solutes and water and remove fluid from the renal interstitium (ascending vasa recta blood flow is almost twice that of descending vasa recta) (Zimmerhackl *et al.* 1985); this process is known as countercurrent exchange mechanism; (d) preservation of a relatively low medullary and papillary blood flow that prevents the removal of solutes (largely sodium chloride and urea) from the renal interstitium; and (e) presence of vasopressin to ensure high water permeability of the collecting duct.

Measurement of urine osmolality (or its imperfect substitute, urine specific gravity) is usually sufficient to assess the renal response to water excess or deprivation. An additional tool introduced for the same purpose, free water clearance, is conceptually cumbersome and lacks practical utility. Free water clearance represents the difference between measured urine volume (per unit time) and the calculated volume required to excrete the solute contained in that urine at a concentration isotonic to serum. A urine more dilute than serum, expected in water excess, exceeds the volume of the calculated isotonic urine, the volume difference being termed positive free water clearance. A urine more concentrated than serum, expected in water depletion, falls short of the volume of the calculated isotonic urine, the volume difference being termed negative free water clearance. The latter term is particularly confusing as there is no gain of water by the kidney in the presence of negative free water clearance, but only a reduction of the water loss required to accomodate the obligatory solute load. In short, the clinical evaluation and management of disorders of water balance do not require assessment of this parameter.

Clinical disorders of water homeostasis

The disorders of sodium and water homeostasis can be classified into three major categories: (a) abnormalities in the size of ECF volume; (b) disturbances in the tonicity of body fluids; and (c) selective deficit or excess of sodium or chloride.

The first group of disorders comprises an enlargement (volume excess or expansion) or a reduction (volume depletion or contraction) in the ECF volume due to a combined and proportional sodium and water excess or deficit, respectively. Disorders of sodium balance are the primary causes of ECF volume excess or depletion. Sodium chloride excess only transiently increases tonicity; the resulting stimulation of thirst and ADH secretion causes water retention, and prevents sustained hypernatraemia. Expansion of ECF volume is the hallmark of this disorder. In an analogous fashion, sodium chloride deficit only transiently decreases tonicity; inhibition of ADH secretion with secondary increase in water excretion prevents sustained hyponatraemia. Depletion of ECF volume is the chief manifestation of this disturbance.

Sustained disturbances in the tonicity of body fluids include increases or decreases in the effective osmolality of body fluids manifested as hypernatraemia or hyponatraemia (hypotonic), respectively. A disproportion between sodium and water content of body fluids underlies hypernatraemia (water content is relatively small for the concomitant sodium content) and hyponatraemia (water content is relatively large for the concomitant sodium content). As hypernatraemia and hyponatraemia are concentration terms, either entity can occur in association with a decreased, normal, or increased sodium content. A primary and isolated disturbance in water balance, deficit or excess, causes hypertonicity (hypernatraemia) or hypotonicity (hyponatraemia), respectively, but does not substantially alter the size of the ECF compartment—the size of this compartment is primarily determined by its sodium content, a variable unaltered in exclusive disturbances of water balance.

A comparison of volume regulation (altered in disorders of sodium balance) and osmoregulation (altered in disorders of water balance) further clarifies important differences between sodium and water homeostasis and their disorders. Whereas effective circulating volume is sensed by receptors in the carotid sinus, atria, and afferent glomerular arteriole in volume regulation, it is serum tonicity that is sensed by hypothalamic osmoreceptors in osmoregulation. Volume regulation is achieved by the control of renal sodium excretion that is mediated by multiple mechanisms, including the sympathetic nervous system, renin–angiotensin–aldosterone, natriuretic peptides, and pressure natriuresis. On the other hand, osmoregulation is accomplished by the control of water balance that is mediated by thirst/water satiety and modulation of renal water excretion via changes in ADH secretion.

In contrast to the first two groups of sodium and water disorders, the third group is characterized by an abnormal relationship between the serum sodium and chloride concentrations. Whereas the serum sodium concentration is generally maintained within the normal limits in these disorders (unless there is an accompanying abnormality of water homeostasis), the serum chloride concentration is either abnormally high or low. The hyperchloraemic type of this form of $[Na^+]/[Cl^-]$ imbalance comprises hyperchloraemic metabolic acidosis and chronic respiratory alkalosis, whereas metabolic alkalosis and chronic respiratory acidosis represent the hypochloraemic type of this imbalance. Importantly, the three major categories of disorders of sodium and water balance described above can coexist in a single patient.

Determinants and measurement of serum sodium concentration

Under normal conditions, the serum sodium concentration is an accurate indicator of serum tonicity because sodium and its anions account for virtually all the effective osmoles present in the ECF (Eq. 2). Thus, it can be assumed that

$$\text{Serum tonicity} \cong 2 \times \text{serum } [Na^+] \tag{3}$$

Because the hydraulic permeability of most cell membranes is very high, water moves freely and rapidly between the ECF and intracellular fluid (ICF) establishing an identical tonicity in the two compartments. In contrast with the ECF, potassium is the major solute responsible for the tonicity of the ICF. Consequently, a predictable relationship exists between serum tonicity on the one hand, and total body 'exchangeable' (i.e. osmotically active) sodium and potassium content (Na_E^+ and K_E^+, respectively) and total body water, on the other, which can be expressed as follows:

$$\text{Serum tonicity} = \frac{2 \times Na_E^+ + 2 \times K_E^+}{\text{Total body water}} \tag{4}$$

where the multiplier 2 accounts for the accompanying anions. Note that the Na_E^+ and K_E^+ determine the size of the ECF and ICF compartment, respectively. Combining Eqs (3) and (4) one can derive Eq. (5), which states that the serum sodium concentration is determined by the ratio of the 'exchangeable' portions of the body's sodium and potassium content to total body water:

$$\text{Serum } [Na^+] \cong \frac{Na_E^+ + K_E^+}{\text{Total body water}} \tag{5}$$

The fundamental relationship embodied in Eq. (5) offers clear insight into a number of clinically important principles: (a) The level of serum sodium is a concentration term that is fixed by the body's 'exchangeable' sodium and potassium content relative to the prevailing total body water. Changes in these variables represent the limited ways through which alterations in serum sodium concentration can occur. (b) Being a concentration term, serum sodium offers no insights into the status of the body's sodium stores; hypernatraemia and hyponatraemia can each occur in the presence of contracted, normal, or expanded sodium stores. Thus, hypernatraemia and hyponatraemia should primarily be viewed as disturbances in water, rather than sodium, balance. (c) Correction of an abnormality in serum sodium concentration entails manipulation of the intake of sodium, potassium, and water relative to their output.

Serum sodium concentration, classically measured by flame photometry, ranges normally from 136 to 145 mmol/l, with an average value of 140 mmol/l. Because water normally comprises 93 per cent of the serum volume, and sodium is restricted to serum water, the average $[Na^+]$ in serum water is approximately 150 mmol/l (140/0.93 = 150). However, measurement of serum $[Na^+]$ by flame photometry has gradually been displaced by the use of the sodium ion-specific electrode, which senses the Na^+ activity in the aqueous phase of serum. At the normal ionic strength of serum water, Na^+ activity is approximately 75 per cent that of $[Na^+]$; because the normal value of $[Na^+]$ in serum water is approximately 150 mmo/l, the normal value of $[Na^+]$ activity is 150 × 0.75 or 112 mmol/l (Maas *et al.* 1985). To avoid major confusion due to the introduction of a new range of normal values, an empirical correction factor is used in the clinical laboratory such that the normal range of $[Na^+]$ remains the same as if the sample were measured by flame photometry. Measurement of serum $[Na^+]$ by means of an ion-specific electrode has now been widely adopted by most clinical laboratories as part of an automated system that performs multiple analysis.

Direct measurement of $[Na^+]$ by the ion-specific electrode has eliminated pseudohyponatraemia. A spurious form of iso-osmolar and isotonic hyponatraemia, pseudohyponatraemia is identified when severe hypertriglyceridaemia or paraproteinaemia increases substantially the solid phase of serum (i.e. decreases the fraction of water in serum volume) and the sodium concentration is measured by means of flame photometry or by an electrode technique involving dilution of the sample. In contrast, the activity of Na^+ measured in an undiluted sample is unaffected by changes in serum water content, and it is automatically corrected by the ion-specific electrode to a concentration based on normal serum water content.

Hyponatraemia

Hyponatraemia is defined as a serum sodium concentration less than 136 mmol/l. Whereas hypernatraemia always denotes hypertonicity, hyponatraemia can be associated with low, normal, or high tonicity.

Dilutional hyponatraemia, by far the most common form of the disorder, is caused by water retention. If water intake exceeds the capacity of the kidney to excrete water, dilution of body solutes ensues with hypo-osmolality and hypotonicity (Fig. 4b, e, f, and g). Hypotonicity, in turn, can lead to cerebral oedema, a potentially life-threatening complication. Hypotonic hyponatraemia can be associated, however, with normal or even high serum osmolality if sufficient amounts of solutes that permeate cell membranes (e.g. urea and ethanol) have been retained (Fig. 4c). Importantly, patients who have hypotonic hyponatraemia but normal or high serum osmolality are as subject to the risks of hypotonicity as are patients with hypo-osmolar hyponatraemia.

Non-hypotonic hyponatraemia

The non-hypotonic hyponatraemias include hypertonic (or translocational) hyponatraemia, isotonic hyponatraemia, and pseudohyponatraemia. Translocational hyponatraemia results from a shift of water from cells to the ECF that is driven by solutes confined in the extracellular compartment (as occurs with hyperglycaemia in uncontrolled DM or retention of hypertonic mannitol); serum osmolality is increased, as is tonicity, the latter causing dehydration of cells (Fig. 4d). Hyperglycaemia is the most common cause of translocational hyponatraemia. An increase of 100 mg/dl (5.6 mmol/l) in the serum glucose concentration decreases serum sodium by approximately 1.6 mmol/l, the end result being a rise in serum osmolality of approximately 2.0 mOsm/kg H_2O.

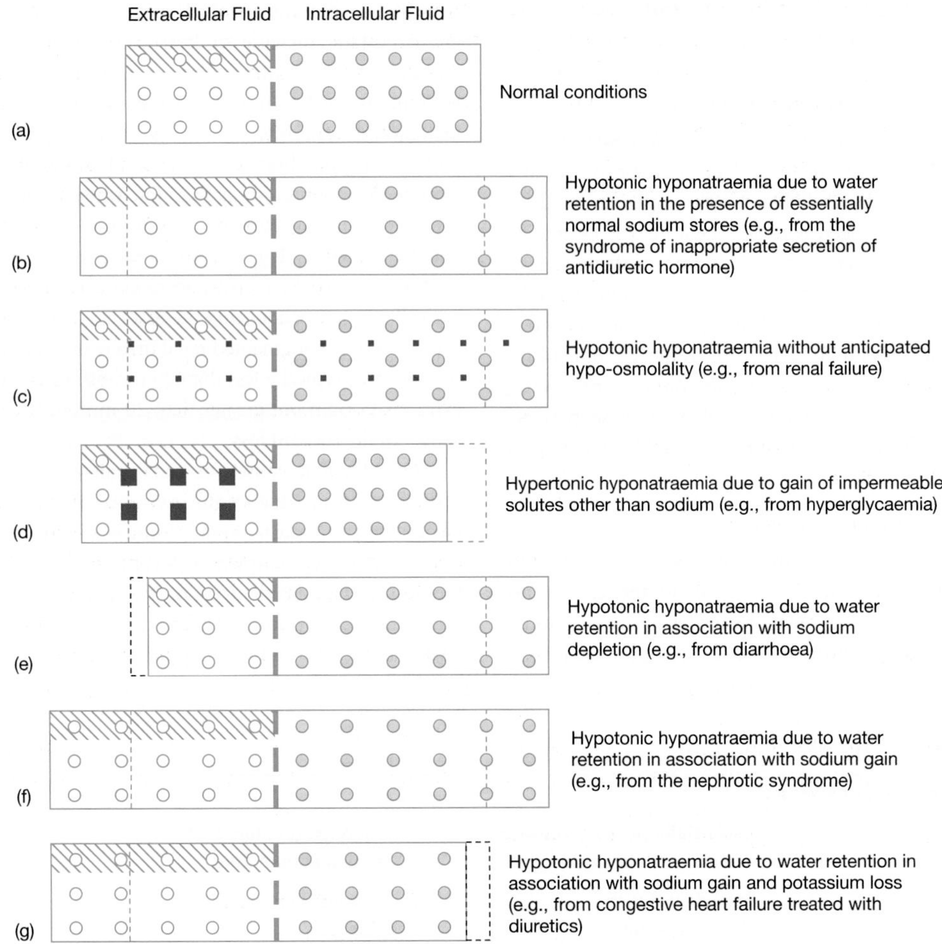

Fig. 4 Extracellular-fluid and intracellular-fluid compartments under normal conditons and during states of hyponatraemia. Normally, the ECF and ICF compartments make up 40 and 60 per cent of total body water, respectively (Panel a). With the syndrome of inappropriate secretion of antidiuretic hormone, the volumes of ECF and ICF expand (although a small element of sodium and potassium loss, not shown, occurs during inception of the syndrome) (Panel b). Water retention can lead to hypotonic hyponatraemia without the anticipated hypo-osmolality in patients who have accumulated ineffective osmoles, such as urea (Panel c). A shift of water from the ICF compartment to the ECF compartment, driven by solutes confined in the ECF, results in hypertonic (translocational) hyponatraemia (Panel d). Sodium depletion (and secondary water retention) usually contracts the volume of ECF but expands the ICF compartment. At times, water retention can be sufficient to restore the volume of ECF to normal or even above-normal levels (Panel e). Hypotonic hyponatraemia in sodium-retentive states involves expansion of both compartments, but predominantly the ECF compartment (Panel f). Gain of sodium and loss of potassium in association with a defect of water excretion, as they occur in congestive heart failure treated with diuretics, lead to expansion of the ECF compartment but contraction of the ICF compartment (Panel g). In each panel, open circles denote sodium, solid circles potassium, large squares impermeable solutes other than sodium, and small squares permeable solutes; the broken line between the two compartments represents the cell membrane, and the shading indicates the intravascular volume.

Hypertonic mannitol, retained in patients with renal insufficiency, has the same effect. In both conditions, the resultant hypertonicity can be aggravated by osmotic diuresis; mitigation of hyponatraemia or frank hypernatraemia can develop, as the total of the sodium and potassium concentrations in the urine falls short of that in serum. Retention in the extracellular space of large volumes of isotonic fluids that do not contain sodium (e.g. isotonic mannitol solution) generates iso-osmolar and isotonic hyponatraemia but no transcellular shifts of water. Massive absorption of isotonic irrigant solutions that are sodium free (e.g. those used during transurethral prostatectomy or for control of uterine bleeding) can cause severe hyponatraemia. Pseudohyponatraemia, as described above, is a spurious form of iso-osmolar and isotonic hyponatraemia that represents a laboratory artefact. Direct measurement of serum sodium with the ion-specific electrode in undiluted sample eliminates this artefact.

Hypotonic hyponatraemia

Hypotonic (dilutional) hyponatraemia is a common clinical problem in hospitalized patients. Although morbidity varies widely in severity, serious complications can arise from the disorder itself as well as from errors in management. Hypotonic hyponatraemia represents an excess of water in relation to existing sodium stores, which can be decreased, essentially normal, or increased (Fig. 4). Retention of water most commonly reflects ingestion of a usual amount of water on the background of impaired renal water excretion; in a minority of cases, it is caused by excessive water intake, with a normal or nearly normal water excretory capacity (Table 2).

Impaired capacity of renal water excretion

Clinical detection of the causes of hypotonic hyponatraemia that are associated with impaired capacity of renal water excretion is greatly facilitated by assessing ECF volume (Table 2). The causes can be categorized into three groups: (a) decreased ECF volume; (b) essentially normal ECF volume; and (c) increased ECF volume (oedema states). Importantly, all conditions of impaired renal excretion of water with the exception of renal failure are characterized by high plasma concentration of vasopressin despite hypotonicity (i.e. non-osmotic stimulation). It must be emphasized, however, that despite the presence of a water excreting defect, hyponatraemia will not develop in these patients unless water intake exceeds the capacity of renal water excretion (plus insensible losses).

Hyponatraemia with decreased ECF volume

It is usually simple to diagnose ECF volume contraction in patients with dilutional hyponatraemia. The patient's history allows the clinician to determine whether sodium loss is of renal or extrarenal origin. Volume depletion can be associated with normal supine blood pressure but an orthostatic fall of the systolic level greater than 15 mm Hg; in addition, an orthostatic increase in heart rate of greater than 15 beats/min and diminished jugular venous pressure can be observed. More severe volume depletion can lead to supine hypotension, reduced tissue perfusion, and diminished skin turgor. Ocular pressure can also decrease and mucous membranes become dry. However, haemodynamic signs of volume depletion are only manifest when volume contraction is quite acute or severe, as retention of water can ameliorate the severity of the volume depletion (Fig. 4e). An increase in serum creatinine and a proportionately greater increase in blood urea nitrogen concentration are typically present evidencing the associated reduction in glomerular filtration rate and augmented renal urea reabsorption. Urine sodium concentration is typically less than 20 mmol/l when volume depletion is of extrarenal origin but greater than 20 mmol/l when the kidneys are the source of the sodium loss.

The principal causes of renal salt-wasting are diuretic agents, osmotic diuresis (due to glucose, urea, or mannitol), adrenal insufficiency, bicarbonaturia, and ketonuria (Table 2). The most common cause of mild hyponatraemia (serum $[Na^+] \geq 130$ mmol/l) is diuretic therapy with a thiazide drug, or less frequently, a loop agent, but clinical evidence of volume depletion might not be present. The mechanisms of diuretic-induced hyponatraemia include ADH release caused

Table 2 Causes of hypotonic hyponatraemia

Impaired capacity of renal water excretion

Decreased volume of extracellular fluid	**Essentially normal volume of extracellular fluid**	**Increased volume of extracellular fluid**
Renal sodium loss	Thiazide diuretics[a]	Congestive heart failure
Diuretic agents	Hypothyroidism	Cirrhosis
Osmotic diuresis (glucose, urea, mannitol)	Adrenal insufficiency	Nephrotic syndrome
Adrenal insufficiency	Syndrome of inappropriate secretion of antidiuretic hormone	Renal failure (acute or chronic)
Cerebral salt-wasting	Postoperative hyponatraemia	Pregnancy
Bicarbonaturia (renal tubular acidosis, disequilibrium stage of vomiting)	Decreased excretion of solutes	
Ketonuria	Beer potomania	
Extrarenal sodium loss	Tea-and-toast diet	
Diarrhoea		
Vomiting		
Blood loss		
Excessive sweating (e.g. in marathon runners)		
Fluid sequestration in 'third space'		
Bowel obstruction		
Peritonitis		
Pancreatitis		
Muscle trauma		
Burns		

Excessive water intake

Primary polydipsia[b]
Dilute infant formula
Sodium-free irrigant solutions (used in hysteroscopy, laparoscopy, or transurethral resection of the prostate)[c]
Accidental intake of large amounts of water (e.g. during swimming lessons)
Multiple tap-water enemas

[a] Sodium depletion, potassium depletion, stimulation of thirst, and impaired urinary dilution are implicated.

[b] Often a mild reduction in the capacity for water excretion is also present.

[c] Hyponatraemia is not always hypotonic.

by volume depletion, decreased fluid delivery to the diluting segment, interference with urinary dilution by the drug, and potassium depletion. Osmotic diuresis from uncontrolled DM, high urea excretion due to high protein feeding, or mannitol administration also produces renal salt wasting; yet renal water losses in excess of sodium plus potassium losses can lead to serum hypertonicity if replacement fluid intake is inadequate. Adrenal insufficiency and isolated mineralocorticoid deficiency cause hypovolaemic hyponatraemia, although in some instances, particularly with isolated glucocorticoid deficiency, patients might have hyponatraemia with an essentially normal ECF volume. Bicarbonaturia secondary to renal tubular acidosis or during the disequilibrium stage of vomiting results in renal sodium loss and impaired water excretion, potentially leading to dilutional hyponatraemia. In diabetic, alcoholic, or fasting ketoacidosis, ketonuria causes obligatory sodium and potassium loss. Cerebral salt wasting, often confused with the syndrome of inappropriate secretion of antidiuretic hormone (SIADH), is characterized by dilutional hyponatraemia, renal loss of sodium chloride, and volume depletion in a patient with intracranial disease (Atkin *et al.* 1996). This syndrome of unclear pathogenesis (natriuresis has been attributed to a brain natriuretic factor or decreased sympathetic activity) is observed most commonly in neurosurgical patients and those suffering a subarachnoid haemorrhage. Cerebral salt wasting usually resolves within a few weeks. Salt-wasting nephropathy refers to a condition of volume depletion and associated hyponatraemia observed in patients with advanced chronic renal insufficiency (glomerular filtration rate < 15 ml/min) receiving a low sodium diet. Renal salt wasting also occurs in the recovery phase of acute tubular necrosis and in post-obstructive diuresis.

The causes of hypotonic hyponatraemia secondary to extrarenal sodium loss include vomiting, diarrhoea, gastrointestinal or other sources of blood loss, excessive sweating (e.g. marathon runners), and fluid sequestration in 'third space' (Table 2). Gastrointestinal fluid losses are the most common causes of ECF volume depletion in clinical practice; they result in hyponatraemia or hypernatraemia depending on the composition of fluid losses and the patient's water intake. The gastrointestinal fluid lost, especially in states of secretory diarrhoea (e.g. cholera), is largely isotonic despite the variable concentration of sodium and potassium (i.e. sodium-rich secretory diarrhoea has a low potassium concentration and vice versa such that the sum of the concentrations of the two electrolytes is approximately constant and isotonic with serum) (Shiau *et al.* 1985). Replacement of gastrointestinal losses with fluid of low electrolyte content causes hyponatraemia.

In contrast to secretory diarrhoeas, most viral and bacterial intestinal infections generate diarrhoeal fluid losses of low electrolyte content (sodium plus potassium concentration between 40 and 100 mmol/l); organic solutes account for the remaining osmoles (Teree *et al.* 1965). Loss of fluid with a low electrolyte content tends to produce hypernatraemia (unless sufficient water replacement is provided). Use of purgative agents for colon cleansing in preparation for colonoscopy can lead to symptomatic hyponatraemia; its pathogenesis probably involves fecal electrolyte loss, impaired water excretion due to ADH release, and a large water intake for cleansing purpose.

Sweating is unlikely to cause sufficient sodium losses to generate hypotonic hyponatraemia unless extreme sodium restriction is in effect. However, the recent popularity of marathon running is responsible for the regular occurrence of cases of acute hyponatraemia (at times severe and symptomatic) due to the dermal loss of sodium in association with aggressive water ingestion (Frizzell *et al.* 1986). Reduced splanchnic blood flow during marathon running might prevent water absorption until completion of the race, when the abrupt absorption of a large amount of water generates hypotonicity. Important causes of fluid sequestration in 'third space' and resultant hypovolaemia include bowel obstruction, peritonitis, pancreatitis, muscle trauma, and burns.

Depletion of potassium accompanies many disorders associated with volume contraction of renal or extrarenal origin, especially diuretic treatment and diarrhoeal diseases. As indicated above, this potassium deficit contributes to the development of hypotonic hyponatraemia (Eq. 5).

Hyponatraemia with essentially normal ECF volume

Thiazide diuretics Some patients with thiazide-induced hyponatraemia appear euvolaemic, their blood pressure is normal or elevated (e.g. when the diuretic has been given to treat hypertension), BUN and serum creatinine are normal, but hypokalaemia is always present and at times severe. The pathogenesis of hyponatraemia includes water retention combined with sodium and potassium losses (Fichman *et al.* 1971). Particularly susceptible are the elderly, especially women. Predisposed individuals develop hyponatraemia within hours after a single dose; body weight increases, probably reflecting stimulation of thirst and impairment of renal water excretion. A rare complication of thiazide administration, this type of hyponatraemia represents one of the most common causes of severe hyponatraemia in adults, given the widespread use of thiazides. Hyponatraemia rapidly corrects upon discontinuation of the drug.

Hypothyroidism Severe hypothyroidism commonly leads to hypotonic hyponatraemia that corrects with thyroid replacement therapy. Patients appear euvolaemic and their laboratory findings are similar to those of the SIADH, excluding thyroid-specific findings (Hanna and Scanlon 1997).

Adrenal insufficiency Patients with Addison's disease (primary adrenal insufficiency) can develop hypovolaemic hyponatraemia due to renal salt wasting. However, some patients with Addison's disease and those with isolated corticotrophin deficiency develop euvolaemic hyponatraemia. Glucocorticoid deficiency increases vasopressin secretion in these patients, as glucocortoids inhibit vasopressin release (Zimmerman *et al.* 1987). Hyperkalaemia is characteristically absent in pure glucocorticoid deficiency but commonly present in other forms of adrenal insufficiency and can be a helpful diagnostic finding. Swift correction of the water excreting defect follows hormonal replacement therapy.

Syndrome of inappropriate secretion of antidiuretic hormone This syndrome represents the most common cause of euvolaemic hypotonic hyponatraemia in clinical practice (Bartter and Schwartz 1967; Verbalis 1995). Vasopressin secretion in patients with SIADH is independent of osmotic or haemodynamic stimuli, resulting in water retention. However, control of sodium balance remains largely intact, urinary sodium excretion reflecting sodium intake. Thus, on physical examination, the ECF volume appears normal, patients being oedema free. Serum $[Na^+]$ is usually between 125 and 135 mmol/l and relatively stable; serum $[Cl^-]$ is also reduced but potassium and total CO_2 are within normal limits. The stability of serum sodium reflects the phenomenon of 'vasopressin escape', which in rats is mediated by a marked decrease in the expression of the aquaporin-2 water channel (Ecelbarger *et al.* 1997). The diagnosis of SIADH rests on the presence of hypotonic hyponatraemia coupled with inappropriate urinary concentration (urine osmolality > 100 mOsm/kg H_2O), clinical euvolaemia, a high urinary $[Na^+]$ (>30 mmol/l) while on a normal sodium intake, normal glomerular filtration rate, and absence of diuretic use, adrenal insufficiency (cortisol deficiency), or hypothyroidism.

In some patients, firming up the diagnosis of SIADH might require evaluation of plasma ADH, and the response to a water load test or volume expansion. Findings consistent with the diagnosis of SIADH include elevated ADH despite serum hypotonicity, inability to decrease urine osmolality to less than 100 mOsm/kg H_2O in response to a water load and to excrete at least 80 per cent of the load within 4 h, and failure to correct the hyponatraemia with volume expansion (e.g. isotonic saline) but improvement after water restriction.

Malignancies, most commonly small-cell lung carcinoma, but also olfactory neuroblastoma and tumours of the pancreas and duodenum, cause SIADH because of ectopic ADH production by the tumour (Kim *et al.* 1996). Conversely, excessive release of ADH of hypothalamic origin is observed in the SIADH associated with various central nervous disorders (acute psychosis, trauma, stroke, haemorrhage, and inflammatory and demyelinating diseases). The mechanisms leading to SIADH in patients with pulmonary disorders are not clear. Human immunodeficiency virus (HIV) infection complicated by pneumocystis carinii pneumonia, central nervous system infections, or malignancies account for a growing number of patients with the SIADH (Vitting *et al.* 1990). Hyponatraemia in symptomatic HIV infection can also result from adrenal insufficiency or volume depletion (e.g. gastrointestinal fluid losses) (Piedrola *et al.* 1996). Table 3 lists the causes of the SIADH.

Drug-induced hyponatraemia Diuretic agents, largely thiazides, represent the drugs responsible for most cases of drug-induced hyponatraemia. However, other drugs can cause hyponatraemia by acting as ADH analogues (e.g. desmopressin, oxytocin), stimulating the release of ADH, potentiating the renal action of ADH, or by unknown mechanisms. Table 1 lists drugs other than diuretics that can cause hyponatraemia.

Postoperative hyponatraemia Postoperative hyponatraemia develops because vasopressin secretion persists in patients receiving excessive amounts of electrolyte-free water (5 per cent dextrose in water, hypotonic saline) (Gowrishankar *et al.* 1998). Pain, severe nausea, and frequently, certain medications trigger vasopressin release. Most patients are clinically euvolaemic and asymptomatic. However, severe symptomatic hyponatraemia can cause lethal complications (Chung *et al.* 1986).

Transient hypotonic hyponatraemia with a mean decrease in serum $[Na^+]$ of about 5 mmol/l has been observed in the first few hours after routine cardiac catherization, but it largely corrects by 24 h. Administration of hypotonic fluids during the procedure together with impaired urine dilution caused by stress, medication, or underlying disease (e.g. heart failure) could explain the hyponatraemia (Aronson 2002).

Hyponatraemia caused by decreased excretion of solutes Low solute excretion limits the maximal urine volume and, therefore, can cause dilutional hyponatraemia if associated with a high water intake (Fox 2002). Prime examples of this type of hyponatraemia are the tea-and-toast diet, observed especially in elderly individuals of poor means, other extreme diets, and beer potomania. If, for example, daily solute excretion is only 100 mOsm, urine output even at maximal urine dilution (50 mOsm/kg H_2O) would be 2 l/day; fluid intake exceeding 2.5 l/day (to account for insensible losses) will cause water retention and hypotonic hyponatraemia. Lack of other dietary intake accounts for the very low solute load in beer potomania (Thaler *et al.* 1998). Refeeding corrects the hyponatraemia.

Hyponatraemia with increased ECF volume

Arterial underfilling in congestive heart failure, cirrhosis, and nephrotic syndrome with severe hypoalbuminaemia can cause hyponatraemia due to excessive ADH secretion (Schrier 1988). This hormonal response is mediated through the carotid baroreceptors that

Table 3 Causes of the syndrome of inappropriate secretion of antidiuretic hornone (SIADH)[a]

Malignancies	Central nervous system disorders	Pulmonary conditions
Pulmonary/mediastinal	Head trauma	Pneumonia
Bronchogenic carcinoma	Acute psychosis	Lung abscess
Mesothelioma	Delirium tremens	Tuberculosis
Thymoma	Mass lesions	Aspergillosis
Digestive system	Tumour; brain abscess; subdural haematoma	Acute respiratory failure
Carcinoma of the pharynx, stomach, duodenum, pancreas	Inflammatory and demyelinating diseases	Positive-pressure ventilation
Genitourinary	Encephalitis; meningitis	Chronic obstructive pulmonary disease
Carcinoma of the uterus, prostate, bladder, ureter	Systemic lupus erythematosus	Cystic fibrosis
Blood/lymphatic	Guillain-Barré syndrome	
Leukaemia, lymphoma	Spinal cord lesions	
Other	Multiple sclerosis	
Ewing tumour	Miscellaneous	
	Stroke	
	Haemorrhage	
	Pituitary stalk section	
	Infection with the human immunodeficiency virus (HIV)	

[a] Many drugs acting through various mechanisms can lead to a syndrome that resembles SIADH (see Table 1).

detect a reduction in arterial stretch or pressure and overcome the inhibitory effect of hypotonicity on vasopressin release.

Congestive heart failure Arterial underfilling caused by the fall in cardiac output in patients with heart failure results in neurohormonal activation (renin–angiotensin, vasopressin, and norepinephrine) that impairs renal water excretion and promotes hypotonic hyponatraemia (Dzau and Hollenberg 1984; Benedict *et al.* 1994). In rats with uncompensated heart failure and hyponatraemia, aquaporin-2 water channels (mRNA and protein level) increase in collecting duct principal cells as a consequence of increased plasma ADH (Xu *et al.* 1997). Hyponatraemia is common in patients with severe congestive heart failure (New York Heart Association classes 3 and 4). In such patients, serum [Na^+] lower than 130 mmol/l prognosticates a short life expectancy unless cardiac function improves (Leier *et al.* 1994). A therapeutic regimen that combines water restriction, an angiotensin-converting enzyme (ACE) inhibitor, and a loop diuretic might improve or correct the hyponatraemia (Dzau and Hollenberg 1984).

Cirrhosis Renal water handling is normal in the early stages of cirrhosis prior to the development of ascites. As the liver disease progresses, ADH secretion increases, thus predisposing to hyponatraemia (Tsuboi *et al.* 1994). At this stage, vasodilation of the splanchnic circulation and possibly additional territories augments ADH release even though ECF volume is substantially increased (Schrier *et al.* 1988). The reduction in renal blood flow observed in advanced cirrhosis (the result of marked sphanchnic vasodilation and neurohormonal activation of the renin–angiotensin and sympathetic nervous systems) appears to have a lesser role in the impaired renal water excretion. The likelihood of developing hyponatraemia increases in patients with cirrhosis who are heavy beer drinkers (beer potomania) or those who develop volume depletion due to aggressive diuretic therapy or large volume paracentesis in the absence of peripheral oedema. A serum [Na^+] less than 130 mmol/l carries a poor prognosis and values lower than 125 mmol/l are found in endstage liver disease. Hyponatraemia in cirrhosis is most commonly asymptomatic although it might worsen hepatic encephalopathy (Papadakis *et al.* 1990).

Nephrotic syndrome Impaired renal water excretion and mild hyponatraemia can be observed in patients with nephrotic syndrome. The pathophysiological mechanism is probably different in patients with preserved renal function (e.g. minimal change nephrotic syndrome) than in those with decreased glomerular filtration rate. Vasopressin release triggered by a decrease in effective circulating arterial volume (i.e. arterial underfilling) appears to be at fault in patients with nephrotic syndrome, severe hypoalbuminaemia, and preserved renal function. Conversely, the renal disease itself probably accounts for the impaired renal water excretion in nephrotic patients with hypofiltration. Aggressive use of diuretics can be responsible for generating severe hyponatraemia in nephrotic patients.

Renal failure Hyponatraemia can occur with advanced acute or chronic renal failure. In these patients, free water excretion is mainly limited by the reduced glomerular filtration rate. As an example, when the glomerular filtration rate is at 10 ml/min (14 l/day) with approximately 20 per cent of filtrate reaching the diluting segments of the nephron, the maximum electrolyte-free water generation is approximately 2.8 l/day. In advanced renal failure, the minimum urine osmolality can be 200–250 mOsm/kg H_2O despite appropriate suppression of ADH secretion; thus, unrestricted water intake might lead to hyponatraemia. The higher minimum urine osmolality is due to increased solute excretion per functioning nephron resulting in osmotic diuresis (Fig. 1). Patients with end-stage renal disease on chronic maintenance haemodialysis commonly have substantial accumulation of ECF in the interdialytic period, but they rarely experience severe hyponatraemia; this probably occurs because water intake results from hypertonicity generated by salt ingestion.

Excessive water intake

The normally large renal capacity for water excretion accounts for the relatively uncommon occurrence of dilutional hyponatraemia due to excessive water intake (Table 2). Complete suppression of ADH release in response to a water load causes water diuresis, with a high urine volume and minimum urine osmolality. In a subject excreting 700 mOsm/day of solute, for example, 14 l of water can be eliminated at a minimum urine osmolality of 50 mOsm/kg H_2O over the course of a day. Increased urine output or polyuria (arbitrarily defined as a urine output > 3 l/day) can reflect water diuresis (due to increased water intake or impaired urinary concentration) or increased solute secretion.

Primary polydipsia

Excessive water intake caused by a primary stimulation of thirst represents the underlying defect in primary polydipsia (compulsive water drinking). If ADH control and the urine dilution mechanism were intact, primary polydipsia should not lead to significant hyponatraemia unless water intake is massive, a situation not frequently encountered. Primary polydipsia is often observed in acutely psychotic patients, particularly those with schizophrenia, and in anxious, middle-aged women. Many of these subjects ingest a moderate to large water load that is compounded by a diminished capacity of renal water excretion. Factors that conspire in generating the hyponatraemia include a central defect in thirst regulation (e.g. the tonicity threshold for thirst is lower than that for ADH release, a reversal of normal), an excessive secretion of ADH or renal response to this hormone, and consequences of therapy for mental disease; some antipsychotic medications impair renal water excretion and induce the sensation of a dry mouth that enhances thirst.

Primary polydipsia also occurs with hypothalamic injury affecting the thirst centre as in infiltrating diseases, including sarcoidosis. Other neurological conditions, such as multiple sclerosis and tuberculous meningitis, can cause polydipsia and polyuria. Patients with isolated primary polydipsia have dilute urine with specific gravity less than 1.005 and osmolality less than 150 mOsm/kg H_2O. If the capacity of renal water excretion is impaired, urine is less than maximally dilute. Water restriction represents the short-term measure for managing the hypotonic state; in patients with severe hyponatraemia, medical supervision of fluid restriction is most important to prevent an excessively rapid correction of hyponatraemia that, by itself, might lead to neurological damage (i.e. central pontine myelinolysis).

Symptomatic hyponatraemia due to an acute water load has also been reported in patients undergoing urinary testing for illegal drugs or preparation for a radiological examination. Concurrent diuretic therapy or ADH release induced by stress or nausea might have played a predisposing role in these otherwise normal individuals. The ingestion of recreational drugs, such as the amphetamine Ecstasy (methylenedioxymethanphetanine or MDMA), can lead to life-threatening hyponatraemia presumably due to a combination of increased water intake and nonosmotic (tonicity independent) ADH release.

Hyponatraemia associated with sodium-free irrigant solutions

Sodium-free flushing solutions containing glycine, sorbitol, or mannitol are used during transurethral resection of the prostate or a bladder tumour, hysteroscopy, or endometrial ablation for control of uterine bleeding (Agarwal and Emmet 1994; Istre *et al.* 1994). As much as 20–30 l of irrigant solutions are used and variable amounts enter the circulation during the procedure leading to hyponatraemia. Risk factors for the development of severe hyponatraemia are prolonged surgery, large tissue resection, and irrigant solution introduced under high pressure. The glycine and sorbitol solutions have a low osmolality (165–200 mOsm/kg H_2O) causing a decrease in serum sodium and tonicity that is greatest immediately following irrigant fluid absorption in the patient's circulation. Both glycine and sorbitol are organic solutes that undergo metabolic degradation leaving behind the free water of the irrigant solution; they are also excreted by the kidney. The manifestations of glycine-associated hyponatraemia include early nausea and, in severe cases, neurological dysfunction, including confusion, muscle twitching, and seizures. The pathogenesis of these symptoms is unclear, but most likely reflects toxicity from glycine or its metabolic products, including ammonia and serine. Hypotonicity might be largely irrelevant, because administration of mannitol to maintain serum tonicity fails to protect from the neurological manifestations.

The diagnosis of irrigant solution-induced hyponatraemia is derived from the clinical history and the demonstration of an osmolal gap (initially it can exceed 30–60 mOsm/kg H_2O).

Other causes of hyponatraemia due to excessive water intake

Multiple tap water enemas in individuals of small body size can cause substantial hyponatraemia. Feeding infants with dilute formula can exceed their renal capacity of water excretion resulting in a hypotonic state. Dilutional hyponatraemia can also result from the accidental intake of large amounts of water during swimming lessons (in a sweet-water swimming pool or lake).

Signs and symptoms of hyponatraemia

The manifestations of hypotonic hyponatraemia are largely related to dysfunction of the central nervous system induced by cerebral oedema. They are more conspicuous when the decrease in the serum sodium concentration is large or rapid (i.e. occurring within a period of hours). Nausea and malaise develop at serum [Na^+] of 120–130 mmol/l. Headache, lethargy, obtundation, and depressed reflexes occur with serum [Na^+] lower than 120 mmol/l. Seizures, coma, permanent brain damage, brain stem herniation, and respiratory arrest and death develop at lower levels of serum sodium concentration. Severe hyponatraemic encephalopathy most often occurs with excessive water retention in patients who are essentially euvolaemic (e.g. those recovering from surgery or those with primary polydipsia); prepubertal children and menstruating women appear to be at particular risk (Arieff *et al.* 1992; Ayus *et al.* 1992).

Hypotonic hyponatraemia causes entry of water derived from the interstitial fluid, vascular compartment, and cerebrospinal fluid into the brain, presumably across a water channel (aquaporin-4). Because the surrounding cranium limits expansion of the brain, intracranial hypertension develops, with a risk of brain injury (Fig. 5). Increased intracranial pressure initially reduces the volume of blood within the vault and of the cerebrospinal fluid; in addition, it promotes the exit of brain ECF into the cerebrospinal fluid compartment (Melton *et al.* 1987). Within hours, brain cells lose potassium, sodium, and chloride

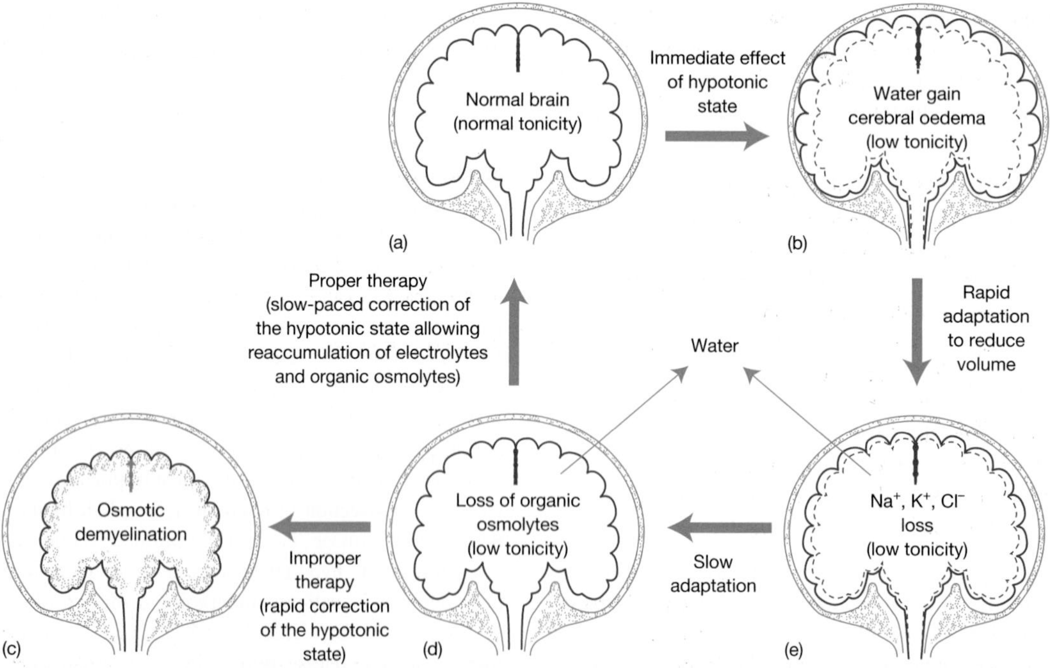

Fig. 5 Effects of hyponatraemia on the brain and adaptive responses. Within minutes after the development of hypotonicity, water gain causes swelling of the brain and a decrease in osmolality of the brain (b). Partial restoration of brain volume occurs within a few hours as a result of cellular loss of electrolytes (rapid adaptation) (c). The normalization of brain volume is completed within several days through loss of organic osmolytes from brain cells (slow adaptation) (d). Low osmolality in the brain persists despite the normalization of brain volume. Proper correction of hypotonicity re-establishes normal osmolality without risking damage to the brain (back to a). Overly aggressive correction of hyponatraemia can lead to irreversible brain damage (osmotic demyelination) (e).

as a result of activation of respective cell membrane channels, thereby promoting partial restoration of cell volume and amelioration of brain swelling (Lien *et al.* 1991). This process is completed via organic solute (osmolytes) loss that occurs as a subsequent step of the volume regulatory response (Fig. 5). Such brain osmolytes include amino acids (glutamine, glutamate, taurine), carbohydrates (myoinositol), and choline compounds (Gullans and Verbalis 1993). The cerebral adaptation to hyponatraemia takes 2–4 days for completion and accounts for the lack of symptoms in many patients with severe chronic hyponatraemia (<120 mmol/l). Nevertheless, brain adaptation is also the source of the risk of central pontine myelinolysis (Fig. 5).

Central pontine myelinolysis

Central pontine myelinolysis or osmotic demyelination is an uncommon but serious condition that can develop one to several days after aggressive treatment of hyponatraemia by any method, including water restriction alone (Tanneau *et al.* 1994; Laureno and Karp 1997). Postoperative patients given large amounts of hypotonic fluids and patients with thiazide-induced hyponatraemia are particularly susceptible. Also, hepatic failure, chronic alcoholism, potassium depletion, and malnutrition increase the risk of this complication. The pathogenesis of this entity remains unclear, but potential mechanisms include ionic overshoot, delayed osmolyte reaccumulation, and disruption of the blood–brain barrier. Presumably, the cellular loss of solutes during adaptation to hyponatraemia increases the risk of damage from shrinkage of the brain in response to a swift elevation in the serum [Na^+] (overly rapid correction of hyponatraemia). Osmotic shrinkage of axons might disrupt interaction with their myelin sheaths inducing demyelination. The demyelination process is often diffuse but sometimes spares the pons. Patients with osmotic demyelination exhibit various neurological manifestations, such as quadriplegia, pseudobulbar palsy, seizures, and coma, and even death. The diagnosis is made by magnetic resonance imaging, a technique more sensitive than CT scanning, although detection of osmotic demyelination with any technique might take 1–2 weeks from the onset of the syndrome (Brunner *et al.* 1990). Outcome is often fatal, while survivors are commonly left with permanent brain damage. Effective treatment has not been identified although promising results in three patients treated with aggressive plasmapheresis have been reported (Bibl *et al.* 1999).

Treatment of hypotonic (dilutional) hyponatraemia

Restriction of electrolyte-free fluid intake to less than the combined fluid losses (urinary, stool, insensible losses) gradually increases the serum [Na^+] and tonicity and should be used in all patients with dilutional hyponatraemia (Adrogué and Madias 2000a; Gross 2001). In patients with hyponatraemia from excessive water intake, simply reducing water ingestion to usual amounts is sufficient to correct the disorder in most cases. In euvolaemic or oedematous patients, reduction of fluid intake to less than 800 ml/day is usually necessary to produce negative water balance. In hypovolaemic patients, isotonic saline infusion corrects the ECF volume depletion and the associated hyponatraemia; yet, electrolyte-free fluid restriction must also be enforced.

The optimal treatment of hypotonic hyponatraemia balances the risks of hypotonicity against those of therapy (Berl 1990). The presence of symptoms and their severity largely determine the pace of correction.

Symptomatic hypotonic hyponatraemia

Patients who have symptomatic hyponatraemia with concentrated urine (osmolality ≥ 200 mOsm/kg H_2O) and clinical euvolaemia or hypervolaemia require infusion of hypertonic saline (Table 4). This treatment provides rapid but controlled correction of hyponatraemia. Hypertonic saline is usually combined with frusemide to limit expansion of the ECF volume. Because frusemide-induced diuresis is equivalent to one-half isotonic saline solution, it aids in the correction of hyponatraemia, as do ongoing dermal and respiratory fluid losses; anticipation of these losses should temper the pace of infusion of hypertonic saline. Obviously, electrolyte-free water intake must be withheld. In addition to hypertonic saline, hormone-replacement therapy should be given to patients with

Table 4 Formula for use in managing hyponatraemia and hypernatraemia and characteristics of infusates

Formula[a]		Clinical use
$\text{Change in serum Na}^+ = \dfrac{[\text{infusate Na}^+ + \text{infusate K}^+] - \text{serum Na}^+}{\text{total body water} + 1}$		Estimate the effect of 1 l of any infusate containing Na^+ and K^+ on serum Na^+
Infusate	**Infusate Na^+ (mmol/l)**	**Extracellular-fluid distribution (%)**
5% Sodium chloride in water	855	100[b]
3% Sodium chloride in water	513	100[b]
0.9% Sodium chloride in water	154	100
Ringer's lactate solution	130	97
0.45% Sodium chloride in water	77	73
0.2% Sodium chloride in 5% dextrose in water	34	55
5% Dextrose in water	0	40

[a] The numerator in the formula is a simplification of the expression (infusate Na^+ − serum Na^+) × 1 l, with the value yielded by the equation in millimoles per litre. The estimated total body water (in litres) is calculated as a fraction of body weight. The fraction is 0.6 in children, 0.6 and 0.5 in non-elderly men and women, respectively, and 0.5 and 0.45 in elderly men and women, respectively. Normally, extracellular and intracellular fluids account for 40 and 60 per cent of total body water, respectively.

[b] In addition to its complete distribution in the extracellular compartment, this infusate induces osmotic removal of water from the intracellular compartment.

suspected hypothyroidism or adrenal insufficiency after blood samples are obtained for diagnostic testing. On the other hand, most patients with hypovolaemia are treated successfully with isotonic saline. Patients with seizures also require immediate anticonvulsant drug therapy and adequate ventilation (Oh *et al.* 1995).

Patients with moderate, symptomatic hyponatraemia, and dilute urine (osmolality < 200 mOsm/kg H_2O) usually require only water restriction and close observation. Examples of such patients are those with isolated primary polydipsia, decreased intake (and excretion) of solutes, or correction of a previously existing water-excretion defect. Severe symptoms (e.g. seizures, coma) call for infusion of hypertonic saline.

There is no consensus about the optimal prescription for treating symptomatic hyponatraemia (Cluitmans and Meinders 1990; Lauriat and Berl 1997; Gross 2001). Nevertheless, correction should be of a sufficient pace and magnitude to reverse in a timely fashion the most serious manifestations of hypotonicity, but should not be so rapid and large as to pose a risk of developing osmotic demyelination. Physiological considerations indicate that a relatively small increase in the serum sodium concentration, of the order of 5 per cent, should substantially reduce cerebral oedema. Even seizures induced by hyponatraemia can be stopped by rapid increases in serum [Na^+] that average only 3–7 mmol/l. Most reported cases of osmotic demyelination occurred after correction in excess of 12 mmol/l per day, but isolated cases occurred after corrections of only 9–10 mmol/l in 24 h or 19 mmol/l in 48 h. Altogether, we recommend a targeted rate of correction that does not exceed 8 mmol/l on any day of treatment (Adrogué and Madias 2000a). Within this target, the initial rate of correction can be 1–2 mmol/l/h for several hours in patients with severe symptoms. Should severe symptoms not respond to correction according to the specified target, we suggest that this limit be cautiously exceeded, as the imminent risks of hypotonicity override the potential risk of osmotic demyelination. Recommended indications for stopping the rapid correction of symptomatic hyponatraemia (regardless of the method used) are cessation of life-threatening manifestations, moderation of other symptoms, or achievement of a serum [Na^+] of 125–130 mmol/l (or even lower if the base-line serum sodium is $<$100 mmol/l). Long-term management of hyponatraemia (described below under asymptomatic hypotonic hyponatraemia) should then be initiated. Should one exceed the recommended target of correction, animal data and a clinical case support the relowering of the serum [Na^+] via administering water and vasopressin to prevent development of osmotic demyelination (Soupart *et al.* 1994, 1999). Although faster rates of correction can be tolerated safely by most patients with acute ($<$48 h) symptomatic hyponatraemia, there is no evidence that such an approach is beneficial (Cheng *et al.* 1990). Moreover, ascertaining the duration of hyponatraemia is usually difficult.

The rate of infusion of the selected solution can be derived expediently by applying a simple formula (Adrogué and Madias 1997) (Table 4). The change in serum [Na^+] induced by the retention of 1 l of a given solution can be estimated as follows:

$$\text{Change in serum Na}^+ = \frac{[\text{infusate Na}^+ + \text{infusate K}^+] - \text{serum Na}^+}{\text{total body water} + 1} \qquad (6)$$

Dividing the change in serum sodium targeted for a given treatment period by the output of this formula determines the volume of infusate required, and hence the rate of infusion. One should use this and other formulae with caution, as it is assumed that the apparent space of distribution of the infused sodium and potassium is total body water, and that no water, sodium, or potassium is lost or gained from the body other than the administered infusate. The apparent space into which administered sodium and potassium distribute might well be smaller than total body water depending on the rate at which the infused electrolytes enter the intracellular compartment. Also, ongoing sodium, potassium, and water losses in gastrointestinal secretions, drainage fluids, or urine during the treatment period cannot be anticipated by Eq. (6) and other formulae. As a general framework, these formulae provide quantitative projections for guiding the repair of abnormalities in serum sodium concentration. Because of uncertainties about the effects of the infusate as well as intercurrent fluid losses, serum [Na^+] should be checked frequently during treatment and the fluid prescription adjusted accordingly. We do not recommend use of the following conventional formula for the correction of hyponatraemia:

$$\text{Sodium requirement} = \text{total body water} \times (\text{desired serum [Na}^+] - \text{current [Na}^+]) \qquad (7)$$

The conventional formula requires a relatively complicated procedure to convert the amount of sodium required to raise the sodium concentration to an infusion rate for the selected solution. Of course, Eq. (7) shares all the limitations described for the recommended formula (Eq. 6). Further, the conventional formula (Eq. 7) underestimates the sodium requirement, as the volume of the infusate retains a considerable fraction of the administered sodium load (volume of infusate multiplied by the final serum [Na^+]). Table 5 depicts illustrative cases of symptomatic hyponatraemia and their management.

Asymptomatic hypotonic hyponatraemia

In some patients with asymptomatic hyponatraemia, the main risk of complications emanates not from the disorder itself, but from its correction phase. This is true of patients who stop drinking large amounts of water and those whose water-excretion defect is repaired (e.g. repletion of ECF volume, discontinuation of offending drugs). If excessive diuresis occurs so that the projected rate of spontaneous correction exceeds that recommended for patients with symptomatic hyponatraemia, hypotonic fluids or desmopressin can be administered.

In contrast, there is no such risk associated with the asymptomatic hyponatraemia that accompanies oedema states or the SIADH because of the prevailing defect of water excretion. Water restriction (to $<$800 ml per day) is the mainstay of long-term management, with the goal being induction of negative water balance. In severe cardiac failure, optimization of haemodynamics by several measures, including the use of ACE inhibitors, can increase excretion of electrolyte-free water and mitigate hyponatraemia. Further, ACE inhibitors enhance the secretion of renal prostaglandins that antagonize the effects of ADH on the collecting tubule. Loop, but not thiazide, diuretics reduce urine concentration and augment excretion of electrolyte-free water, thereby permitting relaxation of fluid restriction. In the SIADH, but not in oedema disorders, loop diuretics should be combined with an abundant sodium intake (in the form of dietary sodium or salt tablets), a treatment that augments water loss. If these measures fail, 600–1200 mg of demeclocycline per day can help by inducing nephrogenic diabetes insipidus (Verbalis 1995). Renal function should be monitored,

Table 5 Managing symptomatic hyponatraemia: illustrative cases

Case No.	Time (h)	Data	Diagnosis/treatment plan	Fluid prescription
1	0	28-year-old woman with stupor and grand-mal seizures 2 days after appendectomy; euvolaemic; weight 67 kg; $[Na^+]$ 113 mmol/l, $[K^+]$ 4.5 mmol/l, Sosm 229 mOsm/kg H_2O, U_{osm} 550 mOsm/kg H_2O	Postoperative hyponatraemia; diazepam 20 mg IV, phenytoin 250 mg IV, laryngeal intubation, mechanical ventilation, withholding of water, frusemide 20 mg IV, 3% NaCl to increase $[Na^+]$ by 3 mmol/l over 2 h	TBW, $0.5 \times 67 = 33.5$ l $\Delta[Na^+] = \frac{513 - 113}{33.5 + 1} = 11.6$ mmol /l per 1 l infusate For a goal of $\Delta[Na^+]$ 3 mmol/l/2 h, $3/11.6 = 0.259$ l/2 h is required, or ~130 ml/h
	2	No further seizure episodes; she responds to pain but not to commands; $[Na^+]$ 116 mmol/l	3% NaCl to increase $[Na^+]$ by 3 mmol/l over 6 h	For a goal of $\Delta[Na^+]$ 3 mmol/l/6 h, $3/11.6 = 0.259$ l/6 h is required, or ~43 ml/h
	8	No seizure activity, patient responds to simple commands; $[Na^+]$ 120 mmol/l	Discontinue 3% NaCl Continue to withhold water Close monitoring	
2	0	60-year-old man with small-cell lung carcinoma, who presents with severe confusion and lethargy; euvolaemic; weight 72 kg; $[Na^+]$ 108 mmol/l, $[K^+]$ 4.0 mmol/l, BUN 8 mg/dl, creatinine 0.6 mg/dl, Sosm 222 mOsm/kg H_2O, U_{osm} 625 mOsm/kg H_2O	Tumour-induced SIADH; withholding of water frusemide 20 mg IV 3% NaCl to increase $[Na^+]$ by 5 mmol/l over 12 h	TBW, $0.6 \times 72 = 43$ l $\Delta[Na^+] = \frac{513 - 108}{43 + 1} = 9.2$ mmol/l per 1 l infusate For a goal of $\Delta[Na^+]$ 5 mmol/l/12 h, $5/9.2 = 0.543$ l/12 h is required, or ~45 ml/h
	12	Mildly lethargic but easily arousable; $[Na^+]$ 114 mmol/l	Discontinue 3% NaCl Continue to withhold water Close monitoring	

Table 5 Continued

Case No.	Time (h)	Data	Diagnosis/treatment plan	Fluid prescription
3	0	70-year-old woman with vomiting and diarrhoea for 4 days, who presents with lethargy but no focal neurologic deficits; hypovolaemic, supine BP 98/58 mmHg; weight 75 kg; $[Na^+]$ 112 mmol/l, $[K^+]$ 2.4 mmol/l, $[HCO_3^-]$ 30 mmol/l, BUN 45 mg/dl, creatinine 1.4 mg/dl, Sosm 242 mOsm/kg H_2O, U_{osm} 650 mOsm/kg H_2O	Hypovolaemic hyponatraemia; potassium depletion; prerenal azotaemia; withholding of water, volume repletion, potassium repletion, increase $[Na^+]$ by no more than 8 mmol/l over 24 h	TBW, 0.45 × 75 = 34 l Selected infusate is 0.9% NaCl containing 30 mmol/l of KCl $\Delta[Na^+] = \frac{(154 + 30) - 112}{34 + 1} = 2.0$ mmol/l per 1 l infusate Administer 1 l/h for the next 2 h
	2	Moderate drowsiness; supine BP 106/64 mmHg; $[Na^+]$ 117 mmol/l, $[K^+]$ 3.1 mmol/l	Withholding of water; continue volume and potassium repletion; note that restoration of ECF volume will eliminate non-osmotic stimulus to ADH release thereby promoting rapid excretion of dilute urine	Switch infusate to 0.45% NaCl containing 30 mmol/l of KCl $\Delta[Na^+] = \frac{(77 + 30) - 117}{34 + 1} = -0.3$ mmol/l per 1 l infusate Administer 100 ml/h for the next 12 h
	6	Mild drowsiness; supine BP 112/68 mmHg; $[Na^+]$ 118 mmol/l, $[K^+]$ 3.2 mmol/l	Despite the formula's estimate that this infusate will not change $[Na^+]$ measurably at 100 ml/h, $[Na^+]$ continues to increase (the sum of sodium and potassium concentrations of the urine must be lower than that of the infusate)	Continue present infusate at 100 ml/h
	12	Minimal drowsiness; supine BP 126/72 mmHg; $[Na^+]$ 119 mmol/l, $[K^+]$ 3.4 mmol/l	Prevent further correction of $[Na^+]$ over the next 12 h	Switch infusate to 5% dextrose containing 30 mmol/l of KCl at a rate matching urinary output

because demeclocycline has nephrotoxic effects, especially in patients with cirrhosis. Moreover, the drug imposes the risk of hypernatraemia in patients who do not take in sufficient water. Management of chronic hyponatraemia will be helped by the anticipated introduction of promising oral agents that antagonize the effect of vasopressin on the V_2 receptor. Encouraging results have been obtained in hyponatraemic patients with cardiac failure, cirrhosis, or the SIADH (Serradeil-Le Gal *et al.* 1996; Saito *et al.* 1997).

Treatment of non-hypotonic hyponatraemia

Corrective measures for non-hypotonic hyponatraemia are directed at the underlying disorder rather than at the hyponatraemia itself. Administration of insulin is the basis of treatment for uncontrolled DM, but deficits of water, sodium, and potassium should also be corrected. Frusemide hastens the recovery of patients who absorb irrigant solutions; if renal function is impaired, haemodialysis is the preferred option.

Common errors in management

Although water restriction ameliorates all forms of hyponatraemia, it is not the optimal therapy in all cases. Hyponatraemias associated with depletion of ECF volume require, in addition to fluid restriction, correction of the prevailing sodium deficit. On the other hand, isotonic saline is unsuitable for correcting the hyponatraemia of the SIADH; if administered, the resulting rise in serum sodium is both small and transient, with the infused salt being excreted in concentrated urine, thereby worsening net retention of water and hyponatraemia. Although uncertainty about the diagnosis occasionally justifies a limited trial of isotonic saline, attentive follow-up is needed to confirm the diagnosis before substantial deterioration occurs. Great vigilance is required to recognize and diagnose hypothyroidism and adrenal insufficiency, as these disorders tend to masquerade as cases of the SIADH. The presence of hyperkalaemia should always alert the physician to the possibility of adrenal insufficiency.

Whereas patients with persistent asymptomatic hyponatraemia require slow-paced management, those with symptomatic hyponatraemia must receive rapid but controlled correction. Prudent use of hypertonic saline can be life-saving, but failure to follow the recommendations for treatment outlined above can cause devastating and even lethal consequences.

Hyponatraemia that is acquired in the hospital is largely preventable. A defect of water excretion can be present on admission, or it can worsen or develop during the course of hospitalization as a result of several antidiuretic influences (e.g. medications, organ failure, and the postoperative state). The presence of such a defect notwithstanding, hyponatraemia will not develop as long as the intake of electrolyte-free water does not exceed the capacity for renal water excretion plus stool and insensible losses. Thus, hypotonic fluids must be supplied carefully to hospitalized patients.

Hypernatraemia

Hypernatraemia, defined as a serum sodium concentration greater than 145 mmol/l, is a common electrolyte disorder. Because sodium is a functionally impermeable solute, it contributes to tonicity and induces the movement of water across cell membranes. Therefore, hypernatraemia invariably denotes hypertonic hyperosmolality and always causes cellular dehydration, at least transiently (Fig. 6). The resultant morbidity can be inconsequential, serious, or even life-threatening. Hypernatraemia frequently develops in hospitalized patients as an iatrogenic condition. Some of its most serious complications result not from the disorder itself but from its inappropriate treatment (Palevsky *et al.* 1996).

Sustained hypernatraemia occurs only when thirst or access to water is impaired. The groups at highest risk are thus patients with altered mental status, intubated patients, infants, and elderly persons. Hypernatraemia in infants usually results from vomiting, a condition that causes hypotonic fluid loss while preventing retention of ingested fluid. In elderly persons, hypernatraemia is usually associated with infirmity or febrile illness (Adrogué and Madias 2000b); the elderly also have thirst impairment. Frail nursing home residents and hospitalized patients are prone to hypernatraemia because they depend on others to satisfy their water requirements. People without access to water, such as those stranded in the desert or on an ocean raft, and those abandoned in a confined space are also at risk of hypernatraemia.

Hypernatraemia represents a deficit of water in relation to the body's sodium stores, which can result from net water loss or hypertonic sodium gain (Table 6). Net water loss accounts for the majority of cases of hypernatraemia. It can occur without associated sodium deficit (pure water loss) or with sodium depletion (hypotonic fluid loss) (Fig. 6). Pure water is lost via dermal, respiratory, or renal routes (Table 6). Contrary to common belief, hypernatraemia caused by pure water loss is associated with a contracted, not normal, ECF volume (Fig. 6a and b), although the ECF contraction is often not clinically evident. In this setting, the sodium content of the ECF remains unaltered, yet one out of each 2.5 l of water loss derives from the ECF compartment. ECF contraction is, of course, magnified when hypernatraemia is caused by hypotonic fluid losses, as sodium content is the primary determinant of the size of the ECF compartment (Fig. 6c). Importantly, hypotonic fluid losses containing both sodium and potassium, as they typically occur during osmotic diuresis and use of cathartics, including lactulose therapy, lead to additional contraction of the ICF compartment (Fig. 6d). Hypertonic sodium gain usually results from clinical interventions or accidental sodium loading (Table 6 and Fig. 6e). The resultant hypernatraemia is associated with ECF expansion together with contraction of the ICF compartment (Fig. 6e).

Hypernatraemia due to pure water loss

Hypodipsia and unreplaced insensible losses

Decreased thirst perception, termed hypodipsia, is common in elderly individuals, but is seldom the sole cause of hypernatraemia due to unreplaced sensible and insensible fluid losses (Robertson 1984). Hypothalamic lesions caused by vascular disease, tumours, or granulomatous disease (e.g. sarcoidosis) also result in hypodipsia, sometimes accompanied by diabetes insipidus. A different entity, known as essential hypernatraemia, is characterized by hypodipsia associated with an upward resetting of the central osmoreceptors. In these patients, water loading inhibits ADH release in response to volume expansion rather than low serum tonicity; thus, administered water is excreted in the urine and hypernatraemia is perpetuated. Although patients with essential hypernatraemia are generally asymptomatic, chlorpropamide administration might moderate the hypernatraemia by enhancing the renal effects of ADH. Patients with primary aldosteronism maintain a stable serum sodium of the order of 143–147 mmol/l. It is presumed that the prevailing mild volume expansion characteristic of this syndrome causes an upward resetting of the osmostat.

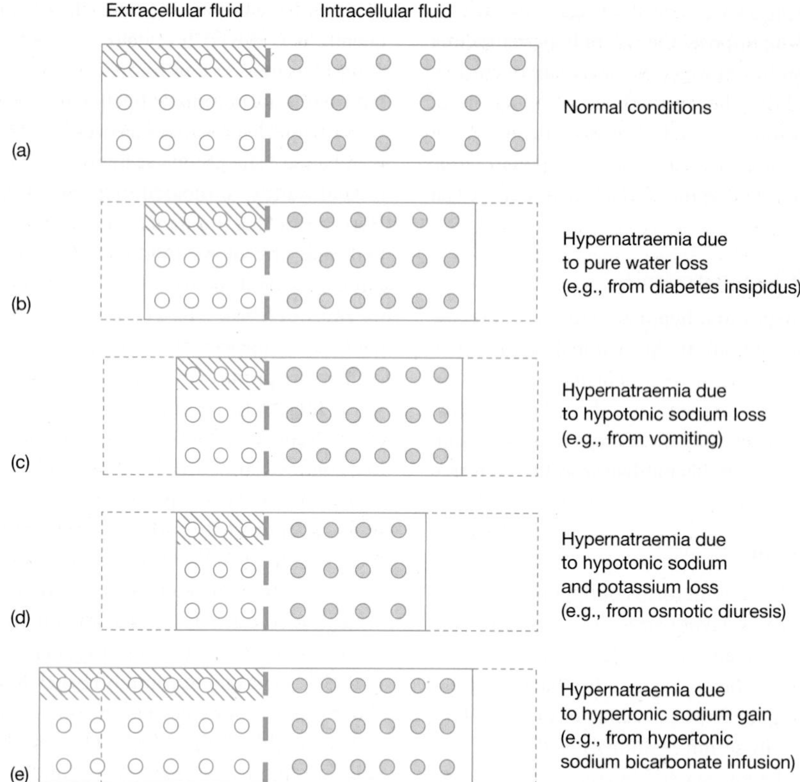

Fig. 6 Extracellular-fluid and intracellular-fluid compartments under normal conditions and during states of hypernatraemia. Normally, the ECF and ICF compartments account for 40 and 60 per cent of total body water, respectively (Panel a). Pure water loss reduces the size of each compartment proportionately (Panel b). Contrary to common belief, the volume of ECF in this setting is reduced, not normal, although the reduction is often not clinically evident. The sodium content of ECF remains unaltered, yet 1 of each 2.5 l of water that is lost is from the ECF compartment. Hypotonic sodium loss causes a relatively larger loss of volume in the ECF compartment than in the ICF compartment (Panel c). Potassium loss in addition to hypotonic sodium loss further reduces the ICF compartment (Panel d). Hypertonic sodium gain results in an increase in ECF but a decrease in ICF (Panel e). In each panel, the open circles denote sodium, and the solid circles potassium; the broken line between the two compartments represents the cell membrane, and the shading indicates the intravascular volume.

Table 6 Causes of hypernatraemia

Net water loss		**Hypertonic sodium gain**
Pure water	**Hypotonic fluid**	
Unreplaced insensible losses (dermal and respiratory)	Renal causes	Hypertonic sodium bicarbonate infusion
Hypodipsia	Loop diuretics	Hypertonic feeding preparation
Central diabetes insipidus	Osmotic diuresis (glucose, urea, mannitol)	Ingestion of sodium chloride
Nephrogenic diabetes insipidus	Polyuric phase of acute tubular necrosis	Ingestion of sea water
	Postobstructive diuresis	Sodium chloride-rich emetics
	Intrinsic renal disease	Hypertonic saline enemas
	Gastrointestinal causes	Intrauterine injection of hypertonic saline
	Vomiting	Hypertonic sodium chloride infusion
	Nasogastric drainage	Hypertonic dialysis
	Enterocutaneous fistula	Primary hyperaldosteronism
	Diarrhoea	Cushing's syndrome
	Use of osmotic cathartic agents (e.g. lactulose)	
	Cutaneous causes	
	Burns	
	Excessive sweating	

Central diabetes insipidus

Diabetes insipidus signifies production of an inappropriately dilute urine and reflects either abnormal release of ADH (i.e. central diabetes insipidus, CDI) or unresponsiveness of the kidney to this hormone (i.e. nephrogenic diabetes insipidus).

CDI results from functional or structural disorders that suppress ADH secretion (Table 7). Ethanol ingestion, anorexia nervosa, acute fatty liver of pregnancy, and correction of supraventricular tachycardia can lead to polyuria caused by transient depression of ADH release. Conversely, structural damage of the sites involved in ADH secretion (i.e. hypothalamic osmoreceptors, the supraoptic or paraventricular nuclei, and the superior portion of the hypothalamic–pituitary tract) accounts for the majority of CDI cases in clinical practice. Incomplete impairment of vasopressin secretion might cause partial forms of the syndrome. Up to one-half of all cases of CDI are idiopathic and most likely due to autoimmune disease (e.g. antibodies against vasopressin-producing cells). Yet, patients with presumed idiopathic CDI can develop an anterior pituitary endocrinopathy years after diagnosis caused by a pituitary or suprasellar tumour, which might have initially caused the CDI. Neurosurgery or trauma to the hypothalamus and neurohypophysis accounts for a significant fraction of cases of CDI; those with severe damage often exhibit the classic triphasic response. The initial phase consists of polyuria that begins within 24 h from the injury and lasts for 4–5 days; it is caused by depression of ADH release. The second phase is oliguric and also lasts for 4–5 days; it is caused by the slow release of ADH stored in the damaged posterior lobe and can lead to excessive water retention. The third phase consists of permanent CDI. Some patients with milder injury have a partial or even total recovery before completing the three phases (Hensen *et al.* 1999). In children, CDI complicates more than 75 per cent of surgical procedures for craniopharyngiomas. Other causes of CDI include primary or secondary tumours of the brain (e.g. lymphoma, leukaemia, lung carcinoma), hypoxic encephalopathy, infiltrative diseases (such as histiocytosis X), postpartum hypopituitarism, and a familial disease (autosomal dominant inheritance). An even less common inherited disease (autosomal recessive) is the Wolfram or DIDMOAD syndrome characterized by CDI, DM, optic atrophy (OA), and deafness (D). In this syndrome, diabetes insipidus results from loss of neurones in the supraoptic nuclei; defects in chromosome 4 and in mitochondrial DNA have been identified (Inoue *et al.* 1998).

CDI typically presents with sudden polyuria (3–7 l/day) and dilute urine (specific gravity < 1.005, urine osmolality < 150 mOsm/kg H_2O). In an alert patient, hypernatraemia is uncommon because of the associated stimulation of thirst and resulting polydipsia. In fact, the typical patient features polyuria and polydipsia and, at most, a serum sodium in the high–normal range. Conversely, in the comatose or postoperative patient, life-threatening hypernatraemia can develop rapidly because of large unreplaced urinary water losses. Marked hypernatraemia develops when a hypothalamic lesion affects both ADH release and thirst.

Table 7 Causes of diabetes insipidus

Central	Nephrogenic
Head trauma	Hereditary
Postoperative	X-linked (V2 receptor)
Hypophysectomy	Autosomal (aquaporin-defect)
Craniopharyngioma	Specific congenital defects
Hypothalamic tumours	Vasopressin V2-receptor mutations
Brainstem tumours	Aquaporin-2 mutations
Primary: dysgerminoma, craniopharngioma, suprasellar pituitary tumours	Acquired
Metastatic: carcinoma of the breast, carcinoma of the lung, lymphoma, leukaemia	Renal disease
Infections	Chronic renal insufficiency
Encephalitis	Polycystic kidney disease
Meningitis	Medullary cystic disease
Tuberculosis	Obstructive uropathy
Syphilis	Pyelonephritis
Vascular	Sickle-cell disease
Aneurysms	Amyloidosis
Brainstem hypoxia	Light-chain disease
Cerebrovascular accidents	Sjögren's syndrome
Sheehan's syndrome (postpartum pituitary haemmorrhage)	Sarcoidosis
Granulomatous disease	Electrolyte disorders
Sarcoidosis	Hypokalaemia
Histiocytosis	Hypercalcaemia
Autoimmune	Drug induced
Vasopressin-neurophysin gene mutations	Lithium
Idiopathic	Demeclocycline
Ethanol ingestion (transient)	Methoxyflurane
	Amphotericin B
	Loop diuretics
	Frusemide
	Ethacrynic acid
	Bumetanide
	Torsemide
	Osmotic diuretics
	Vasopressin antagonists

Hereditary nephrogenic diabetes insipidus (see also Chapter 5.6)

Hereditary (congenital) nephrogenic diabetes insipidus is an uncommon disorder characterized by normal ADH secretion but resistance to its water-retaining action (Bichet *et al.* 1997). Two forms of the disorder can be encountered, an X-linked dominant defect (usual form) and an autosomal recessive form (rare). The X-linked form is fully expressed almost exclusively in males (who experience marked polyuria that is resistant to vasopressin), whereas the female carriers are usually asymptomatic; occasionally, female carriers become severely symptomatic (especially during pregnancy when placental vasopressinase diminishes serum ADH). The responsible genetic defect involves mutations or deletions in the V2 receptor that result in impaired antidiuretic, vasodilator, and procoagulant responses to vasopressin. The autosomal recessive disorder, observed more frequently in consanguineous marriages, results from a postreceptor defect involving the aquaporin-2 gene. In contrast to patients with the X-linked defect, these patients exhibit normal extrarenal V2 receptor-mediated responses, including vasodilatory and procoagulant (i.e. release from endothelial cells of factor VIIIc and von Willebrand's factor) effects (Hochberg *et al.* 1997).

Acquired nephrogenic diabetes insipidus

A relatively common defect, acquired nephrogenic diabetes insipidus results from a variety of conditions that impair the renal concentrating ability because of resistance of the collecting tubule to ADH or disruption of the countercurrent mechanism; such disruption can originate from several causes, including decreased sodium chloride reabsorption in the thick ascending limb (medullary portion) or injury of the renal medulla itself. Renal diseases, electrolyte disorders (hypercalcaemia, hypokalaemia), lithium toxicity and other drugs, gestational diabetes insipidus, and dietary abnormalities represent the most important causes of acquired nephrogenic diabetes insipidus.

Renal disease The modest reduction in renal concentrating capacity observed in the elderly and in patients with non-oliguric acute or chronic renal insufficiency is usually not sufficient to generate polyuria, but might produce nocturia (in subjects not drinking at or near bedtime). Maximum urine osmolality limited to only 350–600 mOsm/kg H_2O obligates a higher urine output to excrete the solute load. The defect reflects, at least in part, increased solute excretion per functioning nephron; in experimental chronic renal failure downregulation of the V2 receptor has been observed due to decreased expression of V2 receptor mRNA (Teitelbaum and McGuiness 1995). A severe water conservation defect, manifest as polyuria, is occasionally associated with some renal diseases, including polycystic kidney disease, medullary cystic disease, chronic obstructive uropathy, sickle-cell disease or trait, amyloidosis, Sjögren's syndrome, and light-chain nephropathy.

Hypercalcaemia Hypercalcaemia and lithium toxicity are the most common causes of symptomatic acquired nephrogenic diabetes insipidus in adults. A persistent increase in serum calcium, more than 11 mg/dl, impairs renal concentration capacity through activation of calcium-sensing receptors in the renal tubules and other functional effects, as well as through calcium deposition in the medulla with secondary tubulointerstitial injury (transient or permanent renal medullary damage). Calcium-sensing receptors are activated in two segments of the renal tubule, the thick ascending limb of the loop of Henle (basolateral membrane) and the inner medullary collecting duct (apical membrane). In the loop of Henle, activation of these receptors closes luminal K^+ channels, with an attendant inhibition of loop reabsorption (sodium chloride, calcium) and a reduction of the medullary osmotic gradient that is normally required for urinary concentration (Wang *et al.* 1996). Further, increased downstream delivery of calcium activates apical calcium-sensing receptors in the inner medullary collecting duct and inhibits the effect of ADH on water permeability. In polyuric hypercalcaemic rats, expression of aquaporin-2 water channels is decreased in renal collecting ducts. A contributory role might also be played by hypercalcaemia-induced generation of prostaglandin E_2 (effect abolished by angiotensin II receptor blockade), which diminishes sodium chloride reabsorption in the thick ascending limb. Normalization of serum calcium usually repairs the nephrogenic diabetes insipidus unless permanent and extensive renal medullary damage had ensued.

Hypokalaemia Severe hypokalaemia caused by potassium depletion impairs the renal concentrating mechanism and stimulates thirst, leading occasionally to polyuria and polydipsia. In experimental animals, the urinary concentrating defect is caused by decreased expression of aquaporin-2 water channels and reduced sodium chloride reabsorption in the thick ascending limb (Marples *et al.* 1996).

Lithium toxicity About 20 per cent of patients receiving long-term treatment with lithium for manic-depressive (bipolar) illness develop symptomatic nephrogenic diabetes insipidus, whereas an additional 30 per cent exhibit milder defects in concentrating capacity. The defect results from lithium entry in collecting duct cells via apical sodium channels and its interference with ADH action. Postulated mechanisms for such interference include reduction of adenylate cyclase activity, decreased density of vasopressin receptors, and downregulation of aquaporin-2 water channels. Polyuria and polydipsia in a patient receiving chronic lithium therapy should not lead to the presumption of nephrogenic diabetes insipidus; these symptoms could reflect other polyuric syndromes, including primary polydipsia, a not uncommon disorder in psychiatric patients.

Pharmacological agents Several drugs other than lithium are uncommon causes of a clinically relevant urinary concentrating defect. Amphotericin B and methoxyflurane (anaesthetic agent) can cause nephrogenic diabetes insipidus possibly related to their renal toxicity (acute renal failure). The same defect is produced by foscarnet and cidofovir, drugs administered to treat cytomegalovirus infection in HIV-infected patients. Demeclocycline, a tetracycline-related antibiotic used in the treatment of SIADH, decreases the responsiveness of the collecting duct to vasopressin. Vasopressin receptor antagonists include drugs under investigation that antagonize the V2 (antidiuretic) receptor and generate a selective water diuresis.

Gestational diabetes insipidus An increase in plasma vasopressinase, the enzyme that degrades vasopressin, is responsible for this transient syndrome that affects some women during the second part of pregnancy. The excess enzyme is released from the placenta. Desmopressin (dDAVP), a pure V2 receptor agonist, is not degraded by the circulating vasopressinase and is thus effective in managing this syndrome.

Dietary abnormalities Chronic ingestion of large volumes of water (primary polydipsia) and osmotic diuresis (e.g. glucosuria) result in medullary solute washout and impaired urinary concentration capacity. A marked decrease in salt and protein intake also impairs urinary concentration, as sodium and urea (product of protein metabolism) account for most of the osmolality of the renal medulla interstitium.

Differential diagnosis of polyuria

Polyuria is defined as a daily urine output greater than 3 l. It is due to water or solute diuresis. Polyuria due to water diuresis is largely caused by three conditions, primary polydipsia, CDI, and nephrogenic diabetes insipidus. In these conditions, urinary solute excretion is within the normal range but urinary osmolality is usually less than 250 mOsm/kg H_2O. Examples of polyuria caused by solute diuresis include osmotic diuresis (glucose in uncontrolled DM, urea in high-protein feedings) and saline diuresis (volume expansion following saline loading or release of bilateral urinary tract obstruction). In solute diuresis, polyuria is driven by the markedly increased urinary solute load; urinary osmolality usually exceeds 300 mOsm/kg H_2O.

Uncontrolled DM is the most common cause of polyuria in the outpatient setting; determination of blood and urine glucose establishes the diagnosis. After ruling out uncontrolled DM, primary polydipsia is the next most commonly observed cause of polyuria; nephrogenic diabetes insipidus is substantially less common and CDI is truly unusual. A history of gradual onset of polydipsia and polyuria points towards primary polydipsia or nephrogenic diabetes insipidus, whereas an abrupt onset is commonly detected in CDI; nocturia and a desire for ice water are also commonly present in CDI. Information regarding use of drugs or previous illness can help establish the diagnosis. Additional tools to determine the cause of polydipsia and polyuria include the response to a standard dehydration test followed, if necessary, by the administration of vasopressin.

Water restriction raises serum tonicity that normally causes release of ADH and an increase in urine osmolality. Once serum tonicity reaches 290 mOsm/kg H_2O, the antidiuretic effect of endogenous ADH is maximal in normal individuals as well as in patients with primary polydipsia, and urine osmolality exceeds 600 mOsm/kg H_2O (Fig. 7). However, the absence of endogenous ADH in patients with CDI or the lack of response to ADH in patients with nephrogenic diabetes insipidus prevents an appropriate increase in urine osmolality.

A standard dehydration test requires (a) withholding all fluids for 3 h prior to the test and for the duration of the test; (b) measurement of the urine volume and osmolality every hour; and (c) measurement of serum $[Na^+]$ and osmolality every 2 h. The water restriction test should be discontinued when the urine osmolality exceeds 600 mOsm/kg H_2O, when urine osmolality remains stable on two to three successive measurements despite a rising serum $[Na^+]$ or osmolality, or when the serum tonicity exceeds 290 mOsm/kg H_2O.

An increase in urine osmolality of more than 600 mOsmol/kg H_2O establishes the diagnosis of primary polydipsia (Fig. 7). Patients with diabetes insipidus, whether central or nephrogenic, fail to reach a urine osmolality level greater than 600 mOsm/kg H_2O in response to a standard water deprivation test (Fig. 7). In addition, their urine osmolality remains stable on two or three successive measurements despite an increasing serum $[Na^+]$ or osmolality, or their serum tonicity might exceed 290 mOsm/kg H_2O. To ascertain the pathogenesis of the failure to concentrate the urine in response to the water deprivation test, 10 μg of dDAVP by nasal inhalation or 5 units of aqueous vasopressin subcutaneously are administered and urine parameters (osmolality and volume) measured. Although urine osmolality might increase modestly in response to ADH in patients with symptomatic nephrogenic diabetes insipidus, it remains below serum osmolality. In contrast, in CDI, it increases to more than 500 mOsm/kg H_2O. Complete CDI is differentiated from the partial form by the urine osmolality prior to and after vasopressin administration; urine osmolality remains lower than 200 mOsm/kg H_2O after water deprivation in complete CDI but increases two- to eightfold after vasopressin; urine osmolality usually reaches 300 mOsm/kg H_2O with water deprivation in partial CDI but the response to vasopressin is small (up to 50 per cent increase in urine osmolality) (Fig. 7). In some instances, the water deprivation test and ADH administration fail to identify the precise cause of polyuria and polydipsia because of a considerable overlap in response and the existence of partial defects in ADH secretion. Measurements of plasma vasopressin are then necessary to establish the diagnosis (Fig. 7). Under rare circumstances, even this step might not be diagnostic and a therapeutic trial with desmopressin is required to establish the cause of polyuria.

Hypernatraemia due to hypotonic fluid loss

Unreplaced hypotonic fluid losses of any origin, renal, gastrointestinal, or cutaneous, generate hypernatraemia, the larger the loss, the greater the expected increase in serum sodium. Renal causes of hypotonic fluid loss include loop diuretics, osmotic diuresis (glucose, urea, and mannitol), postobstructive diuresis, polyuric phase of acute tubular necrosis, and intrinsic renal disease. As previously noted, sustained hypernatraemia develops only if thirst or water access is impaired. Patients with uncontrolled DM and large osmotic diuresis caused by glucosuria usually have hyponatraemia rather than hypernatraemia. When hypernatraemia and hyperglycaemia coexist, the patient is usually severely dehydrated and comatose.

Gastrointestinal causes of hypernatraemia include vomiting, nasogastric drainage, enterocutaneous fistula, diarrhoea, and use of osmotic cathartic agents (e.g. lactulose). Vomiting results in loss of hypotonic fluid (gastric juice has $[Na^+]$ of 20–80 mmol/l and $[K^+]$ of 5–20 mmol/l); coupled with inability to retain oral water intake, vomiting has the potential for generating substantial hypernatraemia.

Diarrhoea has variable effects on serum sodium as previously described (see hypotonic hyponatraemia secondary to gastrointestinal fluid losses). Because of a limited ability to communicate thirst, severe

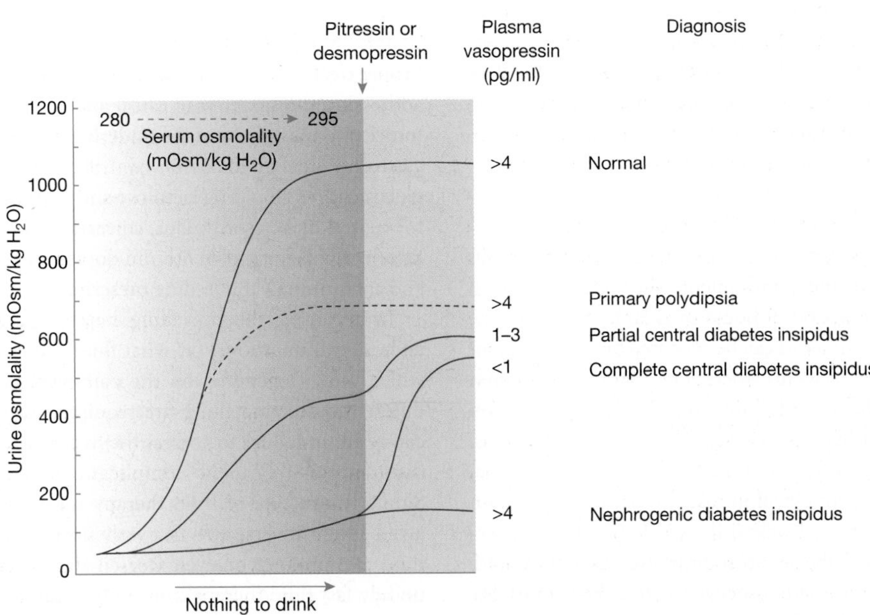

Fig. 7 Response to water deprivation before and after vasopressin administration in normal subjects and in patients with various types of polyuria and polydipsia. (Modified from Valtin, H. *Renal Dysfunction*, Boston: Little Brown, 1979.)

diarrhoea is a common cause of hypernatraemia in infants. Also, diarrhoea can give rise to hypernatraemia in elderly individuals due to the associated hypodipsia. By contrast, unless the gastrointestinal losses are massive or confusion is present, diarrhoea in adults does not cause hypernatraemia. Certain osmotic agents, including sorbitol in managing drug intoxications or lactulose in treating hepatic encephalopathy, commonly generate hypernatraemia in the obtunded or comatose patient given insufficient electrolyte-free fluid.

Excessive fluid loss from the skin or lungs can occur because of fever, exercise, or exposure to high temperature, and leads to hypernatraemia if thirst or access to water is impaired. Insensible fluid loss from the skin or lung occurs by evaporation and, therefore, amounts to pure water loss predisposing to a hypertonic state. Sweat is also a hypotonic fluid ($[Na^+]$ 30–100 mmol/l and $[K^+]$ 5–20 mmol/l), therefore predisposing to hypernatraemia. However, as described before for the case of marathon runners, aggressive water intake makes hyponatraemia a more common clinical problem in individuals performing physical exercise than is hypernatraemia.

Hypernatraemia due to hypertonic sodium gain

Severe or extreme hypernatraemia with $[Na^+]$ greater than 175 mmol/l can be induced by the ingestion or infusion of hypertonic sodium-containing solutions. Hypertonic sodium ingestion can reflect human error involving substitution of sodium chloride for sugar in a paediatric feeding formula, forced ingestion with adverse intent or as a religious ritual, medical prescription of hypertonic saline as an emetic or gargle, accidental ingestion of large quantities of sodium chloride by infants, children, and demented adults, or ingestion of sea water. Partial absorption of hypertonic saline enemas has the same effect. Similarly, severe hypernatraemia develops following the intravenous infusion of hypertonic sodium bicarbonate in the management of severe metabolic acidosis of any cause, including repeated bouts of cardiac arrest, the intrauterine injection of hypertonic saline to induce abortion, and hypertonic haemodialysis (accidental use of dialysate with inordinately high sodium concentration). Assuming reasonably preserved renal function, hypernatraemia caused by hypertonic sodium gain corrects itself swiftly because the prevailing sodium excess is lost in the urine; administration of a loop diuretic and replacement of urine with electrolyte-free water can aid management. Excessively rapid correction of the hypernatraemia should be avoided, especially in asymptomatic patients, as it might reduce the likelihood of full recovery.

Clinical manifestations of hypernatraemia

Signs and symptoms of hypernatraemia largely reflect central nervous system dysfunction and are more prominent when the increase in serum $[Na^+]$ occurs over a period of hours or is large. In adults, the clinical expression of hypernatraemia can be obscured by a concomitant disease (e.g. cerebrovascular accident) whereas in infants and children signs and symptoms of this disorder are usually evident. Common symptoms in infants include hyperpnoea, muscle weakness, restlessness, a characteristic high-pitched cry, insomnia, lethargy, and even coma. Convulsions are typically absent except in cases of inadvertent sodium loading or aggressive rehydration. Unlike infants, elderly patients generally have few symptoms until the serum sodium exceeds 160 mmol/l. Values greater than 180 mmol/l are associated with a high mortality rate, especially in adults. Intense thirst, present initially, dissipates as the disorder progresses and is absent in patients with hypodipsia. The level of consciousness is correlated with the severity of the hypernatraemia. Muscle weakness, confusion, and coma are sometimes manifestations of coexisting disorders rather than of the hypernatraemia itself.

Most outpatients with hypernatraemia are either very young or very old. Unlike hypernatraemia in outpatients, hospital-acquired hypernatraemia affects patients of all ages. The clinical manifestations are even more elusive in hospitalized patients who often have pre-existing neurological dysfunction. As in children, rapid sodium loading in adults can cause convulsions and coma. In patients of all ages, orthostatic hypotension and tachycardia reflect marked hypovolaemia.

Hypernatraemia and the attendant hypertonicity elicit water abstraction from the brain resulting in its shrinkage (Fig. 8a and b). The reduction in cerebral volume can cause rupture of blood vessels that bridge the skull and the brain causing cerebral bleeding, subarachnoid haemorrhage, and permanent neurological damage or death. Within hours, however, an adaptive response ensues aimed at restoring brain volume towards baseline and accounts for the gradual improvement of symptomatology. Solute gain by the brain recalls lost water causing brain volume restitution. Electrolyte entry (sodium, potassium, and chloride) within the first few hours is responsible for the initial phase of this adaptation (Fig. 8c), whereas intracellular accumulation of organic solutes (known as idiogenic osmoles or organic osmolytes) completes the process (Fig. 8d). Hypertonicity-induced reduction in cell volume stresses the cytoskeleton, which activates a specific protein kinase; this kinase promotes protein phosphorylation causing activation of transporters that mediate solute uptake by brain cells (Galcheva-Gargova *et al.* 1994). The major brain organic osmolytes include glutamate, glutamine, taurine, and myo-inositol. This adaptation notwithstanding, restitution of brain volume does not correct brain hyperosmolality (Gullans and Verbalis 1993). In fact, this persistent hyperosmolality might induce life-threatening cerebral oedema during corrective hypotonic fluid administration (Fig. 8e).

The mortality rate varies widely according to the severity and the rapidity of onset of hypernatraemia. Separating the contribution to mortality of hypernatraemia itself from that caused by underlying illnesses is a vexing problem.

Management of hypernatraemia

Proper treatment of hypernatraemia requires a two-pronged approach: addressing the underlying cause and repairing the prevailing hypertonicity. Management of the underlying cause includes interruption of gastrointestinal fluid losses; control of pyrexia, hyperglycaemia and glucosuria, withholding lactulose and diuretics, prescription of dDAVP for central diabetes insipidus, correction of hypercalcaemia and hypokalaemia, adjustment of lithium dosage and possible use of amiloride, and correction of the feeding prescription.

In repairing the prevailing hypernatraemia, the clinician must address two questions: (a) what fluid should be administered? (b) At which rate? Depending on the pathogenesis of the hypernatraemia, different correction fluids are required. Inappropriate fluid selection can result in failure to correct the hypernatraemia, aggravation of the disorder, or treatment complications (e.g. pulmonary oedema). Similarly, the rate of fluid therapy must be properly determined to avoid severe adverse effects; overly slow administration of the correct fluid can prolong or even worsen the hypertonic state, whereas an unduly fast fluid therapy can result in cerebral oedema, seizures, permanent neurological damage, and even death.

In patients with acute hypernatraemia ($<$48 h in duration as seen in accidental sodium loading) rapid correction improves the prognosis

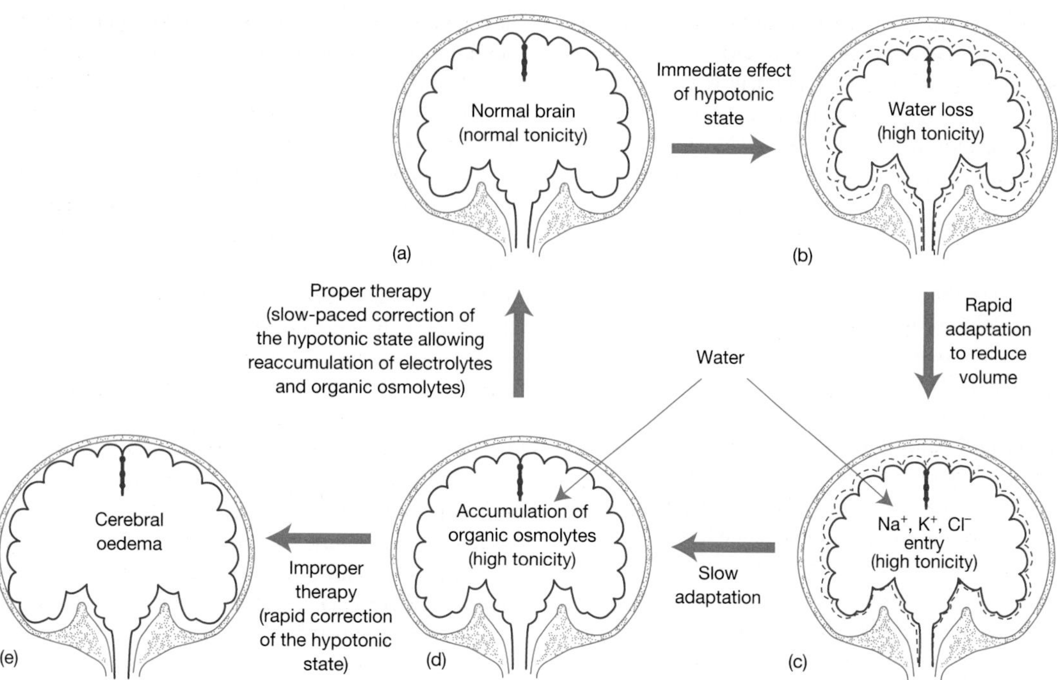

Fig. 8 Effects of hypernatraemia on the brain and adaptive responses. Within minutes after the development of hypertonicity, loss of water from brain cells causes shrinkage of the brain and an increase in osmolality (b). Partial restitution of brain volume occurs within a few hours as electrolytes enter the brain cells (rapid adaptation) (c). The normalization of brain volume is completed within several days as a result of the intracellular accumulation of organic osmolytes (slow adaptation) (d). The high osmolality persists despite the normalization of brain volume. Slow correction of the hypertonic state re-establishes normal brain osmolality without inducing cerebral oedema, as the dissipation of accumulated electrolytes and organic osmolytes keeps pace with water repletion (back to a). In contrast, rapid correction may result in cerebral oedema as water uptake by brain cells outpaces the dissipation of accumulated electrolytes and organic osmolytes. Such overly aggressive therapy carries the risk of serious neurological impairment due to cerebral oedema (e).

without increasing the risk of cerebral oedema, because accumulated electrolytes are rapidly extruded from brain cells. Reduction of the serum sodium by 1 mmol/l/h is appropriate. In patients with hypernatraemia of longer or unknown duration, a slower pace of correction is prudent because the full dissipation of accumulated brain solutes requires several days (Fig. 8). Reduction of serum sodium should thus not exceed 0.5 mmol/l/h to prevent cerebral oedema and convulsions. We recommend a targeted reduction in serum sodium of 10 mmol/l per day for all patients with hypernatraemia except those in whom the disorder has developed over a period of hours, the eventual goal being 145 mmol/l (Adrogué and Madias 2000b). Allowance must be made for ongoing losses of hypotonic fluids, whether obligatory or incidental. In addition, patients with seizures require prompt anticonvulsant therapy and adequate ventilation.

The preferred route for administering fluids is the oral route or a feeding tube; if neither is feasible or the likelihood of proper gastrointestinal absorption is questionable, fluids should be given intravenously. If the latter is not possible, fluids might be given subcutaneously (hypodermoclysis) (Challiner *et al.* 1994).

Among available fluids, only hypotonic fluids are suitable, including pure water, 5 per cent dextrose, 0.2 per cent sodium chloride ('one-quarter' isotonic saline), and 0.45 per cent sodium chloride (one-half isotonic saline). Their composition and fractional distribution in the ECF compartment are presented in Table 4. The choice of the hypotonic infusate impacts directly on the rate of fluid administration, the more hypotonic the lower the required rate of infusion. Because the risk of cerebral oedema increases with the volume of infusate, the volume should be restricted to that required to correct hypertonicity. Except in cases of frank circulatory compromise, 0.9 per cent sodium chloride (isotonic saline) is unsuitable for managing hypernatraemia.

After selecting the appropriate fluid, the physician must determine the rate of infusion. The simple formula presented in managing hyponatraemia (Eq. 6) is also applicable in treating hypernatraemia and estimates the change in serum sodium caused by the retention of 1 l of any infusate (Adrogué and Madias 1997). The required volume, and hence the infusion rate, is determined by dividing the change in serum sodium targeted for a given period by the value obtained from the formula. As previously emphasized, because of uncertainties about the effects of infusate as well as ongoing fluid losses, serum [Na$^+$] should be checked at frequent intervals during treatment. The following conventional formula for correction of hypernatraemia, should not be used:

$$\text{Water deficit} = \text{TBW} \times \left(\frac{\text{current serum } [\text{Na}^+]}{140} - 1\right) \qquad (8)$$

Although this formula provides an adequate estimate of the water deficit in patients with hypernatraemia caused by pure water loss, it underestimates the deficit in patients with hypotonic fluid loss (Fig. 6c and d). Further, it does not provide information on the differential impact of solutions of variable sodium concentration on the patient's hypernatraemia. For example, depending on whether a hypernatraemic patient is euvolaemic or hypovolaemic, repair of the disorder requires the administration of free water (i.e. 5 per cent dextrose in water) or sodium-containing solutions (e.g. isotonic saline, half-isotonic saline, or 'one-quarter' isotonic saline), respectively. This shortcoming is avoided by utilizing the recommended formula (Eq. 6). Table 8 depicts illustrative causes of severe hypernatraemia and their management.

Common errors in management

Isotonic saline is unsuitable for correcting hypernatraemia. Consider a 50-year-old man with a serum [Na^+] of 162 mmol/l and a body weight of 70 kg [estimated volume of total body water, 42 l (0.6 × 70)]. Retention of 1 l of 0.9 per cent sodium chloride will decrease serum [Na^+] by only 0.2 mmol/l ([154 − 162]/[42 + 1] = −0.2). Although the sodium concentration of the infusate is less than the patient's serum [Na^+], it is not sufficiently low to alter the hypernatraemia substantially. Furthermore, ongoing hypotonic fluid losses might outpace the administration of isotonic saline, aggravating the hypernatraemia. The sole indication for administering isotonic saline to a patient with hypernatraemia is depletion of ECF volume that is sufficient to cause substantial haemodynamic compromise. Even in this case, after a limited amount of isotonic saline has been administered to stabilize the patient's circulatory status, a hypotonic fluid (i.e. 0.2 or 0.45 per cent sodium chloride) should be substituted to restore normal haemodynamic values while correcting the hypernatraemia. If a hypotonic fluid is not substituted for isotonic saline, the ECF volume might become seriously overloaded.

Extreme care must be taken to avoid excessively rapid correction or overcorrection of hypernatraemia, with its attendant risk of iatrogenic cerebral oedema. Selecting the most hypotonic infusate that is suitable for the particular type of hypernatraemia ensures the administration of the least amount of fluid. Appropriate allowances for ongoing fluid losses must be made. Most important, the fluid prescription should be reassessed at regular intervals in the light of laboratory values and the patient's clinical status.

Long-term therapy of hypernatraemia

Patients suffering from conditions that predispose to the development of hypernatraemia require implementation of long-term therapy.

Primary hypodipsia Daily determination of body weight can help early detection of hypodipsia-induced dehydration in the elderly. In addition, adherence to a daily fluid-intake schedule promotes prevention and management of hypernatraemia in primary hypodipsia. Risk factors for dehydration include age more than 85 years, female gender, bedridden status, laxative use, chronic infections, more than four chronic disorders, and intake of more than four medications (Lavizzo-Mourrey *et al.* 1988). Consideration of the risk factors present in a given patient should aid prescription and implementation of measures against dehydration. In case of associated defect in vasopressin secretion, specific management is required.

Central diabetes insipidus Most patients with CDI have a normal or only mildly elevated serum sodium because of concurrent stimulation of thirst. They develop hypernatraemia only if thirst or access to water is impaired. Management aims primarily at the control of polyuria by hormone replacement therapy. The vasopressin analogue, desmopressin (also known as dDAVP, 1-desamino-8-D-arginine vasopressin) is usually administered as an intranasal spray once or twice a day (dose range, 5–20 μg) (Richardson and Robinson 1985). Desmopressin is also available as a tablet for oral intake with the daily maintenance dose ranging from 0.1 to 0.8 mg in divided doses. Water retention and development of hyponatraemia is an important potential risk to the use of desmopressin in CDI. Consequently, the minimum dose of the drug that is sufficient to control polyuria should be prescribed in association with continued patient education about water balance.

An additional tool to reduce urine output (i.e. from several litres per day in partial CDI or severe nephrogenic diabetes insipidus, and 10–15 l per day in severe CDI) is to restrict salt and protein intake. If, for example, the patient's maximal urine osmolality is 150 mOsm/kg H_2O and the daily obligatory solute load is reduced to 450 mmol/day, then the daily urine output reaches 3 l/day (450/150 = 3).

Less expensive non-hormonal drugs can be used to control polyuria in CDI, including chlorpropamide, carbamazepine, clofibrate, thiazide diuretics, or non-steroidal anti-inflammatory drugs (NSAIDs). Chlorpropamide, an oral hypoglycaemic agent, has been widely used to enhance the renal response to ADH or desmopressin and to stimulate ADH release. Carbamazepine, an antiseizure agent, increases the response to ADH, and clofibrate (lipid-lowering drug) increases ADH release. The above three drugs can reduce urine output by as much as 50 per cent. Hydrochlorothiazide and NSAID can limit polyuria independent of ADH and are therefore used either in CDI or nephrogenic diabetes insipidus.

Nephrogenic diabetes insipidus A mild form of nephrogenic diabetes insipidus is relatively common in elderly patients or those who have a renal disease that decreases modestly the maximum concentrating capacity. Nocturia develops but is generally not severe enough to result in polyuria. Conversely, symptomatic polyuria due to nephrogenic diabetes insipidus is most frequently the result of hypercalcaemia or chronic lithium use in adults or of an X-linked hereditary nephrogenic diabetes insipidus in children.

Therapy of symptomatic nephrogenic diabetes insipidus is primarily aimed at the correction of the underlying disorder whenever possible, or at the discontinuation of the toxic drug. Correction of hypercalcaemia usually improves or fully reverses the renal dysfunction; discontinuation of lithium therapy can eradicate or ameliorate lithium-induced nephrogenic diabetes insipidus. Lithium administration can increase plasma parathyroid hormone and rarely cause hypercalcaemia, which, in turn, exacerbates the lithium-induced urine concentrating defect.

If lithium therapy must continue, the concurrent administration of amiloride, a potassium-sparing diuretic, might improve mild to moderate urinary concentrating defects. Amiloride closes sodium channels in collecting tubule cells and reduces renal lithium accumulation. This measure is ineffective in patients with severe urinary concentrating defects. Amiloride therapy can cause volume depletion with an attendant increase in proximal lithium reabsorption requiring a reduction in daily lithium dosage.

If the underlying disease cannot be corrected, a number of generic measures can be applied to patients with nephrogenic diabetes insipidus to limit urine output. They include a decreased solute load (i.e. adherence to a low-sodium chloride and low-protein diet), diuretics, and NSAIDs. Diuretic agents, mostly thiazides, such as hydrochlorothiazide, 25 mg once or twice daily, coupled with a low-sodium chloride intake can reduce urine volume by about 50 per cent. They induce mild volume depletion, which in turn increases proximal fluid reabsorption and limits water delivery to the collecting tubule. A combination of thiazide and amiloride potentiates the overall effect and has the additional advantage of reducing thiazide-induced potassium losses. A loop diuretic might help diabetes insipidus by decreasing sodium chloride transport in the

Table 8 Managing severe hypernatraemia: illustrative cases

Case no.	Time (h)	Data	Diagnosis/treatment plan	Fluid prescription
1	0	80-year-old man with severe obtundation, fever, and tachypnoea; decreased skin turgor, dry mucous membranes, supine BP 137/80 mmHg without orthostatic changes; weight 64 kg $[Na^+]$ 166 mmol/l, $[K^+]$ 4.0 mmol/l, Sosm 345 mOsm/kg H_2O	Hypernatraemia due to unreplaced water losses 5% dextrose to reduce $[Na^+]$ by 10 mmol/l over 24 h	TBW, $0.5 \times 64 = 32$ l $\Delta[Na^+] = \frac{0 - 166}{32 + 1} = 5.0$ mmol /l per 1 l infusate For a goal of $\Delta[Na^+]$ 10 mmol/l/24 h, 10/5 = 2 l/24 h are required Adding 1.5 l to compensate for ongoing, obligatory water losses over the 24 h period 2 + 1.5 = 3.5 l/24 h are required or 146 ml/h
	6	Mental status unchanged; haemodynamically stable $[Na^+]$ 164 mmol/l	Treatment plan unchanged Close monitoring	Continue present infusate at 146 ml/h
	12	Moderate obtundation haemodynamically stable. $[Na^+]$ 160 mmol/l, glucose 110 mg/dl, Sosm 335 mOsm/kg H_2O	Treatment plan unchanged Watch for hyperglycaemia Close monitoring	Continue present infusate at 146 ml/h
2	0	48-year-old woman with bout of gastroenteritis, who presents with fever and moderate obtundation; decreased skin turgor, supine BP 110/70 mm; standing BP 100/65 mmHg; weight 60 kg $[Na^+]$ 156 mmol/l, $[K^+]$ 3.0 mmol/l, $[HCO_3^-]$ 28 mmol/l Sosm 325 mOsm/kg H_2O	Hypernatraemia due to hypotonic fluid losses; potassium depletion. Volume repletion, potassium repletion, 0.45% NaCl containing 20 mmol of KCl per litre to decrease $[Na^+]$ by 10 mmol/l over 24 h	TBW, $0.5 \times 60 = 30$ l $\Delta[Na^+] = \frac{(77 + 20) - 156}{30 + 1} = 1.9$ mmol/l per 1 l infusate For a goal of $\Delta[Na^+]$ 10 mmol/l/24 h 10/1.9 = 5.3 l/24 h are required Adding 2 l to compensate for ongoing fluid losses over the 24 h period, 5.3 + 2 = 7.3 l/24 h are required or ≅ 300 ml/h
	8	Mild obtundation, haemodynamically stable. $[Na^+]$ 154 mmol/l, $[K^+]$ 3.2 mmol/l	Unsatisfactory pace of correction Switch infustate to 0.2% NaCl containing 20 mmol of KCl per litre to decrease $[Na^+]$ by 6 mmol/l over 12 h	$\Delta[Na^+] = \frac{(34 + 20) - 154}{30 + 1} = -3.2$ mmol /l per 1 l infusate For a goal of $\Delta[Na^+]$ 6 mmol/l/12 h 6/3.2 = 1.9 l/24 h are required Adding 1 l to compensate for ongoing fluid losses over the 12 h period, 1.9 + 1 = 2.9 l/12 h are required or ≅ 240 ml/h
	20	Mildly somnolent, haemodynamically stable. $[Na^+]$ 149 mmol/l, $[K^+]$ 3.4 mmol/l	Pace of correction satisfactory	Continue present infusate at 240 ml/h

thick ascending limb of the loop of Henle. Because renal prostaglandins antagonize the action of ADH, inhibition of their renal synthesis by NSAIDs (e.g. indomethacin) can help control polyuria. Combination of NSAID and a thiazide diuretic can be used for increased effectiveness. Finally, exogenous vasopressin (i.e. dDAVP) can be of benefit in patients with inadequate response to other therapeutic agents; in fact, most patients with nephrogenic diabetes insipidus do not have complete resistance to vasopressin.

References

(Entries marked with an asterisk comprise useful general reading.)

Abramow, M., Beauwens, R., and Cogan, E. (1987). Cellular events in vasopressin action. *Kidney International Supplement* **21**, S56–S66.

*__Adrogué, H. J. and Madias, N. E.__ (1997). Aiding fluid prescription for the dysnatremias. *Intensive Care Medicine* **23**, 309–316.

*__Adrogué, H. J. and Madias, N. E.__ (2000a). Hyponatremia. *New England Journal of Medicine* **342**, 1581–1589.

*__Adrogué, H. J. and Madias N. E.__ (2000b). Hypernatremia. *New England Journal of Medicine* **342**, 1493–1499.

Agarwal, R. and Emmett, M. (1994). The post-transurethral resection of prostate syndrome: therapeutic proposals. *American Journal of Kidney Diseases* **24**, 108–111.

*__Agre, P.__ (2000). Aquaporin water channels in kidney. *Journal of the American Society of Nephrology* **11**, 764–777.

Arieff, A. I., Ayus, J. C., and Fraser, C. L. (1992). Hyponatraemia and death or permanent brain damage in healthy children. *British Medical Journal* **304**, 1218–1222.

Aronson, D. *et al.* (2002). Hyponatremia as a complication of cardiac catheterization: a prospective study. *American Journal of Kidney Diseases* **40**, 940–946.

Atkin, S. L. *et al.* (1996). Hyponatraemia secondary to cerebral salt wasting syndrome following routine pituitary surgery. *European Journal of Endocrinology* **135**, 245–247.

*__Ayus, J. C., Wheeler, J. M., and Arieff, A. I.__ (1992). Postoperative hyponatremic encephalopathy in menstruant women. *Annals of Internal Medicine* **117**, 891–897.

*__Bartter, F. C. and Schwartz, W. B.__ (1967). The syndrome of inappropriate secretion of antidiuretic hormone. *American Journal of Medicine* **42**, 790–806.

Baylis, P. H. (1987). Osmoregulation and control of vasopressin secretion in healthy humans. *American Journal of Physiology* **253**, R671–R678.

Benedict, C. R. ***et al.*** **for the SOLVD Investigators** (1994). Relation of neurohumoral activation to clinical variables and degree of ventricular dysfunction: a report from the Registry of Studies of Left Ventricular Dysfunction. *Journal of the American College of Cardiology* **23**, 1410–1420.

*__Berl, T.__ (1990). Treating hyponatremia: damned if we do and damned if we don't. *Kidney International* **37**, 1006–1018.

Bibl, D. *et al.* (1999). Treatment of central pontine myelinolysis with therapeutic plasmapheresis (letter). *Lancet* **353**, 1155.

Bichet, D. G., Oksche, A., and Rosenthal, W. (1997). Congenital nephrogenic diabetes insipidus. *Journal of the American Society of Nephrology* **8**, 1951–1958.

Bichet, D. G. *et al.* (1988). Hemodynamic and coagulation responses to 1-desamino [8-D-arginine] vasopressin in patients with congenital nephrogenic diabetes insipidus. *New England Journal of Medicine* **318**, 881–887.

Bie, P. *et al.* (1986). Cardiovascular and endocrine responses to head-up tilt and vasopressin infusion in humans. *American Journal of Physiology* **251**, R735–R741.

Bonvalet, J. P., Pradelles, P., and Farman, N. (1987). Segmental synthesis and actions of prostaglandins along the nephron. *American Journal of Physiology* **253**, F377–F387.

Brunner, J. E. *et al.* (1990). Central pontine myelinolysis and pontine lesions after rapid correction of hyponatremia: a prospective magnetic resonance imaging study. *Annals of Neurology* **27**, 61–66.

Challiner, Y. C. *et al.* (1994). A comparison of intravenous and subcutaneous hydration in elderly acute stroke patients. *Postgraduate Medical Journal* **70**, 195–197.

Cheng, J. C. *et al.* (1990). Long-term neurological outcome in psychogenic water drinkers with severe symptomatic hyponatremia: the effect of rapid correction. *American Journal of Medicine* **88**, 561–566.

Chou, C. L. *et al.* (1999). Reduced water permeability and altered ultrastructure in thin descending limb of Henle in aquaporin-1 null mice. *Journal of Clinical Investigation* **103**, 491–496.

Chung, H. M. *et al.* (1986). Postoperative hyponatremia: a prospective study. *Archives of Internal Medicine* **146**, 333–336.

Cluitmans, F. H. M. and Meinders, A. E. (1990). Management of severe hyponatremia: rapid or slow correction? *American Journal of Medicine* **88**, 161–166.

Deen, P. M. *et al.* (1994). Requirement for human renal water channel aquaporin-2 for vasopressin-dependent concentration of urine. *Science* **264**, 92–95.

Dzau, V. J. and Hollenberg, N. K. (1984). Renal response to captopril in severe heart failure: role of furosemide in natriuresis and reversal of hyponatremia. *Annals of Internal Medicine* **100**, 777–782.

Ecelbarger, C. A. *et al.* (1997). Role of renal aquaporins in escape from vasopressin-induced antidiuresis in rats. *Journal of Clinical Investigation* **99**, 1852–1863.

Fichman, M. P. *et al.* (1971). Diuretic-induced hyponatremia. *Annals of Internal Medicine* **75**, 853–863.

Fox, B. D. (2002). Crash diet potomania. *Lancet* **359**, 942.

Frizzell, R. T. *et al.* (1986). Hyponatremia and ultramarathon running. *Journal of the American Medical Association* **255**, 772–774.

Galcheva-Gargova, Z. *et al.* (1994). An osmosensing signal transduction pathway in mammalian cells. *Science* **265**, 806–808.

Gennari, F. J. Hypo–hypernatraemia: disorders of water balance. In *Oxford Textbook of Clinical Nephrology* 2nd edn., pp. 175–200. Oxford: Oxford University Press, 1998.

Gowrishankar, M. *et al.* (1998). Acute hyponatremia in the perioperative period: insights into its pathophysiology and recommendations for management. *Clinical Nephrology* **50**, 352–360.

*__Gross, P.__ (2001). Treatment of severe hyponatremia. *Kidney International* **60**, 2417–2427.

Gullans, S. R. and Verbalis, J. (1993). Control of brain volume during hyperosmolar and hypoosmolar conditions. *Annual Review of Medicine* **44**, 289–301.

Hanna, F. W. and Scanlon, M. F. (1997). Hyponatremia, hypothyroidism, and role of arginine-vasopressin. *Lancet* **350**, 755–756.

Harris, H. W., Jr., Strange, K., and Ziedel, M. (1991). Current understanding of the cellular biology and molecular structure of antidiuretic hormone-stimulated water transport pathway. *Journal of Clinical Investigation* **88**, 1–8.

Hebert, R. L., Jacobson, H. R., and Breyer, M. D. (1990). PGE2 inhibits AVP-induced water flow in cortical collecting ducts by protein kinase C activation. *American Journal of Physiology* **259**, F318–F325.

Hensen, J. *et al.* (1999). Prevalence, predictors and patterns of postoperative polyuria and hyponatraemia in the immediate course after transsphenoidal surgery for pituitary adenomas. *Clinical Endocrinology (Oxford)* **50**, 431–439.

Hochberg, Z. *et al.* (1997). Autosomal recessive nephrogenic diabetes insipidus caused by an aquaporin-2 mutation. *Journal of Clinical Endocrinology and Metabolism* **82**, 686–689.

Inoue, H. *et al.* (1998). A gene encoding a transmembrane protein is mutated in patients with diabetes mellitus and optic atrophy (Wolfram syndrome). *Nature Genetics* **20**, 143–148.

Istre, O. *et al.* (1994). Postoperative cerebral oedema after transcervical endometrial resection and uterine irrigation with 1.5% glycine. *Lancet* **344**, 1187–1189.

Kim, J. K. *et al.* (1996). Osmotic and non-osmotic regulation of arginine vasopressin (AVP) release, mRNA, and promoter activity in small cell lung carcinoma (SCLC) cells. *Molecular and Cellular Endocrinology* **123**, 179–186.

Laureno, R. and Karp, B. I. (1997). Myelinolysis after correction of hyponatremia. *Annals of Internal Medicine* **126**, 57–62.

Lauriat, S. M. and Berl, T. (1997). The hyponatremic patient: practical focus on therapy. *Journal of the American Society of Nephrology* **8**, 1599–1607.

Lavizzo-Mourrey, R., Johnson, J., and Stalley, P. (1988). Risk factors for dehydration among elderly nursing home residents. *Journal of the American Geriatrics Society* **36**, 213–218.

Leier, C. V., Dei Cas, L., and Metra, M. (1994). Clinical relevance and management of the major electrolyte abnormalities in congestive heart failure: hyponatremia, hypokalemia, and hypomagnesemia. *American Heart Journal* **128**, 564–574.

Lien, Y. H., Shapiro, J. L., and Chan, L. (1991). Study of brain electrolytes and organic osmolytes during correction of chronic hyponatremia: implications for the pathogenesis of central pontine myelinolysis. *Journal of Clinical Investigation* **88**, 303–309.

Lindheimer, M. D., Marron, W. M., and Davison, J. M. (1989). Osmoregulation of thirst and vasopressin release in pregnancy. *American Journal of Physiology* **257**, F159–F169.

Maas, A. H. J. *et al.* (1985). Ion-selective electrodes for sodium and potassium: a new problem of what is measured and what should be reported. *Clinical Chemistry* **31**, 482–485.

Mann, J. F. E. *et al.* (1987). Thirst and the renin–angiotensin system. *Kidney International Supplement* **21**, S27–S34.

Marples, D. *et al.* (1996). Hypokalemia-induced downregulation of aquaporin-2 water channel expression in rat kidney medulla and cortex. *Journal of Clinical Investigation* **97**, 1960–1968.

Melton, J. E. *et al.* (1987). Volume regulatory loss of Na, Cl and K from rat brain during acute hyponatremia. *American Journal of Physiology* **252**, F661–F669.

*Oh, M. S., Kim, H. J., and Carroll, H. J. (1995). Recommendations for treatment of symptomatic hyponatremia. *Nephron* **70**, 143–150.

Oliet, S. H. and Bourque, C. W. (1993). Mechanosensitive channels transduce osmosensitivity in supraoptic neurons. *Nature* **364**, 341–343.

Palevsky, P. M., Bhagrath, R., and Greenberg, A. (1996). Hypernatremia in hospitalized patients. *Annals of Internal Medicine* **124**, 197–203.

Papadakis, M. A., Fraser, C. L., and Arieff, A. I. (1990). Hyponatraemia in patients with cirrhosis. *Quarterly Journal of Medicine* **76**, 675–688.

Piedrola, G. *et al.* (1996). Clinical features of adrenal insufficiency in patients with acquired immunodeficiency syndrome. *Clinical Endocrinology* **45**, 97–101.

Richardson, D. W. and Robinson, A. G. (1985). Desmopressin. *Annals of Internal Medicine* **103**, 228–239.

Robertson, G. L. (1984). Abnormalities of thirst regulation. *Kidney International* **25**, 460–469.

Robertson, G. L. (1987). Physiology of ADH secretion. *Kidney International Supplement* **21**, S20–S26.

Robertson, G. L. Regulation of vasopressin secretion. In *The Kidney: Physiology and Pathophysiology* 2nd edn. (ed. D.W. Seldin and G. Giebisch), pp. 1595–1613. New York: Raven Press, 1992.

Saito, T. *et al.* (1997). Acute aquaresis by the nonpeptide arginine vasopressin (AVP) antagonist OPC-31260 improves hyponatremia in patients with syndrome of inappropriate secretion of antidiuretic hormone (SIADH). *Journal of Clinical Endocrinology and Metabolism* **82**, 1054–1057.

Sands, J. M. and Kokko, J. P. (1996). Current concepts of the countercurrent multiplication system. *Kidney International Supplement* **57**, S93–S99.

Sasaki, S. *et al.* (1994). Cloning, characterization, and chromosomal mapping of human aquaporin of collecting duct. *Journal of Clinical Investigation* **93**, 1250–1256.

*Schrier, R. W. (1988). Pathogenesis of sodium and water retention in high-output and low-output cardiac failure, nephrotic syndrome, cirrhosis and pregnancy. *New England Journal of Medicine* **319**, 1065–1072 and 1127–1134.

Schrier, R. W. *et al.* (1988). Peripheral arterial vasodilation hypothesis: a proposal for the initiation of renal sodium and water retention in cirrhosis. *Hepatology* **8**, 1151–1157.

Serradeil-Le Gal, C. *et al.* (1996). Characterization of SR 121463A, a highly potent and selective, orally active vasopressin V2 receptor antagonist. *Journal of Clinical Investigation* **98**, 2729–2738.

Shiau, Y. F. *et al.* (1985). Stool electrolyte and osmolality measurements in the evaluation of diarrheal disorders. *Annals of Internal Medicine* **102**, 773–775.

Soupart, A. *et al.* (1994). Prevention of brain demyelination in rats after excessive correction of chronic hyponatremia be serum sodium lowering. *Kidney International* **45**, 193–200.

Soupart, A. *et al.* (1999). Therapeutic relowering of the serum sodium in a patient after excessive correction of hyponatremia. *Clinical Nephrology* **51**, 383–386.

Sugimoto, T. *et al.* (1994). Molecular cloning and functional expression of a cDNA encoding the human V1b vasopressin receptor. *Journal of Biological Chemistry* **269**, 27088–27092.

Tanneau, R. S. *et al.* (1994). High incidence of neurologic complications following rapid correction of severe hyponatremia in polydipsic patients. *Journal of Clinical Psychiatry* **55**, 349–354.

Teitelbaum, I. and McGuiness, S. (1995). Vasopressin resistance in chronic renal failure. Evidence for the role of decreased V2 receptor mRNA. *Journal of Clinical Investigation* **96**, 378–385.

Teree, T. M. *et al.* (1965). Stool losses and acidosis in diarrheal disease of infancy. *Pediatrics* **36**, 704–713.

Thaler, S. M., Teitelbaum, I., and Berl, T. (1998). 'Beer potomania' in non-beer drinkers: effect of low dietary solute intake. *American Journal of Kidney Diseases* **31**, 1028–1031.

Thompson, C. J., Burd, J. M., and Baylis, P. H. (1991). Reproducibility of osmotic and nonosmotic tests of vasopressin secretion in men. *American Journal of Physiology* **260**, R533–R539.

Tsuboi, Y. *et al.* (1994). Therapeutic efficacy of the non-peptide AVP antagonist OPC-31260 in cirrhotic rats. *Kidney International* **46**, 237–244.

Verbalis, J. G. Inappropriate antidiuresis and other hypoosmolar states. In *Principles and Practice of Endocrinology and Metabolism* (ed. K. G. Becker). Philadelphia: Lippincott, 1995.

Vitting, K. E. *et al.* (1990). Frequency of hyponatemia and nonosmolar vasopressin release in the acquired immunodeficiency syndrome. *Journal of the American Medical Association* **263**, 973–978.

Wang, W. H., Lu, M., and Hebert, S. C. (1996). Cytochrome P-450 metabolites mediate extracellular Ca (2+)-induced inhibition of apical K+ channels in the TAL. *American Journal of Physiology* **271**, C103–C111.

Xu, D. L. *et al.* (1997). Upregulation of aquaporin-2 water channel expression in chronic heart failure rat. *Journal of Clinical Investigation* **99**, 1500–1505.

Yared, A., Kon, V., and Ichikawa, I. (1985). Mechanism of preservation of glomerular perfusion and filtration during acute extracellular fluid volume depletion. Importance of intrarenal vasopressin–prostaglandin interaction for protecting kidneys from constrictor action of vasopressin. *Journal of Clinical Investigation* **75**, 1477–1487.

Zimmerhackl, B., Robertson, C. R., and Jamison, R. L. (1985). Fluid uptake in the renal papilla by vasa recta estimated by two methods simultaneously. *American Journal of Physiology* **248**, F347–F353.

Zimmerman, E. A., Ma, L. Y., and Nilaver, G. (1987). Anatomical basis of thirst and vasopressin secretion. *Kidney International Supplement* **21**, S14–S19.

2.2 Hypo–hyperkalaemia

Richard L. Tannen and Kenneth R. Hallows

Potassium homeostasis

Body potassium content and distribution

Potassium is the major intracellular cation in the body. Its plasma concentration normally ranges from 3.4 to 4.6 mmol/1; it is approximately 0.4 mmol/1 greater in serum, because of K^+ release from cellular components during clot formation, whereas the intracellular concentration is estimated to be approximately 150 mmol/1.

As outlined in Fig. 1, the high intracellular concentration of K^+ is maintained through several factors that govern K^+ uptake and release from the intracellular compartment. K^+ uptake into the cell is mediated by Na^+,K^+-ATPase, a pump that couples the energy of ATP hydrolysis to the electrogenic extrusion of sodium and uptake of potassium, with a stoichiometry of three Na^+ to two K^+ ions for each ATP hydrolyzed. In steady-state conditions, the rate of active K^+ uptake through the pump is counterbalanced by passive K^+ losses through various leak pathways. The negative intracellular voltage generated by the electrogenic pump serves to retard, whereas the high chemical gradient (intracellular K^+ greater than extracellular K^+) promotes K^+ leakage from the cell. The rate of this leakage is modulated by the electrochemical driving force, and by the permeability characteristics of the membrane, which are determined primarily by ion-selective K^+ channels. These channels are physiologically regulated by a variety of intracellular mediators.

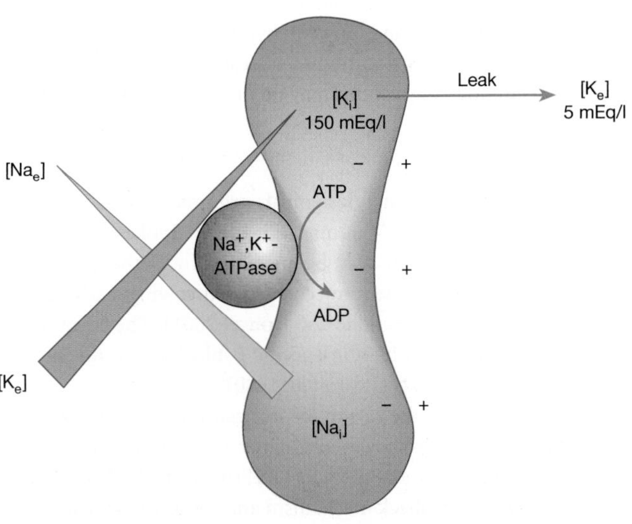

Fig. 1 Regulation of intracellular K^+. Potassium uptake by cells is actively driven by Na^+,K^+-ATPase. Leak-back into the extracellular space is opposed by the electrical gradient (cell interior—negative), favoured by the chemical gradient [intracellular K^+ (K_i^+) > extracellular K^+ (K_e^+)] and modulated by the permeability characteristics of the membrane. [From Kokko, J.P. and Tannen, R.L. (1986). *Fluids and Electrolytes*. Philadelphia: Saunders (with permission).]

The normal total body potassium content depends predominantly on muscle mass (Pierson *et al.* 1984). As shown in Table 1, it is maximal in young adults, declines progressively with age, and is less in women than men because of a lower ratio of muscle mass to fat.

More than 90 per cent of total body potassium is located in the intracellular compartment, mainly in muscle (60–75 per cent). Only 1.4 per cent of the total body K^+ is contained within the water space of the extracellular fluid, with the remainder of extracellular K^+ sequestered in bone.

The defence of extracellular K^+ concentration is sustained by factors that regulate transcellular K^+ distribution and by the kidney, which dictates the body K^+ balance. A hepatic sensor of oral K^+ intake that can modify renal K^+ excretion may also play a role in sustaining K^+ balance (Morita *et al.* 2000).

Transcellular potassium distribution

The transmembrane K^+ gradient largely determines the resting membrane potential of cells. Therefore, alterations in the transcellular distribution of K^+ can profoundly affect critical neuromuscular functions. A variety of factors, listed in Table 2, modulate the distribution of potassium between the intracellular (K_i^+) and extracellular (K_e^+) fluid compartments (Sterns *et al.* 1981; Sterns and Spital 1987). They alter the K_i^+/K_e^+ ratio by modifying either the pump or the leakage mechanisms that dictate intra- and extracellular K^+ concentrations. Some of

Table 1 Total body K^+ content (mmol/kg)

Age (years)	Male	Female
10	37	37
20	58	45
40	52	40
60	48	37
80	45	33

Adapted from data of Pierson *et al.* (1984).

Table 2 Factors that modify transcellular K^+ distribution

Acid–base status
Blood pH
Plasma HCO_3 concentration
Pancreatic hormones
Insulin
Glucagon
Catecholamines
β-Adrenergic
α-Adrenergic
Aldosterone
Plasma osmolality
Exercise
Cellular K^+ content

Adapted with permission from Tannen (1990).

them serve as essential, acute defence mechanisms to counteract life-threatening hypo- or hyperkalaemia.

Acid–base status

Alkalaemia promotes whereas acidaemia diminishes K^+ uptake by cells. The activation of the ATP-dependent K^+ channels by a reduction in intracellular pH appears to account for the acid–base effects on transcellular K^+ distribution (Standen 1992), but inhibition of the Na^+–K^+ pump by intracellular acidosis may also play a part (Ehrenfeld *et al.* 1992).

The quantitative impact of various acid–base perturbations on the plasma K^+ concentration is rather variable (Adrogue and Madias 1981). Metabolic acidosis produced by mineral acids, that is, hyperchloraemic acidosis, results in an average increment in plasma K^+ of 0.7 mmol for each 0.1 pH unit. By contrast, in dogs with metabolic acidosis produced by the acute infusion of organic acids such as β-hydroxybutyric acid, and in humans with lactic acidosis secondary to seizures, the plasma K^+ is unaltered by the acidaemia (Orringer *et al.* 1977; Oster *et al.* 1978). Some studies suggest that stimulation of insulin release by organic acids may counteract the hyperkalaemic properties of the acidaemia (Adrogue *et al.* 1985). It has also been postulated that organic acids are more cell permeant and thus less likely to cause a shift of K^+ out of cells due to an enhanced ability of the organic anion to accompany H^+ into cells (Graber 1993).

The response to respiratory acidosis depends on both the severity and duration of the abnormality; nevertheless, the increment in plasma K^+ is less than with metabolic acidosis and averages approximately 0.1 mmol/l per 0.1 pH unit.

Alkalaemia produced by metabolic alkalosis decreases the plasma K^+ concentration by an average of 0.3 mmol/l per 0.1 pH unit. A high concentration of bicarbonate, independent of alkalaemia, also reduces the plasma K^+ concentration by an average of 0.1 mmol/l for each 1.0 mmol/l increment under hyperkalaemic conditions. Acute respiratory alkalosis, in contrast to previously accepted views, increases rather than decreases plasma K^+ concentration by 0.2 mmol/l per 0.1 pH unit, as a result of enhanced α-adrenergic activity (Krapf *et al.* 1995).

The effect of pH on intracellular K^+ is not similar in all tissues (Hall and Cameron 1981). In animals subjected to respiratory acidosis, cardiac muscle accumulates K^+ concurrently with losses from skeletal muscle.

Pancreatic hormones

Insulin stimulates cellular uptake of K^+ by activating the Na^+–K^+ pump (Bia and DeFronzo 1981; Sterns and Spital 1987) through activation of the pump isoform containing an $\alpha2$ catalytic subunit located in muscle and adipocytes (Marette *et al.* 1993). Consistent with the known intrinsic tyrosine kinase activity of the insulin receptor, such insulin-induced stimulation of Na^+–K^+ pump activity appears to result from phosphorylation of the α-subunit at Tyr-10 (Feraille *et al.* 1999). Insulin affects K^+ transport independently of glucose uptake. Indeed, uraemic patients with impaired glucose tolerance have normal insulin-mediated uptake of K^+ (Alvestrand *et al.* 1984).

Insulin release by the pancreas is itself mediated by the plasma K^+ concentration: a high K^+ concentration stimulates whereas a low K^+ concentration inhibits insulin secretion (Bia and DeFronzo 1981; Sterns *et al.* 1981). Although the magnitude of the change in plasma K^+ required to alter the release of insulin is controversial, there appears to be a K^+–insulin feedback control mechanism that defends the plasma K^+ within the pathological, and possibly the physiological, range of concentrations. Enhanced pancreatic insulin secretion in the face of hyperkalaemia could result from a hyperkalaemia-induced net depolarization of pancreatic β cells, which would promote Ca^{2+} entry into the cells and subsequent insulin release (Henquin 2000).

Glucagon increases the plasma K^+ concentration independently of changes in plasma glucose and insulin, whereas a high plasma K^+ concentration can stimulate glucagon release (Massara *et al.* 1980). Although this relation would seem to impair K^+ homeostasis, when viewed in the context of simultaneous changes in insulin it may have an important regulatory function (Knochel 1977). Thus, concurrent stimulation of glucagon and insulin release by an elevated K^+ concentration can defend K^+ and prevent hypoglycaemia, provided that insulin alters the K^+ translocation to a greater degree than glucagon. Experiments in dogs suggest this may be the case (Hiatt *et al.* 1986).

Catecholamines

Similar to insulin, β_2-adrenergic agonists promote cellular K^+ uptake by activating the Na^+–K^+ pump (Silva and Spokes 1981). This Na^+–K^+ pump activation may be mediated by both cyclic AMP-dependent and -independent mechanisms involving activation of protein kinases A and C (Feraille and Doucet 2001). The effect on K^+ translocation is inhibited by non-specific β-blocking agents, but not by selective β_1-antagonists (Rosa *et al.* 1980).

Modest increases in the serum K^+ concentration do not alter the release of catecholamines; however, a higher concentration may stimulate secretion by the adrenal medulla (DeFronzo *et al.* 1981). Thus, a K^+–catecholamine feedback mechanism analogous to the insulin–K^+ interaction may also have a protective role in the defence against life-threatening hyperkalaemia.

The effects of α-adrenergic agonists on transcellular K^+ distribution are variable depending on the tissue and α-receptor subtype. Stimulation of kidney proximal tubule Na^+ transport in response to noradrenaline occurs primarily via stimulation of the Na^+–K^+ pump in basolateral membranes, which is mediated at least in part by

α1-adrenergic receptors (Feraille and Doucet 2001). Similarly, α1-adrenergic receptor-mediated stimulation in Na^+–K^+ pump activity has been reported in heart muscle and brain, both through intracellular Ca^{2+}-dependent mechanisms (Wang *et al.* 1998; Mallick *et al.* 2000). However, α2-adrenergic receptors appear to have either no effect (in rats and dogs) or an inhibitory effect (in rabbits) on Na^+ transport (and by implication Na^+–K^+ pump activity) in the kidney proximal tubule (Feraille and Doucet 2001). By contrast, in earlier studies involving healthy human volunteers, the α-agonist phenylephrine accentuated the hyperkalaemia produced by KCl infusion or by exercise, and these effects were counteracted by the α-antagonist phentolamine (Williams *et al.* 1984, 1985). Thus, on a whole-body level, it appears that the net effect of non-specific α-adrenergic stimulation is to provoke a net shift of K^+ out of cells, although the relevant tissues, cell types and precise cellular mechanisms remain to be clarified.

Aldosterone

Data from *in vivo* and *in vitro* experiments suggest that aldosterone may alter transcellular K^+ distribution; however, none of the studies is completely conclusive (Cox *et al.* 1978). *In vitro* studies have shown that aldosterone can stimulate Na^+–K^+ pump activity in muscle by enhancing Na^+ influx (Adler 1970; Wehling 1995; Mihailidou *et al.* 1998). The extrarenal tolerance to an acute K^+ load, induced by a high-K^+ diet, is abolished by adrenalectomy (Alexander and Levinsky 1968; DeFronzo *et al.* 1980). However, this might be explained by alterations in catecholamine metabolism or, alternatively, by a heretofore unrecognized renal effect related to a flaw in the design of these experiments (Spital and Sterns 1989). Alterations in the ${K_i}^+/{K_e}^+$ ratio produced by aldosterone could reflect a direct hormonal effect on the translocation of K^+, but, alternatively, the ratio might be altered as a result of K^+ depletion (Young and Jackson 1982). Perhaps the most compelling finding is that exogenous deoxycorticosterone acetate enhanced, and spironolactone impaired, disposal of an acute K^+ load in dialysis patients (Sugarman and Brown 1988). However, although K^+ excretion in the stool was unmodified in this study, acute alterations in colonic K^+ secretion cannot be excluded with certainty.

Osmolality

Hyperosmolality, produced by either mannitol infusion or by hyperglycaemia in diabetic individuals, increases the plasma K^+ concentration (Makoff *et al.* 1971; Cox *et al.* 1978). K^+ leaves the cells as a result of solvent drag and/or increased ${K_i}^+$ secondary to cellular dehydration. Each 10 mOsm/kg increase in plasma osmolality raises plasma K^+ concentration by an average of 0.6 mmol/l, but this should be seen as a rough guideline only (Moreno *et al.* 1969).

Exercise

Recurrent contraction results in K^+ egress from muscle. With modest amounts of exercise the high K^+ concentration of extracellular fluid in the local environment produces vasodilatation and thereby increases regional blood flow (Sejersted and Sjogaard 2000). Vigorous, sustained exercise increases the plasma K^+ concentration modestly, but severe hyperkalaemia can result from exhaustive exercise. Physical training increases the Na^+,K^+-ATPase activity of skeletal muscle (Knochel *et al.* 1985). This adaptation reduces the magnitude of exercise-induced hyperkalaemia by increasing the capacity of skeletal muscle to take up K^+ again.

Cellular potassium content

Intracellular K^+ concentration affects the intra- to extracellular K^+ ratio (Tannen 1983). With K^+ depletion, K^+ loss from the extracellular compartment is proportionately greater than from the intracellular space, thereby increasing the ${K_i}^+/{K_e}^+$ ratio. By contrast, with K^+ retention this ratio is reduced below normal. These changes produce hyperpolarization with K^+ depletion and depolarization with hyperkalaemia (Knochel 1981), as expected given the resultant changes in the Nernst equilibrium potential for K^+. However, with very severe K^+ depletion, pathological phenomena occur which diminish membrane polarization (Knochel 1981) through as yet undefined mechanisms.

Potassium balance

With a standard Western diet the daily ingestion of K^+ ranges from 0.75 to 1.25 mmol/kg body weight. However, K^+ balance can be sustained with intakes as high as 5.0–10.0 mmol/kg. The kidney is dominant in sustaining K^+ balance. More than 90 per cent of K^+ is excreted in the urine and the remainder is eliminated in the stool. When the glomerular filtration rate (GFR) is substantially compromised (<30 ml/min), the absolute magnitude as well as the proportion of K^+ excreted via the faecal route is increased (Hayes *et al.* 1967; Panese *et al.* 1987).

Gastrointestinal transport

Secretion by the colon accounts for the majority of K^+ eliminated in the stool. Both the proximal and distal portions of the colon secrete K^+, but the transport mechanisms and the response to various stimuli differ between these two segments (Ornt *et al.* 1987; Kunzelmann and Mall 2002).

Proximal colon reabsorbs Na^+ and secretes K^+ predominantly via transcellular mechanisms, but also by a paracellular, voltage-dependent pathway. Aldosterone enhances these transports without effects on either transmural potential difference or short-circuit current.

Distal colon can either reabsorb or secrete K^+. Aldosterone also increases Na^+ absorption and K^+ secretion by this segment together with a raised transmural potential difference. In contrast to proximal colon, these effects are inhibited by amiloride. The enhanced capacity to secrete K^+ in response to a high-K^+ diet is more prominent in the distal colon, whereas the diminution in K^+ secretion in response to a low-K^+ diet is more prominent in the proximal colon. The different K^+ transport systems involved and their control have been described in detail in a recent review (Kunzelmann and Mall 2002).

Renal transport (Fig. 2)

Potassium is freely filtered by the glomerulus and reabsorbed along the course of the proximal convoluted tubule and thick ascending limb of the loop of Henle (Giebisch 1998). Either reabsorption or secretion can occur as fluid traverses the proximal straight tubule. Nevertheless, in superficial cortical nephrons, approximately 90 per cent of filtered K^+ has been reabsorbed by the early distal tubule. Regulation of K^+ excretion depends primarily on factors that influence potassium secretion, and less commonly reabsorption, at distal nephron sites including the terminal portion of the distal convoluted tubule, and the cortical and medullary collecting duct.

At a cellular level, K^+ secretion by the principal cells of the distal tubular epithelium is dictated by the model shown in Fig. 3 (Muto 2001).

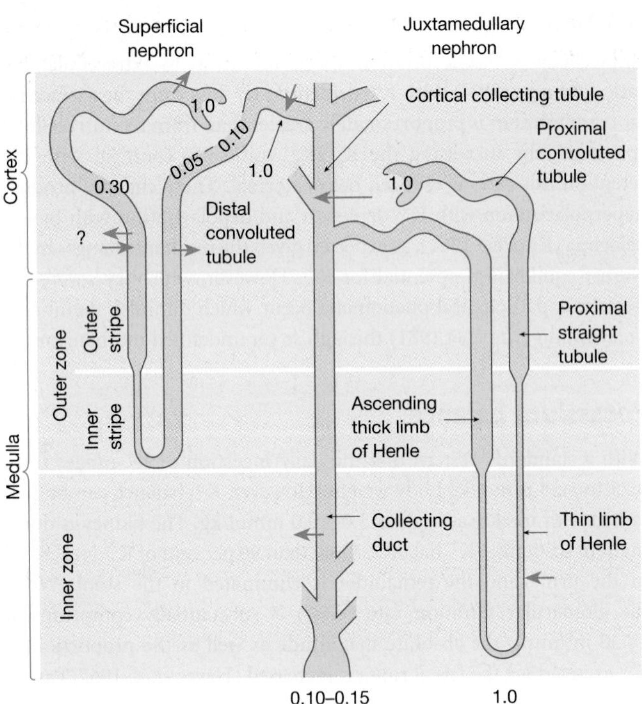

Fig. 2 Sites of K^+ handling by the nephron. Fractional delivery of K^+ under conditions of normal dietary K^+ intake is depicted for both superficial and juxtamedullary nephrons. Values are given at those sites where general agreement exists based on micropuncture experiments in the rat. Arrows show the predominant directions of net K^+ movement at varying sites along the tubule. [From Massry, S.G. and Glassock, R.J. (1983). *Textbook of Nephrology*. Baltimore: Williams and Wilkins (with permission).]

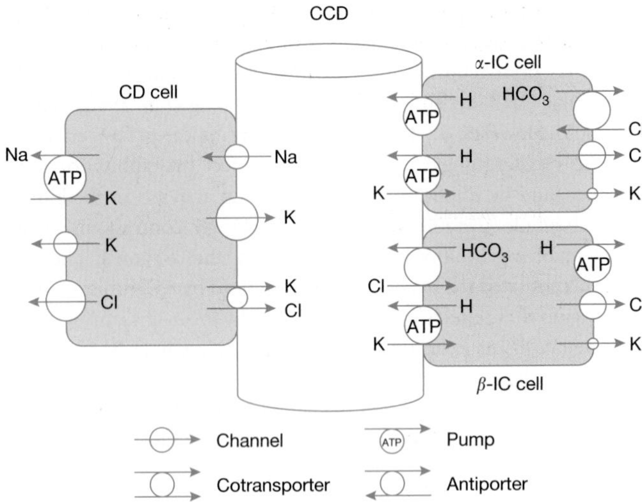

Fig. 3 Major transport systems in the collecting duct of the distal nephron in rabbits. The principal cells secrete K^+ into the tubular fluid. K^+ uptake across the peritubular membrane is driven actively by Na^+,K^+-ATPase, which extrudes Na^+ and takes up K^+ at the basolateral membrane. K^+ movement from the cell into the tubular fluid occurs through apically located K^+ channels and is driven by an electrochemical gradient that favours secretion. K^+ also can be secreted via an electroneutral KCl secretory mechanism in the cortical collecting duct. The α-intercalated cells reabsorb K^+ via H^+,K^+-ATPase situated in the apical membrane with an attendant proton secretion. They also secrete protons via H^+-ATPase located in the apical membrane. K^+ exits from the basolateral membrane through low-conductance K^+ channels and also, at least, in mice, through a KCl cotransporter (Boettger *et al.* 2002). In β-intercalated cells, the K^+ transport pathways are the same, but the membrane locations of the H^+-ATPase and Cl^-/HCO_3^- exchanger are reversed, allowing net HCO_3^- secretion into the lumen. [From Muto, S. (2001). Potassium transport in the mammalian collecting duct. *Physiological Reviews* **81**, 85–116 (with permission).]

Active K^+ uptake across the basolateral membrane is mediated by the Na^+–K^+ pump. K^+ leaves the cell across the apical membrane. Transport by the apical membrane is passive via K^+ channels and is governed by the prevailing electrochemical gradient. These channels, determining the permeability characteristics of the membrane, are controlled by regulatory mechanisms. K^+ channels in the basolateral membrane govern the rate of back-leakage into the blood.

Potassium reabsorption by the α-intercalated cells of the distal nephron is accompanied by proton secretion. Both processes are mediated by a H^+,K^+-ATPase located on the apical membrane (Wingo and Cain 1993).

In some situations, reduced K^+ absorption by the loop of Henle may contribute to heightened urinary elimination of K^+ (Jamison 1987). Furthermore, juxtamedullary nephrons handle K^+ in a different fashion than do superficial nephrons (Jamison 1987). In these segments, K^+ absorbed by the thick ascending limb and outer medullary collecting duct is secreted by the straight proximal tubule and upper portion of the descending limb of the loop of Henle. This medullary recycling sustains a high K^+ concentration in the inner medulla and may contribute to the regulation of K^+ excretion in two ways. First, a high medullary K^+ concentration decreases Na^+ reabsorption by the thick ascending limb and thereby promotes K^+ secretion by enhancing the rate of Na^+ delivery to more distal nephron sites. Second, a high K^+ concentration in the medullary interstitium may impede K^+ reabsorption by the inner medullary collecting duct.

Whereas the role of medullary recycling in governing K^+ excretion requires further definition, various factors that alter distal K^+ secretion (Table 3) and thereby urinary elimination have been well characterized. It is important to appreciate that it is rare for one of these factors to be modified in isolation, so K^+ excretion is usually the aggregate result of several complementary or competing stimuli.

Plasma K^+ concentration

Potassium secretion across the distal tubular epithelium is directly proportional to the prevailing plasma K^+ concentration. An elevation in peritubular K^+ concentration activates the Na^+,K^+-ATPase pump (Feraille and Doucet 2001), lowering intracellular $[Na^+]$ and raising intracellular $[K^+]$, which, in turn, lead to an increase in apical Na^+ conductance along with increases in both basolateral and apical K^+ conductance through ROMK (Muto *et al.* 1999). The combination of these events stimulates K^+ secretion by increasing the driving force for K^+ secretion and the conductance across the plasma membrane. The effect of plasma K^+ concentration on urinary elimination can be masked when fractional K^+ excretion is considered, because the K^+ excretion rate per unit GFR is divided by the prevailing plasma K^+ concentration.

Table 3 Factors that modify K^+ secretion by the distal nephron

Plasma K^+ concentration
Flow rate
Sodium
Transepithelial potential difference
Anions
Adrenal hormones Aldosterone Glucocorticoids
Acid–base factors System pH Ammonia
Other hormones Vasopressin Catecholamines Insulin
Dietary K^+ intake

Adapted with permission from Tannen (1990).

Flow rate

Potassium secretion by the distal nephron is directly proportional to the rate of fluid delivery to this site (Muto 2001). As secretion across the apical membrane is governed by the chemical gradient, increased delivery of fluid stimulates the secretory process by lowering K^+ concentration in the tubular fluid (Malnic *et al.* 1989). The effect of flow is most prominent at the distal convoluted tubule, but can also be detected at the cortical collecting duct in the lower range of flow rates.

Sodium

Increased Na^+ delivery modestly enhances distal K^+ secretion in rats at lower tubular flow rates. This enhanced K^+ secretion is amiloride sensitive, suggesting that it depends on apical epithelial Na^+ channel (ENaC) activity (Malnic *et al.* 1989). Consistent with this hypothesis, it has been shown that a low Na^+ concentration (<30 mmol/l) can impair K^+ secretion by the cortical collecting duct in rats (Good *et al.* 1984). At high rates of Na^+ delivery, however, it is unclear whether enhanced K^+ secretion can be explained by increased luminal $[Na^+]$ *per se* or whether it is the result of the generally concomitant increased flow rate.

Adrenal hormones

Aldosterone is considered the dominant regulatory hormone for K^+, although this concept has recently been challenged (Rabinowitz 1996). It interacts with both Na^+ and K^+ by feedback to sustain K^+ homeostasis (Young *et al.* 1976a). Aldosterone stimulates K^+ secretion by the cortical collecting duct by increasing: (a) the number of Na^+–K^+ pumps (Na^+,K^+-ATPase activity) in the basolateral membrane, (b) the electrochemical driving force across the apical membrane secondary to enhanced electrogenic transport of Na^+, and (c) the K^+ permeability of the apical membrane (Muto 2001; Stockand 2002). K^+ secretion by the principal, but not the intercalated, cells of the cortical collecting duct is affected by aldosterone.

Under normal conditions, changes in Na^+ intake are accompanied by reciprocal changes in plasma aldosterone, so that K^+ homeostasis is preserved despite alterations in Na^+ and fluid delivery to the distal nephron (Young *et al.* 1984). Plasma K^+ also directly regulates aldosterone secretion by the adrenal glands (Rainey 1999). The direct correlation between plasma K^+ and aldosterone concentrations functions as a feedback control mechanism to sustain K^+ homeostasis during changes in K^+ intake.

Glucocorticoids are kaliuretic by a mechanism that involves increased GFR and fluid delivery to the distal nephron (Field *et al.* 1984; Muto 2001).

Vasopressin (ADH)

ADH stimulates Na^+ reabsorption and K^+ secretion by the distal convoluted tubule and cortical collecting duct (Field *et al.* 1984; Schafer 1994). This effect, which is mediated by activation of Na^+ and K^+ channels in the apical membrane and by an increase in Na^+,K^+-ATPase activity, potentiates the effect of aldosterone on K^+ secretion. It is prominent in the rat, but marginal in the rabbit (Muto 2001).

A water–ADH analogous to the Na^+–aldosterone feedback mechanism might sustain K^+ homeostasis (Field *et al.* 1984). The ingestion of large amounts of water increases fluid delivery to the distal nephron and simultaneously decreases plasma ADH, thereby sustaining a normal rate of K^+ excretion; hydropenia, which stimulates ADH secretion, acts in the opposite fashion.

Transepithelial potential difference

As would be anticipated from the cellular model of K^+ transport considered above, an increase in lumen electrical negativity stimulates K^+ secretion. The decrease in K^+ secretion produced by the K^+-sparing diuretic amiloride results from a diminution in the transepithelial potential difference; however, the importance of this potential difference in governing K^+ excretion under physiological circumstances remains to be elucidated.

Anions

Increased excretion of poorly reabsorbable anions, such as sulfate, enhances K^+ secretion by several possible mechanisms, including an increase in fluid and Na^+ delivery to the distal nephron, and an increase in transepithelial potential difference. In addition, a decrease in chloride concentration of tubular fluid stimulates the net K^+ secretion by the distal convoluted tubule by a mechanism that is independent of the aforementioned factors, perhaps through the activation of an electroneutral KCl secretory pathway (Ellison *et al.* 1987; Wingo 1989).

Systemic pH

Acidaemia inhibits and alkalaemia stimulates distal K^+ secretion by altering K^+ uptake across the basolateral membrane and by modulating the K^+ permeability of the apical membrane (Muto 2001). Despite these pH-mediated effects, chronic acid–base disorders are not accompanied by the anticipated changes in K^+ balance because other factors that alter K^+ secretion are perturbed simultaneously (Gennari and Cohen 1975). The one exception is chronic metabolic alkalosis, which is accompanied almost universally by K^+ depletion; however, mechanisms other than the effect of the alkaline pH on K^+ secretion probably account for maintenance of an enhanced K^+ clearance.

Ammonia

Increased rates of renal ammonia production and excretion decrease K^+ secretion at a nephron site beyond the distal convoluted tubule (Tannen 1977; Jaeger *et al.* 1983) in both animals and man. *In vitro* studies with the isolated, perfused kidney indicate that the K^+-sparing effect is related directly to ammonium excretion and can be of considerable magnitude (Sastrasinh and Tannen 1981). Possible mechanisms include competition between NH_4^+ and K^+ for basolateral transport by Na^+,K^+-ATPase (Wall *et al.* 2002) and ammonia stimulation of the apical H^+,K^+-ATPase (Frank *et al.* 2000). As K^+ depletion stimulates, whereas hyperkalaemia depresses, renal ammoniagenesis, the K^+–NH_3 inter-relation may function as another closed-loop feedback mechanism for the regulation of K^+ excretion.

Dietary K^+ intake

Chronic alterations in dietary K^+ intake profoundly modify the renal capacity to either excrete or conserve K^+. There are accompanying changes in K^+ transport by the colonic epithelium, which are analogous to the modifications in K^+ handling by the distal portions of the nephron. The processes of cellular K^+ uptake also adapt to the amount of dietary K^+ ingested.

High-K^+ diet

An acute K^+ load, lethal to anephric animals on a normal K^+ diet, can be tolerated by animals previously adapted to a high-K^+ intake (Alexander and Levinsky 1968). The validity of this observation has been questioned (Spital and Sterns 1986). Recent studies of K^+-supplemented animals with intact kidneys have confirmed an enhanced muscle K^+ uptake due to an increased Na^+,K^+-ATPase in skeletal muscle (Blachley *et al.* 1986; Bundgaard *et al.* 1997).

The colon also adapts its capacity to secrete K^+ under conditions of increased dietary K^+ (Hayslett and Binder 1982), mainly in its distal portion as a result of an increased number of Na^+–K^+ pumps in the basolateral membrane and of apical K^+ channels (Sandle and Butterfield 1999). Although the enhancement of K^+ secretion can occur independently of aldosterone, full expression of this adaptive phenomenon requires the concurrent increase in aldosterone produced by a high-K^+ intake (Foster *et al.* 1985).

The principal cells in the cortical and medullary collecting ducts adapt to a high-K^+ diet in a fashion analogous to those of the colon (Muto 2001). They show an increase in the number of Na^+–K^+ pumps in the basolateral membrane, an increase in ROMK K^+ channels that enhance K^+ conductance of the apical membrane, and an increase in apical ENaC Na^+ channels enhancing the Na^+ entry step; all of which increase the capacity to secrete K^+ (Palmer and Frindt 1999). Although the adaptation in K^+ secretion can occur independently of aldosterone, full expression of the enhanced capacity for K^+ transportation requires an increase in hormone concentrations (Muto 2001). The adapted kidney excretes up to 10–20 times more K^+ than the normal kidney.

Low-K^+ diet

Changes in the cellular mechanisms for K^+ uptake are more complex in response to a low-K^+ diet than to a high-K^+ diet. K^+ depletion decreases the number of Na^+–K^+ pumps in skeletal muscle, but erythrocytes and cardiac muscle show an increase in Na^+,K^+-ATPase activity (Thompson *et al.* 1999). Therefore, erythrocytes and cardiac muscle tend to sustain their intracellular K^+ concentrations during K^+ depletion, whereas skeletal muscle serves as the primary source of K^+ loss. The diminution in Na^+–K^+ pumps in skeletal muscle also slows the rate of cellular K^+ uptake during the reparative process. Thus, K^+-depleted individuals cannot dispose of a K^+ load as readily as normal individuals. The colon reduces the secretory and increases the reabsorptive capacity for K^+ upon ingestion of a low-K^+ diet (Ornt *et al.* 1987). These effects are more prominent in the proximal than the terminal portions of the distal colon. Although the specific cellular mechanisms involved and the part played by aldosterone in the colonic adaptation to a low-K^+ diet have not been fully delineated, upregulation of the β-subunit of the colonic H^+,K^+-ATPase and increased expression of this pump in apical membranes may play an important role (Sangan *et al.* 1999).

The kidney responds to a low-K^+ diet with an enhanced capacity to conserve K^+ (Ornt *et al.* 1987). This conservation results from both a decrease in K^+ secretion and an increase in K^+ reabsorption at sites beyond the distal convoluted tubule. A low-K^+-induced decrease in aldosterone seems to be required for the development of maximal K^+-conserving capacity. The increase in K^+ reabsorption is mediated by a K^+ depletion-induced increase in renal H^+,K^+-ATPase activity (Wingo and Cain 1993; Silver and Soleimani 1999). Various H^+,K^+-ATPase alpha subunit isoforms have been identified in the distal nephron and may be involved in this K^+ depletion-induced increase in K^+ reabsorption (Caviston *et al.* 1999).

Hypokalaemia

Hypokalaemia can result either from a shift of K^+ into cells or from depletion of cellular K^+ stores. In some circumstances, transcellular shifts occur together with K^+ depletion, so that changes in the plasma K^+ do not portray the degree of cellular K^+ depletion. For example, with diabetic ketoacidosis, factors that shift K^+ out of cells produce normal or even elevated concentrations of plasma K^+ despite substantial K^+ depletion. Conversely, high concentrations of catecholamine superimposed on K^+ depletion can produce a lower plasma K^+ than anticipated from the magnitude of the K^+ depletion. In the absence of transcellular shifts, the plasma K^+ is a reasonable reflection of the magnitude of the K^+ deficit, as shown in Fig. 4.

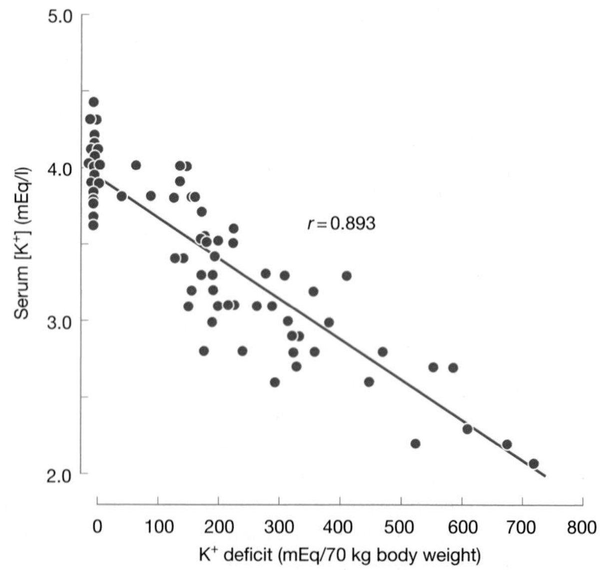

Fig. 4 Relation between serum K^+ and the magnitude of K^+ depletion. The data represent the effect of uncomplicated potassium depletion on plasma K^+ concentration and are derived from the result of balance studies in 24 individuals. [From Sterns *et al.* (1981), with permission of Williams and Wilkins, Baltimore.]

In Fig. 4, a linear relation is depicted up to a K^+ deficit of approximately 700 mmol; however, the kinetics are probably curvilinear with more severe degrees of depletion, as plasma K^+ concentrations of less than 2.0 mmol/l usually reflect deficits of 1000 or more mmoles. It is also important to recognize that a decrease in total body potassium, as assessed, for example, with a counter for total body K^+, does not necessarily indicate a state of K^+ depletion. As K^+ is the major intracellular cation, loss of muscle mass will be accompanied by proportional losses in total body K^+ stores. K^+ depletion is present only when the K^+ loss occurs independently of changes in body mass and thereby produces a decrease in the intracellular concentration of K^+.

Clinical sequelae

Hypokalaemia produced by either K^+ depletion or by a shift of potassium into cells increases the K_i^+/K_e^+ ratio. The resultant hyperpolarization of the membrane increases the threshold for initiation, and interferes with the termination, of an action potential (Knochel 1981). Hence, a variety of neuromuscular functions can be impaired by hypokalaemia. K^+ depletion also decreases the intracellular K^+ concentration with an attendant intracellular acidosis, and thereby interferes with both K^+- and pH-dependent intracellular processes (Adler and Fraley 1977). Therefore, it is not surprising that a large number of abnormalities, outlined in Table 4, result from hypokalaemic states.

Cardiac complications

Cardiac manifestations are amongst the most serious complications of hypokalaemia. Hypokalaemia-induced alterations in the electrocardiogram include flattening of the T-wave, depression of the ST segment, and the development of prominent U-waves, which can give the impression of a prolonged QT interval (Johansson and Larsson 1982). In addition, actual prolongation of the QT interval can be produced by hypokalaemia (Tan *et al.* 1995). These changes, typically observed with serum K^+ of less than 3.0 mmol/l, provide a diagnostic clue to the presence of hypokalaemia. The long QT interval can predispose patients with hypokalaemia to the Torsade de Pointes form of ventricular tachycardia (Tan *et al.* 1995).

The widely recognized precipitation of digitalis intoxication by hypokalaemia can result in a variety of life-threatening arrhythmias (Aronson 1983). Furthermore, hypokalaemia, independently of concurrent digitalis therapy, can induce ventricular arrhythmias, ranging from unifocal, premature beats to tachycardia or fibrillation. Although there is controversy as to whether the mild hypokalaemia that typically accompanies diuretic therapy poses a risk for the development of ventricular arrhythmias, there is convincing evidence that sufficiently severe K^+ depletion promotes ventricular irritability. Furthermore, clinical findings suggest that mild hypokalaemia may be arrhythmogenic in the presence of underlying cardiac disease, and clearly indicate a strong correlation between hypokalaemia and the development of ventricular tachycardia or fibrillation during the acute phase of myocardial infarction (Tannen 1985, 1989). Furthermore hypokalaemia appears to increase the likelihood of perioperative arrhythmias (Wahr *et al.* 1999). In contrast with animal experiments, myocardial function in humans appears well preserved despite significant degrees of K^+ depletion (serum K^+ 2.4–2.9 mmol/l) (O'Regan *et al.* 1985; Shapiro *et al.* 1998).

Table 4 Sequelae of K^+ depletion

Cardiac
Digitalis intoxication
Ventricular arrhythmias
Neuromuscular
Intestinal hypomotility
Paralysis
Rhabdomyolysis
Renal
Impaired blood flow and GFR
Interstitial nephritis
Cyst formation
Fluids and electrolytes
Polyuria–polydipsia
Increased NH_3 production
Metabolic alkalosis
Chloride wasting
Oedema
Hypercalciuria
Phosphaturia
Endocrine
Low aldosterone
High renin
Increased prostaglandins
Glucose intolerance
Growth retardation
Haemodynamics
Hypertension

Neuromuscular function

Hypokalaemia impairs intestinal motility and can produce symptoms ranging from constipation to frank ileus (Welt *et al.* 1960). Similarly, symptoms in skeletal muscle can range from weakness to actual paralysis, which has a predilection for the extremities, but can also result in life-threatening respiratory impairment (Knochel 1981). Paralysis appears to develop when the transmembrane voltage of skeletal muscle falls to values lower than may be predicted from the K_i^+/K_e^+ ratio (Knochel 1981). A recent study found that insulin-mediated stimulation of sarcolemma ATP-sensitive K^+ channels is impaired in hypokalaemic rats, and this correlated with the development of muscle depolarization and paralysis (Tricarico *et al.* 1999).

Severe K^+ depletion can produce rhabdomyolysis. Increases in creatine phosphokinase activity indicative of muscle injury are usually detectable with K^+ less than 3.0 mmol/l (Knochel 1981). The susceptibility to rhabdomyolysis after severe exercise may result from the absence of the vasodilatation normally induced by the egress of K^+ from muscle, but low-K^+-induced changes in glycogen metabolism and decreased activity of the Na^+–K^+ pump may also play a part.

Renal effects

Functional decreases in renal blood flow and GFR, secondary to increases in vasoconstrictor, prostaglandins, and angiotensin II, are induced by severe K^+ depletion (Linas and Dickmann 1982). K^+-depleted rats develop a characteristic swelling, hyperplasia, and prominent cytoplasmic granulation of the cells lining the medullary collecting duct (Muehrcke and Rosen 1964). These changes, which mostly reflect an increase in the luminal surface area of the intercalated cells, correlate with their enhanced capacity to reabsorb K^+ by a luminal H^+,K^+-ATPase (Elger *et al.* 1992). In humans, the dominant lesion is vacuolization of the proximal convoluted tubule, but changes in the collecting duct may have been overlooked because of the limited availability of pathological renal medullary tissue (Relman and Schwartz 1958). Severe, prolonged K^+ depletion can result in a chronic interstitial nephritis with the development of chronic renal failure (Bock *et al.* 1978; Tolins *et al.* 1987). It has been suggested that a low-K^+-induced acceleration of renal ammoniagenesis may account for the tubulointerstitial injury by virtue of the complement-activating potential of ammonia (Tolins *et al.* 1987). More recent studies have attributed the renal damage to intrarenal hypoxia mediated by the intrarenal generation of vasoconstrictors including angiotensin II. Of interest, the development of tubulointerstitial injury was mitigated by administration of an angiotensin II-receptor antagonist (Suga *et al.* 2002). K^+-depleted patients also exhibit a propensity for renal cyst formation (Torres *et al.* 1990).

Fluid and electrolyte disorders

Polyuria and polydipsia are well-recognized sequelae of K^+ depletion. Polydipsia is mediated by the interaction of increased concentrations of angiotensin II with receptors in the subfornical organ of the brain (Saikaley *et al.* 1986). Increased thirst precedes the development of a renal concentrating defect, which further contributes to the polyuric state (Berl *et al.* 1977). The vasopressin-resistant abnormality in renal concentration is attributable to a decrease in medullary tonicity along with impaired water permeability of the collecting duct (Martin and Schrier 1998). The decrease in medullary tonicity is contributed to by impaired choride transport by the thick ascending limb produced by decreased expression and activity of the Na^+–K^+–$2Cl^-$ cotransporter, downregulation of ROMK, and potentially by increased arachidonic acid metabolites; by increased medullary blood flow; by a decrease in aldolase reductase that impairs the accumulation of medullary osmolytes; and by a decrease in urea transporters (Martinez-Maldonado and Opava-Stitzer 1977; Nakanishi *et al.* 1996; Amlal *et al.* 1998; Mennitt *et al.* 2000; Gu *et al.* 2001; Kim *et al.* 2001). A defect in the cyclic AMP-dependent water permeability along with decreased expression of the aquaporin-2 water channel accounts for the impaired water permeability of the collecting duct (Raymond *et al.* 1985; Marples *et al.* 1996; Martin and Schrier 1998; Amlal *et al.* 2000b). Whether excessive production of prostaglandins contribute to the abnormalities in the renal concentrating mechanism is unresolved (Raymond *et al.* 1987).

Potassium depletion accelerates renal ammoniagenesis by altering metabolism in a fashion akin to the changes observed with chronic metabolic acidosis; however, increased ammoniagenesis may not be attributable entirely to the intracellular acidosis produced by K^+ depletion (Tannen 1977, 1989). The heightened production of ammonia elevates the urine pH by increasing urinary buffering capacity, and enhances the capacity to excrete an acid load. As indicated previously, it may contribute to the development of tubulointerstitial injury. Finally, increased renal ammoniagenesis can precipitate hepatic coma in predisposed individuals.

In humans, uncomplicated depletion of K^+ can produce metabolic alkalosis (Hernandez *et al.* 1987). The alkalaemic effect appears to involve interplay with sodium homeostasis and is potentiated by volume contraction. In part this may result from the additive effects of K^+ depletion and aldosterone on proton secretion by distal nephron intercalated cells—potassium depletion stimulating H^+-ATPase and H^+,K^+-ATPase and aldosterone stimulating H^+-ATPase (Eiam-Ong *et al.* 1993b; Bailey *et al.* 1998; Nakamura *et al.* 1999; Silver *et al.* 2000) In the absence of volume contraction, very severe K^+ depletion is required to provoke metabolic alkalosis of significant clinical magnitude. The alkalosis-producing tendency of K^+ depletion can be accounted for by several factors, including enhanced bicarbonate uptake by the proximal tubule, mediated by an increase in the Na^+/H^+ antiporter and basolateral Na^+–HCO_3^- cotransporter (Amemiya *et al.* 1999; Amlal *et al.* 2000a) as well as the distal nephron, and by increased renal ammonia production (Tannen 1987a). A defect in chloride reabsorption, which is produced by severe K^+ depletion, might also contribute to the development of metabolic alkalosis (Garella *et al.* 1970; Luke *et al.* 1978). Impaired chloride reabsorption can involve the entire nephron, but it is most pronounced in the thick ascending limb and distal tubule, where it is accompanied by decreased expression and activity of Na^+–K^+–$2Cl^+$ and the Na^+–Cl^- cotransporters (Amlal *et al.* 1998).

Sodium retention sufficient to produce oedema can be induced by K^+ depletion (Krishna *et al.* 1987). Hyponatraemia has been attributed to diuretic-induced depletion of K^+, but the specific pathogenetic role of hypokalaemia in this setting is unresolved (Fichman *et al.* 1971). Patients with combined hyponatraemia and hypokalaemia appear to be at increased risk for the osmotic demyelination syndrome following correction of hyponatraemia (Lohr 1994). K^+ deprivation increases urinary calcium and phosphorus excretion and results in a modest decrease in plasma calcium along with an increase in concentrations of parathyroid hormone and $1,25(OH)_2D_3$ (Sebastian *et al.* 1990; Krishna and Kapoor 1991; Sebastian *et al.* 1994; Lemann 1999). The hypercalciuria results from K^+-depletion mediated sodium retention and extracellular volume expansion (Lemann 1999); it predisposes towards bone loss and renal calculi (Cirillo *et al.* 1994; Sebastian *et al.* 1994).

Endocrine effects

Potassium depletion increases plasma renin activity by effects on the renal myogenic receptors as well as on the macula densa (Linas 1981; Luke *et al.* 1982). Aldosterone secretion, however, is reduced as a result of a direct, low-K^+-mediated effect on its biosynthesis by the adrenal gland (Sealey and Laragh 1974). Studies in humans and animals are conflicting in regard to the influence of hypokalaemia on renal prostaglandin synthesis; in general, the evidence appears to favour an accelerated, vasodilatory, prostaglandin production in K^+-depleted humans (Dunn 1981).

Insulin secretion by the pancreas is impaired by K^+ depletion (Gordon 1973). Typically, mild glucose intolerance is observed, but on occasion severe hyperglycaemia can develop.

Growth retardation is a well-established result of K^+ depletion, mediated by reductions in both the growth hormone receptor and in IGF-I (Flybjerg *et al.* 1991; Hochberg *et al.* 1995; Hsu *et al.* 1997).

Systemic haemodynamics

Potassium depletion lowers systemic vascular resistance. Sensitivity to the vasoconstrictive effects of both angiotensin II and vasopressin is decreased, whereas the response to noradrenaline is unimpaired (Paller and Linas 1982; Tannen 1983; Murray and Paller 1986). The abnormal response to angiotensin II appears to involve a postreceptor defect mediated by an altered inositol phosphate pathway (Paller *et al.* 1984).

Although the decrease in systemic vascular resistance is accompanied by an increase in cardiac output under basal conditions, the exercise-induced increase in cardiac output is subnormal (Knochel *et al.* 1978).

Blood pressure is lowered in both normotensive and hypertensive animals by K^+ depletion (Paller and Linas 1982; Tannen 1983, 1987b). However, mild K^+ depletion elevates rather than decreases blood pressure in both normotensive and hypertensive humans (Kaplan *et al.* 1985; Lawton *et al.* 1990; Krishna and Kapoor 1991).

Aetiology

Hypokalaemia can be produced either by a shift of K^+ from the extra- to intracellular compartment (transcellular shift) or by actual K^+ depletion. Both processes can occur simultaneously.

Transcellular shifts (Table 5)

The various factors that mediate transcellular shifts of K^+ have been elaborated upon in an earlier section.

Alkalaemia translocates K^+ into cells. Increased concentrations of insulin, whether endogenously generated by administration of a glucose load to individuals with a normal pancreas, or produced by exogenous administration, lower the plasma K^+. β_2-Adrenergic agonists (e.g. adrenaline, salbutamol, terbutaline, fenoterol) are used clinically to treat asthma and to halt premature labour. Intravenous as well as inhalational routes of administration rapidly produce hypokalaemia by shifting K^+ into cells, and reductions to less than 3.0 mmol/l can occur (Conci *et al.* 1984; Braden *et al.* 1997). The hypokalaemic effect is more pronounced in the presence of underlying K^+ depletion. The endogenous release of catecholamines, associated with a variety of acute illnesses, accounts for the transient hypokalaemia often observed when patients are admitted to a hospital (Struthers and Reid 1984) or in patients with acute myocardial infarction, head trauma, and delirium tremens, or after open heart surgery (Madias *et al.* 2000).

Intoxications with several agents can produce hypokalaemia by altering transcellular distribution. Both acute and chronic theophylline toxicity induce hypokalaemia by several possible mechanisms including increases in catecholamines and insulin, and a direct elevation of cAMP mediated through inhibition of phosphodiesterase (Hall *et al.* 1984; Bertino *et al.* 1987). In view of the cardiac arrhythmias that can accompany excess theophylline, hypokalaemia is a serious consequence. β-Blocking drugs may be useful in the treatment of this complication (Kearney *et al.* 1985).

Table 5 Hypokalaemia from redistribution

Alkalaemia
Excessive insulin
Excessive β-adrenergic catecholamines
Intoxications Theophylline Barium Toluene Chloroquine
Calcium-channel blockers
Hypokalaemic periodic paralysis

Poisoning from the ingestion of acid-soluble barium salts produces profound hypokalaemia (<2.0 mmol/l) and flaccid paralysis involving the respiratory muscles (Roza and Berman 1971). Barium selectively blocks K^+ channels, thereby impeding K^+ egress from cells, while the uptake mechanism is unimpaired. In addition to supportive measures, parenteral administration of K^+ is indicated to increase the plasma concentration.

Toluene intoxication, produced by sniffing paint or glue, is accompanied by hypokalaemia and hypophosphataemia (Streicher *et al.* 1981). Although both proximal and distal renal tubular acidosis, and increased urinary hippurate excretion with resultant renal K^+ wasting can be produced by toluene, the data suggest that the hypokalaemia may also be mediated by redistribution of K^+ into cells (Carlisle *et al.* 1991).

Acute chloroquine intoxication frequently is associated with hypokalaemia within a few hours after ingestion (Clemessy *et al.* 1995). Blockade of potassium channels has been suggested as a potential mechanism for this effect.

Calcium channel-blocking drugs enhance cellular uptake of an acute potassium load, presumably by inhibiting calcium-activated K^+ channels (Sugarman and Kahn 1986). They also reduce the interdialytic increase in K^+ in patients on haemodialysis (Solomon and Dubey 1992). However, hypokalaemia has been reported infrequently with standard clinical use of these medications (Trost and Weidmann 1988; Minella and Schulman 1991). As calcium channel-blocking agents also have potential hyperkalaemic properties by impairing adrenal aldosterone secretion, the absence of uniform changes in K^+ homeostasis is not surprising.

Both hereditary and acquired forms of hypokalaemic periodic paralysis produce hypokalaemia by an acute shift of K^+ into cells, which is accompanied by the development of flaccid paralysis. With the autosomal-dominant disorder, which results from a mutation in the dihydropyridine receptor of the calcium channel, the recurrent paralytic attacks can be provoked by various factors that can perturb K^+ homeostasis, including a high carbohydrate intake, exertion, administration of adrenaline, and a high-Na^+ diet (Fontaine *et al.* 1996; Ptacek 1998). Treatment with acetazolamide, perhaps by producing chronic metabolic acidosis or, as suggested recently, by activating calcium-activated K^+ channels improves the weakness between attacks and reduces the incidence of paralytic attacks (Ptacek 1998; Tricarico *et al.* 2000).

The acquired disorder is a complication of thyrotoxicosis and has a predilection for individuals of oriental heritage (Ptacek 1998; Manoukian *et al.* 1999). The increase in skeletal muscle Na^+,K^+-ATPase and the increased catecholamine concentrations produced by excessive amounts of thyroid hormone, which both predispose towards an intracellular shift of potassium, may account for the development of this syndrome in thyrotoxic patients. In contrast to the hereditary form, therapy with β-adrenergic-blocking drugs is useful in mitigating the paralytic episodes (Ptacek 1998).

Potassium depletion (Table 6)

Potassium depletion can result from excessive renal losses, or from either inadequate intake or losses from extrarenal sites, usually the gastrointestinal tract. With the so-called extrarenal forms of depletion of more than 5-day duration, the kidney should show an appropriate degree of K^+ conservation demonstrated by a urinary K^+ concentration

Table 6 Causes of K^+ depletion

Extrarenal (urine K^+ < 20 mmol/day)	**Renal (urine K^+ > 20 mmol/day)**
Inadequate intake	Renal tubular acidosis
Copious perspiration	Diabetic ketoacidosis
Gastrointestinal losses	Chloride depletion
Diarrhoea	Vomiting/gastric suction
Laxative abuse	Diuretics
Villous adenoma	Bartter's syndrome
	Gitelman's syndrome
	Mineralocorticoid excess states
	Liddle's syndrome
	Glucocorticoid excess
	Magnesium depletion
	Antibiotic therapy
	Leukaemia
	Interstitial nephritis—immune related
	Diuretic conditions

below 20 mmol/day. If a spot urine is analysed, a potassium : creatinine ratio of less than 20 mmol/g or a fractional potassium excretion below 6 per cent would be expected, although these diagnostic indices have not undergone rigorous clinical testing. Urinary K^+ concentration can be a misleading index of K^+ excretion because K^+ depletion typically produces polyuria. Although the cause of K^+ depletion is usually obvious, segregation into extrarenal and renal causes, along with an assessment of the concurrent acid–base status, provide a useful framework for the diagnosis of hypokalaemia of uncertain aetiology.

Extrarenal K^+ depletion

Inadequate K^+ ingestion can produce modest deficits in the range of 250–300 mmol. This can occur with a complete fast, unaccompanied by K^+ supplementation, or occasionally in elderly patients on a 'tea and toast' diet. K^+ intake may be relatively inadequate when cell mass increases rapidly (Lawson *et al.* 1972). Decrease in the serum K^+ to less than 2.8 mmol/l has been described as a complication of the treatment of severe megaloblastic and iron-deficiency anaemias. Transfusions of frozen erythrocytes, which are depleted of K^+, can also result in a rapid decline in the serum K^+ (Rao *et al.* 1980).

Prolonged vigorous physical conditioning in a hot climate can produce substantial K^+ depletion as a result of copious K^+ losses by perspiration (Knochel *et al.* 1972). This clinical syndrome, documented in military recruits undergoing basic training, is unusual in that serum K^+ remains normal and urinary K^+ excretion rates high, despite a substantial K^+ deficit. The mechanisms accounting for the unanticipated alterations in the transcellular distribution of K^+ and in renal K^+ handling are unexplained. Rhabdomyolysis is an important complication of the K^+ depletion in this setting.

The most common cause of extrarenal K^+ depletion is loss from the gastrointestinal tract. Diarrhoea, regardless of its cause, produces K^+ depletion, which is usually accompanied by hyperchloraemic metabolic acidosis as a result of the concurrent loss of bicarbonate or bicarbonate precursors in the diarrhoeal fluid (Agarwal *et al.* 1994). However, some secretory diarrhoeas can produce chloride depletion and a resultant metabolic alkalosis. Patients with ureterosigmoidostomies typically develop K^+ depletion, because increased fluid delivery resulting from urination into the colon stimulates K^+ secretion by this segment of the gut (Agarwal *et al.* 1994). Hyperchloraemic metabolic acidosis is also a manifestation of this condition and results from bicarbonate secretion and urinary ammonium absorption by the colonic epithelium. Laxative abuse produces excessive faecal elimination of K^+ without concurrent losses of bicarbonate. Thus, normal acid–base homeostasis is typically preserved (Schwartz and Relman 1953). Metabolic alkalosis, along with inappropriate losses of urinary K^+, has been described in association with laxative abuse, but concurrent diuretic abuse should be considered with this clinical presentation (Fleischer *et al.* 1969). *Melanosis coli* provides a clue to surreptitious laxative abuse. Measurements of stool electrolytes, magnesium, and chemical analysis for phenolphthalein, senna, anthraquinones, and bisacodyl help establish the diagnosis (Topazian and Binder 1994; Phillips *et al.* 1995).

Villous adenomas of the rectum secrete a watery, mucus-containing fluid of high-K^+ content. The acid–base picture described with this rare disorder has been highly variable, ranging from metabolic acidosis to metabolic alkalosis (Babior 1966).

Excessive losses of K^+ from the gastrointestinal tract have been found with geophagia of certain types of clay that have K^+-binding properties (Gonzales *et al.* 1982). By contrast, river-bed clay, which is high in K^+, can produce hyperkalaemia in patients with impaired renal function (Gelfand *et al.* 1975).

Potassium depletion of renal aetiology

Renal tubular acidosis (RTA) (see also Chapter 5.4) Both distal (type I) and proximal (type II) renal tubular acidosis can present with hyperchloraemic metabolic acidosis in association with hypokalaemia and renal K^+ wasting. K^+ depletion is a particularly prominent component of distal tubular acidosis; its manifestations, including weakness and paralysis, can sometimes be the presenting symptoms. Increased rates of distal fluid delivery produced by an acidosis-mediated inhibition of proximal Na^+ reabsorption, in combination with secondary hyperaldosteronism produced by volume contraction, contribute to renal K^+ wasting (Sebastian *et al.* 1971b, 1976). In addition, the defect in proton transport by the distal nephron further accentuates K^+ secretion. Correction of the metabolic acidosis and volume contraction with bicarbonate usually alleviates the excessive kaliuresis, but in some instances the high rates of urinary K^+ excretion persist (Sebastian *et al.* 1971b). If distal RTA were due to a defect in H^+,K^+-ATPase, impaired K^+ reabsorption would produce renal K^+ wasting (Dafnis *et al.* 1992).

Although a minority of patients with proximal tubular acidosis present with hypokalaemia, it is a frequent accompaniment of alkali replacement therapy for the disorder. As the defect in bicarbonate reabsorption from the proximal tubule dictates the need for large quantities of alkali, the ensuing high rates of delivery of sodium bicarbonate to the distal nephron provide a potent stimulus for K^+ secretion (Sebastian *et al.* 1971a, 1976). Whether a defect in K^+ reabsorption at more proximal nephron sites also contributes to the excessive kaliuresis in patients with proximal tubular acidosis is unknown.

As would be anticipated, treatment with carbonic anhydrase inhibitors, which impair proton secretion by both the proximal and distal nephrons, also results in hypokalaemia.

Diabetic ketoacidosis The other acidotic disorder associated with renal K^+ wasting is diabetic ketoacidosis, although hyperosmolar coma without ketosis also is accompanied by K^+ depletion (Adrogue *et al.* 1986). The osmotic diuresis produced by glycosuria, along with the stimulus to K^+ secretion of the elevated excretion of ketoanion, produce a kaliuresis. Despite severe K^+ depletion, diabetic ketoacidosis typically presents with a normal plasma K^+ concentration. The combination of insulin deficiency, metabolic acidosis, and hyperosmolarity accounts for the shift of potassium from the intra- to extracellular fluid compartment (Adrogue *et al.* 1986). Once adequate urine flow is established, K^+ replacement is an important component of treatment.

Chloride depletion Metabolic alkalosis is a prominent component of the K^+ depletion syndromes produced by both chloride-depleting stimuli and by states of mineralocorticoid excess.

A variety of conditions can produce chloride depletion; they all result in a similar clinical picture consisting of hypokalaemic metabolic alkalosis, renal K^+ wasting, contraction of the extracellular fluid volume, and intense urinary chloride conservation (so long as chloruretic drugs are absent) (Schwartz *et al.* 1968). The inappropriate kaliuresis produced by chloride depletion could result from high concentrations of aldosterone secondary to volume contraction, the kaliuretic effect of the associated metabolic alkalosis, and/or the heightened stimulus for K^+ secretion produced by a low chloride concentration in distal tubular fluid (Kassirer *et al.* 1967; Seldin and Rector 1972; Luke 1974; Ellison *et al.* 1987). Although it may play a part in certain clinical circumstances, hyperaldosteronism is not required for K^+ depletion to develop; however, the relative pathophysiological importance of the last two phenomena has not been resolved definitively (Kassirer *et al.* 1967; Luke 1974).

The most common causes of chloride depletion are losses of fluid from the upper gastrointestinal tract by vomiting or gastric drainage, and diuretic therapy (Schwartz *et al.* 1968). Other disorders with chloride depletion include the posthypercapneic state, congenital chloride-wasting diarrhoea, and certain secretory diarrhoeal conditions, sweat chloride losses in patients with cystic fibrosis, and inadequate chloride intake in infants.

Losses of upper gastrointestinal fluids, which have a high HCl content, by vomiting or gastric drainage produce chloride and proton depletion (Kassirer and Schwartz 1966). During the generation of the disorder a portion of the bicarbonate produced by the loss of acid is eliminated in the urine along with K^+. This diminishes the magnitude of the alkalosis, but accounts for the development of the K^+ depletion. The development of chloride depletion is accompanied by urinary chloride conservation, with chloride excretion rates typically less than 10 mmol/day. Despite the ingestion of a diet that generates acid, and the intake of Na^+ and K^+ as non-chloride salts, so long as chloride depletion is sustained, the alkalosis, the volume contraction, and the K^+ depletion are not corrected. Instead, the protons, Na^+, and K^+ are eliminated in the urine. When KCl is provided, chloride is avidly retained along with K^+, and a bicarbonate diuresis ensues, so correcting the metabolic alkalosis. Shifts of Na^+ from the intra- to extracellular compartment contribute to re-expansion of the extracellular fluid volume.

Diuretics that act on the thick ascending limb of the loop of Henle (e.g. frusemide, bumetanide, ethacrynic acid) or the distal convoluted tubule (e.g. thiazides, chlorthalidone) result in K^+ depletion (Kassirer and Harrington 1977; Tannen 1985). The kaliuretic stimulus, in part, results from an increase in salt and water delivery to distal nephron sites that are primed for K^+ secretion by the secondary hyperaldosteronism induced by the volume-contracting effects of diuretic drugs. Chloride depletion produced by urinary chloride losses combined with a restricted chloride intake (i.e. a low-salt diet) also contributes to the development and maintenance of hypokalaemia (Schwartz *et al.* 1968). Correction of the K^+ deficit requires therapy specifically with KCl; other non-chloride salts of K^+ are ineffective in this setting. Urinary chloride excretion is high if assessed during the time that diuretics are being taken; however, intense chloride conservation is demonstrable once therapy is discontinued.

Typically, the values of the serum K^+ stabilize after the first 1–2 weeks of diuretic therapy (Kassirer and Harrington 1977; Tannen 1985). The decrement in plasma K^+ concentration averages 0.6 mmol/l with standard doses of thiazide diuretics and 0.3 mmol/l with standard doses of frusemide (Morgan and Davidson 1980). The K^+ deficit is about 5 per cent of total body storage. However, in approximately 10 per cent of patients, the serum K^+ decreases to less than 3.0 mmol/l. The possibility of undiagnosed primary hyperaldosteronism should always be considered in hypertensive patients who develop diuretic-induced hypokalaemia of this magnitude. Moderate Na^+ restriction and use of the smallest effective drug dosage help to minimize the extent of K^+ depletion.

Normal K^+ homeostasis can be maintained by the use of KCl supplements or by concurrent treatment with the K^+-sparing diuretics amiloride or triamterene. There is general agreement that K^+ maintenance therapy is indicated in patients whose serum K^+ decreases to less than 3.0 mmol/l, who are receiving digitalis preparations, or who are at risk for the development of hepatic coma.

There is considerable controversy concerning the advisability of K^+ maintenance therapy in other diuretic-treated patients. Some believe it is contraindicated because the risks of mild hypokalaemia are modest, whereas the treatment is costly and incurs the risk of hyperkalaemia and other drug-related side-effects (Kassirer and Harrington 1977; Harrington *et al.* 1982; Tannen 1985, 1989). Others are concerned about the risks of life-threatening ventricular arrhythmias, supported by evidence suggesting an increase in sudden death in patients treated with K^+-losing diuretics (Siscovick *et al.* 1994; Grobee and Hoes 1995; Laragh and Sealey 2001). In view of the evidence suggesting that this risk is heightened in individuals with underlying cardiac disease, K^+ maintenance therapy seems appropriate in this subset of patients. K^+ maintenance therapy is also reasonable in patients who develop symptoms that could be secondary to K^+ depletion.

Bartter's and Gitelman's syndromes Bartter's and Gitelman's syndromes are genetic renal K^+ wasting disorders, caused by mutations that impair chloride reabsorption by the thick ascending limb and the distal convoluted tubule, respectively. They are characterized by normotension and hypokalaemic metabolic alkalosis in association with renal potassium and chloride wasting (see Chapter 5.5). Surreptitious diuretic abuse must be considered in any adult who presents with features of either of these syndromes (Jamison *et al.* 1982). Loop-acting diuretics, which mimic Bartter's syndrome and thiazide diuretics, which mimic Gitelman's syndrome, can produce an identical clinical picture, with altered chloride reabsorption and associated renal K^+ wasting and depletion. All such patients should undergo urinary screens for diuretics and some may require evaluation in a metabolic ward for conclusive diagnosis. Other aberrant behaviour resulting in

K^+ depletion, such as surreptitious vomiting or laxative abuse, can usually be readily distinguished from diuretic abuse by measurements of urinary chloride (low in vomiting) and urinary potassium (low in laxative abuse) (Veldhuis *et al.* 1979). Sometimes multiple abuses coexist and pose a considerable diagnostic challenge.

Mineralocorticoid excess A primary increase in mineralocorticoid concentration due either to endogenous production or exogenous administration produces hypokalaemic metabolic alkalosis in association with hypertension. Hypertension results from the Na^+-retaining and volume-expanding properties of mineralocorticoids. K^+ depletion results from renal K^+ wasting produced by high rates of salt and water delivery to a distal nephron that is primed for accelerated K^+ secretion by high concentrations of mineralocorticoid. Na^+ restriction can reverse the tendency for K^+ wasting. Metabolic alkalosis appears to be caused predominantly by severe K^+ depletion, but the high amounts of mineralocorticoid could have an additive effect (Kassirer *et al.* 1967, 1970; Hulter *et al.* 1978; Tannen 1987a). In contrast to chloride depletion, volume-expanded patients with states of mineralocorticoid excess have copious quantities of chloride in the urine. Therefore, measurement of urinary chloride is useful for distinguishing between these two broad subsets of hypokalaemic metabolic alkalosis. Determinations of plasma renin activity, aldosterone, the ratio of aldosterone to renin and cortisol are useful to distinguish between the various types of mineralocorticoid excess, as outlined in Table 7.

Although it was previously thought that approximately 80 per cent of cases of primary hyperaldosteronism present with hypokalaemia, recent improvements in diagnosis of this condition suggest that the incidence of hypokalaemia may be substantially lower (Litchfield and Dluhy 1995; Stowasser and Gordon 2000). Increased recognition of several familial forms of primary hyperaldosteronism may also account for different phenotypic manifestations of this disorder. In normokalaemic patients, a low serum K^+ can often be unmasked by increasing the Na^+ intake (Litchfield and Dluhy 1995). K^+ depletion and often hypertension are corrected by treatment with spironolactone (Litchfield and Dluhy 1995). Patients with glucocorticoid-remediable hyperaldosteronism, a hereditary condition caused by a chimeric 11-β-hydroxylase/aldosterone synthase gene, which renders aldosterone secretion ACTH responsive, are typically normokalaemic but develop severe hypokalaemia when treated with thiazide diuretics (Dluhy and Lifton 1995; Lifton 1996). Secondary hyperaldosteronism resulting from renal vascular disease of either the major or small vessels can also present as hypertension in combination with hypokalaemia (Corry and Tuck 1995). The rare renin-producing tumours are an additional cause of secondary hyperaldosteronism associated with hypertension and hypokalaemia (Corvol *et al.* 1988). These are typically benign haemangiopericytomas of the juxtaglomerular apparatus, but non-renal malignant neoplasms that secrete renin have also been reported. It is of interest that only the hypertensive types of secondary hyperaldosteronism appear to cause K^+ depletion.

Hypokalaemia also occurs with several entities associated with high concentrations of mineralocorticoids other than aldosterone. With these conditions, both plasma aldosterone and renin activity are suppressed. Both acquired and congenital deficiencies of the enzyme 11-β-hydroxysteroid dehydrogenase, which confers mineralocorticoid specificity to the mineralocorticoid receptor by metabolizing cortisol, permit cortisol to activate the receptor and produce a clinical picture of mineralocorticoid excess (see Chapter 5.5). Liquorice as well as the drug carbenoxolone have mineralocorticoid activity, which results from inhibition of the enzyme 11-β-hydroxysteroid dehydrogenase. In addition to liquorice contained in sweets, unusual sources such as chewing tobacco and proprietary medicines have produced hypokalaemia (Blachley and Knochel 1980). Liddle's syndrome, a rare familial illness with autosomal-dominant inheritance, mimics a state of mineralocorticoid excess by a gain of function mutation in the amiloride-inhibitable ENaC sodium channel in the distal nephron (see Chapter 5.5). Recently, an activating mutation in the mineralocorticoid receptor, which results in hypertension and hypokalaemia with suppressed renin and aldosterone levels, has been described (see Chapter 5.5). The adrenogenital syndromes in children are characterized by low cortisol and overproduction of desoxycorticosterone. Hypokalaemia occurs frequently in adults but rarely in children with 17-α-hydroxylase deficiency and in approximately 25 per cent of children with 11-β-hydroxylase deficiency (Biglieri 1995; Mantero *et al.* 1995). Familial glucocorticoid resistance, produced by mutations of the glucocorticoid receptor, presents with high cortisol levels and also can manifest elevated concentrations of steroids with mineralocorticoid activity that produce hypokalaemia (Arai and Chrousos 1995).

Table 7 Mineralocorticoid excess states

High aldosterone	Low aldosterone and PRA
Low PRA (high ratio aldo/PRA)	*Normal cortisol*
Primary hyperaldosteronism	Exogenous mineralocorticoid
Glucocorticoid-remediable aldosteronism	11-β-HSD deficiency
	Congenital
High PRA	Liquorice
Renovascular disease	Carbenoxolone
Main renal arteries	Liddle's syndrome
Small vessels	MR activation mutation
Renin secretory tumour	*Low cortisol*
	Adrenogenital syndrome
	17-α-Hydroxylase deficiency
	11-β-Hydroxylase deficiency
	High cortisol
	Familial glucocorticoid resistance

PRA, plasma renin activity; HSD, hydroxysteroid dehydrogenase; MR, mineralocorticoid receptor.

Glucocorticoid excess Approximately one-third of cases of Cushing's syndrome have K^+ depletion, and hypokalaemia is most frequent in patients with ectopic ACTH production (Prunty *et al.* 1963). Glucocorticoid-mediated increases in GFR and fluid delivery to the distal nephron probably account for the tendency to K^+ wasting, but recent studies suggest that activation of mineralocorticoid receptors by very high cortisol levels may also play a role in the ectopic ACTH syndrome (Stewart *et al.* 1995).

Magnesium depletion Regardless of its cause, magnesium depletion can produce renal K^+ wasting (Solomon 1987). This may result from an increase in aldosterone, but the precise pathophysiology is unresolved (Carney *et al.* 1981; Francisco *et al.* 1981). Magnesium depletion also alters the transcellular distribution of K^+. Reduced intracellular K^+ concentration may result from a decrease in Na^+,K^+-ATPase activity (Kjeldsen and Norgaard 1987). Whether hypomagnesaemia accounts for the K^+ depletion accompanying diuretic therapy is controversial (Ryan 1987; Solomon 1987). Recent evidence that K^+ depletion produces renal magnesium wasting complicates the cause and effect relationship between hypokalaemia and hypomagnesaemia (Quamme 1997). Nevertheless, when magnesium and potassium depletion coexist, replenishment of the magnesium stores is required to correct the disordered K^+ metabolism.

Other causes of renal K^+ depletion High doses of sodium penicillin can produced hypokalaemia because of the high excretion rates of the anionic penicillin molecule (Brunner and Frick 1968). Aminoglycosides can produce both potassium and magnesium wasting by the kidney, through an undefined mechanism (Cronin *et al.* 1980). Hypokalaemia is frequent with acute leukaemia (Pickering and Catovsky 1973). Spurious determinations of K^+ from a high white-cell count, or actual K^+ depletion because of rapid cellular proliferation or as a complication of antibiotic or tumoricidal therapy, may account for this finding. High urinary lysozyme, which appears to be kaliuretic, may also play a part (Muggia *et al.* 1969; Mason *et al.* 1975). Interstitial nephritis in the setting of other autoimmune diseases can also present as a K^+ losing disorder (Wrong *et al.* 1993). Finally, any condition associated with a persistent diuresis may result in K^+ depletion. This can occur with use of the osmotic diuretics mannitol or glycerol, or in the diuretic states following relief of urinary obstruction or recovery from acute tubular necrosis.

Therapy

Therapy is usually required only for replacement of K^+ deficits and not for hypokalaemia that results from transcellular redistribution, because this is usually transitory. Therapeutic issues relevant to particular conditions have been addressed earlier; therefore, this section will focus on broad guidelines for treatment.

Replenishment of K^+ deficit requires consideration of the type of K^+ salt to be used, as well as the route and the rate of replacement.

The chloride salt of potassium (KCl) can correct any K^+ deficit and is an absolute requirement with chloride depletion such as with diuretic therapy or losses of upper gastrointestinal fluids. Bicarbonate or preparations containing bicarbonate precursors (gluconate, citrate, acetate) are indicated when a metabolic acidosis and K^+ deficit coexist. Similarly, phosphate compounds are useful when there is a concomitant phosphate deficit, as, for example, with diabetic ketoacidosis.

Potassium chloride is available in both liquid and tablet forms. Liquid preparations are least expensive and safest; however, they have an unpleasant taste. Therefore, tablets are more widely used for chronic K^+ replacement. Slow-release, wax matrix, and microencapsulated preparations are available, and the microcapsules appear to have fewer gastrointestinal side-effects. Although slow-release preparations are relatively safe, they can produce ulceration of the intestinal tract, a particular risk when intestinal motility is impaired. The K^+-sparing diuretics amiloride or triamterene are effective alternatives to KCl supplementation for patients receiving diuretics.

When feasible, K^+ should be given by the oral rather than intravenous route. Furthermore, with the exception of certain emergent conditions, slow rather than rapid K^+ replacement is preferable. Under most circumstances, administration of 40–120 mmol/day is adequate. With life-threatening hypokalaemic complications, such as paralysis, malignant ventricular arrhythmias, or digitalis intoxication, more rapid intravenous therapy (from 10 to as high as 40 mmol/h) may be appropriate, and cardiac monitoring in an intensive-care unit is advisable (Kruse *et al.* 1994; Weiner and Wingo 1997). In addition, it is preferable for K^+ to be given in solutions that do not contain glucose, since the stimulation of insulin release can potentially lower serum K^+ levels due to intracellular shifts (Weiner and Wingo 1997).

Hyperkalaemia from overzealous K^+ therapy is a life-threatening complication. Hence, a conservative approach to K^+ replacement is recommended under all circumstances.

Hyperkalaemia

Hyperkalaemia can result from a shift of K^+ from the intra- to extracellular fluid compartment or from excessive K^+ retention, which almost always implies a defect in the renal elimination of K^+. Several phenomena can spuriously elevate the serum K^+.

Clinical sequelae (Table 8)

Hyperkalaemia, regardless of its cause, depolarizes excitable tissues by decreasing the K_i^+/K_e^+ ratio; it also impairs recovery of an action potential by increasing the K^+ conductance (Seldin *et al.* 1963). This can result in life-threatening cardiac events.

Cardiac complications

Changes in cardiac conduction induced by high K^+ concentrations are reflected by the electrocardiogram and generally parallel the degree of hyperkalaemia (Surawicz 1967). The earliest changes are tenting of the T-wave, which can progress to P-wave flattening, prolongation of the PR interval, and widening of the QRS complex, with development of a deep S-wave. The ultimate risk is development of a sine-wave pattern or ventricular fibrillation with ineffective cardiac contraction.

Hyperkalaemia also alters conduction of implanted pacemakers (Barold *et al.* 1987; Varriale and Manolis 1987).

Table 8 Sequelae of hyperkalaemia

Cardiac
Impaired conduction
Ventricular fibrillation
Pacemaker dysfunction
Flaccid paralysis
Fluids and electrolytes
Decreased ammonia production
Metabolic acidosis
Natriuresis
Endocrine
High aldosterone
Low renin
Increased prostaglandin $F_{2\alpha}$ excretion
Increased kallikrein excretion
Increased insulin, glucagon
Haemodynamic
Decreased blood pressure
Decreased stroke

Neurological complications

A flaccid paralysis resembling the Guillain–Barré syndrome can result from hyperkalaemia, but typically cardiac toxicity precedes neuromuscular manifestations (Pollen and Williams 1963).

Fluid and electrolytes

Hyperkalaemia decreases the renal production and medullary accumulation of ammonia thereby impeding ammonia secretion. This leads to the development of metabolic acidosis, referred to as type IV renal tubular acidosis (Szylman *et al.* 1976; Sebastian *et al.* 1977; Tannen 1977; Hulter *et al.* 1983; Sastrasinh and Tannen 1983; DuBose 1997). A high K^+ intake is also natriuretic (Tannen 1977).

Endocrine effects

Hyperkalaemia directly stimulates adrenal aldosterone secretion and decreases renin secretion by an effect on the macula densa (Tannen 1983). Sometimes the natriuretic effect of high levels of K^+ overrides the direct, K^+-mediated effects on renin so that plasma renin activity is elevated rather than depressed (Miller *et al.* 1975; Young *et al.* 1976b). A high K^+ intake also selectively increases urinary excretion of prostaglandin $F_{2\alpha}$ and of kallikrein/kinin system mediators (Nasjletti *et al.* 1985; Vio and Fueroa 1987; Jin *et al.* 1999). Both insulin and glucagon secretion are stimulated by hyperkalaemia (Knochel 1977; Bia and DeFronzo 1981).

Haemodynamics

A high-K^+ diet decreases blood pressure both in animal models of hypertension and in hypertensive humans (Tannen 1983, 1987b; Morris *et al.* 1999; He and MacGregor 2001; Sacks *et al.* 2001). The natriuresis induced by a high-K^+ diet plays a significant part in reducing blood pressure and the magnitude of blood pressure reduction by K^+ is greater at a higher Na^+ intake (Linas 1991; He and MacGregor 2001; Sacks *et al.* 2001). Other possible mechanisms include renin suppression, baroreceptor or central neurogenic mechanisms, or a vasodilatory effect related, in part, to an increase in nitric oxide production (Tobian 1988; Zhou *et al.* 1999) and upregulation of the kallikrein/kinin system (Jin *et al.* 1999).

Both animal and human studies also suggest that a high-K^+ diet may protect against the development of stroke and of hypertensive-mediated renal injury by a mechanism distinct from its antihypertensive properties (Khaw and Barrett-Connor 1987; Tobian 1988; He and Whelton 1999; Iso *et al.* 1999; Bazzano *et al.* 2001). The stroke-protective effect may be related to cerebral vasodilatation (Chrissobolis *et al.* 2002).

Aetiology of hyperkalaemia (Table 9)

Spurious hyperkalaemia

Tight or prolonged application of a tourniquet, especially if combined with exercise of the limb, can increase the K^+ concentration of the venous blood sample because of K^+ egress from muscle and its haemoconcentration (Don *et al.* 1990). K^+ release from all the cellular elements after the blood sample is obtained can increase the serum concentration. Haemolysis is the most common phenomenon involving erythrocytes, but more rarely either acquired or hereditary abnormalities in erythrocyte permeability can elevate the serum K^+, if it is not separated promptly from the red cells (Stewart *et al.* 1979; Ho-Yen and Pennington 1980; Haines *et al.* 2001). The release of K^+ from platelets

Table 9 Aetiology of hyperkalemia

Spurious	Redistribution	Renal
Ischaemic blood drawing	Acidosis	Renal failure (severe)
Haemolysis	Insulin deficiency	Aldosterone deficiency
Abnormal erythrocytes	Hyperosmolality	Addison's disease
Thrombocytosis	β-Adrenergic blockade	Enzymatic defects
Leucocytosis	Drugs	Adrenogenital syndrome
	Arginine HCl	Aldosterone synthase I or II
	Succinylcholine	Isolated aldosterone deficiency
	Digitalis	Hyporeninaemic hypoaldosteronism
	Fluoride	HIV disease
	Lithium?	Drugs
	Hyperkalaemic	Prostaglandin synthetase inhibitors
	Periodic paralysis	ACE inhibitors
	Exercise	Angiotensin II receptor antagonists
	Malignant hyperthermia	Heparin
	Parathyroid hormone	Cyclosporin/tacrolimus
		Tubular dysfunction
		Acquired disorders
		Pseudohypoaldosteronism (Types I and II)
		K^+-sparing drugs
		Spironolactone
		Epithelial Na^+ channel blockers
		Amiloride/triamterene
		Trimethoprim
		Pentamidine
		Nafamostat mesilate

during clotting accounts for the higher concentration in serum than plasma, and can be substantial when the platelet count is elevated to more than $1 \times 10^6/mm^3$ (Graber *et al.* 1988). Plasma specimens circumvent this problem. Severe leucocytosis (over $2 \times 10^5/mm^3$) can result in sufficient egress of K^+ from white blood cells stored in the cold for spurious elevation of the K^+ determination (Bronson *et al.* 1966). Furthermore, with storage at room temperature, K^+ uptake by leucocytes can produce spurious hypokalaemia (Adams *et al.* 1981; Masters *et al.* 1996). Thus, prompt separation of plasma from the cellular elements is required to obtain valid plasma K^+ determinations especially in leukaemic patients.

Transcellular shifts

Acidosis, as discussed previously, produces egress of K^+ from cells. The increase in the plasma K^+ concentration is greater with metabolic than respiratory acidosis, and occurs only with hyperchloraemic but not organic acid-induced forms of metabolic acidosis. As stimulation of insulin release by organic acids appears to account for this divergent response, diabetic ketoacidosis produces K^+ redistribution in a fashion comparable to mineral acid-induced metabolic acidosis (Adrogue *et al.* 1986).

Hyperglycaemia produces hyperkalaemia in diabetic patients by the combined effects of hyperosmolarity and insulin deficiency on transcellular K^+ distribution (Cox *et al.* 1978). Other hyperosmolar conditions can also increase the plasma K^+ concentration, whereas insulin deficiency predisposes diabetic patients to severe abnormalities of K^+ from a variety of other mechanisms that can provoke hyperkalaemia.

Although β-adrenergic blockers typically increase K^+ modestly (0.1–0.2 mmol/l), when other homeostatic mechanisms for K^+ are deranged the hyperkalaemia can be more prominent (Carlsson *et al.* 1978; Williams *et al.* 1985). For example, the predialysis plasma K^+ concentration is increased on average by 1.0 mmol/l and exercise-induced hyperkalaemia is substantially worsened with propranolol therapy (Arrizabalaga *et al.* 1983; Yang *et al.* 1986).

Several drugs can produce hyperkalaemia by altering the transcellular distribution of K^+. Infusion of 30 g of the cationic amino acid arginine HCl increases plasma K^+ by 0.5–1.0 mmol/l and can produce life-threatening hyperkalaemia in individuals with deranged K^+ metabolism (Bushinsky and Gennari 1978). Succinylcholine, and other depolarizing muscle relaxants, increase the K^+ permeability of muscle (Thapa and Brull 2000). The K^+ concentration typically increases by 0.5–1.0 mmol/l, but in patients with burns or neuromuscular diseases hyperkalaemia can be more severe. Digitalis preparations diminish cellular K^+ uptake by inhibiting the Na^+–K^+ pump. Substantial hyperkalaemia can accompany digitalis intoxication (Smith *et al.* 1981). Fluoride intoxication appears to increase the plasma K^+ concentration by provoking leakage from the intracellular compartment (McIvor *et al.* 1985). The associated hypocalcaemia enhances the cardiac risks of fluoride-induced hyperkalaemia. It has been suggested that lithium might cause hyperkalemia, but the clinical data are sparse (Goggans 1980).

Hyperkalaemic periodic paralysis is a rare, autosomal-dominant, hereditary disorder due to a mutation in the adult of voltage-gated, muscle sodium channel. It presents with intermittent paralytic episodes accompanied by hyperkalaemia (Fontaine *et al.* 1996; Ptacek 1998). The attacks last from minutes to hours and can be induced by exercise, ingestion of excessive K^+, exposure to cold, or high cortisol concentrations. Increased serum K^+ typically ranges from 6.0 to 8.0 mmol/l, and peaked T-waves are the only associated electrocardiographic abnormality. Therapy with thiazide diuretics are useful for preventing paralytic attacks (Fontaine *et al.* 1996; Ptacek 1998). Although exercise-related increases in the plasma K^+ are usually modest, increases to 7.0 mmol/l occur during acute, maximal physical performance and concentrations as high as 10.0 mmol/l have been reported with prolonged exhaustive exercise such as in marathons (Knochel *et al.* 1985; Sterns and Spital 1987; Sejersted and Sjogaard 2000). Exercise-induced hyperkalaemia is accentuated by β-adrenergic blockade, α-adrenergic agonists, and in patients with chronic renal failure (Carlsson *et al.* 1978; Huber and Marquard 1985; Williams *et al.* 1985).

Malignant hyperthermia, a syndrome provoked by some inhalated anaesthetic agents in individuals with an inherited disorder of muscle metabolism that results in elevated intracellular calcium, can produce excessive K^+ loss from muscle (Loke *et al.* 1998). Significant hyperkalaemia has accompanied this syndrome in patients with chronic renal failure (Murakawa *et al.* 1988; San Juan *et al.* 1988; Simons and Goldman 1988).

Parathyroid hormone excess impairs cellular K^+ uptake in both normal animals and in those with renal failure, apparently by increasing the intracellular calcium concentration and activating calcium-dependent K^+ channels (Sugarman and Kahn 1988; Massry 1990).

Excessive potassium retention

Hyperkalaemia can be produced by excessive K^+ intake, as, for example, by overzealous intravenous infusion, massive oral ingestion with suicidal intent, or endogenous release from cell lysis during therapy of Burkitt lymphoma; however, in most circumstances, K^+ retention occurs because of a deficit in renal elimination (Kaplan 1969; Illingworth and Proudfoot 1980).

Defective urinary excretion of K^+ has three major causes: (a) an inadequate number of functioning nephron units, that is, renal failure; (b) hypoaldosteronism; (c) defective tubular K^+ secretion. The diagnostic evaluation of hyperkalemic patients without severe renal failure (GFR > 20 ml/min) typically involves the measurement of plasma renin and aldosterone concentrations along with a determination of either fractional potassium excretion (FEK) or of the distal transtubular potassium gradient (TTKG). FEK (urine–plasma ratio (U/P) of potassium divided by U/P creatinine) needs to be assessed in relation to GFR to determine whether renal secretion of potassium is impaired. The TTKG, which is determined by dividing U/P potassium concentration by U/P osmolality to correct for water abstraction by the medullary collecting duct, provides an indirect measure of the K^+ concentration gradient and thereby of K^+ transport by the cortical collecting duct (West *et al.* 1986; Halperin and Kamel 1998). It does not require comparison to GFR but there is no clear evidence that its diagnostic accuracy exceeds the assessment of FEK. In a hyperkalemic patient, a TTKG lesser than 8 implies an abnormal K^+ secretory response due to either hypoaldosteronism or a primary defect in tubular K^+ secretion. The accuracy of the TTKG is compromised during polyuria or excretion of a dilute urine (Ethier *et al.* 1990; DuBose 1997; Chacko *et al.* 1998; Halperin and Kamel 1998).

Renal failure

Hyperkalaemia poses a major, life-threatening risk to patients with acute oliguric renal failure; an electrocardiogram to evaluate this complication is one of the initial steps in the management of this condition. Depending on the severity of the insult, hyperkalaemia can also occur with non-oliguric acute renal failure.

The risk of hyperkalaemia is magnified in catabolic patients, in whom the daily increment in the plasma K^+ averages 0.7 mmol/l or more, in contrast to 0.3–0.5 mmol/l in non-catabolic patients with oliguric acute renal failure (Schrier 1979).

If K^+ intake is normal, chronic renal failure does not produce significant hyperkalaemia until the GFR is less than 5 ml/min (Van Ypersele de Strihou 1977; Mitch and Wilcox 1982) although milder elevations in K^+ may be present with less severe declines in GFR (Gennari and Segal 2002). K^+ balance is sustained because the remaining functional nephrons and the colon adapt their capacity to secrete K^+ in the same fashion as with a high K^+ diet (Gennari and Segal 2002). Upregulation of angiotensin II receptors may play a role in colon adaptation (Hatch *et al.* 1998). Adaptation is detectable when the GFR is reduced to one-third of normal, is maximal at a GFR of less than 10 ml/min, and accounts for 10–20 mmol/day of the K^+ elimination (Hayes *et al.* 1967; Panese *et al.* 1987).

Whereas these adaptive processes can prevent hyperkalaemia when K^+ intake is normal, the capacity to defend against an increased K^+ load is compromised with renal failure (Perez *et al.* 1983). Excessive K^+ intake or release from endogenous stores, such as from the cellular destruction associated with trauma, rhabdomyolysis, or bleeding in the gastrointestinal tract, can provoke life-threatening hyperkalaemia. Removal of the colon also compromises the ability to sustain K^+ homeostasis in patients with chronic renal failure (Raju *et al.* 1980).

Although it has been thought that intracellular K^+ concentration is diminished in patients with chronic renal failure (Van Ypersele de Strihou 1977; Mitch and Wilcox 1982) a recent review has highlighted evidence suggesting a good correlation between plasma and intracellular K+ concentrations (Gennari and Segal 2002).

Hypoaldosteronism

Hypoaldosteronism, especially when combined with a decrease in GFR and/or a reduction in the delivery of salt and fluid to the distal nephron, can substantially impair urinary K^+ excretion. Diminished levels of aldosterone result from either a primary defect in the adrenal gland or from an abnormality in the renin–angiotensin II mechanism for stimulating aldosterone secretion (Vaamonde *et al.* 1981). As a result of the decline in renin and aldosterone, along with the fall in GFR, elderly patients are at increased risk to develop hyperkalaemia (Mulkerrin *et al.* 1995; Biswas and Mulkerrin 1997; Rodriguez-Puyol 1998).

Acquired primary adrenal insufficiency, or Addison's disease, results in abnormal gluco- and mineralocorticoid production. Hyperkalaemia, detected in approximately half of these patients at the time of diagnosis, is accentuated by Na^+ restriction, and is a critical complication of acute adrenal crisis, when hypotension further compromises the mechanism of K^+ secretion (Smith *et al.* 1984). Three forms of the adrenogenital syndrome result in mineralocorticoid deficiency with associated hyperkalaemia (Pang 1997). Seventy-five per cent of patients have the most severe classic form of C-21 hydroxylase deficiency, with a mutation of the *CYP21B* gene that completely inactivates 21 hydroxylase activity. They present with salt wasting and hyperkalaemia secondary to defective biosynthesis of aldosterone (Merke *et al.* 2002). Prominent salt wasting and hyperkalaemia can also occur with 3-β-OH-dehydrogenase deficiency and is universally observed with deficiency of the steroidogenic acute regulatory (StaR) protein as a result of impaired aldosterone biosynthesis (Pang 1997).

An autosomal-recessive, selective defect in aldosterone biosynthesis occurs with deficiency in aldosterone synthase I or II, the enzymes responsible for the conversion of corticosterone to aldosterone (Peter *et al.* 1999). Usually, these patients present during infancy with typical features of aldosterone deficiency, but some children only exhibit defective growth. On occasion, the diagnosis is uncovered in adults. Selective, acquired aldosterone deficiency has been described in patients with normal renal function, as well as in a small percentage with underlying chronic renal disease (Schambelan *et al.* 1980; Williams *et al.* 1983; Kokko 1985). The aetiology of these abnormalities is unclear.

Approximately two-thirds of the hyperkalaemic patients with chronic renal failure and a GFR that should be sufficient to maintain normokalaemia manifest the syndrome of hyporeninaemic hypoaldosteronism (Arruda *et al.* 1980; DeFronzo 1980; Schambelan *et al.* 1980). Tubulointerstitial forms of renal disease predominate in this population and diabetes mellitus is commonly present. This syndrome has also been reported in patients infected with the human immunodeficiency virus; however, AIDS patients also can develop hyperkalaemia due to adrenal insufficiency, treatment with drugs that impair K^+ excretion (pentamidine or trimethoprim) and, possibly, an abnormality in K^+ redistribution (Tannen 1996; Caramelo *et al.* 1999; Eledrisi and Verghese 2001).

Hyporeninaemic hypoaldosteronism is characterized by low plasma renin activity unresponsive to Na^+ restriction or frusemide, low plasma and urinary aldosterone, hyperkalaemia, and hyperchloraemic metabolic acidosis (type IV renal tubular acidosis). Fractional K^+ excretion is low for the existing GFR, TTKG is low, and the response to kaliuretic stimuli is blunted. Mineralocorticoid replacement with fludrocortisone (0.2 mg/day) for 2 weeks usually returns the plasma K^+ to normal.

Decreased renin secretion may result from pathological involvement of the juxtaglomerular apparatus (DeFronzo 1980; Phelps *et al.* 1980). Other explanations, for which there is experimental support, include defective prostacyclin production and disordered conversion of inactive (prorenin) to active renin, which is a well-documented complication of diabetes mellitus (Hsueh 1984; Nadler *et al.* 1986). Chronic subtle expansion of extracellular fluid volume with increased concentrations of atrial natriuretic peptide also has been suggested as a cause, as plasma renin activity may be increased by prolonged Na^+ restriction or diuretic therapy (Oh *et al.* 1974; Perez *et al.* 1977; Clark *et al.* 1992; Chan *et al.* 1998). Acute salt restriction, however, can worsen hyperkalaemia in these patients by diminishing the distal delivery of Na^+ without a concurrent rise in aldosterone. Although the hypoaldosteronism is presumed to result from the low plasma renin activity; most patients have subnormal aldosterone secretory responses to both angiotensin II and ACTH infusions (DeFronzo 1980). This would be consistent with either an atrial natriuretic peptide mediated or some other direct suppressive influence on aldosterone secretion.

The hyperchloraemic metabolic acidosis primarily results from hyperkalaemic-induced suppression of renal ammonia production and excretion (Hulter *et al.* 1983; Maher *et al.* 1984; Rastogi *et al.* 1985; Batlle 1986; DuBose 1997). Aldosterone deficiency itself could also participate by impairing proton secretion by the distal nephron.

Therapy for hyporeninaemic hypoaldosteronism includes the avoidance of drugs that can cause hyperkalaemia, and appropriate dietary K^+ restriction. Measures to increase urinary excretion of K^+, such as the use of thiazide or frusemide diuretics, can be useful. Alternatively, the K^+–Na^+ exchange-resin sodium polystyrene sulfonate can be used to increase elimination from the gut, but patient compliance with chronic use of this medication is difficult to achieve. If given, it should be accompanied by laxatives to prevent faecal impaction. Although mineralocorticoid replacement effectively treats the hyperkalaemia, Na^+ retention and worsening hypertension are potentially unacceptable side-effects.

Drug-induced hypoaldosteronism results from interference with the renin–angiotensin–aldosterone axis or from direct effects on the adrenal gland. Prostaglandin synthetase inhibitors produce hyporeninaemic hypoaldosteronism by interfering with prostacyclin-mediated renin secretion (Tan *et al.* 1979; Kutyrina *et al.* 1982). A reduction in GFR and distal Na^+ delivery, as well as inhibition of distal tubule apical K^+ channels, may also contribute (Perazella 2000). Approximately one-fourth of patients with chronic renal failure treated with indomethacin develop hyperkalaemia (Zimran *et al.* 1985). Use of the renal-sparing, non-steroidal sulindac may lessen this complication (Nesher *et al.* 1988). Although not specifically documented hyperkalaemia also is a likely risk of cyclooxygenase-2-selective inhibitors (Brater 1999; Khan *et al.* 2002).

Angiotensin-converting enzyme inhibitors, such as captopril and enalapril, as well as angiotensin II receptor antagonists produce hyperkalaemia by impairing angiotensin-II-mediated secretion of aldosterone (Atlas *et al.* 1979; Textor *et al.* 1982; Perazella 2000). Hyperkalaemia is a well-documented complication of the immunosuppressive drugs cyclosporin and tacrolimus (Adu *et al.* 1983; Bantle *et al.* 1985; United States Multicenter 1994; Lee 1997). The mechanism may involve drug-induced hyporeninaemic hypoaldosteronism, but direct impairment of aldosterone secretion and primary effects on the renal tubule including inhibition of Na^+,K^+-ATPase activity and of apical K^+ channels have been reported (Ling and Eaton 1993; Tumlin and Sands 1993).

Heparin, including the low-molecular weight form, directly impairs adrenal synthesis of aldosterone by inhibiting the enzyme 18-hydroxylase. Doses as low as 10,000 units/day reduce aldosterone secretion (Sherman and Ruddy 1986; Canova *et al.* 1997). As with most other hyperkalaemic stimuli, clinically important elevations in the plasma K^+ are detected only when more than one homeostatic mechanism for K^+ is deranged (Shemer *et al.* 1983; Edes and Sunderrajan 1985; Durand *et al.* 1988).

Defective tubular secretion

A minority of hyperkalaemic patients with chronic renal failure and an adequate GFR have normal aldosterone and plasma renin activity and, apparently, a primary defect in the K^+ secretory function of the distal nephron. They typically have tubulointerstitial types of renal diseases such as obstructive uropathy, renal transplants, sickle-cell disease, lupus erythematosus, amyloidosis, and medullary sponge kidney, all of which can also produce hyporeninaemic hypoaldosteronism (Luke *et al.* 1969; DeFronzo *et al.* 1977a,b, 1979; Batlle *et al.* 1981; Green *et al.* 1984). The K^+ secretory defect in obstructive uropathy results from a decrease in Na^+,K^+-ATPase coupled with a decrease in activity of the apical Na^+ channel and K^+ conductance (Kimura and Mujais 1990; Eiam-Ong *et al.* 1993a; Hwang *et al.* 1993; Muto *et al.* 1993).

In contrast to patients with hyporeninaemic hypoaldosteronism, the hyperkalaemia is unresponsive to mineralocorticoid replacement therapy. Furthermore, the hyperchloraemic metabolic acidosis is usually accompanied by an inability to lower the urine pH appropriately, which, in combination with hyperkalaemic suppression of ammoniagenesis, may contribute to the acidosis (Rastogi *et al.* 1985; Batlle 1986; Schlueter *et al.* 1992).

Two categories of congenital abnormalities manifest hyperkalaemia secondarily to defective tubular function. Classic pseudohypoaldosteronism (type I) most frequently is an autosomal-dominant disorder that results from loss of function mutations in the genes encoding the ENaC sodium channel (Chang *et al.* 1996; Hummler *et al.* 1997; Warnock 2002). It typically presents in infancy with classical features of aldosterone deficiency despite high concentrations of aldosterone. Its severity diminishes during maturation. Multiple organs including the respiratory tract can be affected (Oberfield *et al.* 1979; Kerem *et al.* 1999; Warnock 2002). A milder autosomal-dominant form of this syndrome does not exhibit other organ system involvement and typically remits with age. It is caused by mutations of the mineralocorticoid receptor gene (Kuhnle *et al.* 1990; Geller *et al.* 1998; Warnock 2002). Aggressive therapy with salt supplementation, and control of hyperkalaemia is effective for both subtypes of this disorder.

So-called type II pseudohypoaldosteronism, originally described by Gordon, presents in late childhood or adulthood and can exhibit an autosomal-dominant mode of transmission (Gordon *et al.* 1970, 1988). These patients have hyperkalaemia, hyperchloraemic acidosis, normal renal function, hypertension, low plasma renin activity, and normal or slightly low aldosterone. The absence of kaliuresis in response to an infusion of NaCl but not of sodium sulfate or bicarbonate, suggests enhanced reabsorption of chloride at a distal nephron site (a so-called chloride shunt) (Schambelan *et al.* 1981). Enhanced reabsorption of chloride could produce volume expansion, hypertension, and suppressed plasma renin activity, and concurrently reduce K^+ secretion by diminishing the transtubular voltage gradient. Altered transcellular transport of chloride or a primary defect in K^+ secretion have also been proposed as potential explanations for this syndrome (Warnock 2002). The discovery of four different genetic loci suggests the likelihood of several variants (Mansfield *et al.* 1997; Disse-Nicodeme *et al.* 2001). Mutations in the genes encoding the WNK kinases that localize to the distal nephron may account for this syndrome (Wilson *et al.* 2001). It is of interest that thiazide diuretics may be uniquely kaliuretic in these patients, although some reports suggest that frusemide is also effective (Spitzer *et al.* 1973).

All K^+-sparing diuretics directly impair K^+ secretion by the distal nephron. Spironolactone, a specific aldosterone antagonist, impairs mineralocorticoid-dependent K^+ secretion. Amiloride and triamterene both block the apical Na^+ channel, impede electrogenic Na^+ reabsorption, decrease the transtubular voltage gradient, and thereby reduce both proton and potassium secretion.

Hyperkalaemia is a hazard with all the K^+-sparing drugs. In general, they should not be used when renal function is significantly impaired (GFR $<$ 30 ml/min), in combination with K^+ supplements, or in other circumstances where the risk of hyperkalaemia is increased.

In addition to the K^+-sparing diuretics other drugs, including trimethoprim, pentamidine, and the serine-protease inhibitor nafamostat mesilate, produce hyperkalaemia by blocking the apical Na^+ channel (Medina *et al.* 1990; Choi *et al.* 1993; Schlanger *et al.* 1994; Kleyman *et al.* 1995; Muto *et al.* 1995). Trimethoprim-induced hyperkalaemia, described initially with administration of high doses to patients with AIDS, also can occur with standard doses (Alappan *et al.* 1996; Marinella 1999).

Therapy

Treatment of hyperkalaemia is dictated by the magnitude of the elevation in the plasma K^+, its electrocardiographic manifestations, and the likelihood of progressive worsening. As it is a life-threatening abnormality, it is wise to err in the direction of overly vigorous management. Prompt and intensive treatment is indicated if the serum K^+ concentration exceeds 6.5 mmol/l, if QRS prolongation is present on the electrocardiogram, or if it seems likely that the condition will rapidly worsen.

The therapies used are outlined in Table 10. Initial steps are designed to counteract cardiac toxicity directly and to shift K^+ into the intracellular compartment (Kunis and Lowenstein 1981; Blumberg *et al.* 1988). Definitive therapy requires removal of excessive potassium from the body.

Calcium counteracts the effect of hyperkalaemia on cardiac conduction. It can be given as the gluconate or chloride salt, and acts almost immediately. Remember that calcium salts will precipitate if mixed with a bicarbonate-containing solution.

Insulin, which must be given in combination with glucose to avoid hypoglycaemia, rapidly promotes cellular uptake of K^+. Despite resistance to the hypoglycaemic effects of insulin, patients with chronic renal failure are fully responsive to its effects on cellular K^+ transport. Sodium bicarbonate has been traditionally viewed as useful in promoting cellular uptake of K^+; however, recent studies have not supported its therapeutic effectiveness, although there is conflicting evidence whether it can act in a synergistic fashion with insulin (Blumberg *et al.* 1988, 1992; Spital 1989; Allon 1995; Allon and Shanklin 1996; Kim 1996).

β-Adrenergic agonists, which also induce cellular K^+ uptake, are useful for the therapy of hyperkalaemia (Yang *et al.* 1986; Montoliu *et al.* 1987; Blumberg *et al.* 1988; Allon and Copkney 1990; Allon and Shanklin 1991; Salem *et al.* 1991; Allon *et al.* 1993; Mocan *et al.* 1993; Liou *et al.* 1994). The one shortcoming is that some patients with renal failure are refractory to the K^+ lowering effects of β-agonists (Blumberg *et al.* 1988; Allon and Copkney 1990; Mocan *et al.* 1993; Liou *et al.* 1994). An advantage is their effectiveness by inhalational as well as intravenous routes of administration (Allon *et al.* 1989; Mocan *et al.* 1993; Liou *et al.* 1994). They act synergistically with insulin to lower the plasma K^+ (Allon and Copkney 1990).

Potassium elimination from the body is usually accomplished by use of the cation-exchange resin sodium polystyrene sulfonate. By retention enema each gram removes approximately 0.5 mmol of K^+, whereas oral administration in combination with sorbitol removes approximately 1.0 mmol/g (Flinn *et al.* 1961). Colonic necrosis has been described in several postoperative uraemic patients subjected to sodium polystyrene sulfonate and sorbitol enemas (Lillemore *et al.* 1987; Wootton *et al.* 1989). Animal experiments suggest that sorbitol may be the offending component. Avoidance of sorbitol and caution in the use of sodium polystyrene sulfonate enemas in this clinical circumstance seem prudent until additional information is forthcoming.

When cation-exchange resin therapy is insufficient or not feasible, dialysis may be required. Haemodialysis is substantially more effective than peritoneal dialysis for the purposes of K^+ removal.

The therapy of chronic, mild hyperkalaemia was addressed in the discussion of the syndrome of hyporeninaemic hypoaldosteronism.

Table 10 Therapy for hyperkalaemia

Drug	Dose	Onset of action
Calcium gluconate	10–30 ml of 10% solution	Few minutes
Glucose and insulin	Glucose: 25–50 g/h by continuous IV drip Regular insulin: 5 units IV every 15 min	15–30 min
Albuterol	0.5 mg IV in 5% dextrose in water over 10–15 min 10–20 mg by nebulized inhaler over 10 min	15–30 min 15–30 min
Sodium polystyrene sulfonate	Enema (50–100 g) Oral (40 g)	60 min 120 min

References

(Entries marked with an asterisk comprise useful general reading.)

Adams, P. C., Woodhouse, K. W., Adele, M., and Parnham, A. (1981). Exaggerated hypokalemia in acute myeloid leukemia. *British Medical Journal* **282**, 1034–1035.

Adler, S. (1970). An extrarenal action of aldosterone on mammalian skeletal muscle. *American Journal of Physiology* **218**, 616–621.

***Adler, S. and Fraley, D. S.** (1977). Potassium and intracellular pH. *Kidney International* **11**, 433–442.

***Adrogue, H. J. and Madias, N. E.** (1981). Changes in plasma potassium concentration during acute acid–base disturbances. *American Journal of Medicine* **71**, 456–467.

Adrogue, H. J., Chap, Z., Ishida, T., and Field, J. B. (1985). Role of the endocrine pancreas in the kalemic response to acute metabolic acidosis in conscious dogs. *Journal of Clinical Investigation* **75**, 798.

Adrogue, H. J., Lederer, E. D., Suki, W. N., and Ekonyan, G. (1986). Determinants of plasma potassium levels in diabetic ketoacidosis. *Medicine* **65**, 163.

Adu, D., Turney, J., Michael, J., and McMaster, P. (1983). Hyperkalaemia in cyclosporin-treated renal allograft recipients. *Lancet* **ii**, 370–372.

***Agarwal, R., Afzalpurkar, R., and Fordtran, J. S.** (1994). Pathophysiology of potassium absorption and secretion by the human intestine. *Gastroenterology* **107**, 548–571.

Alappan, R., Perazella, M. A., and Buller, G. K. (1996). Hyperkalemia in hospitalized patients treated with trimethoprim-sulfamethoxazole. *Annals of Internal Medicine* **124**, 316–320.

Alexander, E. A. and Levinsky, N. G. (1968). An extrarenal mechanism of potassium adaptation. *Journal of Clinical Investigation* **47**, 740–748.

Allon, M. and Copkney, C. (1990). Albuterol and insulin for treatment of hyperkalemia in hemodialysis patients. *Kidney International* **38**, 869–872.

Allon, M. and Shanklin, N. (1991). Adrenergic modulation of extrarenal potassium disposal in men with end-stage renal disease. *Kidney International* **40**, 1103–1109.

Allon, M., Dunlay, R., and Copkney, C. (1989). Nebulized albuterol for acute hyperkalemia in patients on hemodialysis. *Annals of Internal Medicine* **110**, 426–429.

Allon, M., Takeshian, A., and Shanklin, N. (1993). Effect of insulin-plus-glucose infusion with or without epinephrine on fasting hyperkalemia. *Kidney International* **43**, 212–217.

***Allon, M.** (1995). Hyperkalemia in end-stage renal disease: mechanisms and management. *Journal of the American Society of Nephrology* **6**, 1134–1142.

Allon, M. and Shanklin, N. (1996) Effect of bicarbonate administration on plasma potassium in dialysis patients: interactions with insulin and albuterol. *American Journal of Kidney Diseases* **28**, 508–514.

Alvestrand, A., Wahren, J., Smith, D., and DeFronzo, R. A. (1984). Insulin-mediated potassium uptake is normal in uremic and healthy subjects. *American Journal of Physiology* **246**, E174–E180.

Amemiya, M., Tabei, K., Kusano, E., Asano, Y., and Alpern, R. J. (1999). Incubation of OKP cells in low-K^+ media increases NHE3 activity after early decrease in intracellular pH. *American Journal of Physiology* **276** (45), C711–C716.

Amlal, H., Wang, Z., and Soleimani, M. (1998). Potassium depletion downregulates chloride-absorbing transporters in rat kidney. *Journal of Clinical Investigation* **101**, 1045–1054.

Amlal, H., Habo, K., and Soleimani, M. (2000a). Potassium deprivation upregulates expression of renal basolateral Na^+–HCO_3^- cotransporter (NBC-1). *American Journal of Physiology* **279**, F279–F543.

Amlal, H., Krane, C. M., Chen, Q., and Soleimani, M. (2000b). Early polyuria and urinary concentrating defect in potassium depletion. *American Journal Physiology* **279**, F655–F663.

*Arai, K. and Chrousos, G. P. (1995). Syndromes of glucocorticoid and mineralocorticoid resistance. *Steroids* **60**, 173–179.

Aronson, J. K. (1983). Digitalis intoxication. *Clinical Science* **64**, 253–258.

Arrizabalaga, P., Montoliu, J., Martinez, V. A., Andreu, L., Lopez-Pedret, J., and Revert, L. (1983). Increase in serum potassium caused by beta-2 adrenergic blockade in terminal renal failure: absence of mediation by insulin or aldosterone. *Proceedings of the European Dialysis and Transplantation Association* **20**, 572–576.

Arruda, J. A. L., Batlle, D. C., Sehy, J. T., Roseman, M. K., Barnowski, R. L., and Kurtzman, N. A. (1980). Hyperkalemia and renal insufficiency: role of selective aldosterone deficiency and tubular unresponsiveness to aldosterone. *American Journal of Nephrology* **1**, 160–167.

Atlas, S. A., Case, D. B., Sealey, J. E., Laragh, J. H., and McKinstry, D. N. (1979). Interruption of the renin–angiotensin system in hypertensive patients by captopril induces sustained reduction in aldosterone secretion, potassium retention and natriuresis. *Hypertension* **1**, 274–280.

Babior, R. M. (1966). Villous adenoma of the colon. Study of a patient with severe fluid and electrolyte disturbances. *American Journal of Medicine* **41**, 615–621.

Bailey, M. A., Fletcher, R. M., Woodrow, D. F., Unwin, R. J., and Walter, S. J. (1998). Upregulation of H^+-ATPase in the distal nephron during potassium depletion: structural and functional evidence. *American Journal of Physiology* **275**, F878–F884.

Bantle, J. P., Nath, K. A., Sutherland, D. E. R., Najarian, J. S., and Ferris, T. F. (1985). Effects of cyclosporine on the renin–angiotensin–aldosterone system and potassium excretion in renal transplant recipients. *Archives of Internal Medicine* **145**, 505.

Barold, S. S., Kalkoff, M. D., Ong, L. S., and Heinle, R. A. (1987). Hyperkalemia-induced failure of atrial capture during dual-chamber cardiac pacing. *Journal of the American College of Cardiology* **10**, 467.

Batlle, D. C. (1986). Sodium dependent urinary acidification in patients with aldosterone deficiency and in adrenalectomized rats: effect of furosemide. *Metabolism* **35**, 852–860.

Batlle, D. C., Arruda, J. A. L., and Kurtzman, N. A. (1981). Hyperkalemic distal renal tubular acidosis associated with obstructive uropathy. *New England Journal of Medicine* **304**, 373–380.

Bazzano, L. A., He, J., Ogden, L. G., Loria, C., Vupputuri, S., Myers, L., and Whelton, P. (2001). Dietary potassium intake and risk of stroke in US men and women. National health and nutrition examination survey I epidemiologic follow-up study. *Stroke* **32**, 1473–1480.

Berl, T., Linas, S. L., Aisenbrey, G. A., and Anderson, R. J. (1977). On the mechanism of polyuria in potassium depletion. The role of polydipsia. *Journal of Clinical Investigation* **60**, 620–625.

Bertino, J. S., Pharm, D., and Walker, J. W. (1987). Reassessment of theophylline toxicity. Serum concentrations, clinical course, and treatment. *Archives of Internal Medicine* **147**, 757.

*Bia, M. J. and DeFronzo, R. A. (1981). Extrarenal potassium homeostasis. *American Journal of Physiology* **240**, F257–F268.

*Biglieri, E. G. (1995). 17α-Hydroxylase deficiency. *Journal of Endocrinological Investigation* **18**, 540–544.

*Biswas, K. and Mulkerrin, E. C. (1997). Potassium homeostasis in the elderly. *Quarterly Journal of Medicine* **90**, 487–492.

Blachley, J. D. and Knochel, J. P. (1980). Tobacco chewer's hypokalemia: licorice revisited. *New England Journal of Medicine* **303**, 784–785.

Blachley, J. D., Crider, B. P., and Johnson, J. H. (1986). Extrarenal potassium adaptation: role of skeletal muscle. *American Journal of Physiology* **251**, F313.

Blumberg, A., Weidmann, P., Shaw, S., and Gnadinger, M. (1988). Effect of various therapeutic approaches on plasma potassium and major regulating factors in terminal renal failure. *American Journal of Medicine* **85**, 507–512.

Blumberg, A., Weidmann, P., and Ferrari, P. (1992). Effect of prolonged bicarbonate administration on plasma potassium in terminal renal failure. *Kidney International* **41**, 369–374.

Bock, K., Cremer, W., and Werner, U. (1978). Chronic hypokalemic nephropathy: a clinical study. *Klinische Wochenschrift* **56** (Suppl. 1), 91–96.

Boettger, T., Hubner, C. A., Maier, H., Rust, M. B., Beck, F. X., and Jentsch, T. J. (2002). Deafness and renal tubular acidosis in mice lacking the K-Cl co-transporter Kcc4. *Nature* **416**, 874–878.

Braden, G. L., von Oeyer, P. T., Germain, M. J., Watson, D. J., and Haag, B. L. (1997). Ritodrine- and terbutaline-induced hypokalemia in preterm labor: mechanisms and consequences. *Kidney International* **51**, 1867–1875.

*Brater, D. C. (1999). Effects of nonsteroidal anti-inflammatory drugs on renal function: focus on cyclooxygenase-2-selective inhibition. *American Journal of Medicine* **107**, 65S–71S.

Bronson, W. R., DeVita, V. T., Carbone, P. P., and Cotlove, E. (1966). Pseudohyperkalemia due to release of potassium from white blood cells during clotting. *New England Journal of Medicine* **274**, 369–375.

Brunner, F. P. and Frick, P. G. (1968). Hypokalemia, metabolic alkalosis, and hypernatremia due to 'massive' sodium penicillin therapy. *British Medical Journal* **4**, 550–552.

Bundgaard, H., Schmidt, T. A., Larsen, J. S., and Kjeldsen, K. (1997). K^+ supplementation increases muscle [Na^+-K^+-ATPase] and improves extrarenal K^+ homeostasis in rats. *Journal of Applied Physiology* **82**, 1136–1144.

Bushinsky, D. A. and Gennari, F. J. (1978). Life-threatening hyperkalemia induced by arginine. *Annals of Internal Medicine* **89**, 632–634.

Canova, C. R., Fischler, M. P., and Reinhart, W. H. (1997). Effect of low-molecular weight heparin on serum potassium. *Lancet* **349**, 1447–1448.

Caramelo, C., Bello, E., Ruiz, E., Rovira, A., Gazapo, R. M., Alcazar, J. M., Martell, N., Ruilope, L. M., Casado, S., and Guerrero, M. F. (1999). Hyperkalemia in patients infected with the human immunodeficiency virus: involvement of a systemic mechanism. *Kidney International* **56**, 198–205.

Carlisle, E. J., Donnelly, S. M., Vasuvattakul, S., Kamel, K. S., Tobe, S., and Halperin, M. L. (1991). Glue-sniffing and distal renal tubular acidosis: sticking to the facts. *Journal of the American Society of Nephrology* **1**, 1019–1027.

Carlsson, E., Fellenius, E., Lundbor, P., and Svensson, L. (1978). Beta-adrenoceptor blockers, plasma-potassium, and exercise. *Lancet* **ii**, 424–425.

Carney, S. L., Wong, N. L. M., and Dirks, J. H. (1981). Effect of magnesium deficiency and excess on renal tubular potassium transport in the rat. *Clinical Science* **60**, 549–554.

Caviston, T. L., Campbell, W. G., Wingo, C. S., and Cain, B. D. (1999). Molecular identification of the renal H^+,K^+-ATPases. *Seminars in Nephrology* **19**, 431–437.

Chacko, M., Fordtran, J. S., and Emmett, M. (1998). Effect of mineralocorticoid activity on transtubular potassium gradient, urinary [K]/[Na] ratio, and fractional excretion of potassium. *American Journal of Kidney Diseases* **32**, 47–51.

Chan, R., Sealey, J. E., Michelis, M. F., Swan, A., Pfaffle, A. E., Devita, M. V., and Zabetakis, P. M. (1998). Renin–aldosterone system can respond to furosemide in patients with hyperkalemic hyporeninism. *Journal of Laboratory and Clinical Medicine* **132**, 229–235.

Chang, S. S., Grunder, S., Hanukoglu, A., Rosler, A., Mathew, P. M., Hanukoglu, I., Schild, L., Lu, Y., Shimkets, R. A., Nelson-Williams, C., Rossier, B. C., and Lifton, R. P. (1996). Mutations in subunits of the epithelial sodium channel cause salt wasting with hyperkalaemic acidosis, pseudohypoaldosteronism type I. *Nature Genetics* **12**, 248–253.

Choi, M. J. *et al.* (1993). Trimethoprim-induced hyperkalemia in a patient with AIDS. *New England Journal of Medicine* **328**, 703–706.

Chrissobolis, S., Ziogas, J., Anderson, C. R., Chu, Y., Faraci, F. M., and Sobey, C. G. (2002). Neuronal NO mediates cerebral vasodilator responses to K^+ in hypertensive rats. *Hypertension* **39**, 880–885.

Cirillo, M. *et al.* (1994). Urinary sodium to potassium ratio and urinary stone disease. *Kidney International* **46**, 1133–1139.

Clark, B. A., Brown, R. S., and Epstein, F. H. (1992). Effect of atrial natriuretic peptide on potassium stimulated aldosterone secretion: potential relevance to hypoaldosteronism in man. *Journal of Clinical Endocrinology and Metabolism* **75**, 399–403.

Clemessy, J. L., Favier, C., Borron, S. W., Hantson, P. E., Vicaut, E., and Baud, F. J. (1995). Hypokalaemia related to acute chloroquine ingestion. *Lancet* **346**, 877–880.

Conci, F., Procaccio, F., and Boselli, L. (1984). Hypokalemia from β_2-receptor stimulation by epinephrine. *New England Journal of Medicine* **310**, 1329.

*__Corry, D. B. and Tuck, M. L.__ (1995). Secondary aldosteronism. *Endocrinology and Metabolism Clinics of North America* **24**, 511–529.

Corvol, P. *et al.* (1988). Seven lessons from seven renin secreting tumors. *Kidney International* **34**, S38–S44.

*__Cox, M., Sterns, R. H., and Singer, I.__ (1978). The defense against hyperkalaemia: the roles of insulin and aldosterone. *New England Journal of Medicine* **299**, 525–532.

Cronin, R. E. *et al.* (1980). Natural history of aminoglycoside nephrotoxicity in the dog. *Journal of Laboratory and Clinical Medicine* **95**, 463–474.

Dafnis, E. *et al.* (1992). Vanadate causes hypokalemic distal renal tubular acidosis. *American Journal of Physiology* **262**, F449–F453.

*__DeFronzo, R. A.__ (1980). Hyperkalemia and hyporeninemic hypoaldosteronism. *Kidney International* **17**, 118–134.

DeFronzo, R. A., Cooke, C. R., Goldberg, M., Cox, M., Myers, A. R., and Agus, Z. S. (1977a). Impaired renal tubular potassium secretion in systemic lupus erythematosus. *Annals of Internal Medicine* **86**, 268–271.

DeFronzo, R. A., Goldberg, M., Cooke, C. R., Barker, C., Crossman, R. A., and Agus, Z. S. (1977b). Investigations into the mechanisms of hyperkalemia following renal transplantation. *Kidney International* **11**, 357–365.

DeFronzo, R. A., Taufield, P. A., Black, H., McPhedran, P., and Cooke, C. R. (1979). Impaired renal tubular potassium secretion in sickle cell disease. *Annals of Internal Medicine* **90**, 310–316.

DeFronzo, R. A., Lee, R., Jones, A., and Bia, M. J. (1980). Effect of insulinopenia and adrenal hormone deficiency on acute potassium tolerance. *Kidney International* **17**, 586–594.

DeFronzo, R. A., Bia, M., and Birkhead, G. (1981). Epinephrine and potassium homeostasis. *Kidney International* **20**, 83–91.

Disse-Nicodeme, S., Desitter, I., Fiquet-Kempf, B., Houot, A., Stern, N., Delahousse, M., Potier, J., Ader, J., and Jeunemaitre, X. (2001). Genetic heterogeneity of familial hyperkalaemic hypertension. *Journal of Hypertension* **19**, 1957–1964.

Dluhy, R. G. and Lifton, R. P. (1995). Glucocorticoid-remediable aldosteronism (GRA): diagnosis, variability of phenotype and regulation of potassium homeostasis. *Steroids* **60**, 48–51.

Don, B. R. *et al.* (1990). Pseudohyperkalemia caused by fist clenching during phlebotomy. *New England Journal of Medicine* **322**, 1290–1292.

Donker, A. J. M. *et al.* (1977). Indomethacin in Bartter's syndrome. *Nephron* **19**, 200–213.

*__DuBose, T. D., Jr.__ (1997). Hyperkalemic hyperchloremic metabolic acidosis: pathophysiologic insights. *Kidney International* **51**, 591–602.

*__Dunn, M. J.__ (1981). Prostaglandins and Bartter's syndrome. *Kidney* **19**, 86–102.

Durand, D. *et al.* (1988). Inducing hyperkalemia by converting by enzyme inhibitors and heparin. *Kidney International* **34** (Suppl. 25), S196–S197.

Edes, T. E. and Sunderrajan, E. V. (1985). Heparin-induced hyperkalemia. *Archives of Internal Medicine* **145**, 1070.

Ehrenfeld, J., Lacoste, I., and Harvey, B. J. (1992). Effects of intracellular signals on Na^+/K^+-ATPase pump activity in the frog skin epithelium. *Biochimica Biophysics Acta* **1106**, 197–208.

Eiam-Ong, S. *et al.* (1993a). H–K-ATPase in distal renal tubular acidosis: urinary tract obstruction, lithium and amiloride. *American Journal of Physiology* **265**, F875–F880.

Eiam-Ong, S., Kurtzman, N. A., and Sabatini, S. (1993b). Regulation of collecting tubule adenosine triphosphatases by aldosterone and potassium. *Journal of Clinical Investigation* **91**, 2385–2392.

*__Eledrisi, M. S. and Verghese, A. C.__ (2001). Adrenal insufficiency in HIV infection: a review and recommendations. *American Journal of the Medical Sciences* **321**, 137–144.

Elger, M., Bankir, L., and Kriz, W. (1992). Morphometric analysis of kidney hypertrophy in rats after potassium depletion. *American Journal of Physiology* **262**, F656–F667.

Ellison, D. H., Velazquez, H., and Wright, F. S. (1987). Mechanisms of sodium, potassium and chloride transport by the renal distal tubule. *Mineral Electrolyte Metabolism* **13**, 422–432.

Ethier, J. H., Kamel, K. S., Magner, P. O., Lemann, J., Jr., and Halperin, M. L. (1990). The transtubular potassium concentration in patients with hypokalemia and hyperkalemia. *American Journal of Kidney Diseases* **15**, 309–315.

Feraille, E., Carranza, M. L., Gonin, S., Beguin, P., Pedemonte, C., Rousselot, M., Caverzasio, J., Geering, K., Martin, P. Y., and Favre, H. (1999). Insulin-induced stimulation of Na^+,K^+-ATPase activity in kidney proximal tubule cells depends on phosphorylation of the alpha-subunit at Tyr-10. *Molecular Biology of the Cell* **10**, 2847–2859.

*__Feraille, E. and Doucet, A.__ (2001). Sodium-potassium-adenosinetriphosphatase-dependent sodium transport in the kidney: hormonal control. *Physiological Reviews* **81**, 345–418.

Fichman, M. P., Vorherr, H., Kleeman, C. R., and Telfer, N. (1971). Diuretic-induced hyponatremia. *Annals of Internal Medicine* **75**, 853–863.

Field, M. J., Stanton, B. A., and Giebisch, G. H. (1984). Differential acute effects of aldosterone, dexamethasone, and hyperkalemia on distal tubular potassium secretion in the rat kidney. *Journal of Clinical Investigation* **74**, 1792–1802.

Fleischer, N., Brown, H., Graham, D. Y., and Delena, S. (1969). Chronic laxative-induced hyperaldosteronism and hypokalemia stimulating Bartter's syndrome. *Annals of Internal Medicine* **70**, 791–798.

Flinn, R. B., Merrill, J. P., and Welzant, W. R. (1961). Treatment of the oliguric patient with a new sodium-exchange resin and sorbitol. *New England Journal of Medicine* **264**, 111–119.

Flybjerg, A., Dorup, I., Everts, M. E., and Orskov, H. (1991). Evidence that potassium deficiency induces growth retardation through reduced circulating levels of growth hormone and insulin-like growth factor I. *Metabolism* **40**, 769–775.

Fontaine, B., Lapie, P., Plassart, E., Tabti, N., Nicole, S., Reboul, J., and Rime-Davoine, C. (1996). Periodic paralysis and voltage-gated ion channels. *Kidney International* **49**, 9–18.

Foster, E. S., Jones, W. J., Hayslett, J. P., and Binder, H. J. (1985). Role of aldosterone and dietary potassium in potassium adaptation in the distal colon of the rat. *Gastroenterology* **88**, 41.

Francisco, L. L., Sawin, L. L., and Dibona, G. F. (1981). Mechanism of negative potassium balance in the magnesium-deficient rat. *Proceedings of the Society for Experimental Biology and Medicine* **168**, 382–388.

Frank, A. E., Wingo, C. S., and Weiner, I. D. (2000). Effects of ammonia on bicarbonate transport in the cortical collecting duct. *American Journal of Physiology* **278**, F219–F226.

Garella, S., Chazan, J. A., and Cohen J. J. (1970). Saline-resistant metabolic alkalosis or chloride-wasting nephropathy. *Annals of Internal Medicine* **73**, 31–38.

Gelfand, M. C., Zarate, A., and Knepshield, J. H. (1975). Geophagia. A cause of life threatening hyperkalemia in patients with chronic renal failure. *Journal of the American Medical Association* **234**, 738–740.

Geller, D. S., Rodriguez-Soriano, J., Boado, A. V., Schifter, S., Bayer, M., Chang, S. S., and Lifton, R. P. (1998). Mutations in the mineralocorticoid receptor gene cause autosomal dominant pseudohypoaldosteronism type I. *Nature Genetics* **19**, 279–281.

*__Gennari, F. J. and Cohen, J. J.__ (1975). Role of the kidney in potassium homeostasis: lessons from acid–base disturbances. *Kidney International* **8**, 1–5.

*__Gennari, F. J. and Segal, A. S.__ (2002). Hyperkalemia: an adaptive response in chronic renal insufficiency. *Kidney International* **62**, 1–9.

*__Giebisch, G. H.__ Cell models of potassium transport in the renal tubule. In *Current Topics in Membranes and Transport*, 28 (ed. G. Giebisch), p. 133. Orlando, FA: Academic Press, 1987.

Goggans, F. C. (1980). Acute hyperkalemia during lithium treatment of manic illness. *American Journal of Psychiatry* **137**, 860–861.

Gonzales, J. J., Owens, W., Ungaro, P. C., Werk, E. E., Jr., and Wentz, P. W. (1982). Clay ingestion: a rare cause of hypokalemia. *Annals of Internal Medicine* **97**, 65–66.

Good, D. W., Velazquez, H., and Wright, F. S. (1984). Luminal influences on potassium secretion: low sodium concentration. *American Journal of Physiology* **246**, F609–F619.

Gordon P. (1973). Glucose intolerance with hypokalemia. Failure of short-term potassium depletion in normal subjects to reproduce the glucose and insulin abnormalities of clinical hypokalemia. *Diabetes* **22**, 544–551.

Gordon, R. D., Geddes, R. A., Pawsey, C. G. K., and O'Halloran, M. W. (1970). Hypertension and severe hypokalemia associated with suppression of renin and aldosterone and completely reversed by dietary sodium restriction. *Australian Annals of Medicine* **4**, 287–294.

Gordon, R. D. *et al.* (1988). A new Australian kindred with the syndrome of hypertension and hyperkalemia has dysregulation of atrial natriuretic factor. *Journal of Hypertension* **6**, S323–S326.

Graber, M. (1993). A model of the hyperkalemia produced by metabolic acidosis. *American Journal of the Kidney Diseases* **22**, 436–444.

Graber, M., Subramani, K., Corish, D., and Schwab, A. (1988). Thrombocytosis elevates serum potassium. *American Journal of Kidney Diseases* **12**, 116–120.

Green J., Szylman, P., Sznajder, I. I., Winaver, J., and Better, O. S. (1984). Renal tubular handling of potassium in patients with medullary sponge kidney. *Archives of Internal Medicine* **144**, 2201–2204.

Gu, R., Wei, Y., Jiang, H., Balazy, M., and Wang, W. (2001). Role of 20-HETE in mediating the effect of dietary K intake on the apical K channels in the mTAL. *American Journal of Physiology* **280**, F223–F230.

Grobbee, D. and Hoes, A. W. (1995). Non-potassium-sparing diuretics and risk of sudden cardiac death. *Journal of Hypertension* **13**, 1539–1545.

Haines, P. G., Crawley, C., Chetty, M. C., Jarvis, H., Coles, S. E., Fisher, J., Nicolaou, A., and Stewart, G. W. (2001). Familial pseudohyperkalaemia Chiswick: a novel congenital thermotropic variant of K and Na transport across the human red cell membrane. *British Journal of Haematology* **112**, 469–474.

Hall, R. J. C. and Cameron, I. R. (1981). Effect of chronic dietary potassium depletion and repletion on cardiac and skeletal muscle structure, electrolytes and pH in the rabbit. *Clinical Science* **60**, 441–449.

Hall, K. W., Dobson, K. E., Dalton, J. G., Ghignone, M. C., and Penner, S. B. (1984). Metabolic abnormalities associated with intentional theophylline overdose. *Annals of Internal Medicine* **101**, 457.

Halperin, M. L. and Kamel, K. S. (1998). Potassium. *Lancet* **352**, 135–140.

Harrington, J. T., Isner, J. M., and Kassirer, J. P. (1982). Our national obsession with potassium. *American Journal of Medicine* **73**, 155–159.

Hatch, M., Freel, R. W., and Vaziri, N. D. (1998). Local upregulation of colonic angiotensin II receptors enhances potassium excretion in chronic renal failure. *Amercian Journal of Physiology* **274**, F275–F282.

Hayes, C. P., Jr., McLeod, M. E., and Robinson, R. R. (1967). An extrarenal mechanism for the maintenance of potassium balance in severe chronic renal failure. *Transactions of the Association of American Physicians* **50**, 207–216.

*__Hayslett, J. P. and Binder, H. J.__ (1982). Mechanism of potassium adaptation. *American Journal of Physiology* **243**, F103–F112.

He, F. J. and MacGregor, G. A. (2001). Beneficial effects of potassium. *British Medical Journal* **323**, 497–501.

He, J. and Whelton, P. K. (1999). What is the role of dietary sodium and potassium in hypertension and target organ injury? *American Journal of the Medical Sciences* **317**, 152–159.

Henquin, J. C. (2000). Triggering and amplifying pathways of regulation of insulin secretion by glucose. *Diabetes* **49**, 1751–1760.

Hernandez, R. E. *et al.* (1987). Dietary NaCl determines severity of potassium depletion-induced metabolic alkalosis. *Kidney International* **31**, 1356.

Hiatt, N., Chapman, L. W., Davidson, M. B., and Mack, H. (1986). Kaluresis independent K-homeostasis: glucagon and b receptor blockade in pancreatectomized dogs. *Hormones and Metabolism Research* **18**, 739–742.

Hochberg, Z., Amit, T., Flyvbjerg, A., and Dorup, I. (1995). Growth hormone (GH) receptor and GH-binding protein deficiency in the growth failure of potassium-depleted rats. *Journal of Endocrinology* **147**, 253–258.

Ho-Yen, D. O. and Pennington, C. R. (1980). Pseudohyperkalemia and infectious mononucleosis. *Postgraduate Medical Journal* **56**, 435–436.

Hsu, F. W., Tsao, T., and Rabkin, R. (1997). The IGF-I axis in kidney and skeletal muscle of potassium deficient rats. *Kidney International* **52**, 363–370.

Hsueh, W. A. (1984). Potential effects of renin activation on the regulation of renin production. *American Journal of Physiology* **247**, F205.

Huber, W. and Marquard, E. (1985). Plasma potassium and blood pH following physical exercise in dialysis patients. *Nephron* **40**, 383.

Hulter, H. N., Sigala, J. F., and Sebastian, A. (1978). K^+ deprivation potentiates the renal alkalosis-producing effect of mineralocorticoid. *American Journal of Physiology* **235**, F298–F309.

Hulter, H. N., Toto, R. D., Ilnicki, I. P., and Sebastian, A. (1983). Chronic hyperkalemic renal tubular acidosis induced by KCL loading. *American Journal of Physiology* **244**, F255–F264.

Hummler, E., Barker, P., Talbot, C., Wang, Q., Verdumo, C., Grubb, B., Gatzy, J., Burnier, M., Horisberger, J., Beermann, F., Boucher, R., and Rossier, B. C. (1997). A mouse model for the renal salt-wasting syndrome pseudohypoaldosteronism. *Proceedings of the National Academy of Sciences of USA* **94**, 11710–11715.

Hwang, S. J. *et al.* (1993). Transport defects of rabbit inner medullary collecting duct cells in obstructive nephropathy. *American Journal of Physiology* **264**, F808–F815.

Illingworth, R. N. and Proudfoot, A. T. (1980). Rapid poisoning with slow-release potassium. *British Medical Journal* **16**, 485–486.

Iso, H., Stampfer, M. J., Manson, J. E., Rexrode, K., Hennekens, C. H., Colditz, G. A., Speizer, F. E., and Willett, W. C. (1999). Prospective study of calcium, potassium, and magnesium intake and risk of stroke in women. *Stroke* **30**, 1772–1779.

Jaeger, P., Karlmark, B., and Giebisch G. (1983). Ammonium transport in rat cortical tubule: relationship to potassium metabolism. *American Journal of Physiology* **245**, F593–F600.

*__Jamison, R. L.__ (1987). Potassium recycling. *Kidney International* **31**, 695.

Jamison, R. L., Ross, J. C., Kempson, R. L., Sufit, C. R., and Parker T. E. (1982). Surreptitious diuretic ingestion and pseudo-Bartter's syndrome. *American Journal of Medicine* **73**, 142–147.

Jin, L., Chao, L., and Chao, J. (1999). Potassium supplement upregulates the expression of renal kallikrein and bradykinin B2 receptor in SHR. *American Journal of Physiology* **276**, F476–F484.

Johansson, B. W. and Larsson, C. (1982). A hypokalemic index ECG as a predictor hypokalemia. *Acta Medica Scandinavica* **212**, 29–31.

Kaplan, M. (1969). Suicide by oral ingestion of a potassium preparation. *Annals of Internal Medicine* **71**, 363–364.

Kaplan, N. M. *et al.* (1985). Potassium supplementation in hypertensive patients with diuretic-induced hypokalemia. *New England Journal of Medicine* **312**, 746–749.

*__Kassirer, J. P. and Harrington, J. T.__ (1977). Diuretics and potassium metabolism: a reassessment of the need, effectiveness and safety of potassium therapy. *Kidney International* **11**, 505–515.

Kassirer, J. P. and Schwartz, W. B. (1966). The response of normal man to selective depletion of hydrochloric acid. Factors in the genesis of persistent gastric alkalosis. *American Journal of Medicine* **40**, 10–18.

Kassirer, J. P., Appleton, F. M., Chzan, J. A., and Schwartz, W. B. (1967). Aldosterone in metabolic alkalosis. *Journal of Clinical Investigation* **46**, 1558–1571.

Kassirer, J. P., London, A. M., Goldman, D. M., and Schwartz, W. B. (1970). On the pathogenesis of metabolic alkalosis in hyperaldosteronism. *American Journal of Medicine* **49**, 306–315.

Kearney, T. E., Manoguerra, A. M., Curtis, G. P., and Ziegler, M. G. (1985). Theophylline toxicity and the beta-adrenergic system. *Annals of Internal Medicine* **102**, 766.

Kerem, E., Bistritzer, R., Hanukoglu, A., Hofmann, T., Zhou, Z., Bennett, W., MacLaughlin, E., Barker, P., Nash, M., Quittell, L., Boucher, R., and Knowles, M. R. (1999). Pulmonary epithelial sodium channel dysfunction and excess airway liquid in pseudohypoaldosteronism. *New England Journal of Medicine* **341**, 156–162.

Khan, K. N. M., Paulson, S. K., Verburg, K. M., Lefkowith, J. B., and Maziasz, T. J. (2002). Pharmacology of cyclooxygenase-2 inhibition in the kidney. *Kidney International* **61**, 1210–1219.

Khaw, K. T. and Barrett-Connor, E. (1987). Dietary potassium and stroke-associated mortality: a 12 year prospective population study. *New England Journal of Medicine* **316**, 235.

Kim, D. U., Jung, J. Y., Kim, Y. H., Cha, J. H., Sands, J. M., Madsen, K. M., and Kim, J. (2001). Effect of prolonged potassium depletion on the expression of urea transporters in rat kidney. *Journal of the American Society of Nephrology* **12**, 17A.

Kim, H. J. (1996). Combined effect of bicarbonate and insulin with glucose in acute therapy of hyperkalemia in end-stage renal disease patients. *Nephron* **72**, 476–482.

Kimmel, P. L. and Goldfarb, S. (1984). Effects of isoproterenol on potassium secretion by the cortical collecting tubule. *American Journal of Physiology* **246**, F804–F810.

Kimura, H. and Mujais, S. K. (1990). Cortical collecting duct Na–K pump in obstructive nephropathy. *American Journal of Physiology* **258**, F1320–F1327.

Kjeldsen, K. and Norgaard, A. (1987). Effect of magnesium depletion on; 3H-ouabain binding site concentration in rat skeletal muscle. *Magnesium* **6**, 55.

Kleyman, T. R., Roberts, C., and Ling, B. N. (1995). A mechanism for pentamidine-induced hyperkalemia: inhibition of distal nephron sodium transport. *Annals of Internal Medicine* **122**, 103–106.

*__Knochel, J. P.__ (1977). Role of glucoregulatory hormones in potassium homeostasis. *Kidney International* **11**, 443–452.

*__Knochel, J. P.__ (1981). Neuromuscular manifestations of electrolyte disorders. *American Journal of Medicine* **72**, 521–535.

Knochel, J. P., Dotin, L. N., and Hamburger, R. J. (1972). Pathophysiology of intense physical conditioning in a hot climate. *Journal of Clinical Investigation* **51**, 242–254.

Knochel, J. P., Foley, F. D., Jr., and Lipscomb, K. (1978). High resting cardiac output with exercise-induced pulmonary edema in the conscious, potassium-deficient dog. *Mineral and Electrolyte Metabolism* **1**, 336–344.

Knochel, J. P., Blachley, J. D., Johnson, J. H., and Carter, N. W. (1985). Muscle cell electrical hyperpolarization and reduced exercise hyperkalemia in physically conditioned dogs. *Journal of Clinical Investigation* **75**, 740.

Kokko, J. P. (1985). Primary acquired hypoaldosteronism. *Kidney International* **27**, 690.

Krapf, R., Caduff, P., Wagdi, P., Staubli, M., and Hulter, H. N. (1995). Plasma potassium response to acute respiratory alkalosis. *Kidney International* **47**, 217–224.

Krishna, G. G. and Kapoor, S. C. (1991). Potassium depletion exacerbates essential hypertension. *Annals of Internal Medicine* **115**, 77–83.

Krishna, G. G., Chusid, P., and Hoeldtke, R. D. (1987). Mild potassium depletion provokes renal sodium retention. *Journal of Laboratory and Clinical Medicine* **109**, 724.

Kruse, J. A., Clark, V. L., Carlson, R. W., and Geheb, M. A. (1994). Concentrated potassium chloride infusions in critically ill patients with hypokalemia. *Journal of Clinical Pharmacology* **34**, 1077–1082.

Kuhnle, U. *et al.* (1990). Pseudohypoaldosteronism in eight families: different forms of inheritance are evidence for various genetic defects. *Journal of Clinical Endocrinology and Metabolism* **70**, 638–641.

Kunis, C. L. and Lowenstein, J. (1981). The emergency treatment of hyperkalemia. *Medical Clinics of North America* **65**, 165–176.

*__Kunzelmann, K. and Mall, M.__ (2002). Electrolyte transport in the mammalian colon: mechanisms and implications for disease. *Physiological Reviews* **82**, 245–289.

Kutyrina, I. M., Androsova, S. O., Warshavskii, V. A., and Tareyeva, I. E. (1982). Effects of indomethacin on the renal function and renin–aldosterone system in chronic glomerulonephritis. *Nephron* **32**, 244–248.

Laragh, J. H. and Sealey, J. E. (2001). K^+ depletion and progression of hypertensive disease or heart failure. The pathogenic role of diuretic-induced aldosterone secretion. *Hypertension* **37**, 806–810.

Lawson, D. H., Murray, R. M., and Parker, J. L. W. (1972). Early mortality in the megaloblastic anaemias. *Quarterly Journal of Medicine* **161**, 1–14.

Lawton, W. J. *et al.* (1990). Effect of dietary potassium on blood pressure, renal function, muscle sympathetic nerve activity, and forearm vascular resistance and flow in normotensive and borderline hypertensive humans. *Circulation* **81**, 173–184.

Lee, D. B. N. (1997). Cyclosporine and the renin-angiotensin axis. *Kidney International* **52**, 248–260.

Lemann, J., Jr. (1999). Relationship between urinary calcium and net acid excretion as determined by dietary protein and potassium: a review. *Nephron* **81** (Suppl. 1), 18–25.

Lifton, R. P. (1996). Molecular genetics of human blood pressure variation. *Science* **272**, 676–680.

Lillemore, K. D., Romolo, J. L., Hamilton, S. R., Pennington, L. R., Burdick, J. F., and Williams, G. M. (1987). Intestinal necrosis due to sodium polystyrene (Kayexalate) in sorbitol enemas: clinical and experimental support for the hypothesis. *Surgery* **101**, 267.

Linas, S. L. (1981). Mechanism of hyperreninemia in the potassium-depleted rat. *Journal of Clinical Investigation* **68**, 347–355.

*__Linas, S. L.__ (1991). The role of potassium in the pathogenesis and treatment of hypertension. *Kidney International* **39**, 771–786.

Linas, S. L. and Dickmann, D. (1982). Mechanism of the decreased renal blood flow in the potassium-depleted conscious rat. *Kidney International* **21**, 757–764.

Ling, B. N. and Eaton, D. C. (1993). Cyclosporin A inhibits apical secretory K^+ channels in rabbit cortical collecting tubule principal cells. *Kidney International* **44**, 974–984.

Liou, H. H. *et al.* (1994). Hypokalemic effects of intravenous infusion or nebulization of salbutamol in patients with chronic renal failure: comparative study. *American Journal of Kidney Diseases* **23**, 266–271.

*__Litchfield, W. R. and Dluhy, R. G.__ (1995). Primary aldosteronism. *Endocrinology and Metabolism Clinics of North America* **24**, 593–612.

Lohr, J. W. (1994). Osmotic demyelination syndrome following correction of hyponatremia: associated with hypokalemia. *American Journal of Medicine* **96**, 408–413.

*__Loke, J. and MacLennan, D. H.__ (1998). Malignant hyperthermia and central core disease: disorders of Ca^{2+} release channels. *American Journal of Medicine* **104**, 470–486.

Luke, R. G. (1974). Effect of adrenalectomy on the renal response to chloride depletion in the rat. *Journal of Clinical Investigation* **54**, 1329–1336.

Luke, R. G., Allison, M. E. W., Davidson, J. F., and Duguid, W. P. (1969). Hyperkalemia and renal tubular acidosis due to renal amyloidosis. *Annals of Internal Medicine* **70**, 1211–1217.

Luke, R. G., Wright, F., Fowler, N., Kashgarin, M., and Giebisch, G. H. (1978). Effects of potassium depletion on renal tubular chloride transport in the rat. *Kidney International* **14**, 414–427.

Luke, R. G., Lyerly, R. H., Anderson, J., Galla, J. H., and Kotchen, T. A. (1982). Effect of potassium depletion on renin release. *Kidney International* **21**, 14–19.

Madias, J. E., Shah, B., Chintalapally, G., Chalavarya, G., and Madias, M. E. (2000). Admission serum potassium in patients with acute myocardial infarction. *Chest* **118**, 904–913.

*Martin, P. and Schrier, R. W. (1998). Role of aquaporin-2 water channels in urinary concentration and dilution defects. *Kidney International* **53** (Suppl. 65), S57–S62.

McIvor, M. E. *et al.* (1985). The manipulation of potassium efflux during fluoride intoxication: implications of therapy. *Toxicology* **37**, 233.

Maher, T., Schambelan, M., Kurts, I., Hulter, H. H., Jones, J. W., and Sebastian, A. (1984). Amelioration of metabolic acidosis by dietary potassium restriction in hyperkalemic patients with chronic renal insufficiency. *Journal of Laboratory and Clinical Medicine* **103**, 432–445.

Makoff, D. L., Da Silva, J. A., and Rosenbaum. B. J. (1971). On the mechanism of hyperkalemia due to hyperosmotic expansion with saline or mannitol. *Clinical Science* **41**, 383–393.

Mallick, B. N., Adya, H. V., and Faisal, M. (2000). Norepinephrine-stimulated increase in Na^+,K^+-ATPase activity in the rat brain is mediated through alpha1A-adrenoceptor possibly by dephosphorylation of the enzyme. *Journal of Neurochemistry* **74**, 1574–1578.

Malnic, G., Berliner, R. W., and Giebisch, G. (1989). Flow dependence of K^+ secretion in cortical distal tubules of the rat. *American Journal of Physiology* **256**, F932–F941.

Manoukian, M. A., Foote, J. A., and Crapo, L. M. (1999). Clinical and metabolic features of thyrotoxic periodic paralysis in 24 episodes. *Archives of Internal Medicine* **159**, 601–606.

Mansfield, T. A., Simon, D. B., Farfel, Z., Bia, M., Tucci, J. R., Lebel, M., Gutkin, M., Vialettes, B., Christofilis, M. A., Kauppinen-Makelin, R., Mayan, H., Risch, N., and Lifton, R. P. (1997). The multilocus linkage of familial hyperkalaemia and hypertension, pseudohypoaldosteronism type II, to chromosomes 1q31–42 and 17p11-q21. *Nature Genetics* **16**, 202–205.

Mantero, F., Opocher, G., Armanini, D., and Filipponi, S. (1995). 11β-Hydroxylase deficiency. *Journal of Endocrinological Investigation* **18**, 545–549.

Marette, A., Krischer, J., Lavoie, L., Ackerley, C., Carpentier, J. L., and Klip, A. (1993). Insulin increases the Na-K-ATPase α_2-subunit in the surface of rat skeletal muscle: morphologic evidence. *American Journal of Physiology* **265**, C1716–C1722.

Marinella, M. A. (1999). Trimethoprim-induced hyperkalemia: an analysis of reported cases. *Gerontology* **45**, 209–212.

Marples, D., Frokiaer, J., Dorup, J., Knepper, M. A., and Nielson, S. (1996). Hypokalaemia-induced down regulation of aquaporin-2 water channel expression in rat kidney medulla and cortex. *Journal of Clinical Investigation* **97**, 1960–1968.

Martinez-Maldonado, M. and Opava-Stitzer, S. Pathophysiology of clinical disorders of urine concentration and dilution. In *Pathophysiology of the Kidney* (ed. N. A. Kurtzman and M. Martinez-Maldonado), pp. 992–1028. Springfield, IL: Thomas, 1977.

Mason, D. Y., Howes, D. T., Taylor, C. R., and Ross, B. D. (1975). Effects of human lysozyme (muramidase) on potassium handling by the perfused rat kidney. A mechanism for renal damage in human monocytic leukaemia. *Journal of Clinical Pathology* **28**, 722–727.

Massara, F., Marteli, S., Cagliero, E., Camanni, F., and Molinatti, G. M. (1980). Influence of glucagon on plasma levels of potassium in man. *Diabetologia* **19**, 414–417.

*Massry, S. G. (1990). Renal failure, parathyroid hormone and extrarenal disposal of potassium. *Mineral and Electrolyte Metabolism* **16**, 77–81.

Masters, P. W., Lawson, N., Marenah, C. B., and Maile, L. J. (1996). High ambient temperature: a spurious cause of hypokalaemia. *British Medical Journal* **312**, 1652–1653.

Medina, I. *et al.* (1990). Oral therapy for *Pneumocystis carinii* pneumonia in the acquired immunodeficiency syndrome—a controlled trial of trimethoprim—sulfamethoxazole versus trimethoprim—dapsone. *New England Journal of Medicine* **323**, 776–782.

Mennitt, P. A., Frindt, G., Silver R. B., and Palmer, L. G. (2000). Potassium restriction downregulates ROMK expression in rat kidney. *American Journal of Physiology–Renal Physiology* **278**, F916–F924.

Merke, D. P., Bornstein, S. R., Avila, N. A., and Chrousos, G. P. (2002). Future directions in the study and management of congenital adrenal hyperplasia due to 21-hydroxylase deficiency. *Annals of Internal Medicine* **136**, 320–334.

Mihailidou, A. S., Buhagiar, K. A., and Rasmussen, H. H. (1998). Na^+ influx and Na^+–K^+ pump activation during short-term exposure of cardiac myocytes to aldosterone. *American Journal of Physiology* **274**, C175–C181.

Miller, P. D., Waterhouse, C., Owens, R., and Cohen, E. (1975). The effect of potassium loading on sodium excretion and plasma renin activity in Addisonian man. *Journal of Clinical Investigation* **56**, 346–353.

Minella, R. A. and Schulman D. S. (1991). Fatal verapamil toxicity and hypokalemia. *American Heart Journal* **121**, 1810–1812.

*Mitch, W. E. and Wilcox, C. S. (1982). Disorders of body fluids, sodium and potassium in chronic renal failure. *American Journal of Medicine* **72**, 536–550.

Mocan, M. Z., Mocan, H. M., Mocan, G., and Borcin, B. (1993). Inhaler salbutamol for acute hyperkalemia in renal failure. *Israel Journal of Medical Science* **29**, 39–41.

Montoliu, J., Lens, X. M., and Revert, L. (1987). Potassium-lowering effect of albuterol for hyperkalemia in renal failure. *Archives of Internal Medicine* **147**, 713.

Moreno, M., Murphy, C., and Goldsmith, C. (1969). Increase in serum potassium resulting from the administration of hypertonic mannitol and other solutions. *Journal of Laboratory and Clinical Medicine* **73**, 291–298.

*Morgan, D. B. and Davidson, C. (1980). Hypokalemia and diuretics: an analysis of publications. *British Medical Journal* **280**, 905–908.

Morita, H., Fujiki, N., Miyahara, T., Lee, K., and Tanaka, K. (2000). Hepatoportal bumetanide-sensitive K^+-sensor mechanism controls urinary K^+ excretion. *American Journal of Physiology* **278**, R1134–R1139.

Morris, R. C., Sebastian, A., Forman, A., Tanaka, M., and Schmidlin, O. (1999). Normotensive salt sensitivity. Effects of race and dietary potassium. *Hypertension* **33**, 18–23.

Muehrcke, R. C. and Rosen, S. (1964). Hypokalemic nephropathy in rat and man A light and electron microscopic study. *Laboratory Investigation* **13**, 1359–1373.

Muggia, F. M., Heinemann, H. O., Farhangi, M., and Osserman, E. F. (1969). Lysozymuria and renal tubular dysfunction in monocytic and myelomonocytic leukemia. *American Journal of Medicine* **47**, 351–366.

Mulkerrin, E., Epstein, F. H., and Clark, B. A. (1995). Aldosterone responses to hyperkalemia in healthy elderly humans. *Journal of the American Society of Nephrology* **6**, 1459–1462.

Murakawa, M., Hatano, Y., Magaribuchi, T., and Mori, K. (1988). Should calcium administration be avoided in treatment of hyperkalemia in malignant hyperthermia? *Anesthesia and Analgesia* **67**, 596–606.

Murray, B. M. and Paller, M. S. (1986). Pressor resistance to vasopressin in sodium depletion, potassium depletion, and cirrhosis. *American Journal of Physiology* **251**, R525.

*Muto, S. (2001). Potassium transport in the mammalian collecting duct. *Physiological Reviews* **81**, 85–116.

Muto, S., Miyata, Y., and Asano Y. (1993). Electrical properties of the rabbit cortical collecting duct from obstructed and contralateral kidneys after unilateral ureteral obstruction. *Journal of Clinical Investigation* **92**, 571–581.

Muto, S., Imai, M., and Asano, Y. (1995). Mechanisms of hyperkalemia caused by nafamostat mesilate. *General Pharmacology* **26**, 1627–1632.

Muto, S., Asano, Y., Seldin, D., and Giebisch, G. (1999). Basolateral Na^+ pump modulates apical Na^+ and K^+ conductances in rabbit cortical collecting ducts. *American Journal of Physiology* **276**, F143–F158.

Nadler, J. L., Lee, F. O., Hsueh, W., and Horton, R. (1986). Evidence of prostacyclin deficiency in the syndrome of hyporeninemic hypoaldosteronism. *New England Journal of Medicine* **314**, 10–15.

Nakamura, S., Amlal, H., Galla, J. H., and Soleimani, M. (1999). NH_4^+ secretion in inner meduallary collecting duct in potassium deprivation: role of colonic H^+,K^+-ATPase. *Kidney International* **56**, 2160–2167.

Nakanishi, T., Yamauchi, A., Yamamoto, S., Sugita, M., and Takamitsu, Y. (1996). Potassium depletion modulates aldose reductase mRNA in rat renal inner medulla. *Kidney International* **50**, 828–834.

Nasjletti, A. *et al.* (1985). High potassium intake selectively increases urinary $PGF_{2\alpha}$ excretion in the rat. *American Journal of Physiology* **248**, F382.

Nesher, G., Zimran, A., and Hershko, C. (1988). Reduced incidence of hyperkalemia and azotemia in patients receiving sulindac compared with indomethacin. *Nephron* **48**, 291–295.

Oberfield, S. E., Levine, L. S., Carey, R. M., Bejar, R., and New, M. I. (1979). Pseudohypoaldosteronism: multiple target organ unresponsiveness to mineralocorticoid hormones. *Journal of Clinical Endocrinology and Metabolism* **48**, 228–234.

Oh, M. S. *et al.* (1974). A mechanism for hyporeninemic hypoaldosteronism in chronic renal disease. *Metabolism* **23**, 1157–1166.

O'Regan, S., Heitz, F., and Davignon, A. (1985). Echocardiographic assessment of left ventricular function in patients with hypokalemia. *Mineral and Electrolyte Metabolism* **11**, 1–4.

***Ornt, D. B., Scandling, J. D., and Tannen, R. L.** (1987). Adaptation for potassium conservation during dietary potassium deprivation. *Seminars in Nephrology* **7**, 193.

Orringer, C. E. *et al.* (1977). Natural history of lactic acidosis after grand-mal seizure. *New England Journal of Medicine* **297**, 796–799.

Oster, J. R., Perez, G. O., and Vaamonde, C. A. (1978). Relationship between blood pH and potassium and phosphorus during acute metabolic acidosis. *American Journal of Physiology* **235**, F345–F351.

Paller, M. S. and Linas, S. L. (1982). Hemodynamic effects of alterations in potassium. *Hypertension* **4** (Suppl. III), 20–26.

Paller, M. S., Douglas, J. G., and Linas, S. L. (1984). Mechanism of decreased vascular reactivity to angiotensin II in conscious, potassium-deficient rats. *Journal of Clinical Investigation* **73**, 79–86.

Palmer, L. G. and Frindt, G. (1999). Regulation of apical K Channels in rat cortical collecting tubule during changes in dietary K intake. *American Journal of Physiology* **277**, F805–F812.

Panese, S. *et al.* (1987). Mechanism of enhanced transcellular potassium-secretion in man with chronic renal failure. *Kidney International* **31**, 1377–1382.

***Perazella, M. A.** (2000). Drug-induced hyperkalemia: old culprits and new offenders. *American Journal of Medicine* **109**, 307–314.

Perez, G. O., Lespier, L. E., Oster, J. R., and Vaamonde, C. A. (1977). Effect of alterations of sodium intake in patients with hyporeninemic hypoaldosteronism. *Nephron* **18**, 259–265.

Perez, G. O., Pelleya, R., Oster, J. R., Kim, D. C., and Vaamonde, C. A. (1983). Blunted kaliuresis after an acute potassium load in patients with chronic renal failure. *Kidney International* **24**, 656–662.

***Pang, S.** (1997). Congenital adrenal hyperplasia. *Endocrinology and Metabolism Clinics of North America* **26**, 853–891.

***Peter, M., Dubuis, M. M., and Sippell, W. G.** (1999). Disorders of the aldosterone synthase and steroid 11-β-hydroxylase deficiencies. *Hormone Research* **51**, 211–222.

Phillips, S., Donaldson, L., Geisler, K., Pera, A., and Kochar, R. (1995). Stool composition in factitial diarrhea: a 6-year experience with stool analysis. *Annals of Internal Medicine* **123**, 97–100.

Pickering, T. G. and Catovsky, D. (1973). Hypokalaemia and raised lysozyme levels in acute myeloid leukaemia. *Quarterly Journal of Medicine* **202**, 677–682.

Pierson, R. N., Jr., Wang, J., Thornton, J. C., Van Itallie, J. B., and Colt, E. W. D. (1984). Body potassium by four-pi; 40_K counting: an anthropometric correction. *American Journal of Physiology* **246**, F234–F239.

Pollen, R. H. and Williams, R. H. (1963). Hyperkalemic neuromusculopathy in Addison's disease. *New England Journal of Medicine* **263**, 273–277.

Prunty, F. T. G. *et al.* (1963). Adrenocortical hyperfunction and potassium metabolism in patients with 'non-endocrine' tumors and Cushing's syndrome. *Journal of Clinical Endocrinology and Metabolism* **23**, 737–746.

***Ptacek, L.** (1998). The familial periodic paralyses and nondystrophic myotonias. *American Journal of Medicine* **104**, 58–70.

***Quamme, G. A.** (1997). Renal magnesium handling: new insights in understanding old problems. *Kidney International* **52**, 1180–1195.

Rabinowitz, L. (1996). Aldosterone and potassium homeostasis. *Kidney International* **49**, 1738–1742.

Rainey, W. E. (1999). Adrenal zonation: clues from 11-β-hydroxylase and aldosterone synthase. *Molecular and Cellular Endocrinology* **151**, 151–160.

Raju, S. F., Kiley, J. E., Johnson, B. B., White, A. R., McCaa, R. E., and Bower, J. D. (1980). Hyperkalemia in a hemodialysis patient without a colon. *Dialysis and Transplantation* **9**, 1086–1088.

Rao, T. L. K., Mathru, M., Salem, M. R., and El-Etra, A. (1980). Serum potassium levels following transfusion of frozen erythrocytes. *Anesthesiology* **52**, 170–172.

Rastogi, S., Bayliss, J. M., Nascimento, L., and Arruda, J. A. L. (1985). Hyperkalemic renal tubular acidosis: Effect of furosemide in humans and in rats. *Kidney International* **28**, 801–807.

Raymond, L. H., Davidson, K. K., and McKinney, T. D. (1985). *In vivo* and *in vitro* studies of urinary concentration ability in potassium-depleted rabbits. *Journal of Clinical Investigation* **76**, 561–566.

Raymond, K. H., Lifschitz, M. D., and McKinney, T. D. (1987). Prostaglandins and the urinary concentrating defect in potassium depleted rabbits. *American Journal of Physiology* **253**, F1113–F1119.

Relman, A. S. and Schwartz, W. B. (1958). The kidney in potassium depletion. *American Journal of Medicine* **24**, 764–773.

***Rodriguez-Puyol, D.** (1998). The aging kidney. *Kidney International* **54**, 2247–2265.

Rosa, R. M. *et al.* (1980). Adrenergic modulation of extrarenal potassium disposal. *New England Journal of Medicine* **302**, 431–434.

Roza, O. and Berman, L. B. (1971). The pathophysiology of barium: P hypokalemic and cardiovascular effects. *Journal of Pharmacology and Experimental Therapeutics* **177**, 433–439.

Ryan, M. P. (1987). Diuretics and potassium/magnesium depletion: directions for treatment. *American Journal of Medicine* **82**, 38–47.

Sacks, F. M., Svetkey, L. P., Wollmer, W. M., Appel, L. J., Bray, G. A., Harsha, D., Obarzanek, E., Conlin, P. R., Miller, E. R., Simons-Morton, D. G., Karanja, N., and Lin, P. (2001). Effects on blood pressure of reduced dietary sodium and the dietary approaches to stop hypertension (DASH) diet. *New England Journal of Medicine* **344**, 3–10.

Saikaley, A., Bichet, D., Kucharczk, J., and Peterson, L. N. (1986). Neuroendocrine factors mediating polydipsia induced by dietary Na, Cl, and K depletion. *American Journal of Physiology* **251**, R1071.

***Salem, M. M., Rosa, R. M., and Batlle, D. C.** (1991). Extrarenal potassium tolerance in chronic renal failure: implications for the treatment of acute hyperkalaemia. *American Journal of Kidney Diseases* **18**, 421–440.

San Juan, A. C., Jr., Wong, K. C., and Port, J. D. (1988). Hyperkalemia after dantrolene and verapamil-dantrolene administration in dogs. *Anesthesia and Analgesia* **67**, 759–762.

Sandle, G. I. and Butterfield, J. (1999). Potassium secretion in rat distal colon during dietary potassium loading: role of pH regulated apical potassium channels. *Gut* **44**, 40–46.

Sangan, P., Kolla, S. S., Rajendran, V. M., Kashgarian, M., and Binder, H. J. (1999). Colonic H^+,K^+-ATPase beta-subunit: identification in apical membranes and regulation by dietary K depletion. *American Journal of Physiology* **276**, C350–C360.

Sastrasinh, S. and Tannen, R. L. (1981). Mechanism by which enhanced ammonia production reduces urinary potassium excretion. *Kidney International* **20**, 326–331.

Sastrasinh, S. and Tannen, R. L. (1983). Effect of potassium on renal NH_3 production. *American Journal of Physiology* **244**, F383–F391.

*__Schafer, J. A.__ (1994). Salt and water homeostasis—is it just a matter of good housekeeping? *Journal of the American Society of Nephrology* **4**, 1933–1950.

Schambelan, M., Sebastian, A., and Biglieri, E. G. (1980). Prevalence, pathogenesis, and functional significance of aldosterone deficiency in hyperkalemic patients with chronic renal insufficiency. *Kidney International* **17**, 89–101.

Schambelan, M., Sebastian, A., and Rector, F. C., Jr. (1981). Mineralocorticoid-resistant renal hyperkalemia without salt wasting (type II pseudohypoaldosteronism): role of increased renal chloride reabsorption. *Kidney International* **19**, 716–727.

Schlanger, L. E., Kleyman, T. R., and Ling, B. N. (1994). K^+-sparing diuretic actions of trimethoprim: inhibition of Na^+ channels in A6 distal nephron cells. *Kidney International* **45**, 1070–1076.

Schlueter, W. *et al.* (1992). On the mechanisms of impaired distal acidification in hyperkalemic renal tubular acidosis: evaluation with amiloride and bumetanide. *Journal of the American Society of Nephrology* **3**, 953–964.

Schrier, R. W. (1979). Acute renal failure. *Kidney International* **15**, 205–216.

Schwartz, W. B. and Relman, A. S. (1953). Metabolic and renal studies in chronic potassium depletion resulting from overuse of laxatives. *Journal of Clinical Investigation* **32**, 258–271.

*__Schwartz, W. B., van Ypersele de Strihou, C., and Kassirer, J. P.__ (1968). Role of anions in metabolic alkalosis and potassium deficiency. *New England Journal of Medicine* **279**, 630–639.

Sealey, J. E. and Laragh, J. H. (1974). A proposed cybernetic system for sodium and potassium homeostasis: coordination of aldosterone and intrarenal physical factors. *Kidney International* **6**, 281–290.

Sebastian, A., McSherry, E., and Morris, R. C., Jr. (1971a). One mechanism of renal potassium wasting in renal tubular acidosis associated with the Fanconi syndrome (type 2 RTA). *Journal of Clinical Investigation* **50**, 231–243.

Sebastian A., McSherry, E., and Morris, R. C., Jr. (1971b). Renal potassium wasting in renal tubular acidosis (RTA). Its occurrence in types I and 2 RTA despite sustained correction of systemic acidosis. *Journal of Clinical Investigation* **50**, 667–678.

Sebastian, A., McSherry, E., and Morris, R. C., Jr. (1976). Impaired renal conservation of sodium and chloride during sustained correction of systemic acidosis in patients with type I, classical renal tubular acidosis. *Journal of Clinical Investigation* **58**, 454–469.

Sebastian, A., Schambelan, M., Lindenfeld, S., and Morris, R. C., Jr. (1977). Amelioration of metabolic acidosis with fludrocortisone therapy in hyporeninemic hypoaldosteronism. *New England Journal of Medicine* **297**, 576–583.

Sebastian, A. *et al.* (1990). Dietary potassium influences kidney maintenance of serum phosphorus concentration. *Kidney International* **37**, 1341–1349.

Sebastian, A. *et al.* (1994). Improved mineral balance and skeletal metabolism in postmenopausal women treated with potassium bicarbonate. *New England Journal of Medicine* **330**, 1776–1781.

*__Sejersted, O. M. and Sjogaard, G.__ (2000). Dynamics and consequences of potassium shifts in skeletal muscle and heart during exercise. *Physiological Reviews* **80**, 1411–1481.

*__Seldin, D. W. and Rector, F. C., Jr.__ (1972). The generation and maintenance of metabolic alkalosis. *Kidney International* **1**, 306–321.

Seldin, D. W., Carter, N. W., and Rector, F. C., Jr. Consequences of renal failure and their management. In *Diseases of the Kidney* 1st edn. (ed. M. B. Strauss and L. G. Welt), pp. 1173–1217. Boston: Little Brown, 1963.

Shapiro, J. I., Banerjee, A., Reiss, O. K., and Elkins, N. (1998). Acute and chronic hypokalemia sensitize the isolated heart to hypoxic injury. *American Journal of Physiology* **274**, H1598–H1604.

Shemer, J., Modan, M., Ezra, D., and Cabili, S. (1983). Incidence of hyperkalemia in hospitalized patients. *Israel Journal of Medical Science* **19**, 659–661.

Sherman, R. A. and Ruddy, M. C. (1986). Suppression of aldosterone production by low-dose heparin. *American Journal of Nephrology* **6**, 165.

Shiffman, F. J., Schiffman, R. L., and Rosa, R. M. (1977). Cellular proliferation and hypokalemia. *Annals of Internal Medicine* **87**, 635–636.

Silva, P. and Spokes, K. (1981). Sympathetic system in potassium homeostasis. *American Journal of Physiology* **241**, F151–F155.

Silver, R. B., Breton, S., and Brown, D. (2000). Potassium depletion increases proton pump (H^+-ATPase) activity in intercalated cells of cortical collecting duct. *American Journal of Physiology* **279**, F195–F202.

Silver, R. B. and Soleimani, M. (1999). H^+-K^+-ATPases: regulation and role in pathophysiological states. *American Journal of Physiology* **276**, F799–F811.

Simons, M. L. and Goldman, E. (1988). A typical malignant hyperthermia with persistent hyperkalaemia during renal transplantation. *Canadian Journal of Anaesthesia* **35**, 409–412.

Siscovick, D. S., Raghunathan, T. E., Psaty, B. M., Koepsell, T. D., Wicklund, K. G., Lin, X., Cobb, L., Rautaharju, P. M., Copass, M. K., and Wagner, E. H. (1994). Diuretic therapy for hypertension and the risk of primary cardiac arrest. *New England Journal of Medicine* **330**, 1852–1857.

Smith, T. W. *et al.* (1981). Treatment of life-threatening digitalis intoxication with digoxin-specific Fab antibody fragments. *New England Journal of Medicine* **307**, 1357–1362.

Smith, S. J. *et al.* (1984). Evidence that patients with Addison's disease are undertreated with fludrocortisone. *Lancet* **i**, 11–14.

Solomon, R. (1987). The relationship between disorders of K^+ and Mg^+ homeostasis. *Seminars in Nephrology* **7**, 253.

Solomon, R. and Dubey, A. (1992). Diltiazem enhances potassium disposal in subjects with end-stage renal disease. *American Journal of Kidney Diseases* **19**, 420–426.

Spital, A. (1989). Bicarbonate in the treatment of severe hyperkalemia. *American Journal of Medicine* **86**, 511–512.

Spital, A. and Sterns, R. H. (1986). Paradoxical potassium depletion: a renal mechanism for extrarenal potassium adaptation. *Kidney International* **30**, 532–537.

Spital, A. and Sterns, R. H. (1989). Extrarenal potassium adaptation: the role of aldosterone. *Clinical Science* **76**, 213–219.

Spitzer, A., Edelmann, C. M., Jr., Goldberg, L. D., and Henneman, P. H. (1973). Short stature, hyperkalemia and acidosis: a defect in renal transport of potassium. *Kidney International* **3**, 251–257.

*__Standen, N. B.__ (1992). Potassium channels, metabolism and muscle. *Experimental Physiology* **77**, 1–25.

*__Sterns, R. H. and Spital, A.__ (1987). Disorders of internal potassium balance. *Seminars in Nephrology* **7**, 206.

*__Sterns, R. H., Cox, M., Fieg, P. U., and Singer, I.__ (1981). Internal potassium balance and the control of the plasma potassium concentration. *Medicine* **60**, 339.

Stewart, G. W., Corrall, R. J. M., Fyffe, J. A., Stockdill, G., and Strong, J. A. (1979). Familial pseudohyperkalemia: a new syndrome. *Lancet* **ii**, 175–177.

Stewart, P. M., Walker, B. R., Holder, G., O'Halloran, D., and Shackleton, C. H. (1995). 11-β-Hydroxysteroid dehydrogenase activity in Cushing's Syndrome: explaining the mineralocorticoid excess state of the ectopic adrenocorticotropin syndrome. *Journal of Clinical Endocrinology and Metabolism* **80**, 3617–3620.

*__Stockand, J. D.__ (2002). New ideas about aldosterone signaling in epithelia. *American Journal of Physiology* **282**, F559–F576.

Stowasser, M. and Gordon, R. D. (2000). Primary aldosteronism: learning from the study of familial varieties. *Journal of Hypertension* **18**, 1165–1176.

Streicher, H. Z., Gabow, P. A., Moss, A. H., Kono, D., and Kaehny, W. D. (1981). Syndromes of toluene sniffing in adults. *Annals of Internal Medicine* **94**, 758–762.

Struthers, A. D. and Reid, J. L. (1984). The role of adrenal medullary catecholamines in potassium homeostasis. *Clinical Science* **66**, 377–382.

Suga, S., Mazzall, M., Ray, P. E., Kang, D., and Johnson, R. J. (2002). Angiotensin II type 1 receptor blockade ameliorates tubulointerstitial injury induced by chronic potassium deficiency. *Kidney International* **61**, 951–958.

Sugarman, A. and Brown, R. S. (1988). The role of aldosterone in potassium tolerance: studies in anephric humans. *Kidney International* **34**, 397–403.

Sugarman, A. and Kahn, T. (1986). Calcium channel blockers enhance extrarenal potassium disposal in the rat. *American Journal of Physiology* **250**, F695.

Sugarman, A. and Kahn, T. (1988). Parathyroid hormone impairs extrarenal potassium tolerance in the rat. *American Journal of Physiology* **254**, F385–F390.

Surawicz, B. (1967). Relationship between electrocardiogram and electrolytes. *American Heart Journal* **73**, 814–834.

Szylman, P., Better, O. S., Chaimowitz, C., and Rosler, A. (1976). Role of hyperkalemia in the metabolic acidosis of isolated hypoaldosteronism. *New England Journal of Medicine* **294**, 361–365.

Tan, H. L., Hou, C. J. Y., Lauer, M. R., and Sung, R. J. (1995). Electrophysiologic mechanisms of the long QT interval syndromes and Torsade de Pointes. *Annals of Internal Medicine* **122**, 701–714.

Tan, S. Y., Shapiro, R., Stockard, H., and Mulrow, P. J. (1979). Indomethacin-induced prostaglandin inhibition with hyperkalemia. *Annals of Internal Medicine* **90**, 783–785.

***Tannen, R. L.** (1977). Relationship of renal ammonia production and potassium homeostasis. *Kidney International* **2**, 453–465.

***Tannen, R. L.** Potassium metabolism. In *Current nephrology* Vol. 6 (ed. H. C. Gonick), pp. 151–186. New York: Wiley, 1983.

***Tannen, R. L.** (1985). Diuretic-induced hypokalemia. *Kidney International* **28**, 998.

***Tannen, R. L.** Potassium metabolism. In *Current Nephrology* Vol. 9 (ed. H. C. Gonick), pp. 359–400. Chicago: Year Book Medical, 1986.

***Tannen, R. L.** (1987a). Effect of potassium on renal acidification and acid–base homeostasis. *Seminars in Nephrology* **7**, 263.

***Tannen, R. L.** (1987b). The influence of potassium on blood pressure. *Kidney International* **32**, S242.

***Tannen, R. L.** (1989). Potassium metabolism. In *Current Nephrology* Vol. 12 (ed. H. C. Gonick), pp. 87–134. St Louis: Year Book.

***Tannen, R. L.** Potassium disorders. In *Fluids and Electrolytes* 3rd edn. (ed. J. P. Kokko and R. L. Tannen), pp. 111–199. Philadelphia: Saunders, 1996.

Textor, S. C., Bravo, E. L., Fouad, F. M., and Tarazi, R. C. (1982). Hyperkalemia in azotemic patients during angiotensin-converting enzyme inhibition and aldosterone reduction with captopril. *American Journal of Medicine* **73**, 719–725.

Thapa, S. and Brull, S. J. (2000). Succinylcholine-induced hyperkalemia in patients with renal failure: an old question revisited. *Anesthesia and Analgesia* **91**, 237–241.

Thompson, C. B., Choi, C., Youn, J. H., and McDonough, A. A. (1999). Temporal responses of oxidative vs. glycolytic skeletal muscles to K^+ deprivation: Na^+ pumps and cell cations. *American Journal of Physiology* **276**, C1411–C1419.

Tobian, L. (1988). Potassium and sodium in hypertension. *Journal of Hypertension* **6** (Suppl. 4), S12–S14.

Tolins, J. P., Hostetter, M. K., and Hostetter, T. H. (1987). Hypokalemic nephropathy in the rat: role of ammonia in chronic tubular injury. *Journal of Clinical Investigation* **79**, 1447–1458.

Topazian, M. and Binder, H. J. (1994). Factitious diarrhea determined by measurement of stool osmolality. *New England Journal of Medicine* **330**, 1418–1419.

Torres, V. E., Young, W. F., Jr., Offord, K. P., and Hattery, R. R. (1990). Association of hypokalemia, aldosteronism, and renal cysts. *New England Journal of Medicine* **322**, 345–351.

Tricarico, D., Capriulo, R., and Camerino, D. C. (1999). Insulin modulation of ATP-sensitive K^+ channel of rat skeletal muscle is impaired in the hypokalaemic state. *Pflugers Archive-European Journal of Physiology* **437**, 235–240.

Tricarico, D., Barbieri, M., and Camerino, D. C. (2000). Acetazolamide opens the muscular $Kca2^+$ channel: a novel mechanism of action that may explain the therapeutic effect of the drug in hypokalemic periodic paralysis. *Annals of Neurology* **48**, 304–312.

Trost, B. N. and Weidmann, P. (1988). Metabolic effects of calcium antagonists in humans, with emphasis on carbohydrate, lipid, potassium, and uric acid homeostasis. *Journal of Cardiovascular Pharmacology* **12** (Suppl. 6), S86–S92.

Tumlin, J. A. and Sands, J. M. (1993). Nephron segment-specific inhibition of Na^+/K^+-ATPase activity by cyclosporin A. *Kidney International* **43**, 246–251.

United States Multicenter FK506 Liver Study Group (1994). A comparison of tacrolimus (FK506) and cyclosporin for immunosuppression in liver transplantation. *New England Journal of Medicine* **331**, 1110–1115.

Vaamonde, C. A., Perez, G. O., and Oster, J. R. (1981). Syndromes of aldosterone deficiency. *Mineral and Electrolyte Metabolism* **5**, 121–134.

***Van Ypersele de Strihou, C.** (1977). Potassium homeostasis in renal failure. *Kidney International* **11**, 491–504.

Varriale, P. and Manolis, A. (1987). Pacemaker Wenckebach secondary to variable latency: an unusual form of hyperkalemic pacemaker exit block. *American Heart Journal* **114**, 189–192.

Veldhuis, J. D., Bardin, C. W., and Demers, L. M. (1979). Metabolic mimicry of Bartter's syndrome by covert vomiting: utility of urinary chloride determinations. *American Journal of Medicine* **66**, 361–363.

Vio, C. P. and Fueroa, C. D. (1987). Evidence for a stimulatory effect of high potassium diet on renal kallikrein. *Kidney International* **31**, 1327–1334.

Wahr, J. A., Parks, R., Boisvert, D., Cumunale, M., Fabian, J., Ramsay, J., and Mangano, D. T. (1999). Preoperative serum potassium levels and perioperative outcomes in cardiac surgery patients. *Journal of the American Medical Association* **281**, 2203–2210.

Wall, S. M., Fischer, M. P., Kim, G., Nguyen, B., and Hassell, K. A. (2002). In rat inner medullary collecting duct, NH_4^+ uptake by the Na^+,K^+-ATPase is increased during hypokalemia. *American Journal of Physiology* **282**, F91–F102.

Wang, Y., Gao, J., Mathias, R. T., Cohen, I. S., Sun, X., and Baldo, G. J. (1998). Alpha-adrenergic effects on Na^+-K^+ pump current in guinea-pig ventricular myocytes. *Journal of Physiology (London)* **509**, 117–128.

***Warnock, D. G.** (2002). Renal genetic disorders related to K^+ and Mg^{2+}. *Annual Review of Physiology* **64**, 845–876.

***Welt, L. G., Holander, W., Jr., and Blythe, W. B.** (1960). The consequences of potassium depletion. *Journal of Chronic Diseases* **2**, 213–254.

Wehling, M. (1995). Nongenomic aldosterone effects: the cell membrane as a specific target of mineralocorticoid action. *Steroids* **60**, 153–156.

***Weiner, I. D. and Wingo, C. S.** (1997). Hypokalemia—consequences, causes, and correction. *Journal of the American Society of Nephrology* **8**, 1179–1188.

West, M. L., Marsden, P. A., Richardson, M. A., Zettle, R. M., and Halperin, M. L. (1986). New clinical approach to evaluate disorders of potassium excretion. *Mineral and Electrolyte Metabolism* **12**, 234–238.

Williams, F. A., Schambelan, M., Biglieri, E. G., and Carey, R. M. (1983). Hypoaldosteronism due to an isolated zona glomerulosa defect. *New England Journal of Medicine* **309**, 1623–1627.

Williams, M. E., Rosa, R. M., Silva, P., Brown, R. S., and Epstein, F. H. (1984). Impairment of extrarenal potassium disposal by α-adrenergic stimulation. *New England Journal of Medicine* **311**, 145–149.

Williams, M. E. *et al.* (1985). Catecholamine modulation of rapid potassium shifts during exercise. *New England Journal of Medicine* **312**, 823–827.

Wilson, F. H., Disse-Nicodeme, S., Choate, K. A., Ishikawa, K., Nelson-Williams, C., Desitter, I., Gurnl, M., Milford, D. V., Lipkin, G. W., Achard, J., Feely, M. P., Dussol, B., Berland, Y., Unwin, R. J., Mayan, H., Simon, D. B., Farfel, Z., Jeunemaitre, X., and Lifton, R. P. (2001). Human hypertension caused by mutations in WNK kinases. *Science* **293**, 1107–1112.

Wingo, C. S. (1989). Potassium secretion by the cortical collecting tubule: effects of Cl gradients and ouabain. *American Journal of Physiology* **256**, F306–F313.

*__Wingo, C. S. and Cain, B. D.__ (1993). The renal H–K-ATPase: physiological significance and role in potassium homeostasis. *Annual Review of Physiology* **55**, 323–347.

Wootton, F. T., Rhodes, D. P., Lee, W. M., and Fitts, C. T. (1989). Colonic necrosis and Kayexalate–sorbitol enemas after renal transplantation. *Annals of Internal Medicine* **111**, 947–949.

Wrong, O. M., Feest, T. G., and Maciver, A. G. (1993). Immune-related potassium-losing interstitial nephritis: a comparison with distal renal tubular acidosis. *Quarterly Journal of Medicine* **86**, 513–534.

Yang, W. C., Huang, T. P., Ho, L. T., Chung, H. M., Chang, Y. L., and Battle, D. C. (1986). Beta-adrenergic-mediated extrarenal potassium disposal in patients with end-stage renal disease: effect of propranolol. *Mineral and Electrolyte Metabolism* **12**, 186.

Young, D. B. and Jackson, T. E. (1982). Effects of aldosterone on potassium distribution. *American Journal of Physiology* **243**, R526–R530.

Young, D. B., McCaa, R. E., Pan, Y. J., and Guyton, A. C. (1976a). Effectiveness of the aldosterone sodium and potassium feedback control system. *American Journal of Physiology* **231**, 945–955.

Young, D. B., McCaa, R. E., Pan, Y. J., and Guyton, A. C. (1976b). The natriuretic and hypotensive effects of potassium. *Circulation Research* **38** (Suppl. II), 84–89.

Young, D. B., Jackson, T. E., Tipayamontri, U., and Scott, R. C. (1984). Effects of sodium intake on steady-state potassium excretion. *American Journal of Physiology* **246**, F772–F778.

Zhou, M., Nishida, Y., Yoneyama, H., Chen, Q., and Kosaka, H. (1999). Potassium supplementation increases sodium excretion and nitric oxide production in hypertensive Dahl rats. *Clinical and Experimental Hypertension* **21**, 1397–1411.

Zimran, A., Kramer, M., Plaskin, M., and Hershko, C. (1985). Incidence of hyperkalaemia induced by indomethacin in a hospital population. *British Medical Journal* **291**, 107.

2.3 Hypo–hypercalcaemia

Neveen A.T. Hamdy and John A. Kanis

Introduction

Disturbances of extracellular calcium homeostasis are frequently encountered during the course of progressive renal failure, dialysis replacement therapy, or after renal transplantation. Hypocalcaemia and hypercalcaemia may be completely asymptomatic, although potentially responsible for a cascade of events leading to increased skeletal and cardiovascular morbidity (Kanis *et al.* 1988; Drueke 1995; Block *et al.* 1998; Slatopolsky 1998; Block and Port 2000; Goodman *et al.* 2000). When severe, they can and do give rise to symptoms, which require treatment in their own right.

The aim of this chapter is to provide an account of the mechanisms giving rise to disturbed calcium homeostasis in uraemia and its consequences, thereby providing a rationale for the interpretation and, where appropriate, the treatment of these abnormalities. The first part of this chapter is devoted to the description of normal physiology against which the abnormalities that arise in uraemia can be set.

Serum calcium and calcium homeostasis

Distribution and function of calcium

Although widely distributed throughout living tissues, the largest amount of calcium (98 per cent) is found in bones. The ability of the skeleton to turnover calcium is essential for growth, for the prevention and healing of fractures, and for remodelling the skeleton in response to physiological and pathological stresses.

Extracellular fluid calcium, only 1 per cent of total body calcium, is critical for normal neuromuscular activity: a fall results in tetany and convulsions, whereas a rise has many adverse effects, including delayed neuromuscular conduction, muscular paralysis, and extraskeletal calcifications.

The intracellular concentration of calcium is considerably less than that in the extracellular fluid, generally by a factor of 100,000 (free extracellular calcium 70–150 nmol/l). Within cells, mitochondria are capable of accumulating large amounts of calcium against electrochemical gradients, but total intracellular concentrations remain extremely low. The activation of many types of cells by hormones or pharmacological agents depends upon increases in intracellular calcium concentration derived from extracellular fluid and perhaps from mitochondrial stores. Changes in cytosolic calcium are critical to signal transduction pathways. These are important regulators of a variety of cell functions including enzyme activity, hormone secretion, glycogen metabolism, muscle contraction, cell division, and exocytosis (Rasmussen and Rasmussen 1990). Many of these functions are achieved by the interaction of intracellular calcium with calcium-binding proteins such as calmodulin or calbindin-D_{28k}, a vitamin D dependent calcium binding protein, present in intestine and kidney (Sooy *et al.* 2000).

Despite the importance of intracellular calcium in a variety of biochemical regulatory processes, and its ultimate dependence on extracellular delivery, there is little evidence that intracellular stores of calcium contribute in any way towards extracellular calcium homeostasis. A single exception is the intracellular concentration of calcium in parathyroid tissue, which is greater than in other cells, increases in response to changes in extracellular calcium concentrations, and determines the secretion rate of parathyroid hormone (PTH) (Nygren *et al.* 1987).

Plasma calcium

The concentration of calcium in plasma is maintained within a narrow range (approximately 2.1–2.6 mmol/l) despite its large movements across gut, bone, kidney, and cells. Changes in the concentration of plasma ionized calcium are usually accompanied by changes in the total amount of calcium in the extracellular fluid, since ionized calcium is passively distributed throughout the extracellular fluid compartment. Within the plasma compartment, approximately 40 per cent of total calcium is bound to proteins, mainly to albumin (90 per cent), in a pH-dependent fashion (Marshall 1976). Large changes in plasma protein concentration, the presence of abnormal proteins, and large shifts in extracellular hydrogen concentration may alter the proportion of bound calcium. A further 5–10 per cent of total plasma calcium is bound to small anions such as citrate, phosphate, and bicarbonate and binding varies with the concentration of these anions. The estimation of total plasma calcium, therefore, may not accurately reflect the ionized calcium concentration (Kanis and Yates 1985; Thode *et al.* 1989). In mild cases of primary hyperparathyroidism, for instance, total calcium may be within the normal laboratory reference range but its ionized fraction may be increased (Ladenson *et al.* 1979; Glendenning *et al.* 1998). Changes in the binding of calcium in plasma occurring as a result of changes in acid–base balance hold important clinical consequences: infusion of alkali into patients with metabolic acidosis increases the binding of calcium to albumin and may cause hypocalcaemic tetany and convulsions due to a decrease in ionized calcium without a change in total plasma calcium (Thode *et al.* 1983).

In the absence of severe acidosis or alkalosis, the amount of albumin is the major determinant of bound calcium. Failure to account for protein binding may result in the erroneous diagnosis of hypercalcaemia in conditions where there is an increased concentration or an abnormality of plasma proteins such as in dehydration, prolonged venous stasis, myeloma, and liver disease. Conversely, total plasma calcium may be low in the hypoproteinaemic states of chronic renal failure, in the nephrotic syndrome, and in patients on continuous ambulatory peritoneal dialysis (CAPD), although the ionized calcium is normal. On the other hand, a normal total plasma calcium may mask true hypercalcaemia in the presence of hypoproteinaemia.

Increased total calcium is measured despite normal or decreased ionized calcium when large amounts of citrated blood products are given, such as during liver transplantation (Bertholf *et al.* 1992). Abnormal binding may also occur in less common circumstances such as following gadodiamide administration during the process of magnetic resonance imaging (MRI), in which case total calcium may be low in the face of a normal ionized calcium (Normann *et al.* 1995).

Many formulas have been proposed for predicting ionized calcium from total plasma calcium, or for 'correcting' the total plasma calcium to a normal protein value (Kanis and Yates 1985). These methods depend on the concurrent measurement of total proteins, albumin, or specific gravity of plasma. None is entirely satisfactory since the affinity of plasma proteins for calcium varies between individuals. A simple, widely used, correction factor for plasma calcium is the subtraction from the total plasma calcium of 0.02 mmol/l (0.08 mg/dl) for every 1 g/l of plasma albumin above 42 g/l, provided that the sample is drawn without venous stasis. The same amount of calcium is added when the plasma albumin is less than 42 g/l (Iqbal *et al.* 1988). In practice, adjusted total serum calcium is closely related to measured ionized calcium concentrations (Conceicao *et al.* 1978), but the strength of these correlations is not sufficient to be of good predictive value in individuals. Ionized plasma calcium, the physiologically relevant calcium fraction, can be measured, but it is by no means certain that it is an adequate gold standard for the biologically active fraction of calcium, particularly in patients with renal failure in whom the dialysable fraction is increased (Kanis and Yates 1985). In studies of populations, the ratio of ionized to total calcium is sufficiently constant so that either measurement may be used. Measurement of ionized calcium is recommended, however, in the investigation of uraemic patients with severe hypoproteinaemic states and in those with marked derangement of acid–base metabolism.

In addition to ionized calcium, the kidney also filters the small proportion (approximately 6 per cent) of total plasma calcium that is complexed with anions. These fractions can be measured by passing plasma through membrane filters, which retain the protein-bound calcium (Tofaletti *et al.* 1977). The measurement of ultrafiltrable calcium is of value when assessing the renal handling of calcium, particularly in chronic renal failure, which is associated with abnormalities in the complexed fraction of calcium.

Movements of calcium

The ionized fraction of plasma calcium is maintained by movements (fluxes) to and from the extracellular fluid. These movements (summarized in Fig. 1) are reviewed briefly below and discussed in detail subsequently.

The body is not a closed system with respect to calcium in the sense that calcium is lost from the body by glomerular filtration, intestinal secretion, and to a lesser extent by sweat, and enters the body by intestinal absorption and renal tubular reabsorption. Calcium balance

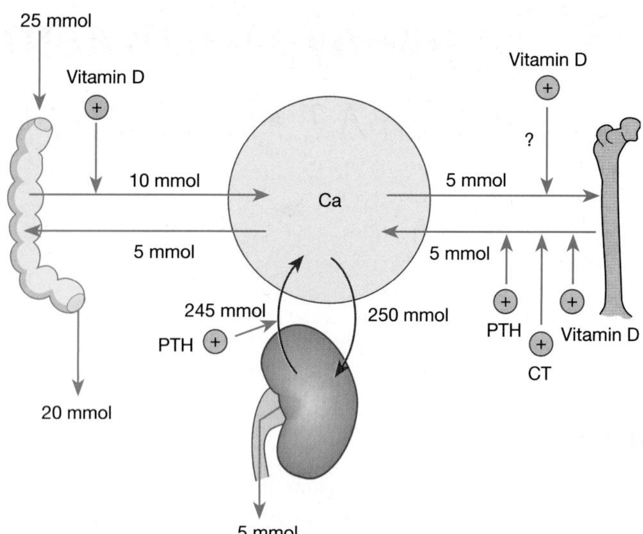

Fig. 1 Major fluxes of calcium (mmol/day) in a healthy adult. Exchange of calcium in the extracellular fluid occurs in bone, gut, and kidney. The net balance for calcium equals the net absorption minus the loss of calcium in faeces and urine, which is zero in a healthy adult. Hormones regulate the major fluxes of calcium: PTH increases renal tubular reabsorption of calcium and bone resorption, calcitonin inhibits bone resorption, and vitamin D augments intestinal absorption of calcium. The precise role of vitamin D in augmenting bone resorption and mineralization *in vivo* is not clear.

is the result of the integrated fluxes across bone, gut, and kidney. These fluxes continually change under the influence of a variety of factors including several hormones and eventually determine, at least in part the extracellular fluid calcium concentration. The hormones responsible for calcium homeostasis can be subdivided into 'controlling' hormones and 'influencing' hormones. The controlling or major calcium-regulating hormones include PTH, calcitonin, and the vitamin D metabolites. The production of these hormones is altered in response to changes in plasma ionized calcium concentrations, and their principal actions are to alter one or more of the bidirectional fluxes shown in Fig. 1. The influencing hormones, which include thyroid hormone, growth hormone, and adrenal and gonadal steroids, also affect calcium homeostasis, but their secretion is determined primarily by factors other than changes in plasma calcium.

Chronic renal failure is associated with abnormalities of all major calcium-regulating hormones and, with the possible exception of intestinal secretion, of all the fluxes of calcium to and from the extracellular fluid. An extreme example is provided by patients on dialysis in whom transfer of calcium to and from the dialysate solution adds an extra bidirectional flux.

Major calcium-regulating hormones

Parathyroid hormone

PTH is a single peptide chain composed of 84 amino acids. The first translation product of PTH: pre-pro-PTH (115 amino acids) is formed in the rough endoplasmic reticulum of the parathyroid chief cells and is converted within seconds to pro-PTH (90 amino acids). Within minutes, pro-PTH is converted to the intact PTH molecule (84 amino acids), which is then stored in secretory granules and is either secreted in response to hypocalcaemic stimuli or degraded within the cell. Intact PTH is cleaved, partly in the liver, into short *N*-terminal biologically active fragments and larger inactive *C*-terminal fragments. In the presence of hypercalcaemia, most of the molecule is degraded into biologically inactive fragments. The kidney is a major site of degradation of PTH. Plasma concentrations of the mid-region and *C*-terminal fragments, normally cleared by the kidney, are characteristically increased in chronic renal failure (Martin *et al.* 1979). The clearance of various fragments of PTH varies according to the dialysis system. In general, CAPD provides more efficient clearance of peptides than haemodialysis, and for any given rate of PTH secretion, values of PTH are less in CAPD patients than in patients undergoing haemodialysis (Hamdy *et al.* 1990a).

Only the first 32–34 amino acids of the PTH molecule (reading from the *N*-terminus) are necessary for biological activity. The two-site 'intact' PTH immunoassays detecting both the amino- and carboxy-terminals of the molecule have significantly improved the interpretation of PTH measurements (Nussbaum *et al.* 1987; Kao *et al.* 1992). However, PTH concentrations, as measured by these intact PTH (1–84) assays, still overestimate the degree of hyperparathyroidism in uraemia (Quarles *et al.* 1992; Wang *et al.* 1995). The loss of the first six amino acids of the PTH molecule leading to a truncated PTH (7–84) fragment eliminates its biological activity but not its immunoreactivity so that it is also measured by most of the commercially available 'intact' PTH assays (Lepage *et al.* 1998; Nguyen-Yamamoto *et al.* 2002). In normal subjects, PTH (7–84) fragments represent 10–20 per cent of the 'intact' PTH concentration as measured by the standard intact PTH, rising to 40–60 per cent in patients with renal failure unable to clear the fragments (John *et al.* 1999; Brossard *et al.* 2002).

Newly developed 'whole PTH' assays, which recognize only the biologically active first six amino acids of the *N*-terminal region of the human PTH molecule, may improve the accuracy of the clinical assessment of parathyroid function (John *et al.* 1999; Gao *et al.* 2001).

Further progress in the field of PTH assays includes the development of 'rapid PTH' assays (Kao *et al.* 1994), useful in the intraoperative evaluation of the successful outcome of a parathyroidectomy procedure, particularly in patients undergoing revision neck surgery (Irvin *et al.* 1999; Sokoll *et al.* 2000).

Parathyroid hormone secretion

The major physiological stimulus for PTH secretion is a reduction in the plasma concentration of ionized calcium, acting within seconds by stimulating the calcium-sensing receptor on parathyroid cells (Brown *et al.* 1994). Lowering extracellular ionized calcium results in the immediate release of PTH from the parathyroid chief cells with an attendant decrease of the intracellular degradation of PTH. Conversely, an increase in plasma ionized calcium above normal suppresses PTH secretion directly, thereby completing a negative feedback loop.

In the longer term, PTH secretion may be modulated by changes in vitamin D metabolism. Through binding to specific receptors in parathyroid tissue, calcitriol directly reduces PTH-mRNA synthesis (Silver 2000) and parathyroid cell proliferation (Szabo *et al.* 1989; Drueke 2000). Calcitriol administration thus suppresses the secretion of PTH to an extent greater than would be anticipated from any change in serum calcium alone in *in vitro* and *in vivo* systems as well as in some clinical situations (Fig. 2) (Slatopolsky *et al.* 1984; Hamdy *et al.* 1989). The number of calcitriol receptors decreases in uraemia (Drueke 1995) particularly when parathyroid hyperplasia is severe (Fukuda *et al.* 1993).

Calcium sensing—the 'calciostat'

Calcium sensing is essential for calcium homeostasis. This is achieved by means of the calcium-sensing receptor (CaR): a G protein-coupled receptor present on parathyroid, kidney, bone marrow, and osteoblast precursor cells (Brown *et al.* 1999). The highest concentration of CaR is in parathyroid cells where it detects exquisite changes in extracellular calcium (first messenger) to which the cells respond by an increase in intracellular calcium (second messenger). Contrary to all other endocrine cells, the parathyroid cell responds to an increase in intracellular calcium by decreasing rather than increasing PTH secretion.

In the kidney, the CaR reaches its highest concentration in the thick ascending limb of the loop of Henle where its activation reduces renal tubular reabsorption of calcium by an effect similar to that of a loop diuretic. Activation of the CaR also reduces 1α-hydroxylase enzyme activity with an attendant decrease in calcitriol production. Stimulation of the CaR also increases the permeability of the distal convoluted tubule to water, leading to a less concentrated urine (Friedman 2000).

In uraemic patients, a substantial reduction in the CaR expression in the parathyroid cells may contribute to the altered 'set-point' for calcium control of PTH secretion observed in end-stage renal failure (Kifor *et al.* 1996).

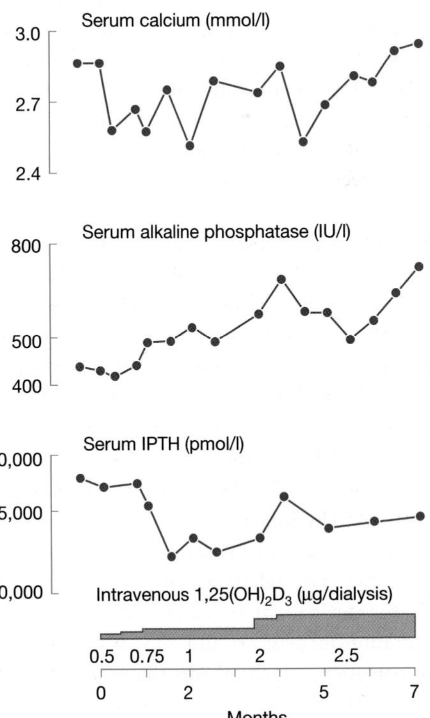

Fig. 2 The effect of intravenous calcitriol after each dialysis session in a hypercalcaemic patient with hyperparathyroidism. The reduction in serum calcium together with that of immunoreactive PTH, suggests a direct effect of calcitriol on parathyroid secretion.

Set-point for calcium control of PTH secretion

The relationship between PTH and serum calcium is best expressed as a sigmoidal curve. The concentration of ionized serum calcium, which decreases maximal PTH concentration by 50 per cent, is defined as the 'set-point' for calcium control of PTH secretion. Minor changes in this set-point produce major changes in PTH secretion at any given level of extracellular calcium. There is, however, a minimal rate of PTH release by the parathyroid cells representing a basal non-suppressible component of PTH secretion (Brown 1991). Set-point differs between normal subjects, but varies less between members of the same family, indicating a genetic component in its determination.

Parathyroid gland function is altered in chronic renal failure (Cundy *et al.* 1988; Felsenfeld and Llach 1993). In uraemic subjects, high ionized calcium concentrations lead to significantly less suppression of PTH secretion than in normal subjects, probably because of parathyroid gland size and intrinsic secretory function of individual parathyroid cells. The basal PTH secretion, expressed as a percentage of maximum PTH secretion, is also considerably greater in dialysis patients than in normal individuals (56 versus 25 per cent). This large, non-suppressible, component of PTH release in uraemic patients with hyperplastic parathyroid glands changes the configuration of the inverse sigmoidal calcium PTH curve leading to a decrease in its slope (Brown 1991).

It has been suggested that the set-point may not be a fixed property in the dialysis patient as it is continuously modified by sustained changes in existing serum calcium. Serum calcium levels vary markedly in dialysis patients, probably as a consequence of impaired calcium regulation via the failed kidneys, of various degrees of calcium loading during dialysis sessions, of the use of calcium-containing phosphate binders but also of different forms of renal osteodystrophy with a variable skeletal capacity to buffer calcium (Felsenfeld and Rodriguez 1996).

Aluminium directly suppresses the secretion of PTH, so that plasma PTH is characteristically, although not invariably, low in patients with aluminium toxicity (Burnatowska-Hledin *et al.* 1983). Serum calcium levels are often raised in patients with aluminium overload, possibly due to an effect of aluminium to decrease the skeletal uptake of calcium. The relative contribution of a direct effect of aluminium on the parathyroid cells and an indirect effect of the high calcium levels to suppress parathyroid secretion is difficult to ascertain in man. Removal of aluminium with desferrioxamine increases the secretion of PTH and decreases serum calcium, but also increases the turnover of calcium in bone (Malluche *et al.* 1984; Ott *et al.* 1986).

The set-point around which calcium stimulates PTH secretion can be modulated by calcitriol (Dunlay *et al.* 1989; Szabo *et al.* 1989; Malberti *et al.* 1992) and by numerous other factors such as magnesium concentration, which have a calcium-like effect on the acute secretion of PTH. Although a high concentration of magnesium in dialysis solutions decreases PTH secretion (Pletka *et al.* 1974), it may also adversely affect visceral metastatic calcification and crystal maturation in bone (Meema *et al.* 1987). In contrast, low dialysate magnesium concentration increases serum PTH but may result in chronic magnesium depletion, which impairs the sensitivity of bone to PTH (Parsons *et al.* 1980).

The set-point for PTH secretion is progressively disturbed in renal failure (Brown *et al.* 1982; Slatopolsky *et al.* 1988; Ramirez *et al.* 1993). For example, restoration of normal serum calcium by haemodialysis may decrease PTH secretion, but escape occurs with time, despite the maintenance of normal serum calcium values (Kanis *et al.* 1988). A similar phenomenon occurs in patients with renal osteodystrophy during long-term treatment with vitamin D derivatives (Ali *et al.* 1993; Hamdy *et al.* 1995) indicating that the change in set-point, which occurs with time, is not solely due to vitamin D deficiency (at least not calcitriol) (Fig. 3). These and other observations reviewed elsewhere (Lopez-Hilker *et al.* 1986; Lloyd *et al.* 1989) suggest that, in uraemia, factors other than serum calcium and calcitriol concentrations influence parathyroid cell growth and secretion.

Actions of parathyroid hormone

The target organs for PTH action include bone, kidney, and gut. The effects of PTH are initiated by its binding to the high affinity Type I PTH cell surface receptor (Juppner 1999).

In the kidney, PTH rapidly increases tubular reabsorption of calcium, particulary at the distal convoluted tubule. Within days, PTH stimulates 1α-hydroxylase activity, thereby increasing 1,25-dihydroxyvitamin D levels and promoting intestinal calcium transport. PTH also reduces the renal tubular reabsorption of phosphate and bicarbonate, thereby lowering plasma phosphate and pH. In the presence of hypocalcaemia, these direct and indirect dynamic effects of PTH on the kidney contribute to raising the extracellular fluid concentration of calcium. Whereas in moderate uraemia, increased secretion of PTH is able to sufficiently stimulate 1α-hydroxylase activity and to increase renal tubular reabsorption of calcium to maintain normal serum calcium levels, these homeostatic responses fail in advanced uraemia.

Most of the skeletal actions of PTH on osteoblasts and osteoclasts are mediated by Gs-activated cyclic adenosine monophosphate (cAMP)/protein kinase A induction (Goltzman 1999). High circulating concentrations of PTH increase both bone resorption and formation. In uncomplicated hyperparathyroidism, the net efflux of calcium from bone is close to zero despite a marked acceleration of bone turnover (Kanis *et al.* 1980). In renal failure the balance between bone formation and resorption is disturbed, generating focal areas of osteosclerosis and osteoporosis, eventually resulting in net bone loss.

The relationship between extracellular calcium concentration and PTH is disturbed in uraemia; this is referred to as 'resistance' to PTH, as increased concentrations of immunoreactive PTH coexist with

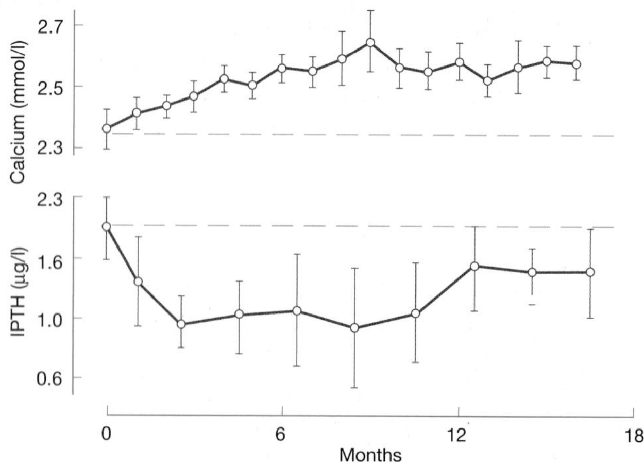

Fig. 3 Sequential changes in plasma calcium (mean ± SEM) and serum immunoreactive PTH in 13 patients treated continuously with alfacalcidol. Note the sustained increase in plasma calcium, but the poorly sustained suppression of immunoreactive PTH.

hypocalcaemia (Massry 1976). PTH injection also fails to raise plasma calcium levels to the same extent in uraemic as in normal subjects. Conversely, the recovery from hypocalcaemia induced by an ethylene diaminetetraacetic acid (EDTA) infusion is delayed in uraemia, despite increases in immunoreactive PTH (Kraut *et al.* 1981). The presence of these phenomena in the early stages of chronic renal failure suggests that skeletal resistance to the calcium-mobilizing action of PTH is important in the pathogenesis of both hypocalcaemia and secondary hyperparathyroidism (Llach *et al.* 1975; Massry 1976). Skeletal resistance to PTH is reversed, at least partially, by pretreatment with calcitriol (Kanis *et al.* 1979). It has been proposed that the skeletal resistance to PTH may be due to the high circulating levels of PTH (7–84) fragments. This might explain the need to maintain higher levels of intact PTH, as measured by currently available commercial assays which detect inactive fragments, to sustain normal bone turnover in patients on dialysis (Slatopolsky *et al.* 2000).

Calcitonin

Calcitonin is a peptide hormone containing 32 amino acid residues with a disulfide bridge between two cysteine residues in positions 1 and 7. The entire sequence is needed for biological activity. Calcitonin is mainly produced in the 'C' cells of the thyroid and also in non-thyroidal sites such as the thymus, the adrenal gland, and possibly the pars intermedia of the pituitary gland (Sexton *et al.* 1999).

Calcitonin inhibits bone resorption, thereby lowering plasma calcium. Its secretion is affected by several agents, including calcium, gastrointestinal hormones such as cholecystokinin, enteroglucagon, and gastrin, β-adrenergic agents, and alcohol. Calcitonin is a calcium-regulating hormone, operating by negative feedback: a rise in plasma calcium stimulates calcitonin secretion, which inhibits bone resorption with an attendant fall in calcium. Conversely, a fall in plasma calcium reduces the secretion of calcitonin leading to an increase in calcium release from bone. Calcitonin also lowers renal tubular reabsorption of calcium (Haas *et al.* 1971), a phenomenon of uncertain clinical significance. These actions of calcitonin complement those of PTH in maintaining extracellular fluid concentration of calcium (Kanis *et al.* 1985; Azria 1989).

The physiological role of calcitonin remains unclear, especially as a deficiency (total thyroidectomy) or excess (medullary carcinoma of the thyroid) is associated with only minor disturbances in skeletal or mineral homeostasis. Still, athyroidal man (supplemented with thyroid hormones) handles a calcium challenge less efficiently than normal subjects (Woodhouse and Barnes 1968), suggesting that calcitonin may influence the speed with which disturbances in calcium homeostasis are corrected.

Calcitonin circulates in a heterogeneous form and is degraded in part by the kidney so that values are difficult to interpret in patients with renal failure (Ardaillou 1975). Interestingly, some, but not all, investigators have found that the secretion rate of calcitonin is lower in patients with hyperparathyroid bone disease than in those without, suggesting that the endogenous secretion of calcitonin may protect against the development of hyperparathyroid bone disease (Kanis *et al.* 1977; Malluche *et al.* 1986).

Vitamin D

Humans normally derive vitamin D_3 (cholecalciferol) from the diet and from the skin by ultraviolet irradiation of 7-dehydrocholesterol. Vitamin D_2 (ergocalciferol) is used as a dietary supplement, particularly in margarine. In many respects the metabolism and actions of vitamin D_2 and D_3 are comparable. Vitamin D undergoes a series of metabolic transformations before exerting biological activity. The first step is its conversion in the liver to calcidiol (25-hydroxy-vitamin D_3), the major circulating vitamin D metabolite and the one most commonly measured clinically to provide an index of nutritional status. There is a marked seasonal variation in plasma calcidiol, with a peak in late summer and a trough in late winter when plasma concentrations commonly approach those associated with vitamin D deficiency status in the United Kingdom. Both sunlight and dietary intake are of crucial importance in maintaining vitamin D status in Northern Europe. The second step in vitamin D metabolism is the further hydroxylation of vitamin D, mainly in the kidney, to either 1,25-dihydroxy-vitamin D_3 (calcitriol) or to 24,25-dihydroxy-vitamin D_3 (secalciferol). The renal metabolism of calcitriol is closely regulated. Production is favoured under conditions of deficiency of vitamin D, calcium, or phosphate and is augmented by a variety of hormones including PTH, oestradiol, prolactin, and growth hormone. Conversely, calcium and phosphate repletion inhibit the synthesis of calcitriol, as does a decrease in PTH. This regulated metabolism qualifies calcitriol as a major calcium-regulating hormone, even though the stimulus for its synthesis is unlikely to be a change in extracellular calcium. Calcitriol can be considered to be the hormonal form of vitamin D in the sense that its production from endocrine tissue (the kidney) is controlled by the calcium and phosphate status of the individual, and that the action of this hormone reverses the stimulus to its secretion. In addition, calcitriol participates in the negative feedback regulation of PTH secretion.

As for other steroid hormones, the genomic mechanism of action of calcitriol is mediated by a receptor of the steroid-nuclear receptor super family: the vitamin D receptor (VDR) (Freedman 1999). Calcitriol induces the vitamin D-dependent calcium binding protein, calbindin, particularly calbindin-D_{28k} which plays a significant role in intestinal absorption and in distal tubular reabsorption of calcium (Sooy *et al.* 2000).

The principal actions of vitamin D are to increase the intestinal absorption of calcium and phosphate and possibly the resorption of calcium from bone. The latter effect, very obvious *in vitro*, is unlikely in humans, at physiological levels. Vitamin D metabolites also directly enhance calcium transport in the distal nephron (Friedman and Gesek 1993; Sooy *et al.* 2000).

Lack of vitamin D in man is associated with defective mineralization of cartilage and bone. It remains to be seen whether mineralization results from a direct effect of vitamin D and its metabolites on bone or is secondary to changes in extracellular fluid concentrations of calcium and phosphate (Kanis *et al.* 1982).

The metabolism of vitamin D is severely compromised in uraemia. Low or undetectable serum values for calcitriol are found in patients with end-stage renal failure who are functionally vitamin D deficient, even in the presence of adequate supplies of calcidiol. This deficiency largely accounts for the intestinal malabsorption seen in end-stage chronic renal failure, one of the main causes of hypocalcaemia, and the major stimulus for PTH secretion. Calcitriol deficiency also directly stimulates PTH mRNA gene expression thus contributing to increased PTH secretion.

In patients with renal failure, large doses of vitamin D may increase the intestinal absorption of calcium, and heal osteomalacia and osteitis fibrosa. The bone disease is 'vitamin D resistant' in the sense that a biological response requires doses of vitamin D far above those required to satisfy the physiological needs of normal individuals whereas it is obtained with physiological quantities of calcitriol or its synthetic analogue alfacalcidol (Kanis *et al.* 1982).

Production of calcitriol is sustained, until renal function is markedly impaired. Plasma calcitriol values may even increase in early renal failure. In advanced uraemia, the decreased synthesis of calcitriol is due to loss of renal tissue and to the inhibitory effects of hyperphosphataemia on the 1α-hydroxylase enzyme. In moderate renal failure, phosphate restriction increases serum values of calcitriol and the intestinal absorption of calcium (Portale *et al.* 1984), an observation suggesting that low levels of calcitriol, occasionally reported in moderate renal failure, reflect an homeostatic response to phosphate retention (Adler *et al.* 1985).

Vitamin D is transported by a specific vitamin D-binding protein (DBP). Patients with protein-losing states such as the nephrotic syndrome and those on CAPD may lose significant amounts of vitamin D binding protein, with a consequent decrease in serum calcidiol and calcitriol (Goldstein *et al.* 1981). In the nephrotic syndrome, these losses may induce intestinal malabsorption of calcium and hypocalcaemia. During CAPD, losses of calcidiol and other metabolites are not expected to affect intestinal absorption of calcium markedly since these patients have largely lost their capacity for 1α-hydroxylation. Indeed, calcium absorption is similar in patients treated by peritoneal dialysis and in those treated by intermittent haemodialysis (Hamdy *et al.* 1990a).

Drugs, such as anticonvulsants and barbiturates, induce hepatic microsomal enzymes potentially increasing the metabolism of calcidiol to inert products (Christensen *et al.* 1981). More importantly, anticonvulsants may block the action of vitamin D metabolites on gut and bone (Jubiz *et al.* 1977; Hahn and Halstead 1979). In moderate renal failure, the administration of these drugs is likely to aggravate intestinal malabsorption of calcium but would have progressively less effect as renal disease progresses. In patients treated with anticonvulsants, larger amounts of 1α-hydroxylated derivatives may thus be required for the treatment of established bone disease due to impaired target tissue responses to vitamin D.

Disturbed calcium transport in uraemia

In a normal adult, intestinal absorption of calcium is closely matched to its renal excretion in order to maintain calcium homeostasis. Both hypo- and hypercalcaemia develop as a result of a change in fluxes across sites of transport for calcium to and from the extracellular fluid. In view of the hormonal abnormalities described above, it is not surprising that chronic renal failure is associated with major disruptions in calcium homeostasis.

Intestine

Unlike calcium fluxes between extracellular fluid and bone and kidney, the intestinal absorption of calcium is episodic, depending upon the delivery of calcium in an absorbable form. The availability of calcium for absorption depends upon many dietary factors, including the presence of phosphate, fatty acids, and phytates, all of which bind calcium and prevent its absorption. Absorption occurs throughout the length of the small intestine, mainly in the duodenum and upper part of the jejunum, and to a lesser extent in the colon.

The influx of calcium depends on both active transport and diffusion processes (Wasserman and Chandler 1985). Active transport of calcium high in the gastrointestinal tract is vitamin D dependent and is saturable. The efficiency of vitamin D-dependent absorption increases with decreasing intakes of calcium. In growing children and in adults taking vitamin D, upper intestinal absorptive efficiency may reach 80 per cent (Kanis and Passmore 1989). At high intakes, the transport mechanism becomes saturated and more calcium becomes available for diffusional transport in the more distal gut (Nordin 1976).

The rate-limiting factor for transcellular calcium transport in the small intestine is the recently cloned apical epithelial calcium channel (ECaC) (Hoenderop *et al.* 1999). ECaC, which is expressed in 1,25-dihydroxy-vitamin D-responsive tissues in the proximal intestine, allows calcium entry in the enterocyte and thus plays the role of the 'gate-keeper' of the vitamin D-dependent active transepithelial intestinal calcium transport (Hoenderop *et al.* 2000).

A significant amount of calcium is lost in the gut through intestinal secretion. There is very little evidence that this is under metabolic control. In the presence of calcium malabsorption, faecal losses of calcium may exceed dietary intake, despite appreciable intestinal calcium absorption.

In uraemia, the progressive loss of vitamin D-dependent transport due to defective calcitriol synthesis has several consequences. First, patients are unable to adapt to changes in calcium demands through vitamin D-induced modulations of calcium transport. Second, the true absorption of calcium is critically load-dependent and the low efficiency of absorption by diffusion limits the usefulness of calcium supplements to increase net intestinal absorption. Relatively high oral doses of calcium can thus be given for phosphate-binding without a high incidence of hypercalcaemia (Slatopolsky *et al.* 1986). In calcium-treated patients, due caution should be exerted with the use of vitamin D derivatives, however, as they restore the active transport component with increased potential for hypercalcaemia to develop.

Bone

Skeletal metabolism is profoundly disturbed in renal failure, resulting in renal osteodystrophy, the spectrum of which is reviewed elsewhere (Kanis *et al.* 1988; Hamdy 1995a; Hruska and Teitelbaum 1995; Slatopolsky 1998) and discussed in Chapter 11.3.9.

In addition to alterations in calcium fluxes across quiescent bone surfaces, it is relevant to consider the general disturbances in skeletal metabolism where these impact significantly on calcium homeostasis. In the adult skeleton, in balance with respect to calcium, the amount of bone resorption and formation are equivalent. Mineral accretion and resorption, although closely related, do not occur at the same anatomical site, at the same time. In the adult, bone remodelling occurs on all bone surfaces and accounts for approximately 95 per cent of skeletal calcium turnover. Early in the remodelling sequence, osteoclasts assemble at a focus on the bone surface to excavate a resorption cavity, removing both mineral and organic matrix. Osteoclasts disappear after completion of this phase. Several days later, bone-forming cells (osteoblasts) are attracted principally to sites of previous resorption. This sequence of events permits the self-repair of bone and is one of the main mechanisms preserving both skeletal mass and architecture (Frost 1966).

Normally, 10–15 per cent of the bone surfaces are engaged in the process of bone remodelling. PTH is one of the major factors influencing the number of bone remodelling sites present at any one time: in severe hyperparathyroidism, such as found in uraemia, up to 100 per cent of the bone surface may be occupied by remodelling events, increasing bone turnover 7–10-fold. This has surprisingly few consequences on extracellular calcium homeostasis, since the amount of bone formed closely matches the amount resorbed. In contrast, this increase in bone turnover may have consequences on the net flux of calcium from bone and thus on bone mass. In the remodelling process, bone formation always follows resorption so that an increase in bone remodelling results in a finite deficit in bone, proportional to the rate of bone turnover. If, during the remodelling sequence, there is an imbalance between the amount of bone resorbed and that formed, in favour of net calcium losses, increases in bone turnover will amplify those losses (Fig. 4). Bone mass has indeed been shown to progressively decrease, particularly at cortical sites, in proportion with the decrease in glomerular filtration rate (GFR) (Rix *et al.* 1999). On the basis of normal fluxes of calcium to and from bone (Fig. 1), a sevenfold increase in bone turnover should deliver an additional 30 mmol/l of calcium to the extracellular fluid, if bone formation (or its mineralization) is markedly impaired. In patients with mild to moderate renal failure, decreasing bone turnover by suppressing PTH secretion with the use of alfacalcidol (Hamdy *et al.* 1995), also prevents the bone loss associated with progressive renal failure (Rix *et al.* 1999).

Mild to moderate aluminium intoxication suppresses osteoblastic activity despite continuing osteoclast activity. Each erosion cavity is thus replaced with an inadequate amount of bone, leading to progressive osteoporosis (Heaf *et al.* 1983). In this case, hypercalcaemia may also be present due to decreased calcium utilization by suppressed osteoblasts. This may occur following a dialysis session, as the skeleton cannot cope with the increased calcium load provided by the dialysis fluid, or as a result of the use of calcium-containing phosphate binders or that of vitamin D metabolites. Severe aluminium intoxication inhibits all elements of bone turnover (Cournot-Witmer *et al.* 1981; DeVernejoul *et al.* 1985).

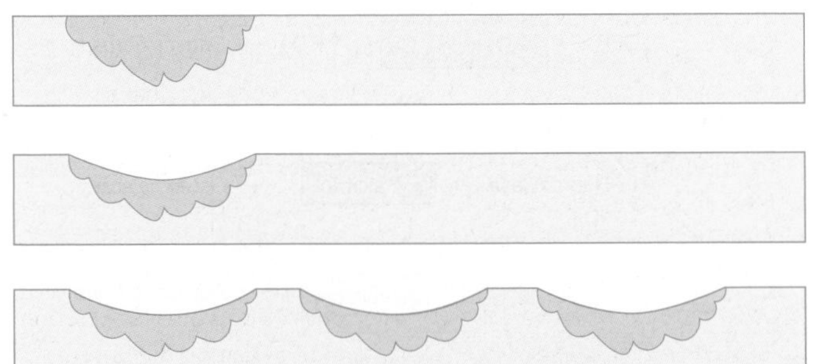

Fig. 4 Schematic diagrams showing the effect of increased bone turnover on bone balance. The upper panel shows a cancellous bone surface where normal bone remodelling is occurring on 10 per cent of the trabecular surface. The centre panel shows a small but finite deficit in mineralized bone. When bone remodelling is increased skeletal losses of calcium from bone are accentuated (lower panel). This is analogous to the increase in bone turnover due to hyperparathyroidism in association with an imbalance in the amount of bone formed compared with that resorbed (e.g. aluminium toxicity). Skeletal losses of calcium are amplified at a rate proportional to the number of bone remodelling units present at any one time.

Kidney

Calcium fluxes across the kidney are much greater than those across gut or bone (Fig. 1). The renal handling of calcium by the kidney is a complex process taking place at different sites in the nephron. This process is reviewed elsewhere (Friedman 2000) and discussed in detail in Chapter 5.1.

In health, approximately 97 per cent of calcium filtered by the kidneys is reabsorbed, mainly under the influence of PTH. The hypercalcaemia of mild hyperparathyroidism is mainly due to increased renal tubular reabsorption of calcium, since fasting calcium excretion is often normal, whereas an increase would be expected if the net flux of calcium from bone to extracellular fluid were augmented (Kanis *et al.* 1980). In many patients with primary hyperparathyroidism, increased bone resorption is matched by an enhanced bone formation since calcium excretion is usually normal. Similarly, in hypoparathyroidism, fasting renal excretion is usually normal despite a low plasma calcium pointing to a decrease in renal tubular reabsorption of calcium.

The way in which uraemia affects renal handling of calcium has not been well characterized. Renal tubular reabsorption of calcium is markedly decreased in uraemia (Cochran and Nordin 1971; Paterson *et al.* 1982), but most patients with significant renal impairment also have an increased secretion of PTH, expected to augment renal tubular reabsorption of calcium. Renal calcium filtration decreases in direct proportion to the decline in GFR. The net result is a decrease in the urinary excretion of calcium often encountered in the course of progressive renal failure.

It has been suggested that vitamin D is required for the normal effects of PTH on renal tubular reabsorption of calcium. Vitamin D is also able to increase renal tubular reabsorption of calcium independently of PTH (Hoenderop *et al.* 2000).

The renal clearance of calcium is closely related to the clearance of sodium and there is evidence for a cotransport mechanism, at least at some sites. Data on the relationship between sodium and calcium transport in normal subjects are scarce, but it is likely that, in renal failure, the increased sodium load per nephron contributes to the decreased renal tubular reabsorption of calcium. The shared sodium and calcium transport mechanism carries significant implications for the management of hypercalcaemia with saline (NaCl) infusions, and may be important in the pathophysiology of severe hypercalcaemia (see later in this chapter).

Disorders of calcium homeostasis in uraemia

Hypo- and hypercalcaemia occur under steady state conditions when abnormalities arise at the sites of calcium exchange with the extracellular fluid, such as:

- Increased or decreased net gastrointestinal absorption
- Increased or decreased net bone resorption
- Increased or decreased renal tubular reabsorption
- Reduction or increase in GFR.

Many examples of the complex interplay between primary pathology and calcium fluxes at other sites are seen in uraemia, and some are reviewed below.

Clinical features of hypo- and hypercalcaemia

The clinical features of hypocalcaemia are specific (Table 1) but uncommon in patients with uraemia. Individual susceptibility is variable, particularly in parathyroidectomized patients in whom tetanic symptoms may develop when serum calcium is at the lower end of the normal range.

The clinical features of hypercalcaemia (Table 2) are non-specific. The susceptibility of individual patients varies also considerably. Common symptoms include lethargy, anorexia, constipation, and, particularly in renal disease, those due to extraskeletal and vascular calcifications. There is growing evidence that the increase in cardiovascular morbidity and mortality observed in dialysis patients (Foley *et al.* 1998) are due to vascular calcifications resulting from hyperphosphataemia, hypercalcaemia, and increased calcium–phosphorus product due to hyperparathyroidism (Block and Port 2000). Nephrocalcinosis is more common in non-PTH-mediated hypercalcaemia than in hyperparathyroidism. Hypercalcaemic features depend in part upon the evolution and the nature of the disorder. Symptoms are more frequent in patients in whom hypercalcaemia develops rapidly.

Neuromuscular symptoms disappear very rapidly with treatment of hypocalcaemia, but the same is not true for hypercalcaemia. Drowsiness, confusion, lethargy, and cranial nerve palsies may persist for many days after the restitution of normal serum calcium concentrations, and the failure of symptoms to improve rapidly with treatment should not be taken as evidence that they are attributable to other underlying disorders.

Table 1 Clinical features of hypocalcaemia

Neurological
Neuromuscular irritability
Paraesthesia
Tetany
Irritability
Convulsions
Intracranial calcification
Papilloedema
Eyes
Cataracts
Cardiovascular
Prolongation of QT interval
Resistance to digoxin

Table 2 Clinical features of hypercalcaemia

Neurological
Lethargy and drowsiness
Confusion, coma
Emotional lability, depression
Cranial nerve palsies
Hypotonia and decreased deep tendon reflexes
Gastrointestinal
Anorexia, vomiting
Constipation
Peptic ulceration
Acute pancreatitis
Visceral calcification
Cardiovascular
Hypertension
Arrhythmias
Sensitivity to digoxin
Renal
Polyuria, polydipsia
Hypercalciuria and nephrolithiasis
Nephrocalcinosis
Impairment of glomerular filtration rate
Other tissues
Soft tissue calcification
Red eye syndrome
Pseudogout
Pruritus

The hypocalcaemia of renal failure

Hypocalcaemia is relatively frequently encountered in the course of progressive renal impairment. The decreased synthetic capacity of the failing kidney to produce calcitriol, and phosphate retention due to progressive decrease in GFR, are the two main mechanisms responsible for the development of hypocalcaemia. Calcitriol deficiency lowers the intestinal absorption of calcium, but the mechanism by which phosphate retention decreases serum calcium is not clear beyond its ability to suppress the 1α-hydroxylase enzyme, further decreasing the production of calcitriol (Fig. 5). The importance of phosphate retention for calcium homeostasis is further demonstrated by the ability of phosphate restriction to increase ionized concentrations of calcium under steady state conditions in both early and advanced renal failure (Portale *et al.* 1984).

Hypocalcaemia is the major stimulus for the secretion of PTH, which in turn decreases renal tubular reabsorption of phosphate, and hence plasma phosphate, but increases plasma calcium (see above). In

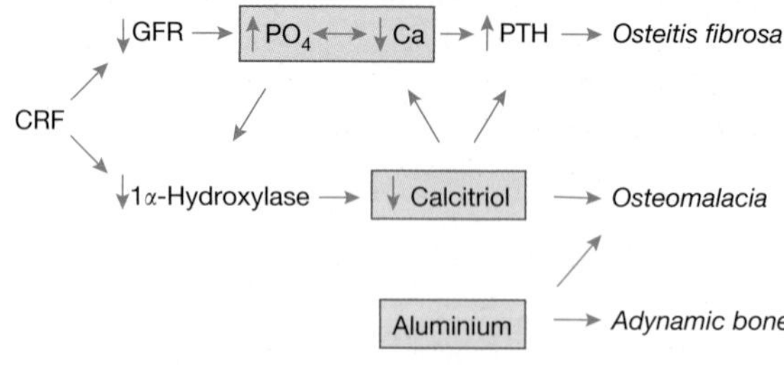

Fig. 5 A simple scheme for the pathogenesis of renal bone disease. Progressive renal failure induces decrements in GFR and synthetic capacity for calcitriol. An increase in plasma phosphate (PO_4) due to the reduction in GFR stimulates the secretion of PTH indirectly by decreasing plasma calcium values. Hyperphosphataemia further inhibits synthesis of calcitriol. Malabsorption of calcium contributes to hypocalcaemia. Hyperphosphataemia and calcitriol deficiency also directly stimulate PTH secretion. During progressive renal failure, plasma calcium and phosphate tend to remain normal (because of the renal and skeletal effects of PTH) at the expense of an increasing secretion rate of PTH. When the compensatory abilities of the kidney are compromised by renal failure, hyperphosphataemia and hypocalcaemia prevail.

the early stages of renal impairment, mineral abnormalities are largely masked by the mobilization of homeostatic mechanisms to maintain serum calcium and phosphate within the normal range at the expense, however, of an ever-increasing secretion rate of PTH (Slatopolsky *et al.* 1972). Up to 75 per cent of asymptomatic patients with a creatinine clearance of less than 50 ml/min demonstrate histological evidence for hyperparathyroid bone disease (Hamdy *et al.* 1995). In advanced renal failure, the number of residual nephrons is not sufficient to lower plasma phosphate, and hyperphosphataemia and hypocalcaemia ensue (Fig. 5).

Hypocalcaemia is rarely florid in slowly progressive uraemia, except in children, in whom the calcium homeostat may be impaired, and in patients with coexisting deficiencies of vitamin D including those with the nephrotic syndrome and urinary losses of vitamin D (see above). Hypocalcaemic crises may be precipitated by the infusion of alkali in severely acidotic patients. Hypocalcaemia is also aggravated by defective dietary intake of calcium, since calcium absorption is largely proportional to dietary intake when the vitamin D endocrine system fails.

Management of hypocalcaemia in chronic renal failure

Control of hyperphosphataemia by dietary restriction of phosphate, the use of phosphate-binding agents such as calcium-containing binders or synthetic polymers such as sevelamer (Renagel) and the judicious and timely use of active metabolites of vitamin D or their analogues such as calcitriol, alfacalcidol, or dihydrotachysterol represent the mainstay of management of hypocalcaemia in chronic renal failure (Ramsdell 1999; Locatelli *et al.* 2002; Malluche *et al.* 2002). Calcitriol and its synthetic analogue alfacalcidol bypass the metabolic block caused by uraemia, but dihydrotachysterol is also biologically active without the necessity for 1α-hydroxylation. Dihydrotachysterol and alfacalcidol undergo hepatic hydroxylation, and the 25-hydroxy derivatives formed in this way are the major circulating forms of these agents. Reasonable starting doses are 1 μg daily for alfacalcidol and calcitriol, and 200 μg daily for dihydrotachysterol. These doses are larger than those generally required to maintain normocalcaemia so that patients with impaired renal function are liable to become hypercalcaemic rapidly if doses are not titrated according to requirements. Alternatively, lower starting doses of the vitamin D derivatives (0.25 or 0.5 μg) may be given with the disadvantage of a slower response. Vitamin D requirements vary in the presence of hyperparathyroid bone disease and decrease while healing progresses (Kanis *et al.* 1979). A major disadvantage with the use of calcidiol and vitamin D is their slow onset and cessation of action so that doses are less readily titrated according to requirements and toxic effects are reversed less rapidly after treatment interruption than with calcitriol, alfacalcidol, or dihydrotachysterol (Kanis and Russell 1977) (Fig. 6).

Serum creatinine rises with the use of 1α-hydroxy-vitamin D and calcitriol, as a consequence of an increased production of creatinine rather than of an impaired GFR. A large double blind placebo-controlled trial in patients with mild to moderate renal failure given up to 1 μg alfacalcidol daily for 2 years disclosed no deleterious effect of vitamin D on the course of progressive renal failure provided that hypercalcaemia is avoided (Hamdy *et al.* 1995). It is currently advocated to use these agents, together with dietary phosphate restriction and phosphate binders, earlier in the course of progressive renal failure than currently practiced, to correct the mineral abnormalities which lead to parathyroid hyperplasia and its inevitable consequences

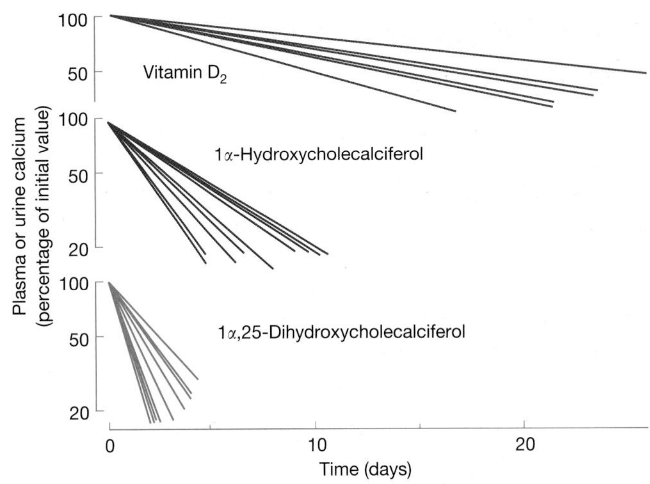

Fig. 6 Rate of reversal of hypercalcaemia and hypercalciuria following cessation of treatment with vitamin D_2, alfacalcidol, and calcitriol. The decrease in plasma or urine calcium was monoexponential. The half-life of reversal of vitamin D poisoning is much shorter with calcitriol and alfacalcidol than with vitamin D.

(Cundy *et al.* 1985; Hamdy 1995b; Felsenfeld 1997; Block and Port 2000; Locatelli *et al.* 2002; Malluche *et al.* 2002).

When renal replacement therapy is initiated, both CAPD and haemodialysis may initially correct disturbances in calcium homeostasis. The use of standard dialysate solutions containing 1.5 mmol/l of calcium results in a positive transfer of calcium to the haemodialysis patient. Serum calcium rises at the end of a dialysis session by 0.15 ± 0.01 mmol/l, and decreases by a similar amount in the interdialytic period. Serum calcium levels are more constant in CAPD patients given a higher, 1.75 mmol/l, dialysate calcium concentration (Bouillon *et al.* 1975). This is partly the reason why hyperparathyroid bone disease is less conspicuous in patients on CAPD than in those on haemodialysis.

The use of standard dialysate solutions and the restoration of serum calcium commonly improve bone disease, presumably as a result of suppression of PTH secretion. Unfortunately, PTH returns subsequently to original values and bone disease recurs despite the maintenance of serum calcium (Fig. 7). This 'escape' is attributed to the fact that each dialysis induced rise in plasma calcium is only transient and that the acute suppression of PTH values is followed by a rebound after termination of haemodialysis. The existence of a similar escape in patients treated with vitamin D, suggests that the fluctuations induced by haemodialysis are not the sole determinants of PTH secretion.

Higher dialysate calcium may induce hypercalcaemia (Drueke *et al.* 1977), and the hope that it might suppress PTH secretion has not been fully realized (Goldsmith *et al.* 1971).

Lower dialysate calcium concentrations may induce a transient hypocalcaemia in patients on CAPD, due to increased peritoneal losses (Hamdy *et al.* 1990a). This effect is poorly sustained as a result of increased calcium efflux from bone. Low dialysate calcium concentrations are thus rarely used in the long-term management of hypercalcaemic patients but have been used to increase the tolerance to vitamin D metabolites (Hamdy *et al.* 1991) and to calcium-containing phosphate binders (Sawyer *et al.* 1988; Morinière *et al.* 1993).

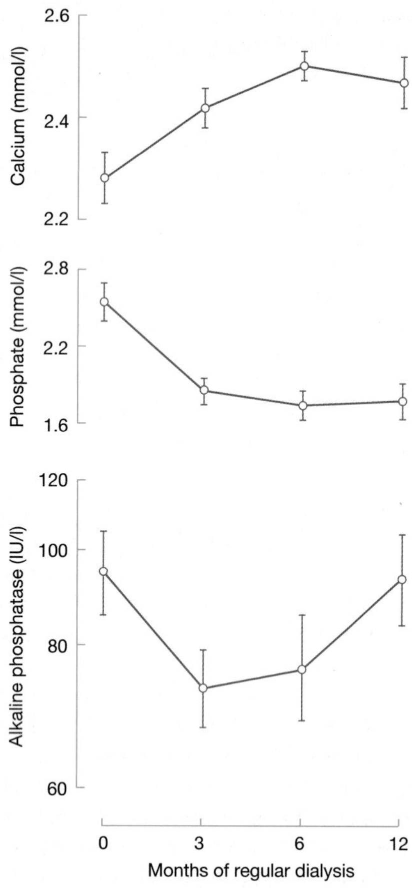

Fig. 7 Sequential changes in plasma biochemistry (mean ± SEM) in a cohort of 20 patients with hyperparathyroid bone disease before and during the first year of regular haemodialysis. None of the patients were receiving any form of vitamin D treatment. Note that the sustained decrease in plasma phosphate and increase in plasma calcium were associated with a marked ($p < 0.02$), but only transient, suppression of alkaline phosphatase activity.

Hypocalcaemia after parathyroidectomy

Hypocalcaemia occurs in 13–30 per cent of cases after parathyroid surgery (Anderberg *et al.* 1981; Kaplan *et al.* 1982). Its causes include excision of all parathyroid tissue, in total parathyroidectomy, transient vascular ischaemia of remaining parathyroid tissue, or suppression of healthy parathyroid tissue by long-term hypercalcaemia after subtotal parathyroidectomy (Dent 1962). In patients with high bone turnover before surgery, parathyroidectomy abruptly interrupts bone resorption while bone formation continues. The attendant extensive remineralization of the skeleton may induce severe hypocalcaemia and hypophosphataemia, occasionally associated with tetany. It may last several weeks, depending on the severity of preoperative hyperparathyroid bone disease (Charhon *et al.* 1985). Fuller Albright was the first to describe these manifestations to which he coined the term 'hungry bone syndrome' (Albright and Reifenstein 1948).

In a large series of patients with primary hyperparathyroidism, 12.6 per cent developed the hungry bone syndrome following surgery. Preoperative clinical and biochemical predictors of severe postoperative hypocalcaemia include severity of hypercalcaemia, serum alkaline phosphatase activity and degree of renal impairment (Brasier and Nussbaum 1988). Hypocalcaemia occurs more rapidly and more markedly in uraemic patients than in patients with primary hyperparathyroidism, even after partial parathyroidectomy because of pre-existing high bone turnover. Patients may remain asymptomatic until the onset of convulsions, which may be associated with multiple fractures because of underlying renal osteodystrophy.

It is often necessary to administer large intravenous doses of calcium (up to 6 g daily), for a number of weeks after surgery, in order to avoid postoperative tetany. Preoperative administration of 1α-hydroxylated derivatives of vitamin D diminishes the degree and duration of postoperative hypocalcaemia (Kanis *et al.* 1979). We routinely treat patients with calcitriol or alfacalcidol for 2 or 3 weeks before surgery with meticulous monitoring of serum calcium, particularly in the presence of coexisting hypercalcaemia. In patients with the most severe hyperparathyroid bone disease, additional short-term treatment with bisphosphonates may prevent severe postoperative hypocalcaemia by decreasing bone turnover preoperatively.

Other causes of hypocalcaemia

Acute renal failure

Some degree of hypocalcaemia occurs in most patients with acute renal failure, particularly in the oliguric phase, probably as a consequence of hyperphosphataemia. This is aggravated by extensive tissue injury or by phosphate infusion during parenteral nutrition. Hypocalcaemia may also occur in the presence of normal or low serum phosphate concentrations.

Hypocalcaemia is noteworthy in acute renal failure due to rhabdomyolysis, as phosphate released by damaged tissue binds large amounts of calcium and causes calcification evident on bone scintigraphy, with eventual long-term morbidity (Esnault *et al.* 1990). Indeed, the finding of hypocalcaemia without recognized muscle damage raises the possibility that the diagnosis has been overlooked, for example, in comatose patients or after an alcohol or heroin overdose (Feinstein *et al.* 1981).

Hypomagnesaemia

Hypomagnesaemia is a rare cause of hypocalcaemia, which should be recognized because the hypocalcaemia is refractory to treatment until magnesium repletion is achieved. Causes of magnesium deficiency are discussed in Chapter 2.5. Those relevant to nephrology include the intrinsic renal tubular disorders (Bartter's syndrome, magnesium wasting, renal tubular acidosis, and the diuretic phase of acute renal failure) as well as use of drugs such as the loop diuretics and aminoglycosides. Magnesium deficiency should be suspected in postparathyroidectomy hypocalcaemia, since the 'hungry bone syndrome' sequesters not only calcium but also magnesium in bone. The cause of the refractory hypocalcaemia is multifactorial: severe hypomagnesaemia impairs the secretion of PTH and inhibits the effects of PTH on target tissues, particularly bone, giving rise to pseudohypoparathyroidism.

Magnesium sulfate may be administered by intravenous infusion, but care is obviously required in the presence of marked renal failure. Parenteral doses vary from 20 to 80 mmol daily. Oral replacement treatment is rarely required, except during the diuretic phase of acute renal failure. Unfortunately, magnesium salts may induce diarrhoea when given by mouth, but magnesium oxide at a dose of 250 or 500 mg four times daily is usually well tolerated.

Hypercalcaemia in renal failure

Both in health and disease, an increase in the net flux of calcium from gut and/or bone will cause hypercalcaemia to an extent dependent upon concurrent changes in tubular reabsorption of calcium and GFR.

In health, the net intestinal influx of calcium to the extracellular fluid is approximately 20 per cent of the dietary intake or 5 mmol daily, whereas the net skeletal flux is zero if the skeleton is in balance for calcium (Fig. 1). Increased intestinal absorption of calcium contributes to the hypercalcaemia associated with vitamin D poisoning and sarcoidosis, and in the context of renal failure in the milk-alkali syndrome and in some patients with autonomous tertiary hyperparathyroidism. An increased intestinal absorption of calcium is unlikely to cause life-threatening hypercalcaemia on its own, unless the dietary intake of calcium is excessive (e.g. milk-alkali syndrome) or in the presence of severe uraemia. Thus an increase in net calcium absorption from 20 to 40 per cent in the presence of a normal calcium diet would result in an additional 8 mmol of calcium distributed principally in the extracellular fluid. Plasma calcium is expected to rise by 0.53 mmol/l or from 2.5 to 3.03 mmol/l. This degree of hypercalcaemia is, however, an overestimation for several reasons. Firstly, other sites for calcium exchange, including protein binding, soft tissue, and bone, buffer the increase. Secondly, the absorbed calcium augments the load of calcium filtered by the kidneys so that, under steady state conditions, a twofold increase in calcium delivery to the extracellular fluid doubles calcium excretion. Consideration of the relationship between plasma calcium and calcium excretion indicates that this should increase plasma calcium from 2.5 to 2.8 mmol/l—an increase of only 0.3 mmol/l. Finally, the increment induced is likely to be even less in patients in whom hyperabsorption is not mediated by hyperparathyroidism, since hypercalcaemia will suppress the secretion of PTH and decrease renal tubular reabsorption of calcium and bone resorption. The sparing effect of decreased renal tubular reabsorption in the face of a hypercalcaemic challenge operates in hypercalcaemia and suggests that calcium delivery into the extracellular fluid must be increased several-fold before severe hypercalcaemia occurs, unless renal function is also abnormal.

The ability of the kidney to alter plasma calcium by changing renal tubular reabsorption of calcium is progressively compromised in patients with uraemia, who become more sensitive to challenges that induce hypercalcaemia. A number of other factors, which impair the buffering capacity of bone, also appear in uraemia. The presence of aluminium in bone decreases the ability of patients to withstand a calcium challenge. Conversely, the presence of hyperparathyroid bone disease increases the buffering capacity of bone, possibly because of the more ready calcium exchange at sites of woven bone formation.

Abnormalities in GFR, renal tubular reabsorption, or intestinal absorption alone are unlikely to cause severe hypercalcaemia, whereas net bone resorption must increase several-fold to raise plasma calcium above 3 mmol/l, provided that other homeostatic mechanisms are operating normally. Hypercalcaemia is therefore rarely the result of a single abnormality, but is usually caused by a combination of factors, often coupled with a failure of normal homeostatic processes.

Hypercalcaemia in dialysis-independent patients

Hypercalcaemia is rare in patients not yet established on dialysis. The coexistence of hypercalcaemia and progressive renal failure raises the possibility of a causal role of the former. Causes of hypercalcaemia are listed in Table 3 according to their frequency in clinical practice.

Sarcoidosis

Sarcoidosis is associated with ectopic and unregulated synthesis of calcitriol by sarcoid tissue in response to sunlight or ingestion of vitamin D (Mason *et al.* 1984). Hypersensitivity to vitamin D occurs despite bilateral nephrectomy, indicating that the increase in serum calcitriol is not mediated by renal 1α-hydroxylation. Augmented intestinal absorption of calcium and hypercalciuria ensue (Papapoulos *et al.* 1979). Hypercalcaemia is rarely observed, however, despite increased intestinal absorption of calcium, as long as renal function is able to clear the calcium load. Extrarenal production of calcitriol and hypercalcaemia can be suppressed within a few days by the administration of corticosteroids (Sandler *et al.* 1984).

Ectopic production of calcitriol is also occasionally seen in patients with tuberculosis (Fuss *et al.* 1988) or lymphoma (Breslau *et al.* 1984) and resolves with treatment of the underlying disorder.

Milk-alkali syndrome

Hypercalcaemia and renal failure may be observed in patients with a chronic high intake of calcium salts or milk and absorbable alkali. This so-called 'milk-alkali syndrome' is now a rarity largely due to the widespread use of non-absorbable antacids and H_2-receptor antagonists in the management of peptic ulcer disease (French *et al.* 1986). The finding of renal failure and hypercalcaemia associated with a metabolic alkalosis should alert the physician to the possible diagnosis. If therapy is delayed, irreversible renal damage may occur despite rehydration and discontinuation of the medication.

Acute renal failure

Hypercalcaemia may occur during the diuretic phase of acute renal failure as the consequence of persistent secondary hyperparathyroidism after the restoration of renal function, analogous to the case

Table 3 Causes of hypercalcaemia

Common
Primary hyperparathyroidism
Neoplasia
Vitamin D toxicity
Thiazide diuretics
Artefactual (prolonged venous stasis, hyperproteinaemia)
Infrequent
Immobilization
Tertiary hyperparathyroidism, particularly in transplant recipients
Sarcoidosis (and other granulomatous diseases)
Hyperthyroidism
Rare
Diuretic phase of acute renal failure
Benign familial hypercalcaemia
Addisonian crisis
Phaeochromocytoma
Milk alkali syndrome
Vitamin A toxicity
Aluminium toxicity
Parenteral nutrition (calcium and aluminium)
Silicon retention

after transplantation (Llach *et al.* 1981). An alternative, or additional, factor is the mobilization of calcium from previous calcification in injured tissues. A similar mechanism probably accounts for the increased frequency with which hypercalcaemia is seen in acute renal failure after an alcohol or heroin overdose. It is important to recall that parenteral nutrition may itself induce hypercalcaemia in patients with acute renal failure. This is most commonly due to high concentrations of calcium, but also rarely due to aluminium contamination of casein, albumin, or purified protein fraction (DeBroe *et al.* 1988).

Hypercalcaemia in dialysis patients

Hypercalcaemia may be observed in over a third of patients on dialysis. Most common causes are liberal use of vitamin D supplementation to treat hyperparathyroidism and the frequent need to use calcium-containing phosphate binders. The decision to stop both vitamin D metabolites and phosphate binders often results in an exacerbation of hyperparathyroidism with a further rise in the calcium–phosphorus product. Hypercalcaemia associated with malignancy needs to be excluded. Other less common causes of hypercalcaemia are listed in Table 3.

Vitamin D toxicity

All vitamin D preparations may induce hypercalcaemia. In the case of calcidiol or the parent compounds, their long half-life precludes the reversal of their biological effects for weeks or months. The advantage of the 1α-hydroxylated derivatives lies in the ease with which doses are titrated according to requirements, and the rapidity with which toxic effects are reversed upon stopping treatment (Kanis and Russell 1977, Fig. 6). The greatest risks of hypercalcaemia with the use of calcitriol and alfacalcidol in the treatment of renal bone disease occur at the start of treatment, particularly in patients with aluminium retention or adynamic bone lesions. In others, the risk increases later, when biochemical responses to treatment are nearing completion. In patients with hyperparathyroidism who respond to treatment, requirements thus progressively decrease with time as bone disease heals and hypercalcaemia usually occurs for the first time when serum activity of alkaline phosphatase decreases towards normal (Kanis *et al.* 1979). It is important to monitor serum calcium in patients treated with active metabolites of vitamin D, as sustained increases in plasma calcium and phosphate are associated with extraskeletal and vascular calcifications (Block *et al.* 1998).

Attempts to return PTH levels to normal in patients on dialysis have been linked with the development of 'adynamic bone lesions', histologically characterized by a low number of osteoblasts and osteoclasts, a very low bone turnover, normal or low PTH levels and low serum alkaline phosphatase activity. Patients with adynamic bone disease tend to develop hypercalcaemia, either spontaneously or following the use of vitamin D metabolites, probably because the calcium buffering capacity of bone is diminished so that calcium challenges such as those of a dialysis treatment, are less efficiently cleared from the extracellular fluid compartment (Kurz *et al.* 1994).

Aluminium intoxication

Adequate treatment of dialysis water has become widely available, so that the ingestion of aluminium-containing phosphate binders is currently the major source of aluminium intoxication (DeBroe *et al.* 1988). This may lead to adynamic bone disease in which case hypercalcaemia is common (see above). This slowly resolves when aluminium sources are eliminated. Alternatively, patients can be treated with desferrioxamine, which chelates aluminium in a form that can be excreted or removed by dialysis. Doses commonly used are 4–6 g weekly in divided doses by intravenous infusion, at the start or towards the end of dialysis treatments. Removal of aluminium increases bone turnover and decreases plasma calcium. Treatment with vitamin D derivatives can then be instituted.

Patients on dialysis may have both aluminium overload and hyperparathyroidism. The use of aluminium-containing phosphate binders after the failure of other binders to control serum phosphate, results in a higher accumulation of aluminium in bone with a high as opposed to low bone turnover. Aluminium is then diffusely distributed throughout the marrow rather than present at the critical mineral–osteoid interface. In such patients, parathyroidectomy should only be considered after appropriate removal of aluminium with desferrioxamine, as failure to do so would result in the postoperative redistribution of aluminium to critical bone surfaces and to a difficult-to-treat low turnover osteomalacia. The mere removal of aluminium may result in a response to treatment with vitamin D although in most cases subsequent parathyroidectomy will be required.

Adynamic bone disease

Marked suppression of bone formation with a propensity to hypercalcaemia is characteristic but not specific for aluminium toxicity (Cohen-Solal *et al.* 1992). Similar findings have been reported in patients treated with calcium salts (Hercz *et al.* 1993), with iron overload (DeVernejoul *et al.* 1982), with diabetes mellitus (Vincenti *et al.* 1984) or after total parathyroidectomy (Charhon *et al.* 1985). Outside the context of aluminium intoxication, the clinical significance of the 'adynamic bone lesion' remains uncertain.

Autonomous 'tertiary' hyperparathyroidism

Patients with markedly hyperplastic glands may not respond to vitamin D and even low doses may induce hypercalcaemia (Nielsen *et al.* 1977; Kanis *et al.* 1979). Moreover, the long-term use of vitamin D is associated with relapse despite the maintenance of normal or high serum calcium concentrations (Sharman *et al.* 1982; Ali *et al.* 1993) (see Fig. 3). In these spontaneously hypercalcaemic patients, parathyroidectomy is the treatment of choice.

Alternative means of modulating PTH secretion or its target organ effects and therefore hypercalcaemia have been sought. The intravenous administration of vitamin D metabolites bypasses the immediate delivery of pharmacological concentrations to the small intestine and delivers proportionately more calcitriol to the parathyroid gland. Indeed, changes in PTH secretion have been observed, independent of those induced by changes in serum calcium, in hypocalcaemic and normocalcaemic patients on dialysis (Slatopolsky *et al.* 1984; Andress *et al.* 1989). A similar effect is observed in hypercalcaemic patients (Hamdy *et al.* 1989), suggesting that such treatments may alter the set point for PTH release. The intravenous administration of vitamin D metabolites may represent an advantage over the oral route in the long term, although this remains to be conclusively established (Morinière *et al.* 1993; Canella *et al.* 1994; Bacchini *et al.* 1997).

Alternative non-calcaemic vitamin D analogues such as 22-oxacalcitriol, 26,27-hexa-fluorocalcitriol, 19-nor-1,25-dihydroxy-vitamin D_2 and 1α-hydroxy-vitamin D_2 did not hold their promise of 'non-calcaemia' and were not found to be superior to calcitriol or alfacalcidol in the long-run (Slatopolsky and Brown 1997).

Low calcium dialysate increases the tolerance to vitamin D metabolites in patients on peritoneal dialysis (Hamdy *et al.* 1991), but its prolonged use without adequate vitamin D supplementation, may result in a negative calcium balance and aggravation of hyperparathyroidism (Argiles *et al.* 1993).

An alternative management of hypercalcaemia associated with high bone turnover due to autonomous hyperparathyroidism is the use of inhibitors of bone resorption, such as the bisphosphonates (Hamdy *et al.* 1987, 1990b; Fleisch 2000). These agents inhibit osteoclast-mediated bone resorption, decreasing calcium (and phosphate) efflux from bone, thereby lowering serum calcium. This is associated with the potential risk of increasing PTH levels by stimulating parathyroid secretion. In the long-term, this may lead to progressive parathyroid hyperplasia. On the other hand, the calcium-lowering effect of bisphosphonates may permit the reintroduction of vitamin D metabolites. These issues remain to be addressed in long-term studies on a large number of patients. In our experience, the ability of bisphosphonates to decrease bone turnover is best exploited in the short-term treatment of dialysis patients with severe autonomous hyperparathyroidism before parathyroidectomy to ensure a smooth postoperative period by decreasing the likelihood of a hungry bone syndrome.

The use of calcimimetic agents appears promising (Antonsen *et al.* 1998; Goodman and Jurner 2002; Nemeth 2002) and studies are currently in progress to address their potential beneficial effects and safety aspects in the uraemic patient.

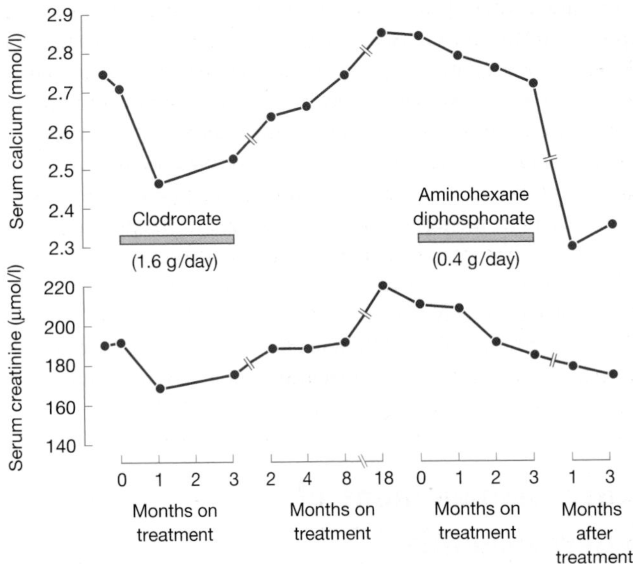

Fig. 8 The effects of bisphosphonate treatment in a patient with hypercalcaemia due to tertiary hyperparathyroidism. This patient had modest renal impairment following renal transplantation. The institution of treatment with the bisphosphonates (clodronate and neridronate) resulted in a small decrease in serum creatinine associated with a reduction in serum calcium. For this reason the subsequent parathyroidectomy was undertaken, and improved renal function was sustained when the serum calcium was normal.

Hypercalcaemia after renal transplantation

Successful renal transplantation is associated with the almost immediate resumption of calcitriol synthesis and restoration of intestinal calcium absorption to normal (Lucas *et al.* 1985). Persistence of pre-existing hyperparathyroidism is the most common cause of post-transplantation hypercalcaemia (Messa *et al.* 1998). Indeed, only one in four patients demonstrates normal PTH levels more than a year after establishment of graft function, due to slow involution of parathyroid hyperplasia but also due to incomplete normalization of renal function. Hypercalcaemia occurs in 9–52 per cent of transplant recipients (Reinhart *et al.* 1998; Torres *et al.* 2002). Widely regarded as benign and transient, it may persist beyond the first year in 5–10 per cent of patients (Massari 1997). When persisting for longer than 2 years post-transplantation, it does not spontaneously resolve (Gonzalez *et al.* 1990). It usually first manifests itself a few weeks after successful establishment of graft function, also coinciding with tapering the dose of corticosteroids required for immunosuppression and may result in graft dysfunction (Torres *et al.* 2002).

The majority of patients with persistent hypercalcaemia have biochemical features consistent with hyperparathyroidism, including a normal fasting urinary excretion of calcium, indicating an increased renal tubular reabsorption of calcium, elevated PTH levels and indices of bone turnover and a decreased renal tubular reabsorption of phosphate (Cundy *et al.* 1983).

Although hypercalcaemia is usually benign, it might, if untreated interfere with graft function. Inhibitors of bone resorption improve graft function in a minority of patients by decreasing serum calcium (Fig. 8). For this reason we commonly give one of the bisphosphonates, such as clodronate 1600 mg daily, to such patients. If renal function improves, partial parathyroidectomy is preferred. Bisphosphonates do not provide a long-term treatment of hypercalcaemia (see above), but do provide a rationale to select patients for parathyroidectomy (Hamdy *et al.* 1987).

Other suggested mechanisms for transient post-transplant hypercalcaemia include the mobilization of skeletal calcium, extraskeletal calcification, and phosphate depletion, resulting in hypophosphataemia. This may develop after transplantation because of persistent hyperparathyroidism, the use of high doses of corticosteroids, that of phosphate binding antacids, or due to primary tubular dysfunction of the allograft (Felsenfeld *et al.* 1986; Torres *et al.* 2002).

Malignant disease, more frequent in the immunosuppressed patient than in healthy subjects, may cause hypercalcaemia due to focal increases in bone resorption or due to secretion of hypercalcaemic factors by the primary tumour: the humoral hypercalcaemia of malignancy (Mundy 1990; Kanis *et al.* 1994; Kanis and McCloskey 1995). In addition to antitumour therapy, rehydration and bisphosphonates reinstate normocalcaemia in some 90 per cent of patients (Hamdy and Papapoulos 2002).

Effect of hypercalcaemia on renal function

In the absence of intrinsic renal disease, hypercalcaemia has important direct effects on renal function, which in turn exacerbate hypercalcaemia. Volume depletion, and calcium-induced renal vasoconstriction impair the GFR in conjunction with a hypercalcaemia-induced reduction in the glomerular ultrafiltration coefficient K_f (Benabe and Martinez-Maldonado 1978). The ability to conserve water is impaired by a calcium-induced resistance to the action of vasopressin (nephrogenic diabetes insipidus) (Suki *et al.* 1969; Levi *et al.* 1983). The decreased tubular sodium delivery augments tubular reabsorption of calcium and further exacerbates hypercalcaemia. Thus, volume depletion and impaired renal function are implicated in the majority of patients with significant hypercalcaemia. Calcium precipitation may result in structural damage, particularly in the renal medulla and in interstitial calcium deposition, chronic inflammation, and interstitial fibrosis, all of which impair the ability to withstand a calcium challenge. These hypercalcaemia-induced renal effects further aggravate its severity. For example, moderate hypercalcaemia due to skeletal metastases may rapidly evolve into a hypercalcaemic crisis without marked changes in the rate of tumour-mediated bone resorption. In myelomatosis a synergistic interaction between hypercalcaemia and Bence Jones proteinuria, may impair glomerular filtration (Smolens *et al.* 1987), accounting for up to 50 per cent of the eventual increment in serum calcium.

Acute management of hypercalcaemia

In the patient with renal failure but not yet on dialysis treatment, the acute management of hypercalcaemia involves first the restoration of extracellular fluid volume (Hosking *et al.* 1981; Harinck *et al.* 1987). This is best achieved by infusing normal saline (0.9 per cent NaCl) rather than dextrose solutions. An adequate saline load decreases renal tubular reabsorption of calcium and decreases uraemia due to pre-renal causes. When profound hypoalbuminaemia is present, restoration of intravascular volume may require the infusion of plasma proteins. Since renal impairment may be irreversible, care should be taken not to overload the cardiovascular system with saline or protein. Potassium or magnesium may need to be supplemented, particularly in patients receiving digoxin, although this should be done with great care in the presence of renal failure. Since in patients with severe hypercalcaemia up to 50 per cent of any increase in serum calcium is attributable to renal causes, adequate volume expansion may be all that is required.

Loop diuretics are used to increase the excretion of sodium and decrease tubular reabsorption of calcium. In patients who are not adequately volume expanded, the resulting increase in salt and water depletion will offset any beneficial effects. Thus diuretics should be used cautiously and many, including us, do not advocate their routine use in the management of hypercalcaemia. Thiazide diuretics increase renal tubular reabsorption of calcium and are occasionally the sole cause of hypercalcaemia (Dent *et al.* 1987). They should be avoided.

Intravenous phosphate lowers serum calcium dramatically, in part through the formation of calcium–phosphate complexes in the extracellular fluid and their subsequent clearance by the reticuloendothelial system. This treatment may entail massive deposition of calcium phosphate including in the kidney. It is particularly hazardous in patients with renal impairment and fatalities have been reported. Intravenous phosphate is no longer an accepted form of treatment for hypercalcaemia.

Specific inhibitors of bone resorption have proved useful in the management of hypercalcaemia refractory to saline alone. Calcitonin, a specific inhibitor of osteoclast activity, increases sodium excretion and decreases renal tubular reabsorption of calcium (Haas *et al.* 1971; Hosking and Gilson 1984). The renal effects probably contribute little to the hypocalcaemic activity. Inhibition of bone resorption generally requires large doses (200 IU every 4 h), and side-effects such as nausea and flushing may be troublesome. Serum calcium decreases rapidly to a nadir reached 4–6 h after a single injection. When calcitonin is given repeatedly, the effect decreases progressively. This tachyphylaxis is attributed to down-regulation of skeletal calcitonin receptors (Tashjian *et al.* 1978).

Bisphosphonates have proved useful in the management of hypercalcaemia due to various causes (Fleisch 2000; Hamdy and Papapoulos 2002). They are usually given by intravenous infusion and repeated daily. The extent of the reduction in serum calcium depends on the dose and type of bisphosphonate used. In malignancy-associated hypercalcaemia, the calcium-lowering response is short-lived. The rate of bone resorption and hence calcaemia returns to initial values within 2–4 weeks of discontinuing treatment if the malignancy is left untreated. Effective doses of various bisphosphonates reflect their difference in potency (Hamdy and Papapoulos 2002). The hypercalcaemia of haematological malignancies, sarcoidosis, and vitamin D toxicity respond slowly to corticosteroids and normalization of serum calcium may require up to 2–3 weeks (Percival *et al.* 1984). Patients with non-haematological malignancies do not respond.

References

Adler, A. J., Ferran, N., and Berlyne, G. M. (1985). Effect of inorganic phosphate on serum ionised calcium concentration *in vitro*: a reassessment of the 'trade-off hypothesis'. *Kidney International* **28**, 932–935.

Albright, F. and Reifenstein, E. C., Jr. *The Parathyroid Glands and Metabolic Bone Disease*. Baltimore, MD: Williams and Wilkins, 1948.

Ali, A. A., Barghese, Z., Moorhead, J. F., Ballod, R. A., and Sweny, P. (1993). Calcium set-point progressively worsens in hemodialysis patients despite conventional oral 1 alpha hydroxy cholecalciferol supplementation. *Clinical Nephrology* **39**, 205–209.

Anderberg, B., Gillquist, J., Larsson, L., and Lundstrom, B. (1981). Complications to subtotal parathyroidectomy. *Acta Chirurgica Scandinavica* **147**, 109–113.

Andress, D. L., Norris, K. C., Coburn, J. W., Slatopolsky, E. A., and Sherrard, D. J. (1989). Intravenous calcitriol in the treatment of refractory osteitis fibrosa of chronic renal failure. *New England Journal of Medicine* **321**, 274–279.

Antonsen, J. E., Sherrard, D. J., and Andress, D. L. (1998). A calcimimetic agent acutely suppresses parathyroid hormone levels in patients with chronic renal failure. *Kidney International* **53**, 223–227.

Ardaillou, R. (1975). Kidney and calcitonin. *Nephron* **15**, 250–260.

Argiles, A. *et al.* (1993). Hemodialysis and hemofiltration, Ca kinetics, and the long-term effects of lowering dialysate calcium concentration. *Kidney International* **43**, 630–640.

Azria, M. *The Calcitonins*. Basel: Karger, 1989.

Bacchini, G. *et al.* (1997). 'Pulse oral' versus intravenous calcitriol therapy in chronic hemodialysis patients. A prospective and randomized study. *Nephron* **77**, 267–272.

Benabe, J. E. and Martinez-Maldonado, M. (1978). Hypercalcemic nephropathy. *Archives of Internal Medicine* **138**, 777–779.

Bertholf, R. L., Bertholf, M. F., Brown, C. M., and Riley, W. J. (1992). Ionized calcium buffering in the transfused anhepatic patient: ab initio calculations of calcium ion concentrations. *Annals of Clinical and Laboratory Science* **22**, 40–50.

Block, G. A. and Port, F. K. (2000). Re-evaluation of risks associated with hyperphosphatemia and hyperparathyroidism in dialysis patients: recommendations for a change in management. *American Journal of Kidney Diseases* **35**, 1226–1237.

Block, G. A., Hulbert-Shearon, T. E., Levin, N. W., and Port, F. K. (1998). Association of serum phosphorus and calcium × phosphate product with mortality risk in chronic hemodialysis patients: a national study. *American Journal of Kidney Diseases* **31**, 607–617.

Bouillon, R., Verberckmoes, R., and DeMoor, P. (1975). Influence of dialysate calcium concentration and vitamin D on serum parathyroid hormone during repetitive dialysis. *Kidney International* **7**, 422–432.

Brasier, A. R. and Nussbaum, S. R. (1988). Hungry bone syndrome: clinical and biochemical predictors of its occurrence after parathyroid surgery. *American Journal of Medicine* **84**, 654–660.

Breslau, N. A., McGuire, J. L., Zerwekh, J. E., and Frenkel, E. P. (1984). Hypercalcaemia associated with increased serum calcitriol levels in three patients with lymphoma. *Annals of Internal Medicine* **100**, 1–7.

Brossard, J. H., Yamamoto, L. N., and D'Amour, P. (2002). Parathyroid hormone metabolites in renal failure: bioactivity and clinical implications. *Seminars in Dialysis* **15**, 196–201.

Brown, E. M. (1991). Extracellular calcium sensing, regulation of parathyroid cell function, and role of calcium and other ions as extracellular (first) messengers. *Physiological Reviews* **71**, 371–411.

Brown, E. M., Wilson, R. E., Eastman, R. C., Pallotta, J., and Marynick, S. P. (1982). Abnormal regulation of parathyroid hormone release by calcium in secondary parathyroidism due to chronic renal failure. *Journal of Clinical Endocrinology and Metabolism* **54**, 172–179.

Brown, E. M., Pollak, M., Riccardi, D., and Hebert, C. S. (1994). Cloning and characterisation of an extracellular Ca^{2+}-sensing receptor from parathyroid and kidney: new insights into the physiology and pathophysiology of calcium metabolism. *Nephrology, Dialysis, Transplantation* **9**, 1703–1706.

Brown, E. M. *et al.* (1999). G-protein coupled, extracellular Ca2+-sensing receptor: a versatile regulator of diverse cellular functions. *Vitamins and Hormones* **55**, 1–71.

Burnatowska-Hledin, M. A., Kaiser, L., and Mayor, G. H. (1983). Aluminium, parathyroid hormone and osteomalacia. *Special Topics in Endocrinology and Metabolism*, **5**, 201–226.

Cannella, G. *et al.* (1994). Evidence of healing of secondary hyperparathyroidism in chronically hemodialysed uremic patients treated with long-term intravenous calcitriol. *Kidney International* **46**, 1124–1132.

Charhon, S. A., Berland, Y. F., Olmer, M. J., Delawari, E., Traeger, J., and Meunier, P. J. (1985). Effects of parathyroidectomy on bone formation and mineralisation in hemodialysed patients. *Kidney International* **27**, 426–435.

Christensen, C. K., Lund, B., Sorensen, O. H., Nielsen, H. E., and Mosekilde, L. (1981). Reduced 1,25-dihydroxyvitamin D and 24,25-dihydroxyvitamin D in epileptic patients receiving combined anticonvulsant therapy. *Metabolic Bone Disease and Related Research* **3**, 17–22.

Cochran, M. and Nordin, B. E. C. (1971). Causes of hypocalcaemia in chronic renal failure. *Clinical Science* **40**, 305–315.

Cohen-Solal, M. E. *et al.* (1992). Non-aluminic adynamic bone disease in non-dialysed uremic patients: a new type of osteopathy due to overtreatment? *Bone* **13**, 1–5.

Conceicao, S. C., Weightman, D., Smith, P. A., Luno, J., Wand, M. K., and Kerr, D. N. S. (1978). Serum ionised calcium concentration: measurement versus calculation. *British Medical Journal* **i**, 1103–1105.

Cournot-Witmer, G. *et al.* (1981). Aluminium localisation in bone from haemodialysed patients: relationship to matrix mineralisation. *Kidney International* **20**, 375–385.

Cundy, T., Kanis, J. A., Heynen, G., Morris, P. J., and Oliver, D. O. (1983). Calcium metabolism and hyperparathyroidism after renal transplantation. *Quarterly Journal of Medicine* **52**, 67–78.

Cundy, T., Hand, D., Oliver, D., Oliver, D. O., Woods, C. G., Wright, F. W., and Kanis, J. A. (1985). Who gets renal bone disease before beginning dialysis? *British Medical Journal* **290**, 271–275.

Cundy, T., Hamdy, N. A. T., and Kanis, J. A. (1988). Factors modifying the secretion and action of parathyroid hormone in renal failure. *Contributions to Nephrology* **64**, 5–15.

DeBroe, M. E., D'Haese, P. C., Elseviers, M. M., Clement, J., Visser, W. J., and Van de Vyver, F. L. Aluminium and end-stage renal failure. In *Proceedings of the International Congress on Nephrology* (ed. A. M. Davison), pp. 1086–1116. London: Baillière Tindall, 1988.

Dent, C. E. (1962). Some problems with hyperparathyroidism. *British Medical Journal* **2**, 1419–1425.

Dent, D. M., Miller, J. L., Klaff, L., and Barron, J. (1987). The incidence and causes of hypercalcaemia. *Postgraduate Medical Journal* **63**, 745–750.

DeVernejoul, M. C. *et al.* (1982). Calcium phosphate metabolism and bone disease in patients with homozygous thalassaemia. *Journal of Clinical Endocrinology and Metabolism* **54**, 276–281.

DeVernejoul, M. C., Marchonis, S., and London, G. (1985). Increased bone aluminium deposition after subtotal parathyroidectomy in dialysed patients. *Kidney International* **27**, 785–791.

Drueke, T. B. (1995). The pathogenesis of parathyroid gland hyperplasia in chronic renal failure. *Kidney International* **48**, 259–272.

Drueke, T. B. (2000). Cell biology of parathyroid gland hyperplasia in chronic renal failure. *Journal of American Society of Nephrology* **11**, 1141–1152.

Drueke, T., Bordier, P. J., Man, N. K., Jungers, P., and Marie, P. (1977). Effect of high dialysate calcium concentration on bone remodelling serum biochemistry and parathyroid hormone in patients with renal osteodystrophy. *Kidney International* **11**, 267–274.

Dunlay, R., Rodriguez, M., Felsenfeld, A., and Llach, F. (1989). Direct inhibitory effect of calcitriol on parathyroid function (sigmoidal curve) in dialysis patients. *Kidney International* **36**, 1093–1098.

Esnault, V., Testa, A., Dupas, B., and Guernel, J. (1990). Major muscle calcifications of the neck after non-traumatic rhabdomyolysis with acute renal failure. *Nephrology, Dialysis, Transplantation* **5**, 461–463.

Feinstein, E. I., Akmal, M., Telfer, N., and Massry, S. G. (1981). Delayed hypercalcemia with acute renal failure associated with non-traumatic rhabdomyolysis. *Archives of Internal Medicine* **141**, 753–755.

Felsenfeld, A. J. (1997). Considerations for the treatment of secondary hyperparathyroidism in renal failure. *Journal of the American Society of Nephrology* **8**, 993–1004.

Felsenfeld, A. J. and Llach, F. (1993). Parathyroid gland function in renal failure. *Kidney International* **43**, 771–789.

Felsenfeld, A. J. and Rodriguez, M. (1996). The set-point for calcium—another view. *Nephrology, Dialysis, Transplantation* **11**, 1722–1725.

Felsenfeld, A. J., Gutman, R. A., Drezner, M., and Llach, F. (1986). Hypophosphataemia in long-term renal transplant recipients: effects on bone histology and 1,25-dihydroxycholecalciferol. *Mineral and Electrolyte Metabolism* **12**, 333–341.

Fleisch, H. *Bisphosphonates: From the Laboratory to the Patient.* London: Academic Press, 2000.

Foley, R. N., Parfrey, P. S., and Sarnak, M. J. (1998). Clinical epidemiology of cardiovascular disease in chronic renal disease. *American Journal of Kidney Diseases* **32** (Suppl. 3), S112–S119.

Freedman L. P. (1999). Increasing complexity of coactivation in nuclear receptor signalling. *Cell* **97**, 5–8.

French, J. K., Holdaway, I. M., and Williams, L. C. (1986). Milk alkali syndrome following over-the-counter antacid self medication. *New Zealand Medical Journal* **99**, 322–323.

Friedman, P. A. (2000). Mechanisms of renal calcium transport. *Experimental Nephrology* **8**, 343–350.

Friedman, P. A. and Gesek, F. A. (1993). Vitamin D accelerates PTH-dependent calcium transport in the distal convoluted tubule. *American Journal of Physiology* **265**, F300–F308.

Frost, H. M. (1966). Relation between bone tissue and cell population dynamics histology and tetracycline labelling. *Clinical Orthopaedics and Related Research* **49**, 65–75.

Fukuda, N. *et al.* (1993). Decreased 1,25-dihydroxyvitamin D3 receptor density is associated with a more severe form of parathyroid hyperplasia in chronic uremic patients. *Journal of Clinical Investigation* **92**, 1436–1443.

Fuss, M. *et al.* (1988). Are tuberculous patients at a great risk from hypercalcaemia? *Quarterly Journal of Medicine* **69**, 869–878.

Gao, P. *et al.* (2001). Development of a novel radioimmunoradiometric assay exclusively for biologically active whole parathyroid hormone 1–84: implications for improvement of accurate assessment of parathyroid function. *Journal of Bone and Mineral Research* **16**, 605–614.

Glendenning, P., Gutteridge, D. H., Retallack, R. W., Stuckey, B. G., Kermode, D. G., and Kent, G. N. (1998). High prevalence of normal total calcium and intact PTH in 60 patients with proven primary hyperparathyroidism: a challenge to current diagnsotic criteria. *Australian and New Zealand Journal of Public Health* **28**, 173–178.

Goldsmith, R. S., Furszyfer, J., Johnson, W. J., Fournier, A. E., and Arnaud, C. D. (1971). Control of secondary hyperparathyroidism during long-term haemodialysis. *American Journal of Medicine* **50**, 692–699.

Goldstein, D. A., Haldimann, B., Sherman, D., Norman, A. W., and Massry, S. G. (1981). Vitamin D metabolites and calcium metabolism in patients with nephrotic syndrome and normal renal function. *Journal of Clinical Endocrinology and Metabolism* **52**, 116–121.

Goltzman, D. (1999). Interactions of PTH and PTHrP with the PTH/PTHrP receptor and downstream signaling pathways: exceptions that provide the rules. *Journal of Bone and Mineral Research* **14**, 173–177.

Gonzalez, M. T. *et al.* (1990). Long-term evaluation of renal osteodystrophy after kidney transplantation: comparative study between intact PTH levels and bone biopsy. *Transplantation Proceedings* **22**, 1407–1411.

Goodman, W. G. and Turner, S. A. (2002). Future role of calcimimetics in end-stage renal disease. *Advances in Renal Replacement Therapy* **9**, 200–208.

Goodman, W. G. *et al.* (2000). Coronary artery calcification in young adults with end-stage renal disease who are undergoing dialysis. *New England Journal of Medicine* **342**, 1478–1483.

Haas, H. G., Dambacher, M. A., Guncaga, J., and Lauffenburger, T. (1971). Renal effects of calcitonin and parathyroid extract in man. *Journal of Clinical Investigation* **50**, 2689–2702.

Hahn, T. J. and Halstead, L. R. (1979). Anticonvulsant drug-induced osteomalacia; alterations in mineral metabolism and response to vitamin D_3 administration. *Calcified Tissue International* **27**, 13–18.

Hamdy, N. A. T. (1995a). The spectrum of renal bone disease. *Nephrology, Dialysis, Transplantation* **10**, S14–S18.

Hamdy, N. A. T. (1995b). The need to treat predialysis patients. *Nephrology, Dialysis, Transplantation* **10** (Suppl. 4), S19–S22.

Hamdy, N. A. T. and Papapoulos, S. E. (2002). Management of malignancy-associated hypercalcaemia. *Clinical Reviews in Bone and Mineral Metabolism* **1**, 65–76.

Hamdy, N. A. T. *et al.* (1987). Clodronate in the medical management of hyperparathyroidism. *Bone* **8** (Suppl.), S69–S77.

Hamdy, N. A. T., Brown, C. B., and Kanis, J. A. (1989). Intravenous calcitriol lowers serum calcium concentrations in uraemic patients with severe hyperparathyroidism and hypercalcaemia. *Nephrology, Dialysis, Transplantation* **4**, 545–548.

Hamdy, N. A. T., Brown, C. B., and Kanis, J. A. (1990a). Mineral metabolism in chronic ambulatory peritoneal dialysis (CAPD). *Contributions to Nephrology* **85**, 100–110.

Hamdy, N. A. T., McCloskey, E. V., Brown, C. B., and Kanis, J. A. (1990b). Effects of clodronate in severe hyperparathyroid bone disease in chronic renal failure. *Nephron* **56**, 6–12.

Hamdy, N. A. T., Boletis, J., Charlesworth, D., Kanis, J. A., and Brown, C. B. (1991). Low calcium dialysate increases the tolerance to vitamin D in peritoneal dialysis. *Contributions to Nephrology* **89**, 190–199.

Hamdy, N. A. T. *et al.* (1995). Effect of alfacalcidol on the natural course of renal bone disease in mild to moderate renal failure. *British Medical Journal* **310**, 358–363.

Harinck, H. I. J. *et al.* (1987). Role of bone and kidney in tumor-induced hypercalcemia and its treatment with bisphosphonate and sodium chloride. *American Journal of Medicine* **82**, 1133–1142.

Heaf, J. G., Nielsen, L. P., and Mogensen, N. B. (1983). Use of bone mineral content determination in the evaluation of osteodystrophy among hemodialysis patients. *Nephron* **35**, 103–107.

Hercz, C. *et al.* (1993). Aplastic osteodystrophy without aluminium: the role of 'suppressed' parathyroid function. *Kidney International* **44**, 860–866.

Hoenderop, J. G. J. *et al.* (1999). Molecular identification of the apical Ca^{2+} channel in 1,25-dihydroxyvitaminD_3-responsive epithelia. *Journal of Biological Chemistry* **274**, 8375–8378.

Hoenderop, J. G. J., Muller, D., Suzuki, M., van Os, C. H., and Bindels, R. (2000). Epithelial calcium channel: gate-keeper of active calcium reabsorption. *Current Opinion in Nephrology Hypertension* **9**, 335–340.

Hosking, D. J. and Gilson, D. (1984). Comparison of the renal and skeletal actions of calcitonin in the treatment of severe hypercalcaemia of malignancy. *Quarterly Journal of Medicine* **53**, 359–368.

Hosking, D. J., Cowley, A., and Bucknall, C. A. (1981). Rehydration in the treatment of severe hypercalcaemia. *Quarterly Journal of Medicine* **200**, 473–481.

Hruska, K. A. and Teitelbaum, S. L. (1995). Renal osteodystrophy. *New England Journal of Medicine* **333**, 166–175.

Iqbal, S. J. *et al.* (1988). Need for albumin adjustments of urgent total serum calcium. *Lancet* **2**, 1477–1478.

Irvin, G. L. *et al.* (1999). Improved success rate in reoperative parathyroidectomy with intraoperative PTH. *Annals of Surgery* **229**, 874–879.

John, M. R. *et al.* (1999). A novel immunoradiometric assay detects full length human PTH but not amino-terminally truncated fragments: implications for PTH measurements in renal failure. *Journal of Clinical Endocrinology and Metabolism* **84**, 4287–4290.

Jubiz, W., Haussler, M. R., McCain, T. A., and Tolman, K. G. (1977). Plasma 1,25-dihydroxyvitamin D levels in patients receiving anticonvulsant drugs. *Journal of Clinical Endocrinology and Metabolism* **44**, 617–621.

Juppner, H. (1999). Receptors for parathyroid hormone and parathyroid hormone-related peptide: exploration of their biological importance. *Bone* **25**, 87–90.

Kanis, J. A. and McCloskey, E. V. Disorders of calcium metabolism and their management. In *Myeloma. Biology and Management* (ed. J. S. Malpas, D. E. Bergesal, and R. A. Kyle), pp. 375–396. Oxford: Oxford Medical Publications, 1995.

Kanis, J. A. and Passmore, R. (1989). Calcium supplementation of the diet—I and II. *British Medical Journal* **296**, 137–140 (see also pp. 205–208).

Kanis, J. A. and Russell, R. G. G. (1977). Rate of reversal of hypercalcaemia induced by vitamin D_3 and its 1α-hydroxylated derivatives. *British Medical Journal* **i**, 78–81.

Kanis, J. A. and Yates, A. J. P. (1985). Measuring serum calcium. *British Medical Journal* **290**, 728–729.

Kanis, J. A. *et al.* (1977). Changes in histological and biochemical indexes of bone turnover after bilateral nephrectomy in patients on haemodialysis. Evidence for a possible role of endogenous calcitonin. *New England Journal of Medicine* **296**, 1073–1079.

Kanis, J. A. *et al.* (1979). Treatment of renal bone disease with 1α-hydroxylated derivatives of vitamin D_3. *Quarterly Journal of Medicine* **48**, 289–322.

Kanis J. A., Cundy, T., Heynen, G., and Russell, R. G. G. (1980). The pathophysiology of hypercalcaemia. *Metabolic Bone Disease and Related Research* **2**, 143–159.

Kanis, J. A., Guilland-Cumming, D. F., and Russell, R. G. G. Comparative physiology and pharmacology of the metabolites and analogues of vitamin D. In *The Endocrinology of Calcium Metabolism* (ed. J. A. Paterson), pp. 321–62. New York, NY: Raven Press, 1982.

Kanis, J. A., Heynen, G., Paterson, A., and Hamdy, N. Endogenous secretion of calcitonin in physiological and pathological conditions. In *Calcitonin* (ed. A. Pecile), pp. 81–88. Amsterdam: Elsevier, 1985.

Kanis, J. A., Cundy, T., and Hamdy, N. A. T. Renal osteodystrophy. In *Metabolic Bone Disease. Clinical Endocrinology and Metabolism* Vol. 2 (ed. T. J. Martin), pp. 193–241. London: Baillière, 1988.

Kanis, J. A., O'Rourke, N., and McCloskey, E. V. (1994). Consequences of neoplasia-induced bone resorption and the use of clodronate. *International Journal of Oncology* **5**, 713–731.

Kao, P. C. *et al.* (1992). Clinical performance of parathyroid immunoradiometric assays. *Mayo Clinic Proceedings* **67**, 637–645.

Kao, P. C., van Herden, J. A., and Taylor, R. L. (1994). Intraoperative monitoring of parathyroid procedures by a 15-minute parathyroid hormone immunochemiluminometric assay. *Mayo Clinic Proceedings* **69**, 532–537.

Kaplan, E. L., Bartlett, S., Sugimoto, J., and Fredland, A. (1982). Relation of postoperative hypocalcaemia to operative techniques: deleterious effect of excessive use of parathyroid biopsy. *Surgery* **92**, 827–834.

Kifor, O. *et al.* (1996). Reduced immunostaining for the extracellular Ca2+-sensing receptor in primary, uremic secondary hyperparathyroidism. *Journal of Clinical Endocrinology and Metabolism* **81**, 1598–1606.

Kraut, J. A. *et al.* (1981). Reduced parathyroid response to acute hypocalcaemia in dialysis osteomalacia. *Clinical Research* **29**, 102A.

Kurz, P. *et al.* (1994). Evidence for abnormal calcium homeostasis in patients with adynamic bone disease. *Kidney International* **46**, 855–861.

Ladenson, J. H., Lewis, J. W., McDonald, J. M., Slatopolsky, E., and Boyd, J. C. (1979). Relationship of free and total calcium in hypercalcemic conditions. *Journal of Clinical Endocrinology and Metabolism* **48**, 393–397.

Lepage, R. *et al.* (1998). A non-(1–84) circulating parathyroid hormone (PTH) fragment interferes significantly with intact PTH commercial assay measurements in uremic samples. *Clinical Chemistry* **44**, 805–809.

Levi, M., Peterson, L., and Berl, T. (1983). Mechanism of concentrating defect in hypercalcaemia. Role of polydipsia and prostaglandins. *Kidney International* **23**, 489–497.

Llach, F., Massry, S. G., Singer, F. R., Kurokawa, K., Kaye, J. H., and Coburn, J. W. (1975). Skeletal resistance to endogenous parathyroid hormone in patients with early renal failure: a possible cause for secondary hyperparathyroidism. *Journal of Clinical Endocrinology and Metabolism* **41**, 339–345.

Llach, F., Felsenfeld, A. J., and Haussler, M. R. (1981). The pathophysiology of altered calcium metabolism in rhabdomyolysis-induced acute renal failure. Interactions of parathyroid hormone, 25-hydroxycholecalciferol, and 1,25-dihydroxycholecalciferol. *New England Journal of Medicine* **305**, 117–123.

Lloyd, H. M., Parfitt, A. M., Jacobi, J. M., Willgoss, D. A., Craswell, P. W., Petrie, J. J. B., and Boyle, P. D. (1989). The parathyroid glands in chronic renal failure: a study of their growth and other properties made on the basis of findings in patients with hypercalcaemia. *Journal of Laboratory and Clinical Medicine* **114**, 358–367.

Locatelli, F. *et al.* (2002). Management of disturbances of calcium and phosphate metabolism in chronic renal insufficiency, with emphasis on the control of hyperphosphataemia. *Nephrology, Dialysis, Transplantation* **17**, 723–731.

Lopez-Hilker, S., Galceran, T., Chan, Y. L., Rapp, N., Martin, K. J., and Slatopolsky, E. (1986). Hypocalcemia may not be essential for the development of secondary hyperparathyroidism in chronic renal failure. *Journal of Clinical Investigation* **78**, 1097–1102.

Lucas, P. A., Brown, R. C., Bloodworth, L., Woodhead, J. S., and Coles, G. A. (1985). Determinants of serum calcium after renal transplantation: the role of 1,25$(OH)_2D_3$. *Proceedings of the European Dialysis and Transplant Association and the European Renal Association* **22**, 1212–1217.

Malberti, F., Surian, M., and Cosci, P. (1992). Effect of chronic intravenous calcitriol on parathyroid function and set point of calcium in dialysis patients with refractory secondary hyperparathyroidism. *Nephrology, Dialysis, Transplantation* **7**, 822–828.

Malluche, H. H., Smith, A. J., Abreo, K., and Faugere, M.-C. (1984). The use of desferrioxamine in the management of aluminium accumulation in bone in patients with renal failure. *New England Journal of Medicine* **311**, 140–144.

Malluche, H. H., Faugere, M. C., Ritz, E., Caillers, G., and Wildberger, D. (1986). Endogenous calcitonin does not protect against hyperparathyroid bone disease in renal failure. *Mineral and Electrolyte Metabolism* **12**, 113–118.

Malluche, H. H., Mawad, H., and Koszewski, N. J. (2002). Update on vitamin D and its newer analogues: actions and rationale for treatment in chronic renal failure. *Kidney International* **62**, 367–374.

Marshall, R. W. Plasma fractions. In *Calcium Phosphate and Magnesium Metabolism. Clinical Physiology and Diagnostic Procedures* (ed. B. E. C. Nordin), pp. 162S–168S. Edinburgh: Churchill Livingstone, 1976.

Martin, K. J., Hruska, K. A., Freitag, J. J., Khlar, S., and Slatopolsky, E. (1979). The peripheral metabolism of parathyroid hormone. *New England Journal of Medicine* **301**, 1092–1098.

Mason, R. S., Frankel, T., Chan, Y. L., Lissner, D., and Posen, S. (1984). Vitamin D conversion by sarcoid lymph node homogenate. *Annals of Internal Medicine* **100**, 59–61.

Massari, P. (1997). Disorders of bone and mineral metabolism after renal transplantation. *Kidney International* **52**, 1412–1421.

Massry, S. G. (1976). Skeletal resistance to the calcaemic action of parathyroid hormone in uraemia: a mechanism for the hypocalcaemia and secondary hyperparathyroidism of chronic renal failure. *Clinical Endocrinology* **5** (Suppl.), 317S–325S.

Meema, H. E., Oreopoulos, D. G., and Rapoport, A. (1987). Serum magnesium level and arterial calcification in end-stage renal disease. *Kidney International* **32**, 388–394.

Messa, P. *et al.* (1998). Persistent secondary hyperparathyroidism after renal transplantation. *Kidney International* **54**, 1704–1713.

Morinière, P. H. *et al.* (1993). Improvement of severe secondary hyperparathyroidism in dialysis patients by intravenous 1α (OH) vitamin D_3, oral $CaCO_3$ and low dialysate calcium. *Kidney International* **43** (Suppl. 41), S121–S124.

Mundy, G. R. (1990). Incidence and pathophysiology of hypercalcaemia. *Calcified Tissue International* **46** (Suppl.), S3–S10.

Nemeth, E. F. (2002). Pharmacological regulation of parathyroid hormone secretion. *Current Pharmaceutical Design* **8**, 2077–2087.

Nguyen-Yamamoto, L. *et al.* (2002). Origin of parathyroid hormone (PTH) fragments detected by intact-PTH assays. *European Journal of Endocrinology* **147**, 123–131.

Nielsen, H. E., Christensen, M. S., Melsen, F., Romer, F. K., and Hansen, H. E. (1977). Effect of 1α-hydroxyvitamin D_3 on parathyroid function in patients with chronic renal failure. *Clinical Endocrinology* **7** (Suppl.), 67–72.

Nordin, B. E. C., ed. *Calcium Phosphate and Magnesium Metabolism. Clinical Physiology and Diagnostic Procedures.* Edinburgh: Churchill Livingstone, 1976.

Normann, P. T., Froysa, A., and Svaland, M. (1995). Interference of gadodiamide injection (OMNISCAN) on the colorimetric determination of serum calcium. *Scandinavian Journal of Clinical and Laboratory Investigation* **55**, 421–426.

Nussbaum, S. R. *et al.* (1987). Highly sensitive two-site immunoradiometric-assay of parathryn, and its clinical utility in evaluating patients with hypercalcemia *Clinical Chemistry* **88**, 1364–1371.

Nygren, P. *et al.* (1987). Bimodal regulation of secretion by cytoplasmic Ca^{2+} as demonstrated by the parathyroid. *FEBS Letters* **213**, 195–198.

Ott, S. M. *et al.* (1986). Changes in bone histology after treatment with desferrioxamine. *Kidney International* **29** (Suppl. 18), S108–S113.

Papapoulos, S. E., Clemens, T. L., Fraher, L. J., Lewin, I. G., Sandler, L. M., and O'Riordan, J. L. H. (1979). 1,25-Dihydroxycholecalciferol in the pathogenesis of the hypercalcaemia of sarcoidosis. *Lancet* **i**, 627–630.

Parsons, V., Papapoulos, S. E., Weston, M. J., Tomlinson, S., and O'Riordan, J. L. H. (1980). The long-term effect of lowering dialysate magnesium on circulating parathyroid hormone in patients on regular haemodialysis therapy. *Acta Endocrinologica (Copenhagen)* **93**, 455–460.

Paterson, A. D., Yates, A. J. P., Cundy, T., Russell, R. G. G., and Kanis, J. A. (1982). Effects of vitamin D on renal tubular reabsorption of calcium in man. *Clinical Science* **63**, 42.

Percival, R. C. *et al.* (1984). The role of glucocorticoids in the management of malignant hypercalcaemia. *British Medical Journal* **i**, 287–289.

Pletka, P., Bernstein, D. S., Hampers, C. L., Merrill, J. P., and Sherwood, L. M. (1974). Relationship between magnesium and secondary hyperparathyroidism during long-term haemodialysis. *Metabolism* **23**, 619–624.

Portale, A. A., Booth, B. E., Halloran, B. P., and Morris, R. C. (1984). Effect of dietary phosphorus on circulating concentrations of 1,25-dihydroxyvitamin D and immunoreactive parathyroid hormone in children with moderate renal insufficiency. *Journal of Clinical Investigation* **73**, 1580–1589.

Quarles, L. D., Lobaugh, B., and Murphy, G. (1992). Intact parathyroid hormone overestimates the presence and severity of parathyroid-mediated osseous abnormalities in uremia. *Journal of Clinical Endocrinology and Metabolism* **75**, 145–150.

Ramirez, J. A. *et al.* (1993). Direct *in vivo* comparison of calcium regulated parathyroid hormone secretion in normal volunteers and patients with secondary hyperparathyroidism. *Journal of Clinical Endocrinology and Metabolism* **76**, 1489–1494.

Ramsdell, R. (1999). Renagel: a new and different phosphate binder. *ANNA J* **26**, 346–347.

Rasmussen, H. and Rasmussen, J. (1990). Calcium as intracellular messenger: from simplicity to complexity. *Current Topics in Cellular Regulation* **31**, 1–109.

Rix, M. *et al.* (1999). Bone mineral density and biochemical markers of bone turnover in patients with predialysis chronic renal failure. *Kidney International* **56**, 1084–1093.

Reinhardt, W. *et al.* (1998). Sequential changes of biochemical bone parameters after kidney transplantation. *Nephrology, Dialysis, Transplantation* **13**, 436–442.

Sandler, L. M., Winearls, C. G., Fraher, L. J., Clemens, T. L., Smith, R., and O'Riordan, J. L. H. (1984). Studies of the hypercalcaemia of sarcoidosis: effect of steroids and exogenous vitamin D_3. *Quarterly Journal of Medicine* **53**, 165–180.

Sawyer, N., Noonan, K., Altman, P., Marsh, F., and Cunningham, J. (1988). High dose calcium carbonate with stepwise reduction in dialysate calcium concentration: effective phosphate control and aluminium avoidance in haemodialysis patients. *Nephrology, Dialysis, Transplantation* **3**, 1–5.

Sexton, P. M., Findlay, D. M., and Martin, T. J. (1999). Calcitonin. *Current Opinion in Chemistry* **6**, 1067–1093.

Sharman, V. L. *et al.* (1982). Long-term experience of alfacalcidol in renal osteodystrophy. *Quarterly Journal of Medicine* **51**, 271–278.

Silver, J. (2000). Molecular mechanisms of secondary hyperparathyroidism. *Nephrology, Dialysis, Transplantation* **15**, S2–S7.

Slatopolsky, E. (1998). The role of calcium, phosphorus and vitamin D metabolism in the development of secondary hyperparathyroidism. *Nephrology, Dialysis, Transplantation* **13** (Suppl. 3), 3–8.

Slatopolsky, E. and Brown, A. J. (1997). Vitamin D and its analogs in chronic renal failure. *Osteoporosis International* **7** (Suppl. 3), S202–S208.

Slatopolsky, E., Weerts, C., Thielan, J., Horst, R., Harter, H., and Martin, K. J. (1984). Marked suppression of secondary hyperparathyroidism by intravenous administration of 1,25-dihydroxycholecalciferol in uremic patients. *Journal of Clinical Investigation* **74**, 2136–2143.

Slatopolsky, E., Weerts, C., Lopez-Hilker, S., Norwood, K., Zink, M., Windus, D., and Delmez, J. (1986). Calcium carbonate as a phosphate binder in patients with chronic renal failure undergoing dialysis. *New England Journal of Medicine* **315**, 157–161.

Slatopolsky, E., Lopez-Hilker, S., Dusso, A., Morrissey, J. J., and Martin, K. J. (1988). Parathyroid hormone secretion: pertubations in chronic renal failure. *Contributions to Nephrology* **64**, 16–24.

Slatopolsky, E. *et al.* (2000). A novel mechanism for skeletal resistance in uremia. *Kidney International* **58**, 753–761.

Smolens, P., Barnes, J. L., and Kreisberg, R. (1987). Hypercalcemia can potentiate the nephrotoxicity of Bence Jones proteins. *Journal of Laboratory and Clinical Medicine* **110**, 460–465.

Sokoll, L. J., Drew, H., and Udelsman, R. (2000). Intraoperative parathyroid hormone analysis: a study of 200 consecutive cases. *Clinical Chemistry* **46**, 1662–1668.

Sooy, K., Kohut, J., and Christakos, S. (2000). The role of calbindin and 1,25-dihydroxyvitamin D3 in the kidney. *Current Opinions in Nephrology and Hypertension* **9**, 341–347.

Suki, W. N., Eknoyan, G., Rector, F. C., and Seldin, D. W. (1969). The renal diluting and concentrating mechanism in hypercalcaemia. *Nephron* **6**, 50–61.

Szabo, A., Merke, J., Beier, E., Mall, G., and Ritz, E. (1989). 1,25$(OH)_2$ vitamin D_3 inhibits parathyroid cell proliferation in experimental uremia. *Kidney International* **35**, 1049–1056.

Tashjian, A. H., Jr., Wright, D. R., Ivey, J. L., and Pont, A. (1978). Calcitonin binding sites in bone. Relationships to biological response and escape. *Recent Progress in Hormone Research* **34**, 285–334.

Thode, J., Fogh-Andersen, N., Wimberley, P. D., Moller Sorensen, A., and Siggard-Andersen, O. (1983). Relation between pH and ionised calcium *in vitro* and *in vivo* in man. *Scandinavian Journal of Clinical and Laboratory Investigation* **165**(Suppl. 43), 79–82.

Thode, J. *et al.* (1989). Comparison of total serum calcium, albumin-corrected total calcium, and ionised calcium in 1213 patients with suspected calcium disorders. *Scandinavian Journal of Clinical Laboratory Investigation* **49**, 217–223.

Tofaletti, J., Savory, J., and Gitelman, H. J. (1977). Continuous flow determination of dialysable calcium in serum. *Clinical Chemistry* **23**, 1258–1263.

Torres, A., Lorenzo, V., and Salido, E. (2002). Calcium metabolism and skeletal problems after transplantation. *Journal of American Society of Nephrology* **13**, 551–558.

Vincenti, F., Arnaud, S. B., and Recker, R. (1984). Parathyroid and bone response of the diabetic patient to uraemia. *Kidney International* **25**, 677–682.

Wang, M. *et al.* (1995). Relationship between 1–84 parathyroid hormone and bone histomorphometric parameters in dialysis patients without aluminium toxicity. *American Journal of Kidney Diseases* **26**, 836–844.

Wasserman, R. H. and Chandler, J. S. Molecular mechanisms of intestinal calcium absorption. In *Bone and Mineral Research* Vol. 3 (ed. W. A. Peck), pp. 181–221. Amsterdam: Elsevier, 1985.

Woodhouse, N. J. Y. and Barnes, N. D. The response of athyroidal patients to calcium infusion. Evidence for an action of calcitonin. In *Calcitonin* (ed. S. Taylor), pp. 361–336. London: Heinemann, 1968.

2.4 Hypo–hyperphosphataemia

Caroline Silve and Gérard Friedlander

Introduction

A normal human body contains approximately 600 g of phosphorus (~23 mol), 85 per cent in the skeleton in crystalline form, 15 per cent in soft tissues, almost exclusively in the form of phosphate esters, and 0.1 per cent in the extracellular fluids, largely in the form of inorganic phosphate anions. In addition to its role in bone mineralization, inorganic phosphate is essential for cellular metabolism. It is a constituent of key organic molecules, such as second messengers (cAMP and cGMP), fuel (ATP), and coenzymes (NAD). It is also a constituent of structural molecules such as phosphoproteins, phospholipids, and nucleic acids. It is involved in most metabolic pathways, either in the form of ATP or coenzymes, or as inorganic phosphate. Enzymatic activities are sensitive to changes in intracellular inorganic phosphate concentration: increased phosphate concentration stimulates the activity of kinases (hexokinase, phosphofructokinase) or glutaminase, while decreased phosphate concentration stimulates 25-OH-cholecalciferol 1α-hydroxylase, AMP-deaminase, and 5′-nucleotidase.

Recently, 'new' functions have been attributed to extracellular inorganic phosphate levels. At physiological extracellular concentrations, phosphate specifically induces osteopontin gene expression and chondrocyte apoptosis. At elevated extracellular concentrations, such as observed in chronic renal insufficiency, phosphate induces vascular smooth muscle cells to differentiate into osteoblast-like cells able to sustain mineralization (Beck *et al.* 2000; Adams *et al.* 2001; Ahmed *et al.* 2001; Giachelli *et al.* 2001).

In order for inorganic phosphate to ensure its physiological roles, it is critical that serum phosphate concentration remains within a physiological range. Serum inorganic phosphate exists as three fractions, protein bound (~10 per cent), complexed to cations (~35 per cent), and ionized (~55 per cent). About 90 per cent of inorganic phosphate is ultrafiltrable, and represents the 'active' form of phosphate. Phosphate homeostasis is closely linked to that of calcium for two main reasons, the concentration of each ion in extracellular fluids is controlled by the concentration of the other, and fixed proportions of both ions are required for physiological bone mineralization. Accordingly, hypophosphataemia is often associated with a defect in bone mineralization, while hyperphosphataemia predisposes to ectopic calcification.

Systemic phosphorus homeostasis depends on intestinal absorption, bone metabolism, and renal excretion. Disorders of phosphate balance and/or distribution in body fluids give rise to hypo- or hyperphosphataemia. The kidney plays the dominant part in maintaining the serum phosphorus concentration. Thus, most disorders associated with an altered phosphate homeostasis in humans result from intrinsic or extrinsic alterations in renal tubular reabsorption and thus of phosphate excretion. The recent molecular identification of phosphate transporters, phosphate transporter regulators, and genes associated with familial and acquired hypo- and hyperphosphataemias has enhanced our understanding of phosphate homeostasis in physiological and pathological situations. Simultaneously, unexpected insights have been shed into regulation of phosphate homeostasis and consequences of its altered metabolism. This chapter is devoted to a description of disorders affecting serum phosphorus balance with the aim of positioning the recently identified actors. The following issues will be addressed: (a) molecular aspects of sodium phosphate cotransporters; (b) physiological basis of phosphate balance; (c) acquired hypo- and hyperphosphataemias; and (d) familial hypo- and hyperphosphataemia.

Given the important new literature to be cited on the subject of 'hypo- and hyperphosphataemias', we refer to book chapters and review articles whenever possible, in order to quote recently published articles.

Molecular aspects of sodium phosphate cotransporters and regulators

Approximately 10 years ago, the search for the transporter involved in renal phosphate homeostasis led to the molecular identification of the first sodium phosphate cotransporter, Npt1. Since then, seven non-homologous $NaPO_4$ cotransporters belonging to four types have been characterized at the molecular level (Tenenhouse *et al.* 1998; Murer *et al.* 2000a,b; Beck and Silve 2001; Werner and Kinne 2001). In this section, we review the main properties of each type (Table 1), with a special emphasis on the type II family, given the importance of Npt2a in renal phosphate regulation.

Type I $NaPO_4$ transporters (Npt1)

Type I $NaPO_4$ transporter is expressed in the kidney, liver, and brain. In the kidney it is expressed in brush border membrane from the three proximal tubule segments. Expression and activity are not regulated by phosphate deprivation or PTH (Murer 2000; Murer *et al.* 2001). Based on recent data it is proposed that Npt1 is a chloride channel and a xenobiotic transporter, and possibly, a $NaPO_4$ cotransporter modulator (Broer *et al.* 1998). In mice, invalidation of Hepatocyte Nuclear Factor 1 alpha (HNF1α) gene is associated with hypophosphataemia and decreased Npt1 mRNA expression in the kidney (Pontoglio *et al.* 2000).

Table 1 Main properties of $NaPO_4$ transporters (adapted from Beck and Silve 2001)

Type	Pi affinity (mM)	Chromosome (human)	Name	Species	Main tissular expression	cDNA (bp)	Protein (aa)	PTH[a]	PO_4[a]	pH[a]	Electrogenic (in oocytes)
I	0.29	6p22	NPT1	Human	RPT[b], liver	1549	467	−	−	−	+
			NPT1	Human	RPT, liver	1794	465				
			Npt1	Mouse	RPT, liver	1885	465				
			NaPi-1	Rat	RPT, liver	1700	465				
			NaPi-1	Rabbit	RPT, liver	1855	465				
IIa	0.1	5q35	NaPi-2	Rat	RPT	2440	637	+	+	+ (↑ at high pH)	+
			NaPi-3	Human	RPT	2554	639				
			NaPi-4	Opossum	RPT	2528	653				
			NaPi-6	Rabbit	RPT	2501	642				
			NaPi-7	Mouse	RPT	2423	637				
IIb	0.05	4p15	Npt2b	Mouse	Intestine, lung	4039	697	−	+ (?)	+	+ (?)
			NAPI-3B	Human	Intestine, lung	2280	690				
			NaPi-IIb	Human	Intestine, lung	4135	689				
IIc	0.07	2 (mouse)		Human	RPT	2020	599	?	+	+ (↑ at high pH)	−
III (PiT-1)	0.025	2q13	GLVR1	Human	Ubiquitous	3220	679	−	+	+ (↓ at high pH)	+
			Glvr1	Mouse	Ubiquitous	3227	681				
			Glvr1	Hamster	Ubiquitous	2040	679				
			RPHO-1	Rat	Ubiquitous	2890	681				
			Pit1	Cat	Ubiquitous	2128	681				
III (PiT-2)	0.025	8p11	Ram1	Hamster	Ubiquitous	1959	652	−	+		+
			Ram1	Rat	Ubiquitous	2287	656				
			GLVR2	Human	Ubiquitous	3175	652				
IV		19q13	BNPI	Rat	Brain	2024	560	−	−	?	− (?)
			hBNPI	Human	Brain	2366	560				
			DNPI	Human	Brain	3946	582				

[a] Regulation by PTH, PO_4, or pH.

[b] RPT: renal proximal tubule.

Type II $NaPO_4$ cotransporters (Npt2)

Soon after Npt1 description, Npt2a (previously designated NaPi-2) was identified and its key role in renal regulation of phosphate homeostasis demonstrated (Murer 2000; Murer *et al.* 2001) (Fig. 1). Two additional subgroups of type II $NaPO_4$ cotransporters are now recognized. Subgroup IIb is mostly expressed in the small intestine and lungs (Hilfiker *et al.* 1998; Murer *et al.* 2001; Xu *et al.* 2002). Subgroup IIc is also expressed in apical membrane of renal proximal tubules and appears to be growth regulated (Segawa *et al.* 2002).

Amino acid comparisons revealed that the three type II $NaPO_4$ subgroups are 36–38 per cent homologous (Murer 2000; Murer *et al.* 2001). Amino acid sequences are ~640 (Npt2a), ~690 (Npt2b), and ~599 (Npt2c) long with eight putative transmembrane domains having the highest predicted homology. Extracellular segments contain putative *N*-linked glycosylation sites, while potential phosphorylation sites for protein kinase A and/or C are detected in intracellular loops and *C*-terminal region. The *C*-terminal regions of Npt2b and 2c but not 2a contain a cluster of cystein residues. The role of the potential phosphorylation sites in the regulation of transporter activity is yet to be clarified. The main specific properties of each Npt2 subgroup are presented in the following paragraphs.

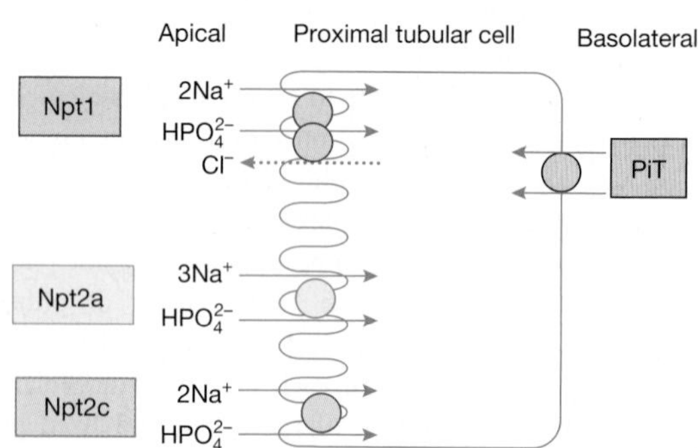

Fig. 1 Renal regulation of phosphate homeostasis.

Npt2a

Npt2a is expressed intensely in proximal tubules, but also detected in brain, osteoclasts, and lung (Murer 2000; Murer *et al.* 2000). Three Npt2a related cDNA (named Npt2aa, ab, and ag) resulting from alternate splicing of the Npt2a gene have been identified (Tatsumi *et al.* 1998). Their role in renal membrane $NaPO_4$ cotransport is not clear. Npt2a protein is exclusively expressed at the apical membrane in proximal tubular cells. Vitamin D receptor-responsive elements (VDRE) and a phosphate response element (PRE) have been identified in NPT2a gene promoter (Taketani *et al.* 1998; Kido *et al.* 1999). Transcription factor muE3 (TFE3) may participate in the transcriptional regulation of the NPT2 gene by dietary Pi.

Npt2a transports three Na^+ ions and one divalent PO_4, which generates a net inward current (one positive charge by cycle) under physiological condition (Murer 2000; Murer *et al.* 2000a,b). The specific pH dependence of Npt2a cotransporter (high transport rates at high pH values) is due to several factors: competition with the final Na^+-interaction steps, preferential interaction with divalent Pi, and effects of protons on the reorientation of the empty carrier. Specific amino acid residues contribute to this pH dependence.

The transporter can function as a monomer. There is at least one functional cysteine bridge in the large extracellular loop and evidence for a second connecting TM 3 and 7. At least one of these S–S bridges has to be intact for a functional transporter. Specific amino acid residues are involved in PTH-dependent internalization and/or apical expression, as well as in the pH dependence.

Npt2a transport properties, with the exception of stoichiometry, reproduce that of phosphate renal reabsorption. Its activity increases with increasing media pH, decreases under the influence of PTH and is regulated by dietary phosphate.

Npt2b

Npt2b protein is found essentially in the apical membrane of upper small intestinal enterocytes and type II pneumocytes. Npt2b mediated phosphate transport is electrogenic. Its pH dependence is opposite to that of Npt2a (Hilfiker *et al.* 1998; Murer *et al.* 2001). Dietary restriction of phosphate stimulates via vitamin D_3 the small intestinal apical Na-P(i) (Katai *et al.* 1999). The age-related decrease in intestinal sodium-dependent Pi absorption is correlated with a decreased NaP(i)-IIb mRNA expression (Xu *et al.* 2002).

Npt2c

At the time of writing only one paper had documented Npt2c (Segawa *et al.* 2002). Its affinity for Pi is 0.07 mM in 100 mM Na^+ and depends on extracellular pH. The type IIc Na/Pi cotransport is electroneutral. In Northern blotting analysis, the type IIc transcript was only expressed in the kidney and more strongly in weaning animals. The type IIc protein is localized at the apical membrane of the proximal tubular cells in superficial and midcortical nephrons of weaning rat kidney. Npt2c could function as a Na/Pi cotransporter in weaning animals, but its role is reduced in adults. It appears to be a growth-related renal Na/Pi cotransporter, which has a high affinity for Pi.

Type III $NaPO_4$ cotransporters

Type III $NaPO_4$ cotransporters have been originally described as cell surface receptors for gibbon ape leukaemia virus (GALV) and murine amphotropic retrovirus (A-MuLV) (Kavanaugh and Kabat 1996). These receptors are highly related phosphate symporters (62 per cent identity in amino acid sequence). Their human homologs are designated PiT1 (GALV receptor, formerly GLVR1) and PiT2 (A-MuLV receptor, formerly GLVR2 or Ram1) (Beck and Silve 2001). PiT1 gene structure is identified and its promoter region has been cloned and analysed in humans, while PiT2 genomic structure is in process. PiT1 and PiT2 sequences are 648 to 681 amino acid long (Salaün 2001) and characteristic of integral membrane proteins. PiTs present 12 putative transmembrane-spanning domains, with extracellular *N*- and *C*-terminal extremities, and a large hydrophilic central intracellular domain (loop 7) (Rodrigues and Heard 1999; Salaün *et al.* 2001) which contains several consensus kinase C and A phosphorylation sites. In contrast to the other types, type III $NaPO_4$ cotransporters are ubiquitous in most species, PiT1 and PiT2 are coexpressed on most cells (although each virus uses only its own receptor to enter cells). They appear to represent a family of housekeeping $NaPO_4$ cotransport systems, but little is known on their role in overall phosphate homeostasis and on their cellular regulation. PiT1 and PiT2 adapt to extracellular phosphate concentration *in vitro*, a feature shared with type II transporters but not type I and IV (Salaün 2001). PiT1 appears to be the only $NaPO_4$ cotransporter expressed in parathyroid glands (at least in the rat). In this tissue, a low PO_4 diet increases PiT1 mRNA, whereas $1,25(OH)_2D$ injected in vitamin D deficient rats augments specifically PiT1 and PiT2 mRNA, respectively, in parathyroid glands and the gut. PiT transcripts are found throughout the kidney. We have observed its location on proximal tubular basal and apical membranes (personal unpublished data). In skeletal tissue PiT1 and PiT2, expressed by osteoblasts and chondrocytes, may play a role in the extracellular matrix mineralization process. Current evidence demonstrate that PiT1 may be an active player in the pathophysiological mechanisms of vascular smooth muscle cell calcifications (Ahmed *et al.* 2001; Giachelli *et al.* 2001) and in the induction of phosphate-mediated osteoblast apoptosis (Adams *et al.* 2001).

Type IV cotransporters

Although originally described as $NaPO_4$ cotransporters, type IV cotransporters function as vesicular glutamate transporters (Fujiyama *et al.* 2001).

Physiological basis of phosphate balance

Four points will be examined: (a) phosphate distribution in body fluids and tissues; (b) its handling by bone; (c) by intestine, and (d) by the kidney.

Phosphate distribution in extracellular fluid

(Stewart and Broadus 1987; Amiel *et al.* 1996; Wesson 1997; Silve and Friedlander 2000; Suki *et al.* 2000)

Phosphorus in body fluids is almost exclusively in the form of phosphate mostly as a constituent of organic molecules, and only a small part as inorganic orthophosphate. Plasma phosphate concentration refers to the concentration of the inorganic moiety, which varies with age, gender, and dietary intake. It is high in babies (2 mmol/l at 1 week) and children until the end of adolescence, probably as a consequence of high and low circulating levels of growth and sex hormones respectively. It averages 1.1 mmol/l (3.4 mg/dl, or 3.4 mg per cent) (normal range 0.77–1.45 mmol/l) in healthy adults. Because plasma phosphate concentration undergoes circadian variations and decreases after glucose ingestion, blood samples should be obtained in the morning, after an overnight fast. Phosphate concentration is greater in red blood cells than in plasma so that, *in vivo* haemolysis may result in hyperphosphataemia. *In vitro* haemolysis during blood sampling or prolonged storage of blood before separation of serum are well-known causes of artefactual hyperphosphataemia. At a physiological plasma pH of 7.4, given a pK'_2 value of 6.8, the ratio of ionic species of phosphate is a 4 : 1 mixture of HPO_4^{2-} and $H_2PO_4^-$. Plasma phosphate represents less than 1/1000 of the intracellular stores, which has two important consequences: first, acute shifts of phosphate between cells and plasma may induce rapid and large variations of plasma phosphate concentration; secondly, chronic negative phosphate balance, related to renal or extrarenal losses, may develop without a significant hypophosphataemia.

Phosphate in cells (other than bone cells)

Phosphate is the most abundant intracellular anion, with a cytoplasmic concentration of about 1 mmol/l as determined by NMR analysis. Little is known about regulation of intracellular phosphate as a function of cell types and, inside cells, of cellular organites. Cellular phosphate uptake occurs against an electrochemical gradient. This uphill transport is achieved in some cells (leucocytes) through anion exchange but, in most cells, by a sodium phosphate cotransport. These 'housekeeping' sodium phosphate cotransporters probably belong to the $NaPO_4$ cotransporter type III family (PiT1 and PiT2) (see above) whose transport activity depends on extracellular inorganic phosphate concentration, and most likely modulates intracellular phosphate concentration.

Bone handling of phosphate

Phosphate in bone

(Stewart and Broadus 1987; Amiel *et al.* 1996)

Phosphate is a major constituent of the mineral phase of bone, 85 per cent of which is crystalline hydroxyapatite, $Ca_{10}(PO_4)_6(OH)_2$, and 15 per cent amorphous calcium phosphate. Cleavage of phosphate esters and inorganic pyrophosphate by alkaline phosphatase from osteoblasts liberates phosphate which combines with calcium and precipitates to form first brushite ($CaHPO_4 \cdot 2H_2O$) at the inception of mineralization. As mineralization progresses, the calcium phosphate molar ratio increases from 1.2 in poorly crystallized hydroxyapatite to 1.67, in parallel with improvement in crystal perfection. Inorganic pyrophosphate is a potent inhibitor of hydroxyapatite formation and dissolution. Recently, ANK, a multipass transmembrane protein likely involved in the transport of intracellular pyrophosphate into extracellular matrix, has been identified (Nurnberg *et al.* 2001; Reichenberger *et al.* 2001). Inhibiting mutations in ANK cause autosomal dominant craniometaphyseal dysplasia (CMD), a disease characterized by marked osteosclerosis of the craniofacial bones, and flared metaphyses of the long bones (Nurnberg *et al.* 2001; Reichenberger *et al.* 2001). It is hypothesized that mutations decrease PPi levels in bone extracellular matrix, which in turn cause increased density and progressive thickening of cranial bones. The role of ANK in non-mineralizing cells remains to be analysed.

Modulation of bone remodelling

Release and uptake of phosphate from and into bone depend on bone formation and resorption. Bone matrix synthesis and mineralization is under the control of the bone forming cells, osteoblasts, while bone resorption is controlled by the bone-degrading cells, osteoclasts. Osteoblasts differentiate from mesenchymal stem cells at sites of bone formation (Aubin 2001), whereas osteoclasts differentiate from haematopoietic mononuclear cells present in peripheral blood and bone marrow (Suda *et al.* 2001). In healthy adults, phosphate flux from bone to extracellular fluid equals the rate of accretion of phosphate in bone (about 7 mmol/day). Serum phosphate concentration is critical to maintain a calcium phosphate ion product for normal mineralization, and independently influences bone resorption. Many hormones and local factors modulate bone formation and resorption (Amiel *et al.* 1996; Canalis and Delany 2002; Conover and Rosen 2002) (Table 2). Hormones exert their effect partly through the release of mediators. For example, the stimulatory effect of growth hormone on bone formation is mediated by insulin-like growth factor 1, and some of the effects of PTH are exerted by transforming growth factor β and insulin-like growth factor 1 (Aubin 2001; Quinn *et al.* 2001; Conover and Rosen 2002). Most hormones or mediators [PTH, 1,25-dihydroxyvitamin D_3, interleukin-1b and -6, tumour necrosis factor (TNF), and prostaglandin E2] modulate osteoclast induced bone resorption only in the presence of osteoblasts, which express specific receptors (Suda *et al.* 2001; Horowitz and Lorenzo 2002). Activated osteoblasts, in turn, secrete other cytokines, and either stimulate existing osteoclasts or induce the formation of new osteoclasts from resident progenitors. One major exception to this general rule is calcitonin, which inhibits osteoclast activity after binding to its receptor expressed on osteoclasts.

Four discoveries have recently changed the comprehension of bone remodelling control. First, a signaling pathway, the RANK (for receptor activating NFKB) system, has been identified (ASBMR and Committee 2000; Suda *et al.* 2001). It comprises three molecules, the RANK ligand, expressed on the surface of osteoblast progenitors and stromal fibroblasts, the RANK receptor expressed on osteoclast progenitors, and a soluble decoy receptor, referred to as osteoprotegerin (OPG) also synthesized by osteoblasts and stromal cells. These molecules are family

Table 2 Hormonal regulation of bone remodelling

	Resorption	Formation
Hormones of mineral metabolism		
PTH	(↑)	↑
$1{,}25(OH)_2$ vitamin D	(↑)	↓(↑)
Calcitonin	↓	0
Other hormones		
Growth hormone	0	↑
Leptin/NPY	0	↓
Glucocorticoids	(↑)	↓
Thyroid hormones	0	↑
Insulin	0	↑
Oestrogens	(↓)	(↓)
Local factors		
RANK ligand/RANK receptor	↑	0
Osteoprotegerin	↓	0
LRP5	0	↑
PTHrP	↑	↑
PGE1	↑	↑
Interleukin-1	↑	(↑)
Interleukin-6	↑	0
IGF1	0	↑
Interferon g	↓	↓
TGFb	↓(↑)	(↑)

↓ denotes decrease, ↑ denotes increase, 0 denotes an action secondary to bone formation and resorption coupling, symbols in parentheses represent indirect actions.

members of the TNF ligand and receptor signalling. Description of the RANK system has provided new insights into the pathway that links osteoblast and osteoclast development. In a process involving cell–cell interactions, RANK ligand binds to RANK receptor and stimulates a signal transduction cascade leading to osteoclast differentiation and activation. Conversely, OPG can bind RANK ligand and inhibit osteoclast differentiation.

Second, leptin has been identified as a potent inhibitor of bone formation acting through the central nervous system in mice (Ducy *et al.* 2000; Amling *et al.* 2001). Neuropeptide Y (NPY) acting via central Y2 receptors may be the downstream modulator of leptin action (Baldock *et al.* 2002). The central control of bone mass and its disorders take place possibly at the level of the arcuate nucleus where NPY neurons express both leptin receptors and Y2 receptors. At least two mechanisms may be involved. Central hypothalamic NPY influence bone metabolism by neuroendocrine effects, and/or by alterations in autonomic neuronal activity. Modulation of bone mass by leptin and activation of Y2 receptors has been associated with changes in trabecular bone; whether cortical bone is similarly affected remains to be confirmed. These observations regarding a central regulatory circuit of bone formation via leptin and/or NPY were established in mice and remain to be proven in humans.

Third, the low-density lipoprotein receptor-related protein 5 (LRP5) plays a key role in the control of bone mass (Patel and Karsenty 2002). Activating and inhibitory mutations in LRP5 gene (chromosome 11q12–13) have been associated respectively, with the high-bone-mass trait (HBM) and the autosomal recessive osteoporosis–pseudoglioma syndrome.

Finally, PTH exerts anabolic effects on bone when administered intermittently at low doses (Neer *et al.* 2001; Fox 2002). Given the exquisite pulsatile secretion of PTH as a function of calcium concentration, this phenomenon has most likely some physiological relevance.

Mechanisms of phosphate transport in bone cells

A sodium-dependent phosphate transport is present in osteoblasts and chondrocytes (Caverzasio and Bonjour 1996; Aubin 2001; Salaün 2001; Suzuki *et al.* 2001). It is believed to play a key role in the mineralization process. It is modulated by extracellular phosphate concentration, stimulated by fluoride, aluminium, insulin, insulin-like growth factor 1 (IGF1), platelet-derived growth factor, TGFb, PTH, and PTHrP, and inhibited by calcitriol. Current evidence demonstrates that osteoblasts and chondrocytes express sodium phosphate cotransporter type III (PiT1 and PiT2), but not type I or II (Palmer *et al.* 1997, 2000; Guicheux *et al.* 2000; Suzuki *et al.* 2000). PiT1 mRNA is more abundant than PiT2 mRNA induced by osteoblast differentiation and by IGF1. Both mRNA are increased by phosphate, an effect attributed to an increased RNA stability.

Sodium-dependent phosphate transport has also been demonstrated in osteoclasts (Gupta *et al.* 2001). It is stimulated by bone particles, an effect that involves the integrin receptor and cell–matrix interactions. The presence of a type II Na-dependent PO_4 transport (Npt2) protein has been reported in avian and mouse osteoclasts. In avian osteoclasts, a larger protein (~95 kDa) than renal NPT2a protein was detected; in mouse osteoclasts, the Npt2 cDNA sequence was identical to that of the proximal tubule. PO_4 limitation and Na-dependent PO_4 cotransport inhibition in osteoclasts diminish bone resorption *in vitro* (Leeuwenburgh *et al.* 2001) an effect mediated by a shortage of ATP. Some of the phosphate released by bone resorption may be taken up by the osteoclasts through Npt2 transport activity and used for ATP production.

Intestinal handling of phosphate

Sites of phosphate absorption

(Stewart and Broadus 1987; Wesson 1997)

The intestinal absorption of phosphate amounts to about 80 per cent of phosphate intake. During vitamin D deficiency or with a diet low in phosphate, net phosphate secretion accounts for a negative balance. The intestine plays a minor role in phosphate homeostasis as a result of its great capacity to absorb phosphate together with a low ability to regulate it. Phosphate is absorbed throughout the intestinal tract. The relative contributions of duodenum, jejunum, and ileum to the overall intestinal phosphate absorption vary with species and experimental conditions. In humans, the greatest transepithelial concentration gradient of inorganic phosphate is achieved in the jejunum.

Regulation of phosphate absorption by the intestine

Phosphate intake

A diet low (0.2 g/100 g) or high in phosphate (7.8 g/100 g), respectively, increases or decreases the fractional duodenal absorption of phosphate in the rat (Amiel *et al.* 1996). The effect of a low-phosphate diet is detected in the intestine only 2 weeks after the alteration of the phosphate supply, but is already maximal in the kidney within 72 h. The intestine therefore plays a minor role in phosphate homeostasis (Fig. 2). A low-phosphate diet increases renal phosphate uptake by the proximal tubular cell and stimulates 1α-hydroxylase activity. The ensuing increase in plasma 1,25-dihydroxy-vitamin D_3 is partly responsible for the increase in fractional phosphate absorption by the intestine.

Vitamin D

1,25-Dihydroxy-vitamin D_3 increases intestinal phosphate absorption. It is thus involved in the intestinal adaptation to a low-phosphate diet (Amiel *et al.* 1996) and accounts for the phosphate malabsorption observed in rickets. 1,25-Dihydroxy-vitamin D_3 acts directly on the mucosal sodium-dependent phosphate cotransport system by increasing its maximal velocity, an effect recently shown to be at least partially mediated in an age-dependant manner by stimulation of the intestinal $NaPO_4$ cotransporter Npt2b gene transcription. Whether this effect results also from changes in the physical state of the lipidic environment of the transporters is not clear.

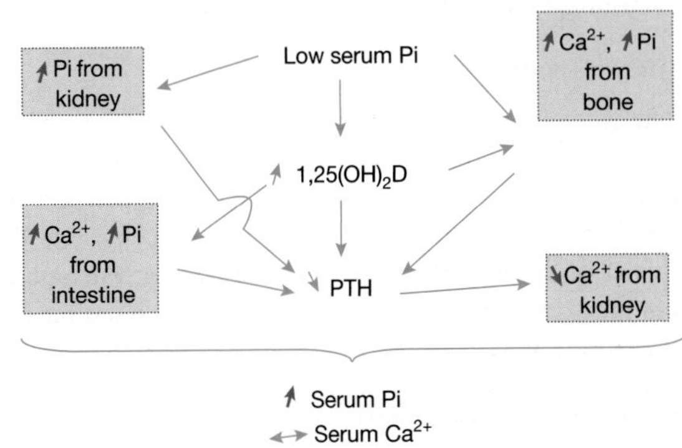

Fig. 2 Phosphate homeostasis.

Parathyroid hormone

Although recently questioned (Nemere and Larsson 2002), the dogma indicates that parathyroid hormone (PTH) controls phosphorus absorption in the small intestine entirely through 1,25-dihydroxy-vitamin D_3.

Calcium intake

Calcium does not influence directly sodium-dependent phosphate transport. The reduced phosphate absorption observed with high calcium intake may be related to the formation of a non-absorbable $CaPO_4$ complex or to a decreased PTH secretion and, in turn, 1,25-dihydroxy-vitamin D_3 formation induced by a positive calcium balance.

Mechanisms of phosphate transport in the intestine

As in the kidney, intestinal phosphate absorption results from two combined processes. The first, located mainly in the jejunum and the ileum, is a passive paracellular diffusion, which follows the concentration gradient. It is quantitatively more important than in proximal renal tubule. The second located mainly in the duodenum, at the luminal mucosal membrane is an active transport against a concentration gradient, which corresponds to a saturable Na^+-dependent process. This cotransport involves two Na^+ ions and carries both the monovalent and divalent forms of phosphate. It is under allosteric regulation by H^+: a low pH decreases its affinity for sodium. Its properties are similar to those reported in the proximal tubular cell of the kidney. The transport protein is an isoform of the Npt2b protein (Murer *et al.* 2001) expressed at the brush border of enterocytes. Its expression, but not mRNA, is increased by $1,25(OH)_2D$ and a low-PO_4 diet. In contrast, $1,25(OH)_2D$ and a low-PO_4 diet increase PiT2 and PiUS (Pi uptake stimulator) mRNA expression (Katai *et al.* 1999; Salaün 2001). Clearly, intestinal absorption of phosphate does not involve Npt2b only, but requires the participation of multiple components.

Renal handling of phosphate

(Amiel *et al.* 1996; Wesson 1997; Murer 2000; Murer *et al.* 2000a,b; Silve and Friedlander 2000)

The close inverse relationship between plasma phosphate concentration and renal phosphate reabsorption demonstrates the major role played by the kidney in the control of phosphate balance. At steady state, the kidney excretes the amount of phosphate absorbed in the intestine (about 20–25 mmol/day on an average diet) by reabsorbing 80–85 per cent of the load filtered at the glomeruli. Three main features determine the role of the kidney in phosphate homeostasis: the saturability of renal phosphate reabsorption, the adaptation of the maximum reabsorptive capacity to the intake, and its rapid and intense hormonal regulation such as that exerted by PTH.

Glomerular filtration

Phosphate is freely filtered by the glomerulus. At pH 7.4, the calculated phosphate concentration in the glomerular ultrafiltrate using the Donnan equilibrium correction factor is about 90 per cent of the phosphate concentration measured in plasma water, close to that of total plasma, a result confirmed experimentally by micropuncture studies in rats. Ultrafilterability of phosphate decreases as the plasma calcium concentration increases.

Urinary excretion of phosphate

On an average diet, 15–20 per cent of the filtered phosphate is excreted. Net phosphate reabsorption displays saturability and reaches a plateau (maximum capacity of transport: $TmPO_4$) when plasma phosphate concentration increases. $TmPO_4$ does not remain constant as the glomerular filtration rate (GFR) varies so that the *Tm* corrected for the GFR (*Tm*/GFR), or renal threshold of phosphate, is preferred. This ratio represents the plasma phosphate concentration above which phosphate appears in the urine. $TmPO_4$/GFR is estimated from plasma and urinary concentrations of phosphate and creatinine in the fasting state from a nomogram (Walton and Bijvoet 1975). It is modulated by numerous factors, such as phosphate content of the diet and PTH levels so that its value must be interpreted in the light of the clinical context.

Tubular localization of phosphate transport

(Amiel *et al.* 1996; Wesson 1997; Knochel 2000; Murer 2000; Murer *et al.* 2000a,b; Silve and Friedlander 2000; Suki *et al.* 2000)

Phosphate reabsorption occurs mainly in the proximal convoluted tubule. About 60–70 per cent of the filtered load is already reabsorbed by the last proximal convolution accessible to micropuncture. A further 5–10 per cent is reabsorbed in the pars recta. The capacity of the pars recta to reabsorb phosphate is greatly enhanced in the absence of PTH. In acutely thyroparathyroidectomized rats, almost all the phosphate leaving the convoluted part is reabsorbed at this site and less than 1 per cent of the filtered load reaches the distal convoluted tubule.

Absolute phosphate reabsorption decreases progressively from the early convolutions to the pars recta, and is greater in juxtamedullary than in superficial nephrons. When reabsorption is analysed per single nephron glomerular filtration rate (at least in rats), the same difference is observed between juxtamedullary and deep nephrons and attributed to anatomical differences, the deep ones containing proportionally more convolutions than the superficial ones, in which the pars recta represents about 40 per cent of the length. However, the turnover of carrier molecules in brush border membranes is greater in superficial than in juxtamedullary nephrons, a feature related to the higher fluidity and lower sphingomyelin content of apical membranes of the superficial nephrons. In parallel with the heterogeneity of phosphate reabsorption along the superficial proximal tubule, the sodium phosphate cotransport system exhibits two kinetic components with similar V_{max} values but different affinities: a high affinity (low K_m) in the early part and a low affinity in the late part. The proximal tubules of the deep nephrons contain only the high affinity system.

Net phosphate reabsorption, about 5–10 per cent of the filtered load, takes place beyond the early convoluted distal tubule, in the connecting tubule cells. The existence of phosphate transport in the collecting tubule is controversial, and, when found, is passive and concerns less than l per cent of the filtered load. Phosphate reabsorption takes place in the thin and thick ascending limb of the loop of Henle, at least '*in vitro*' as indicated by tubule microperfusion studies performed in rodents.

Cellular and molecular mechanisms of phosphate transport

The vectorial transcellular phosphate transport through proximal tubular epithelium is a two-step process, uphill apical Na-dependent uptake and downhill basolateral diffusional or facilitated efflux. The apical entry of phosphate depends tightly on the activity of Na^+,K^+-ATPase and, therefore, on oxidative phosphorylation, highlighting the link between phosphate transport and cellular metabolism. The coexistence in the proximal tubule of similar systems, involving glucose and amino acids, explains why phosphate reabsorption is reduced when glucose or amino acid loads are increased in the tubular luminal fluid.

In contrast, provision of substrates for mitochondrial respiration specifically increases phosphate reabsorption while glucose reabsorption is little modified. When phosphate supply is limited, glycolysis and oxidative phosphorylation compete for phosphate utilization (Crabtree effect).

Apical entry of phosphate

(Amiel *et al.* 1996; Knochel 2000; Murer 2000; Murer *et al.* 2000a,b; Suki *et al.* 2000)

The apical uptake of phosphate is under the control of a sodium phosphate cotransport whose main properties have been characterized.

Apical sodium phosphate cotransport is affected by pH, by alterations in the ratio of divalent (HPO_4^{2-}) to monovalent ($H_2PO_4^-$) forms, and by an allosteric effect of protons on the cotransporter (Murer 2000; Murer *et al.* 2000a,b). At pH 7.4: (a) the divalent (HPO_4^{2-}) form is preferentially reabsorbed; (b) the cotransport system is electroneutral; (c) alterations in H^+ concentration change the affinity of the carrier for Na^+ (K_mNa = 70 mmol/l at pH 7.4 and 190 mmol/l at pH 6.4). Thus, phosphate reabsorption is less affected by pH with increasing Na concentrations, implying that phosphate transport is more sensitive to intracellular pH (associated with a low sodium concentration) than to luminal pH (associated with a high sodium concentration). Both allosteric regulation and the existence of a preferentially reabsorbed form of phosphate fit with the effect of pH on phosphate transport: luminal acidification decreases phosphate binding to the carrier and thus decreases phosphate reabsorption; conversely, cellular acidification increases phosphate release from the carrier into the cytosol and thus increases phosphate reabsorption. Alkalinization has the opposite effect.

Npt2a

Most of the transport properties described above are reproduced in heterologous Npt2a expression experiments. Changes in Npt2a protein expression parallel alterations in proximal phosphate handling, documenting its physiological importance. Npt2a protein and mRNA expression are regulated by PTH and dietary phosphate content (Murer 2000; Murer *et al.* 2000a,b, 2001; Silve and Friedlander 2000; Suki *et al.* 2000). The key role of NPT2a in the regulation of phosphate homeostasis has been conclusively demonstrated by targeted inactivation of the Npt2a gene in mice (Npt2a$^{-/-}$ mice) (Beck *et al.* 1998). These mice suffer a severe renal phosphate wasting, which cannot be compensated by an increased expression in other $NaPO_4$ transporters in the homozygous mice. Although current evidence designate Npt2a activity as the rate limiting and regulated step in renal phosphate reabsorption, the role of other transporters is not excluded (Fig. 1). Accordingly, brush border membrane vesicles (BBMV) from Npt2a$^{-/-}$ mice retain 30 per cent of the $NaPO_4$ cotransport activity of BBMV from wild-type mice (Hoag *et al.* 1999). Little is known about the third member (Npt2c) of the type II sodium phosphate cotransporter family whose expression is observed exclusively in renal proximal tubules and is regulated by growth (Segawa *et al.* 2002). The role of the Npt type III, expressed mainly at the basolateral membrane of proximal tubular cells, is not defined. Finally, Npt2b (mRNA) is also expressed in the distal kidney.

Basolateral transport of phosphate

Little is known on the basolateral transport of phosphate. Phosphate is released at the basolateral side mainly by passive diffusion along the electrochemical gradient. Two other mechanisms have been proposed. The first involves an anion exchanger but has been observed in the rat but not in the rabbit. The second involves a sodium-dependent cotransport, the kinetics of which differ from that of the apical membrane. Whether it relies on a Npt type III cotransporter is unclear. It should be emphasized that an active phosphate transport at the basolateral membrane would be oriented toward entry into the cell and would therefore not be involved in transepithelial phosphate reabsorption but would rather oppose it. This cotransport might provide phosphate to the cell under conditions of limited luminal phosphate availability and could explain why the impairment of pars recta function provoked by phosphate depletion can be prevented by the supply of phosphate at the basolateral side.

Regulation of phosphate renal excretion

Three main topics will be considered: adaptation of urinary phosphate excretion to phosphate content of the diet; hormonal modulation of phosphate transport by PTH, vitamin D, and other hormones; and, finally, non-hormonal modulation of phosphate transport (acid–base status, calcium, extracellular fluid volume). FGF23 and its role in phosphate homeostasis will be described in the section on 'familial hypophosphataemia'.

Regulation of phosphate excretion and more recently, of Npt2a expression, have been extensively studied both *in vitro* and *in vivo*. Comparison of '*in vivo*' and '*in vitro*' experiments yield similar conclusions regarding the role of dietary phosphate content and PTH but are conflicting for most other regulators, such as calcitriol, and thus underline their complexity.

Phosphate content of the diet

The phosphate content of the diet is a main regulator of renal phosphate reabsorption. In animals fed a low-phosphate diet (<0.02 per cent w/w), urinary phosphate excretion declines to about 1 per cent of the filtered load together with an increase in fractional reabsorption of phosphate and $TmPO_4$/GFR. This adaptation occurs without substantial changes in phosphataemia, but results from specific modifications of the apical sodium phosphate cotransport, since glucose transport is unaffected in BBMV studies (Amiel *et al.* 1996; Wesson 1997). Transepithelial reabsorption of glucose is, however, affected by the decreased ATP synthesis associated with phosphate depletion. A low phosphate intake increases the V_{max} but not the Km value of phosphate transport, a finding suggesting either an activation (or recruitment) of pre-existing transport units or an increased turnover of operating transport units, or *de novo* protein synthesis, or both.

Adaptation to the phosphate content of the diet probably involves more than one mechanism, depending on whether dietary phosphate restriction or excess is acute or chronic. Acute adaptations to dietary phosphate deprivation or excess occur within 2 hours (Ritthaler *et al.* 1999; Riccardi *et al.* 2000), are PTH-independent and do not require protein synthesis (Murer *et al.* 1999; Murer 2000; Murer *et al.* 2000a,b). Acute and chronic adaptations may also involve an increased fluidity enhancing the turnover of cotransport units in brush border membranes (Amiel *et al.* 1996).

Dissimilar mechanisms probably underly *in vivo* chronic adaptation to low-phosphate diet in the absence of substantial changes in phosphataemia and *in vitro* adaptation to phosphate deprivation, triggered by a drastic decrease of extracellular phosphate concentration. In both cases intracellular steps leading to overexpression of sodium phosphate cotransporters remain to be identified.

The adaptation of tubular phosphate reabsorption to a low-phosphate diet also occurs in other situations requiring increased cellular availability of phosphate, such as growth, pregnancy, and lactation.

Parathyroid hormone

PTH is a major hormonal regulator of renal phosphate handling (Biber *et al.* 2000). Patients with hyper- and hypoparathyroidism have respectively a reduced and an increased phosphate threshold. Administration of parathyroid extract or of the synthetic 1–34 fragment of PTH increases phosphate excretion, whereas acute parathyroidectomy in the rat reduces phosphate excretion from about 20 per cent to less than 1 per cent of the filtered load within 1 h, with a concomitant rise of the *Tm*/GFR.

PTH binds to specific receptors located on the surface of target cells. Two distinct PTH receptors have been identified, both of which belong to the B family of G protein coupled receptors (Mannstadt *et al.* 1999). The first, denominated PTH/PTHrP receptor or PTHR1 is equally activated by both PTH and PTHrP. The second receptor, PTHR2, is probably not involved in renal phosphate reabsorption. Its native ligand is not PTH but rather the tuberoinfundibular peptide of 39 residues (TIP 39) (Usdin *et al.* 2000).

PTHR1 mediates the endocrine actions of PTH in the kidney and bone, and therefore plays a critical role in calcium phosphate homeostasis. PTHR1 is highly expressed in the kidney at the site known to be a PTH target, that is, the basolateral membrane of cortical epithelial cells and is also detected on apical surfaces. PTH is predominantly cleared from the circulation by glomerular filtration and degradation in the proximal tubules. Megalin, a multifunctional endocytic receptor in proximal tubular cells, is involved in the renal catabolism of PTH and potentially antagonizes the luminal PTHR1 activity in these cells (Hilpert *et al.* 1999).

After PTH binding, PTHR1 stimulates two signalling pathways, the adenylate-cAMP-protein kinase A and the phospholipase C-calcium-protein kinase C systems. Although both pathways are involved in the inhibition of NaPi cotransport by PTH, the former predominates whereas the latter may contribute to the fine tuning of phosphate reabsorption (Mannstadt *et al.* 1999; Murer *et al.* 2000a,b; Silve and Friedlander 2000). It has been demonstrated that apical PTH receptors may preferentially initiate the effect through a PKC-dependent mechanism (Traebert *et al.* 2000). This result is particularly interesting in view of the recent demonstration that direct binding of PTHR1 to NHERF2 selectively transfers signalling from adenylate cyclase to phospholipase C pathways in WT PS 120 fibroblasts (Mahon *et al.* 2002).

PTH action on phosphate transport can be modulated: 1,25-dihydroxy-vitamin D_3 plays a permissive role in the phosphaturic action of PTH, while α_2-adrenergic agonists and serotonin inhibit the PTH-induced increase of cellular cAMP concentration. The phosphaturic response to PTH is blunted by a low-phosphate diet, an effect located beyond the production of cAMP, implicating perhaps the cytosolic concentration of nicotinamide adenine dinucleotide (NAD) since *in vivo* administration of nicotinamide restores it. Glucocorticoids, metabolic acidosis, dopamine, and 1,25-dihydroxy-vitamin D_3, also restore the phosphaturic effect of PTH through an unknown mechanism (Stewart and Broadus 1987; Amiel *et al.* 1996; Silve and Friedlander 2000; Suki *et al.* 2000).

As already stated, cAMP produced in response to PTH by proximal cells acts as an intracellular second messenger. In addition to its direct effect on the activity of the transporter, cAMP may act indirectly on phosphate transport by stimulating gluconeogenesis (Amiel *et al.* 1996). Cytosolic NAD, the concentration of which is increased by gluconeogenesis, has been proposed to be the effector of the inhibition of phosphate reabsorption.

Part of the cAMP generated in response to PTH enters the proximal tubule luminal fluid so that, under normal conditions, its urinary excretion is about twice the filtered load. Hence the use of urinary cAMP for the clinical evaluation of the parathyroid status. Nephrogenous cAMP, expressed in nanomoles per deciliters of glomerular filtration, offers an efficient discriminative tool to distinguish hypoparathyroid, normal, and hyperparathyroid groups (Stewart and Broadus 1987). Urinary cAMP is also often expressed as a rate, per unit milligram of creatinine. Nephrogenous cAMP has been shown to be more than a marker of PTH activity: it also contributes to the phosphaturic effect of the hormone. Extracellular cAMP is metabolized into adenosine which is taken up into tubular cells through dipyridamole-sensitive carriers (Friedlander *et al.* 1992; Bankir *et al.* 2002). Interestingly, dipyridamole reduces Pi excretion in man (Prie *et al.* 1998).

Molecular mechanisms and post-transcriptional regulation of the proximal tubule Npt2a transporter in response to PTH and dietary Pi

Renal Pi reabsorption is mainly regulated in midcortical and superficial nephrons which, under basal conditions, express less Npt2a than juxtamedullary nephrons. Under chronic low or high Pi intakes, the distribution patterns of BBM Npt2a protein and mRNA abundance are congruent. In contrast, after switch from one diet to the other, changes in Npt2a protein abundance in the BBM preceed by several hours changes in mRNA (Ritthaler *et al.* 1999; Riccardi *et al.* 2000). Increase in Npt2a expression in BBM is associated with presynthesized Npt2a protein translocation from intracellular stores to the BBM, through a process which requires an intact microtubular network. PTH and high PO_4 diet induce a rapid endocytosis of Npt2a cotransporters via clathrin-coated vesicles and its accumulation in the subapical endocytotic apparatus, resulting in a reduction in the number of cotransporters expressed at the apical membrane (Murer *et al.* 1999; Hernando *et al.* 2000, 2001). The transporter is subsequently delivered to lysosomes and degraded without recycling to the apical membrane. These events account for the PTH induced decrease in the V_{max} of the transporter with no change in its affinity.

The fact that Npt2a protein is strictly apically addressed together with its controlled regulated endocytosis suggest that Npt2a interacts with scaffolding and/or anchoring proteins (Custer *et al.* 1997; White *et al.* 1998; Schell *et al.* 1999). Candidates are the Na/H-exchanger NHE3 associated regulatory factor NHERF-1 and multidrug resistance proteins. Indeed, NHERF-1 invalidation by homologous recombination results in renal phosphate leak related to impaired adressing of NPT2a to the apical membrane, whereas apical NHE3 localization is not affected (Shenolikar *et al.* 2002). P-glycoprotein (Pgp) 1 (MDR1) has been indirectly shown to increase the proximal tubule Pi uptake and NPT2 translocation to the apical membrane in rats (Prie *et al.* 2001a). In addition, PDZ-proteins such as PDZK1 (also called NaPi-Cap1 or diphor-1 for dietary phosphate regulator 1), localized in the microvilli, and NaPi-Cap2, localized in the subapical compartment of proximal tubular cells most likely interact with the Npt2a *C*-terminus extremity (Murer *et al.* 2000a,b; Hernando *et al.* 2002).

PTH not only induces an acute, selective retrieval of Npt2a from apical membrane, but also determines a chronic regulation of Npt2a mRNA. Parathyroidectomy increases Npt2a mRNA within 2–4 days, whereas PTH infusion to parathyroidectomized rats reduces the abundance of Npt2a mRNA. Whether PTH also regulates Npt1 and 3 remains to be determined.

Vitamin D

The effect of the active metabolite of vitamin D, 1,25-dihydroxycholecalciferol or calcitriol, on renal phosphate reabsorption has been evaluated in numerous studies, both *in vivo* and *in vitro* (Amiel *et al.* 1996). Results are conflicting as a result of the difficulty to exclude indirect effects of alterations in plasma concentrations of phosphate, calcium and PTH (Friedlaender *et al.* 2001). In rats, for instance, low doses of 1,25-dihydroxy-vitamin D_3, do not change plasma calcium but increase phosphate reabsorption whereas larger doses raise phosphataemia (due to increased intestinal absorption) and decrease phosphate reabsorption. In rats fed a low-phosphate diet, 1,25-dihydroxy-vitamin D increases phosphate excretion independently of cAMP.

The interaction of 1,25-dihydroxy-vitamin D_3 with PTH in the regulation of renal phosphate transport is also unclear (Amiel *et al.* 1996). The phosphaturic effect of PTH, blunted by vitamin D deficiency, is restored by administration of 1,25-dihydroxy-vitamin D_3 with an attendant rise in urinary excretion of cAMP, suggesting an improved PTH stimulation of adenylate cyclase. Thus, rather than directly inhibiting phosphate transport, vitamin D could exert a permissive action on the phosphaturic effect of PTH. Moreover, a feedback loop links the circulating concentrations of PTH and 1,25-dihydroxy-vitamin D_3: PTH stimulation of renal lα-hydroxylase increases plasma levels of 1,25-dihydroxy-vitamin D_3, which in turn inhibits PTH secretion. The lack of inhibition of PTH secretion due to low circulating 1,25-dihydroxy-vitamin D_3 is one element of the hyperparathyroidism secondary to renal insufficiency. Thus, although calcitriol is not mandatory for renal adaptation to a low-phosphate diet, it clearly participates since:

(1) calcitriol synthesis is stimulated by a decrease of extracellular phosphate concentration (Zhang *et al.* 2002).

(2) insulin-like growth factor 1, the synthesis of which is increased by phosphate restriction, stimulates calcitriol synthesis through a calcium-dependent mechanism (Menaa *et al.* 1995).

(3) calcitriol potentiates the stimulatory effect of insulin-like growth factor 1 on phosphate transport (Condamine *et al.* 1994).

1,25-Dihydroxy-vitamin D_3 increased PO_4 transport in brush border membrane vesicles and in a subclone of cultured OK cells, suggesting that this effect is located '*in vivo*' in the proximal tubule. Furthermore, it has been demonstrated both *in vivo* and *in vitro*, that Npt2a is a target of 1,25-dihydroxy-vitamin D_3 regulation (Taketani *et al.* 1998). This observation is in agreement with the presence of VDRE in Npt2a promoter sequence. Just as for the effects of 1,25-dihydroxy-vitamin D on renal phosphate excretion, the effects of 1,25-dihydroxy-vitamin D on Npt2a are not observed in all experimental settings (Fernandes *et al.* 1997), indicating that although calcitriol clearly regulates phosphate homeostasis, its contribution *in vivo* varies as a function of the mineral metabolism status.

FGF23

FGF23 has been recently identified as the gene directly associated with tumour induced osteomalacia, with hypophosphataemia due to renal phosphate leak and with ADHR. It may be a key factor in the regulation of tubular phosphate reabsorption (see below).

Stanniocalcins

Stanniocalcins are two peptides produced locally in the kidney. They may serve important paracrine regulatory functions in renal phosphate handling (Ishibashi and Imai 2002). STC-1 might stimulate proximal tubular PO_4 reabsorption, whereas STC-2 might exert the opposite function.

Other hormones

(Amiel *et al.* 1996)

Glucocorticoids have a phosphaturic effect *in vivo* when given chronically at pharmacological doses; *in vitro*, 10^{-9} M dexamethasone reduces PO_4 uptake by tubular proximal cells. They inhibit phosphate transport in renal cells through a stimulation of protein kinase C independent of a modulation of Na^+–H^+ exchange (Vrtovsnik *et al.* 1994; Xan *et al.* 2000). A decrease in rat renal brush border membrane Npt2a transporter mRNA and protein abundance and glycosphingolipid composition has been demonstrated (Levi *et al.* 1995). A maturation decrease in Npt2a protein abundance might be mediated by glucocorticoids (Prabhu *et al.* 1997).

Thyroxine (Euzet *et al.* 1996; Alcalde *et al.* 1999) and growth hormone (Bianda *et al.* 1997; Tenenhouse *et al.* 1998) probably increase the phosphate needs of the organism, which may explain the observed increase in phosphate uptake by the brush border membranes. Growth hormone, in part through insulin-like growth factor 1, increases phosphate transport both *in vivo* and *in vitro*. Insulin decreases phosphate excretion and blunts the phosphaturic effect of PTH in dog and rat. A direct effect of insulin on phosphate transport has been suggested in BBMV studies. Moreover, insulin stimulates the renal PTH-dependent 1α-hydroxylase activity in diabetic rats. In other '*in vitro*' models, epidermal growth factor (EGF) and transforming growth factors α and β inhibit phosphate transport. EGF decreases the abundance of Npt2 mRNA both *in vivo* and *in vitro* (Arar *et al.* 1999), but in contrast, stimulates phosphate reabsorption in microperfused proximal tubules (Amiel *et al.* 1996).

Some hormones shown to be phosphaturic *in vivo* do not have a direct effect on phosphate transport: calcitonin raises plasma phosphate concentrations in thyroparathyroidectomized rats, increases fractional phosphate excretion (from 5 to 10 per cent), probably through to the concomitant increase in the filtered load. Pharmacological concentrations of glucagon increase urinary excretion of phosphate as a likely consequence of an increased plasma concentration of cAMP (see above).

Mediators

Dopamine and serotonin, two bioactive amines synthesized within proximal tubular cells, from L-dopa and tryptophan respectively, are paracrine modulators of phosphate transport. Dopamine is phosphaturic while serotonin has the opposite effects (Friedlander 1998; de Toledo *et al.* 1999). As pointed out previously, dopamine restores the phosphaturic effect of PTH during dietary phosphate restriction. Dopamine synthesis increases during extracellular fluid expansion, and may thus play a role in the concomitant hyperphosphaturia. Catecholamines, through α_2-adrenergic receptors, are also antiphosphaturic. The availability of pharmacological modulators of the synthesis and degradation of these amines may prove useful in the modulation of phosphate reabsorption.

Non-hormonal factors

Acid–base status (Amiel *et al.* 1996; Murer *et al.* 2000a,b) Chronic metabolic acidosis increases phosphate excretion, through an increased filtered load and a reduced tubular reabsorptive capacity: in BBMV from rats with chronic acidosis, V_{max} is significantly decreased, although the affinity is normal. Respiratory alkalosis decreases fractional excretion of phosphate. This effect does not result from an intrinsic modification of the tubular epithelium since *T*m/GFR remains unchanged, but rather from the hypophosphataemia induced by the shift of phosphate towards the muscle. Conversely, respiratory acidosis is associated with hyperphosphataemia and an increased phosphate excretion.

Proximal luminal acidification and alkalinization decrease and increase phosphate reabsorption, respectively '*in vivo*' in agreement with '*in vitro*' evidence of allosteric regulation of the sodium dependent cotransporter by protons.

Long-term acid or alkali loading decrease and increase respectively the renal cortical abundance of the proximal Npt2a (Ambuhl *et al.* 1998; Kim *et al.* 2000).

Plasma calcium concentration (Amiel *et al.* 1996) In intact animals, modifications of the plasma calcium concentration influence phosphate reabsorption through changes in PTH secretion. In the absence of PTH, increasing plasma calcium concentration augments phosphate reabsorption. The achieved plasma level of calcium seems critical. Whether modifications of the intracellular calcium concentration are involved is not clear: administration of calcium ionophores, which facilitate calcium entry into the cell, increases phosphate reabsorption whereas luminal calcium has been reported to have a direct stimulatory effect on phosphate transport in the proximal tubule.

Extracellular volume expansion Extracellular volume expansion inhibits phosphate tubular reabsorption. In intact animals, this effect is PTH dependent as saline infusion decreases calcium plasma concentration and stimulates PTH secretion. In parathyroidectomized animals, extracellular volume expansion still inhibits phosphate reabsorption. The molecular aspects of the effects of extracellular volume expansion on phosphate tubular reabsorption have not been studied.

Acquired hypo- and hyperphosphataemias

Acquired hypophosphataemia

Definition of hypophosphataemia and phosphate depletion

Plasma phosphate concentration may fall below 0.75 mmol/l in the absence of phosphate depletion as a consequence of an acute shift of phosphate from extracellular fluid to cells. Such transient movements are observed following administration of glucose or other nutrients that enter the glycolytic pathway. Similarly, acute hyperventilation-related respiratory alkalosis stimulates glycolysis at the phosphofructokinase step and may induce hypophosphataemia (Crook 1997). However, hypophosphataemia is most frequently associated with chronic phosphate depletion, which is responsible for the symptoms described below. Any superimposed phosphate shift from extracellular fluid to cells aggravates the clinical picture and may lead to life-threatening situations.

Clinical picture

Pathophysiological basis

Most symptoms of hypophosphataemia and phosphate depletion are due to decreased availability of intracellular ATP and an impaired oxygen delivery to tissues (Crook and Swaminathan 1996; Subramanian and Khardori 2000; Haglin 2001). ATP depletion results from both decreased synthesis and increased breakdown. Phosphate depletion decreases ATP synthesis as a consequence of an impaired synthesis of 1,3-diphosphoglycerate and 2,3-diphosphoglycerate. In erythrocytes, the concentration of 2,3-diphosphoglycerate modulates the affinity of haemoglobin for oxygen, shifting the oxyhaemoglobin dissociation curve to the right. Depletion of both ATP and 2,3-diphosphoglycerate increases the affinity of haemoglobin for oxygen, with an attendant decreased delivery of oxygen to tissues, impaired oxidative phosphorylation and impaired ATP production. ATP production by oxidative phosphorylation is further impaired as the little phosphate available within the cell is used primarily for glycolysis (Crabtree effect). Two phenomena augment the breakdown of ATP: the stimulation of AMP deaminase by phosphate depletion accelerates conversion of AMP to inosine-5′-monophosphate, whereas the stimulation of 5′-nucleotidase increases catabolism of the nucleotide pool.

The progressive depletion of ATP and 2,3-diphosphoglycerate may be clinically silent for a long time: signs and symptoms develop during exacerbation of hypophosphataemia caused by an acute shift of phosphate from extracellular fluid to cells. This may occur as a consequence of refeeding previously phosphate-depleted patients, as phosphate is utilized for early steps of glycolysis. Plasma concentrations may then decline to values below 0.3 mmol/l.

Signs and symptoms

(Hodgson and Hurley 1993; Subramanian and Khardori 2000)

These are summarized in Table 3.

Causes of acquired hypophosphataemia and phosphate depletion

Phosphate depletion occurs as a consequence of decreased phosphate intake or intestinal absorption (Table 4), increased urinary excretion, or both. Chronic depletion *per se* results in mild to moderate hypophosphataemia which may evolve into severe hypophosphataemia as a conequence of superimposed acute shifts of phosphate from extracellular fluid to cells (Table 5). This happens frequently in some complex diseases, discussed below.

Hypophosphataemia consecutive to increased urinary excretion of phosphate

Impaired tubular function Impaired proximal reabsorption augments the urinary excretion of phosphate, in the Fanconi syndrome (see also Chapter 5.3). It is then associated with decreased reabsorption of glucose, amino acids, and bicarbonate. In adults, the Fanconi syndrome may be induced by toxic agents (heavy metals such as lead, mercury, or cadmium), drugs (outdated tetracycline, aminoglycosides, maleic acid, streptozotocin, 6-mercaptopurine), or may be associated with other diseases, including disorders of protein metabolism (multiple myeloma, amyloidosis, Sjögren's syndrome), metabolic disorders (secondary hyperparathyroidism, vitamin D deficiency), and renal diseases (nephrotic syndrome, renal transplantation). Proximal reabsorption is also disturbed during recovery from ureteral obstruction or acute tubular

Table 3 Signs and symptoms of hypophosphataemia

Tissue	Abnormality	Mechanism involved (other than ATP depletion)
Kidney	↓ Phosphate excretion	↓ Filtered load ↑ Proximal and distal reabsorption
	↑ Ca and Mg excretion	↑ Filtered load ↓ Readsorption (loop of Henle)
	Glycosuria, bicarbonaturia	
	Metabolic hyperchloraemic acidosis (RIA) (severe phosphate depletion)	↓ Excretion of titratable acidity and ammonia
	↑ Plasma [1,25$(OH)_2$D]	↑ 1α Hydroxylase activity
	Hypercalcaemia	↑ Bone turnover and intestinal calcium absorption
Bone	↑ Resorption Osteomalacia (long-term hypophosphataemia) Osteopathy with ↓ osteoblastic surfaces Osteitis fibrosa (when hypophosphataemia due to primary hyperparathyroidism	↑ Osteoclastic activity
Gastrointestinal tract	↑ Phosphate, Ca, and Mg absorption Anorexia, nausea, vomiting gastric atony, ileus	↑ Vitamin D synthesis
Nervous system		
CNS	Metabolic encephalopathy (confusion, paraesthesia, seizures, coma)	
Nerves	↓ Tendon reflexes	
Skeletal muscles	Proximal myopathy (atrophy, myalgia, ↓ nerve conduction velocity) Diaphragm dysfunction with hypoventilation Rhabdomyolysis, only in extreme hypophosphataemia, that is, shift superimposed on chronic phosphate depletion	↑ [Ca]i leading to activation of lysosomal enzymes
Heart	↑ Left ventricular end-diastolic pressure, ↓ stroke work and contractility	↓ Cellular content of phosphate, glycogen, glucose-6-phosphate, phospholipids, creatine phosphate
Blood cells		
Red blood cells	↓ P_{50} value for O_2 Haemodialysis (plasma phosphate < 0.2 mmol/l)	
Leucocytes	↓ Chemotaxis, phagocytosis, and antibacterial activity (contribution to bacterial and fungal infection)	Impaired function of cytoskeleton
Platelets	Thrombocytopenia, increased size, ↓ half-life, impaired clot retraction	
Others	Impaired glucose homeostasis	↑ Insulin response to glucose ↓ Tissue sensitivity to insulin

Table 4 Causes of hypophosphataemia related to decreased intestinal intake or increased gastrointestinal losses

Cause	Mechanism
Decreased intake	Phosphate intake < 5 mmol/day [obligatory faecal loss of (5–8 mmol/day) during artificial feeding (association with antacids or anabolism)]
Phosphate-binding agents	Aluminium or magnesium hydroxide, aluminium carbonate gels (severe phosphate depletion when prolonged treatment with low phosphate intake)
Vitamin D deficiency	In children: ↓ intake or intestinal absorption or hepatic 25-hydroxylation
Malabsorption	↓ Absorption of phosphate and vitamin D
Glucocorticoid excess	Spontaneous or iatrogenic Cushing syndromes: direct effect on intestinal mucosa and ↓ effect of vitamin D metabolites
Upper gastrointestinal losses	Vomiting, nasogastric suction (rarely cause severe phosphate depletion)

necrosis. An isolated renal phosphate leak with moderate hypophosphataemia is occasionally seen in adults with either nephrolithiasis or bone loss depending on the calcitriol status (Prie *et al.* 2001b). Loss of function mutation in Npt2a gene have been identified in this content (see below) (Prié *et al.* 2002).

Exaggerated PTH secretion Primary and secondary hyperparathyroidism may lead to phosphate depletion and hypophosphataemia. Primary hyperparathyroidism is usually associated with moderate hypophosphataemia, because the increased urinary loss of phosphate is balanced by phosphate mobilization from bone and by an increased

Table 5 Causes of shift of inorganic phosphate from extracellular fluid to cells

Cause	Mechanism
Respiratory alkalosis	↑ Intracellular pH with ↑ glycolysis (stimulation of phosphofructokinase) and ↑ phosphate uptake
Heat stroke	Respiratory alkalosis?
Nutrient effects	
Glucose	When insulin administered concomitantly, ↑ cellular glucose and phosphate uptake, moderate hypophosphataemia because of feedback inhibition of glucokinase by glucose-6-phosphate
Fructose	Severe hypophosphataemia (no feedback inhibition of fructokinase)
Hyperalimentation	Refeeding syndrome after malnutrition or starvation
Hormones	
Insulin	Promotes glycolysis
Glucagon	Indirect effect, related to hyperglycaemia-induced insulin release
β-Adrenergic agonists	Indirect effect, related to hyperglycaemia-induced insulin release
Vitamin D	Shift of phosphate to bone in the treatment of rickets or osteomalacia
Others	In condensing bone metastases of prostatic or breast carcinoma

intestinal absorption. Hypophosphataemia is associated with hypercalcaemia, increased plasma immunoreactive PTH, and increased excretion of nephrogenic cAMP. Increased bone resorption for that is, osteitis fibrosa cystica is evidenced as subperiostal bone resorption on finger X-rays. The increased calcium × phosphate product in the urine and plasma may result in nephrolithiasis, metastatic calcifications, and nephrocalcinosis.

Secondary hyperparathyroidism results from chronic hypocalcaemia of any origin and is associated with low plasma phosphate concentration, except in chronic renal insufficiency.

Paraneoplasic 'hyperparathyroidism' also called pseudohyperparathyroidism and humoral hypercalcaemia of malignancy is a paraneoplasic syndrome characterized by the biochemical signs of hyperparathyroidism, in the absence of detectable PTH levels. It is caused by the tumoral production of a PTH-related peptide (see below) (Pizurki *et al.* 1991).

Other endocrine disorders Increased phosphate excretion results from the infusion of large amounts of glucagon perhaps as the consequence of enhanced hepatic release of cAMP but has not been reported in chronic states of hyperglucagonaemia, such as glucagonoma or burns.

Insulin stimulates proximal reabsorption of phosphate. Increased phosphate excretion is thus likely to contribute to the depletion observed in insulin-dependent diabetes mellitus.

Acute glucocorticoids increases phosphate excretion through decreased proximal reabsorption. Long-term glucocorticoid treatment also increases excretion: this may be due to phosphate depletion together with decreased intestinal absorption. By contrast, mineralocorticoids do not affect phosphate excretion.

Renal transplantation Following successful renal transplantation, proximal tubular dysfunction with decreased phosphate reabsorption and low plasma phosphate has been described and may persist for months. Possible causal factors include persistent secondary hyperparathyroidism, glucocorticoid therapy, and intrinsic tubular dysfunction of the graft.

Tumour-associated hypophosphataemia Increased phosphate excretion with hypophosphataemia is observed in two different paraneoplasic syndromes, called humoral hypercalcaemia of malignancy (HHM) and tumour-induced osteomalcia (TIO). Hypophosphataemia in HHM is caused by the secretion of PTHrP by the tumour (Strewler 2000). PTH and PTHrP share partial amino acid sequence homology within their amino-terminal portion, activate the same receptor (PTHR1) in bone and kidney and have largely indistinguishable biological properties with regard to the regulation of adult mineral ion homeostasis: hypophosphataemia is associated with hypercalcaemia and increased levels of $1,25(OH)_2D$. Although PTHrP was initially discovered as the cause of the humoral hypercalcaemia of malignancy syndrome, its most prominent physiological role is to control endochondral bone formation.

In contrast, in TIO, increased urinary phosphate excretion is associated with normal plasma calcium concentration, and low 1,25-dihydroxy-vitamin D_3. TIO aetiopathogenesis is discussed with genetic hypophosphataemia.

Diuretics and extracellular volume status Volume contraction induced by diuretics tends to blunt the phosphaturic effect of acetazolamide, thiazides, and, to a lesser extent, furosemide or ethacrynic acid. Volume expansion increases phosphate excretion, and occurs during hypersecretion or administration of mineralocorticoids, liquorice intoxication, or saline infusion. Sodium bicarbonate infusion induces hyperphosphaturia through both volume expansion and competition between bicarbonate and phosphate in the proximal tubule.

Hypophosphataemia consecutive to decreased phosphate intake and gastrointestinal loss of phosphate

These conditions are summarized in Table 4.

Hypophosphataemia consecutive to shift of inorganic phosphate from extracellular fluid to cells

These conditions are summarized in Table 5.

Two examples of hypophosphataemia of multiple causes: alcoholism and diabetes mellitus

Severe hypophosphataemia develops during a treatment-induced acute shift of phosphate into cells superimposed upon pre-existing depletion.

Alcoholism Phosphate depletion is caused by decreased intake, related to vomiting, malnutrition, and malabsorption; these factors also account for vitamin D deficiency and impaired calcium absorption. Secondary hyperparathyroidism may further augment the renal excretion of phosphate. Ethanol *per se* may cause phosphate loss from muscle cells. Glucose infusions, hyperventilation, and increased catecholamine secretion caused by alcohol withdrawal and the anabolic phase contribute to the acute shift of phosphate to cells during treatment.

Diabetes mellitus Hypophosphataemia is common during recovery from ketoacidosis. Pre-existing phosphate depletion results from increased urinary excretion related to polyuria (osmotic diuresis). Insulin deficiency and metabolic acidosis cause a negative cellular balance for phosphate through catabolism, reduced phosphorylation, reduced glycolysis, and cleavage of phosphate from organic molecules within cells. Hypophosphataemia develops at the onset of insulin therapy, when glucose and, hence, phosphate are taken up in the cells and is perpetuated by the resumption of anabolism.

Treatment of hypophosphataemia

(Knochel 2000)

Besides treatment of the underlying cause, treatment of symptomatic hypophosphataemia includes the provision of phosphate. In patients solely on parenteral nutrition or in life-threatening situations, it should be given intravenously (15–25 mmol of potassium phosphate per 1000 kcal of alimentation fluid or 0.3–0.6 mmol phosphorus per kg body weight and per day). In most other situations, oral supplementation is used: 1–3 g/day of phosphorus usually given as sodium, potassium, or ammonium phosphate. Provision of the daily requirement in divided doses prevents diarrhoea and improves intestinal absorption. Discontinuation of antacid therapy, when possible, facilitates phosphate repletion.

In patients with renal phosphate leak, oral supplementation is often associated with vitamin D. This may lead to phosphate precipitation and thus to renal stones or nephrocalcinosis. Dipyridamole, which prevents adenosine uptake by proximal tubular cells (see above), reduces urinary phosphate excretion, and may therefore decrease or even suppress the need for oral supplementation (Prie *et al.* 1998).

Hyperphosphataemia

Definition

A plasma phosphate concentration above 1.45 mmol/l in adults is considered as hyperphosphataemia. Much higher concentrations may be reached, up to four times this value. Spurious hyperphosphataemia may result from haemolysis during blood sampling or during storage. Hyperphosphataemia is often asymptomatic; clinical features and presymptomatic biological effects depend on the context. An acute increase in plasma phosphate is characteristically accompanied by a reduction in plasma calcium and its own symptomatology (Sutters *et al.* 1996). When plasma phosphate rise is chronic, hypocalcaemia is corrected by compensatory mechanisms, calcium phosphate then precipitates in tissues. This is observed in several syndromes discussed below: chronic renal failure with secondary hyperparathyroidism or aluminium intoxication, vitamin D intoxication, tumoral calcinosis, and, rarely, thyrotoxicosis.

Clinical picture

The calcium phosphate concentration product (Ca × P) is a major determinant of the fate of metastatic calcium deposits in experimental models and in patients with chronic renal failure. A Ca × P of 70 (in mass units) or 5.6 (in SI units) is the threshold above which metastatic calcification develops. Reported thresholds vary over a wide range and the therapeutic target should be lower than 5.6.

Large calcium phosphate deposits around joints are unsightly, limit mobility but cause surprisingly few symptoms. Conjunctival and corneal calcifications are common on routine examination of patients on regular dialysis but initially asymptomatic. Their rapid increase, for example during vitamin D therapy causes hypercalcaemic peak, and is accompanied by inflammation of the conjunctiva and soreness ('uraemic red eye'). Calcification of the myocardium decreases left ventricular function and may cause arrhythmias. Calcific aortic stenosis, developing on previously normal valves, causes the usual features of that disease and has proved fatal.

The most severe symptoms associated with hyperphosphataemia occur in the syndrome of acute calciphylaxis, characterized by the rapid progression of metastatic calcification in subcutaneous sites and small vessels, leading to painful necrosis of skin and subcutaneous fat with occasional exposition of large areas of skeletal muscle in severe cases. It is a hazard of vitamin D and calcium carbonate treatment, best avoided by careful monitoring of plasma calcium and phosphate levels.

Hyperphosphataemia in chronic renal failure causes symptoms by several other mechanisms discussed elsewhere in this textbook (Edwards 2002). It is the major trigger for the onset of hyperparathyroidism in early chronic renal failure, with eventual bone pain, pathological fractures, growth retardation, proximal myopathy and, to a limited extent, anaemia.

Causes, prevention, and treatment of acquired hyperphosphataemia

Causes

They are listed in Table 6 [see (Thatte *et al.* 1995) for review]. Several are discussed below: acute and chronic renal failure, tumoral calcinosis, vitamin D intoxication, and tumour lysis syndrome.

Acute renal failure Hyperphosphataemia is characteristic in the oliguric and early diuretic phases of acute tubular necrosis, when GFR is depressed. It is often accentuated by acidosis and hypercatabolism due to infection, trauma and, more conspicuously, haemolysis and rhabdomyolysis. In rhabdomyolysis, it is accompanied by hypocalcaemia and metastatic calcification during the oliguric phase and hypercalcaemia in the late diuretic phase. Metastatic calcification also occurs during acute renal failure of other causes in experimental animals and in man (Ibels and Alfrey 1981). It is best prevented by the control of plasma phosphate through adequate dialysis though in practice it is seldom symptomatic in the absence of rhabdomyolysis.

Chronic renal failure In early renal failure, plasma phosphate is maintained in the normal range by an increase in plasma PTH. At GFR below 20 ml/min, plasma phosphate rises despite increasing hyperparathyroidism. At a GFR below 10 ml/min, hyperphosphataemia is almost universal in northern European patients whose diet is fairly high in protein and dairy products (Block 2000). Therapy tries to maintain normal plasma phosphate levels to prevent the complications discussed in the previous section. Phosphate intake should be reduced by avoiding or restricting milk and cheese, eggs, meat, fish, and cereals. This leaves a rather monotonous diet, particularly for patients with other dietetic restrictions such as diabetics. Consequently, phosphate restriction is usually combined with the prescription of phosphate binders.

During regular haemodialysis plasma phosphate declines rapidly during the first hour as phosphate is cleared from the extracellular pool; thereafter, phosphate removal is limited by equilibration across cell membranes. Consequently, if hyperphosphataemia is resistant to dietary advice and prescription of phosphate binders, lengthening dialysis time and increasing the frequency of dialysis are better options than increasing dialyser surface area or blood flow, despite their high penalty in convenience and cost.

Tumoral calcinosis Large masses of encapsulated, amorphous calcium phosphate may develop around the major joints, particulary

Table 6 Causes of acquired hyperphosphataemia

Cause	Mechanism
↓ Urinary phosphate excretion	
Renal failure	Acute renal failure may be associated with, but not causative of hyperphosphataemia In chronic renal failure, plasma phosphate concentration increases when GFR $<$ 20 ml/min (in early stage of chronic renal failure, secondary hyperparathyroidism decreases phosphate reabsorption)
Hypoparathyroidism	Acquired: after destruction of parathyroid glands (surgery, radiotherapy, haemochromatosis, cancer metastases) or idiopathic
Acromegaly	Increased proximal phosphate reabsorption
Tumoral calcinosis	Calcium and phosphate tumour-like depositions (hips, elbows, shoulders) ↑ Intestinal calcium and phosphate absorption [due to ↑ (vitamin D) and ↑ renal absorption (despite normal PTH)]
↑ Phosphate intake	Phosphate-rich enemas and laxatives
Shift of phosphate to extracellular fluid	From red blood cells (haemolysis), skeletal muscle cells (rhabdomyolysis), cancer cells (onset of chemotherapy in lymphoma and lymphoblastic leukaemia) Therapeutic use of diphosphonates Hyperthyroidism

shoulders, elbows, wrists, hips, and knees, in patients with chronic renal failure and severe hyperparathyroidism, in vitamin D intoxication, and in the milk-alkali syndrome (Thatte *et al.* 1995; Block 2000). However, 'tumoral calcinosis' usually refers to a rare disease in which similar lesions develop in young adults who have not taken vitamin D and usually have a normal renal function (see familial hyperphosphataemia below).

Vitamin D intoxication Common clinical features are essentially those of hypercalcaemia and may include chronic renal failure and metastatic calcifications (Marriott 1997; Lee *et al.* 1999; Koutkia *et al.* 2001). Serum calcium is often very high while serum phosphate is normal or moderately elevated. The effect on bone varies from osteopenia on radiographs to dense bones resembling osteopetrosis. As a consequence of the long half-life of vitamin D, hypercalcaemia, hyperphosphataemia, and their consequences subside only over several months after withdrawal of the drug.

Life-threatening hypercalcaemia requires rehydration, saline, and furosemide infusion, and if necessary dialysis. Lesser degrees of intoxication respond to a low-calcium diet, corticosteroids, and calcitonin.

Tumour lysis syndrome The rapid response of acute leukaemia, lymphomas, and other rapidly growing tumours to chemotherapy may be followed by acute renal failure, usually attributed to hyperuricaemia accompanied by showers of urate crystals in the urine; it can be prevented by prophylactic administration of allopurinol and adequate hydration before chemotherapy (Jeha 2001). In a few patients, mainly affected by Burkitt's lymphoma, acute renal failure develops in the absence of hyperuricaemia, together with a peak of hyperphosphataemia (4–5 mmol/l) within a few days after initiation of chemotherapy and remits when serum phosphate is restored to normal by dialysis. Urine becomes milky at the height of hyperphosphaturia. Hypocalcaemia and other metabolic consequences including potentially lethal hyperkalaemia, accompany the rapid involution of this highly sensitive tumour.

Prevention and treatment of hyperphosphataemia

The strategies of prevention and treatment of hyperphosphataemia in advanced renal failure have been summarized above and are detailed in other chapters. Reduction of dairy products and meat in the diet cannot lower dietary phosphorus below 700–900 mg/day, so that administration of phosphate binders is necessary in severe renal failure. Calcium carbonate is preferred, as a phosphate binder, to aluminium hydroxide and aluminium carbonate in order to avoid aluminium retention and toxicity but may lead to hypercalcaemia and metastatic calcifications. A newly developed calcium- and aluminium-free phosphate binder, sevelamer hydrochloride (RenaGel), reduces serum phosphate without altering serum Ca in haemodialysis patients and is thus promising treatment (Amin 2002; Chertow *et al.* 2002). Recent therapeutic advances include the development of calcimimetics to control PTH secretion and non-calcaemic vitamin D analogues (Edwards 2002).

Familial hypo- and hyperphosphataemias

Hypophosphataemias

Genetic hypophosphataemias are separated into three groups according to the cause of the decreased phosphate reabsorption by the proximal tubule: (a) primary defect in phosphate reabsorption; (b) defect in a gene which controls $NaPO_4$ reabsorption; and (c) defects of phosphate tubular transport as part of complex disorders (Table 7).

Familial hypophosphataemias caused by a primary decrease in sodium phosphate cotransport activity in the proximal tubule

To this day, mutations in the NPT2a gene have been excluded in the classical form of familial hypophosphataemias (Miller and Portale 1999; Econs and White 2000) but found in unrelated adult patients with hypophosphataemia associated with osteoporosis or renal stone disease (Prié *et al.* 2002). Interestingly, two familial forms, X-linked hypophosphataemic rickets (XLH) and autosomal dominant hypophosphataemic rickets (ADHR), and one acquired form, TIO, share a similar phenotype characterized by rickets and/or osteomalacia and an

Table 7 Genetic forms of hypophosphataemia: inheritance, gene, and gene defect hypophosphataemias[a]

	Abbreviation	Inheritance/ chromosome localization	Gene	Defect in gene function
With a primary defect of renal phosphate reabsorption				
With abnormal vitamin D metabolism[b]				
X-linked hypophosphataemic rickets	XLH	X-D/sporadic/Xp22.1	PHEX	Loss
Autosomal dominant hypophosphataemic rickets	ADHR	AD/12p13	FGF23	Gain
Tumour induced osteomalacia	TIO	*Acquired*	FGF23	Overproduction
Hypophosphataemic bone disease	HBD	ND	?	?
With normal vitamin D metabolism[c]				
Isolated autosomic dominant hypophosphataemia autosomal	IADH	AD/sporadic/5q35	Npt2a	Gain
hereditary hypophosphataemic rickets with hypercalciuria	HHRH	AR		?
With hypercalciuric nephrolithiasis				
X-linked recessive hypophosphataemic rickets and Dent's disease	XRHR	X-R/X	CLCN5	Loss
With a defect in a gene which controls tubular phosphate reabsorption				
Increased PTH/PTHR1 signalling pathway				
Jansen-type metaphyseal chondrodysplasia	JMC	3p22–21	PTHR1	Gain
Familial hyperparathyroidism				
Multiple endocrine neoplasia type 1	MEN 1	AD/11q13	Menin	Loss
Hyperparathyroidism–jaw tumour syndrome	HPTJT/HPRT2	AD/1q21–23	?	
Familial hypocalciuric hypercalcaemia	FHH	AD/3q13	CaR	Loss
Neonatal severe primary hyperparathyroidism	NSHPT	AR/3q13	CaR	Loss
Decreased 1,25(OH)$_2$ vitamin D/VDR signalling pathway				
Vitamin D dependent rickets type 1[d]	VDDR type 1	AR/12q14	P450	Loss
Vitamin D dependent rickets type 2	VDDR type 2	AR/12q12–14	VDR	Loss

[a] Hypophosphataemias associated with type 1 and 2 tubular acidosis (familial Fanconi syndromes) are not presented in the table.

[b] Hypophosphataemia is associated with normal calcaemia and calciuria, high normal PTH, and low levels of 1,25(OH)$_2$ vitamin D relative to phosphataemia.

[c] Hypophosphataemia is associated with normal calcaemia, hypercalciuria, normal PTH, appropriate levels of 1,25(OH)$_2$ vitamin D, and lithiasis or osteoporosis. Hypercalciuria is explained by the increased intestinal calcium absorption due to the increased or high normal 1,25(OH)$_2$ vitamin D levels.

[d] Also called pseudo-vitamin D deficient rickets.

abnormal vitamin D metabolism (Miller and Portale 1999; Econs and White 2000). These phenotypic similarities suggest that the pathogenesis of ADHR, XLH, and TIO includes the dysregulation of a shared phosphate regulating pathway. This pathway could involve an abnormal regulation of Npt2a activity by a putative humoral phosphaturic factor named phosphatonin. This hypothesis has been recently confirmed by the identification of FGF23 as the gene mutated in ADHR and overexpressed in TIO, suggesting that FGF23 is the humoral factor, phosphatonin.

In the following section, the main characteristics of the familial hypophosphataemias caused by a primary decrease in sodium phosphate cotransport activity in the proximal tubule with or without abnormal vitamin D metabolism and rickets are summarized with special emphasis on aetiopathogenesis.

With abnormal vitamin D metabolism and rickets

This group includes at least three diseases: XLH, ADHR, and hypophosphataemic bone disease (HBD). TIO, although acquired, will be discussed with ADHR, given their phenotypic similarities. The hallmark of these diseases is isolated renal phosphate wasting with inappropriately normal calcitriol concentration. Their clinical and biochemical abnormalities largely overlap (Econs and White 2000).

X-linked hypophosphataemic rickets XLH is the most common form of vitamin D resistant rickets, with an incidence of approximatey 1/20,000 live births. It is inherited as an X-linked dominant trait. Clinical and biological signs are variable in intensity, probably because of the variable expression of the normal allele. The gene mutated in XLH, named PHEX, an abbreviation for PHosphate-regulating gene with homology to endopeptidases located on the X-chromosome (HYP and Consortium 1995) encodes a membrane-associated metalloprotease of the M13 family, which includes neutral endopeptidase 24.11, endothelin converting enzymes 1 and 2, and the Kell blood group of antigen (Turner and Tanzawa 1997). PHEX is mainly expressed in bone but not in the kidney, so that a humoral mechanism has been postulated to explain why its mutations decrease tubular phosphate reabsorption (Econs and Francis 1997; Sabbagh *et al.* 2000; Holm *et al.* 2001; Liu *et al.* 2001). The prevailing hypothesis suggests that PHEX normally inactivates the putative humoral phosphaturic factor phosphatonin, and that loss of function mutations in PHEX increases circulating levels of phosphatonin in XLH. Reported sporadic cases represent new mutations. Early diagnosis, possible in children of known families, leads to early treatment and the prevention of severe bone disease.

Autosomal dominant hypophosphataemic rickets and oncogenic osteomalacia The clinical manifestations of ADHR are usually severe, similar but more variable than those observed in XLH (Econs and McEnery 1997). ADHR transmission is autosomal dominant. Incomplete penetrance, delayed onset, and loss of phenotype have been reported. FGF23 is the gene mutated in ADHR (ADHR and Consortium 2000). Missense mutations affect one of two closely spaced arginine residues (R176 and R179) present within a potential subtilisin-like proprotein convertase minimum consensus cleavage site (RXXR motif). It has been speculated that FGF23 is a circulating factor with an important role in phosphate homeostasis and that a gain of function mutation causes the ADHR phenotype.

The clinical manifestations of TIO, a rare paraneoplastic syndrome, include bone pain, fractures, fatigue, and proximal muscle weakness, with severe hypophosphataemia caused by low phosphate reabsorption and inappropriately normal 1,25$(OH)_2$D concentration (Econs and White 2000). The underlying tumours are usually benign, mostly of mesenchymal origin (haemangiopericytomas, fibromas, angiosarcomas). The invariable cure of hypophosphataemia after tumour resection has led to the hypothesis of the secretion of a humoral phosphaturic factor (phosphatonin) (Seufert *et al.* 2001) TIO tumours express FGF23 gene and protein (Shimada *et al.* 2001). Several lines of evidence have definitely identified FGF23 as the factor secreted by tumours to cause hypophosphataemia: (a) FGF23 cDNA has been cloned from a haemangiopericytoma causing TIO, (b) administration of full-length recombinant FGF23 decreases serum phosphate concentrations in mice, and (c) continuous production of FGF23 in nude mice following implantation of FGF23-producing Chinese Hamster Ovary (CHO) cells reproduce the clinical, biochemical, and histological features of TIO.

Hypophosphataemic bone disease Hypophosphataemic bone disease (HBD) is a rare disease characterized by renal phosphate wasting, short stature, and lower extremity deformity, thus similar to ADHR, although most reported cases do not display radiographic evidence of rickets (Econs and White 2000). In the light of the incomplete penetrance observed in ADHR, it is possible that HBD and ADHR are not distinct entities.

FGF23, a phosphaturic hormone It has been proposed that FGF23 is a phosphate-regulating hormone secreted by one or several tissues, with a native, phosphaturic action (Strewler 2001; Silve and Beck 2002). The level of FGF23 in blood could be determined, at least in part, by the rate of its inactivation by cleavage by PHEX protease at the ^{179}Arg/^{180}Ser site. Overproduction of FGF23 by tumours as in TIO, mutations that prevent its cleavage by PHEX, as in ADHR, or mutations that inactivate PHEX, as in XLH, would all increase the level of active FGF23, with attendant hyperphosphaturia, hypophosphataemia, and rickets/osteomalacia. This attractive scheme requires clarification of a number of points concerning the role of FGF23 in the control of phosphate and vitamin D metabolisms.

With normal vitamin D metabolism regulation

Isolated autosomic dominant hypophosphataemia with osteoporosis or lithiasis: Npt2a mutation Isolated hypophosphataemia due to a decreased renal phosphate reabsorption associated with high normal circulating 1,25$(OH)_2$ vitamin D levels and hypercalciuria has been reported in patients with urolithiasis or bone demineralization (Prie *et al.* 2001b). This phenotype is compatible with a loss of function of Npt2a gene (Beck *et al.* 1998). Two distinct mutations in the Npt2a gene at the heterozygous state have been recently identified in two individuals with hypophosphataemia, one with recurrent urolithiasis and the other with bone demineralization (Prié *et al.* 2002). Both mutations result in an impaired function of the mutated transporters. Coexpression of the mutant proteins and wild type Npt2a protein alters the wild type NPT2a function, indicating a dominant negative effect of the mutated transporter. NPT2a plays thus a major role in phosphate homeostasis in humans. The identification of functional variants of the NPT2a gene in patients with hypophosphataemia associated with either urolithiasis or bone demineralization demonstrate that a defect in renal phosphate reabsorption is a genetic component contributing to the pathogenesis of these two common diseases.

Autosomal recessive hypophosphataemic rickets with hypercalciuria (hereditary hypophosphataemic rickets with hypercalciuria) This disease is characterized by increased renal phosphate clearance with hypophosphataemia, hyperabsorptive hypercalciuria, low PTH and increased 1,25$(OH)_2$D serum level. Although this phenotype is reminiscent of that observed in Npt2a invalidated mice, mutation in Npt2a and Npt1 genes have been excluded in the affected families (Jones *et al.* 2001; van den Heuvel *et al.* 2001). The aetiology and the inheritance pattern of this disease are under investigation: intracellular proteins regulating Npt2a activity, such as Diphor-1 and PiUS (discussed in a previous section) are potential candidate ARHR/HHRH genes.

With hypercalciuric nephrolithiasis: X-linked recessive hypophosphataemic rickets and Dent's disease

X-linked recessive hypophosphataemic rickets (XLRH) and Dent's disease are two out of four disorders defined as hereditary hypercalciuric nephrolithiasis, caused by mutation in a chloride channel CLCN5 (Table 7) (Piwon *et al.* 2000). The two other disorders are X-linked recessive nephrolithiasis (XRN) and the idiopathic low molecular weight proteinuria of Japanese children (JILMWP) (Thakker 2000). All four renal tubular disorders are characterized by low molecular weight proteinuria (LMWP), hypercalciuria, nephrocalcinosis, nephrolithiasis, and renal failure. Other renal proximal tubular defects, which include aminoaciduria, phosphaturia, glycosuria, kaliuresis, uricosuria, and an acquired impairment of urinary acidification, may also occur. Hypophosphataemia with rickets has been a particular feature of Dent's disease and XLRH. The common genetic aetiology (CLCN5 mutations) and the phenotypic similarities between these two syndromes indicate that they are variants of one disorder. It has been proposed that the CLCN5 gene controls both apical receptor-mediated and fluid phase proximal tubular endocytosis.

Familial hypophosphataemias caused by a defect in a gene controlling $NaPO_4$ reabsorption

In these disorders, phosphate transport is intrinsically normal but hypophosphataemia is the consequence of another genetic defect.

Defect in PTHR1 signalling pathway

Jansen-type metaphyseal chondrodysplasia Jansen-type metaphyseal chondrodysplasia is characterized by hypophosphataemia and hypercalcaemia, with normal or undetectable plasma concentrations of PTH or PTHrP. It is associated to autosomal dominant mutations in the PTHR1 gene causing constitutional activation of the receptor (Jüppner *et al.* 2002).

Familial hyperparathyroidism The diagnosis of familial hyperparathyroidism rests on calcium metabolism abnormalities and increased serum PTH levels (Larsson 2000; Marx 2000) although hypophosphataemia is usually present. The main forms are summarized in Table 7.

Defect in 1,25$(OH)_2$ vitamin D/VDR signalling pathway

(Malloy *et al.* 1999; Miller and Portale 1999; and Chapter 5.2)

Vitamin D dependent rickets (VDDR) comprise two distinct autosomal recessive rare genetic disorders caused by a renal 1α-hydroxylase defect (type 1) or by a defect in the structure and function of the vitamin D receptor (VDR) gene leading to an end-organ resistance to 1,25-dihydroxy-vitamin D_3 (type 2). In both, rickets due to a primary calcium deficiency develop in children despite usual supplementation with vitamin D. The defective VDR activation impairs calcium and phosphate absorption and leads to hypocalcaemia and consequent hyperparathyroidism with hyperphosphaturia.

Type 1 vitamin D dependent rickets It is associated with mutations in the vitamin D 1α hydroxylase gene, P4501a. Severe rickets appear before the age of 1 year. Hypophosphataemic myopathy is frequently present with eventual tetany and convulsions. The disease is characterized by frequent severe pulmonary infections due to muscle weakness, deficient T-cell function, and macrophage cytotoxicity. 1,25-dihydroxy-vitamin D_3 levels are undectable. Treatment rests on 1,25-dihydroxy-vitamin D_3 or 1α hydroxy-vitamin D supplementation.

Type 2 vitamin D dependent rickets This disorder is related to several distinct defects in the VDR gene. Loss of the VDR function as a ligand inducible transcriptional factor are caused by point mutations in the VDR gene, which, depending on their location, affect DNA binding, hormone binding, and/or heterodimerization with the retinoid X receptors. The clinical features are not correlated with the type of mutation. 1,25-dihydroxy-vitamin D_3 levels are extremely high. Approximately half of the patients, usually the more severely affected, present alopaecia. Treatment includes calcium plus high doses of calciferol analogues or extremely high oral or intravenous doses of calcium in patients resistant to maximal doses of all calciferols.

Familial hypophosphataemia caused by a defective phosphate tubular transport as part of complex disorders

Familial Fanconi syndromes (Chapter 5.3)

Familial Fanconi syndromes include: type 2 (proximal) renal acidosis, metabolic bone disease, with rickets in children or osteomalacia in adults, and hypophosphataemic myopathy. They can be inherited or associated with other inherited metabolic diseases (Amiel *et al.* 1996; Broyer 1997; Niaudet 1998; Sayer and Pearce 2001; Neiberger *et al.* 2002).

Type I renal tubular acidosis (Chapter 5.4)

Type I renal tubular acidosis are rare autosomal dominant disorders characterized by a primary defect of distal tubular acidification and a normal proximal tubular function (Amiel *et al.* 1996; Lemann *et al.* 2000; Igarashi *et al.* 2002).

Hyperphosphataemias

Familial hyperphosphataemias regroup rare and heterogeneous disorders which are due to either a deficiency in PTH production (hypoparathyroidism) or a resistance of target tissues to the effects of PTH. The latter can result from either loss of function mutation in the PTHR1 gene (Blomstrand lethal chondrodysplasia), or from a defect in another gene involved in the PTHR1 signalling pathway (pseudohypoparathyroidism or PHP). Clinical findings are observed in infancy or childhood.

Hypoparathyroidism

Main forms of familial hypoparathyroidism are presented in Table 8 (Gunther *et al.* 2000; Ding *et al.* 2001; Thakker 2001; Van Esch and Devriendt 2001).

Blomstrand lethal chondrodysplasia

Blomstrand lethal chondrodysplasia (BLC) is a rare recessive condition caused by homozygote or compound heterozygote loss of function mutations in the PTHR1 gene. Lethality is attributed to a defect in endochondral bone ossification associated with the lack of PTHrP effects in cartilage (Jüppner *et al.* 2002).

Table 8 Genetic forms of hyperphosphataemia: inheritance, gene, and gene defect

	Name	Inheritance/ chromosome	Protein	Defect in gene function
Hypoparathyroidism				
Autoimmune	APECED[a]	AR/21q22.3	AIRE[b]	Loss
Due to developmental defect				
Complex	Di George/CATCH[c] 22	AD/22q11	Microdeletion	Loss
	Kenny–Caffey/Sanjad–Sakati	AR/1q42–43	?	
	HDR[d]	AR/10p15	GATA3	Loss
Isolated	FIH[e]	AR/6p23–24	GCMB	Loss
	XLHPT	X-R/Xp27–2p25	Insertion–deletion	Loss?
Due to defects in PTH secretion	FIH	AD/11	PTH/prepro	Loss
		AR/11	PTH/signal peptide	Loss
		AD/3q13.3q21	CaR	Gain
PTH resistance				
Blomstrand chondrodysplasia	BLC	AR/3p21–22	PTHR1	Loss
Pseudohypoparathyroidism	Type 1A	AD-Mat+Pat/20q13.3	GNAS1	Loss/imprinting
	Type 1B	AD-Mat/20q13.3	GNAS1	Loss/imprinting
	Type 1C	?	?	
	Type 2	?		
Tumoral calcinosis	HTC	AD/?	?	

[a] APECED: autoimmune polyendocrinopathy–candidiasis–ectodermal dystrophy.

[b] AIRE: autoimmune regulator.

[c] CATCH: cardiac defect, abnormal facies, thymic hypoplasia, T-cell deficiency, cleft palate, hypoparathyroidism.

[d] HRD: hypoparathyroidism, sensorineural deafness, and renal insufficiency.

[e] FIH: familial isolated hypoparathyroidism.

Table 9 Clinical forms of pseudohypoparathyroidism (PHP)

Signs	PHP 1A	PHP 1B	PPHP	PHPIC	PHP 2
AHO[a]	+	−	+	+	−
↓ Gs activity RBC[b]/Fb[c]	+	−	+	ND	−
Hypocalcaemia/hyperphosphataemia	+	+	−	+	+
Renal resistance to PTH					
cAMP	+	+	−	+	−
PO_4	+	+	−	+	+
Other hormonal resistance (TSH, glucagon)	+	−	− (?)	ND	−
Inheritance	Mat[d] + Pat	Mat	Pat		?
Gene defect	Gsa	Gsa	Gsa	Renal adenyl cyclase (?)	

[a] AHO: Albright hereditary osteodystrophy.

[b] RBC: red blood cells.

[c] Fb: skin fibroblasts.

[d] Mat, maternal; pat, paternal.

Pseudohypoparathyroidism

PHP is a group of heterogeneous diseases whose cardinal feature is renal resistance to PTH (Levine 2000). It is characterized by hypocalcaemia, hyperphosphataemia, and low 1,25-dihydroxy-vitamin D levels, despite a normal renal function. A variety of abnormalities can be present in some, but not all, patients with PHP, including Albright's hereditary osteodystrophy (AHO), resistance to other peptide hormones, increased bone resorption, and hypercalciuria. Responses generated through the adenylate cyclase pathway are used routinely to study parathyroid function in patients, so that this pathway has been explored thoroughly in PHP. The current classification of PHP into two types is the result of such investigations.

The clinical and biological findings are summarized in Table 9.

Pseudohypoparathyroidism type 1

Type 1 PHP is characterized by a decreased stimulation of urinary cAMP excretion after PTH infusion. It is further divided into types 1A, 1B, and 1C. PHP type 1A presents with AHO, a characteristic set of somatic features which regroups short stature, brachydactyly, and subcutaneous ossification and signs of resistance to other hormones that act through the stimulation of adenylate cyclase. Isolated PTH resistance without a somatic phenotype is called PHP type 1B (PHP1B). The hormonal resistance and the dysmorphy in type 1A PHP are maternally and paternally inherited, respectively. Both type 1A and B have been associated with a defect in the Gsalpha protein gene GNAS1 (Jüppner *et al.* 1998; Liu *et al.* 2000; Weinstein *et al.* 2002). In families with PHP1A some members have the somatic phenotype AHO without PTH resistance, a paradoxical paternally inherited condition termed pseudopseudohypoparathyroidism (PPHP). The complex pattern of inheritance and clinical heterogeneity of the clinical forms of PHP/PPHP are attributed to a tissue specific imprinting of Gsa gene expression, only the maternal allele of Gsa being expressed in the renal proximal tubule (Hayward *et al.* 1998; Weinstein *et al.* 2002).

In a minority of patients with AHO and resistance to multiple hormones, Gs and Gi function are normal (PHPIC) (Levine 2000). Other defects in the PTH coupling mechanisms may thus be present, one of which could be a defective activation of the adenylate cyclase catalytic subunit by a normal Gs protein. Finally, some patients present an apparent dissociation between immunoreactive and bioactive PTH, suggesting the presence of an abnormal PTH or antagonist. The nature of this putative inhibitor awaits characterization.

There is no curative treatment for PHP; symptomatic treatment with calcitriol reduces hypocalcaemia.

Pseudohypoparathyroidism type 2

This disease is extremely rare, poorly understood, and characterized by a lack of cellular response to increased cellular cAMP induced by PTH. An interaction of cellular calcium and cAMP has been suggested since correction of hypocalcaemia restores the PTH-induced phosphaturia (Levine 2000).

Hyperphosphataemic tumoral calcinosis

Hyperphosphataemic tumoral calcinosis (HTC) is a rare autosomal dominant metabolic disorder characterized by the presence of ectopic calcinosis and hyperphosphataemia, caused by an elevated renal phosphate reabsorption threshold and elevated serum 1,25-dihydroxy-vitamin D levels (Jayaraj and Lyles 2000). PTH levels are normal. Soft tissue periarticular masses are the best-known component of the disease; however, it is variably expressed. The genetic defect is not identified.

References

Adams, C. S. *et al.* (2001). Matrix regulation of skeletal cell apoptosis. Role of calcium and phosphate ions. *Journal of Biological Chemistry* **276**, 20316–20322.

ADHR and Consortium (2000). Autosomal dominant hypophosphataemic rickets is associated with mutations in FGF23. The ADHR Consortium. *Nature Genetics* **26**, 345–348.

Ahmed, S. *et al.* (2001). Calciphylaxis is associated with hyperphosphatemia and increased osteopontin expression by vascular smooth muscle cells. *American Journal of Kidney Diseases* **37**, 1267–1276.

Alcalde, A. I. *et al.* (1999). Role of thyroid hormone in regulation of renal phosphate transport in young and aged rats. *Endocrinology* **140**, 1544–1551.

Ambuhl, P. M. *et al.* (1998). Regulation of renal phosphate transport by acute and chronic metabolic acidosis in the rat. *Kidney International* **53**, 1288–1298.

Amiel, C. *et al.* Hypo-hyperphosphatemia. In *Oxford TextBook of Clinical Nephrology* (ed. A. Davison, S. Cameron, J. P. Grunfeld, C. Ponticelli, E. Ritz, and C. Winearls), pp. 249–269. Oxford: Oxford University Press, 1996.

Amin, N. (2002). The impact of improved phosphorus control: use of sevelamer hydrochloride in patients with chronic renal failure. *Nephrology, Dialysis, Transplantation* **17**, 340–345.

Amling, M. *et al.* (2001). Central control of bone mass: brainstorming of the skeleton. *Advances in Experimental Medicine and Biology* **496**, 85–94.

Arar, M. *et al.* (1999). Epidermal growth factor inhibits Na-Pi cotransport in weaned and suckling rats. *American Journal of Physiology* **276**, F72–F78.

ASBMR and Committee (2000). Proposed standard nomenclature for new tumor necrosis factor family members involved in the regulation of bone resorption. The American Society for Bone and Mineral Research President's Committee on Nomenclature. *Journal of Bone and Mineral Research* **15**, 2293–2296.

Aubin, J. E. (2001). Regulation of osteoblast formation and function. *Reviews in Endocrine & Metabolic Disorders* **2**, 81–94.

Baldock, P. A. *et al.* (2002). Hypothalamic Y2 receptors regulate bone formation. *Journal of Clinical Investigation* **109**, 915–921.

Bankir, L. *et al.* (2002). Extracellular cAMP inhibits proximal reabsorption: are plasma membrane cAMP receptors involved? *American Journal of Physiology. Renal, Fluid and Electrolyte Physiology* **282**, F376–F392.

Beck, L. and Silve, C. (2001). Molecular aspects of phosphate homeostasis in mammals. *Nephrologie* **22**, 149–159.

Beck, G. R., Jr., Zerler, B., and Moran, E. (2000). Phosphate is a specific signal for induction of osteopontin gene expression. *Proceedings of the National Academy of Sciences of the United States of America* **97**, 8352–8357.

Beck, L. *et al.* (1998). Targeted inactivation of Npt2 in mice leads to severe renal phosphate wasting, hypercalciuria, and skeletal abnormalities. *Proceedings of the National Academy of Sciences of the United States of America* **95**, 5372–5377.

Bianda, T. *et al.* (1997). Effects of short-term insulin-like growth factor-I or growth hormone treatment on bone turnover, renal phosphate reabsorption and 1,25 dihydroxyvitamin D3 production in healthy man. *Journal of Internal Medicine* **241**, 143–150.

Biber, J. *et al.* (2000). Parathyroid hormone-mediated regulation of renal phosphate reabsorption. *Nephrology, Dialysis, Transplantation* **15** (Suppl. 6), 29–30.

Block, G. A. (2000). Prevalence and clinical consequences of elevated Ca × P product in hemodialysis patients. *Clinical Nephrology* **54**, 318–324.

Broer, S. *et al.* (1998). Chloride conductance and Pi transport are separate functions induced by the expression of NaPi-1 in Xenopus oocytes. *Journal of Membrane Biology* **164**, 71–77.

Broyer, M. (1997). Infantile cystinosis. *Revue du Praticien* **47**, 1550–1553.

Canalis, E. and Delany, A. M. (2002). Mechanisms of glucocorticoid action in bone. *Annals of the New York Academy of Sciences* **966**, 73–81.

Caverzasio, J. and Bonjour, J. P. (1996). Characteristics and regulation of Pi transport in osteogenic cells for bone metabolism. *Kidney International* **49**, 975–980.

Chertow, G. M., Burke, S. K., and Raggi, P. (2002). Sevelamer attenuates the progression of coronary and aortic calcification in hemodialysis patients. *Kidney International* **62**, 245–252.

Condamine, L. *et al.* (1994). Local action of phosphate depletion and insulin-like growth factor 1 on *in vitro* production of 1,25-dihydroxyvitamin D by cultured mammalian kidney cells. *Journal of Clinical Investigation* **94**, 1673–1679.

Conover, C. and Rosen, C. The role of insulin like growth factors and binding proteins in bone cell biology. In *Principles of Bone Biology* (ed. J. Bilezikian, L. G. Raisz, and G. A. Rodan), pp. 801–816. San Diego, San Francisco, New York, Boston, London, Sydney, Tokyo: Academic Press, 2002.

Crook, M. (1997). Importance of plasma phosphate determination. *Journal of the International Federation of Clinical Chemistry* **9**, 16–17, 110–113.

Crook, M. and Swaminathan, R. (1996). Disorders of plasma phosphate and indications for its measurement. *Annals of Clinical Biochemistry* **33** (Pt 5), 376–396.

Custer, M. *et al.* (1997). Identification of a new gene product (diphor-1) regulated by dietary phosphate. *American Journal of Physiology* **273**, F801–F806.

de Toledo, F. G. *et al.* (1999). Gamma-L-glutamyl-L-DOPA inhibits Na(+)-phosphate cotransport across renal brush border membranes and increases renal excretion of phosphate. *Kidney International* **55**, 1832–1842.

Ding, C., Buckingham, B., and Levine, M. A. (2001). Familial isolated hypoparathyroidism caused by a mutation in the gene for the transcription factor GCMB. *Journal of Clinical Investigation* **108**, 1215–1220.

Ducy, P. *et al.* (2000). Leptin inhibits bone formation through a hypothalamic relay: a central control of bone mass. *Cell* **100**, 197–207.

Econs, M. J. and Francis, F. (1997). Positional cloning of the PEX gene: new insights into the pathophysiology of X-linked hypophosphatemic rickets. *American Journal of Physiology* **273**, F489–F498.

Econs, M. J. and McEnery, P. T. (1997). Autosomal dominant hypophosphatemic rickets/osteomalacia: clinical characterization of a novel renal phosphate-wasting disorder. *Journal of Clinical Endocrinology and Metabolism* **82**, 674–681.

Econs, M. and White, K. Inherited phosphate wasting disorders. In *Osteoporosis and Metabolic Bone Disease* (ed. M. Econs), pp. 111–132. Totowa, NJ: Humana Press, 2000.

Edwards, R. M. (2002). Disorders of phosphate metabolism in chronic renal disease. *Current Opinion in Pharmacology* **2**, 171–176.

Euzet, S., Lelievre-Pegorier, M., and Merlet-Benichou, C. (1996). Effect of 3,5,3′-triiodothyronine on maturation of rat renal phosphate transport: kinetic characteristics and phosphate transporter messenger ribonucleic acid and protein abundance. *Endocrinology* **137**, 3522–3530.

Fernandes, I. *et al.* (1997). Abnormal sulfate metabolism in vitamin D-deficient rats. *Journal of Clinical Investigation* **100**, 2196–2203.

Fox, J. (2002). Developments in parathyroid hormone and related peptides as bone-formation agents. *Current Opinion in Pharmacology* **2**, 338–344.

Friedlaender, M. M. *et al.* (2001). Vitamin D reduces renal NaPi-2 in PTH-infused rats: complexity of vitamin D action on renal P(i) handling. *American Journal of Physiology. Renal, Fluid and Electrolyte Physiology* **281**, F428–F433.

Friedlander, G. (1998). Autocrine/paracrine control of renal phosphate transport. *Kidney International* **65** (Suppl.), S18–S23.

Friedlander, G. *et al.* (1992). Mechanisms whereby extracellular adenosine 3′,5′-monophosphate inhibits phosphate transport in cultured opossum kidney cells and in rat kidney. Physiological implication. *Journal of Clinical Investigation* **90**, 848–858.

Fujiyama, F., Furuta, T., and Kaneko, T. (2001). Immunocytochemical localization of candidates for vesicular glutamate transporters in the rat cerebral cortex. *Journal of Comparative Neurology* **435**, 379–387.

Giachelli, C. M. *et al.* (2001). Vascular calcification and inorganic phosphate. *American Journal of Kidney Diseases* **38**, S34–S37.

Guicheux, J. *et al.* (2000). A novel *in vitro* culture system for analysis of functional role of phosphate transport in endochondral ossification. *Bone* **27**, 69–74.

Gunther, T. *et al.* (2000). Genetic ablation of parathyroid glands reveals another source of parathyroid hormone. *Nature* **406**, 199–203.

Gupta, A. *et al.* (2001). Identification of the type II Na(+)-Pi cotransporter (Npt2) in the osteoclast and the skeletal phenotype of Npt2−/− mice. *Bone* **29**, 467–476.

Haglin, L. (2001). Hypophosphataemia: cause of the disturbed metabolism in the metabolic syndrome. *Medical Hypotheses* **56**, 657–663.

Hayward, B. E. *et al.* (1998). Bidirectional imprinting of a single gene: GNAS1 encodes maternally, paternally, and biallelically derived proteins. *Proceedings of the National Academy of Sciences of the United States of America* **95**, 15475–15480.

Hernando, N. *et al.* (2000). PTH-induced downregulation of the type IIa Na/P(i)-cotransporter is independent of known endocytic motifs. *Journal of the American Society of Nephrology* **11**, 1961–1968.

Hernando, N. *et al.* (2001). Molecular determinants for apical expression and regulatory membrane retrieval of the type IIa Na/Pi cotransporter. *Kidney International* **60**, 431–435.

Hernando, N. *et al.* (2002). PDZ-domain interactions and apical expression of type IIa Na/Pi cotransporters. *Proceedings of the National Academy of Sciences of the United States of America* **99**, 11957–11962.

Hilfiker, H. *et al.* (1998). Characterization of a murine type II sodium phosphate cotransporter expressed in mammalian small intestine. *Proceedings of the National Academy of Sciences of the United States of America* **95**, 14564–14569.

Hilpert, J. *et al.* (1999). Megalin antagonizes activation of the parathyroid hormone receptor. *Journal of Biological Chemistry* **274**, 5620–5625.

Hoag, H. M. *et al.* (1999). Effects of Npt2 gene ablation and low-phosphate diet on renal Na(+)/phosphate cotransport and cotransporter gene expression. *Journal of Clinical Investigation* **104**, 679–686.

Hodgson, S. F. and Hurley, D. L. (1993). Acquired hypophosphatemia. *Endocrinology and Metabolism Clinics of North America* **22**, 397–409.

Holm, I. A. *et al.* (2001). Mutational analysis and genotype–phenotype correlation of the PHEX gene in X-linked hypophosphatemic rickets. *Journal of Clinical Endocrinology and Metabolism* **86**, 3889–3899.

Horowitz, M. and Lorenzo, J. A. Local regulators of bone: IL-1, TNF, Lymphotoxin, Interferon-g, IL-8, IL-10, IL-4, the LIF/IL-6 family, and additional cytokines. In *Principles of Bone Biology* (ed. J. Bilezikian, L. G. Raisz, and G. A. Rodan), pp. 961–978. San Diego: Academic Press, 2002.

HYP and Consortium (1995). A gene (PEX) with homologies to endopeptidases is mutated in patients with X-linked hypophosphatemic rickets. The HYP Consortium. *Nature Genetics* **11**, 130–136.

Ibels, L. S. *et al.* (1981). Calcification in end-stage kidneys. *American Journal of Medicine* **71**, 33–37.

Igarashi, T. *et al.* (2002). Unraveling the molecular pathogenesis of isolated proximal renal tubular acidosis. *Journal of the American Society of Nephrology* **13**, 2171–2177.

Ishibashi, K. and Imai, M. (2002). Prospect of a stanniocalcin endocrine/paracrine system in mammals. *American Journal of Physiology. Renal, Fluid and Electrolyte Physiology* **282**, F367–F375.

Jayaraj, K. and Lyles, K. Genetics of tumoral calcinosis. In *Osteoporosis and Metabolic Bone Disease* (ed. M. Econs), pp. 153–161. Totowa, NJ: Humana Press, 2000.

Jeha, S. (2001). Tumor lysis syndrome. *Seminars in Hematology* **38**, 4–8.

Jones, A. *et al.* (2001). Hereditary hypophosphatemic rickets with hypercalciuria is not caused by mutations in the Na/Pi cotransporter NPT2 gene. *Journal of the American Society of Nephrology* **12**, 507–514.

Jüppner, H., Schipani, E., and Silve, C. Jansen's metaphyseal chondrodysplasia and Blomstrand's lethal chondrodysplasia: two genetic disorders caused by PTH/PTHrP receptor mutations. In *Principles of Bone Biology* (ed. J. Bilezikian, L. G. Raisz, and G. A. Rodan), pp. 1117–1136. San Diego: Academic Press, 2002.

Jüppner, H. *et al.* (1998). The gene responsible for pseudohypoparathyroidism type Ib is paternally imprinted and maps in four unrelated kindreds to chromosome 20q13.3. *Proceedings of the National Academy of Sciences of the United States of America* **95**, 11798–11803.

Katai, K. *et al.* (1999). Regulation of intestinal Na+-dependent phosphate co-transporters by a low-phosphate diet and 1,25-dihydroxyvitamin D3. *Biochemical Journal* **343** (Pt 3), 705–712.

Kavanaugh, M. P. and Kabat, D. (1996). Identification and characterization of a widely expressed phosphate transporter/retrovirus receptor family. *Kidney International* **49**, 959–963.

Kido, S. *et al.* (1999). Identification of regulatory sequences and binding proteins in the type II sodium/phosphate cotransporter NPT2 gene responsive to dietary phosphate. *Journal of Biological Chemistry* **274**, 28256–28263.

Kim, G. H. *et al.* (2000). Long-term regulation of renal Na-dependent cotransporters and ENaC: response to altered acid-base intake. *American Journal of Physiology. Renal, Fluid and Electrolyte Physiology* **279**, F459–F467.

Knochel, J. Clinical and physiologic phosphate disturbances. In *The Kidney*. (ed. D. Seldin and G. Giebisch), pp. 1905–1933. Philadelphia: Lippincott Williams-Wilkins, 2000.

Koutkia, P., Chen, T. C., and Holick, M. F. (2001). Vitamin D intoxication associated with an over-the-counter supplement. *New England Journal of Medicine* **345**, 66–67.

Larsson, C. (2000). Dissecting the genetics of hyperparathyroidism—new clues from an old friend. *Journal of Clinical Endocrinology and Metabolism* **85**, 1752–1754.

Lee, K. W. *et al.* (1999). Iatrogenic vitamin D intoxication: report of a case and review of vitamin D physiology. *Connecticut Medicine* **63**, 399–403.

Leeuwenburgh, S. *et al.* (2001). Osteoclastic resorption of biomimetic calcium phosphate coatings *in vitro*. *Journal of Biomedical Materials Research* **56**, 208–215.

Lemann, J., Jr. *et al.* (2000). Acid and mineral balances and bone in familial proximal renal tubular acidosis. *Kidney International* **58**, 1267–1277.

Levi, M. *et al.* (1995). Dexamethasone modulates rat renal brush border membrane phosphate transporter mRNA and protein abundance and glycosphingolipid composition. *Journal of Clinical Investigation* **96**, 207–216.

Levine, M. A. (2000). Clinical spectrum and pathogenesis of pseudohypoparathyroidism. *Reviews in Endocrine & Metabolic Disorders* **1**, 265–274.

Liu, S., Guo, R., and Quarles, L. D. (2001). Cloning and characterization of the proximal murine Phex promoter. *Endocrinology* **142**, 3987–3995.

Liu, J. *et al.* (2000). A GNAS1 imprinting defect in pseudohypoparathyroidism type IB. *Journal of Clinical Investigation* **106**, 1167–1174.

Mahon, M. J. *et al.* (2002). Na(+)/H(+) exchanger regulatory factor 2 directs parathyroid hormone 1 receptor signalling. *Nature* **417**, 858–861.

Malloy, P. J., Pike, J. W., and Feldman, D. (1999). The vitamin D receptor and the syndrome of hereditary 1,25-dihydroxyvitamin D-resistant rickets. *Endocrine Reviews* **20**, 156–188.

Mannstadt, M., Juppner, H., and Gardella, T. J. (1999). Receptors for PTH and PTHrP: their biological importance and functional properties. *American Journal of Physiology* **277**, F665–F675.

Marriott, B. M. (1997). Vitamin D supplementation: a word of caution. *Annals of Internal Medicine* **127**, 231–233.

Marx, S. J. (2000). Hyperparathyroid and hypoparathyroid disorders. *New England Journal of Medicine* **343**, 1863–1875.

Menaa, C. *et al.* (1995). Insulin-like growth factor I, a unique calcium-dependent stimulator of 1,25-dihydroxyvitamin D3 production. Studies in cultured mouse kidney cells. *Journal of Biological Chemistry* **270**, 25461–25467.

Miller, W. L. and Portale, A. A. (1999). Genetic causes of rickets. *Current Opinion in Pediatrics* **11**, 333–339.

Murer, H. *et al.* (1999). Posttranscriptional regulation of the proximal tubule NaPi-II transporter in response to PTH and dietary P(i). *American Journal of Physiology* **277**, F676–F684.

Murer, H. *et al.* (2000a). Proximal tubular phosphate reabsorption: molecular mechanisms. *Physiological Reviews* **80**, 1373–1409.

Murer, H., Kaissling, B., Forster, I., and Biber, J. Cellular mechanisms in proximal tubular handling of phosphate. In *The Kidney* (ed. D. Seldin and G. Giebisch), pp. 1870–1884. Philadelphia: Lippincott Williams-Wilkins, 2000b.

Murer, H. *et al.* (2001). Molecular mechanisms in proximal tubular and small intestinal phosphate reabsorption. *Molecular Membrane Biology* **18**, 3–11 (plenary lecture).

Neer, R. M. *et al.* (2001). Effect of parathyroid hormone (1–34) on fractures and bone mineral density in postmenopausal women with osteoporosis. *New England Journal of Medicine* **344**, 1434–1441.

Neiberger, R. E. *et al.* (2002). Renal manifestations of congenital lactic acidosis. *American Journal of Kidney Diseases* **39**, 12–23.

Nemere, I. and Larsson, D. (2002). Does PTH have a direct effect on intestine? *Journal of Cell Biochemistry* **86**, 29–34.

Niaudet, P. (1998). Mitochondrial disorders and the kidney. *Archives of Disease in Childhood* **78**, 387–390.

Nurnberg, P. *et al.* (2001). Heterozygous mutations in ANKH, the human ortholog of the mouse progressive ankylosis gene, result in craniometaphyseal dysplasia. *Nature Genetics* **28**, 37–41.

Palmer, G., Bonjour, J. P., and Caverzasio, J. (1997). Expression of a newly identified phosphate transporter/retrovirus receptor in human SaOS-2 osteoblast-like cells and its regulation by insulin-like growth factor I. *Endocrinology* **138**, 5202–5209.

Palmer, G. *et al.* (2000). Transforming growth factor-beta stimulates inorganic phosphate transport and expression of the type III phosphate transporter Glvr-1 in chondrogenic ATDC5 cells. *Endocrinology* **141**, 2236–2243.

Patel, M. S. and Karsenty, G. (2002). Regulation of bone formation and vision by LRP5. *New England Journal of Medicine* **346**, 1572–1574.

Piwon, N. *et al.* (2000). ClC-5 Cl^--channel disruption impairs endocytosis in a mouse model for Dent's disease. *Nature* **408**, 369–373.

Pizurki, L. *et al.* (1991). Stimulation by parathyroid hormone-related protein and transforming growth factor-alpha of phosphate transport in osteoblast-like cells. *Journal of Bone and Mineral Research* **6**, 1235–1241

Pontoglio, M. *et al.* (2000). HNF1alpha controls renal glucose reabsorption in mouse and man. *EMBO Reports* **1**, 359–365.

Prabhu, S. *et al.* (1997). Effect of glucocorticoids on neonatal rabbit renal cortical sodium-inorganic phosphate messenger RNA and protein abundance. *Pediatric Research* **41**, 20–24.

Prie, D. *et al.* (1998). Dipyridamole decreases renal phosphate leak and augments serum phosphorus in patients with low renal phosphate threshold. *Journal of the American Society of Nephrology* **9**, 1264–1269.

Prie, D. *et al.* (2001a). P-glycoprotein inhibitors stimulate renal phosphate reabsorption in rats. *Kidney International* **60**, 1069–1076.

Prie, D. *et al.* (2001b). Frequency of renal phosphate leak among patients with calcium nephrolithiasis. *Kidney International* **60**, 272–276.

Prié, P. *et al.* (2002). Nephrolithiasis and osteoporosis associated with hypophosphatemia caused by mutations in the type 2a sodium phosphate cotransporter. *New England Journal of Medicine* **347**, 983–991.

Quinn, J. M. *et al.* (2001). Transforming growth factor beta affects osteoclast differentiation via direct and indirect actions. *Journal of Bone and Mineral Research* **16**, 1787–1794.

Reichenberger, E. *et al.* (2001). Autosomal dominant craniometaphyseal dysplasia is caused by mutations in the transmembrane protein ANK. *American Journal of Human Genetics* **68**, 1321–1326.

Riccardi, D. *et al.* (2000). Dietary phosphate and parathyroid hormone alter the expression of the calcium-sensing receptor (CaR) and the Na+-dependent Pi transporter (NaPi-2) in the rat proximal tubule. *Pflugers Archiv: European Journal of Physiology* **441**, 379–387.

Ritthaler, T. *et al.* (1999). Effects of phosphate intake on distribution of type II Na/Pi cotransporter mRNA in rat kidney. *Kidney International* **55**, 976–983.

Rodrigues, P. and Heard, J. M. (1999). Modulation of phosphate uptake and amphotropic murine leukemia virus entry by posttranslational modifications of PIT-2. *Journal of Virology* **73**, 3789–3799.

Sabbagh, Y., Jones, A. O., and Tenenhouse, H. S. (2000). PHEXdb, a locus-specific database for mutations causing X-linked hypophosphatemia. *Human Mutation* **16**, 1–6.

Salaün, C., ed. Structure du récepteur du rétrovirus murin amphotrope/transporteur de phosphate PiT-2: topologie, assemblages quaternaires et modulations in situ par le phosphate, Paris: Université Paris VI Pierre et Marie Curie, 2001.

Salaün, C., Rodrigues, P., and Heard, J. M. (2001). Transmembrane topology of PiT-2, a phosphate transporter-retrovirus receptor. *Journal of Virology* **75**, 5584–5592.

Sayer, J. A. and Pearce, S. H. (2001). Diagnosis and clinical biochemistry of inherited tubulopathies. *Annals of Clinical Biochemistry* **38**, 459–470.

Schell, M. J. *et al.* (1999). PiUS (Pi uptake stimulator) is an inositol hexakisphosphate kinase. *FEBS Letter* **461**, 169–172.

Segawa, H. *et al.* (2002). Growth-related renal type II Na/Pi cotransporter. *Journal of Biological Chemistry* **277**, 19665–19672.

Seufert, J. *et al.* (2001). Octreotide therapy for tumor-induced osteomalacia. *New England Journal of Medicine* **345**, 1883–1888.

Shenolikar, S. *et al.* (2002). Targeted disruption of the mouse NHERF-1 gene promotes internalization of proximal tubule sodium phosphate cotransporter type IIa and renal phosphate wasting. *Proceedings of the National Academy of Sciences of the United States of America* **99**, 11470–11475.

Shimada, T. *et al.* (2001). Cloning and characterization of FGF23 as a causative factor of tumor-induced osteomalacia. *Proceedings of the National Academy of Sciences of the United States of America* **98**, 6500–6505.

Silve, C. and Beck, L. (2002). Is FGF23 the long sought after phosphaturic factor phosphatonin? *Nephrology, Dialysis, Transplantation* **17**, 958–961.

Silve, C. and Friedlander, G. Renal Regulation of Phosphate excretion. In *The Kidney* (ed. D. Seldin and G. Giebisch), pp. 1885–1904. Philadelphia: Lippincott Williams-Wilkins, 2000.

Stewart, A. and Broadus, A. Mineral Metabolism. In *Endocrinology and Metabolism* (ed. P. Felig, J. D. Baxter, A. E. Broadus, and L. A. Frohmn), pp. 1317–1453. New York: McGraw-Hill Book Company, 1987.

Strewler, G. J. (2000). The physiology of parathyroid hormone-related protein. *New England Journal of Medicine* **342**, 177–185.

Strewler, G. J. (2001). FGF23, hypophosphatemia, and rickets: has phosphatonin been found? *Proceedings of the National Academy of Sciences of the United States of America* **98**, 5945–5946.

Subramanian, R. and Khardori, R. (2000). Severe hypophosphatemia. Pathophysiologic implications, clinical presentations, and treatment. *Medicine (Baltimore)* **79**, 1–8.

Suda, T. *et al.* (2001). The molecular basis of osteoclast differentiation and activation. *Novartis Foundation Symposium* **232**, 235–247; discussion 47–50.

Suki, W., Lederer, E. D., and Rouse, D. Renal transport of calcium, magnesium, and phosphate. In *The Kidney* (ed. B. BM), pp. 520–574. Philadelphia: W.B. Saunders, 2000.

Sutters, M., Gaboury, C. L., and Bennett, W. M. (1996). Severe hyperphosphatemia and hypocalcemia: a dilemma in patient management. *Journal of the American Society of Nephrology* **7**, 2056–2061.

Suzuki, A. *et al.* (2000). Stimulation of sodium-dependent phosphate transport and signaling mechanisms induced by basic fibroblast growth factor in MC3T3-E1 osteoblast-like cells. *Journal of Bone and Mineral Research* **15**, 95–102.

Suzuki, A. *et al.* (2001). Stimulation of sodium-dependent inorganic phosphate transport by activation of Gi/o-protein-coupled receptors by epinephrine in MC3T3-E1 osteoblast-like cells. *Bone* **28**, 589–594.

Taketani, Y. *et al.* (1998). Regulation of type II renal Na+-dependent inorganic phosphate transporters by 1,25-dihydroxyvitamin D3. Identification of a vitamin D-responsive element in the human NAPi-3 gene. *Journal of Biological Chemistry* **273**, 14575–14581.

Tatsumi, S. *et al.* (1998). Identification of three isoforms for the Na+-dependent phosphate cotransporter (NaPi-2) in rat kidney. *Journal of Biological Chemistry* **273**, 28568–28575.

Tenenhouse, H. S. *et al.* (1998). Differential expression, abundance, and regulation of Na+-phosphate cotransporter genes in murine kidney. *American Journal of Physiology* **275**, F527–F534.

Thakker, R. V. (2000). Pathogenesis of Dent's disease and related syndromes of X-linked nephrolithiasis. *Kidney International* **57**, 787–793.

Thakker, R. V. (2001). Genetic developments in hypoparathyroidism. *Lancet* **357**, 974–976.

Thatte, L. *et al.* (1995). Review of the literature: severe hyperphosphatemia. *The American Journal of the Medical Sciences* **310**, 167–174.

Traebert, M. *et al.* (2000). Luminal and contraluminal action of 1–34 and 3–34 PTH peptides on renal type IIa Na-P(i) cotransporter. *American Journal of Physiology. Renal, Fluid and Electrolyte Physiology* **278**, F792–F798.

Turner, A. J. and Tanzawa, K. (1997). Mammalian membrane metallopeptidases: NEP, ECE, KELL, and PEX. *FASEB Journal* **11**, 355–364.

Usdin, T. B. *et al.* (2000). New members of the parathyroid hormone/parathyroid hormone receptor family: the parathyroid hormone 2 receptor and tuberoinfundibular peptide of 39 residues. *Frontiers in Neuroendocrinology* **21**, 349–383.

van den Heuvel, L. *et al.* (2001). Autosomal recessive hypophosphataemic rickets with hypercalciuria is not caused by mutations in the type II renal sodium/phosphate cotransporter gene. *Nephrology, Dialysis, Transplantation* **16**, 48–51.

Van Esch, H. and Devriendt, K. (2001). Transcription factor GATA3 and the human HDR syndrome. *Cellular and Molecular Life Sciences* **58**, 1296–1300.

Vrtovsnik, F. *et al.* (1994). Glucocorticoid inhibition of Na-Pi cotransport in renal epithelial cells is mediated by protein kinase C. *Journal of Biological Chemistry* **269**, 8872–8877.

Walton, R. J. and Bijvoet, O. L. (1975). Nomogram for derivation of renal threshold phosphate concentration. *Lancet* **2**, 309–310.

Weinstein, L. S., Chen, M., and Liu, J. (2002). Gs(alpha) mutations and imprinting defects in human disease. *Annals of the New York Academy of Sciences* **968**, 173–197.

Werner, A. and Kinne, R. K. (2001). Evolution of the Na-P(i) cotransport systems. *American Journal of Physiology. Regulatory, Integrative and Comparative Physiology* **280**, R301–R312.

Wesson, L. G. (1997). Homeostasis of phosphate revisited. *Nephron* **77**, 249–266.

White, K. E. *et al.* (1998). A PDZ domain-containing protein with homology to diphor-1 maps to human chromosome 1q21. *Annals of Human Genetics* **62** (Pt 4), 287–290.

Xan, H. J., Kim, D. H., and Park, S. H. (2000). Regulatory mechanisms of Na/Pi cotransporter by glucocorticoid in renal proximal tubule cells: involvement of cAMP and PKC. *Kidney & Blood Pressure Research* **23**, 1–9.

Xu, H. *et al.* (2002). Age-dependent regulation of rat intestinal type IIb sodium phosphate cotransporter by 1,25-(OH)(2) vitamin D(3). *American Journal of Physiology. Cell Physiology* **282**, C487–C493.

Zhang, M. Y. *et al.* (2002). Dietary phosphorus transcriptionally regulates 25-hydroxyvitamin D-1alpha-hydroxylase gene expression in the proximal renal tubule. *Endocrinology* **143**, 587–595.

2.5 Hypo–hypermagnesaemia

John H. Dirks

Normal magnesium metabolism

Magnesium is the second most abundant intracellular cation in the body (Dirks *et al.* 1996; Yu 2000). Normal serum Mg^{2+} concentration is 1.7–2.3 mg/dl or 0.75–1.00 mmol/l (1.3–1.9 mEq/l) of which 70–80 per cent is ultrafiltrable, 60–70 per cent being ionized and 10 per cent complexed to citrate, bicarbonate, and phosphate (Dirks *et al.* 1996) (Table 1). About 20–30 per cent of serum Mg^{2+} is bound to protein, largely albumin. The percentage varies with albumin concentration, and requires correction as serum albumin falls. Serum ionized Mg^{2+} as measured by Mg^{2+}sensitive electrodes can range from 0.45 to 0.67 mmol/l. The total Mg^{2+} in the extracellular fluid represents only 1 per cent of total body Mg^{2+} (around 24 gm or 1000 mmol). The largest portion of Mg^{2+} is found in mineralized bone (50–60 per cent); 40–50 per cent resides in cells, chiefly in muscle tissue and also in soft tissue cells. About half the bone storage of Mg^{2+} is slowly available for exchange with the extracellular fluid. Cellular Mg^{2+} concentration ranges from 10 to 12 mmol/l, but recent intracellular measurements have demonstrated that free ionized Mg^{2+} in cells is approximately 0.5 mmol, the remainder being bound to intracellular macromolecules, membranes, and enzymes. Mg^{2+} affects intracellular function including the transport of K^+ and Ca^{2+}, and modulates signal transduction, energy metabolism, and cell proliferation. Intracellular Mg^{2+} plays a critical role in the function of many intracellular enzymes such as Na^+,K^+-ATPase. The free intracellular Mg^{2+} concentration is approximately equal to the extracellular fluid Mg^{2+} concentration, so there is little concentration gradient. A hallmark of total cellular Mg^{2+} concentration is that it equilibriates very slowly with changes in ionized extracellular fluid Mg^{2+}, a process involving hours to days or weeks. Therefore, it is difficult to assess Mg^{2+}stores from tissue Mg^{2+} measurement when serum Mg^{2+} changes.

Table 1 Summary of magnesium facts

Magnesium chemistry
Atomic number 12
Mass 24 Da
1 mmol = 24 mg
1 mEq = 12 mg
Serum
1.7–2.3 mg/dl
0.75–1.00 mmol/l
1.3–1.9 mEq/l
Ionized 60–70%
Complexed 10%
Protein bound 20–30%

Overall, body Mg^{2+} homeostasis is shown in Fig. 1 (Quamme *et al.* 1980; Suki *et al.* 2000; Yu 2001). The average daily Mg^{2+} intake in North America is approximately 300–360 g or 12–14 mmol, obtained primarily from vegetables, grain cereals, fish, and meat. Intake in females is somewhat lower at 280–300 mg. It is often considered that the average daily Mg^{2+} intake in Western populations is currently at a low limit for maintaining balance, health, and well being. This may be particularly true for neonates, infants undergoing surgery, and the ageing population, especially old people in chronic care institutions. The intestinal tract reabsorbs 30–50 per cent of normal Mg^{2+} intake but absorption can vary from a low of 20 per cent to a high of 70–80 per cent during severe Mg^{2+} deficiency depending on body intake and need. The active vitamin D metabolite, calcitriol, has not been conclusively shown to augment Mg^{2+} reabsorption whereas it does not result in a specific increase in intestinal reabsorption of Ca^{2+} and PO_4^{2-}. Magnesium is also secreted into the colon, partially offsetting overall absorption and this accounts for significant losses during acute and chronic diarrhoea especially with a loss of large volume of fluids (Hodgkinson *et al.* 1979).

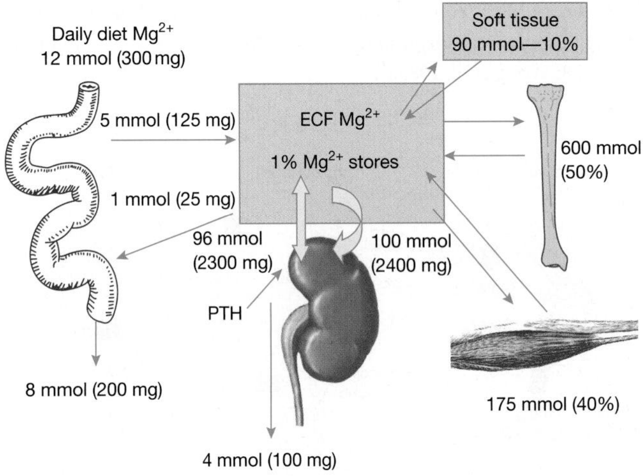

Fig. 1 A schematic diagram of normal magnesium metabolism showing the relationship of the extracellular fluid (ECF) ionized Mg^{2+} concentration to diet and gastrointestinal (GI) absorption to various tissues with percentage of body stores of Mg^{2+} in the body and to the kidney.

The overall intestinal absorption of 100 mg of Mg^{2+} is then balanced by a similar amount of Mg^{2+} renal excretion. The role of Mg^{2+} is widely discussed in the literature in terms of its relationship to a variety of chronic diseases, including diabetes mellitus (White *et al.* 1993), thrombotic disorders, atherosclerosis, coronary artery disease, hypertension, asthma, Sudden Infant Death Syndrome, and migraine and will not be discussed here (Al-Rasheed *et al.* 2000; Alamoudi 2001). Further, Mg^{2+} is used extensively in the treatment of acute and chronic cardiac disease with generally positive results, but the data remain inconclusive concerning the benefits of Mg^{2+} in reducing morbidity and mortality (Alamoudi 2000, 2001; Agus *et al.* 2001).

Renal magnesium reabsorption

Approximately 100 mmol Mg^{2+} is filtered in 24 h. Seventy to eighty per cent of this serum Mg^{2+} is filtered at the glomerulus, about 3 per cent or about 4 mmol (100 mg) is excreted in the urine, and approximately 96 mmol is reabsorbed by the renal tubules. The amount excreted can vary considerably from less than 1 mmol during a state of marked hypomagnesaemia and Mg^{2+} depletion to a value close to the filtered load during extreme hypermagnesaemia. Net tubular secretion of Mg^{2+} has not been demonstrated in the mammalian nephron. Normal Mg^{2+} reabsorption is illustrated in Fig. 2. The proximal convoluted tubules reabsorb 10–15 per cent of the filtered Mg^{2+}, the thick ascending limb (TAL) of the loop of Henle absorbs 60–70 per cent and 10–15 per cent is infused into the distal nephron, the latter determining the final amount of Mg^{2+} excreted. Figure 2 contrasts Na^+ and Ca^{2+} reabsorption with Mg^{2+} reabsorption and indicates relatively lower Mg^{2+} reabsorption in the proximal tubule and relatively higher Mg^{2+} absorption in the TAL, with similar reabsorption rates in the distal nephron. However, as will be discussed, Mg^{2+} and Ca^{2+} have a competitive interaction in the TAL, causing a reduction in each other's reabsorption (Sutton *et al.* 1996; Yu 2001; Satoh and Romero 2002).

Previously, it was concluded that there was a transport maximum (T_m) for magnesium reabsorption, but this turned out to be a fortuitous occurrence of increased proximal tubule and decreased TAL Mg^{2+} transport at high rates of Mg^{2+} infusion resulting in progressively higher serum Mg^{2+} concentrations. However, it is useful to consider an apparent tubular reabsorption maximum (Massry *et al.* 1969; Quamme *et al.* 1978; Wong *et al.* 1983a).

The proximal tubule permeability to Mg^{2+} is low and the overall reabsorption appears to depend passively on salt and water reabsorption. Magnesium reabsorption in the proximal tubule is influenced by the extracellular fluid volume that is reduced by volume expansion and increased by volume contraction. Proximal reabsorption also varies with luminal Mg^{2+} concentration. Osmotic diuretics such as mannitol reduce proximal Mg^{2+} reabsorption. As Mg^{2+} concentration rises, relatively more is reabsorbed. Reabsorption is more complete in hypomagnesaemia.

The major site of Mg^{2+} reabsorption is the TAL of the loop of Henle. Figure 3 illustrates the percentage of the delivered load reabsorbed during Mg^{2+} infusion in the perfused loop of Henle. Figure 4(a) shows Mg^{2+} is passively reabsorbed via the paracellular channels due to a lumen-positive transepithelial gradient generated by the luminal Na^+–K^+–$2Cl^-$ (or NKCC2) cotransporter and potassium recycling into the lumen. Magnesium reabsorption can readily be reduced by loop diuretics such as frusemide which inhibits the luminal Na^+–K^+–$2Cl^-$ cotransporter and reduces the lumen-positive potential, thus, in turn, reducing the passive flux across the paracellular channel. Figure 4(a) illustrates that Ca^{2+} is similarly passively reabsorbed in the TAL. It is now known that Ca^{2+} is regulated by the paracellular tight junction protein Paracellin-1, a member of the claudin family. This new information solves an interesting set of relationships between Ca^{2+} and Mg^{2+} excretion, so that hypercalcaemia or hypermagnesaemia can increase the excretion of both divalent ions (Fig. 3). This mechanism has been elucidated with the discovery of a calcium sensitive receptor (CaSR) on the basilar side of the TAL cell, sensitive to increased extracellular fluid Ca^{2+} or Mg^{2+} concentration, which activates the Ca^{2+} receptor. The receptor, in turn, activates cyclic AMP, or the arachidonic acid cascade to inhibit the luminal Na^+–K^+–$2Cl^-$ cotransporter and the apical potassium channel (ROMK), reducing the transepithelial positive potential and resulting in hypercalciuria and hypermagnesuria as passive Mg^{2+} and Ca^{2+} reabsorption across the paracellular pathway is progressively reduced. Recent information may also suggest some interaction between Ca^{2+} and Mg^{2+} at the level of the paracellular channel as the initial loop of Paracellin-1 is highly negatively charged, but specific details are not available as yet. Hypocalcaemia and hypomagnesuria can have the opposite effect on the Ca^{2+} sensor by deactivating the receptor, and relatively increasing transport across the TAL eliciting a more favourable positive potential and resulting in more complete Ca^{2+} or Mg^{2+} retention due to relatively greater passive reabsorption of Ca^{2+} and Mg^{2+} as illustrated in Fig. 4(a).

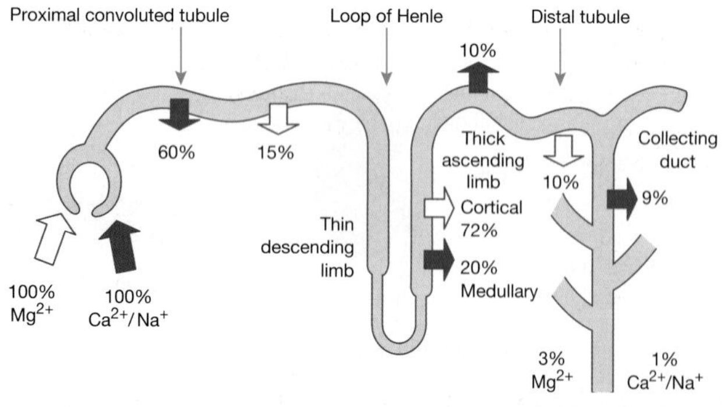

Fig. 2 A schematic nephron showing the relative rate of reabsorption of Mg^{2+} or Na^+/Ca^{2+} across the proximal convoluted tubular thick ascending limb of the loop of Henle and the distal convoluted tubule (DCT).

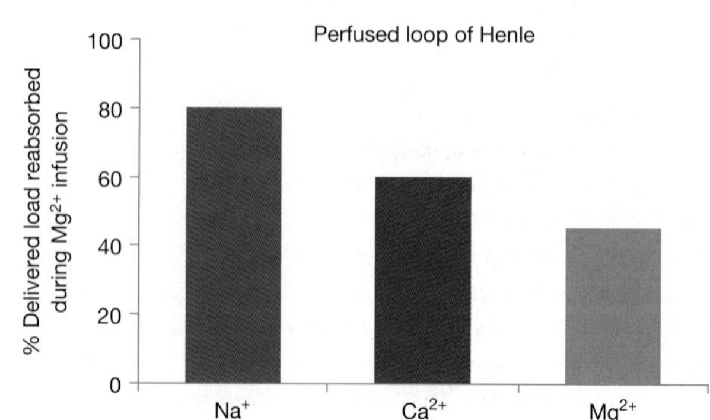

Fig. 3 Effect of Mg^{2+} infusion in the thick ascending limb (TAL) or Na^+, Ca^{2+}, and Mg^{2+} reabsorption as a percentage of the delivered load.

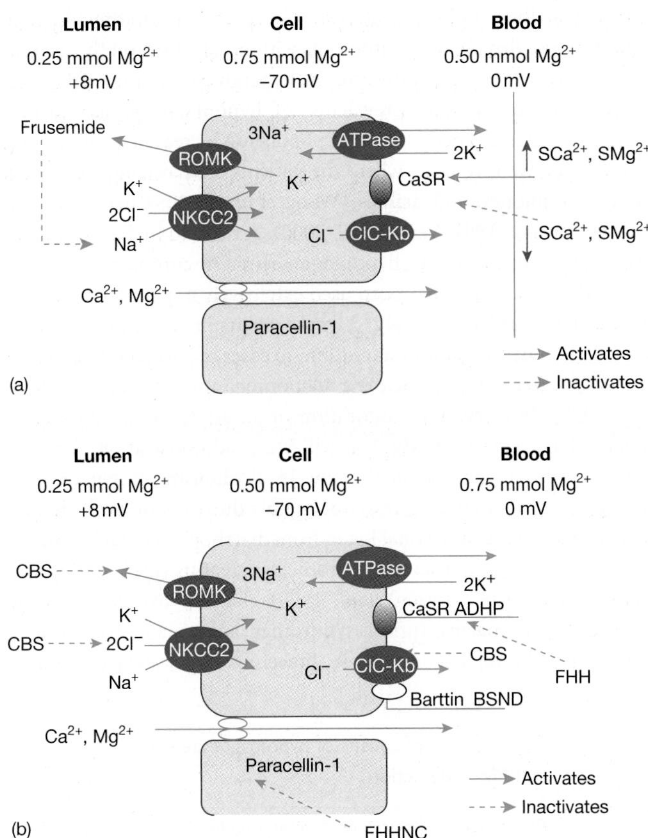

Fig. 4 A cellular model of Mg^{2+} handling in the thick ascending limb (TAL) demonstrating the luminal NKCC2 and ROMK transporter; the basilar Na^+,K^+-ATPase transport, the chloride channel (ClC-Kb), the calcium sensitive receptor (CaSR), and the paracellular Paracellin-1 (PCLN-1): (a) demonstrates the inhibitory effect of frusemide on NKCC2 and the inhibitory and activating effects of serum Ca^{2+} and Mg^{2+} concentrations affecting the sensitivity of CaSR and hence the absorption of Ca^{2+} and Mg^{2+}; (b) illustrates the inherited tubule disorders that affect TAL transporters and receptors. The acronyms for the inherited disorders are noted in Table 5.

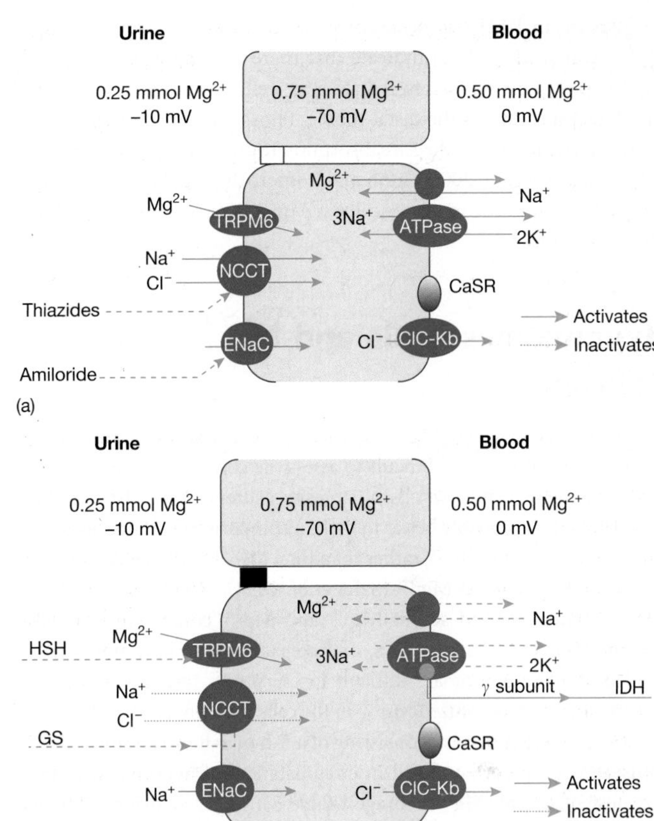

Fig. 5 A cellular model of magnesium handling in the distal convoluted tubule demonstrating the luminal thiazide sensitive Na^+–Cl^- transporter (NCCT), the luminal Mg^{2+}–Ca^{2+} channel TRPM6, the Na^+ channel ENaC, and the basilar Na^+,K^+-ATPase pump, the Mg^{2+}/Na^+ exchange and the chloride channel (ClC-Kb). (a) Depicts the normal function and inhibiting site of thiazide diuretics and amiloride; (b) depicts current understanding of inherited Mg^{2+} disorders and the site of affected mutations. The acronyms are noted in Table 5.

In the distal convoluted tubule, or DCT [Fig. 5(a)] (Quamme 1997), Mg^{2+} reabsorption is still significant and represents the fine control of Mg^{2+} excretion. Overall, distal Mg^{2+} reabsorption is transcellular and active. At the lumen, Mg^{2+} is passively absorbed on the luminal side due to favourable electrochemical gradients into the cell and passage via a Mg^{2+}–TRPM6 channel. Mg^{2+} is then discharged at the basilar side via a Mg^{2+}–Na^+ exchange process, dependent on the activity of Na^+,K^+-ATPase. The response of the calcium sensors to serum Mg^{2+} and Ca^{2+} concentrations may also affect net transcellular Mg^{2+} transport (Cole *et al.* 2000a). The complete details of Mg^{2+} reabsorption in the DCT are as yet undetermined. In particular, diffusion across the luminal membrane requires further investigation (Dai *et al.* 2001).

Table 2 lists the factors that can cause major changes in Mg^{2+} excretion alongside those that induce modest minor changes. Important changes include variation in extracellular fluid volume, serum Ca^{2+} and Mg^{2+} concentrations, and acid–base disturbances.

A variety of hormones including parathyroid hormone (PTH), calcitonin, vasopressin, prostaglandins, glucagon, insulin, and others increase TAL and DCT Mg^{2+} reabsorption with a minimum or no

Table 2 List of factors that increase and decrease Mg^{2+} excretion or, conversely decrease and increase tubular Mg^{2+} reabsorption

Increase	**Decrease**
Hypermagnesaemia	Hypomagnesaemia and Mg^{2+} depletion
Hypercalcaemia	Hypocalcaemia
Volume expansion	Volume contraction
Diuretics: loop, thiazide, osmotic	Diuretics: amiloride, spironolactone
Metabolic acidosis	Metabolic alkalosis
Phosphate depletion	Hyperparathyroidism
Carbohydrate, protein, alcohol ingestion	Hypothyroidism
Toxic	
Cisplatin	
Aminoglycosides	

effect on NaCl reabsorption (Dai *et al.* 1998a,b). In tissue culture, aldosterone increases distal Mg^{2+} transport (Dai *et al.* 1998b). Unlike Ca^{2+}, no hormone has been clearly identified as playing a significant physiological role in regulating serum Mg^{2+} concentration although an increase in PTH has been correlated with a decrease in ionized Mg^{2+}. Dai *et al.* (1997c) indicate that there are important effects of chronic metabolic acidosis in reducing, as well as alkalosis in increasing Mg^{2+} reabsorption in the distal tubule. Phosphate depletion has been shown to reduce distal Mg^{2+} reabsorption (Sutton *et al.* 1996; Dai *et al.* 1997c; Agarwal *et al.* 2000; Satoh and Romero 2002). Dai *et al.* (1997a) found that Amiloride increases cellular Mg^{2+} reabsorption by blocking the Na^{+} channel.

Hypomagnesaemia and Mg^{2+} deficiency

Hypomagnesaemia and Mg^{2+} deficiency are terms often used interchangeably as it remains difficult to assess the correlation between lowered serum Mg^{2+} and lower tissue stores measurements of Mg^{2+} (Alfrey *et al.* 1974). It is probably better to make a comparison with tissue Mg^{2+} using ionized serum Mg^{2+} rather than total Mg^{2+} that includes protein bound and complexed Mg^{2+} (Saha *et al.* 1998). However, correlation between lower ionized serum Mg^{2+} and Mg^{2+} content in red cells, mononuclear cells, lymphocytes, and skeletal muscle have not usually yielded good results or are difficult to carry out. Ideally, one should obtain a measure of ionized Mg^{2+} in the cells (Martini *et al.* 2001).

A Mg^{2+} retention test, consisting of a 5-h or 1-h intravenous Mg^{2+} infusion is frequently utilized in circumstances of hypomagnesaemia as a test of overall Mg^{2+} storage (Table 3). Mg^{2+} deficient patients retain a greater fraction of an intravenously administered level of Mg^{2+} and excrete relatively less Mg^{2+} in the urine over a time period than do normal patients (Ryzen *et al.* 1985). The Mg^{2+} retention test is not valid in patients who have renal Mg^{2+} wasting. There is considerable overlap between normal and moderately Mg^{2+} deficient patients. Therefore, the Mg^{2+} retention test is usually more suitable for clinical research studies than in clinical practice. The detection of low serum Mg^{2+} concentration remains the best working tool to assess Mg^{2+} deficiency; particularly when considered in the context of urine Mg^{2+} excretion (Carney *et al.* 1980). If serum Mg^{2+} is low in the presence of urine Mg^{2+} of less than 0.5–1 mmol or 12–24 mg/day, a dietary deficiency or abnormally low gastrointestinal reabsorption is the likely cause. If urine Mg^{2+} is above 1.0 mmol or 24 mg/day, renal wasting is the likely cause of hypomagnesaemia and Mg^{2+} deficiency.

Aetiology of Mg^{2+} deficiency

Table 4 lists the causes of Mg^{2+} deficiency including low Mg^{2+} intake, reduced gastrointestinal absorption, increased renal Mg^{2+} wasting as well as clinical situations with multifactoral causes (Dacey 2001). Hypomagnesaemia may occur due to redistribution of Mg^{2+} between extracellular fluid and tissue stores, as occurs with noradrenaline or insulin release driving Mg^{2+} into cells without an effect on the overall Mg^{2+} balance. Hypomagnesaemia in hyperglycaemia may delay the disposal of glucose. The prevalence of hypomagnesaemia reaches 10–15 per cent in a general inpatient population increasing to 50–70 per cent in intensive care units where the patients are receiving parenteral therapy, antibiotics, and dialysis (Wong *et al.* 1983b; Chernow *et al.* 1989; Aglio *et al.* 1991; Verive *et al.* 2000). A twofold higher mortality rate has been attributed to hypomagnesaemia in coronary care units where Mg^{2+} treatment has been used extensively in patients with cardiovascular disorders. Low Mg^{2+} intake occurs in geographic areas of general malnutrition and in starvation, in cases of parenteral nutrition with Mg^{2+} free fluid, nasogastric suctioning, and alcoholism (Elisaf *et al.* 1995). In starvation, restoration of an adequate dietary Mg^{2+} intake will correct serum Mg^{2+} as will Mg^{2+} administration in Mg^{2+} deficiency due to parenteral therapy. In alcoholism, 25 per cent or more patients are hypomagnesaemic mainly due to poor Mg^{2+} intake but also due to gastrointestinal losses from diarrhoea, acute renal Mg^{2+} wasting, and associated acute or chronic pancreatitis (Dick *et al.* 1969; Bohmer *et al.* 1982; Ryzen *et al.* 1990). Table 4 lists an array of gastrointestinal malabsorption syndromes accompanied by Mg^{2+} deficiency including coeliac disease, bowel fistulae, watery diarrhoea,

Table 3 List of considerations for the evaluation of body Mg^{2+} status

Serum Mg^{2+} concentration
Cellular measurements
Mg^{2+} retention test
Urine Mg^{2+} excretion as related to low serum Mg^{2+}

Table 4 List of causes of hypomagnesaemia and Mg^{2+} depletion

Redistribution (extracellular to cells—no tissue Mg^{2+} deficiency)
Catecholamine excess states
Insulin administration
Acute respiratory alkalosis
Reduced intake
Starvation, malnutrition, alcoholism
Reduced gastrointestinal absorption
Specific Mg^{2+} malabsorption
Generalized malabsorption syndromes
Extensive bowel resections, fistula
Chronic diarrhoea, laxative abuse
Renal
Inherited Mg^{2+} tubular defects (see Table 5)
Drug-induced tubular defects
Cisplatin, amphotericin, pentamidine
Aminogycosides, cyclosporin, foscarnet
Renal tubular acidosis
Diabetic ketoacidosis, hyperalimentation
Diuretic therapy
Diuretic phase of acute tubular necrosis
Postobstructive diuresis
Hyperaldosteronism
Hypercalcaemia and hyperparathyroidism
Postrenal transplant
General
Chronic alcoholism
Acute pancreatitis
Major burns
Hungry bone syndrome (postparathyroidectomy)
Syndrome of inappropriate ADHP secretion
Excessive lactation and sweating

and various steatorrhoeas (LaSala *et al.* 1985). Short bowel due to surgical procedures for obesity may lead to major symptomatic Mg^{2+} depletion (Dyckner *et al.* 1982a; Fagan *et al.* 2001). A rare disease, primary infantile hypomagnesaemia is a recessively inherited intestinal defect in Mg^{2+} absorption (Friedman *et al.* 1967; Paunier *et al.* 1968; Larner *et al.* 2001; Kantorovich *et al.* 2002). The disorder usually presents in early infancy with tetany or seizures accompanied by severe hypomagnesaemia and hypocalcaemia. The hypocalcaemia is secondary to hypomagnesaemia, which can suppress the normal secretion of PTH and can be associated with bone resistance to PTH. Such infants usually respond to high dose oral or parenteral Mg^{2+} supplementation, even though diarrhoea is readily provoked. Slow Mg^{2+} administration using nocturnal nasogastric feeding has been successfully instituted mitigating the attendant diarrhoea (Cole *et al.* 2000b). Recent studies indicate that renal Mg^{2+} wasting may also be present as Mg^{2+} infusion results in a higher than expected Mg^{2+} excretion. A mutation has recently been identified in the gene for the mucosal Mg^{2+} channel TRPM6 in both the intestine and the distal tubule (Jin-no *et al.* 1999; Schlingmann *et al.* 2002).

In acute pancreatitis, saponification with Mg^{2+} and Ca^{2+} from necrotic fat tissue may account for low Mg^{2+}. Cutaneous losses following major burns or excess loss of sweat during long distance running can deplete body Mg^{2+} storage. Lactation can lead to Mg^{2+} deficiency.

In all instances of extrarenal Mg^{2+} loss leading to hypomagnesaemia and Mg^{2+} deficiency, urine Mg^{2+} excretion is low and reflects avid renal retention of Mg^{2+}.

Renal Mg^{2+} wasting

Hypomagnesaemia accompanied by an inappropriately high rate of renal Mg^{2+} excretion indicates renal Mg^{2+} wasting. A 24-h urine with more than 1 mmol of Mg^{2+} (24 mg) coincident with a serum Mg^{2+} less than 0.53 mmol/l (1.3 mg/dl) points to renal wasting conditions. Table 4 summarizes the causes of renal Mg^{2+} wasting due to polyuric states as in diabetic ketoacidosis with severe hyperglycaemia, postobstructive diuresis with high excretion of urea, the recovery phase of acute tubular necrosis, ATN, and osmotic diuresis due to mannitol infusion. More commonly, extracellular fluid expansion, if sustained, increases Mg^{2+} excretion along with other electrolytes such as potassium. Similarly, hyperalimentation can cause Mg^{2+} deficiency if Mg^{2+} replacement is neglected. Secondary sustained volume expansion due to mineralocorticoid excess such as in primary hypoaldosteronism or due to various causes of the syndrome of inappropriate antidiuretic hormone (SIADH) can also induce modest Mg^{2+} wasting. Following correction of metabolic acidosis, hypomagnesaemia may result from Mg^{2+} shifts into cells. Renal Mg^{2+} wasting occurs in distal tubular acidosis (Bianchetti *et al.* 1993). Loop diuretics such as frusemide increase Mg^{2+} and Ca^{2+} excretion and can lead to mild Mg^{2+} deficiency. Thiazide diuretics inhibit the neutral NaCl transporter in the DCT and during acute diuresis Mg^{2+} excretion can increase sufficiently to cause hypomagnesaemia. Hypomagnesaemia tends to wear off as the diuretic action of thiazide dissipates.

Inherited tubular disorders

While rare, the number of inherited tubular Mg^{2+} disorders is increasing providing new insights into the normal transport of Mg^{2+} (Cole *et al.* 2000a; Sayer *et al.* 2001; Konrad *et al.* 2003). These inherited disorders are listed in Table 5, and are depicted for nephron sites in Figs 4(b) and 5(b) for the DCT.

Abnormalities of the TAL

The TAL transporters' disorders (see also Chapter 5.5)

Classical Bartter's syndrome (CBS) (see Chapter 5.4) with salt depletion, hyperreninaemia, hyperaldosteronism, and hypokalaemic metabolic alkalosis, but normal blood pressure is due to any one of three inactivating mutations in the TAL: the apical luminal Na^+–K^+–$2Cl^-$ cotransporters (BSC-1); the apical inwardly rectifying K^+ channel (ROMK-1); or the basilar Cl^- channel (ClC-Kb) (Simon *et al.* 1996a,b, 1997; Zelikovic *et al.* 2003). All mutations cause hypercalciuria, but only one-third of patients are magnesuric and hypomagnesaemic. The difference between Ca^{2+} and Mg^{2+} excretions remain unclear. Vasodilator prostaglandins (E2 and prostacyclin) released in Bartter's syndrome may account for normal blood pressure and increased Mg^{2+} reabsorption in the distal nephron. Antenatal Bartter's syndrome with sensineural deafness and marked salt loss at birth, hypercalciuria and nephrocalcinosis is due to a gene mutation in a protein, Bartin, a β-subunit of the basilar chloride channel (ClC-Kb) (Dai *et al.* 2001). Hypomagnesaemia does not occur in antenatal Bartter's syndrome (BSND) (Sayer *et al.* 2001; Konrad *et al.* 2003).

Calcium sensor receptor disorders

Normally, hypermagnesaemia and hypercalcaemia directly induce renal Mg^{2+} and Ca^{2+} wasting by activating the TAL Ca^{2+} sensors so as to reduce paracellular Mg^{2+} and Ca^{2+} passage (Pollack *et al.* 1993). This may be offset by increased DCT Mg^{2+} reabsorption due to PTH. In familial hypocalciuric hypercalcaemia (FHH), an autosomal recessive disease, inactivating mutations in the Ca^{2+} receptors of the parathyroid gland and the DTAL result in hypercalcaemia, hypermagnesaemia,

Table 5 List of inherited tubular disorders that affect Mg^{2+} excretion according to nephron sites

Thick ascending limb
TAL transporters
In Classic Bartter's syndrome (CBS)
Mutations in TAL transporters: NKCC2, ROMK, and ClC-Kb
Antenatal Bartter's syndrome with sensorineural deafness (BSND)
Mutation in Bartin at ClC-Kb
Calcium sensor receptor disorders (CaSR)
Activating mutations
Autosomal dominant hypoparathyroidism (ADHP)
Inactivating mutations
Familial hypocalciuric hypercalcaemia (FHH)
Paracellin-1 (PCLN-1)
Familial hypomagnesaemia with hypercalciuria and nephrocalcinosis (FHHNC)
Distal convoluted tubule
Gitelman's syndrome (GS)
Mutations in thiazide sensitive cotransporter (NCCT)
Isolated dominant hypomagnesaemia with hypocalciuria (IDH)
Mutation in δ-subunit of ATPase
Hypomagnesaemia with secondary hypocalcaemia (HSH)
Mutation in TRPM6–Mg^{2+} channel

hypocalciuria, and hypomagnesuria (Kristiansen *et al.* 1985; Pollack *et al.* 1993). In FHH, a higher serum Ca^{2+} or Mg^{2+} is required to sensitize the receptor. The parathyroid glands may be enlarged, but a parathyroidectomy does not help. The infantile autosomal dominant form causes hyperparathyroidism with hypercalcaemia, hypercalciuria, polyuria, and magnesuria. On the other hand, activating mutations of the Ca^{2+} sensors cause autosomal dominant hypoparathyroidism (ADHP) (Pollack *et al.* 1994; Pearce *et al.* 1996). Such patients are mildly hypomagnesaemic due to Mg^{2+} wasting. Calcimimetic agents restore CaSR sensitivity in patients with primary and secondary hyperparathyroidism and further investigation is required to determine the role of calcimimetics in FHH (Coburn *et al.* 1999).

Paracellin disorders

Considerable interest is focused on familial hypomagnesaemic hypercalciuria with nephrocalcinosis (FHHNC), which consists of polyuria, hypermagnesuria, hypomagnesaemia, and hypercalciuria with severe nephrocalcinosis (Nicholson *et al.* 1995; Praga *et al.* 1995; Torralbo *et al.* 1995; Simon *et al.* 1998, 1999; Al-Makadma 2000; Benigno *et al.* 2000; Monkawa *et al.* 2000; Blanchard *et al.* 2001; Weber *et al.* 2001; Wolf *et al.* 2002). This autosomal recessive disease is associated with urinary tract infections, nephrolithiasis, hyperuricaemia, hypokalaemia, and acidosis. Patients progress to chronic and eventually endstage renal failure due to nephrocalcinosis, interstitial fibrosis, and glomerular sclerosis. Recently, the deficit has been traced to the tight junction protein of the paracellular channels of TAL with an inactivating mutation in Paracellin-1, a member of the tight junction claudin 16 family. Ca^{2+} and Mg^{2+} movement across the paracellular channels is impaired with an attendant hypercalciuria and magnesuria. An array of mutations has been described. Treatment with thiazide and Mg^{2+} salts appears to be of no significant benefit. A successful renal transplant can cure the disease.

Abnormalities of the DCT

Gitelman's syndrome (see also Chapter 5.5)

The classical inherited disorder of DCT transporters is Gitelman's syndrome. It closely resembles Bartter's syndrome (Gitelman *et al.* 1966; Simon *et al.* 1996; Kamel *et al.* 1998; Schultheis *et al.* 1998; Barakat 2001; Schepkens *et al.* 2001). Both demonstrate the biochemical features of a response to volume contraction reflected by elevated serum renin, aldosterone, and angiotensin concentrations accompanied by hypokalaemic metabolic alkalosis, and normal blood pressure. Gitelman's syndrome differs from Bartter's syndrome in that the patients are always hypocalciuric (similar to chronic thiazide treatment) and, almost universally, hypermagnesuric, resulting in chronic hypomagnesaemia in almost 100 per cent of patients. An inactivating mutation in the luminal thiazide sensitive NaCl transport (NCCT or TSC) has been identified as the cause of Gitelman's syndrome. Hypocalciuria is explained by the increased Ca^{2+} reabsorption as the distal tubule cell is hyperpolarized due to reduced transport of NCCT allowing increased diffusion of Ca^{2+} into the cell and increased basilar reabsorption via Na^{+}–Ca^{2+} exchange or Ca^{2+}ATPase. Mg^{2+} reabsorption is similarly increased in cell cultures in the presence of thiazide, but this does not occur clinically in Gitelman's syndrome leaving the explanation of increased Mg^{2+} excretion unclear. The Mg^{2+} loss in Gitelman's syndrome is greater than during thiazide diuresis, suggesting the involvement of additional mechanisms. Some have suggested backflux across paracellular channels but the DCT has no paracellin. Altered function of the Ca^{2+}–Mg^{2+} channel TRPM6 is a possible explanation (Schlingmann *et al.* 2002). Gitelman's syndrome is considered a mild disease, but patients report chronic symptoms such as nocturia and paresthesias (Cruz *et al.* 2001).

Isolated dominant hypomagnesaemia with hypocalciuria

Recently, variants of Gitelman's syndrome reported in the Netherlands and Turkey (Schultheis *et al.* 1998; Meij *et al.* 2000; Kantorovich *et al.* 2002; Pantanetti *et al.* 2002) have been attributed to a mutation in the FXYD2 coding for the γ-subunit of Na^{+},K^{+}-ATPase. The syndrome of isolated dominant hypomagnesaemia with hypocalcaemia resembles Gitelman's syndrome despite the absence of metabolic alkalosis, elevated serum levels of renin, aldosterone, or angiotensin. In Turkey, a glycogenolysis II syndrome has been reported with hypomagnesaemia, hypercalcaemia, hypocalciuria, and osteopenia, again without the stigmata of volume depletion. The mechanism of the selective tubular disorder leading to hypomagnesaemia in these newly described conditions is currently unknown (Oktenli 2000).

Hypomagnesaemia with secondary hypocalcaemia

In some patients with primary infantile Mg^{2+} hypomagnesaemia (HSH), renal Mg^{2+} wasting may occur, which may result in seizures as well as other central nervous system abnormalities. A common deficit in the lumen Mg^{2+} channel and a mutation in TPRM6 were recently discovered (Schlingmann *et al.* 2002). It is noteworthy that high oral Mg^{2+} intake restored serum Mg^{2+} overcoming, in part, the defective Mg^{2+} channel (Walder *et al.* 2002). Further, Meij *et al.* (2003) recently described a new distal Mg^{2+} transport deficit not accounted for by the gene mutations known to be involved in Mg^{2+} transport (Meij *et al.* 2003). The exploration of genetic Mg^{2+} and Ca^{2+} disorders using molecular techniques and genetic probes is clearly increasing our fundamental understanding of cellular Mg^{2+} and Ca^{2+} transport with the prospect of new insights into inherited and acquired disease and the possibilities of more precise diagnosis and new treatment.

Drug induced tubular defects

Cisplatin is widely used for solid germinal cell tumours. Up to 90–100 per cent of patients develop hypomagnesaemia during prolonged treatment (Mavichak *et al.* 1985, 1988; Shah *et al.* 1991; Lajer *et al.* 1999; Lord 1999). Renal magnesuria often persists for a long time after Cisplatin is stopped but usually the hypomagnesaemia is mild and asymptomatic. Hypocalciuria also develops so that there is a strong resemblance to Gitelman's syndrome and to a dysfunction of the thiazide-sensitive neutral NaCl transporter. The Cisplatin analogue Carboplatin is less nephrotoxic (Ettinger *et al.* 1994). Amphotericin (Barton *et al.* 1984), the standard therapy for systemic fungal infections, can cause distal renal tubular acidosis with Mg^{2+} and K^{+} loss. Aminoglycosides cause Mg^{2+} and K^{+} wasting with hypomagnesaemia, hypocalcaemia, hypokalaemia, and tetany (Elliott *et al.* 2000). Renal Mg^{2+} wasting can occur after approximately 2 weeks and is dose related, but not specifically correlated with the occurrence of acute renal failure (the other major renal toxicity due to aminoglycosides). All aminoglycoside antibiotics including gentamicin, tobramycin, and amikacin, as well as neomycin, can produce renal Mg^{2+} wasting. Careful monitoring of therapeutic levels has reduced the incidence of aminoglycoside induced acute renal failure and renal Mg^{2+} wasting. Intravenous pentamidine frequently causes Mg^{2+} wasting (Mani 1992). Foscarnet, used to treat cytomegalovirus and chorioretinitis, can induce reversible renal Mg^{2+} wasting with hypocalcaemia and hypomagnesaemia (Palestine *et al.* 1991; Huycke *et al.* 2000). Renal transplant patients infrequently have Mg^{2+} depletion (Mazzaferro *et al.* 2002). Cyclosporin A can cause renal Mg^{2+} wasting as well as hypomagnesaemia and may account for periodic serious central nervous system symptoms like ataxia, tremor, depression, and dysphasia observed in patients treated with higher doses of cyclosporin (June *et al.* 1985; Barton *et al.* 1987; Vannini *et al.* 1999; Miura *et al.* 2002). Cyclosporin causes more severe neurotoxicity in the presence of a distal tubular deficit such as Gitelman's syndrome (Al-Rasheed *et al.* 2000; Miura *et al.* 2002). Tubulointerstitial nephropathy occasionally causes Mg^{2+} wasting. Overall, the astute clinician is always on the lookout for newer causes of Mg^{2+} loss and Mg^{2+} elevation (Scott *et al.* 1996).

General causes

In patients with hyperparathyroidism and severe osteitis fibrosa, requiring parathyroidectomy, a 'hungry bone syndrome' can occur rapidly after surgery with severe hypomagnesaemia, hypocalcaemia, and hypophosphataemia. The sudden decrease in circulatory PTH stops bone resorption, but bone formation continues so that Ca^{2+} and Mg^{2+} quickly enter the bone resulting in hypocalcaemia and hypomagnesaemia. Urgent and often massive parenteral Ca^{2+} and Mg^{2+} replacement is necessary until bone formation slows. It should be noted that hypomagnesaemia in childhood can lead to bone loss. Chronic alcoholism is perhaps the most common reason for Mg^{2+} deficiency and is due to poor Mg^{2+} intake, gastrointestinal losses due to diarrhoea, pancreatitis, and renal wasting due to tubular dysfunction that later resolves (Elisaf *et al.* 1995). Low dialysis bath fluids for both haemodialysis and peritoneal dialysis can bring about hypomagnesaemia, as can plasma exchange or continuous dialysis procedure. In cancer with chemotherapy, such as mycosis fungoides, serum levels of both Mg^{2+} and Ca^{2+} may be low (Morgan *et al.* 2002).

Clinical manifestations of Mg^{2+} deficiency

Clinical consequences of Mg^{2+} depletion are listed in Table 6 for cardiac, neuromuscular, central nervous system, and metabolic systems. Many patients with hypomagnesaemia are entirely asymptomatic for prolonged periods of time. Coexistent hypokalaemia and hypocalcaemia may induce several similar symptoms and signs such as enhanced neuromuscular irritability, making it difficult to know what to attribute specifically to hypomagnesaemia.

Table 6 List of clinical consequences of Mg^{2+} depletion

Cardiovascular
Ventricular arrhythmias: premature ventricular contractions
Increased susceptibility to digoxin arrhythmias
Ventricular tachycardia: Torsade de Pointes. Ventricular fibrillation
Atrial arrhythmias (rare): atrial fibrillation and atrial tachycardia
Hypertension
Coronary artery spasm
Sudden death
Neuromuscular
Weakness
Muscle fasciculations
Tremors and tetany
Positive Chvostek's and Trousseau's signs
Central nervous system
Apathy, depression
Anxiety
Delirium
Convulsions
Psychosis
Vertigo, nystagmus
Coma
Metabolic—responsive only to magnesium therapy
Refractory hypocalcaemia
Refractory hypokalaemia

Cardiovascular system

Mg^{2+} is an obligatory cofactor for the Na^+,K^+-ATPase responsible for pumping K^+ into the cell and hyperpolarizing the cell membrane. With Mg^{2+} deficiency, Na^+,K^+-ATPase function is impaired and intracellular K^+ falls. The relatively depolarized cell membrane is more predisposed to ectopic excitation and tachyarrhythmias. Further, the repolarization is delayed as demonstrated in electrocardiogram recordings, including prominent T-waves, U-waves, and prolonged QT or QU intervals (Loeb *et al.* 1968; Seller *et al.* 1970; Bashour *et al.* 1973; Chen *et al.* 1982; Ramee *et al.* 1985). Many studies suggest that hypomagnesaemia predisposes to tachyarrhythmia, particularly ventricular, and specifically to Torsades de Pointes and ventricular fibrillation (Table 6). In such cases, Mg^{2+} replacement is urgent (Agus *et al.* 2001). Digitalis toxicity-related arrhythmia is also unmasked by Mg^{2+} depletion. The true risk for arrhythmia among patients with hypomagnesaemia has not yet been defined. Several studies support the theory that patients are two to three times more likely to develop arrhythmia during the first two hospitalized days if they are hypomagnesaemic. Dyckner and Wester (1982b) presented two cases of ventricular tachycardia (VT) which received magnesium infusions that resulted in a significantly high retention of magnesium, VT attacks disappeared permanently in one case and temporarily in the other case according to skeletal muscle biopsies and blood samples taken before and after the Mg^{2+} infusion. Potassium depletion is a frequent associated disorder.

Neuromuscular system

Mg^{2+} blocks plasma membrane 2-type Ca^{2+} channels and intracellular Ca^{2+} release and is critical for sarcoplasmic reticular Ca^{2+}-ATPase, essential for muscle contraction in the presence of lower Mg^{2+} when an increase in skeletal muscle contractibility and delayed relaxation occurs. Enhanced neuromuscular irritability with tremor, muscle twitching, Trousseau's and Chvostek's signs, and obvious tetany are undoubtedly associated with hypomagnesaemia. The copresence of hypocalcaemia and hypokalaemic metabolic alkalosis exacerbates neuromuscular irritability.

Central nervous system (CNS) changes

Hypomagnesaemia may trigger an array of CNS symptoms including generalized, multi-focal, or clonic–tonic seizures. A loud noise can be a trigger stimulus. Other manifestations can be anxiety, depression, ataxia, psychosis, and coma as described in the literature in the case of hypomagnesaemic patients on cyclosporin. These symptoms improve after Mg^{2+} replacement (Fiset *et al.* 1996; Sutton *et al.* 1996; Schlingmann *et al.* 2002). The neuromuscular syndromes are more common in malabsorption and alcoholism but relate to the severity and the acuity of the hypomagnesaemia. Other electrolyte abnormalities such as hypokalaemia and hypocalcaemia may play a contributing role.

Metabolic disturbance

Hypokalaemia and potassium depletion are frequently associated with Mg^{2+} deficiency (Whang *et al.* 1985; Wong *et al.* 1985). In this situation, K^+ deficiency cannot be corrected until the Mg^{2+} deficiency is repaired. Hypomagnesaemia can reduce intracellular K^+ and also increase renal K^+ wasting. Hypocalcaemia occurs frequently in hypomagnesaemic patients and is not corrected until serum Mg^{2+} is restored. PTH response to a hypocalcaemic stimulus is impaired, circulatory levels of PTH and calcitriol are low, and the bone is resistant to PTH and vitamin D. The reason for inappropriately low PTH secretion is ascribed to an increase in the α-subunit of G proteins. Within 24 h of Mg^{2+} replacement, hypocalcaemia is corrected, and serum PTH levels rise.

Treatment of Mg^{2+} deficiency (Table 7)

Mg^{2+} deficiency should be prevented by supplementation in patients whose dietary intake is low or who are receiving parenteral nutrition without sufficient Mg^{2+}. Magnesium oxide pills (140 mg) three to four times per day supply 85 g of absorbable Mg^{2+} per tablet or 255–340 mg/day. A comparable parenteral maintenance dose is 8–10 mEq/day. Asymptomatic hypomagnesaemic patients can readily be treated, unless renal wasting is present in which case additional Mg^{2+} is required.

Table 7 An outline for the treatment of Mg^{2+} deficiency

Prevention: supplementation
If intake reduced or parenteral nutrition
Increase diet Mg^{2+}, or oral MgO, 140 mg 2–4 times per day
Mild deficiency
140 mg MgO 3–4 times per day
Amiloride 5–10 mg/day
Symptomatic
Urgent
1–2 g intravenous $MgSO_4 \cdot 7H_2O$ (2 ml = 1 g equivalent to 8 mEq or 100 mg of Mg^{2+}) in D/W, repeat if necessary; then slow intravenous infusion
Less urgent
48–64 mEq (6–8 g) intravenous in the first 24–48 h and followed by 24–32 mEq/day (3–4 g) for next 2–6 days

Generally, treatment is based on the degree of Mg^{2+} deficiency, urgency of clinical presentation, and state of renal function. Oral replacement is used for mild cases and for replacement of continuing Mg^{2+} losses once magnesium deficiency has been corrected. All oral Mg^{2+} salts eventually cause diarrhoea. Magnesium hydroxide and magnesium oxide are most generally used. The oral Mg^{2+} dose is titrated against Mg^{2+} losses in the stool and in patients with major Mg^{2+} malabsorption, high oral doses may be required (Adhiyaman *et al.* 2001). In renal Mg^{2+} wasting disorders, potassium-sparing diuretics such as amiloride and triamterene frequently reduce Mg^{2+} excretion to some extent resulting in milder Mg^{2+} wasting (Devane *et al.* 1981). The inactivation of the ENaC, or sodium channels, hyperpolarizes the distal tubule cell leading to increased Mg^{2+} reabsorption. Spironolactones can provoke a similar Mg^{2+} retaining response. Hypokalaemia and potassium depletion may need to be corrected concurrently. Potassium magnesium citrate has been used to correct both deficiencies (Ruml 1999; Pak 2000).

Intravenous replacement

The standard treatment of hospitalized patients relies on $MgSO_4 \cdot 7H_2O$. Each 2-ml ampoule of a 50 per cent solution contains 100 g (8 mEq) of elemental Mg^{2+}. The infusion rate is directly related to the urgency of the clinical situation. Rapid intravenous administration of 2–4 ml $MgSO_4$ in 50–100 ml saline or D/W is given over 2–5 min for a patient with cardiac arrhythmia or seizures, and repeated, if necessary. Thereafter, a slower rate of infusion is required as Mg^{2+} slowly moves into cells and half the administered dose is excreted in the urine. Thus, slower Mg^{2+} replacement allows better body Mg^{2+} retention. In a symptomatic patient, a deficit of 1–2 mEq/kg body weight is assumed and $MgSO_4$ is administered in progressively decreasing amounts over successive days beginning with 64 mEq (8 g) in the first 24 h and then 32 mEq (4 g) over the next 2–6 days. Mg^{2+} replacement is continued for 1–2 days after attaining normal serum Mg^{2+} so as to insure continued tissue repletion. In the presence of significant renal Mg^{2+} wasting, intravenous replacement should be augmented as much of the supplement is promptly expelled in the urine. If the glomerular filtration rate (GFR) is reduced, the Mg^{2+} infusion rate needs to be reduced by 25–50 per cent and serum Mg^{2+} should be measured frequently. Symptoms of hypermagnesaemia during replacement are demonstrated clinically by hypotension, signs of vasodilation such as facial flushing, and signs of neurogenic blockade with hyporeflexia and atrioventricular block (A–V block). Serum Ca^{2+} may fall as diffusible calcium sulfate is formed and excreted in the urine. In addition, urinary K^+ losses may result in hypokalaemia. Therefore, it may be necessary to slow Mg^{2+} correction and correct with $MgCl_2$. Serum Ca^{2+} and K^+ levels also may require correction.

Hypermagnesaemia

The body, with a normal kidney function, has a remarkable ability to increase Mg^{2+} excretion in response to a Mg^{2+} load. Very quickly, Mg^{2+} reabsorption is reduced in the TAL and DCT and only a modest increase in serum Mg^{2+} results. When renal function is reduced, hypermagnesaemia can readily appear. Mild elevations of serum Mg^{2+} occur in patients in intensive care units and dialysis centres. The causes of

Table 8 List of causes of hypermagnesaemia

Potentially serious
Renal failure–GFR < 30 ml/min
Acute
Chronic
Plus excess Mg^{2+} intake
Antacids, cathartics and enemas
Parenteral Mg overdose (e.g. preeclampsia)
Dialysis—accidental high bath Mg^{2+}
Mild to modest
Familial hypocalciuric hypercalcaemia
Hyperparathyroidism
Hypothyroidism
Lithium treatment
Addison's disease

hypermagnesaemia are listed in Table 8. Usually, hypermagnesaemia is mild in chronic as well as acute renal failure. When residual GFR is less than 30 ml/min and when magnesium intake is increased sharply due to large amounts of Mg^{2+}containing cathartics, enemas, or parenteral infusion or other sources, very serious hypermagnesaemia may develop (Ditzler 1970; Qureshi *et al.* 1996). The use of $MgSO_4$ in patients with preeclampsia and eclampsia has worked well. However, serum hypermagnesaemia can occur in the patient and the newborn, symptoms develop and treatment becomes urgent. Other common causes of hypermagnesaemia with benign clinical manifestations include primary hyperparathyroidism, hypothyroidism, Addison's disease, and lithium therapy (Christiansen *et al.* 1976).

Marked hypermagnesaemia is a serious and often fatal condition. Early symptoms and signs become evident at serum Mg^{2+} levels of 4–6 mg/dl and include hypotension, nausea, vomiting, and facial flushing. Higher levels of Mg^{2+} depress neuromuscular transmission of cardiac conduction and sympathetic ganglia. The hypermagnesaemic patient progresses to flaccid muscle paralysis, hyporeflexia, bradycardia, respiratory depression, coma, and cardiac arrest as serum Mg^{2+} rises to 10.0–20 mg/dl (5–10 mmol/l.) The cardiovascular toxic effects reflect a sequence of peripheral vasodilation and hypotension. Smooth muscle paralysis may occur in the small intestine and bladder. The electrocardiographic changes demonstrate prolonged PR, QRS, and QT intervals with non-specific T-wave changes resulting in bradycardia and heart block, culminating in asystolic cardiac arrest and death (Berns *et al.* 1976). These effects result from inhibition of acetylcholine release and are antagonized by Ca^{2+} salts, an important emergency treatment.

Treatment

Mild asymptomatic hypermagnesaemia requires no treatment except the removal of obvious extra sources of Mg^{2+} intake. A careful evaluation of unusual Mg^{2+} sources is often necessary. The return to normal serum Mg^{2+} is rapid due to renal Mg^{2+} excretion. Symptomatic elevations in serum Mg^{2+} with cardiovascular toxicity require acute intravenous administration of calcium gluconate, as the antagonist of Mg^{2+}. Injections of intravenous Ca^{2+} over a period of 5 min are repeated again if necessary. Simultaneously, renal Mg^{2+} excretion can be enhanced with forced volume expansion and intravenous administration of frusemide increasing Mg^{2+} excretion to approach that filtered. Careful replacement of urine losses of NaCl and K^+ are required. In an urgent situation, one should move rapidly to institute haemodialysis or peritoneal dialysis with a very low or zero bath Mg^{2+}. Dialysis rapidly reduces serum Mg^{2+} by 1/3 to 1/2 over 3.5 h. Repeated or continuous dialyses may be necessary (Kelber *et al.* 1994).

It is very important that all parenteral infusions and injections of Mg^{2+} and all Mg^{2+} containing medications be stopped at the beginning of treatment. Treatment of hypermagnesaemia is usually successful, but a significant number of deaths do occur every year as hypermagnesaemia may not be recognized early enough or the inadvertent source of Mg^{2+} is more than can be coped with. Our understanding of the role of Mg^{2+}, its disorders, and its treatment continues to advance.

References

(Entries marked with an asterisk comprise useful general reading.)

Adhiyaman, V., Adhiyaman, S., and Vaishnavi, A. (2001). Life-threatening hypomagnesemic hypocalcemia and hypokalemia in celiac disease. *American Journal of Gastroenterology* **96**, 3473 (letter).

Agarwal, R. and Knochel, J. P. Hypophosphatemia and hyperphosphatemia. In *Brenner and Rector's The Kidney* 6th edn. Vol. 1 (ed. Barry M. Brenner), pp. 1071–1125. Philadelphia, PA: W.B. Saunders Company, 2000.

Aglio, L. S. *et al.* (1991). Hypomagnesemia is common following cardiac surgery. *Journal of Cardiothoracic and Vascular Anesthesia* **5**, 201–208.

Agus, M. S. D. and Agus, Z. S. (2001). Cardiovascular actions of magnesium. *Critical Care Clinics* **17**, 175–186.

Alamoudi, O. S. B. (2000). Hypomagnesemia in stable asthmatics: prevalence, correlation with severity and hospitalization. *European Respiratory Journal* **16**, 427–431.

Alamoudi, O. S. B. (2001). Electrolyte disturbances in patients with chronic, stable asthma: effect of therapy. *Chest* **120**, 431–436.

*__Alfrey, A. C., Miller, N. L., and Butkus, D.__ (1974). Evaluation of body magnesium stores. *Journal of Laboratory & Clinical Medicine* **84**, 153–162.

Al-Makadma, A. K. (2000). Familial hypomagnesemia hypercalciuria with nephron calcinosis and high myopia. *Current Pediatric Research* **4**, 23–28.

Al-Rasheed, A. K. *et al.* (2000). Cyclosporine A neurotoxicity in a patient with idiopathic renal magnesium wasting. *Pediatric Neurology* **23**, 353–356.

Barakat, A. J. (2001). Gitelmans syndrome (familial hypokalemia–hypomagnesemia). *Journal of Nephrology* **14**, 43–47.

Barton, C. H. *et al.* (1984). Renal magnesium wasting associated with amphotericin B therapy. *American Journal of Medicine* **77**, 471–474.

Barton, C. H. *et al.* (1987). Hypomagnesemia and renal magnesium wasting in renal transplant recipients receiving cyclosporine. *American Journal of Medicine* **83**, 693–699.

Bashour, T., Rios, J. C., and Gorman, P. A. (1973). U wave alternans and increased ventricular irritability. *Chest* **64**, 377–379.

*__Benigno, V.__ *et al.* (2000). Hypomagnesaemia-hypocalciuria-nephrocalcinosis: a report of nine cases and a review. *Nephrology, Dialysis, Transplantation* **15**, 605–610.

Berns, A. S. and Kollmeyer, K. R. (1976). Magnesium-induced bradycardia. *Annals of Internal Medicine* **85**, 760–761 (letter).

Bianchetti, M. G., Oetliker, O. H., and Lutschg, J. (1993). Magnesium deficiency in primary distal tubular acidosis. *Journal of Pediatrics* **122**, 833 (Comment. Letter).

*__Blanchard, A.__ *et al.* (2001). Paracellin-1 is critical for magnesium and calcium reabsorption in the human thick ascending limb of Henle. *Kidney International* **59**, 2206–2215.

Bohmer, T. and Mathiesen, B. (1982). Magnesium deficiency in chronic alcoholic patients uncovered by an intravenous loading test. *Scandinavian Journal of Clinical and Laboratory Investigation* **42**, 633–636.

Carney, S. L. *et al.* (1980). Effect of magnesium deficiency on renal magnesium and calcium transport in the rat. *Journal of Clinical Investigation* **65**, 180–188.

Chen, W. C. U. *et al.* (1982). ECG changes in early stage of magnesium deficiency. *American Heart Journal* **104**, 1115–1116 (letter).

Chernow, B. *et al.* (1989). Hypomagnesemia in patients in postoperative intensive care. *Chest* **95**, 391.

Christiansen, C. and Baastrup, P. C. (1976). Transbol I: lithium, hypercalcemia, hypermagnesemia, and hyperparathyroidism. *Lancet* **2** (7992), 969 (letter).

*Coburn, J. W. *et al.* (1999). Calcium-sensing receptor and calcimimetic agents. *Kidney International* **56** (Suppl. S73), S52–S58.

*Cole, D. E. C. and Quamme, G. A. (2000a). Inherited disorders of renal magnesium handling. *Journal of American Society of Nephrology* **11**, 1937–1947.

Cole, D. E. C., Kooh, S. W., and Vieth, R. (2000b). Primary infantile hypomagnesaemia: outcome after 21 years and treatment with continuous nocturnal nasogastric magnesium infusion. *European Journal of Pediatrics* **159**, 38–43.

Cruz, D. N. *et al.* (2001). Gitelmans syndrome revisited: an evaluation of symptoms and health-related quality of life. *Kidney International* **59**, 710–717.

*Dacey, M. J. (2001). Hypomagnesemic disorders. *Critical Care Clinics* **17**, 155–173.

Dai, L. *et al.* (1997a). Mechanisms of amiloride stimulation of Mg^{2+} uptake in immortalized mouse distal convoluted tubule cells. *American Journal of Physiology* **272** (2 Pt 2), F249–F256.

Dai, L. *et al.* (1997b). Phosphate depletion diminishes Mg^{2+} uptake in mouse distal convoluted tubule cells. *Kidney International* **51**, 1710–1718.

Dai, L. *et al.* (1997c). Acid-base changes alter Mg^{2+} uptake in mouse distal convoluted tubule cells. *American Journal of Physiology* **272** (6 Pt 2), F759–F766.

Dai, L. *et al.* (1998a). Aldosterone potentiates hormone-stimulated Mg^{2+} uptake in distal convoluted tubule cells. *American Journal of Physiology* **274** (2 Pt 2), F336–F341.

Dai, L. *et al.* (1998b). Glucagon and arginine vasopressin stimulate Mg^{2+} uptake in mouse distal convoluted tubule cells. *American Journal of Physiology* **274** (2 Pt 2), F328–F335.

Dai, L. *et al.* (2001). Magnesium transport in the renal distal convoluted tubule. *Physiological Review* **81**, 51–84.

Devane, J. and Ryan, M. P. (1981). The effects of amiloride and triamterene on urinary magnesium excretion in conscious saline-loaded rats. *British Journal of Pharmacology* **72**, 285–289.

Dick, M., Evans, R. A., and Watson, L. (1969). Effect of ethanol on magnesium excretion. *Journal of Clinical Pathology* **22**, 152–153.

Ditzler, J. W. (1970). Epsom-salts poisoning and a review of magnesium-ion physiology. *Anesthesiology* **32**, 378–380.

Dyckner, T. *et al.* (1982a). Magnesium deficiency following jejunoileal bypass operations for obesity. *Journal of the American College of Nutrition* **1**, 239–246.

Dyckner, T. and Wester, P. O. (1982b). Magnesium deficiency contributing to ventricular tachycardia: two case reports. *Acta Medica Scandinavica* **212**, 89–91.

Elisaf, M. *et al.* (1995). Pathogenetic mechanisms of hypomagnesemia in alcoholic patients. *Journal of Trace Elements in Medicine and Biology* **9**, 210–214.

Elliott, C., Newman, N., and Madan, A. (2000). Gentamicin effects on urinary electrolyte excretion in healthy subjects. *Clinical Pharmacology and Therapeutics* **67**, 16–21.

Ettinger, L. J. *et al.* (1994). A phase II study of carboplatin in children with recurrent or progressive solid tumors. *Cancer* **73**, 1297–1301.

Fagan, C. and Phelan, D. (2001). Severe convulsant hypomagnesaemia and short bowel syndrome. *Anaesthesia and Intensive Care* **29**, 281–283.

Fiset, C. *et al.* (1996). Hypomagnesemia: characterization of a model of sudden cardiac death. *Journal of the American College of Cardiology* **27**, 1771–1776.

Friedman, M., Hatcher, G., and Watson, L. (1967). Primary hypomagnesaemia with secondary hypocalcaemia in an infant. *Lancet* **1** (7492), 703–705.

Gitelman, H. J., Graham, J. G., and Welt, L. G. (1966). A new familial disorder characterized by hypokalemia and hypomagnesemia. *Transactions of the Association of American Physicians* **79**, 221–235.

Hodgkinson, A., Marshall, D. H., and Nordin, B. E. (1979). Vitamin D and magnesium absorption in man. *Clinical Science* **57**, 121–123.

Huycke, M. M. *et al.* (2000). A double-blinded placebo-controlled crossover trial of intravenous magnesium sulfate for foscarnet-induced ionized hypocalcemia and hypomagnesemia in patients with AIDS and cytomegalovirus infection. *Antimicrobial Agents and Chemotherapy* **44**, 2143–2148.

Jin-no, Y. *et al.* (1999). Primary hypomagnesemia caused by isolated magnesium malabsorption: atypical case in adult. *Internal Medicine* **38**, 261–265.

June, C. H. *et al.* (1985). Profound hypomagnesemia and renal magnesium wasting associated with the use of cyclosporine for marrow transplantation. *Transplantation* **39**, 620–624.

Kamel, K. S. *et al.* (1998). Studies on the pathogenesis of hypokalemia in Gitelman's syndrome: role of bicarbonaturia and hypomagnesemia. *American Journal of Nephrology* **18**, 42–49.

Kantorovich, V. *et al.* (2002). Genetic Heterogeneity in familial and magnesium wasting. *Journal of Clinical Endocrinology and Metabolism* **87**, 613–617.

Kelber, J. *et al.* (1994). Acute effects of different concentrations of dialysate magnesium during high-efficiency dialysis. *American Journal of Kidney Diseases* **24**, 453–460.

Konrad, M. and Weber, S. (2003). Recent advances in molecular genetics of hereditary magnesium-losing disorders. *Journal of the American Society of Nephrology* **14**, 249–260.

Kristiansen, J. H., Brochner, Mortensen, J., and Pedersen, K. O. (1985). Familial hypocalciuric hypercalcaemia. I, Renal handling of calcium, magnesium and phosphate. *Clinical Endocrinology* **22**, 103–116.

Lajer, H. and Daugaard, G. (1999). Cisplatin and hypomagnesemia. *Cancer Treatment Reviews* **25**, 47–58.

Larner, A. J. *et al.* (2001). Isolated familial hypomagnesaemia with novel neurological features: causal link or chance concurrence. *European Journal of Neurology* **8**, 495–499.

LaSala, M. A. *et al.* (1985). Magnesium metabolism studies in children with chronic inflammatory disease of the bowel. *Journal of Pediatrics Gastroenterology and Nutrition* **4**, 75–81.

Loeb, H. S. *et al.* (1968). Paroxysmal ventricular fibrillation in two patients with hypomagnesemia: treatment by transvenous pacing. *Circulation* **37**, 210–215.

Lord, R. C. C. (1999). Cisplatin-induced hypomagnesemia. *Medical Biochemistry* **1**, 247–249.

Mani, S. (1992). Pentamidine-induced renal magnesium wasting. *AIDS* **6**, 594–595 (letter).

*Martini, L. A. and Wood, R. J. (2001). Assessing magnesium status: a persisting problem. *Nutrition in Clinical Care* **4**, 332–337.

Massry, S. G., Coburn, J. W., and Kleeman, C. R. (1969). Renal handling of magnesium in the dog. *American Journal of Physiology* **216**, 1460–1467.

Mavichak, V. *et al.* (1985). Studies on the pathogenesis of cisplatin-induced hypomagnesemia in rats. *Kidney International* **28**, 914–921.

Mavichak, V. *et al.* (1988). Renal magnesium wasting and hypocalciuria in chronic cis-platinum nephropathy in man. *Clinical Science* **75**, 203–207.

Mazzaferro, S. *et al.* (2002). Ionized and total serum magnesium in renal transplant patients. *Journal of Nephrology* **15**, 275–280.

Meij, I. C. *et al.* (2000). Dominant isolated renal magnesium loss is caused by misrouting of the Na^+,K^+-ATPase gamma-subunit. *Nature Genetics* **26**, 265–266.

Meij, I. C. *et al.* (2003). Exclusion of mutations in FXYD2, CLDN16 and SLC12A3 in two families with primary renal Mg^{2+} loss. *Nephrology, Dialysis, Transplantation* **18**, 512–516.

Miura, K. *et al.* (2002). Role of hypomagnesemia in chronic cyclosporine nephropathy. *Transplantation* **73**, 340–347.

Monkawa, T. *et al.* (2000). Novel mutations in thiazide-sensitive Na–Cl cotransporter gene of patients with Gitelmans syndrome. *Journal of the American Society of Nephrology* **11**, 65–70.

Morgan, M., Maloney, D., and Duvic, M. (2002). Hypomagnesemia and hypocalcemia in mycosis fungoides: a retrospective case series. *Leukemia & Lymphoma* **43**, 1297–1302.

Nicholson, J. C. *et al.* (1995). Familial hypomagnesemia–hypercalciuria leading to end-stage renal failure. *Pediatric Nephrology* **9**, 74–76.

Oktenli, C. (2000). Renal magnesium wasting, hypomagnesemic–hypocalcemia, hypocalciuria and osteopenia in a patient with glycogenosis type II. *American Journal of Nephrology* **20**, 412–417.

Pak, C. Y. C. (2000). Correction of thiazide-induced hypomagnesemia by potassium–magnesium citrate from review of prior trials. *Clinical Nephrology* **54**, 271–275.

Palestine, A. G. *et al.* (1991). A randomized, controlled trial of foscarnet in the treatment of cytomegalovirus retinitis in patients with AIDS. *Annals of Internal Medicine* **115**, 665–673.

Pantanetti, P. *et al.* (2002). Severe hypomagnesaemia-induced hypocalcaemia in a patient with Gitelmans syndrome. *Clinical Endocrinology* **56**, 413–418.

Paunier, L. *et al.* (1968). Primary hypomagnesemia with secondary hypocalcemia in an infant. *Pediatrics* **41**, 385–402.

Pearce, S. H. *et al.* (1996). A familial syndrome of hypocalcemia with hypercalciuria due to mutations in the calcium-sensing receptor. *New England Journal of Medicine* **335**, 1115–1122.

***Pollack, M. R.** *et al.* (1993). Mutations in the human Ca(2^+)-sensing receptor gene cause familial hypocalciuric hypercalcemia and neonatal severe hyperparathyroidism. *Cell* **75**, 1297–1303.

***Pollack, M. R.** *et al.* (1994). Autosomal dominant hypocalcemia caused by a Ca(2^+)-sensing receptor gene mutation. *Nature Genetics* **8**, 303–307.

Praga, M. *et al.* (1995). Familial hypomagnesemia with hypercalciuria and nephrocalcinosis. *Kidney International* **47**, 1419–1425.

Quamme, G. A. (1997). Renal magnesium handling: new insights in understanding old problems. *Kidney International* **52** (5), 1180–1195.

Quamme, G. A. and Dirks, J. H. (1980). Intraluminal and contraluminal magnesium on magnesium and calcium transfer in the rat nephron. *American Journal of physiology* **238**, F187–F198.

Quamme, G. A. *et al.* (1978). Magnesium handling in the dog kidney: a micropuncture study. *Pflugers Archiv—European Journal of Physiology* **377**, 95–99.

Qureshi, T. and Melonakos, T. K. (1996). Acute hypermagnesemia after laxative use. *Annals of Emergency Medicine* **28**, 552–555.

Ramee, S. R. *et al.* (1985). Torsades de Pointes and magnesium deficiency. *American Heart Journal* **109**, 164–167.

Ruml, L. A. (1999). Effect of varying doses of potassium–magnesium citrate on thiazide induced hypokalemia and magnesium loss. *American Journal of Therapeutics* **6**, 45–50.

Ryzen, E. and Rude, R. K. (1990). Low intracellular magnesium in patients with acute pancreatitis and hypocalcemia. *Western Journal of Medicine* **152**, 145.

Ryzen, E. *et al.* (1985). Parenteral magnesium tolerance testing in the evaluation of magnesium deficiency. *Magnesium* **4**, 137–147.

Saha, H. *et al.* (1998). Serum ionized versus total magnesium in patients with chronic renal disease. *Nephron* **80**, 149–152.

Satoh, J. and Romero, M. F. (2002). Mg^{2+} transport in the kidney. *BioMetals* **15** (3), 285–296.

Sayer, J. A. and Pearce, S. H. (2001). Diagnosis and clinical biochemistry of inherited tubulopathies. *Annals of Clinical Biochemistry* **38**, 459–470.

Schepkens, H. and Lameire, N. (2001). Gitelmans syndrome: an overlooked cause of chronic hypokalemia and hypomagnesemia in adults. *Acta Clinica Belgica* **56**, 248–254.

Schlingmann, K. P. *et al.* (2002). Hypomagnesemia with secondary hypocalcemia is caused by mutations in TPRM6, a new member of the TPRM gene family. *Nature Genetics* **31**, 166–170.

Schultheis *et al.* (1998). Phenotype resembling Gitelmans syndrome in mice lacking the apical Na^+–Cl^- cotransporter of the distal convoluted tubule. *Journal of Biological Chemistry* **273**, 29150–29155.

Scott, V. L. *et al.* (1996). Ionized hypomagnesemia in patients undergoing orthotopic liver transplantation: a complication of citrate intoxication. *Liver Transplantation & Surgery* **2**, 343–347.

Seller, R. H. *et al.* (1970). Digitalis toxicity and hypomagnesemia. *American Heart Journal* **79**, 57–68.

Shah, G. M. and Kirschenbaum, M. A. (1991). Renal magnesium wasting associated with therapeutic agents. *Mineral & Electrolyte Metabolism* **17**, 58–64.

Simon, D. B. *et al.* (1996a). Bartter's syndrome, hypokalaemic alkalosis with hypercalciuria, is caused by mutations in the Na–K–2Cl cotransporter NKCC2. *Nature Genetics* **13**, 183–188.

***Simon, D. B.** *et al.* (1996b). Genetic heterogeneity of Bartter's syndrome revealed by mutations in the K^+ channel, ROMK. *Nature Genetics* **14**, 152–156.

Simon, D. B. *et al.* (1996c). Gitelman's variety of Bartter's syndrome, inherited hypokalaemic alkalosis, is caused by mutations in the thiazide-sensitive Na–Cl cotransporter. *Nature Genetics* **12**, 24–30.

Simon, D. B. *et al.* (1997). Mutations in the chloride channel gene, CLCNKB, cause Bartter's syndrome type III. *Nature Genetics* **7**, 171–178.

Simon, D. B. *et al.* (1998). The molecular basis of renal magnesium wasting: familial hypomagnesemia with nephrocalcinosis (abstract). *Journal of the American Society of Nephrology* **9**, 559A.

***Simon, D. B.** *et al.* (1999). Paracellin-1, a renal tight junction protein required for paracellular Mg^{2+} resorption. *Science* **285**, 103–106.

***Suki, W. N., Lederer, E. D., and Rouse, D.** Renal transport of calcium, magnesium, and phosphate. In *Brenner and Rector's The Kidney* 6th edn. Vol. 1 (ed. Barry M. Brenner), pp. 520–574. Philadelphia, PA: W.B. Saunders Company, 2000.

Sutton, R. A. L and Dirks, J. H. Disturbances of calcium and magnesium metabolism, In *Brenner and Rector's The Kidney* 5th edn. Vol. 1, pp. 1038–1085. Philadelphia, PA: W.B. Saunders Company, 1996.

Torralbo, A. *et al.* (1995). Renal magnesium wasting with hypercalciuria, nephrocalcinosis and ocular disorders. *Nephron* **69**, 472–475.

Vannini, S. D. P. *et al.* (1999). Permanently reduced plasma ionized magnesium among renal transplant recipients on cyclosporine. *Transplant International* **12**, 244–249.

Verive, M. J. *et al.* (2000). Evaluating the frequency of hypomagnesemia in critically ill patients by using multiple regression analysis and a computer-based neural network. *Critical Care Medicine* **28**, 3534–3539.

Walder, R. Y. *et al.* (2002). Mutation of TPRM6 causes familial hypomagnesemia with secondary hypocalcemia. *Nature Genetics* **31**, 171–174.

***Weber, S.** *et al.* (2001). Novel paracellin-1 mutations in 25 families with familial hypomagnesemia with hypercalciuria and nephrocalcinosis. *Journal of American Society of Nephrology* **12**, 1872–1881.

***Whang, R.** *et al.* (1985). Magnesium depletion as a cause of refractory potassium repletion. *Archives of Internal Medicine* **145**, 1686–1689.

White, J. R. and Campbell, R. K. (1993). Magnesium and diabetes: a review. *Annals of Pharmacotherapy* **27**, 775–780.

Wolf, M. T. *et al.* (2002). Follow-up of five patients with FHHNC due to mutations in the Paracellin-1 gene. *Pediatric Nephrology* **17**, 602–608.

Wong, N. L., Dirks, J. H., and Quamme, G. A. (1983a). Tubular reabsorptive capacity for magnesium in the dog kidney. *American Journal of Physiology* **244**, F78–F83.

Wong, E. T. *et al.* (1983b). A high prevalence of hypomagnesemia and hypermagnesemia in hospitalized patients. *American Journal of Clinical Pathology* **79**, 348–352.

Wong, N. L. *et al.* (1985). Enhanced distal absorption of potassium by magnesium-deficient rats. *Clinical Science* **69**, 625–630.

***Yu, A. S. L.** Disturbances of magnesium metabolism. In *Brenner and Rector's The Kidney* 6th edn. Vol. 1, pp. 1055–1070. Philadelphia, PA: W.B. Saunders Company, 2000.

Yu, A. S. L. (2001). Evolving concepts in epithelial magnesium transport. *Current Opinion in Nephrology and Hypertension* **10**, 649–653.

Zelikovic, I. *et al.* (2003). A novel mutation in the chloride channel gene, CLC-NKB, as a cause of Gitelman and Bartter syndromes. *Kidney International* **63**, 24–32.

2.6 Clinical acid–base disorders

Biff F. Palmer, Robert G. Narins, and Jerry Yee

Introduction

To ensure that cellular enzymes function normally acid–base status is carefully regulated to maintain the arterial pH between 7.35 and 7.45. Similarly, intracellular pH, although varying from cell to cell, is maintained generally between 7.0 and 7.3. This regulation occurs in the setting of continuous production of acidic metabolites and is accomplished by intracellular and extracellular buffering processes in conjunction with respiratory and renal regulatory mechanisms. The first part of this chapter provides a brief overview of normal acid–base homeostasis. The remainder of the chapter is devoted to the clinical entities that give rise to metabolic acidosis and metabolic alkalosis.

Net acid production (see also Chapter 5.4)

Under normal circumstances humans are confronted by an ongoing acid challenge. The normal diet contains components which upon metabolism are converted to acids or alkali. Amino acids such as lysine and arginine are metabolized to acids, while the amino acids glutamate and aspartate, and organic anions such as acetate and citrate, yield alkali upon metabolism. Sulfur-containing amino acids (methionine and cysteine) are metabolized to H_2SO_4, and organophosphates are metabolized to H_3PO_4, both strong acids. In general, animal foods are rich in proteins and organophosphates which provide a net acid diet, while plant foods are richer in organic anions which provide more of an alkaline load. In addition to acid/alkali produced from metabolism of the diet, there is a small daily production of organic acids such as acetic acid, lactic acid, and pyruvic acid from metabolism. Lastly, there is a small amount of acid generated by the excretion of alkali into the stool. Under normal circumstances, daily net acid production is approximately 1 mmol of H^+ per kilogram body weight.

Buffer systems in the regulation of pH

The most immediate defense against addition of acid or alkali to the body is provided by intracellular and extracellular buffers. Buffer systems serve to minimize the change in pH during the addition of acid or alkali, but do not, by themselves, remove acid/alkali from the body. The most important of these buffer systems in the extracellular fluid (ECF) is the HCO_3^-/CO_2 system. The pivotal role of this system stems from the abundance of each of its two components. The HCO_3^-/CO_2 system is an open buffer system, which means that each member of the buffer pair can enter or leave the system. A closed buffer system, by contrast, is one in which neither member of the buffer pair can enter or leave, such that the concentration of total buffer is fixed. In the case of the HCO_3^-/CO_2 buffer system, the CO_2 concentration is maintained by respiratory control and the kidney regulates the HCO_3^- levels. Addition of acid leads to conversion of HCO_3^- to CO_2 according to the reaction:

$$HA + NaHCO_3 \leftrightarrow NaA + H_2O + CO_2. \quad (1)$$

HCO_3^- is consumed, but respiratory compensation allows for the excretion of the CO_2 produced. The acid also stimulates renal alkali synthesis in an attempt to limit the fall in HCO_3^- levels. The net result is that this open buffer minimizes any change in pH.

While the HCO_3^-/CO_2 system is the most important ECF buffer, other buffers such as serum proteins and phosphate ions also participate in the maintenance of a stable pH. During metabolic acidosis, the skeleton becomes a major buffer source as acid-induced dissolution of bone apatite releases alkaline calcium salts and HCO_3^- into the ECF.

Within the intracellular compartment, pH is also tightly regulated. Intracellular pH is maintained by intracellular buffers such as haemoglobin in red cells, cellular proteins, organophosphate complexes, and bicarbonate, as well as HCO_3^-/CO_2 transport mechanisms which serve to transport acid and alkali into and out of the cell.

Respiratory system in regulation of pH

While buffers minimize the changes in pH upon acid/alkali addition, they do not serve to remove the acid or alkali from the body. This is accomplished by the lungs and kidneys working in concert. The lungs regulate the CO_2 tension, while the kidneys regulate the HCO_3^- concentration. While the HCO_3^-/CO_2 buffer system is not the only buffer system, all buffer systems in the extracellular space are in a steady-state at a common pH. Because the concentration of HCO_3^- is far greater than that of other buffers, changes in the HCO_3^-/CO_2 buffer pair can easily titrate other buffer systems and thus establish the pH. To understand how the lungs and kidneys function in concert, it is instructive to review the Henderson–Hasselbalch equation:

$$pH = 6.1 + \log([HCO_3^-] \div (0.03 \times Pco_2)). \quad (2)$$

From Eq. (2), it can be seen that pH is determined by the ratio of HCO_3^- to CO_2. Any condition associated with similar fractional changes in the concentrations of these components will not alter pH. Thus, if HCO_3^- and CO_2 concentrations are both halved (the ratio remaining constant), blood pH will not change.

The lungs serve to defend pH by altering alveolar ventilation which serves to control the P_{CO_2} of body fluids. An increase in non-volatile acid production lowers blood pH and HCO_3^- concentration, which stimulates the respiratory centre to increase alveolar ventilation and thereby lower the P_{CO_2}. The decrease in blood pH will be less than that which would have occurred in the absence of respiratory compensation. If the fractional change in CO_2 tension was similar to that in HCO_3^- concentration, blood pH would not change. However, respiratory compensations generally do not return blood pH to normal, and thus the fractional change in CO_2 tension will be less than that in HCO_3^- concentration.

There is a highly predictable degree of respiratory compensation that is provoked by a given decrease in HCO_3^- concentration. If the P_{CO_2} is higher or lower than predicted for a given level of hypobicarbonataemia, a primary respiratory acidosis or alkalosis must be superimposed. Several formulas are available that accurately predict what the P_{CO_2} should be for a given low HCO_3^- concentration. One such formula predicts that in stable steady-state of metabolic acidosis, the P_{CO_2} appropriate to the degree of hypobicarbonataemia equals 8 plus the product of 1.5 and the serum HCO_3^- (i.e. total CO_2) concentration.

$$P_{CO_2}\ (\text{mmHg}) = 1.5 \times [HCO_3^-] + 8 \pm 2. \quad (3)$$

Although the interval has not been precisely defined, it appears to take 12–36 h of stable acidosis for the P_{CO_2} to achieve its nadir. Use of this formula prior to achievement of the steady-state—that is, while the HCO_3^- concentration is at its nadir but while the P_{CO_2} is still decreasing towards its nadir—gives the false impression that the P_{CO_2} is inappropriately high for the measured serum HCO_3^- concentration.

Similar precision in predicting the appropriateness of the P_{CO_2} may be achieved by knowing that in steady-state metabolic acidosis the P_{CO_2} declines by 1.1–1.4 mmHg for each 1 mmol/l decrease in serum HCO_3^- concentration. Thus, a decline of 10 mmol/l in serum HCO_3^- concentration, from the normal value of 25 mmol/l to the abnormal value of 15 mmol/l, should lower the P_{CO_2} by 11–14 mmHg (i.e. from the normal value of 40 mmHg to between 26 and 29 mmHg).

A useful feature of the mathematics relating P_{CO_2}, HCO_3^- concentration, and pH is that in steady state, pure metabolic acidosis, the P_{CO_2} (in mmHg) equals 100 times the last two digits of the pH. For example, when the pH is 7.30 the P_{CO_2} will approximate 30 mmHg. Finally, in steady-state metabolic acidosis, addition of the number 15 to the measured serum HCO_3^- concentration yields the P_{CO_2} and the last two digits of the pH. This formula closely estimates the P_{CO_2} over a serum HCO_3^- range of 12–40 mmol/l.

When the P_{CO_2} is too high or too low for a given low serum HCO_3^- concentration, a mixed respiratory–metabolic acid–base disorder must be present. Thus, by knowing what the P_{CO_2} should be for any given degree of metabolic acidosis (i.e. decrease in HCO_3^- concentration), the physician can determine whether the respiratory response is appropriate. This powerful diagnostic tool can unveil a primary respiratory acid–base disorder that is superimposed on a primary metabolic acidosis. Unsuspected pneumonia, pulmonary embolus, salicylism, or other causes of respiratory alkalosis or acidosis may be first suspected only after a careful review of the blood gases.

According to current concepts, the change in serum HCO_3^- concentration is transmitted only slowly to the interstitium of the brainstem, where it signals chemoreceptors located below the surface of the medulla oblongata. Activated receptors translate this chemical message into a change in respiration by signalling other neurones in the medullary respiratory centre, which in turn, alter phrenic nerve activity and, subsequently, alveolar ventilation. The time required to maximize respiration is a function of the speed with which the acidity of plasma can be transmitted to the interstitial fluid of the brainstem. Because changes in systemic HCO_3^- concentration are even more slowly transferred to the cerebrospinal fluid (CSF) than they are to the interstitium of the brain, respiration is stimulated and the P_{CO_2} is decreased well before any change in CSF bicarbonate concentration is measurable. Unlike HCO_3^-, which can penetrate the blood–brain barrier only slowly, arterial P_{CO_2}, instantaneously makes itself felt in the CSF. Thus the early stages of systemic acidosis and acidaemia cause a paradoxical alkalinization of the CSF, which is due to the asynchronous fall in P_{CO_2} and HCO_3^- concentration in the CSF; that is, the $P_{CO_2}/[HCO_3^-]$ ratio decreases. In time, the spinal fluid acidifies as the HCO_3^- concentration declines in proportion to that in blood.

During the reparative phase of metabolic acidosis, when the serum HCO_3^- concentration is increasing, a paradoxical acidification of the CSF occurs. The improving HCO_3^- concentration signals the medullary respiratory centre to reduce the rate of ventilation. Because the increasing P_{CO_2} gains access to the CSF faster than does HCO_3^-, a transient 'respiratory' acidification occurs.

Renal regulation of pH

While buffer systems and respiratory excretion of CO_2 can provide partial defense of hydrogen ion activity, the kidneys provide the ultimate defense against addition of non-volatile acids to the body's fluids. The titration of the body's buffer systems would lead to their eventual depletion if no means were available for excretion of the non-volatile acids generated by net acid production.

The kidney's role in the regulation of non-volatile acid–base balance includes two components: (a) reclamation of filtered HCO_3^- and (b) simultaneous regeneration of HCO_3^- consumed by net acid production and excretion of the acid. The kidneys filter approximately 4000 mmol of HCO_3^- a day, excretion of which would rapidly lead to severe metabolic acidosis. Thus, the kidney must reclaim this filtered bicarbonate. This process of reclamation requires that renal epithelial cells secrete protons to convert the poorly reabsorbable luminal HCO_3^- to the readily absorbable CO_2 (Alpern 1990). This process simply prevents bicarbonaturia from occurring but does not rid acid from the body. Following reclamation, the kidney must then secrete an additional 1 mmol/kg/day of hydrogen ions into the tubular lumen. This process can be viewed most simply as follows. In the cell, H_2CO_3 (derived from hydrated CO_2) separates into H^+ and HCO_3^-; the former is secreted into the tubular lumen while the latter is returned to the systemic circulation via the renal veins. This regenerates the HCO_3^- used to buffer the net acid production (Eq. 1). Secreted hydrogen ions are buffered by titratable buffers, and by NH_3 and are excreted. If the luminal protons were reabsorbed they would titrate the HCO_3^- added to the renal veins and so negate any acid–base benefits from this secretory process. Understanding the latter point highlights the importance of renal buffers to the process of renal HCO_3^- regulation.

To maintain acid–base balance, the kidney must excrete net acid at a rate equal to the rate of extrarenal net acid production

(~1.0 mmol/kg/day). The rate of net acid excretion (NAE) is given by the equation:

$$NAE = (U_{NH_4} \times V) + (U_{TA} \times V) - (U_{HCO_3} \times V), \quad (4)$$

where $U_{NH_4} \times V$ is the rate of ammonium excretion, $U_{TA} \times V$ is the rate of titratable acid excretion, and $U_{HCO_3} \times V$ is the rate of HCO_3^- excretion.

As shown above, the processes of HCO_3^- reclamation and regeneration are both accomplished by the same general mechanism—acidification of the tubule fluid along the nephron. The proximal tubule lowers luminal pH from 7.3 to approximately 6.7, and thus reclaims the major portion of filtered HCO_3^-. The thick ascending limb and distal nephron contribute by reclaiming any remaining HCO_3^- that escapes the proximal tubule. Bicarbonate regeneration begins in the proximal tubule with titration of filtered buffers, but the key component occurs in the collecting duct where the final urinary acidification leads to titration of ammonia, phosphate, and other titratable buffers.

Systemic effects of metabolic acidosis

Before discussing specific conditions associated with metabolic acidosis, a brief overview of the systemic effects of acidosis will be provided (Table 1). Abnormalities of systemic pH may effect wide-ranging changes in tissue and organ function. The symptoms and signs shared by many of the metabolic acidoses relate to these generalized effects; other specific effects of the individual disease entities add to the complexity of presentation.

The clinical features of the metabolic acidoses are strongly influenced by the rate and magnitude of the fall in pH. As with many metabolic disorders, those developing rapidly are far more likely to produce dramatic signs and symptoms than are the more slowly developing disorders. For example, in chronic renal failure the serum HCO_3^- concentration and blood pH progressively decline over months to years, eventually reaching steady-state values of 18 mmol/l and 7.30, respectively. Patients usually show no symptoms from these modest changes. In acute renal failure, however, the same chemical abnormalities may develop over a period of hours to days, in which case symptoms almost always are present.

Table 1 Systemic effects of metabolic acidosis

Cardiovascular
Heart: bradycardia, arrhythmias, decreased contractility
Vascular: arteriolar vasodilation, increased venous tone, increased pulmonary venous tone
Pulmonary
Ventilation: Kussmaul respiration
Oxygen delivery: increased in acute acidosis (Bohr effect), normal in chronic acidosis (decreased 2,3 diphosphoglyceric acid)
Gastrointestinal
Gastric distention
Decreased motility
Renal
Natriuretic effect
Hypercalciuria
Metabolic/hormonal
Protein wasting
Increased catecholamine secretion
Increased mobilization of calcium from bone
Haematological
Leucocytosis

Cardiac effects

The heart rate responds biphasically to increasing degrees of acidaemia. Tachycardia is frequently observed as blood pH falls from 7.40 to 7.10. This increasing heart rate is caused by the acid-stimulated release of epinephrine from the adrenal medulla (Wildenthal *et al.* 1968). Predictably, the use of β-adrenergic blocking agents prevents this effect otherwise seen with progressive acidaemia. As blood pH falls below 7.10, the heart rate progressively slows, exacerbated by β-adrenergic blocking drugs. The pathogenesis of severe acidaemia-induced bradycardia is uncertain. Potential mechanisms include an inhibition of catecholamine-induced chronotropy and/or the accumulation of acetylcholine via inhibition of acetylcholinesterase (Mitchell *et al.* 1972). Systemic acidosis may also predispose to the development of ventricular fibrillation. The more malignant ventricular arrhythmias complicating the metabolic acidoses may be related in part to concomitant abnormalities in potassium, magnesium, or phosphorus.

Severe acidaemia impairs myocardial contractility (Mitchell *et al.* 1972). Impaired contraction results from the algebraic sum of the opposing actions of acid. Acid exerts both a negative inotropic effect directly on the heart and an indirect positive inotropic effect, by stimulating the release of epinephrine. As blood pH falls from 7.40 to 7.20, the negative inotropic effect of acid and the positive inotropic effect of released catecholamines offset each other and leave myocardial contraction largely unscathed. As blood pH falls below 7.20, the negative inotropic effect of acidosis becomes progressively more apparent.

Vascular effects

The countervailing effects of low pH and increasing concentrations of catecholamines leave arteriolar tone largely unchanged until pH values falls below 7.20. While a variety of *in vivo* and *in vitro* systems have been used to demonstrate these aforementioned effects, studies of the perfused human forearm have most convincingly demonstrated the net vasodilator effect of low pH (Kontos *et al.* 1968). The hypotension complicating severe metabolic acidosis is frequently characterized by warm, well-perfused peripheral tissues, giving rise to the term 'warm shock'.

Advancing acidaemia causes sustained venoconstriction (Sharpey-Schafer *et al.* 1965). Venous smooth muscle contracts in the presence of increasing concentrations of protons and may persistently respond to catecholamines, despite the severe acidaemia. Constriction of peripheral veins reduces their reservoir function, forcing more blood centrally and increasing the workload of the heart. Therapy with alkali diminishes the elevated pressures in the ventricle and pulmonary artery. This centralization of blood volume from increasing degrees of acidaemia adds to the heart's burden when myocardial contraction is impaired. It follows that congestive heart failure is one of the dreaded results of unchecked severe acidaemia.

Animal and human data, on balance, indicate that increasing acidaemia progressively reduces cardiac output. This appears to be the outcome of decreased myocardial contraction combined with a progressive slowing of heart rate. The exacerbating effects of increasing central blood volume and the tendency to ventricular arrhythmias together cause the lethal haemodynamic effects complicating advanced degrees of metabolic acidosis. In general, it appears that the myocardium is less vulnerable when blood pH is maintained above 7.20, which broadly corresponds to a blood HCO_3^- concentration greater than 10 mmol/l (assuming that respiratory compensation is appropriate).

Pulmonary effects

Increasing degrees of hypobicarbonataemia stimulate respiration, allowing the salutary effect of hypocapnia to mitigate the degree of acidaemia (see above). This chronic increase in ventilation is often difficult for even the most careful observer to identify in patients with chronic metabolic acidosis, because small increases in the rate and depth of ventilation enable the lungs to enhance their clearance of CO_2 from the blood. Acute, severe metabolic acidoses, however, cause hyperpnaea (i.e. increased tidal volume) and modest degrees of tachypnaea (i.e. rapid respiration).

A variety of metabolic and physicochemical effects of acidosis may strikingly alter the transport and delivery of oxygen to peripheral tissues. Two offsetting and synchronous effects of acidosis are important to tissue oxygenation. The Bohr effect describes the interaction of hydrogen ions with haemoglobin. Increased concentrations of protons within the microenvironment of the red blood cell (RBC) instantaneously decrease the affinity of haemoglobin for oxygen, thereby facilitating tissue oxygenation. Alkalinization has an immediate and opposite effect. An offsetting effect of pH on haemoglobin–oxygen binding is more slowly mediated by induced changes in RBC glycolysis. Increasing acidaemia slows glycolysis and over a period of 12–36 h depletes erythrocytes of some intermediates, most notably 2,3-diphosphoglyceric acid (DPG), a compound which, like acid, decreases haemoglobin's affinity for oxygen. Alkalinization has an equal and opposite influence on the rate of glycolysis, which is also slowly mediated.

It follows that acute acidosis beneficially affects tissue oxygenation by eliciting the Bohr effect. However, the progressive depletion of RBC DPG over time nullifies this benefit of acidosis. In a similar fashion, acute alkalinization may abruptly depress tissue oxygenation; but in time, increasing RBC concentrations of DPG re-establish normal tissue oxygen delivery: the rapid onset of increased haemoglobin affinity for oxygen is offset by the slower buildup of DPG. From the aforementioned observations, it has been argued that the rapid administration of alkali to patients with chronic metabolic acidosis may result in transient tissue hypoxia. The chronically acidotic patient has normal tissue oxygenation, resulting from the offsetting actions of low pH and RBC depletion of DPG. Excessively rapid therapy with large amounts of alkali, may remove the beneficial Bohr effect while erythrocytes remain depleted of phosphorylated intermediates. During this transient phase, haemoglobin affinity for oxygen may increase to the point of depriving tissues of much-needed oxygen.

Gastrointestinal effects

Experimentally induced systemic acid–base perturbations alter gastrointestinal motility, absorption, secretion, and structural integrity. The difficulties inherent in studying the various functions of the gastrointestinal tract, especially in sick, acidotic patients, have left it uncertain whether data derived from animal studies are translatable to humans. A variety of functional gastrointestinal complaints and physical findings are seen in the majority of patients presenting with acute diabetic ketoacidosis. Abdominal pain, distension, nausea, and vomiting are often prominent and occasionally so severe as to suggest an acute abdominal emergency. These symptoms and signs are quickly reversed by appropriate therapy of ketoacidosis. Since these findings often complicate the initial presentation of type 1 diabetes, it is unlikely to be caused by pre-existing neuropathic changes. The ready reversibility of all signs and symptoms also belies the possibility of chronic underlying disease. It is not yet clear whether these symptoms are related to the acidosis itself, the ketogenesis, or other complicating fluid–electrolyte and biochemical changes accompanying the ketoacidosis.

Although much work has been done to define the basis for the negative inotropism and disordered arteriolar and venous muscle tone in severe metabolic acidosis, surprisingly little has been done to clarify the effects of acid–base changes on gastrointestinal tone and motility. Muscle strips from the lower oesophagus and stomach, when bathed in acidotic media, demonstrated decreased amplitude and frequency of spontaneous contraction (Schulze–Delrieu and Lepsien 1982). As with the heart, acidosis may alter the net accumulation of free Ca^{2+} inside cells and thereby disrupt normal tone and contraction.

Intestinal muscle tone and contractility, as in the heart and stomach, appear adversely affected by systemic acidosis. Rabbit taenia coli muscle preparations demonstrate decreased sensitivity to cholinergic stimulation when incubated in even mildly acidotic media (Lofqvist and Nilsson 1981). Although no convincing data show that these observations also hold for the human colon, it is tempting to speculate that some of the intestinal manifestations of chronic acid–base abnormalities are mediated by such changes.

Renal effects

Proximal renal tubule NaCl reabsorption is impaired by acute metabolic acidosis but is rapidly normalized with repair of the hypobicarbonataemia. This effect is at least partly due to impairment of the passive portion of proximal renal tubule sodium reabsorption. Under normal conditions filtered $NaHCO_3$ is reabsorbed along with isoosmotic amounts of water in the earliest segments of the proximal tubule. Because sodium is reabsorbed with proportionate amounts of water while disproportionately more HCO_3^- is reabsorbed, the residual tubular filtrate has an unchanged sodium concentration but a lower HCO_3^- concentration. Unreabsorbed Cl^- is now dispersed in a smaller volume of glomerular filtrate, thereby increasing the chloride concentration above that of the parent plasma. The high chloride concentration and the favourable lumen-to-plasma gradient stimulate the passive absorption of the anion. The positive luminal charge resulting from disproportionate reabsorption of anionic chloride then facilitates passive sodium reabsorption.

With acute metabolic acidosis the serum HCO_3^- concentration, and therefore the filtered load of bicarbonate, decrease to lower levels. Since the filtered load of $NaHCO_3$ is diminished, its absolute reabsorption in the earliest portion of the proximal tubule falls, thereby rendering unfavourable the generation of the passive forces required for non-active NaCl chloride reabsorption. Accordingly, more NaCl is delivered distally, a portion of which escapes into the final urine, effecting the natriuresis of acute acidosis.

Calcium metabolism

Approximately half of circulating Ca^{2+} is bound to serum albumin and so is biologically inactive. Cationic Ca^{2+} is normally bound to anionic carboxyl groups of various proteins. With increasing degrees of acidaemia, protons replace Ca^{2+} on protein, thereby increasing the ionized, biologically active form of calcium. This ionized fraction is now freely filtered at the glomerulus. Thus, acidaemia tends to increase the filtered load of calcium.

Parathyroid hormone (PTH) plays an important role in mediating bone buffering of accumulating acid loads (Arruda *et al.* 1980). Parathyroidectomized animals become more hypobicarbonataemic from a given acid load than do intact controls. Treatment with exogenous PTH restores normal bone buffering. These studies underscore the importance of PTH and bone in regulating acid–base homeostasis. Acidosis exerts an inhibitory effect on the proximal tubular enzyme 1α-hydroxylase. The pathophysiologic significance of acidosis-induced inhibition of vitamin D activation is not yet clear.

It is well known that increasing burdens of acid are absorbed and buffered by bone. Pioneering studies by Lemann and coworkers demonstrated a close stoichiometry between positive hydrogen balance and negative Ca^{2+} balance in human volunteers ingesting excessive acid loads (Litzow *et al.* 1967). These studies led to the view that entering hydrogen ions titrated bone carbonates, thereby protecting the serum HCO_3^- concentration at the expense of the slow dissolution of bone. These data have been further extrapolated to suggest that the chronic metabolic acidosis complicating advanced renal disease plays a significant role in uraemic osteodystrophy. The mechanism by which acidosis dissolves bone may in part be related to increased sensitivity to the effects of PTH (Beck and Webster 1976).

Metabolic acidosis inhibits the tubular reabsorption of calcium. The overall effects of acute and chronic metabolic acidosis vary as to the site of this inhibition and whether hypercalciuria results. During acute metabolic acidosis proximal Ca^{2+} reabsorption is inhibited but because distal Ca^{2+} reabsorption is simultaneously stimulated, no net change in Ca^{2+} excretion occurs. During chronic metabolic acidosis the proximal reabsorption of Ca^{2+} is stimulated while distal reabsorption is inhibited, resulting in hypercalciuria (Sutton *et al.* 1979). Thus, some chronic metabolic acidoses (excluding those associated with renal failure) are characterized by the increased flow of Ca^{2+} from bone into the extracellular space, where the low pH causes less Ca^{2+} to be bound to protein. The increased concentration of ionized calcium, in turn, increases its glomerular filtration. Since net tubular Ca^{2+} reabsorption is decreased, the increased filtered load is translated into striking degrees of hypercalciuria. Distal renal tubular acidosis is the major form of chronic metabolic acidosis associated with such large increments in Ca^{2+} excretion. Although the mechanism by which systemic acidosis impairs Ca^{2+} absorption is unknown, it appears to be independent of systemic arterial pH.

Hormonal effects

Catecholamine secretion during metabolic acidosis plays a prominent role in the response of myocardial contraction and arteriolar dilatation. Increased plasma catecholamine levels not only reflect the general stress of metabolic acidosis but appear to be a specific response elicited by acidified ECF. When the adrenal gland is perfused with an acidified fluid, catecholamine secretion is specifically stimulated. While aldosterone secretion is clearly increased in metabolic acidosis, it is uncertain whether this is a specific effect of acidosis or is secondary to associated hyperkalaemia or adrenocorticotropic hormone (ACTH) release.

Protein wasting

The kidney responds to increases in the daily acid burden by increasing NAE largely through an enhanced synthesis of ammonia buffer. The kidney extracts amino acid precursors, strips their nitrogen, and recycles the remaining carbon skeleton in the form of CO_2 and glucose. Glutamine serves as the prime renal ammoniagenic precursor. It therefore follows that during periods of acid stress, the kidney's ability to enhance proton excretion depends on an increasing supply of glutamine and increased renal capacity to extract the glutamine and convert it to ammonia buffer. Endogenous and exogenous proteins serve as a ready source of glutamine. Thus it appears that acidosis simultaneously stimulates endogenous protein breakdown, ensuring delivery of glutamine to the kidney. Stimulation of renal ammoniagenesis by acidosis then enhances the conversion of the amino acid to the needed ammonia buffer. The acidosis induced whole body protein degradation is an important cause of malnutrition when the acidosis is prolonged (Movilli *et al.* 1998).

Metabolic acidosis (see also Chapter 5.4)

The development of metabolic acidosis can be traced to renal or extrarenal processes. Extrarenal processes include increased endogenous acid production and accelerated extrarenal loss of bicarbonate. The renal processes rest on a primary defect in renal acidification despite no increase in extrarenal hydrogen ion production. Metabolic acidosis of renal origin occurs because either the renal synthesis of new HCO_3^- is insufficient to regenerate that lost in buffering normal endogenous acid production [as in distal renal tubular acidosis (RTA) or advanced renal failure], or because a significant fraction of filtered HCO_3^- is lost (as occurs in proximal RTA). In either condition, effective extracellular volume is reduced and as a result the avidity for renal chloride reabsorption derived from the diet is increased, causing a hyperchloraemic metabolic acidosis.

The biochemical features of a metabolic acidosis include a low pH, a reduced HCO_3^- concentration, and an appropriate reduction in the $P\text{CO}_2$, reflecting respiratory compensation. A low HCO_3^- concentration alone is not diagnostic of metabolic acidosis because it may also result from the renal compensation for chronic respiratory alkalosis. Measurement of the arterial pH easily differentiates between these two possibilities.

Once metabolic acidosis is confirmed, calculation of the serum anion gap is a useful step in the differential diagnosis of the disorder. The anion gap is equal to the difference between the plasma concentrations of the major cation (Na) and the major measured anions ($Cl^- + HCO_3^-$) and reflects the charge difference between unmeasured anions and unmeasured cations.

$$\text{Anion gap} = [Na^+] - ([Cl^-] + [HCO_3^-]). \quad (5)$$

The normal value of the anion gap is approximately 10 ± 2 mmol/l. In interpreting the anion gap one must remember that the total charge of anions must equal the total charge of cations. As a result, a fall in the serum HCO_3^- concentration must be offset by a rise in the concentration of other anions. If the anion accompanying excess H^+ is chloride, then the decrease in the serum HCO_3^- concentration is matched by an equal rise in the serum Cl^- concentration. The acidosis is classified as a normal anion gap or hyperchloraemic metabolic acidosis. By contrast, if excess H^+ is accompanied by a non-chloride anion, then the decrease in HCO_3^- concentration is balanced by a rise in the concentration of the unmeasured anion and the Cl^- concentration remains the same. In this setting the acidosis is said to be a high anion gap metabolic acidosis. Table 2 lists the causes of metabolic acidosis according to the prevailing value for the anion gap.

A useful method to distinguish extrarenal and renal causes of metabolic acidosis is to measure urinary ammonium excretion (Halperin *et al.* 1988). Extrarenal causes of metabolic acidosis are associated with an appropriate increase in NAE primarily reflected by high levels of urinary ammonium excretion. By contrast, NAE and urinary ammonium levels are low in metabolic acidosis of renal origin. Unfortunately, measurement of urinary ammonium is not commonly available in clinical medicine. However, one can indirectly assess the amount of urinary ammonium present by calculating the urinary anion gap (UAG):

$$\text{UAG} = (U_{\text{Na}} + U_{\text{K}}) - U_{\text{Cl}}. \qquad (6)$$

Under normal circumstances the UAG is positive with values ranging from 30 to 50 mmol/l. A negative value for the UAG suggests the presence of increased renal excretion of an unmeasured cation, that is, a cation other than Na^+ or K^+. One such cation is NH_4^+. Metabolic acidosis of extrarenal origin is associated with a marked increase in urinary NH_4^+ excretion and, therefore, a large negative UAG. If the acidosis is of renal origin, urinary NH_4^+ excretion will be minimal and the UAG will usually be positive. Calculation of the UAG is not useful when there is increased excretion of Na^+ coupled to a non-chloride anion. For example, in diabetic ketoacidosis the UAG may remain positive, despite an appropriate increase in urinary NH_4^+ excretion due to the increased urinary excretion of sodium ketoacid salts.

In contrast to urinary NH_4^+ excretion, measurement of urine pH cannot reliably distinguish acidosis of renal or extrarenal origin. For example, an acid urine pH does not necessarily indicate an appropriate increase in NAE. With a significant reduction in the availability of ammonium to serve as a buffer, only a small amount of distal H^+ secretion will lead to a maximal reduction in urine pH. In this setting the pH of the urine is acid but the quantity of H^+ excretion is insufficient to meet daily acid production. By contrast, alkaline urine does not necessarily imply a renal acidification defect. In conditions where availability of NH_4^+ is not limiting, distal H^+ secretion can be massive and yet the urine remains relatively alkaline due to the buffering effects of NH_4^+.

Table 2 Classification of metabolic acidosis

Hyperchloraemic normal anion gap acidosis
Renal origin
Proximal renal tubular acidosis (Type II RTA)
Hypokalaemic distal renal tubular acidosis (Type I RTA)
Hyperkalaemic distal renal tubular acidosis (Type IV RTA)
Renal tubular acidosis of renal insufficiency (GFR usually >15–20 ml/min)
Extrarenal origin
Diarrhoea
Gastrointestinal-ureteral connections
External loss of pancreatic or biliary secretions
High anion gap metabolic acidosis
Renal origin
Uremic acidosis (GFR usually < 15–20 ml/min)
Extrarenal origin
Lactic acidosis
Diabetic ketoacidosis
Starvation ketoacidosis
Alcoholic ketoacidosis
Poisoning
Salicylate
Ethylene glycol
Methanol
Paraldehyde

Hyperchloraemic normal anion gap metabolic acidosis

A hyperchloraemic, normal anion gap, metabolic acidosis can be of renal or extrarenal origin. Metabolic acidosis of renal origin is the result of several types of abnormalities in tubular H^+ transport. The RTA of renal insufficiency is characterized by a normal anion gap acidosis, however, with severe reductions in the glomerular filtration rate (GFR) a high anion gap metabolic acidosis eventually develops. At this point the acidosis is often referred to as 'uraemic acidosis.' Metabolic acidosis of extrarenal origin is most commonly due to gastrointestinal HCO_3^- losses. Other common causes include the external loss of biliary and pancreatic secretions and ureteral diversion procedures.

Renal origin

Proximal renal tubular acidosis (Type II RTA)

Type II RTA is extensively discussed in Chapter 5.4. Under normal circumstances approximately 90 per cent of the filtered load of HCO_3^- is reabsorbed in the proximal tubule. Serum HCO_3^- concentration is maintained slightly below the threshold at which bicarbonaturia develops. When it exceeds 26–28 mmol/l, the excess HCO_3^- is appropriately excreted in the urine. In proximal RTA, the threshold for HCO_3^- reabsorption is reduced and results in a self-limited bicarbonaturia. A portion of the filtered HCO_3^- escapes reabsorption in the proximal tubule, thereby overwhelming the capacity of the distal nephron to reabsorb it. The resulting bicarbonaturia causes hypobicarbonataemia, with an attendant decrease of the filtered load of alkali despite the development of systemic acidaemia; the urine pH remains relatively alkaline due to the presence of HCO_3^- in the urine. Eventually, a new steady state is reached at which point the reduced filtered load of HCO_3^- matches the reduced tubular reabsorptive capacity and bicarbonaturia ceases. At this point, the delivery of HCO_3^- to the distal nephron may be abnormally increased, but it is of a magnitude that can be reabsorbed by the distal nephron. The urine is acidified to a pH of less than 5.5, and NAE equals endogenous acid production, although at a lower serum HCO_3^- concentration. In the steady state, the serum HCO_3^- concentration is usually in the range of 16–18 mmol/l.

One of the characteristic findings in proximal RTA is the presence of hypokalaemia. The development of hypokalaemia is the result of renal K^+ wasting due to the coupling of increased aldosterone levels and increased distal Na^+ delivery. The loss of $NaHCO_3$ in the urine leads to volume depletion which in turn activates the renin–angiotensin–aldosterone system. Under the influence of aldosterone, some portion of the increased Na^+ delivered in the distal tubule is reabsorbed leading to increased K^+ secretion. In the steady state, when virtually all the filtered HCO_3^- is reabsorbed in the proximal and distal nephron, renal K^+ wasting is minimal and the degree of hypokalaemia tends to be mild. By contrast, treatment of metabolic acidosis with $NaHCO_3$ improves the acidosis but worsens the degree of hypokalaemia. An increase in the filtered concentration of HCO_3^- above the reabsorptive threshold of the kidney augments the excretion of $NaHCO_3$ and $KHCO_3$.

Proximal RTA may occur as an isolated defect in acidification, but more commonly occurs in the setting of widespread dysfunction of the proximal tubule (Fanconi syndrome). In addition to decreased HCO_3^- reabsorption, patients with the Fanconi syndrome show evidence of impaired reabsorption of glucose, phosphate, uric acid, amino acids, and low molecular weight proteins. A variety of inherited and acquired disorders have been associated with the development of Fanconi syndrome and proximal RTA (Table 3). The most common inherited cause is cystinosis. Adults with the Fanconi syndrome most commonly have a dysproteinaemic condition such as multiple myeloma.

Unlike distal RTA, proximal RTA is not associated with nephrolithiasis or nephrocalcinosis. However, skeletal abnormalities are commonly present in these patients. Osteomalacia can develop as a result of chronic hypophosphataemia due to renal phosphate wasting. In addition, these patients may have a deficiency of the active form of vitamin D due to an inability to convert 25-hydroxyl-vitamin D_3 to 1,25-dihydroxy-vitamin D_3 in the proximal tubule. In adults, osteopenia may be present due to acidosis-induced demineralization of bone.

The diagnosis and the treatment of proximal RTA is reviewed in detail in Chapter 5.4.

Table 3 Causes of proximal (Type II) renal tubular acidosis (see also Chapter 5.4, Table 4)

Not associated with the Fanconi syndrome
Sporadic
Familial
Disorder of carbonic anhydrase
Drugs: acetazolamide, sulfanilamide
Carbonic anhydrase II deficiency
Associated with Fanconi syndrome
Selective (no systemic disease present)
Sporadic
Familial
Generalized (systemic disorder present)
Genetic disorders
Cystinosis
Wilson's disease
Hereditary fructose intolerance
Lowe's syndrome
Metachromatic leukodystrophy
Dysproteinaemic states
Myeloma kidney
Light chain deposition disease
Primary and secondary hyperparathyroidism
Drugs or toxins
Outdated tetracycline
Ifosfamide
Gentamicin
Streptozotocin
Lead
Cadmium
Mercury
Tubulointerstitial disease
Posttransplant rejection
Balkan nephropathy
Medullary cystic disease

Hypokalaemic distal renal tubular acidosis (Type I RTA)

Type I RTA is reviewed in Chapter 5.4. In contrast to proximal RTA, patients with distal RTA do not acidify their urine, despite severe metabolic acidosis. This disorder is due to a reduction in net H^+ secretion in the distal nephron resulting in impairment in HCO_3^- regeneration. As a result these patients are in a state of persistent positive acid balance requiring bone buffers to prevent severe systemic acidaemia. The pathophysiological basis for this defect could be the result of either impaired H^+ secretion (secretory defect) or an abnormally permeable distal tubule resulting in increased back-leak of normally secreted H^+ (gradient defect).

Patients with distal RTA exhibit low rates of ammonium secretion given the degree of systemic acidaemia. In part, the decreased secretion is due to the failure to trap NH_4 in the tubular lumen of the collecting duct due to the inability to lower the pH of the fluid. In addition, there is likely impairment in the medullary transfer of ammonium due to the presence of interstitial disease. Interstitial disease is frequently present in such patients due to an associated underlying disease or as a result of nephrocalcinosis or hypokalaemia-induced interstitial fibrosis.

Unlike proximal RTA, these patients frequently manifest evidence of nephrolithiasis and nephrocalcinosis. This predisposition to renal calcification is due to a number of factors. First, urinary Ca^{2+} excretion is high secondary to acidosis-induced bone mineral dissolution. This increase in urinary Ca^{2+} excretion is made worse by the low intraluminal concentration of HCO_3^- in the distal nephron. Normally, HCO_3^- acts to increase distal calcium absorption. Systemic acidaemia lowers the luminal concentration of HCO_3^- in the distal nephron so that Ca^{2+} absorption is decreased and urinary Ca^{2+} excretion is further augmented. The increased Ca^{2+} excretion is more likely to result in supersaturation of the urine due to the presence of an alkaline pH. The high urine pH decreases the solubility of calcium phosphate complexes. Stone formation is further enhanced as a result of low urinary citrate excretion. Citrate is metabolized to HCO_3, and thus its reabsorption contributes to correction of metabolic acidosis. Unfortunately urinary citrate serves as the major Ca^{2+} chelator in the urine, and thus its enhanced reabsorption in acidosis predisposes to nephrolithiasis and nephrocalcinosis.

Distal RTA may occur as a primary disorder, either idiopathic or inherited, but most commonly occurs in association with a systemic disease (Table 4). There is a particularly striking association with hypergammaglobulinaemic states. Several drugs and toxins have also been linked with the development of this disorder.

The diagnosis and the treatment of distal RTA is detailed in Chapter 5.4.

Hyperkalaemic distal renal tubular acidosis (Type IV RTA)

Type IV RTA is presented in detail in Chapter 5.4. It is characterized by a disturbance in distal nephron function that impairs renal excretion of both H^+ and K^+ resulting in a hyperchloraemic normal anion gap

Table 4 Causes of hypokalaemic distal (Type I) renal tubular acidosis (see also Chapter 5.4, Table 6)

Primary
Idiopathic
Familial
Secondary
Autoimmune disorders
Hypergammaglobulinaemia
Sjogren's syndrome
Primary biliary cirrhosis
Systemic lupus erythematosus
Genetic diseases
Ehlers–Danlos syndrome
Marfan's syndrome
Hereditary elliptocytosis
Drugs and toxins
Amphotericin B
Toluene
Disorders with nephrocalcinosis
Hyperparathyroidism
Vitamin D intoxication
Idiopathic hypercalciuria
Tubulointerstitial disease
Obstructive uropathy
Renal transplantation

Table 5 Causes of hyperkalaemic distal (Type IV) renal tubular acidosis (see also Chapter 5.4, Table 8)

Mineralocorticoid deficiency
Low renin, low aldosterone
Diabetes mellitus
Drugs
Non-steroidal anti-inflammatory agents
Cyclosporin A, tacrolimus
β-Blockers
High renin, low aldosterone
Adrenal destruction
Congenital enzyme defects
Drugs
Angiotensin-converting enzyme inhibitors
Angiotensin II receptor blockers
Heparin
Ketoconazole
Abnormal cortical collecting duct
Absence or defective mineralocorticoid receptor
Drugs
Spironolactone
Triamterene
Amiloride
Trimethoprim
Pentamidine
Chronic tubulointerstitial disease

acidosis and hyperkalaemia (DuBose 1997). The syndrome is usually associated with mild to moderate renal insufficiency, but, the magnitude of hyperkalaemia and acidosis are disproportionately severe for the observed degree of renal insufficiency. While hypokalaemic distal (Type I) RTA is also a disorder of distal nephron acidification, this disorder can be distinguished from Type I RTA on the basis of several important characteristics. First, they are obviously separable on the basis of serum K^+ concentration. Second, in Type IV RTA mild to moderate chronic renal failure is almost always present, whereas in Type I RTA renal function is often normal or only mildly impaired. Third, in most cases of Type IV RTA the urine pH, measured during spontaneous acidosis, is appropriately low (<5.5), whereas urine pH during spontaneous or induced acidosis in Type I RTA fails to decrease appropriately (>5.5). Fourth, metabolic acidosis in Type IV RTA is mild with plasma HCO_3^- concentration rarely less than 15 mmol/l, but in Type I RTA, acidosis is often severe with plasma HCO_3^- concentrations less than 15 mmol/l. It should be remembered that Type IV RTA is a much more common form of RTA and is, therefore, more likely to be encountered, particularly in adult patients.

The pathophysiological basis for this disorder can either be a deficiency in circulating aldosterone or a disease of the cortical collecting duct. In either case a defect in distal H^+ secretion develops. Impaired Na^+ reabsorption in the principal cell decreases the luminal electronegativity of the cortical collecting duct. Impaired distal acidification results from the decreased driving force for H^+ secretion into the tubular lumen. H^+ secretion is further impaired in this segment as well as in the medullary collecting duct either as a result of the loss of the direct stimulatory effect of aldosterone on H^+ secretion or an abnormality in the H^+-secreting cell.

Decreased luminal electronegativity in the cortical collecting duct also impairs renal K^+ excretion. Hyperkalaemia aggravates the defect in distal acidification by decreasing the amount of ammonia available to act as a urinary buffer (Hulter *et al.* 1977). Hyperkalaemia limits the availability of ammonia in two ways. First, it decreases ammonia production in the proximal tubule. Second, ammonium transport in the thick ascending limb is inhibited because the large increase in luminal K^+ concentration effectively competes with ammonium for transport on the Na–K–2Cl cotransporter and apical K^+ channel. Thus, NAE decreases as a result of limited buffer availability for titration of secreted hydrogen ions.

The differential diagnosis of Type IV RTA can be divided into those conditions associated with decreased circulating levels of aldosterone and conditions associated with impaired function of the cortical collecting duct (Table 5). Perhaps the most common disease associated with Type IV RTA in adults is diabetes mellitus. In these patients, primary NaCl retention leads to volume expansion and suppression and atrophy of the renin-secreting juxtaglomerular apparatus (Sebastian *et al.* 1977).

Similarly, several commonly used drugs such as non-steroidal anti-inflammatory agents, angiotensin-converting enzyme inhibitors, and heparin can lead to decreased mineralocorticoid activity. Impaired function of the cortical collecting duct can be a feature of structural damage to the kidney as in interstitial renal disease or result from use of certain drugs.

Diagnosis and treatment of a Type IV RTA is reviewed in detail in Chapter 5.4.

Renal tubular acidosis of renal insufficiency

Metabolic acidosis is a consistent feature of chronic renal insufficiency. It results from the failure of the tubular acidification process to excrete the normal daily acid load. As functional renal mass is reduced by disease, ammonium production and H^+ secretion by the remaining nephrons increase but eventually fail to keep pace with daily acid production. NAE does not match daily endogenous acid production and a hyperchloraemic normal anion gap acidosis develops as the GFR falls below 30–40 ml/min. With more advanced renal failure (GFR <15–20 ml/min) the acidosis changes predominantly to the high anion gap variety.

Titratable acid excretion (primarily a function of distal phosphate delivery) remains normal in patients with mild to moderate renal insufficiency. Two factors are responsible for the continued normal absolute phosphate delivery to the distal nephron. First, fractional reabsorption of phosphate in the proximal tubule is reduced by secondary hyperparathyroidism. Second, as renal failure progresses, serum phosphate increases and the filtered load of phosphate declines less than does the GFR. The principal defect in NAE is the inability to excrete adequate amounts of ammonium in the urine, despite increased production of ammonium per remaining nephron; overall production is decreased as a result of a severe skrinkage of total renal mass. In addition, less ammonium is delivered to the medullary interstitium secondary to disrupted medullary anatomy (Buerkert *et al.* 1983). The ability to lower the urinary pH remains intact because distal nephron H^+ secretion is less impaired than NH_3 excretion. Quantitatively, however, the total amount of secreted H^+ secretion is reduced and the urine pH is acidic as a consequence of very little buffer in the urine. The lack of NH_4 in the urine is reflected by a positive value for the UAG.

When GER falls below 10–15 ml/min, phosphate and other anions (sulfate and organic acids) accumulate in the serum and convert the acidosis to the high anion gap variety.

Correction of the metabolic acidosis in patients with renal insufficiency is relatively easy to achieve by administering an amount of alkali equal to daily acid production. Treatment with 0.5–1.5 mmol/kg/day of $NaHCO_3$ will raise the serum HCO_3^- level above 20 mmol/l in most cases. To prevent volume overload, loop diuretics are often used in conjunction with alkali therapy. Eventually the acidosis becomes refractory to medical therapy and dialysis must be initiated. Recent evidence suggests that metabolic acidosis in the setting of renal failure needs to be aggressively treated. Chronic acidosis has been associated with metabolic bone disease and may lead to an accelerated catabolic state in patients with chronic renal failure (Alpern and Sakhaee 1997).

In summary, a defect in any one of the normal mechanisms of renal acidification will give rise to a hyperchloraemic normal anion gap metabolic acidosis. The acidosis of renal insufficiency can be associated with an increased anion gap when the GFR is markedly reduced; however, the underlying defect in renal acidification remains the same. Examination of the urine pH, the serum K^+ concentration, and determining whether there is evidence of widespread proximal tubular dysfunction are tools that can be used to distinguish the various causes of metabolic acidosis thought to be of renal origin.

Extrarenal origin

Diarrhoea

Intestinal secretions beyond the stomach including the pancreas and biliary tract are often rich in bicarbonate. Their accelerated loss leads to metabolic acidosis. The resultant volume loss signals the kidney to increase the reabsorption of salt. Renal retention of NaCl combined with the intestinal loss of $NaHCO_3$ generates a hyperchloraemic, normal anion gap metabolic acidosis. In response to the systemic acidaemia the kidney markedly increases NAE, mainly through an increased urinary excretion of ammonium. Hypokalaemia, as a result of gastrointestinal losses, and the low serum pH both stimulate the synthesis of ammonia in the proximal tubule. The increase in availability of ammonia to act as a urinary buffer allows for a maximal increase in H^+ secretion by the distal nephron.

Examination of the urine pH in diarrhoea can be misleading in the evaluation of the appropriateness of the renal response to systemic acidaemia. In fact, urine pH during chronic diarrhoeal states may be persistently greater than 6.0, despite systemic acidaemia. In this regard, a patient who presents with hypokalaemic, hyperchloraemic metabolic acidosis with a urine pH greater than 5.5 could either have a diarrhoeal disorder or a hypokalaemic RTA. Distinction between these two possibilities is best achieved by a careful clinical history except in a patient with surreptitious laxative abuse and by the determination of the UAG. In diarrhoea, the relatively high urine pH is associated with a negative UAG because most of the augmented NH_4^+ is excreted in the urine as NH_4Cl. In hypokalaemic distal RTA, the urine pH is relatively high due to the inability to secrete H^+ in the distal nephron. In steady-state proximal RTA also, the pH is relatively high. In both conditions, the urinary excretion of ammonia is very low and the UAG is positive.

Gastrointestinal–ureteral connections

Surgical diversion of the ureters into an isolated segment of the gastrointestinal (GI) tract (serving as a 'new' urinary bladder) is oftentimes used in the treatment of patients with neurological bladder abnormalities or urological tumours to replace the dysfunctional native bladder. It can be associated with a hyperchloraemic, normal anion gap metabolic acidosis developing through several mechanisms. First, NH_4^+ and Cl^- in the urine may simply be reabsorbed by the intestine. The NH_4^+ is then metabolized in the liver to NH_3 and H^+. Second, urinary Cl^- may be reabsorbed in exchange for HCO_3^- through activation of the Cl^-/HCO_3^- exchanger on the intestinal lumen. In some patients, a renal defect in acidification can develop and exacerbate the degree of acidosis. Such a defect may result from tubular damage due to pyelonephritis or increased colonic pressures.

The main factors that influence the development and severity of acidosis are the length of time the urine remains in contact with the bowel segment and the total surface area of bowel exposed to urine. In patients with a ureterosigmoid anastamosis, the acidosis tends to be more common and severe as compared to patients with an ileal conduit. The latter procedure was purposefully designed to minimize the time and area of contact between urine and intestinal surface. Patients with this procedure who develop an acidosis should be examined for the possibility of an ileal loop obstruction since this would lead to an increase in contact time between the urine and the intestinal surface.

High anion gap metabolic acidosis

Lactic acidosis

One of the most common causes of a high anion gap metabolic acidosis is lactic acidosis. Lactic acid is the end product in the anaerobic metabolism of glucose. The last step in this pathway is the reversible reduction of pyruvic acid by lactic acid dehydrogenase and NADH to lactic acid:

$$\text{Pyruvate} + \text{NADH} + H^+ \Leftrightarrow \text{Lactate} + \text{NAD}^+. \qquad (7)$$

Under normal conditions, the reaction is shifted towards the right such that the normal lactate/pyruvate ratio is approximately 10 : 1. The reactants in this pathway are inter-related as follows:

$$\text{Lactate} = K \times \frac{[\text{Pyruvate}] \times [\text{NADH}] \times [\text{H}^+]}{[\text{NAD}^+]}. \tag{8}$$

On the basis of this relationship it is evident that lactate can increase for three reasons. First, as a consequence of increased pyruvate production alone so that the lactate/pyruvate ratio remains normal. An isolated increase in pyruvate production is seen, for example, in the settings of intravenous glucose or epinephrine infusions, in respiratory or metabolic alkalosis. Lactate levels in these conditions are only minimally elevated, rarely exceeding 5 mmol/l. Second, lactate can increase as a result of an increased NADH/NAD$^+$ ratio. The lactate/pyruvate ratio can increase markedly and the absolute values for the concentrations of lactate and pyruvate may be very elevated. Finally, lactate concentrations can increase when both pyruvate production and NADH/NAD$^+$ ratio are increased. This is usually the case in severe lactic acidosis.

Under normal circumstances virtually all tissues metabolize glucose via the glycolytic pathway and generate lactate with the majority of lactate production occurring in brain, erythrocytes, and skeletal muscle. In turn, lactate is extracted predominately by the liver and renal cortex and is either reconverted to glucose or becomes fuel for oxidation for CO_2 and H_2O. This dynamic relationship between lactate and glucose is termed the Cori cycle. Its importance is evident when the normal daily production of lactate (15–30 mmol/kg/day, equivalent to 15–30 mmol/ of H$^+$/kg/day) is considered. The quantitative importance of this pathway in disposing of the proton load produced during glycolysis should be compared with the 1 mmol/kg/day daily NAE by the kidney. Furthermore, it is apparent that even if the Cori Cycle is only mildly disrupted, with lactate production exceeding its consumption, a devastating metabolic acidosis can rapidly develop.

Lactic acidosis is generated whenever lactic acid production exceeds utilization (Madias 1986). The resulting accumulation of serum lactate is most commonly accompanied by hypobicarbonataemia and systemic acidaemia as well as by an increased anion gap. This imbalance can result from lactic acid's overproduction, underutilization, or both. Severe exercise is an example in which lactic acidosis can develop because its production overwhelms the normal capacity to utilize it. The short-lived nature of the acidosis in these conditions suggests that a concomitant defect in lactic acid utilization is present in most conditions of sustained and severe lactic acidosis.

A partial list of the disorders associated with the development of lactic acidosis is given in Table 6. It has been proposed that these disorders can be separated into two major types. *Type A lactic acidosis* includes tissue underperfusion or acute hypoxia as seen in patients with cardiopulmonary failure, severe anaemia, haemorrhage, hypotension, sepsis, and carbon monoxide poisoning. *Type B lactic acidosis* develops without evidence of overt hypoperfusion or hypoxia, in patients with a variety of disorders such as congenital defects in glucose or lactate metabolism, diabetes mellitus, liver disease, effects of drugs and toxins, and neoplastic diseases. It should be pointed out that in clinical practice many patients often exhibit features of Type A and Type B lactic acidosis simultaneously.

Lactic acid has two optical isomers, the D and L forms. Lactic acidosis is mostly due to L-lactic acid since the lactate dehydrogenase enzyme present in mammalian cells synthesizes only the L-isomer. In human beings, the trivial quantities of D-lactate that appear in blood and the urine are absorbed from food, or produced in the GI tract by certain lactobacilli. Experimental infusions of the two isomers have revealed that D-lactate is cleared more slowly than its enantiomer and that it significantly prolongs the half-life of the normal L-lactate.

Table 6 Causes of lactic acidosis

Type A (tissue underperfusion and/or hypoxia)
Cardiogenic shock
Septic shock
Haemorrhagic shock
Acute hypoxia
Carbon monoxide poisoning
Anaemia
Type B (absence of hypotension and hypoxia)
Hereditary enzyme deficiency (e.g. glucose 6-phosphatase)
Drugs or toxins
Phenformin
Antiretroviral drugs (e.g. Stavudine)
Cyanide
Salicylate
Ethylene glycol
Methanol
Systemic disease
Liver failure
Malignancy

D-lactic acidosis can develop in patients with short bowel syndromes who develop overgrowth of D-lactic acid-producing bacteria. Manifestations of this disorder tend to be neurological in nature. Weakness, ataxia, slurred speech, and confusion are often combined with bizarre behaviour. These findings do not necessarily correlate with blood levels of D-lactate suggesting that other absorbed bacterial products may contribute to the neuropathology. Use of a D-lactate dehydrogenase enzyme assay is required to make the diagnosis of D-lactic acidosis in a patient with a high anion gap in whom routine L-lactate levels are normal and no other cause for the metabolic disorder is evident. Oral administration of poorly absorbable antibiotics has proved beneficial in eliminating the pathological bacteria responsible for the genesis of this disorder.

The primary goal in the therapy of lactic acidosis is correction of the underlying disorder. Every attempt should be made to restore tissue perfusion and oxygenation when they are compromised.

Although the role of alkali in the treatment of lactic acidosis is somewhat controversial, we believe that HCO_3^- should be administered when the systemic pH falls to less than 7.10 as haemodynamic instability becomes much more likely with severe acidaemia. However, attempts to normalize the pH or HCO_3^- concentration should be avoided.

Diabetic ketoacidosis

Diabetic ketoacidosis is a metabolic condition characterized by the accumulation of acetoacetic acid and β-hydroxybutyric acid. The development of ketoacidosis is primarily the result of insulin deficiency and a relative or absolute increase in glucagon concentration. These hormonal changes increase fatty acid mobilization from adipose tissue and at the same time alter the oxidative machinery of the liver such that delivered fatty acids are primarily metabolized into ketoacids. In addition, peripheral glucose utilization is impaired and the gluconeogenic pathway in the liver is maximally stimulated. The resultant hyperglycaemia leads to an osmotic diuresis and volume depletion.

Blood ketoacids accumulate when the rate of hepatic ketoacid generation exceeds peripheral utilization. The H^+ accumulation in the ECF destroys HCO_3^- while the ketoacid anion concentration rises. The reduction in serum HCO_3^- concentration approximates the increase in anion gap initially. The degree to which the anion gap is elevated will depend on the rapidity, severity, and duration of the ketoacidosis as well as the status of the ECF volume. While an increased anion gap acidosis is the most common chemical disturbance seen in diabetic ketoacidosis, a hyperchloraemic normal anion gap acidosis is oftentimes present depending upon the stage of the disease process. In the earliest stages of ketoacidosis, when extracellular volume is near normal, ketoacid anions are rapidly excreted by the kidney as sodium and potassium salts. Their excretion is equivalent to the loss of potential bicarbonate. This urinary loss, while the kidney retains dietary NaCl, results in a hyperchloraemic normal anion gap acidosis.

As ketogenesis accelerates and volume depletion worsens, a larger proportion of the ketoacid anions is retained within the body, thus increasing the anion gap. Treatment terminates ketoacid production and transforms the high anion gap metabolic acidosis back into a hyperchloraemic normal anion gap acidosis. Restoration of ECF volume augments the renal excretion of the sodium salts of the ketoacid anions. This loss of 'potential bicarbonate' combined with the retention of administered NaCl accounts for the redevelopment of the hyperchloraemic normal anion gap acidosis. In addition, K and Na, administered in solutions containing NaCl and KCl, enter cells in exchange for H^+, which renders the intravenous therapy tantamount to administering HCl. The reversal of the hyperchloraemic acidosis is accomplished over several days as the deficit in HCO_3^- is replenished by the kidney.

Acidosis can be severe with HCO_3^- reductions to 5 mmol/l or less. Ketoacids can be identified by crushed nitroprusside tablets or reagent strips. However, this test can be misleading in assessing the severity of ketoacidosis as it only detects the presence of acetone and acetoacetate but does not react with β-hydroxybutyrate. Acetoacetic acid and β-hydroxybutyric acid are interconvertible with the NADH/NAD$^+$ ratio being the primary determinant as to which moiety predominates. In the setting of a high ratio, formation of β-hydroxybutyric acid is favoured and the nitroprusside test will become less positive or even negative, despite significant ketoacidosis. This situation can occur when ketoacidosis is accompanied by lactic acidosis or in the setting of alcoholic ketoacidosis. During treatment, the NADH/NAD$^+$ ratio tends to decline favouring the formation of acetoacetic acid. As a result, the nitroprusside test becomes more strongly positive during treatment even though the body burden of ketoacids is declining.

Treatment of diabetic ketoacidosis involves the use of insulin and intravenous fluids to correct volume depletion. Deficiencies in potassium and Mg^{2+} are common and therefore these electrolytes are typically added to intravenous solutions. Alkali therapy is generally not required because administration of insulin leads to the conversion of ketoacid anions into HCO_3^- and allows partial correction of the acidosis. However, HCO_3^- therapy may be indicated in patients who present with severe acidaemia ($pH < 7.1$).

Starvation ketoacidosis

Abstinence from food can lead to a mild high anion gap metabolic acidosis secondary to increased production of ketoacids. This disorder is similar to diabetic ketoacidosis in that starvation leads to relative insulin deficiency and glucagon excess. As a result there is increased mobilization of fatty acids and at the same time the liver is 'programmed' to oxidize fatty acids to ketoacids. With prolonged starvation, the blood ketoacid level can approach 5–6 mmol/l. The serum HCO_3^- concentration rarely falls to values less than 18 mmol/l. More fulminant ketoacidosis is aborted by the fact that ketone bodies stimulate the pancreatic islets to release insulin so that lipolysis is held in check. This break in the ketogenic process is notably absent in insulin dependent diabetics. There is no specific therapy indicated in this disorder.

Alcoholic ketoacidosis

Ketoacidosis develops in patients with a history of chronic ethanol abuse, decreased food intake, and often a history of nausea and vomiting. As with starvation ketosis, a decrease in the insulin/glucagon ratio leads to accelerated fatty acid mobilization and alters the enzymatic machinery of the liver to favour ketoacid production. However, there are features unique to this disorder that differentiates it from simple starvation ketosis. First, alcohol withdrawal combined with volume depletion and starvation markedly increase the levels of circulating catecholamines. As a result, the peripheral mobilization of fatty acids exceeds that typically found with starvation alone and can lead to marked ketoacid production and severe metabolic acidosis. Second, the metabolism of alcohol leads to accumulation of NADH and an increased NADH/NAD$^+$ ratio reflected by a higher β-hydroxybutyrate to acetoacetate ratio. As previously mentioned, the nitroprusside reaction may be diminished by this redox shift, despite the presence of severe ketoacidosis. Treatment is centred on the administration of glucose. Glucose leads to the rapid resolution of the acidosis because stimulation of insulin release leads to diminished fatty acid mobilization from adipose tissue as well as decreased hepatic output of ketoacids. Associated deficiencies in K^+, Mg^{2+}, and phosphorus require therapy.

Poisoning

Salicylate

Aspirin (acetylsalicylic acid) is one of the most widely available therapeutic agents and is associated with the largest number of accidental or intentional poisonings. At toxic concentrations, salicylate uncouples oxidative phosphorylation and leads to overproduction of lactic and other organic acids. In children, ketoacid production may also be increased. The accumulation of lactic acid, salicylic acid, ketoacids, and other organic acids produce a high anion gap metabolic acidosis. Simultaneously, salicylate directly stimulates the respiratory centre. Increased ventilation lowers the $P\text{CO}_2$ causing respiratory alkalosis. Children primarily manifest a high anion gap metabolic acidosis with toxic salicylate levels while the respiratory alkalosis is most evident in adults. When coexistent, both effects become additive in lowering serum HCO_3^- values but are offsetting each other in terms of the final pH. Thus, such a patient with a salicylate-induced mixed metabolic acidosis and respiratory alkalosis, may for example, have a HCO_3^- level of 12 mmol/l and a $P\text{CO}_2$ of 20 mmHg, a set of values which fixes arterial pH at 7.40. In addition to conservative management, the initial goal of therapy is to correct systemic acidaemia and to alkalinize the urine. By increasing systemic pH, the ionized fraction of salicylic acid increases and, as a result, accumulation of the drug in the central nervous system (CNS) decreases. Similarly, an alkaline urine pH increases urinary excretion because the ionized fraction of the drug is poorly reabsorbed by the tubule. At serum concentrations of greater than 80 mg/dl or in the setting of severe clinical toxicity, haemodialysis can be used to accelerate the removal of the drug from the body.

Ethylene glycol

Ethylene glycol is a clear aliphatic diol with a pleasant odour and a warm, sweet taste. It is used as a solvent for paints and plastics, in hydraulic brake fluid, in ink, and for softening cellophane and is the principal component (usually 95 per cent) of motor vehicle antifreeze. Its ready availability, accounts for many cases of ethylene glycol poisoning (Davis *et al.* 2002), especially in desperate alcoholics.

After rapid absorption through the stomach, this highly water-soluble compound distributes evenly throughout bodily tissues. The elimination half-life is 3–5 h. The kidney filters and passively reabsorbs the compound, with nearly 20 per cent of a dose of 1 mg/kg body weight excreted unchanged in the urine. Hepatic metabolism, catalysed by the enzyme alcohol dehydrogenase, accounts for nearly all the rest of this drug's elimination. Ethylene glycol metabolism follows several pathways. Small amounts (3–10 per cent) of oxalic acid and an even smaller amount of hippuric acid are generated. Oxalic acid is formed through glycoaldehyde, glycolate, and glyoxylate, with consequent generation of NADH, the reduced form of the pyridine nucleotide NAD^+. These metabolites are more toxic than their parent compound. The increase in the cellular $NADH/NAD^+$ ratio augments lactic acid production from pyruvic acid. Glycolic acid accounts for most of the increment in the anion gap in experimental and human poisonings associated with ethylene glycol.

In the absence of prompt therapy, a dose of 1.0–1.5 mg/kg of body weight of ethylene glycol is lethal for an average-sized adult. The range of reported lethal doses is very large, and survival of substantially larger ingestions has been documented. Toxic symptoms and the degree of metabolic acidosis closely parallel the plasma level of glycolic acid (Gabow *et al.* 1986). As the affinity of hepatic alcohol dehydrogenase for alcohol is 100 times greater than its affinity for ethylene glycol, ethanol therapy has been used to slow ethylene glycol's metabolism to its more toxic byproducts. In fact, concurrent ingestion of ethanol with ethylene glycol may delay the onset of the latter's toxicity.

The clinical features of ethylene glycol poisoning are well characterized. Patients tend to pass through three distinct stages of toxicity. The initial findings are those of CNS depression, ataxia (which is dose-dependent), slurred speech and stupor (with modest ingestion), and coma and convulsions (when larger quantities have been consumed). This first stage usually lasts for up to 12 h, but may be prolonged for days; metabolic acidosis becomes evident and mortality rates are high during this initial phase.

The second stage of toxicity is characterized by cardiopulmonary failure with tachypnoea, tachycardia, rales, a ventricular gallop rhythm, cyanosis, and even mild hypertension. Whether the pulmonary oedema is simply a function of toxic myocardial depression or whether non-cardiac causes also contribute has not been clarified. The last stage is marked by oliguric or anuric acute renal failure and may be heralded by flank pain in awake and responsive patients. Renal function recovery is partial or complete, but may take several months (Jacobsen *et al.* 1982).

Cytotoxic effects of ethylene glycol's metabolites and the deposition of calcium oxalate account for the renal failure. Some patients pass directly from the first to the third stage, avoiding cardiopulmonary disorders. Ethylene glycol ingestion increases both the anion and osmolal gaps (see Eq. 9). In addition to glycolate, lactate may contribute to the increased anion gap. Hypoxia, hypotension, and altered tissue redox ratios contribute to the lactic acidosis. The urinary sediment reveals either the acicular (needle-shaped) crystals of calcium oxalate monohydrate or its more familiar octahedrals (i.e. the 'envelopes') of calcium oxalate dihydrate. Rarely the monohydrate takes on the shape of a dumbbell. Crystalluria, may be absent in patients presenting soon after ingestion, because maximum production of oxalate does not occur until 8 h after ingestion. Repeated urinalyses may be necessary to reveal emerging crystalluria. The degree of hypobicarbonataemia is roughly equal to the circulating level of glycolate and to the increment in the anion gap. Hypocalcaemia and leucocytosis are also reported. Lumbar puncture usually shows a mild pleocytosis, normal glucose concentration, and mild-to-moderate increases in protein.

Ethylene glycol levels can be roughly approximated from the difference between the measured and calculated serum osmolalities (see also Chapter 2.1). The electrolyte and non-electrolyte contribution to normal serum osmolality is almost entirely accounted for by the sum of sodium and its accompanying anions, and by urea and glucose:

$$\begin{aligned}\text{Calculated osmolality} = {} & 2 \times [\text{Na}]\ (\text{mmol/l}) \\ & + \text{BUN}\ (\text{mg/dl})/2.8 \\ & + \text{Glucose}\ (\text{mg/dl})/18. \end{aligned} \tag{9}$$

Doubling the serum sodium concentration accounts for the electrolyte component of serum osmolality, dividing the BUN and glucose by 2.8 and 18, respectively, converts them from mass units to milliosmoles per litre. The calculated serum osmolality should agree with the value estimated by freezing point depression to within 10 mOsm/l. To the extent that the measured osmolality exceeds the calculated value by more than 10 mOsm/l, some circulating non-electrolyte solute not accounted for by urea or glucose is causing the disparity. Most drugs do not contribute to an osmolal gap, because they are of high molecular weight and are taken in small amounts. Ethylene glycol, however, can cause this osmolal gap. Because its molecular weight is only 62 mg/mmol, each 62 mg/100 ml of circulating ethylene glycol increases the osmolal gap by 10 mOsm/l. Patients may enter the hospital many hours after ingesting ethylene glycol so that the parent compound is fully catabolized, allowing the blood ethylene glycol level to approach zero while glycolic acid levels remain high. The acid does not add to the osmolal gap, because its proton is lost with HCO_3^- in the titration process; the glycolate simply replaces lost alkali. Thus, at this stage, the osmolal gap is normal, while the anion gap is increased.

Exposure to toxins has most likely occurred when a high anion gap acidosis is unassociated with azotaemia or with ketoacidosis or lactic acidosis. If the osmolal gap is also increased, then ethylene glycol or methanol is most likely the culprit. The typical clinical picture of ethylene glycol toxicity, in the presence of a high anion gap acidosis and an osmolal gap, is highly characteristic. Demonstration of leucocytosis, hypocalcaemia, and calcium oxalate crystalluria, and, finally, the finding of ethylene glycol in the blood, confirm the diagnosis. Autopsy often reveals calcium oxalate deposition in the vessels and meninges of the brain and kidney tubules (Pons and Custor 1946). In surviving patients, calcium oxalate crystals have been shown to persist in the kidney for months.

Ethylene glycol is very rapidly absorbed from the stomach, so that gastric lavage, though it should be attempted, may be of limited benefit.

Therapy is directed at the acidaemia and the prevention of further metabolism of ethylene glycol. A loading dose of 0.6–1.0 g of ethanol per kilogram of body weight should be given over 1 h and followed by a maintenance infusion of 10–20 g/h so as to maintain a blood ethanol level of 100 mg/100 ml, a concentration at which it effectively competes with ethylene glycol for hepatic alcohol dehydrogenase. Haemodialysis and peritoneal dialysis have both been used to remove these highly dialysable toxins. Rebound increases in ethylene glycol levels may occur after dialysis is stopped, making it critically important to continue therapy for at least 24 h after plasma levels of ethylene glycol become unmeasurable. To prevent dangerous toxicity, haemodialysis should be instituted immediately if there is clinical or laboratory evidence of extreme exposure. Though haemodialysis more efficiently removes ethylene glycol, peritoneal dialysis is an effective alternative and should be initiated if haemodialysis is unavailable.

To avoid the difficulties of monitoring and maintaining therapeutic ethanol levels, some authors have recommended adding the alcohol directly to the dialysate bath (100 mg/100 ml). To enhance renal oxalate excretion, the ECF volume should be kept appropriately expanded and diuretics given to achieve and maintain a brisk diuresis. 4-methylpyrazole (4-MP, fomepizole) inhibits alcohol dehydrogenase more potently than does ethanol, thereby more effectively preventing the conversion of ethylene glycol to its toxic metabolites (Mycyk and Leikin 2003). Moreover, the metabolism of ethanol is slower than that of 4-MP; this indicates that the latter has a more rapid onset of action than alcohol. Because it also inhibits the metabolism of ethanol, coadministration of 4-MP with ethanol is not recommended. Lastly, 4-MP administration eliminates the variability associated with the metabolism of ethanol, particularly during administration of haemodialysis, making it the drug of choice in ethylene glycol toxicity, despite its significantly greater cost over an ethanol infusion.

If the osmolal gap is repeatedly normal in a patient known to have ingested ethylene glycol many hours earlier, one may assume very low blood glycol levels. Ethanol therapy becomes unnecessary at this point, since the alcohol's only therapeutic purpose is to prevent conversion of the parent compound into its more toxic products. Dialysis is still indicated for removal of the toxic metabolites.

Methanol

Methyl alcohol (methanol) is a clear liquid with a molecular weight of 32. Its odour is distinctly different from that of ethanol, but its presence may be masked by impurities added during its production or by the many liquids with which it is miscible. In illicit alcoholic beverages, the cheaper methanol may be substituted for the more expensive ethanol. This widely available toxin is found in many solvents, cleaners, shellacs, and varnishes, and is added to industrial ethanol-containing solutions to 'denature' them, that is, to render them poisonous. Toxic exposure to methanol can occur by several routes, including ingestion, inhalation, and absorption from the skin. However, with better industrial safety standards, inhalation and skin absorption are now infrequent, and most toxicities derive from ingestion. Still, recent reports have documented sporadic cases and outbreaks of sometimes lethal methanol intoxication from skin absorption such as the application of methanol-soaks to the skin of febrile children.

Methanol poisoning from ingestion has occurred both sporadically and in epidemics (Davis *et al.* 2002). In addition to denatured alcohol, other sources of methanol include certain antifreeze preparations, car windshield cleaners, Sterno (flammable heating compound), and, most recently, diluents used for photocopy machines. The most frequently cited lethal dose is 30 ml of absolute methanol, but patients have been known to survive after ingesting 500 ml; others have died after taking as little as 15 ml of a 10 per cent solution. Despite aggressive therapy, mortality from methanol poisoning continues to approximate 20 per cent and is related to both duration and severity of the ensuing acidosis.

Methanol has an apparent volume of distribution similar to that of ethanol (0.6–0.7 l/kg body weight). It diffuses readily into lipid-containing tissues. Its highest concentrations are found within the kidney, liver, and gastrointestinal tract. Within the optic nerve and the vitreous humor it produces visual impairment and blindness. Formate is primarily responsible for the ocular toxicity. At least 25 per cent of a methanol dose is eliminated by the lungs and only 3–5 per cent is excreted unchanged in the urine. Methanol is metabolized mainly in the liver by alcohol dehydrogenase, at a rate that is independent of serum levels and only one-seventh as rapid as that of ethanol. This enzyme catalyzes methanol's sequential conversion to formaldehyde and formic acid. The latter's oxidation to CO_2 and water is folate-dependent. In rhesus monkeys, methanol-induced formic acidosis can be prevented by pretreatment with folic acid or 5-formyl tetrahydrofolate (McMartin *et al.* 1975). This vitamin dependency of formate metabolism has led to speculation that malnourished alcoholics may not readily clear formic acid.

Elimination kinetics depends on the quantity of methanol absorbed. The serum half-life at low dosages is 14–20 h, and at higher dosages 24–30 h. Blocking alcohol dehydrogenase by ethanol extends the half-life to 30–35 h.

The byproducts of methanol metabolism, principally formaldehyde and formic acid, account for the clinical manifestations of toxicity. Unmetabolized methanol exerts little toxic effect. Indeed, despite the fact that serum methanol levels peak within 1–2 h of ingestion, symptoms and signs develop after a lag time of 8–30 h. This lag time correlates well with the time required for the toxic accumulation of formic acid.

Acutely exposed patients develop CNS and GI system symptoms. Headache, confusion, vertigo, and lethargy are common. Blurred vision, blindness, photophobia, and a feeling of 'being in a snowfield' are visual complaints in half of the cases of epidemic toxicity. Dilated pupils, constriction of the visual fields, retinal oedema, and hyperaemia, blurring, and loss of cupping of the optic disk may be seen. Normal eyegrounds, despite the presence of other toxic manifestations, may result from subtoxic repeated exposures. Euphoria, which frequently accompanies ethanol ingestion, is not a feature of methanol intoxication.

Abdominal pain may obtain from pancreatitis, with consequent hyperamylasaemia, from mucosal irritation of the GI tract, or from swelling of the kidney. Notably, the hyperamylasaemia usually represents salivary isoamylase, levels of which are often elevated in alcoholics. CNS symptoms rarely occur at levels below 20 mg/100 ml, but because formate accounts for the bulk of toxicity, peak levels must be gauged with respect to a given individual's symptoms. Ocular symptoms usually are not manifested at levels less than 100 mg/100 ml. A peak level of more than 50 mg/100 ml indicates serious poisoning. Fatalities in untreated patients generally occur with levels of 15–200 mg/100 ml, but mortality and also, ocular toxicity correlate best with the degree of metabolic acidosis secondary to the accumulation of formic acid. All signs are potentially reversible with prompt initiation of therapy; however, severe sequelae, such as blindness and Parkinsonism, may occur if treatment is delayed.

A high anion gap metabolic acidosis, due to formic acid accumulation, occurs with severe toxicity. Lactic acidosis and ketoacidosis occasionally complicate methanol toxicity. Formate seems to account for the entire increment in the anion gap in the early stages of the acidosis and in patients with mild exposure. More severely intoxicated patients are likely to develop ketosis and/or lactic acidosis.

Methanolaemia increases the osmolal gap. Each 100 mg/l (i.e. each 10 mg/100 ml) of methanol contributes 3.2 mOsm/l. Ethanol levels should be obtained, since ethanol is frequently consumed with methanol and also adds to the osmolal gap. In patients ingesting sufficient ethanol with methanol, the osmolal gap often increases disproportionately more than the increment in the anion gap. This is due to ethanol's slowing of methanol metabolism, which at once maintains a higher methanol level, increasing the osmolal gap, while the reduced rate of formate accrual minimizes any increase in the anion gap.

The laboratory findings in methanol intoxication include hyperamylasaemia, increased circulating levels of various liver enzymes, proteinuria, glycosuria, and, occasionally, haematuria. Autopsy findings have revealed a variety of diffuse multisystemic changes. The CNS pathology includes ganglion cell degeneration of the retina, and cerebral oedema and haemorrhage showing a striking predilection for symmetrical involvement of the putamen. Miscellaneous changes that are consistently found include pulmonary congestion, fatty lever, haemorrhagic pancreatitis, and acute tubular necrosis.

It is generally accepted that mortality and the potential for irreversible ophthalmopathy parallel the duration and the severity of the metabolic acidosis. In a large series the mortality rate was 50 per cent when the serum HCO_3^- concentration was less than 10 mmol/l (Bennett *et al.* 1953). Additionally, ocular toxicity seems to correlate with the degree of acidosis. It is not possible to predict whether acute visual impairment will persist or will improve with therapy. Thus, once the diagnosis is strongly suspected, therapy should be initiated promptly. Gastric lavage and/or administration of ipecac is indicated for patients presenting within 2 h of methanol ingestion, but may be still useful after longer periods if the patient has impaired GI motility, as may be seen with coma or with ingestion of drugs that impair motility.

Folate, as leucovorin, should be administered intravenously, especially because alcoholic patients often are malnourished and ineffectively utilize folic acid, potentially prolonging the elimination half-life of formic acid. Sodium bicarbonate should be infused in doses appropriate to sustain the arterial pH above 7.20. The haemodynamic consequences of severe acidosis may impair tissue perfusion, and superimpose lactic acidosis on the methanol-induced formic acidosis. Appropriate alkali therapy in conjunction with ECF volume expansion protects against this vicious circle.

As in the case of ethylene glycol toxicity (see above), ethanol also reduces the rate of methanol metabolism by more aggressively competing for binding to alcohol dehydrogenase. Thus ethanol therapy should be instituted immediately in patients with metabolic acidosis, methanol levels exceeding 20–30 mg/100 ml, or other clinical signs of toxicity. As with ethylene glycol toxicity, 4-MP is also the drug of choice for methanol intoxication (Mycyk and Leikin 2003).

Dialysis remains one of the mainstays of therapy in methanol toxicity. Due to their small molecular size and water solubility, methanol and formic acid are efficiently removed by haemodialysis. Although the clearance of formate is less than that of methanol, its volume of distribution is much less than methanol's. Thus, the plasma half-life of formic acid is shorter than that of methanol in a haemodialysed patient. As haemodialysis is eight times more effective than peritoneal dialysis in clearing methanol, peritoneal dialysis should be used only if haemodialysis is unavailable. Because ethanol is also cleared with dialysis, infusion rates of ethanol should be increased, or ethanol should be added to the dialysate bath.

Dialysis should be initiated for methanol intoxication when any of the following indications is observed: known ingestion of at least 30 ml of absolute methanol; a blood methanol level of 50 mg/100 ml or more; the presence of a high anion gap metabolic acidosis; or mental, visual, or funduscopic changes attributable to methanol. Dialysis should be continued until the methanol level has been reduced to less than 25 mg/100 ml. As in ethylene glycol toxicity 4-MP can be used as the primary treatment (Brent *et al.* 1999).

Paraldehyde

Paraldehyde, is a low-molecular-weight cyclic polyether of polymerized acetaldehyde. It is a colourless liquid with a strong, unpleasant odour. It is prone to spontaneous decomposition when stored unprotected from light and air. Paraldehyde, still used as a sedative and as an antiseizure medication, may be given orally, parenterally, or rectally. Regardless of its route of administration, 7 per cent is excreted by the lungs within 4 h, with an additional 4–21 per cent eventually being exhaled. The remainder is metabolized chiefly by the liver; little to none appears in the urine. It is catabolized, in sequence, to acetaldehyde, acetic acid, and, finally, CO_2, and water. Liver disease retards this oxidation. Disulfiram administration has been shown to slow paraldehyde metabolism in animals.

Despite more than a century of therapeutic use, paraldehyde-associated acidosis was first recognized only in the 1950s. Toxicity typically occurred in patients consuming large quantities of ethanol, who were often addicted to paraldehyde as well. It is presumed that a tachyphylaxis to paraldehyde-induced narcosis allowed patients to remain awake while continuing their ingestion.

Presenting symptoms of intoxicated patients include nausea and vomiting, abdominal pain, and lethargy. Most patients have ingested considerable quantities of paraldehyde up to the time of admission, presenting with the unmistakable, offensive odour of the drug. Paraldehyde administration to ethanol-intoxicated patients can be dangerous (Burstein 1943).

Findings on presentation include mild-to-moderate dehydration, hypotension, Kussmaul respirations, and heme-positive gastric contents or stool. The lungs are usually clear to auscultation, but paraldehyde induced non-cardiogenic pulmonary oedema can occur.

The laboratory findings include hyperkalaemia, striking leucocytosis, and an increased anion gap metabolic acidosis. Although acetate, pyruvate, lactate, and the measurable ketone, acetoacetate, have been excluded, the offending acid has not been identified. It is quite possible, if not likely, that β-hydroxybutyric acidosis accounts for the paraldehyde-associated increased anion gap.

The oxidation of paraldehyde generates reduced pyridine nucleotide, which in turn stimulates conversion of acetoacetate to the nitroprusside-negative β-hydroxybutyric acid. This chemical sequence acts to cloud the diagnosis. Until recently no cases of paraldehyde-associated acidosis have been reported in more than a decade; it is during that period that the entity of β-hydroxybutyric acidosis became appreciated. Older literature suggested that the increased anion gap acidosis was the result of ingestion of the acetic acid formed from decomposed paraldehyde; however, when dogs were fed fresh and decomposed paraldehyde preparations, there was no difference in the otherwise trivial high anion gap acidosis that developed. Despite the proposed accumulation of nitroprusside-negative β-hydroxybutyrate as the unmeasured anion, a patient may in fact show positive ketones in serum. It should be remembered that acetaldehyde gives a false-positive nitroprusside reaction (pseudoketosis); this should be borne in mind when one considers the significance of ketonaemia (Hadden and Metzner 1969).

If a normal anion gap acidosis develops, RTA, linked to paraldehyde, should be considered. In addition to the problems associated with acidosis and pulmonary oedema, the clinical course of paraldehyde toxicity may be further complicated by acute renal failure.

Therapy should be directed at the acidosis and hypotension induced by paraldehyde intoxication and include intravenous administration of saline solution to correct fluid deficits, and HCO_3^- administration to correct acidaemia. Removal of paraldehyde by dialysis has not been documented; however, dialysis may be required to treat sodium overload from HCO_3^- administration in severely acidaemic, oliguric patients.

Metabolic alkalosis

Metabolic alkalosis is characterized by an increase in pH and an increase of plasma HCO_3^- concentration with compensatory hypoventilation. It is the most common acid–base disturbance encountered in hospitalized patients. Perturbations of either renal or extrarenal physiological processes may result in metabolic alkalosis. The most frequent cause is loss of gastric HCl, and if renal function is adequate, this alkalosis promptly responds to treatment by Cl^- containing solutions. Because Cl^- depletion accompanies many but not all forms of metabolic alkalosis, the disorder can be divided into those forms that are 'chloride-responsive' and those that are 'chloride-resistant'.

When determining the cause and treatment plan for a particular metabolic alkalosis, one must define the pathophysiological disturbance that generated the alkalosis and the mechanisms that maintain it. The latter point is particularly noteworthy because, unlike in metabolic acidosis, metabolic alkalosis may be perpetuated, despite correction of the initiating factors that are no longer operative. To generate metabolic alkalosis, a loss of acid or a gain of alkali must first accrue with primary elevation of the plasma HCO_3^-. To maintain the alkalosis, the renal mechanisms that restore normobicarbonataemia must be contravened by Cl^- deficiency and other forces, which will be described below.

Systemic effects of metabolic alkalosis (Table 7)

Cardiac effects

Metabolic alkalosis exerts a positive inotropic effect whose magnitude is small. A vasodilatory action on coronary and peripheral vessels has been observed in animal models, but not convincingly in man. Recent experimental observations in the pulmonary vasculature point to a role for nitric oxide as a mediator of the vasodilatory response to alkalaemia (see Section on 'Vascular effects'). Myocardial contractility during metabolic alkalosis *in vivo* has also not been sufficiently and systematically documented to the point where an effect of alkalosis can be presumed.

Table 7 Systemic effects of metabolic alkalosis

Cardiovascular
Heart: arrhythmias, especially in chronic obstructive pulmonary disease
Vascular: arteriolar vasodilation
Pulmonary
Ventilation: hypoventilation
Oxygen delivery: decreased in acute alkalosis (Bohr effect)
Renal
Antinatriuretic effect
Nervous system
Peripheral: neuromuscular irritability
Central: confusion, lethargy, seizures

Vascular effects

Alkalaemia can be associated with vasodilation. In the human pulmonary artery, endothelial nitric oxide synthase activity is induced by alkalinization (Yamaguchi *et al.* 1996; Gordon *et al.* 1999, 2003; Mizuno *et al.* 2002). Vasodilation follows the liberation of the potent vasodilator, nitric oxide, thereby decreasing pulmonary vascular resistance and offsetting, at least in part, the hypoxia of extreme metabolic alkalosis.

Pulmonary effects

Compensatory hypoventilation occurs in metabolic alkalosis. The anticipated degree of compensation is variable. However, an elevation in $P\text{CO}_2$ of 0.5–0.7 mmHg is anticipated for each 1 mmol/l increment of serum HCO_3^-. The acute reduction of extracellular H^+ concentration (rise in pH, i.e. alkalaemia) induces chemoreceptors in the medulla of the brain to diminish respiratory drive, and thereby raise the $P\text{CO}_2$. Acutely, alkalaemia also shifts the haemoglobin dissociation curve for oxygen leftward, increasing haemoglobin's affinity for oxygen, and thereby reducing oxygenation of tissues. Chronically, however, the RBC content of the glycolytic intermediate, 2,3-DPG, decreases. Because the 2,3-DPG *increases* the affinity of haemoglobin for oxygen, in the chronic state, the alkaline pH and the diminished DPG levels offset each other, allowing tissue oxygen delivery to normalize.

In addition, the hypoventilatory response associated with metabolic alkalosis has been associated with aggravation of hypoxaemia in patients with chronic obstructive pulmonary disorders, with marked hypercapnia occurring in selected instances (i.e. $P\text{CO}_2$ exceeding 60 mmHg). Hypercapnia beyond that expected in uncomplicated metabolic alkalosis, defines the coexistence of a primary respiratory acidosis. In such instances, correction of the metabolic alkalosis is imperative as this treatment has been shown to have a salutary effect on hypoxaemia in patients with chronic obstructive pulmonary disease (Bear *et al.* 1977). Lastly, cardiac dysrhythmias may be exacerbated in patients with chronic obstructive pulmonary disease, particularly those with hypoxaemia.

Renal effects

Proximal tubule cells are more sensitive to changes in peritubular pH than are more distal tubular cells. Net HCO_3^- absorption declines in the proximal tubule when peritubular fluid pH increases during metabolic alkalosis (Chan *et al.* 1982; Sasaki *et al.* 1982). The mechanisms underpinning the attempts of the proximal tubule to correct the hyperbicarbonataemia include reduced apical Na^+/H^+ antiporter activity and increased basolateral Cl^-/HCO_3^- exchange. The net effect of these adaptations is a reduction in proximal HCO_3^- reabsorption and loss of HCO_3^- into the distal nephron, resulting in an alkaline urine. This process continues until the decline in serum HCO_3^- concentration and the filtered load of alkali falls below the proximal tubular threshold for HCO_3^- reabsorption, at which point the final urine becomes bicarbonate-free. The urine at this time is relatively devoid of NH_3 buffer due to the reduced ammoniagenesis caused by Cl^- depletion, alkaline pH, and ECF contraction.

Hypokalaemia frequently accompanies metabolic alkalosis. In the intact animal, a reduction in extracellular K^+ concentration weakly acidifies the kidney (Adam *et al.* 1986). In the proximal tubule, it is presumed that this acidification drives $Na^+/3HCO_3^-$ symporter activity to augment HCO_3^- reabsorption (Adam *et al.* 1986). The latter process is facilitated during K^+ depletion due to enhanced apical Na^+/H^+ exchanger activity. In the outer medulla, K^+ deficits induce an increase in type A intercalated cells, which house apical H^+-ATPases and H^+, K^+-ATPases as well as a basolateral Cl^-/HCO_3^- exchanger (Madsen and Fischer 1986). Overactivity of these, particularly the latter, has been postulated to conserve K^+ at the expense of maintaining HCO_3^- reabsorption during alkalosis. The type B intercalated cell of the cortical collecting duct has an apical Cl^-/HCO_3^- exchanger and is even more stimulated than the type A cell during Cl^- depletion (Luke and Levitin 1967). The relative lack of luminal Cl^- results in a lack of HCO_3^- secretion, and downstream medullary collecting duct cells reabsorb any remaining luminal HCO_3^- (Gifford *et al.* 1990; Verlander *et al.* 1992). After Cl^- is restored, bicarbonaturia occurs with Cl^- reabsorption, repairing the alkalosis. Lastly, Cl^- reabsorption has long been shown to be diminished during K^+ deficiency, apparently as a result of the downregulation of specific Cl^- transporters (Galla *et al.* 1991). Alkalosis is then perpetuated by the Cl^- deficit as tubuloglomerular feedback increases proximal absorption of a HCO_3^--rich ultrafiltrate.

Nervous system

Metabolic alkalosis may present with the same clinical features associated with hypocalcaemia and will be discussed in this context. The plasma ionized Ca^{2+} concentration is rapidly reduced by alkalaemia as Ca^{2+} ions become albumin-bound. The relative insufficiency for Ca^{2+} to participate in normal central and peripheral nervous system function may then manifest as mental confusion, lethargy, paresthesias, and neuromuscular irritability, with muscle cramping, tetany and even seizures. The alkalosis also retards oxygen delivery (see above), enhances acetylcholine release at nerve endings, and stimulates citrate formation in neural tissues. Citrate complexes with Ca^{2+} and further diminishes its biological activity. These chemical forces all conspire to enhance neuromuscular excitability.

Table 8 Causes of metabolic alkalosis

Extrarenal aetiologies
Gastric loss of HCl
Gastric suction
Vomiting
Anorexia nervosa/bulimia
Gastrocystoplasty
Faecal loss of HCl
Congenital chloridorrhoea
Villous adenoma
Laxative abuse
Clay ingestion
Cystic fibrosis
Renal aetiologies
Diuretics
Posthypercapnoeic alkalosis
Magnesium depletion
Penicillin therapy
Potassium depletion
Tubule channel disorders
Bartter's syndrome
Gitelman's syndrome
Liddle's syndrome
Alkali loads
Exogenous alkali loads
Milk-alkali syndrome
Metabolic alkalosis in haemodialysis
Treatment of Haemorrhage
Endogenous alkali loads
Post-therapy of organic acidosis
Refeeding alkalosis
Disorders characterized by mineralocorticoid excess
Low renin, high aldosterone
Primary aldosteronism
Glucocorticoid-remediable aldosteronism
Low renin, low aldosterone
Inhibition of 11β-hydroxysteroid dehydrogenase
Apparent mineralocorticoid excess syndrome
Cushing's syndrome
Congenital adrenal hyperplasia
High renin, high aldosterone
Renin-secreting tumours
Renovascular hypertension
Malignant hypertension

Extrarenal origin (Table 8)

Gastric hydrochloric acid loss

This chloride-responsive alkalosis is divisible into two phases: an *acute generative phase* that creates the 'new' HCO_3^- and adds it to the blood, and a *chronic steady-state phase* that maintains the alkalosis, preventing the renal excretion of the alkali.

Active gastric suction, repetitive emesis such as occurs in anorexia nervosa/bulimia, gastrocystoplasty, or gastric loss of H^+ from any other cause produces a net addition of HCO_3^- to the plasma. The concomitant Cl^- depletion fosters ECF volume contraction with secondary increases of renin, angiotensin, and aldosterone. The consequent angiotensin II-mediated enhancement of HCO_3^- reabsorption along with the diminished GFR and associated K^+ deficiency all sustain a higher serum HCO_3^- level. When the degree of hyperbicarbonataemia causes the filtered load of alkali to exceed the newly increased reabsorptive capacity, bicarbonaturia resumes, holding the sum at its new higher value. This resumption of HCO_3^- loss obligates the excretion of both Na^+ and K^+, the latter provoked by hyperaldosteronism. The urine becomes relatively acidic though after active Cl^- loss stops and the plasma HCO_3^- is sustained at its new level. During this, *chronic steady-state phase* urinary Na^+, HCO_3^-, and Cl^- losses are low. Urinary Cl^- levels are typically less than 10–20 mmol/l.

The metabolic alkalosis is correctable simply by restoring Cl^- in adequate amounts, as a normal saline solution (Kassirer and Schwartz 1966; Rosen *et al.* 1988). All K^+ deficits should be promptly and concurrently treated with KCl. The addition of a selective H_2 antagonist or a proton pump inhibitor can be utilized to reduce gastric H^+ losses when nasogastric suction must absolutely be continued or after gastrocystoplasty.

Faecal chloride loss

Congenital chloridorrhoea

This autosomal-recessive disorder is caused by a mutation of the 'downregulated in adenoma' (DRA) gene that encodes an anionic transporter involved in ileal and colonic Cl^- transport (Byeon *et al.* 1998; Etani *et al.* 1998). Affected individuals have defective colonic Cl^- reabsorption, whereas their cation exchanger (Na^+ reabsorbed for H^+ secreted) functions normally. The result is that HCl accumulates in the lumen, attracting NH_3 and forming NH_4Cl. The loss of H^+ allows HCO_3^- to accumulate in the blood. A copious Cl^- rich diarrhoea is a constant feature of the syndrome. The stool Cl^- concentration exceeds the sum of the concentration of cations, Na^+ and K^+. This 'cation gap' reflects the presence of excreted NH_4^+ that accompanies some of the stool Cl^-. As with gastric Cl^- loss, the ECF volume contraction invokes secondary hyperaldosteronism that worsens the metabolic alkalosis generated by HCl losses. In addition, hypokalaemia is a frequent feature of the disorder.

Treatment consists of aggressive repletion of K^+ and Cl^- by dietary supplementation. Antidiarrhoeal agents are not effective in congenital chloridorrhoea. The diminution of gastric HCl secretion by proton pump inhibition may reduce stool Cl^- losses, thereby decreasing the alkalosis in some individuals (Aichbichler *et al.* 1997).

Villous adenoma

The normal colonic effluent is typically alkaline. In scattered cases of villous adenoma, however, metabolic alkalosis has been present. It had been previously postulated that these particular tumours secreted an acid-rich solution; however, it is more likely that metabolic alkalosis results from the obligatory K^+ depletion caused by the adenomatous secretion. Intriguingly though, the DRA protein is expressed to a lesser degree in some colonic adenomas, which would lend credence to the theory that villous adenomas produce metabolic alkalosis via secretion of a Cl^--rich fluid. Surgical resection cures this form of metabolic alkalosis.

Laxative abuse

Cathartic abuse may present as metabolic alkalosis. Urinary K^+ concentrations are characteristically depressed in this often surreptitious disorder of HCl depletion. In one study, the diagnosis of factitious diarrhoea was established in 17 per cent of patients presenting with at least 4 weeks of watery stools (de Wolff *et al.* 1981). An examination of the urine, plasma, and stool for phenolphthalein, senna, cascara, magnesium, and bisacodyl may establish the diagnosis (Phillips *et al.* 1995). Alkalosis recedes upon discontinuation of laxatives and reconstitution of the ECF volume.

Clay ingestion

A highly unusual form of hypokalaemic alkalosis occurs during geophagia of red clay. The clay binds K^+ in the GI tract. Treatment only requires the discontinuation of this form of pica (Gonzalez *et al.* 1982; Severance *et al.* 1988).

Cystic fibrosis

Extreme losses of Cl^- in sweat can lead to metabolic alkalosis (Arvanitakis and Lobeck 1973; Beckerman 1979; Pedroli *et al.* 1995; Bates *et al.* 1997; Mauri *et al.* 1997). In cystic fibrosis, mutations of the cystic fibrosis transmembrane regulator gene, which encodes an outwardly secreting Cl^- channel, produce excessive cutaneous Cl^- losses on a continuous basis. In the absence of sufficient dietary salt ingestion, metabolic alkalosis may ensue and will be sustained in the presence of ongoing ECF volume contraction. Gene therapy of this disorder will hopefully become a therapy that will reverse the various manifestations of this disease. For now, vigilance in maintaining salt balance is the treatment of choice for such patients.

Renal origin

Diuretics

Chloruretic agents such as the loop and thiazide diuretics produce ECF volume contraction. The reduction of the ECF space in the absence of any loss of total body HCO_3^- or even with a small increase in NAE and new HCO_3^- synthesis, increases the concentration of serum HCO_3^-. This chloride-responsive alkalosis is usually modest: re-expansion of the ECF volume induces bicarbonaturia with reversal of the alkalosis. Associated K^+ losses should, of course, also be repaired.

Posthypercapnic alkalosis

This chloride-responsive alkalosis occurs in patients with prolonged respiratory acidosis whose serum HCO_3^- concentration is increased as the consequence of the metabolic compensation of their primary respiratory disorder. Renal adaptation to chronic hypercapnia leads to chloruresis from increased NAE and heightened HCO_3^- reabsorption, both of which offset in part the respiratory acidosis. The chloruresis obligates loss of Na^+ and K^+ with an attendant, frequent depletion of these cations. Rapid improvement of the respiratory condition(s) reduces the P_{CO_2} faster than the concentration of HCO_3^-, causing a transient 'posthypercapnic' metabolic alkalosis. Alkalosis is then maintained by ECF volume contraction and K^+ depletion as well as, to a small extent, by the increased proximal tubular acidification of the urine, initiated during chronic adaptation to respiratory acidosis. Posthypercapnic alkalosis is generally seen in patients with chronic obstructive pulmonary disease, pulmonary hypertension, and right-sided heart failure. Such patients are often oedematous (i.e. the interstitial fluid space expands, despite a reduction in the 'effective intravascular volume') and may require acetazolamide to induce a $NaHCO_3^-$ diuresis and the retention of dietary Cl^-. Improvement in the right-sided heart function from prolonged hypoxic pulmonary vasoconstriction, will secondarily improve the GFR and further enhance the corrective bicarbonaturia.

Magnesium deficiency

Prolonged deprivation of magnesium-containing foodstuff or sustained hypermagnesuria are the principal causes of hypomagnesaemia. Associated alkalosis may result from augmented distal acidification, via induction of a hyperreninaemic hyperaldosteronism. Hypomagnesaemia from starvation; diuretic therapy; chronic losses from osmotic diuresis in uncontrolled diabetics; tubular damage from aminoglycosides, amphotericin, foscarnet, or cisplatin therapy (Bianchetti *et al.* 1991); burns; malabsorption; and chronic diarrhoeal disorders often synergizes with a more obvious clinical disorder to aggravate alkalosis further.

Hypomagnesaemia is frequently accompanied by hypokalaemia from ongoing intracellular K^+ wasting and kaliuresis (Whang *et al.* 1967, 1985) due to reduced Na^+,K^+-ATPase function. Repair of K^+ deficits thus requires prior correction of the Mg^{2+} deficit. Loss of Mg^{2+} also impairs the secretion of PTH and produces skeletal resistance to its effects.

Penicillin therapy

The administration of very large amounts of anionic penicillin or penicillin-type antibiotic (carbenicillin, ampicillin) may induce metabolic alkalosis (Brunner and Frick 1968; Klastersky *et al.* 1973). The presence of non-reabsorbable anions in the distal nephron increases the luminal electronegativity and, thus, H^+ and K^+ secretion and excretion. A reduction in chloride-dependent HCO_3^- secretion in the cortical collecting duct may also favour H^+ secretion. This sequence of events would be expected to occur in patients with ECF volume depletion with typical urinary Cl^- concentrations less than 30 mmol/l and secondary hyperaldosteronism. Due to the changing spectrum of antibiotic therapy, penicillin-induced alkalosis is now rare.

Potassium depletion

Pure K^+ depletion in the absence of obvious ECF contraction, a rare cause of metabolic alkalosis, has been clearly demonstrated in the intact animals and in humans with very large deficits in potassium (i.e. $>$400 mmol). The alkalosis is usually of modest degree because there is a disproportionate degree of NaCl retention, unless NaCl intake is concomitantly restricted (Jones *et al.* 1982; Hernandez *et al.* 1987; Amlal *et al.* 1998). In animals, a hypokalaemia-induced reduction in GFR maintains the alkalotic state, but the mechanism in man has not been as clearly delineated. However, correction of this alkalosis requires K^+ repletion as it is resistant to NaCl administration.

Tubule channel disorders (see Chapter 5.5)

Bartter's syndrome

Bartter's syndrome encompasses a group of autosomal recessive disorders characterized by chloride-resistant alkalosis and normal or low blood pressure (Stein 1985). The disorder typically presents prenatally, during infancy, or during early childhood. Hypokalaemia is often prominent and may lead to vascular hyporesponsiveness with impaired response to pressor agents, extreme muscular weakness with paralysis, and impaired urinary concentrating ability from 'kaliopenic nephropathy'. Moreover, the hypokalaemia may induce secretion of vasodilatory prostaglandins, particularly PGE_2. The excessive prostaglandin production further impairs urinary concentrating ability and lowers blood pressure, in association with enhanced kinin production (Fujita *et al.* 1982; Stein 1985). Cyclo-oxygenase inhibition with non-steroidal anti-inflammatory agents successfully restores vascular responsiveness in patients with Bartter's syndrome.

First characterized by Bartter as a childhood disorder of metabolic alkalosis, with ECF volume contraction, hypokalaemia, and hypercalciuria (and occasionally, nephrocalcinosis), the disorder has now been subcategorized into at least three distinct disorders detailed in Chapter 5.5 (Bettinelli *et al.* 1992; Simon *et al.* 1996a,b, 1997; Kurtz 1998; Konrad *et al.* 2000; Birkenhager *et al.* 2001; Estevez *et al.* 2001; Lorenz *et al.* 2002).

The differential diagnosis of hypokalaemic alkalosis with ECF volume contraction should always include Bartter's syndrome, which must be distinguished from vomiting-induced alkalosis and diuretic abuse. In vomiting, the urine Cl^- is typically depressed in contradistinction to the continually elevated levels seen in Bartter's syndrome (Veldhuis *et al.* 1979). With diuretic abuse, the urinary Cl^- may be high or low, depending upon how recently the diuretic was administered. A urinary screen for thiazides and loop-active agents will confirm the diagnosis of diuretic abuse (Jamison *et al.* 1982). The surreptitious abuse of laxatives may mimic Bartter's syndrome, and testing the stool for phenolphthalein may disclose this self-induced cause of metabolic alkalosis (Jamison *et al.* 1982).

Treatment of Bartter's syndrome has met with extremely variable success. Restoration of K^+ stores to normal, Mg repletion, correction of ECF volume deficits, and treatment with amiloride, propranolol, enalapril, spironolactone, and prostaglandin inhibitors have all been tried with limited success (Griffing *et al.* 1982; Hene *et al.* 1987; Morales *et al.* 1988).

Gitelman's syndrome (see Chapter 5.5)

Like Bartter's syndrome, this disorder is associated with a chloride-resistant metabolic alkalosis, hypokalaemia, and normotension. Often misrepresented as an adult *forme fruste* of Bartter's syndrome, Gitelman's syndrome features hypomagnesaemia attributable to urinary Mg^{2+} wasting and hypocalciuria (Simon *et al.* 1996c). ECF volume depletion is generally milder than that encountered in Bartter's syndrome. Nephrocalcinosis is not a characteristic feature because hypercalciuria is absent. Because the biochemical and clinical features of Gitelman's syndrome mimic those induced by thiazide diuretics, the thiazide-sensitive cotransporter (TSC) gene was chosen as a candidate gene for this disorder (Simon *et al.* 1996a). Indeed, it has now been clearly shown that this form of metabolic alkalosis results from mutation of this NaCl cotransporter (De Jong *et al.* 2002).

Liddle's syndrome (see also Chapter 5.5)

The alkalosis is generated in this autosomal-dominant abnormality by hyper-absorption of Na^+ through the epithelial Na^+ channel (ENaC) of the inner medullary collecting duct (Botero-Velez *et al.* 1994; Canessa *et al.* 1994; Hansson *et al.* 1995; Goulet *et al.* 1998; Abriel *et al.* 1999; De Jong *et al.* 2002). The gain-of-function mutation of ENaC, which occurs infrequently as a sporadic mutation (Yamashita *et al.* 2001), increases secretion of K^+ and H^+ via enhanced Na^+ reabsorption and renders the patient hypokalaemic and hyperbicarbonataemic. ECF volume expansion and hypertension are constant features; plasma renin activity and aldosterone levels are suppressed. Treatment of these generally young individuals includes a Na-restricted diet and blockade of ENaC with agents such as amiloride.

Alkali loads

Exogenous alkali loads

Milk-alkali syndrome

The milk-alkali syndrome was previously seen mainly in patients with peptic ulcer disease treated with calcium-based antacids and milk. In this disorder, a triad of forces was operative: metabolic alkalosis, hypercalcaemia, and renal functional impairment. Initially, an exogenous base is given as orally administered calcium carbonate or milk and Cl is lost usually secondary to vomiting; however, the milk-alkali syndrome can occur in the absence of vomiting. The ECF volume contraction decrease the filtered load of HCO_3^-, thereby maintaining alkalosis. In addition, hypercalcaemia, from both increased Ca^{2+} intake and from volume depletion, stimulates renal HCO_3^- reabsorption, thereby worsening the alkalosis. Indeed, the elevation of the serum HCO_3^- becomes a function of the daily 'dose' of HCO_3^-. In fact, metabolic alkalosis with HCO_3^- levels as great as 40 mmol/l has been documented in individuals who ingested up to 1600 mmol of HCO_3^- daily, although generally, the HCO_3^- level does not exceed 33–36 mmol/l. Plasma Ca^{2+} concentrations are concomitantly elevated, but generally to levels less than 16 mg/dl.

The combination of alkalosis and hypercalcaemia produces soft tissue calcifications, particularly of the cornea and kidney. The alkaline urine characteristic of milk-alkali patients and hypercalciuria provide an optimal milieu for the development of nephrocalcinosis from Ca^{2+} phosphate stones. Hypocalciuria occurs later and is apparent at the time of diagnosis during presentation for renal failure. Hypercalcaemia also invokes anorexia, nausea, and vomiting, and nephrogenic diabetes insipidus, all of which may contribute to further ECF volume depletion and reduction in GFR. Despite the severity of alkalosis, plasma K^+ concentrations usually do not fall below 3 mmol/l. Treatment of milk-alkali syndrome includes salt repletion and discontinuation of the ingested alkali. Presently, treatment of acid peptic disease by proton pump inhibitors or H_2 antagonists has effectively prevented this problem.

Metabolic alkalosis in haemodialysis

A variant of the milk-alkali syndrome is seen in the haemodialysis patients given calcium carbonate or calcium acetate to bind dietary phosphorus. When these HCO_3^- equivalents are administered in large amounts, alkalaemia results because the dialytic infusion of HCO_3^- is often sufficient to offset the daily metabolic production of acid. Typically, dialysate HCO_3^- concentrations are 35–40 mmol/l and the average venous total CO_2 content preceding dialytic therapy is often in the normal or near-normal range (22–26 mmol/l).

Treatment of haemorrhage

The acute and massive addition of citrated RBCs in patients with significant blood loss can lead to hyperbicarbonataemia with metabolic alkalosis. The hepatic conversion of citrate to HCO_3^- in the face of ECF volume depletion adds an alkaline load to the plasma during a period of Na^+ avidity and lowered GFR, thereby maintaining the alkalosis. Similarly, the addition of large quantities of lactated Ringer's solution in these circumstances to augment the plasma volume aggravates the alkalaemia, following conversion of lactate ions to HCO_3^-.

Endogenous alkali loads

Post-therapy of organic acidosis

This form of alkalosis usually follows treatment with exogenous HCO_3^- of diabetic ketoacidosis, alcoholic ketoacidosis, or lactic acidosis. In these three disorders, ketone or lactate anions that have not undergone renal excretion can be rapidly oxidized to HCO_3^- once the primary cause of the acidosis has been eliminated (e.g. insulin therapy or restoration of circulatory sufficiency). The regenerated HCO_3^- from residual organic anions, plus that which was administered exogenously and any 'new' HCO_3^- resulting from enhanced NAE, for example, increased ammoniagenesis, summate to increase the plasma HCO_3^- into the alkalotic range. The alkalaemia is perpetuated by concurrent ECF volume depletion and hypokalaemia and rectified by prompt reversal of these abnormalities. In diabetic ketoacidosis, the administration of saline precludes the above sequence from occurring. Indeed, overly zealous volume expansion depletes such patients of ketone-anions, replacing them with Cl^-, and thereby replacing a high anion gap metabolic acidosis with a hyperchloraemic metabolic acidosis, albeit of lesser severity.

Refeeding alkalosis

Metabolic alkalosis may occur following carbohydrate, but not protein or fat loading, of patients who had been fasting and have developed an attendant ketoacidosis. Hepatic conversion of ketone bodies to HCO_3^- with concomitantly enhanced ammoniagenesis and new HCO_3^- formation combine during the refeeding period to produce a net alkalosis during the period of Na^+ avidity that typifies caloric starvation. An increase in renal HCO_3^- reabsorption may sustain the alkalosis during carbohydrate refeeding. This effect stems from increased reabsorption attributable to the increased glucose load. Lastly, sodium acetate or potassium acetate is frequently added to total parenteral nutrition solutions and adds an exogenous load of alkali that sums to the reconverted HCO_3^- and new renal HCO_3^- loads.

Disorders characterized by mineralocorticoid excess

Low plasma renin activity with high aldosterone levels

Primary aldosteronism

All forms of primary aldosteronism are characterized by ECF volume expansion and low plasma renin activity (Ganguly 1998). Aldosterone engages the cytosolic type 1 mineralocorticoid receptor in collecting duct cells, which has a high affinity for the mineralocorticoid and for cortisol, and the hormone–receptor complex translocates to the nucleus to initiate the synthesis of proteins that produce the syndrome of mineralocorticoid excess. Aldosterone not only increases the open channel probability of the apical principal cell epithelial Na^+ channel but enhances basolateral Na^+,K^+-ATPase activity and translocation of more Na^+,K^+-ATPases and apical K^+ channels to their respective loci of action (Eiam-Ong *et al.* 1993). The summation of the actions of these effectors produces Na^+ retention with ECF volume expansion and hypertension, kaliuresis, and increased NAE. The latter, in conjunction with sustained hypokalaemia, generates and sustains metabolic alkalosis. Despite ECF volume expansion, patients are not oedematous and 'escape' from hypermineralocorticoidism, perhaps through a decreased abundance of the thiazide-sensitive Na–Cl cotransporter (Wang *et al.* 2001).

Causes of primary aldosteronism include mainly adenomatous hypersecretion, adrenal hyperplasia, glucocorticoid-remediable aldosteronism, ACTH-producing tumours, and rarely, adrenal carcinoma. In primary aldosteronism attributable to bilateral glandular hyperplasia (micro- or macronodular), a circadian rhythm of aldosterone may be demonstrable, with morning levels increasing under the influence of ACTH and falling later during the evening. By contrast, with adenomas, morning aldosterone levels are generally lower than evening levels. Aside from evaluation of the circadian pattern of aldosterone, other diagnostic screening tests for the primary disorder may include the plasma aldosterone-to-renin ratio, urinary aldosterone levels and the response of the secretion of renin and aldosterone to NaCl loading (Ganguly 1998). After the suspicion of primary aldosteronism is raised, more definitive manoeuvres such as computed tomography, adrenal ^{131}I-labelled 19-iodocholesterol uptake and adrenal venous sampling ('the gold standard') should be carried out before surgical intervention is contemplated.

After the diagnosis of hyperaldosteronism is established, treatment with spironolactone or epleronone to block the type 1 mineralocorticoid receptor or a K^+-sparing diuretic such as amiloride should be initiated. Appropriate surgery will abolish the alkalosis and hypokalaemia. Hypertension, however, frequently does not remit and its severity remains a function of the degree of vascular resistance and cardiac hypertrophy that remain postsurgically.

Glucocorticoid-remediable aldosteronism

Glucocorticoid-remediable aldosteronism, also referred to as familial hyperaldosteronism type 1, results from an autosomal dominant disorder that produces gene chimerism (Rich *et al.* 1992). Gene fusion of the CYP11B1 (11β-hydroxylase) promoter to the coding sequence of the CYP11B2 (aldosterone synthase) gene permits aldosterone, corticosterone, and cortisol precursor synthesis to be regulated by ACTH. The biochemical profile of this disorder is unique, with highly elevated levels of 18-oxotetrahydrocortisol and 18-hydroxycortisol being characteristic features. Treatment with exogenous glucocorticoid suppresses ACTH secretion and ameliorates the severe hypertension and variable degree of hypokalaemia that characterize afflicted patients, generally by the age of 21 years.

Low plasma renin activity with low aldosterone levels

Inhibition of 11β-hydroxysteroid dehydrogenase (see Chapter 5.5)

The glycyrrhetinic acid contained in particular chewing tobacco, carbenoxolone, licorice, or certain confections can produce a hypermineralocorticoid-like syndrome (White *et al.* 1994). This chemical compound suppresses the activity of the cortical collecting duct isoform of the principal cell enzyme, 11β-hydroxysteroid dehydrogenase. This enzyme normally inactivates cortisol, which can activate the mineralocorticoid receptor, to cortisone, which cannot activate this receptor (Mune *et al.* 1995). Normally, promiscuous occupation of the distal tubule type 1 mineralocorticoid receptor by cortisol is prevented by the dehydrogenase. However, unrestrained cortisol-mediated receptor activation (during inhibition of the enzyme) produces hypermineralocorticoidism, with concomitant suppression of plasma renin activity and aldosterone. Diuretic therapy has often been prescribed for the accompanying Na^+ retention in this disorder, thereby aggravating hypokalaemia to the point of paralysis or rhabdomyolysis. Treatment requires withdrawal of the offending agent and repair of K^+ deficits.

Apparent mineralocorticoid excess syndrome (see Chapter 5.5)

Licorice-like in its clinical manifestations, but differing in its age of onset, this autosomal-recessive disorder presents as juvenile hypertension. There is accompanying hypokalaemic metabolic alkalosis. The cause of this disorder is a loss-of-function mutation of 11β-hydroxysteroid dehydrogenase located at aldosterone-sensitive sites in the collecting tubules, thereby permitting the type 1 mineralocorticoid receptor to persistently engage its ligand, cortisol, instead of inactivating it to cortisone (Mune *et al.* 1995). A greatly depressed urine cortisone-to-cortisol ratio is a *sine qua non*. As with carbenoxolone- or glycyrrhetinic acid-induced inhibition of 11β-hydroxysteroid dehydrogenase, plasma renin activity and aldosterone will be depressed from ECF volume expansion. The differential diagnosis therefore also includes Liddle's syndrome, a mineralocorticoid-producing tumour (e.g. DOC-producing tumour) and aetiologies marked by ACTH hypersecretion.

Cushing's syndrome

Cushing's syndrome is produced by excessive endogenous glucocorticoid production or exogenous administration of glucocorticoid, often for a non-endocrinological disorder. ACTH-dependent Cushing's syndrome results from pituitary adenomatous hypersecretion of ACTH (Cushing's disease), ectopic tumour production of ACTH or a CRH-producing tumour (Newell-Price *et al.* 1998). ACTH-independent Cushing's syndrome is produced by autonomous glucocorticoid hypersecretion from an adrenal adenoma or carcinoma or by adrenal micro- or macronodular hyperplasia. Iatrogenic Cushing's syndrome occurs during prolonged glucocorticoid administration by the oral, topical, or inhaled routes (Ruiz-Maldonado *et al.* 1982; Nutting and Page 1995). The latter syndrome may also occur during treatment with medroxyprogesterone acetate, a long-acting progestin with mild glucocorticoid activity, or more rarely, from factitious administration.

Normally, plasma cortisol levels are nearly 100-fold higher than those for aldosterone. However, cortisol does not usually produce a mineralocorticoid effect because of its rapid degradation by 11β-hydroxysteroid dehydrogenase. Therefore, unless the capacity of the dehydrogenase is overwhelmed, glucocorticoid excess cannot produce hypermineralocorticoidism. In Cushing's syndrome, continual occupancy of the type 1 mineralocorticoid receptor induces the hypermineralocorticoid state with ECF volume expansion, metabolic alkalosis, and hypokalaemia. However, in non-iatrogenic Cushing's syndrome, there may be further provocation of alkalosis by the enhancement of NAE and NH_4^+ production by non-aldosterone mineralocorticoids such as desoxycorticosterone and corticosterone. Some evidence suggests that ACTH may suppress 11β-hydroxysteroid dehydrogenase activity, thereby imparting a greater mineralocorticoid potency to the glucocorticoid. This effect of ACTH would also explain the constancy of severe hypokalaemia in patients with ectopic production of ACTH.

Establishment of the aetiology of Cushing's syndrome rests first on the demonstration of hypercortisolism. Exogenous and factitious Cushing's syndrome must be excluded (Cizza *et al.* 1996). Self-administration of glucocorticoids presents clinicians with a notoriously difficult diagnosis and may require evaluation of the urine for synthetic steroids by high-pressure liquid chromatography (Lin *et al.* 1997). First, high urinary cortisol levels should be documented in a 24-h urine collection. It should be followed by a dexamethasone suppression testing to determine whether cortisol overproduction is dependent upon ACTH hypersecretion. If suppression is not achieved, the source of ACTH should be pinpointed by other diagnostic procedures.

Treatment of cortisol overproduction by adrenal tumours is surgical extirpation of the affected gland. However, ectopic ACTH secretion may not be treated so simply. In such cases, metyrapone or aminoglutethimide should be added to inhibit adrenal steroidogenesis. Selective destruction of the adrenal cortical layers, zonas fasiculata and reticularis, by mitotane will abolish hypercortisolism when surgery cannot be carried out. Aldosterone production, however, will remain after this chemical adrenalectomy.

Congenital adrenal hyperplasia

Two forms of congenital adrenal hyperplasia produce a hypertensive form of metabolic alkalosis. Hypersecretion of ACTH is due to deranged production of cortisol with consequent overproduction of a variety of non-aldosterone mineralocorticoid precursors (White *et al.* 1987).

In 11β-hydroxylase deficiency, there is excessive production of 11-deoxycorticosterone and adrenal androgens. The potent mineralocorticoid effect of 11-deoxycorticosterone produces early onset hypertension and mild metabolic alkalosis while the androgens induce virilization in females or ambiguous genitalia in males. In 17α-hydroxylase deficiency, the absence of this enzyme impedes sex steroid and cortisol production followed by enhanced secretion of 17-deoxysteroids, including pregnenolone, progesterone, deoxycorticosterone, and corticosterone. Hypogonadism thus occurs in the face of hypertensive hypokalaemic alkalosis from the mineralocorticoid effects of the latter two hormones. Treatment of either of these two types of congenital adrenal hyperplasia relies on the suppression of elevated ACTH levels with an exogenous glucocorticoid, which lowers the overproduction of mineralocorticoid precursors.

High plasma renin activity and high aldosterone levels

Renin-secreting tumours

Primary renin secretion from several different types of tumours has been described. Hemangiopericytomas or juxtaglomerular apparatus tumours are the best known (Kihara *et al.* 1968); however, renin hypersecretion from renal cell harmartomas, nephroblastomas, and carcinomas has also been documented (Mitchell *et al.* 1970; Hirose *et al.* 1974; Hollifield *et al.* 1975). Secondary hyperaldosteronism with hypertension from ECF volume expansion and hypokalaemia may be accompanying features, but metabolic alkalosis is generally mild. Definitive treatment for this disorder is surgical.

Renovascular hypertension

The association of hypertension and hypokalaemia in renovascular hypertension from whichever cause stands out more so than the induction of metabolic alkalosis. In fact, no statistically significant difference in mean plasma total CO_2 content was found in a large study that compared 175 patients with renovascular hypertension to its control group of essential hypertensive patients (Simon *et al.* 1972). However, the degree of chronic renal failure in many patients may have produced an offsetting metabolic acidosis to the extent that a primary increment in HCO_3^- concentration was masked.

Malignant hypertension

Severe hypertension with elevated renin and aldosterone levels has been minimally studied in terms of metabolic alkalosis (McCaa *et al.* 1979). In a single study of 15 patients, the plasma total CO_2 content was 29 mmol/l, just 3 mmol/l above that of a control group with non-malignant hypertension, and the mean plasma K^+ concentration was 3.6 mmol/l. No systematic study of the electrolytic composition following treatment of affected individuals has been performed and the treatment in some instances would be expected to obfuscate the data (e.g. treatment with diuretics).

References

Abriel, H. *et al.* (1999). Defective regulation of the epithelial Na^+ channel by Nedd4 in Liddle's syndrome. *Journal of Clinical Investigation* **103**, 667–673.

Adam, W. R., Koretsky A. P., and Weiner, M. W. (1986). 31P–NMR *in vivo* measurement of renal intracellular pH: effects of acidosis and K^+ depletion in rats. *American Journal of Physiology* **251**, F904–F910.

Aichbichler, B. W., Zerr, C. H., Santa Ana, C. A., Porter, J. L., and Fordtran, J. S. (1997). Proton-pump inhibition of gastric chloride secretion in congenital chloridorrhea. *New England Journal of Medicine* **336**, 106–109.

Alpern, R. J. (1990). Cell mechanisms of proximal tubule acidification. *Physiological Reviews* **70**, 79–114.

Alpern, R. J. and Sakhaee, K. (1997). The clinical spectrum of chronic metabolic acidosis: homeostatic mechanisms produce significant morbidity. *American Journal of Kidney Diseases* **29**, 291–302.

Amlal, H., Wang, Z., and Soleimani, M. Potassium depletion downregulates chloride-absorbing transporters in rat kidney. *Journal of Clinical Investigation* **101**, 1045–1054.

Arruda, J. A. *et al.* (1980). Parathyroid hormone and extrarenal acid buffering. *American Journal of Physiology* **239**, F533–F538.

Arvanitakis, S. N. and Lobeck, C. C. (1973). Metabolic alkalosis and salt depletion in cystic fibrosis. *Journal of Pediatrics* **82**, 535–536.

Bates, C. M., Baum, M., and Quigley, R. (1997). Cystic fibrosis presenting with hypokalemia and metabolic alkalosis in a previously healthy adolescent. *Journal of the American Society of Nephrology* **8**, 352–355.

Bear, R. *et al.* (1977). Effect of metabolic alkalosis on respiratory function in patients with chronic obstructive lung disease. *Canadian Medical Association Journal* **117**, 900–903.

Beck, N. and Webster, S. K. (1976). Effects of acute metabolic acidosis on parathyroid hormone action and calcium mobilization. *American Journal of Physiology* **230**, 127–131.

Beckerman, R. C. (1979). Metabolic alkalosis in infants with cystic fibrosis. *Pediatrics* **64**, 389.

Bennett, I. L. *et al.* (1953). Acute methyl alcohol poisoning: a review based on experiences in an outbreak of 323 cases. *Medicine* **32**, 431.

Bettinelli, A. *et al.* (1992). Use of calcium excretion values to distinguish two forms of primary renal tubular hypokalemic alkalosis: Bartter and Gitelman syndromes. *Journal of Pediatrics* **120**, 38–43.

Bianchetti, M. G., Kanaka, C., Ridolfi-Luthy, A., Hirt, A., Wagner, H. P., and Oetliker, O. H. (1991). Persisting renotubular sequelae after cisplatin in children and adolescents. *American Journal of Nephrology* **11**, 127–130.

Birkenhager, R. *et al.* (2001). Mutation of BSND causes Bartter syndrome with sensorineural deafness and kidney failure. *Nature Genetics* **29**, 310–314.

Botero-Velez, M., Curtis, J. J., and Warnock, D. G. (1994). Brief report: Liddle's syndrome revisited—a disorder of sodium reabsorption in the distal tubule. *New England Journal of Medicine* **330**, 178–181.

Brent, J. *et al.* (1999). Fomepizole for the treatment of ethylene glycol poisoning. Methylpyrazole for Toxic Alcohols Study Group. *New England Journal of Medicine* **340**, 832–838.

Brunner, F. P. and Frick, P. G. (1968). Hypokalaemia, metabolic alkalosis, and hypernatraemia due to 'massive' sodium penicillin therapy. *British Medical Journal* **4**, 550–552.

Buerkert, J., Martin, D., Trigg, D., and Simon, E. (1983). Effect of reduced renal mass on ammonium handling and net acid formation by the superficial and juxtamedullary nephron of the rat. Evidence for impaired reentrapment rather than decreased production of ammonium in the acidosis of uremia. *Journal of Clinical Investigation* **71**, 1661–1675.

Burstein, C. L. (1943). The hazard of paraldehyde administration. *Journal of American Medical Association* **121**, 187.

Byeon, M. K., Frankel, A., Papas, T. S., Henderson, K. W., and Schweinfest, C. W. (1998). Human DRA functions as a sulfate transporter in Sf9 insect cells. *Protein Expression and Purification* **12**, 67–74.

Canessa, C. M. *et al.* (1994). Amiloride-sensitive epithelial Na^+ channel is made of three homologous subunits. *Nature* **367**, 463–467.

Chan, Y. L., Biagi, B., and Giebisch, G. (1982). Control mechanisms of bicarbonate transport across the rat proximal convoluted tubule. *American Journal of Physiology* **242**, F532–F543.

Cizza, G. *et al.* (1996). Factitious Cushing syndrome. *Journal of Clinical Endocrinology and Metabolism* **81**, 3573–8577.

Davis, L. E. *et al.* (2002). Methanol poisoning exposures in the United States: 1993–1998. *Journal of Toxicology. Clinical Toxicology* **40**, 499–505.

De Jong, J. C., Van Der Vliet, W. A., Van Den Heuvel, L. P., Willems, P. H., Knoers, N. V., and Bindels, R. J. (2002). Functional expression of mutations in the human NaCl cotransporter: evidence for impaired routing mechanisms in Gitelman's syndrome. *Journal of the American Society of Nephrology* **13**, 1442–1448.

de Wolff, F. A., de Haas, E. J., and Verweij, M. (1981). A screening method for establishing laxative abuse. *Clinical Chemistry* **27**, 914–917.

DuBose, T. D., Jr. (1997). Hyperkalemic hyperchloremic metabolic acidosis: pathophysiologic insights. *Kidney International* **51**, 591–602.

Eiam-Ong, S., Kurtzman, N. A., and Sabatini, S. (1993). Regulation of collecting tubule adenosine triphosphatases by aldosterone and potassium. *The Journal of Clinical Investigation* **91**, 2385–2392.

Estevez, R. *et al.* (2001). Barttin is a Cl^- channel beta-subunit crucial for renal Cl^- reabsorption and inner ear K^+ secretion. *Nature* **414**, 558–561.

Etani, Y. *et al.* (1998). A novel mutation of the down-regulated in adenoma gene in a Japanese case with congenital chloride diarrhea. Mutations in brief no. 198. *Human Mutation* **12**, 362 (Online).

Fujita, T., Ando, K., Sato, Y., Yamashita, K., Nomura, M., and Fukui, T. (1982). Independent roles of prostaglandins and the renin–angiotensin system in abnormal vascular reactivity in Bartter's syndrome. *American Journal of Medicine* **73**, 71–76.

Gabow, P. A., Clay, K., Sullivan, J. B., and Lepoff, R. (1986). Organic acids in ethylene glycol intoxication. *Annals of Internal Medicine* **105**, 16–20.

Galla, J. H., Gifford, J. D., Luke, R. G., and Rome, L. (1991). Adaptations to chloride-depletion alkalosis. *American Journal of Physiology* **261**, R771–R781.

Ganguly, A. (1998). Primary aldosteronism. *New England Journal of Medicine* **339**, 1828–1834.

Gifford, J. D., Sharkins, K., Work, J., Luke, R. G., and Galla, J. H. (1990). Total CO_2 transport in rat cortical collecting duct in chloride-depletion alkalosis. *American Journal of Physiology* **258**, F848–F853.

Gonzalez, J. J., Owens, W., Ungaro, P. C., Werk, E. E., Jr., and Wentz, P. W. (1982). Clay ingestion: a rare cause of hypokalemia. *Annals of Internal Medicine* **97**, 65–66.

Gordon, J. B., Halla, T. R., Fike, C. D., and Madden, J. A. (1999). Mediators of alkalosis-induced relaxation in pulmonary arteries from normoxic and chronically hypoxic piglets. *American Journal of Physiology* **276**, L155–L163.

Gordon, J. B. *et al.* (2003). What leads to different mediators of alkalosis–induced vasodilation in isolated and *in situ* pulmonary vessels? *American Journal of Physiology. Lung Cellular and Molecular Physiology*. **284**, L799–L807.

Goulet, C. C., Volk, K. A., Adams, C. M., Prince, L. S., Stokes, J. B., and Snyder, P. M. (1998). Inhibition of the epithelial Na^+ channel by interaction of Nedd4 with a PY motif deleted in Liddle's syndrome. *Journal of Biological Chemistry* **273**, 30012–30017.

Griffing, G. T., Komanicky, P., Aurecchia, S. A., Sindler, B. H., and Melby, J. C. (1982). Amiloride in Bartter's syndrome. *Clinical Pharmacology and Therapeutics* **31**, 713–718.

Hadden, J. W. and Metzner, R. J. (1969). Pseudoketosis and hyperacetaldehydemia in paraldehyde acidosis. *American Journal of Medicine* **47**, 642–647.

Halperin, M. L., Richardson, R. M., Bear, R. A., Magner, P. O., Kamel, K., and Ethier, J. (1988). Urine ammonium: the key to the diagnosis of distal renal tubular acidosis. *Nephron* **50**, 1–4.

Hansson, J. H. *et al.* (1995). A de novo missense mutation of the beta subunit of the epithelial sodium channel causes hypertension and Liddle syndrome, identifying a praline-rich segment critical for regulation of channel activity. *Proceedings of the National Academy of Sciences of the United States of America* **92**, 11495–11499.

Hene, R. J., Koomans, H. A., Dorhout Mees, E. J., vd Stolpe, A., Verhoef, G. E., and Boer, P. (1987). Correction of hypokalemia in Bartter's syndrome by enalapril. *American Journal of Kidney Diseases* **9**, 200–205.

Hernandez, R. E., Schambelan, M., Cogan, M. G., Colman, J., Morris, R. C., Jr., and Sebastian, A. (1987). Dietary NaCl determines severity of potassium depletion-induced metabolic alkalosis. *Kidney International* **31**, 1356–1367.

Hirose, M., Arakawa, K., Kikuchi, M., Kawasaki, T., and Omoto, T. (1974). Primary reninism with renal hamartomatous alteration. *Journal of the American Medical Association* **230**, 1288–1292.

Hollifield, J. W., Page, D. L., Smith, C., Michelakis, A. M., Staab, E., and Rhamy, R. (1975). Renin-secreting clear cell carcinoma of the kidney. *Archives of Internal Medicine* **135**, 859–864.

Hulter, H. N., Ilnicki, L. P., Harbottle, J. A., and Sebastian, A. (1977). Impaired renal H^+ secretion and NH_3 production in mineralocorticoid-deficient glucocorticoid-replete dogs. *American Journal of Physiology* **232**, F136–F146.

Jacobsen, D., Ostby, N., and Bredesen, J. E. (1982). Studies on ethylene glycol poisoning. *Acta Medica Scandinavica* **212**, 11–15.

Jamison, R. L., Ross, J. C., Kempson, R. L., Sufit, C. R., and Parker, T. E. (1982). Surreptitious diuretic ingestion and pseudo-Bartter's syndrome. *American Journal of Medicine* **73**, 142–147.

Jones, J. W., Sebastian, A., Hulter, H. N., Schambelan, M., Sutton, J. M., and Biglieri, E. G. (1982). Systemic and renal acid–base effects of chronic dietary potassium depletion in humans. *Kidney International* **21**, 402–410.

Kassirer, J. P. and Schwartz, W. B. (1966). Correction of metabolic alkalosis in man without repair of potassium deficiency. A re-evaluation of the role of potassium. *American Journal of Medicine* **40**, 19–26.

Kihara, I., Kitamura, S., Hoshino, T., Seida, H., and Watanabe, T. (1968). A hitherto unreported vascular tumor of the kidney: a proposal of 'juxtaglomerular cell tumor'. *Acta Pathologica Japonica* **18**, 197–206.

Klastersky, J., Vanderklen, B., Daneau, D., and Mathiew, M. (1973). Carbenicillin and hypokalemia. *Annals of Internal Medicine* **78**, 774–775.

Konrad, M. *et al.* (2000). Mutations in the chloride channel gene CLCNKB as a cause of classic Bartter syndrome. *Journal of the American Society of Nephrology* **11**, 1449–1459.

Kontos, H. A., Richardson, D. W., and Patterson, J. L., Jr. (1968). Vasodilator effect of hypercapnic acidosis on human forearm blood vessels. *American Journal of Physiology* **215**(6), 1403–1405.

Kurtz, I. (1998). Molecular pathogenesis of Bartter's and Gitelman's syndromes. *Kidney International* **54**, 1396–1410.

Lin, C. L., Wu, T. J., Machacek, D. A., Jiang, N. S., and Kao, P. C. (1997). Urinary free cortisol and cortisone determined by high performance liquid chromatography in the diagnosis of Cushing's syndrome. *Journal of Clinical Endocrinology and Metabolism* **82**, 151–155.

Litzow, J. R., Lemann., J., Jr., and Lennon, E. J. (1967). The effect of treatment of acidosis on calcium balance in patients with chronic azotemic renal disease. *Journal of Clinical Investigation* **46**, 280–286.

Lofqvist, J. and Nilsson, E. (1981). Influence of acid–base changes on carbachol- and potassium-induced contractions of taenia coli of the rabbit. *Acta Physiologica Scandinavica* **111**, 59–68.

Lorenz, J. N. *et al.* (2002). Impaired renal NaCl absorption in mice lacking the ROMK potassium channel, a model for type II Bartter's syndrome. *Journal of Biological Chemistry* **277**, 37871–37880.

Luke, R. G. and Levitin, H. (1967). Impaired renal conservation of chloride and the acid–base changes associated with potassium depletion in the rat. *Clinical Science* **32**, 511–526.

Madias, N. E. (1986). Lactic acidosis. *Kidney International* **29**, 752–774.

Madsen, K. M. and Tisher, C. C. (1986). Structural–functional relationship along the distal nephron. *American Journal of Physiology* **250**, F1–F15.

Mauri, S., Pedroli, G., Rudeberg, A., Laux-End, R., Monotti, R., and Bianchetti, M. G. (1997). Acute metabolic alkalosis in cystic fibrosis: prospective study and review of the literature. *Mineral and Electrolyte Metabolism* **23**, 33–37.

McCaa, C. S., Langford, H. G., Cushman, W. C., and McCaa, R. E. (1979). Response of arterial blood pressure, plasma renin activity and plasma aldosterone concentration to long-term administration of captopril in patients with severe, treatment-resistant malignant hypertension. *Clinical Science* **57**, 371s–373s.

McMartin, K. E., Makar, A. B., Martin, G., Palese, M., and Tephly, T. R. (1975). Methanol poisoning. I. The role of formic acid in the development of metabolic acidosis in the monkey and the reversal by 4-methylpyrazole. *Biochemical Medicine* **13**, 319–333.

Mitchell, J. D., Baxter, T. J., Blair-West, J. R., and McCredie, D. A. (1970). Renin levels in nephroblastoma (Wilms' tumour). Report of a renin secreting tumour. *Archives of Disease in Childhood* **45**, 376–384.

Mitchell, J. H., Wildenthal, K., and Johnson, R. L., Jr. (1972). The effects of acid–base disturbances on cardiovascular and pulmonary function. *Kidney International* **1**, 375–389.

Mizuno, S., Demura, Y., Ameshima, S., Okamura, S., Miyamori, I., and Ishizaki, T. (2002). Alkalosis stimulates endothelial nitric oxide synthase in cultured human pulmonary arterial endothelial cells. *American Journal of Physiology. Lung Cellular and Molecular Physiology* **283**, L113–L119.

Morales, J. M. *et al.* (1988). Long-term enalapril therapy in Bartter's syndrome. *Nephron* **48**, 327.

Movilli, E. *et al.* (1998). Correction of metabolic acidosis increases serum albumin concentrations and decreases kinetically evaluated protein intake in haemodialysis patients: a prospective study. *Nephrology, Dialysis, Transplantation* **13**, 1719–1722.

Mune, T., Rogerson, F. M., Nikkila, H., Agarwal, A. K., and White, P. C. (1995). Human hypertension caused by mutations in the kidney isozyme of 11 beta-hydroxysteroid dehydrogenase. *Nature Genetics* **10**, 394–399.

Mycyk, M. B. and Leikin, J. B. (2003). Antidote review: fomepizole for methanol poisoning. *American Journal of Therapeutics* **10**, 68–70.

Newell-Price, J., Trainer, P., Besser, M., and Grossman, A. (1998). The diagnosis and differential diagnosis of Cushing's syndrome and pseudo-Cushing's states. *Endocrine Reviews* **19**, 647–672.

Nutting, C. M. and Page, S. R. (1995). Iatrogenic Cushing's syndrome due to nasal betamethasone: a problem not to be sniffed at! *Postgraduate Medical Journal* **71**, 231–232.

Pedroli, G. *et al.* (1995). Chronic metabolic alkalosis: not uncommon in young children with severe cystic fibrosis. *American Journal of Nephrology* **15**, 245–250.

Phillips, S., Donaldson, L., Geisler, K., Pera, A., and Kochar, R. (1995). Stool composition in factitial diarrhea: a 6-year experience with stool analysis. *Annals of Internal Medicine* **123**, 97–100.

Pons, C. A. and Custor, R. P. (1946). Acute ethylene glycol poisoning. A clinico-pathologic report of 18 fatal cases. *The American Journal of Medical Sciences* **211**, 544–554.

Rich, G. M., Ulick, S., Cook, S., Wang, J. Z., Lifton, R. P., and Dluhy, R. G. (1992). Glucocorticoid-remediable aldosteronism in a large kindred: clinical spectrum and diagnosis using a characteristic biochemical phenotype. *Annals of Internal Medicine* **116**, 813–820.

Rosen, R. A., Julian, B. A., Dubovsky, E. V., Galla, J. H., and Luke, R. G. (1988). On the mechanism by which chloride corrects metabolic alkalosis in man. *American Journal of Medicine* **84**, 449–458.

Ruiz-Maldonado, R., Zapata, G., Lourdes, T., and Robles, C. (1982). Cushing's syndrome after topical application of corticosteroids. *American Journal of Diseases of Children* **136**, 274–275.

Sasaki, S., Berry, C. A., and Rector, F. C., Jr. (1982). Effect of luminal and peritubular $HCO_3^{(-)}$ concentrations and PCO_2 on $HCO_3^{(-)}$ reabsorption in rabbit proximal convoluted tubules perfused in vitro. *Journal of Clinical Investigation* **70**, 639–649.

Schulze-Delrieu, K. and Lepsien, G. (1982). Depression of mechanical and electrical activity in muscle strips of opossum stomach and esophagus by acidosis. *Gastroenterology* **82**, 720–724.

Sebastian, A., Schambelan, M., Lindenfeld, S., and Morris, R. C., Jr. (1977). Amelioration of metabolic acidosis with fludrocortisone therapy in hyporeninemic hypoaldosteronism. *New England Journal of Medicine* **297**, 576–583.

Severance, H. W. Jr., Holt, T., Patrone, N. A., and Chapman, L. (1988). Profound muscle weakness and hypokalemia due to clay ingestion. *Southern Medical Journal* **81**, 272–274.

Sharpey-Schafer, E. P., Semple, S. J., Halls, R. W., and Howarth, S. (1965). Venous constriction after exercise; its relation to acid–base changes in venous blood. *Clinical Science* **29**, 397–406.

Simon, D. B. *et al.* (1996a). Genetic heterogeneity of Bartter's syndrome revealed by mutations in the K^+ channel, ROMK. *Nature Genetics* **14**, 152–156.

Simon, D. B., Karet, F. E., Hamdan, J. M., DiPietro, A., Sanjad, S. A., and Lifton, R. P. (1996b). Bartter's syndrome, hypokalaemic alkalosis with hypercalciuria, is caused by mutations in the Na–K–2Cl cotransporter NKCC. *Nature Genetics* **13**, 183–188.

Simon, D. B. *et al.* (1996). Gitelman's variant of Bartter's syndrome, inherited hypokalaemic alkalosis, is caused by mutations in the thiazide-sensitive Na–Cl cotransporter. *Nature Genetics* **12**, 24–30.

Simon, D. B. *et al.* (1997). Mutations in the chloride channel gene, CLCNKB, cause Bartter's syndrome type III. *Nature Genetics* **17**, 171–178.

Simon, N., Franklin, S. S., Bleifer, K. H., and Maxwell, M. H. (1972). Clinical characteristics of renovascular hypertension. *Journal of the American Medical Association* **220**, 1209–1218.

Stein, J. H. (1985). The pathogenetic spectrum of Bartter's syndrome. *Kidney International* **28**, 85–93.

Sutton, R. A., Wong, N. L., and Dirks, J. H. (1979). Effects of metabolic acidosis and alkalosis on sodium and calcium transport in the dog kidney. *Kidney International* **15**, 520–533.

Veldhuis, J. D., Bardin, C. W., and Demers, L. M. (1979). Metabolic mimicry of Bartter's syndrome by covert vomiting: utility of urinary chloride determinations. *American Journal of Medicine* **66**, 361–363.

Verlander, J. W., Madsen, K. M., Galla, J. H., Luke, R. G., and Tisher, C. C. (1992). Response of intercalated cells to chloride depletion metabolic alkalosis. *American Journal of Physiology* **262**, F309–F319.

Wang, X. Y. *et al.* (2001). The renal thiazide-sensitive Na–Cl cotransporter as mediator of the aldosterone-escape phenomenon. *Journal of Clinical Investigation* **108**, 215–222.

Whang, R., Morosi, H. J., Rodgers, D., and Reyes, R. (1967). The influence of sustained magnesium deficiency on muscle potassium repletion. *Journal of Laboratory and Clinical Medicine* **70**, 895–902.

Whang, R., Flink, E. B., Dyckner, T., Wester, P. O., Aikawa, J. K., and Ryan, M. P. (1985). Magnesium depletion as a cause of refractory potassium repletion. *Archives of Internal Medicine* **145**, 1686–1689.

White, P. C., New, M. I., and Dupont, B. (1987). Congenital adrenal hyperplasia. *New England Journal of Medicine* **316**, 1519–1524.

White, P. C., Curnow, K. M., and Pascoe, L. (1994). Disorders of steroid 11 beta-hydroxylase isozymes. *Endocrine Reviews* **15**, 421–438.

Wildenthal, K., Mierzwiak, D. S., Myers, R. W., and Mitchell, J. H. (1968). Effects of acute lactic acidosis on left ventricular performance. *American Journal of Physiology* **214**, 1352–1359.

Yamaguchi, K. *et al.* (1996). Endothelial modulation of pH-dependent pressor response in isolated perfused rabbit lungs. *American Journal of Physiology* **270**, H252–H258.

Yamashita, Y. *et al.* (2001). Two sporadic cases of Liddle's syndrome caused by de novo ENaC mutations. *American Journal of Kidney Diseases* **37**, 499–504.

3

The patient with glomerular disease

3.1 The renal glomerulus—the structural basis of ultrafiltration

Marlies Elger and Wilhelm Kriz

The correct name for the structure to be described is 'renal corpuscle'; 'glomerulus' strictly refers only to the tuft of glomerular capillaries (glomerular tuft). However, the use of the term glomerulus for the entire corpuscle is widely accepted.

A renal corpuscle is made up of a tuft of specialized capillaries supplied by an afferent arteriole, drained by an efferent arteriole, and enclosed in Bowman's capsule (Figs 1 and 2). The entire tuft of capillaries is covered by the epithelial cells (podocytes), representing the visceral layer of Bowman's capsule. At the vascular pole, the visceral layer of Bowman's capsule becomes the parietal layer, which is a simple squamous epithelium. At the urinary pole the parietal epithelium abruptly transforms to the epithelium of the proximal tubule. The space between both layers of Bowman's capsule is called the urinary space; at the urinary pole this passes into the tubule lumen. The glomerular basement membrane (GBM) lies at the interface between the glomerular capillaries and the podocytes. At the vascular pole, the GBM becomes the multilayered basement membrane of the parietal epithelium of Bowman's capsule.

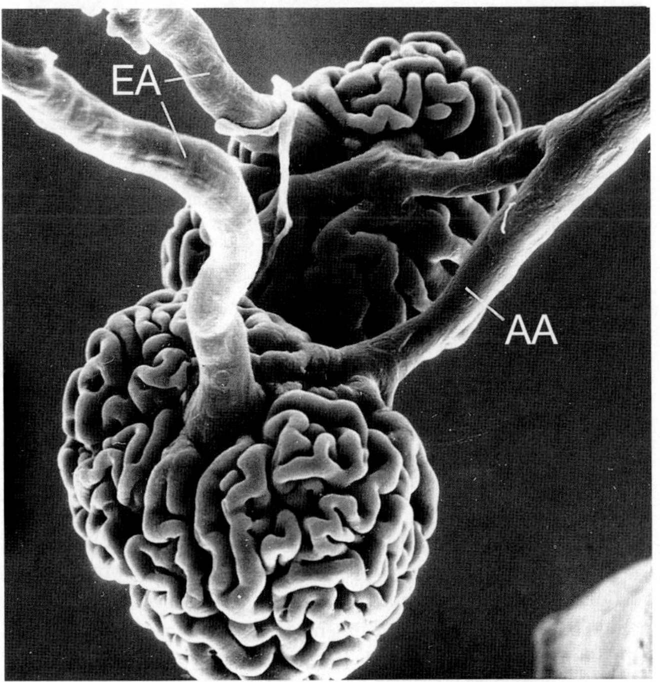

Fig. 1 Scanning electron micrograph showing a vascular cast of two juxtamedullary glomeruli (rat). Each capillary tuft is supplied by an afferent arteriole (AA) which, on the surface of the tuft, immediately divides into several branches. Efferent arterioles (EA) emerge out of the centre of the tuft. 400×.

Renal corpuscles are the starting points of the nephrons. Thus, the number of nephrons exactly correlates with the number of renal corpuscles—in humans, this is about one million in each kidney, in the rat about 30,000 per kidney. Renal corpuscles are roughly spherical in shape, with a diameter of approximately 200 μm in humans, and about 120 μm in the rat. Juxtamedullary renal corpuscles are generally somewhat larger (by about 20 per cent) than midcortical and superficial corpuscles (Tisher and Brenner 1989; Kriz and Kaissling 1992).

The glomerular tuft—a 'wonder net'

At the entrance to Bowman's capsule the afferent arteriole divides into several (three to five) primary capillary branches (Figs 1 and 3) (Yang and Morrison 1980). Each of these branches gives rise to a capillary network (glomerular lobule) which runs toward the urinary pole, turns back towards the vascular pole and unites with tributaries from the other lobules to form the efferent arteriole. The separation into lobules is not strict; near the vascular pole anastomoses are found interconnecting the lobules, but they are not formed between the afferent and efferent portions of the same lobule (Winkler *et al.* 1991). The efferent arteriole develops deep within the centre of the glomerular tuft from the confluence of tributaries from all lobules.

Thus, in contrast to the afferent arteriole, the efferent arteriole has an intraglomerular segment. Upon leaving the glomerulus, the efferent arteriole is closely associated with the extraglomerular mesangium. The intraglomerular segment is completely surrounded by mesangium; a smooth muscle layer is gradually established until the efferent arteriole leaves the extraglomerular mesangium.

Topography of a glomerular lobule—glomerular capillaries are unique

The capillary network, together with the mesangium, is surrounded by the visceral epithelial cells and the GBM, which indent deeply to follow the surface of the lobules. The individual capillaries are—along their entire length—attached to the mesangium, which constitutes the axis of a glomerular lobule. The mesangial interface comprises only

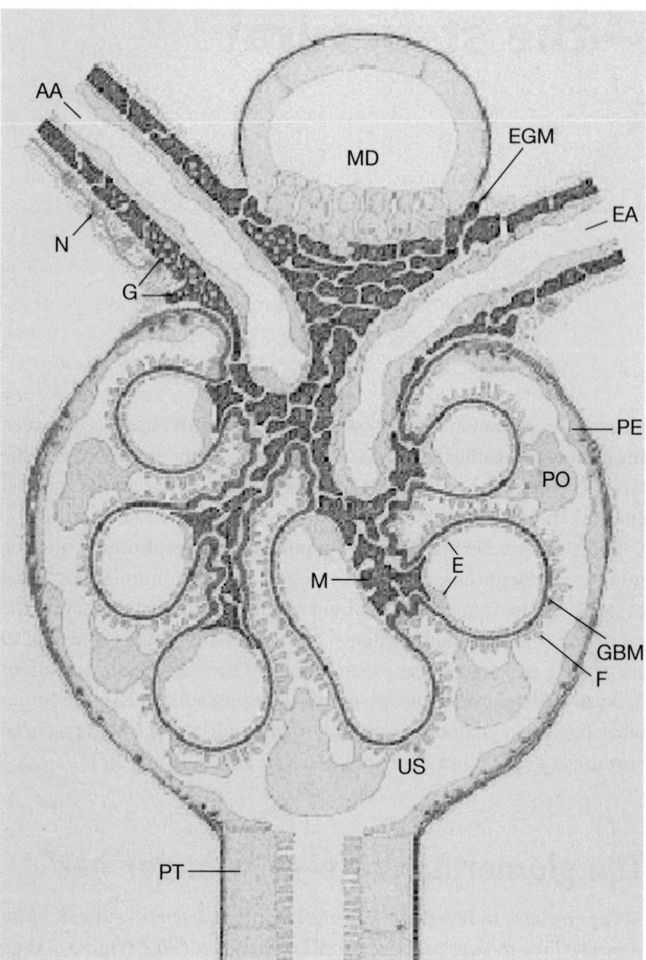

Fig. 2 Diagram of a longitudinal section through a renal corpuscle and the juxtaglomerular apparatus (JGA). The capillary tuft consists of a network of specialized capillaries, which are outlined by a fenestrated endothelium (E). At the vascular pole an afferent arteriole (AA) enters and an efferent arteriole (EA) leaves the tuft. The capillary network is surrounded by Bowman's capsule, comprising two different epithelia: the visceral and the parietal epithelium. The visceral epithelium consisting of highly branched podocytes (PO) directly follows—together with the glomerular basement membrane (GBM)—the surface of the capillaries and the mesangium (M). At the vascular pole, the visceral epithelium and the GBM are reflected into the parietal epithelium (PE) of Bowman's capsule (and its basement membrane), which passes over into the epithelium of the proximal tubule (PT) at the urinary pole. Mesangial cells (M) are situated in the axes of glomerular lobules. At the vascular pole the glomerular mesangium is continuous with the extraglomerular mesangium (EGM), consisting of cells and matrix. The EGM, together with the terminal portion of the afferent arteriole containing the granular cells (G), the efferent arteriole, and the macula densa (MD), establish the JGA. All cells that are suggested to be of smooth muscle origin are shown in a dark colour. F, foot processes; N, sympathetic nerve terminals; US, urinary space.

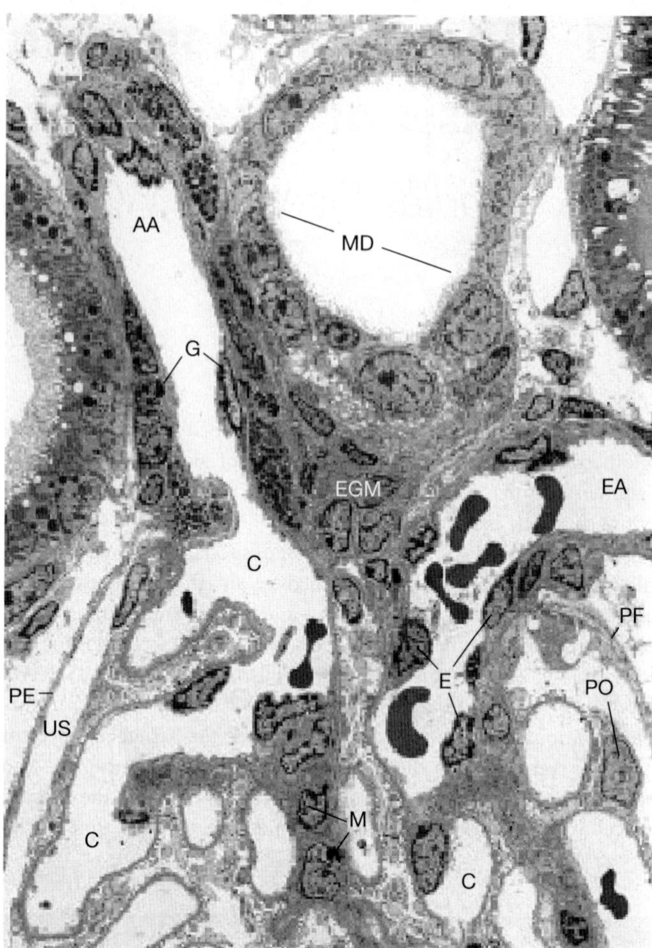

Fig. 3 Longitudinal section through the glomerular vascular pole showing both arterioles and the juxtaglomerular apparatus (JGA) (rat). At the entrance into the glomerulus, the afferent arteriole (AA) immediately branches into capillaries (C). The efferent arteriole (EA) usually arises deeper in the tuft and can be identified by the high number of endothelial cells (E) at the exit from the glomerulus. The macula densa (MD) of the thick ascending limb is in contact with the extraglomerular mesangium (EGM) and the glomerular arterioles. The media of the AA contains granular cells (G). M, mesangial cells; PE, parietal epithelium; PO, podocytes; US, urinary space. Electron micrograph (1300×).

a small portion of the capillary circumference. The major part of the endothelial tube is in close contact with the GBM (pericapillary part) and the layer of interdigitating foot processes of the visceral epithelium. This part of the capillary wall represents the actual filtering surface (Fig. 4). Thus, the GBM and the visceral epithelium of Bowman's capsule do not form complete envelopes around individual capillaries; the wall of the glomerular capillaries, therefore, has two portions: a peripheral portion, which bulges into Bowman's space and is covered by the glomerular basement membrane and the visceral epithelium of Bowman's capsule (podocytes), and a much smaller juxtamesangial portion, which only consists of the endothelium (without an underlying GBM) directly abutting the mesangium.

At the points where the capillaries come into contact with the mesangium, the GBM and the podocyte layer deviate from a pericapillary course and cover the mesangium; these points have been called mesangial angles. Therefore, two parts of the GBM and the visceral

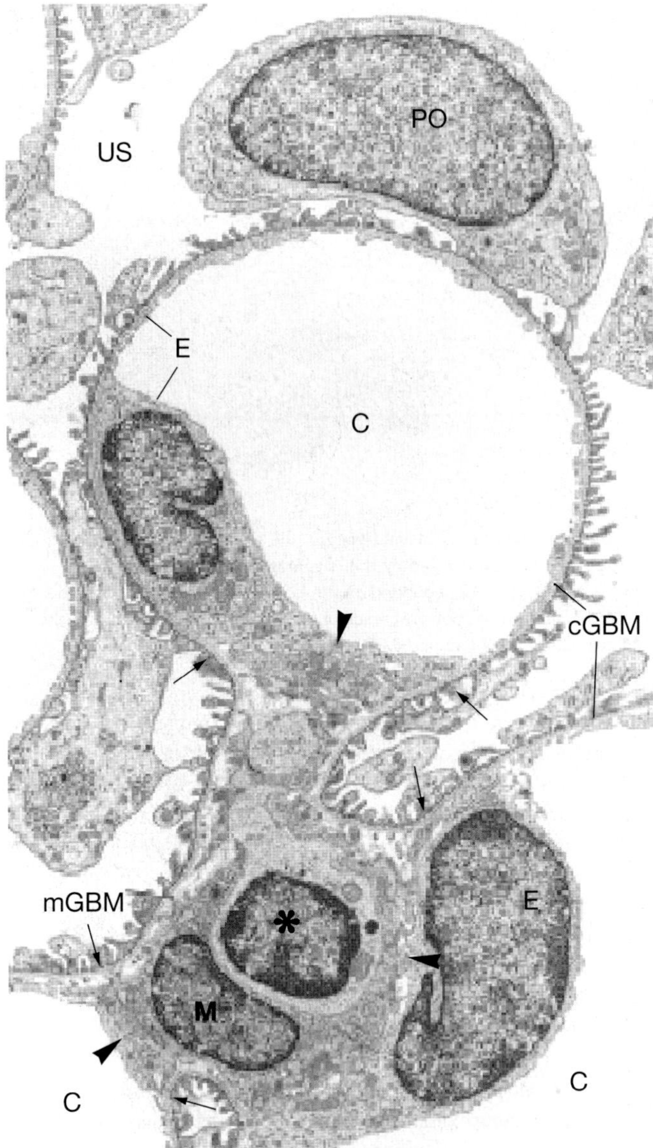

Fig. 4 Part of a glomerular lobule (rat), showing the arrangement of structures in the glomerular tuft. The capillary (C) is outlined by a flat fenestrated endothelium (E). The podocyte layer (PO) and the glomerular basement membrane (GBM) do not encircle the capillary completely, they form a common surface cover around the entire lobule. In the peripheral portion of the capillary the filtration barrier is formed (see also Fig. 5). Two subdomains of the GBM are delineated from each other by mesangial angles (arrows): the pericapillary GBM (cGBM) faced by the podocyte and endothelial layer, and the perimesangial GBM (mGBM) bordered by the podocyte layer and the mesangium. Within the mesangium two types of mesangial cells are shown: contractile mesangial cells proper (M) and a cell (*) that is probably a macrophage that has invaded the mesangium. Note the intimate relationships between the endothelium and the mesangium (arrowheads). US, urinary space. 6100×.

epithelium can be distinguished: a pericapillary part and a perimesangial part. The pericapillary part of the GBM is smooth and follows the outline of the capillary, whereas the perimesangial part is irregular in thickness and is frequently wrinkled.

Capillary endothelium—a perforated, highly charged structure

The capillary tube is made up of fenestrated endothelial cells (Fig. 4). The cell bodies are often located close to the mesangial axis. They contain the usual organelles; the endothelial cytoskeleton consists mainly of intermediate filaments and microtubules; individual fenestrations are lined by clusters of microfilaments (Vasmant *et al.* 1984).

The flat fenestrated parts of the cells comprise about 60 per cent of the capillary surface. They are characterized by round to oval pores 50–100 nm in diameter (Fig. 5). These pores occupy about 13 per cent of the capillary surface in the rat (Bulger *et al.* 1983); in absolute terms, the total area of all pores in a rat glomerulus amounts to about 22 mm^2 (Larsson and Maunsbach 1980). Unlike fenestrated endothelium at other sites, glomerular endothelial pores lack a diaphragm, they are open. Pores bridged by diaphragms in glomerular capillaries are only found along the outflow segment (Elger *et al.* 1991).

Vascular endothelial growth factor (VEGF) plays a pivotal role in angiogenesis. During organogenesis, VEGF is expressed in epithelia adjacent to developing endothelial tubes. In the kidney, VEGF expression persists in podocytes of adult glomeruli (Breier *et al.* 1992) and the glomerular endothelium and the peritubular capillaries are one of the few normal adult tissues in which the VEGF receptor can be detected (Feng *et al.* 2000). Analysis of knockout mice demonstrates that $VEGF_{164}$ and $VEGF_{188}$ isoforms are essential for normal ingrowth and survival of glomerular capillaries and, thereby, normal glomerular filtration (Mattot *et al.* 2002). VEGF also plays a role in glomerular vascular pathology. VEGF isoform 165, the most abundant isoform in man, and $VEGF_{121}$ are beneficial for endothelial glomerular injury associated with various glomerulonephritides, thrombotic microangiopathies, or renal transplant rejection. $VEGF_{165}$ aptamer led to a reduction of glomerular endothelial regeneration and an increase in endothelial cell death (Ostendorf *et al.* 1999; Suga *et al.* 2001). In experimental diabetes, blockage of VEGF improves early renal dysfunction by decreasing hyperfiltration, albuminuria, and glomerular hypertrophy (De Vriese *et al.* 2001).

The *luminal membrane* of endothelial cells carries a thick surface coat (up to 60 nm) and filamentous plugs as thick as 90 nm filling the endothelial pores (Rostgaard and Qvortrup 2002). This cell coat is negatively charged due to the presence of polyanionic glycoproteins (Horvat *et al.* 1986), including the sialoglycoprotein podocalyxin, which represents the major surface polyanion of glomerular endothelial as well as epithelial cells (Sawada *et al.* 1986).

Endothelial cells are active participants in processes controlling coagulation, inflammation, and immune processes, and an aberration in the controlling mechanisms may contribute to the development of disease within the glomerulus (Savage 1994, 1998). Renal endothelial cells share an antigen system with cells of the monocyte/macrophage lineage; they express surface antigens of the class II histocompatibility antigens. Similar to platelets, glomerular endothelial cells contain components of the coagulation pathway and are capable of binding factors IXa and Xa, and of synthesizing, releasing, and binding von Willebrand factor (factor VIII) (Wiggins *et al.* 1989).

In most forms of kidney disease, renal leucocyte infiltration is prominent, leading to focal accumulation at sites of injury. In the glomerular endothelium—as the site of first contact of infiltrating leucocytes and transmigration—cytokines such as IL-1β and chemokines

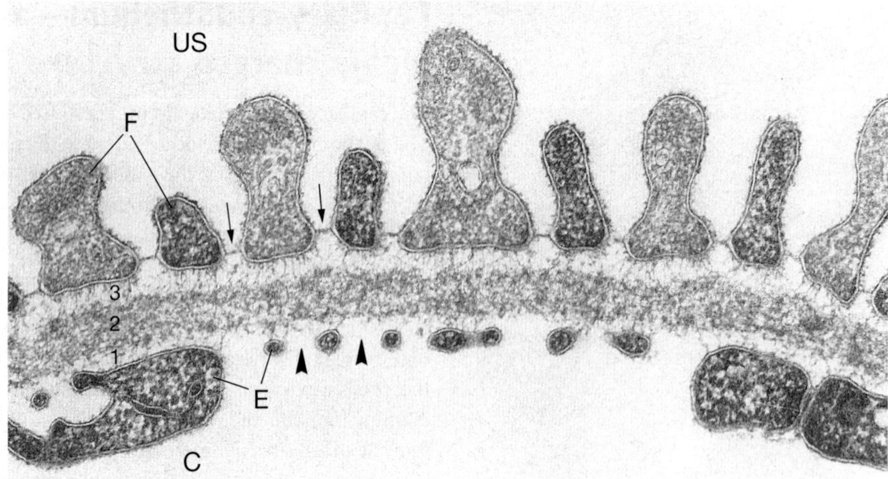

Fig. 5 Filtration barrier. The peripheral part of the glomerular capillary wall comprises the fenestrated endothelial layer (E), the glomerular basement membrane, and the interdigitating foot processes (F). The filtration slits between the foot processes are bridged by thin diaphragms (long arrows). Arrowheads point to the endothelial pores. The glomerular basement membrane shows a lamina densa (2) bounded by the lamina rara interna (1) and the lamina rara externa (3). In this picture, tannic acid staining allows discrimination between the alternating foot processes of two neighbouring podocytes: the more densely stained processes belong to one cell, and the others to the neighbouring cell. C, capillary lumen. 60,000×.

such as the monocyte chemoattractant MCP-1 are produced. They stimulate expression of endothelial lectins (E- and P-selectins), believed to mediate early rolling interaction between leucocytes and endothelium, as well as the expression of endothelial adhesion molecules like ICAM-1 that serve as ligands for integrins in the membrane of the inflammatory cells (Schlöndorff *et al.* 1997; Rabb *et al.* 1998). Fractalkine, a recently described chemotactic adhesin located on glomerular and peritubular endothelia at sites of inflammation, binds to a specific receptor (CX_3CR) that is not shared by any other chemokine. It triggers the adhesion of mononuclear cells under physiological flow conditions (Fong *et al.* 1998; Cockwell *et al.* 2002). Glomerular endothelial cells synthesize and release endothelin-1 and endothelium-derived relaxing factor (EDRF) (Ott *et al.* 1993; Herman *et al.* 1998).

Visceral epithelium—filtration slits are formed by interdigitating foot processes

The visceral epithelial layer of Bowman's capsule consists of highly differentiated cells, the podocytes (Bulger and Hebert 1988; Tisher and Brenner 1989; Kriz and Kaissling 1992). The podocytes are attached to the GBM, which is mainly synthesized by these cells (Striker and Striker 1985; Abrahamson 1987).

In the developing glomerulus, the visceral epithelium consists of simple polygonal cells. In rat, mitotic activity of these cells is completed soon after birth, along with the cessation of the formation of new nephrons (Nagata *et al.* 1993), and the final number of podocytes is determined. In humans, this point is reached during prenatal life. Differentiated podocytes appear to be unable to replicate (Fries *et al.* 1989; Nagata and Kriz 1992; Kriz 2002), thus, in the adult degenerated podocytes cannot be replaced. In response to an extreme stimulation (long-term treatment with FGF-2) the nucleus may undergo mitotic division; however, the cells are not able to complete cell division (cytokinesis), resulting in binucleated cells (Kriz *et al.* 1995b).

Podocytes have a voluminous cell body, which bulges into the urinary space (Figs 6 and 7). Long primary processes emerge from the cell body and extend towards the capillaries, to which they affix by their distal portions that fall apart into numerous secondary processes (foot processes). The foot processes of neighbouring podocytes regularly interdigitate with each other, leaving between them meandering slits (filtration slits), which are bridged by a very thin membrane (slit membrane or slit diaphragm).

Podocytes are polarized epithelial cells with a luminal (apical) and an abluminal (basal) cell membrane domain. The basal domain corresponds to the sole plates of the foot processes, which are embedded into the GBM up to approximately 60 nm. The border between basal and luminal membrane is represented by the slit diaphragm.

The *luminal membrane*, including the slit diaphragm, is covered by a thick surface coat, which is rich in sialoglycoproteins that are responsible for the high negative surface charge of podocytes. They include podoendin (Huang and Langlois 1985), SGP115/107 (Mendrick and Rennke 1988), and podocalyxin (Kerjaschki *et al.* 1984; Sawada *et al.* 1986), which via the linker protein NHERF2 (Na^+/H^+-exchanger regulatory factor 2) and ezrin is attached to the actin cytoskeleton. The surface charge of podocytes contributes to the maintenance of the interdigitating pattern of the foot processes. In response to neutralization of the surface charge by cationic substances (e.g. protamine sulfate, poly-L-lysin), the glomerular epithelium undergoes a series of changes, including retraction of foot processes and formation of tight junctions between adjacent foot processes (Seiler *et al.* 1977; Andrews 1988).

The *abluminal membrane* contains the specific anchor systems used to connect podocytes to the GBM (see below). The many receptor proteins are generally found on the entire surface of podocytes; they include those for angiotensin II (AT1 and AT2; Nitschke *et al.* 2000; Sharma *et al.* 2001), noradrenaline ($\alpha 1$; Huber *et al.* 1998), acetylcholine (M5; Nitschke *et al.* 2001), prostaglandin (Bek *et al.* 1999), ATP (Fischer *et al.* 2001), endothelin (ETA; Rebibou *et al.* 1992; Spath *et al.* 1995),

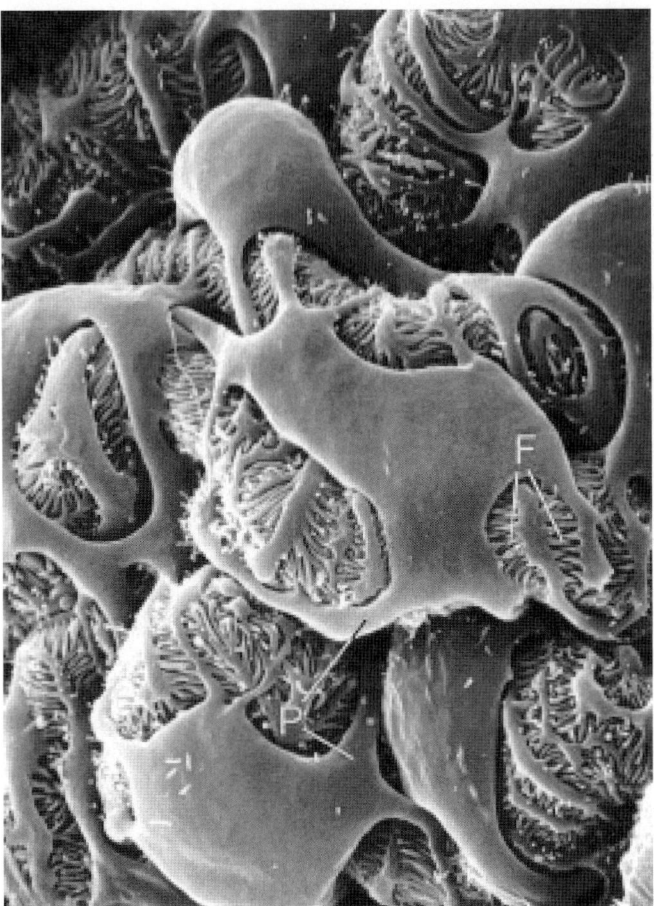

Fig. 6 Scanning electron micrograph of rat glomerular capillaries. The urinary side of the capillary is covered by the highly branched podocytes. The interdigitating system of primary (P) and secondary (F) processes lines the entire surface of the glomerular basement membrane and proceeds also beneath the cell bodies (see Fig. 7). In between the interdigitating foot processes (F) of neighbouring cells the filtration slits are spared. 3300×.

ANP (Zhao *et al.* 1994), PTH/PTHrP (Amizuka *et al.* 1997; Endlich *et al.* 2001b), TGFβ (Yamamoto *et al.* 1998), IL-4/IL-13 (Van Den Berg *et al.* 2000), FGF2 (Ford *et al.* 1997), C3b-receptor (Kazatchkine *et al.* 1982), and gp330/megalin (Kerjaschki and Farquhar 1983). Megalin, a glycoprotein of 330 kDa (Saito *et al.* 1994) is a major podocyte antigen of rat Heymann nephritis.

The cell body contains a prominent nucleus, a well-developed Golgi apparatus, abundant rough and smooth endoplasmic reticulum, prominent lysosomes, and mitochondria (Fig. 7a). In contrast to the cell body, the cell processes contain only a few organelles. The organelles in the cell body indicate a high level of anabolic as well as catabolic activity. In addition to the work necessary to sustain structural integrity of these specialized cells, most, if not all, components of the GBM are synthesized by the podocytes (Abrahamson 1987). Podocytes regularly contain large membrane-bound bodies filled with a proteinaceous material, frequently arranged in layers (Thoenes 1967). Their membrane is continuous with that of the endoplasmic reticulum. The relevance of these bodies is unknown.

The cell contains a well-developed cytoskeleton. In the cell body and the primary processes, microtubules and intermediate filaments (vimentin, desmin) dominate (Fig. 7b) (Bachmann *et al.* 1983; Vasmant *et al.* 1984; Andrews 1988; Drenckhahn and Franke 1988; Kriz *et al.* 1995a). Microfilament bundles containing actin, myosin, and α-actinin are found in the primary processes and in the foot processes (Trenchev *et al.* 1976; Andrews 1988; Drenckhahn and Franke 1988).

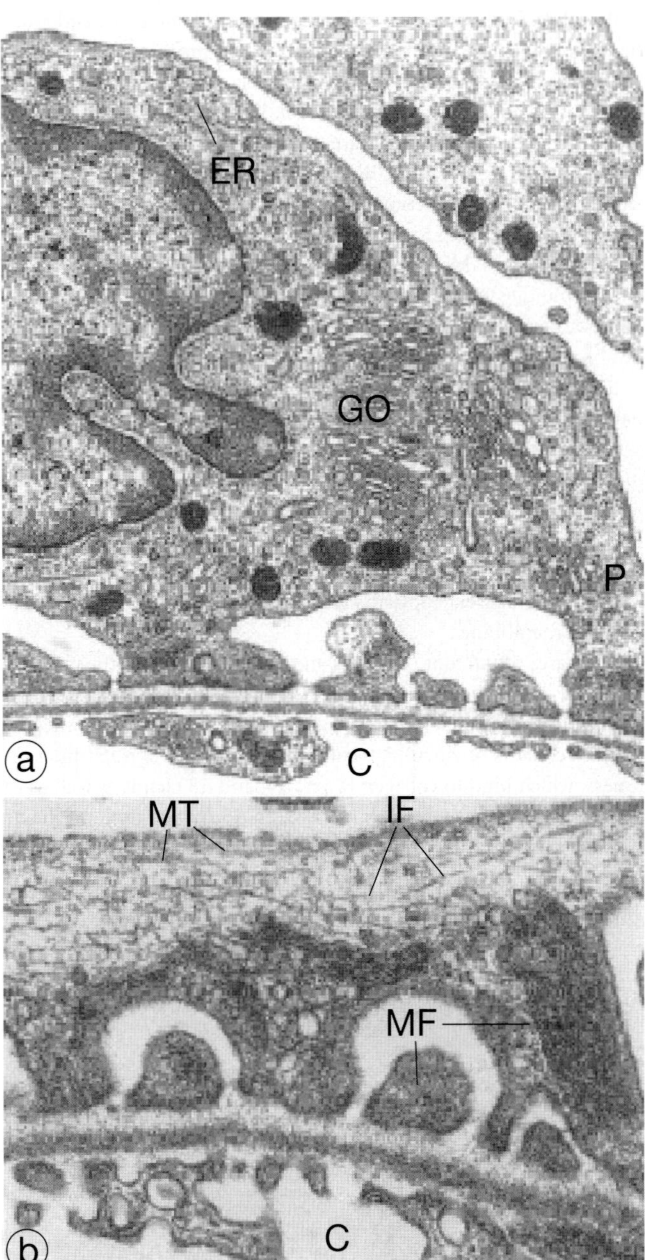

Fig. 7 (a) Electron micrograph showing part of a podocyte cell body anchored via processes to the glomerular basement membrane. The majority of these processes are foot processes. The others are ridge-like bases of the cell body and distal portions of primary processes (P). Note the prominent Golgi apparatus (GO); also rough endoplasmic reticulum (ER) is fairly abundant. C, capillary lumen. 25,000×. (b) Primary and secondary processes of podocytes showing cytoskeletal elements. Intermediate filaments (IF) and microtubules (MT) are abundant in the primary processes; thick bundles of microfilaments (MF) are located in the foot processes. C, capillary lumen. 46,000×.

Bundles of microtubules and intermediate filaments extend from the cell body to the distal end of the primary processes. The microtubules are of mixed polarity, which appears to be essential for process formation of podocytes (Kobayashi *et al.* 1998). As intracellular transport systems the microtubules are probably involved in the transport of substances (e.g. for the GBM) to the peripheral parts of the cell. Another important function of the microtubules and intermediate filaments may be found in their cytoskeletal properties in relation to mechanical forces. Microtubules resist compression of their long axis and, as bundles interconnected by microtubule-associated proteins, withstand bending forces. Intermediate filaments, on the other hand, are able to resist tensile forces (Wang *et al.* 1993).

In the cell body and the primary processes, actin-containing microfilaments are seen in a thin layer underlying the apical cell membrane (Drenckhahn and Franke 1988). In the foot processes, prominent bundles of microfilaments run longitudinally in the middle and upper portion. At the transition to the primary processes, the microfilaments form loops roughly parallel to the turning point of the slit and extend into the adjacent process of the same cell (Fig. 8). They appear to anchor in the dense cytoplasm associated with the inner aspect of the basal cell membrane.

The bases of the foot processes and the distal parts of the primary processes from which the foot processes originate are firmly attached to the GBM, mediated by integrins and dystroglycans. The integrin complex consists of vinculin, paxillin, and talin, and of $\alpha3\beta1$ integrin dimers, which bind to collagen IV $\alpha3$, $\alpha4$, and $\alpha5$ chains as well as to laminin 11, a heterotrimer composed of $\alpha5/\beta2/\gamma1$ laminin chains (Miner 1999; Kreidberg and Symons 2000). The dystroglycan complex (Durbeej *et al.* 1998; Raats *et al.* 2000a; Regele *et al.* 2000) consists of the cytoplasmic adaptor protein utrophin, of the transmembranous β-dystroglycan, and of the extracellular matrix-binding α-dystroglycan which is a receptor for agrin and laminin $\alpha5$ chains.

On the one hand, dystroglycans and integrins are thought to coordinate the formation of a polygonal network of laminin in basement membranes (Schwarzbauer 1999); thus, cell matrix contacts in podocyte foot processes may be crucially involved in maintenance of GBM substructure and hence may participate in the barrier function. On the other hand, outside-in signalling via these systems quite obviously influences the function of the cytoskeleton which, in cases of derangements of the GBM, may lead to foot-process effacement (see below). The filtration slits are the site of convective fluid flow through the visceral epithelium. The total length of the filtration slit in a rat glomerulus amounts to about 50 cm (Kriz *et al.* 1995a; Mundel and Kriz 1995). Since the slit has a rather constant width of 30–45 nm, the total area of the slit membrane approximates 20×10^3 μm^2, comprising about 10–13 per cent of the peripheral capillary surface.

The structure and biochemical composition of the slit membrane are still incompletely understood. Chemically fixed and tannic acid treated tissue reveals a zipper-like structure with a row of 'pores', of dimensions approximately 4×14 nm, on either side of a central bar (Rodewald and Karnovsky 1974). In quick-frozen tissue, a more homogeneous structure with only a central bar is apparent (Hora *et al.* 1990). Proteins that establish the slit membrane include nephrin, Neph1, p-cadherin, and FAT. Presently, it is not clear how these proteins participate in the molecular organization of this structure. The cytoplasmic tails of these proteins allow a dynamic connection of the

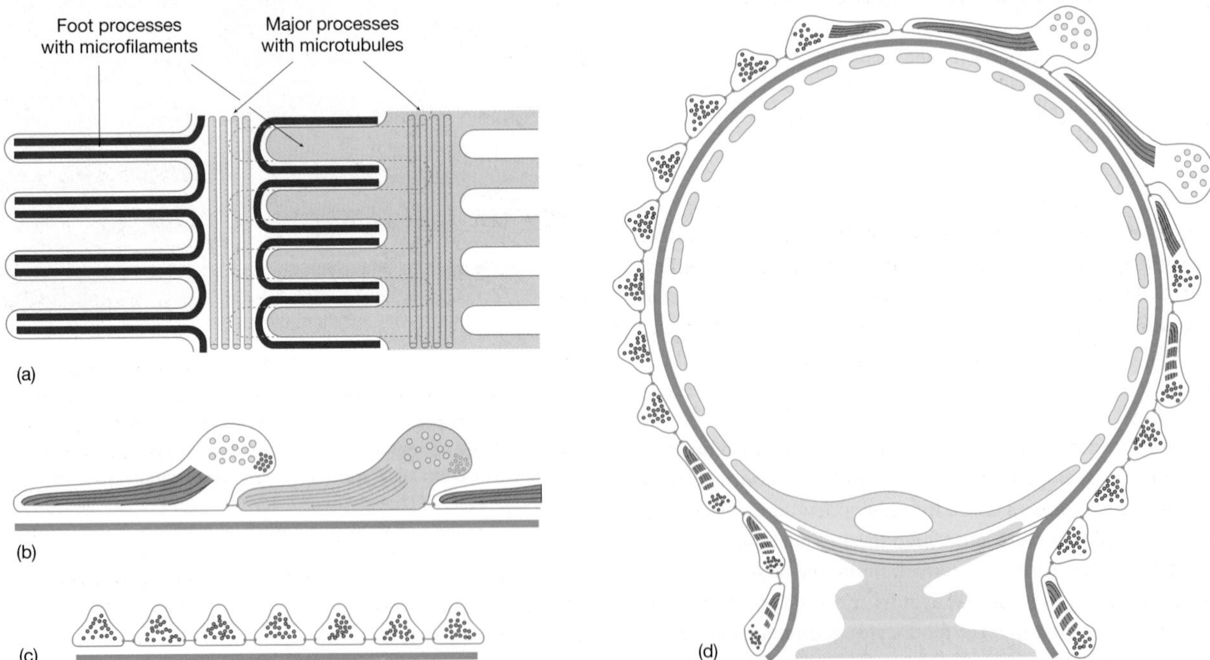

Fig. 8 Arrangement of cytoskeletal elements in podocyte processes: (a) view from above; (b) section of foot processes parallel and (c) perpendicular to the longitudinal axis of foot processes. Two major processes (one in white, one in yellow) with their foot processes are shown. The actin filaments (red) of foot processes form continuous loops which end in the foot process sole plates. At their bend they are in close association with microtubules (green) that run longitudinally in the major processes. (d) Scheme of a cross-section through a capillary loop. The foot processes that contain a complete actin-based contractile apparatus, cover the outer aspect of the GBM and may serve to counteract the elastic distension of the GBM. After Mundel and Kriz (1995).

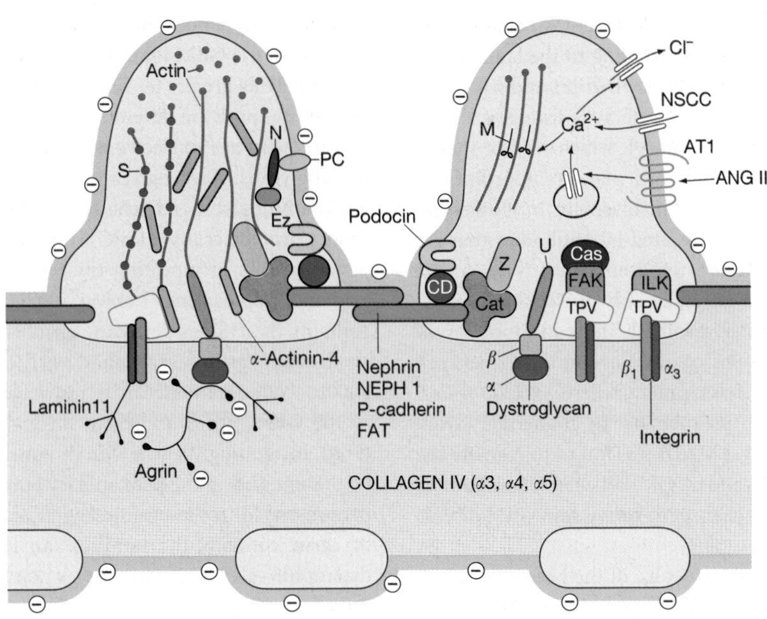

Fig. 9 Schematic drawing of the molecular equipment in podocyte foot processes: Cas, p130Cas; Cat, catenins; CD, CD2-associated protein; Ez, ezrin; FAK, focal adhesion kinase; ILK, integrin-linked kinase; M, myosin; N, NHERF2; NSCC, non-selective cation channel; PC, podocalyxin; S, synaptopodin; TPV, talin, paxillin, vinculin; U, utrophin; Z, ZO1. Proteins presently known to participate in the molecular structure of the slit membrane include nephrin, NEPH1, P-cadherin, and FAT. See text for further explanations.

slit membrane to the cytoskeleton. Proteins that mediate and/or regulate this connection include ZO1, α-, β-, γ-catenins, podocin, CD2AP, and α-actinin 4. Figure 9 summarizes some main features of the molecular organization of podocyte foot processes (modified after Endlich *et al.* 2001a).

Functional relevance of podocytes

It is difficult to precisely define the function of podocytes; they are still a mysterious cell type. In our view, podocytes are best understood as a modified type of a pericyte with specialized intercellular junctions, that is, the slit diaphragm; thus, as a supportive cell that, in addition, controls paracellular permeability. The foot processes contain an actin-based contractile system anchored to the outer aspect of the GBM (i.e. to the capillary wall). Thereby, foot processes correspond to the contractile processes of pericytes elsewhere in the body, counteracting the distension of the capillary wall.

The supportive function of podocytes is based on the firm connection of the contractile apparatus in foot processes to the basement membrane. Podocytes (like processes of pericytes at many places) do not encircle the capillary completely (as do smooth muscle cells of arterioles), thus, podocytes (like pericytes) can perform their wall-stabilizing function only in conjunction with the GBM. As will be described below, the basic supportive structure of a glomerular capillary wall is represented by the GBM cylinder, which opens towards the mesangium like a tyre to the rim and a mesangial cell that bridges this gap by a contractile cell process. Thus, basically, the GBM together with the mesangial bridge form a complete cylinder which is able to develop wall tension and thus to resist distension. In addition, however, the GBM must be regarded as an elastic structure (Welling *et al.* 1995), which will distend when transmural pressure gradients rise. The foot processes probably act as numerous small patches counteracting local expansion of the GBM. Moreover, podocyte processes filling the niches of GBM infoldings contribute to the stabilization of the GBM-folding pattern by interconnecting opposing portions of the GBM (Kriz *et al.* 1995a).

Glomerular basement membrane—the backbone of the glomerular tuft

The GBM represents the skeletal backbone of the glomerular tuft (Fig. 4). In transmission electron micrographs of traditionally fixed tissue, the GBM appears as a trilaminar structure made up of a lamina densa bounded by two less dense layers—the lamina rara interna and externa (Fig. 5). In humans, the thickness of the GBM ranges from 300 to 370 nm (Steffes *et al.* 1983); in children it may be considerably thinner (Morita *et al.* 1988). In rats and other experimental animals, the thickness is between 110 and 190 nm (Rasch 1979; Bulger and Hebert 1988).

In accordance with basement membranes at other sites, the major components of the GBM include type IV collagen, heparan sulfate proteoglycans, and laminin (Mohan and Spiro 1986; Timpl and Dziadek 1986). Types V and VI collagen, and entactin have also been demonstrated. On the other hand, the GBM has many unique properties, notably a distinct spectrum of type IV collagen and laminin isoforms (Couchman *et al.* 1994; Miner 1999b).

At least six different type IV collagen genes have been cloned, which encode the $\alpha 1$ to $\alpha 6$ chains, respectively, of type IV collagen. The distribution of $\alpha 3$ (IV) and $\alpha 4$ (IV) chains, which are located in the lamina densa, differs from that of the classical $\alpha1$ (IV) and $\alpha2$ (IV) found in the subendothelial space (corresponding to the lamina rara interna) and in the mesangium. This suggests that $\alpha3$ and $\alpha4$, along with $\alpha5$, form a network that is separate from that consisting of $\alpha1$ and $\alpha2$ chains (Sanes *et al.* 1990). The $\alpha3$ and $\alpha4$, which replace the $\alpha1$ and $\alpha2$ chains during maturation of the GBM, play an important role in GBM function, as derived from their involvement in glomerular disease: Goodpasture's syndrome is mediated by antibodies that are targeted to the $\alpha3$ (IV) chain; in Alport's syndrome, mostly $\alpha3$–$\alpha5$ are all absent, caused by mutations in generally only one of the responsible genes (Hudson *et al.* 1994; Tryggvason 1995). As in Alport's syndrome, GBM deterioration begins postnatally, only the $\alpha1/\alpha2$ network is essential for normal glomerular development, whereas the $\alpha3/\alpha4/\alpha5$ network is essential for long-term maintenance of glomerular structure (Harvey *et al.* 1998). Recently, LMX1B was found to regulate the coordinated expression of $\alpha3$ (IV) and $\alpha4$ (IV) collagen (Morello *et al.* 2001). A point mutation in the $\alpha4$ chain gene causes thin GBM disease (Monnens 2001).

Current models picture the basic structure of the basement membrane as a three-dimensional network of collagen type IV. Monomers of type IV collagen consist of a triple helix of length 400 nm which, at its carboxy-terminal end, has a large non-collagenous globular domain called NC1. At the amino terminus, the helix possesses a triple helical rod (60 nm) in length, the 7S domain. Interactions between the 7S domains of two triple helices or the NC1 domains of four triple helices allow collagen type IV monomers to form dimers and tetramers. In addition, triple helical strands interconnect by lateral associations via binding of NC1 domains to sites along the collagenous region (Fig. 9) (Timpl and Dziadek 1986; Yurchenco and Ruben 1987). These interactions between type IV collagen triple helices result in a flexible, nonfibrillar polygonal assembly that is considered to provide mechanical strength to the basement membrane and to serve as a scaffold for alignment of other matrix components (Pihlajaniemi 1996).

Cell attachment to the GBM is mediated by glycoproteins such as fibronectin, laminin, and entactin. Laminin is the major noncollagenous glycoprotein in basement membranes and it plays a key role in mediating the differentiation of adjacent epithelia. It represents a growing family of α, β, and γ chains, which form $\alpha\beta\gamma$ cruciforms or Y-shaped heterotrimers (Burgeson *et al.* 1994). Five α chains, three β chains, and three γ chains have been found that assemble to form twelve known isoforms. In the GBM, $\alpha5$, $\beta2$, and $\gamma1$, which refer to laminin 11, as well as $\beta1$ have been detected. Laminin 11 is highly restricted in the kidney, as it is found only in the GBM and the arteriolar basement membranes. Mice lacking $\beta2$ develop massive proteinuria and foot process effacement, and die during early postnatal life (Hansen and Abrass 1999; Miner 1999). Laminin is thought to bind directly or via entactin (Katz *et al.* 1991) to type IV collagen as well as to integrin and non-integrin cell surface receptors of endothelial and epithelial cells, thereby interconnecting cells and basement membrane. For instance, $\alpha3\beta1$ plays a major role in adhesion of glomerular endothelial cells to collagen, and $\alpha5\beta1$ is the major fibronectin receptor on these cells (Adler and Eng 1993) (see also above).

The relative amount of components varies between basement membranes of different sources. The GBM contains more type IV collagen and less laminin than does the renal tubular basement membrane (Brees *et al.* 1995). Because of covalent cross-linking, the type IV collagen network provides a stronger scaffolding to render the basement membrane more resilient and permanent than a laminin polymer (Yurchenco and Cheng 1994). The higher content of type IV collagen in the GBM than in the tubular basement membrane may be indicative of a greater tensile strength of the GBM adapted to the high transmural pressure differences at this site.

The GBM has an electronegative charge, due mainly to polyanionic proteoglycans. Proteoglycans consist of a core protein to which glucosaminoglycan side chains are attached. With respect to heparan sulfate proteoglycans (HSPG), these side chains are heparan sulfates, which consist of repeating disaccharide units containing an uronic acid and glucosamine (Kanwar 1984; Noonan *et al.* 1991). The GBM contains the HSPGs perlecan, agrin, collagen XVIII, and others with small core proteins (Farquhar 1991; Halfter *et al.* 1998; Raats *et al.* 2000b). Whereas perlecan is restricted to the subendothelial aspect of the GBM, agrin is present throughout the width of the mature GBM. Interestingly, agrin with its entire molecule structure appears to be present only in the pericapillary portion, the *C*-terminus cannot be demonstrated in the perimesangial portion. Because the *C*-terminus of agrin contains the binding site for α-dystroglycan, the agrin–dystrophin–glycoprotein complex that links the GBM to the cytoskeleton of the podocyte may only be important in the pericapillary GBM involved in ultrafiltration (Raats *et al.* 2000a). Aggregation of proteoglycan molecules results in the formation of a meshwork that is kept highly hydrated by water molecules trapped in the interstices of the matrix. HSPGs within the GBM may act as an anticlogging agent to prevent hydrogen bonding and adsorption of anionic plasma proteins and maintain an efficient flow of water through the membrane (Kanwar 1984). In addition, they are important for binding growth factors and their receptors. In several forms of proteinuric glomerulopathies, such as systemic lupus erythematosus, minimal change disease and diabetic nephropathy, changes occur in the heparan sulfate side chains of agrin that may be related to the development of proteinuria. The mechanisms for alterations in heparan sulfate, which can lead to reduced heparan sulfate function comprise the masking by immune complexes, depolymerization by radicals (oxygen and nitrogen), degradation by enzymes such as elastase, and biochemical changes like the degree of sulfation (Raats *et al.* 2000b).

Filtration barrier—filtration occurs along an extracellular pathway

The filtration barrier is composed of (a) the endothelium with large open pores, (b) the dense network of the GBM, and (c) the slit diaphragms between the podocyte foot processes.

Compared with the barrier established in capillaries elsewhere in the body, there are at least two outstanding characteristics of the filtration barrier in the glomerulus: the permeability for water, small solutes, and ions is extremely high, while the permeability for plasma proteins of the size of albumin and larger is very low.

The high hydraulic permeability is obviously explained by the fact that filtration occurs along extracellular routes. All components of this route, the endothelial pores, the highly hydrated GBM, and the slit membrane can be expected to be quite permeable for water and small solutes. The hydraulic conductance of the individual layers of the filtration barrier is difficult to examine. In a mathematical model of glomerular filtration, the hydraulic resistance of the endothelium was predicted to be small, whereas the GBM and filtration slits each contributed roughly one-half of the total hydraulic resistance of the capillary wall (Drumond and Deen 1994).

In experimental pathological models as well as in human glomerulopathies such as membranous nephropathy or minimal change nephropathy, foot process effacement with a drastic reduction of the filtration slit length is a prominent feature. This decrease in slit length (or slit frequency) is correlated with a decrease in the ultrafiltration coefficient, K_f (Kiberd 1992; Guasch and Myers 1994). The decrease in frequency of filtration slits not only causes a decrease in total slit membrane area, that is, in the crucial filtration area, but also causes an increase in the average path length for the filtrate through the GBM, thereby explaining the decreased hydraulic permeability in these nephropathies (Drumond *et al.* 1994).

The barrier function for macromolecules is based on the size, shape, and charge of the respective molecule (recently reviewed in Daniels 1993; Daniels *et al.* 1993; Deen *et al.* 2001); the relevance of each of these parameters is in debate. The latest thinking is that the proximal portions of the barrier (endothelium, GBM) are responsible for the charge selectivity, whereas the slit membrane represents the size/shape barrier (Deen *et al.* 2001). Negatively charged molecules are accumulated throughout the entire depth of the filtration barrier, including the surface coats of endothelial and epithelial cells, and the high content of negatively charged HSPG in the GBM. Polyanionic macromolecules in the plasma, such as plasma proteins, are repelled by these assemblies of negatively charged molecules, establishing an electronegative shield. Removal or blocking of the negative charge in experimental models results in proteinuria. Selectively reduced renal proteoglycan synthesis is correlated with proteinuria in diabetic mice (Farquhar 1991).

The size/shape selectivity for macromolecules of the filtration barrier is established by the slit membrane; details on how the slit membrane performs this function are unknown. Uncharged macromolecules up to an effective radius of 1.8 nm pass freely through the filter. Larger compounds are more and more restricted (indicated by their fractional clearances which progressively decrease), and are totally restricted at effective radii of more than 4.0 nm. The term 'effective radius' is an empirical value, measured in artificial membranes, which takes into account the shape of macromolecules and attributes a radius to non-spherical molecules. Plasma albumin has an effective radius of 3.6 nm; without the repulsion due to the negative charge, plasma albumin would pass through the filter in considerable amounts (Deen *et al.* 1979). The importance of the slit diaphragm for size selectivity is evidenced by experiments with ferritin (radius 6.1 nm). Whereas anionic ferritin particles accumulate at the level of endothelial fenestrae and the subendothelial space, cationized ferritin penetrates the lamina densa and accumulates beneath the slit diaphragm.

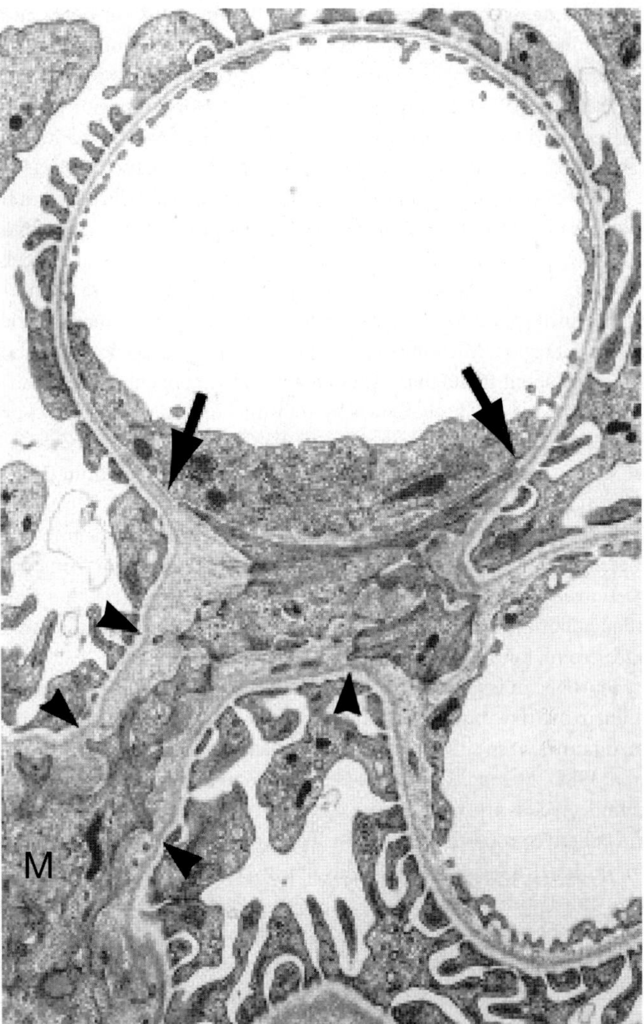

Fig. 10 Glomerular capillary and mesangium. In the juxtacapillary region, long mesangial cell processes extend between opposite mesangial angles, where they are fixed to the GBM (arrows). In the axial region, finger-like processes connect the mesangial cells to the perimesangial glomerular basement membrane (arrowheads). Note bundles of microfilaments in the cell processes. M, mesangial cell. 13,000×.

Mesangium—maintenance of the structural integrity of the tuft

The mesangium occupies the axial region of a glomerular lobule and consists of mesangial cells and the surrounding mesangial matrix (Figs 4 and 10), first described by Zimmermann (1929). Since the ultrastructural characterization of the mesangium in the early sixties (Latta *et al.* 1960; Farquhar and Palade 1962), mesangial cells have been in the forefront of glomerular research. They are generally believed to form a supporting framework that maintains the structural integrity of the glomerular tuft.

The mesangial matrix consists mostly of basement membrane components (Karkavelas and Kefalides 1988). At variance to the GBM it contains the $\alpha1$ and $\alpha2$ chains of type IV collagen, the $\beta1$ chain of laminin, considerable amounts of fibronectin, chondroitin sulfate proteoglycan, the small leucine-rich proteoglycans biglycan and decorin and the heparan sulfate proteoglycans perlecan, bamacan, and collagen type XVIII (Border *et al.* 1989; Couchman *et al.* 1994; Miner 1999); in addition, microfibrillar proteins are abundant (Gibson *et al.* 1989; Sterzel *et al.* 2000).

Mesangial cells are considered to be contractile cells that have a common origin with smooth muscle cells. They are irregular in shape, with numerous cytoplasmic processes that contain prominent assemblies of microfilaments (Fig. 10). With immunocytochemistry, these microfilaments have been shown to contain actin, myosin, and α-actinin (Kreisberg *et al.* 1985; Drenckhahn and Franke 1988). Moreover, the mesangial cells are electrically coupled by gap junctions (Pricam *et al.* 1974). Mesangial cells possess receptors for angiotensin II, vasopressin, atrial natriuretic factor, and prostaglandins (among others) (Sraer *et al.* 1974; Dworkin *et al.* 1983; Stockand and Sansom 1998).

The GBM is the primary effector site of mesangial cell contraction (Sakai and Kriz 1987; Kriz *et al.* 1990). Mesangial cells are connected extensively with the GBM, either by direct apposition of mesangial cell processes (focal adhesions) or by microfibrils (Fig. 10). These connections, which appear to be mechanically strong, are found throughout the mesangial region. Microfibrils are unbranched non-collagenous, tubular structures about 15 nm thick. They are a major component of the mesangial matrix, as has been shown by transmission electron microscopy after tannic acid staining (Mundel *et al.* 1988) and by immunocytochemistry using antibodies against microfibrillar proteins derived from elastic tissue (Gibson *et al.* 1989). Microfibrils are generally coated by fibronectin (Schwartz *et al.* 1985). The high content of fibronectin within the mesangium (Madri *et al.* 1980) may be related to the need for firm connections between the different structures; first, for the interconnection of microfibrils, giving a firm mechanical support to the mesangial matrix; and second, for the adhesion of mesangial cells to the GBM.

Fibronectin is involved in the connection between actin and extracellular matrix components, including type IV collagen of basement membranes, at specific adhesion sites, called focal adhesions (Burridge *et al.* 1988). Mesangial cells have been shown to form focal adhesions in culture (Woods and Couchman 1992; Petermann *et al.* 1993). Moreover, the adhesive properties of mesangial cells to the substrate are dependent on $\alpha 3\beta 1$ integrin, which binds fibronectin to the termini of actin filaments (Cosio *et al.* 1990).

Mesangial cell-to-GBM contacts are found along the entire perimesangial GBM. The intracellular actin filament bundles are arranged in such a way that segments of the GBM located on opposing sides of the mesangium are interconnected. These connections are most prominent at mesangial angles consisting of tongue-like mesangial processes which establish a bridge between both mesangial angles of the GBM (Figs 10–12) (Sakai and Kriz 1987).

Evidence for the importance of these connections for the structural integrity of the tuft was obtained by selective destruction of the mesangium by experimental application of antibody against the cell surface antigen Thy 1 (Paul *et al.* 1984; Bagchus *et al.* 1986). In this situation, the mesangial region as well as the mesangial—endothelial interface is greatly enlarged, leading to a partial 'unfolding' of glomerular capillaries associated with capillary ballooning (Lemley *et al.* 1992), and profound changes in the glomerular haemodynamics (Blantz *et al.* 1991).

The large pressure gradient across the GBM is obviously a crucial challenge to the glomerulus. The distending forces acting on the GBM have to be counterbalanced by inwardly directed forces. Due to the fixation of the GBM to the mesangium at the mesangial angles, outwardly directed pressure will stretch the GBM, which—as an elastic structure—develops wall tension in response. The mesangial cells interconnecting opposing parts of the GBM, need to resist these expansile forces. Therefore, a major role of the contractile apparatus of the mesangial cells may be static in nature, operating by isometric or minute isotonic contractions. Whether mesangial contraction also plays a role in the regulation of glomerular haemodynamics is still a matter of debate. Because the mesangial–endothelial interface comprises only a small part of the capillary circumference, a contraction of mesangial cell processes at this site would lead to minor changes in the capillary diameter.

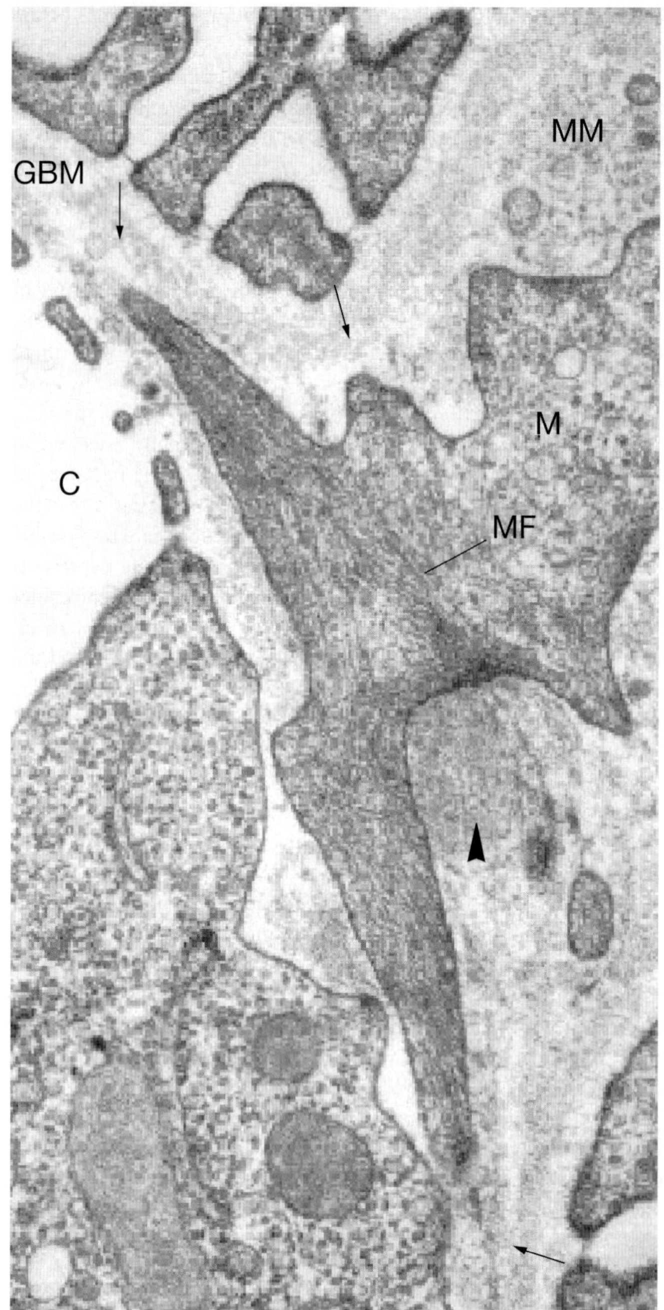

Fig. 11 Juxtacapillary portion of mesangium showing tongue-like mesangial processes fixed to the GBM at the mesangial angles (arrows). Note the rich equipment of mesangial processes with bundles of microfilaments (MF) which are attached to the cell membrane. The mesangial matrix (MM) contains abundant microfibrils (arrowhead). C, capillary lumen. 61,200×.

In addition to their contractile ability, mesangial cells are phagocytic. They have been shown to take up particulate tracers (Farquhar and Palade 1962) as well as immune complexes, which may accumulate within the mesangial region in glomerular diseases (reviewed by

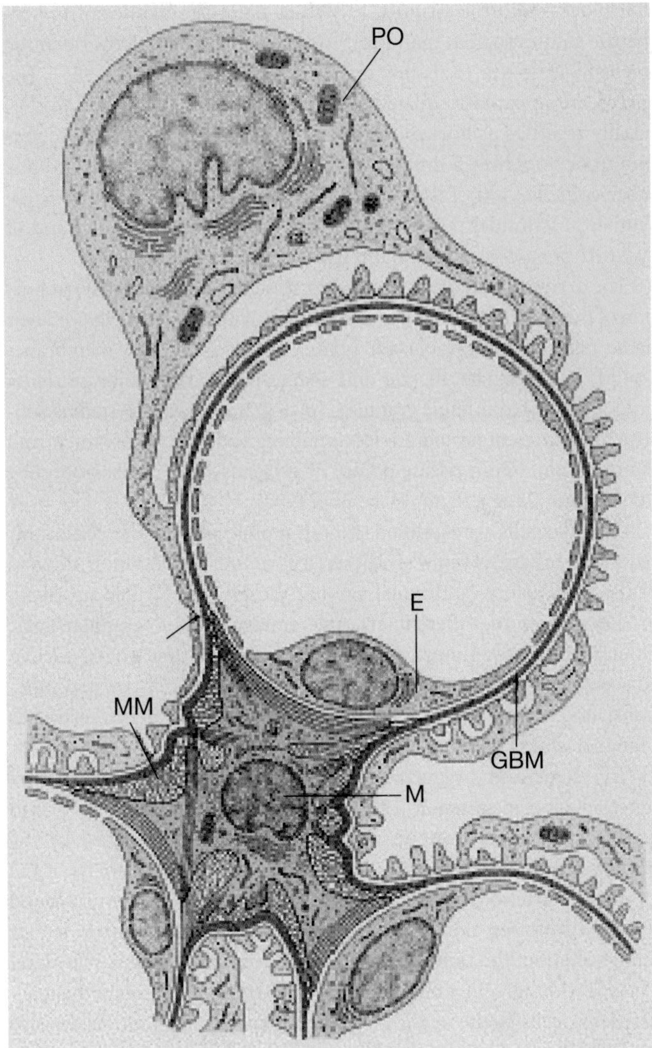

Fig. 12 Schematic showing the filtration barrier as well as the centrolobular position of a mesangial cell (M) and its relationships to the glomerular capillaries and to the glomerular basement membrane (GBM). The glomerular capillary consists of a fenestrated endothelium (E). The peripheral portion of the capillary is surrounded by the GBM which, at the mesangial angles (arrow), deviates from the pericapillary course and covers the mesangium. The interdigitating system of the podocyte (PO) foot processes forms the distal layer of the filtration barrier. Connections between mesangial cell processes and the GBM are prominent at mesangial angles, and are also numerous along the perimesangial GBM. Many of these connections are mediated by microfibrils which are a major constituent of the mesangial matrix (MM). Thus, a mechanical firm linkage of the perimesangial GBM to the contractile apparatus of the mesangial cells is established [modified after Kriz and Kaissling (1992)].

Schlondorff 1987). A small subpopulation of cells (3–7 per cent) is bone marrow derived; they represent macrophages that have invaded the mesangium.

Parietal epithelium

The parietal layer of Bowman's capsule consists of squamous epithelial cells resting on a basement membrane (Figs 2 and 3). The flat cells are polygonal, with a central cilium and few microvilli. Parietal cells are filled with bundles of actin filaments running in all directions (Pease 1968). Within the cells surrounding the vascular pole, the actin filaments are very dense and located within cytoplasmic ridges that run in a circular fashion around the glomerular entrance. The recent finding of muscarinic receptors on the parietal epithelium (Lebrun *et al.* 1992) suggests that the contractile tone of these cells is subject to regulation.

The basement membrane is, at variance to the GBM, composed of several dense layers separated by translucent layers and contains bundles of fibrils ('microligaments'; Mbassa *et al.* 1988). Collagen $\alpha1$, $\alpha2$, $\alpha5$, and $\alpha6$ (type IV) chains prevail in this basement membrane (Miner 1999). Recent studies suggest a role of type XIV collagen in the organization of the multilayered basement membrane of Bowman's capsule. This is an interstitial collagen that can bind to proteoglycans from basement membranes. It is speculated that type XIV collagen could act as a spacer or binding element in the formation of fibril bundles in this basement membrane (Lethias *et al.* 1994). In contrast to the GBM, the predominant proteoglycan of this basement membrane is a chondroitin sulfate proteoglycan, and the laminin isoforms 1 and 10 prevail (Couchman *et al.* 1994; Miner 1999b). The transition from the GBM to the basement membrane of Bowman's capsule borders the glomerular entrance. This transitional region is mechanically connected to the smooth muscle cells of the afferent and efferent arterioles as well as to extraglomerular mesangial cells (see below).

Extraglomerular mesangium—a closure device of the glomerular entrance

At the vascular pole of the glomerulus the mesangium passes through the opening of Bowman's capsule and continues into the extraglomerular mesangium (Barajas *et al.* 1989; Barajas 1997) (Figs 2 and 3). The extraglomerular mesangium represents a solid complex of cells and matrix that is neither penetrated by blood vessels nor lymphatic capillaries.

The extraglomerular mesangium is located in the cone-shaped space between the two glomerular arterioles and the macula densa cells of the thick ascending limb and, laterally, faces the renal interstitium. Extraglomerular mesangial cells are flat and elongated, separating into bunches of long cell processes at their poles (Spanidis and Wunsch 1979). They are arranged in several layers, parallel to the base of the macula densa. The cells are embedded in a matrix similar in appearance and composition as the mesangial matrix; however, microfibrils are comparably rarely found. Affixation of macula densa cells to the extraglomerular mesangium appears to be mediated by $\beta6$-integrin, which is known to associate with αv to form the fibronectin binding heterodimer $\alpha v\beta6$ (Breuss *et al.* 1993).

Although direct evidence is lacking, extraglomerular mesangial cells can be expected to be contractile for several reasons. First, they contain prominent bundles of microfilaments containing F-actin in their processes. Second, like intraglomerular mesangial cells, they have strong structural similarities with arteriolar smooth muscle cells and granular cells, suggesting that they are all of the same origin. Third, these cells are all extensively coupled by gap junctions (Pricam *et al.* 1974; Taugner *et al.* 1978). Fourth, high amounts of heat shock protein 25 (HSP25) are present in glomerular and, especially, in extraglomerular mesangial cells. Phosphorylation and redistribution of HSP25 are increased by angiotensin II-induced contraction of mesangial cells, and these processes are apparently mediated by a p38MAP kinase including signalling pathway. HSP25/27, which is believed to be a mediator of sustained smooth muscle cell contraction, might be a component of the contraction machinery in the glomerular and extraglomerular cells (Müller *et al.* 1999). The contractile processes of extraglomerular mesangial cells are connected to the basement membrane of Bowman's capsule and to the walls of both glomerular arterioles. As a whole, the extraglomerular mesangium interconnects all structures of the glomerular entrance. The extraglomerular mesangium can be regarded as a closure device of the glomerular entrance, maintaining its structural integrity against the distending forces exerted on the entrance by the high intra-arteriolar and intraglomerular pressure (Elger *et al.* 1998). A function of the extraglomerular mesangium for the recruitment of mesangial cells has been proposed. In anti-Thy-1 glomerulonephritis, the cellular population of the mesangium apparently occurs from the extraglomerular mesangium (Hugo *et al.* 1997).

Juxtaglomerular apparatus—intersection of local and systemic regulation

The juxtaglomerular apparatus (JGA) is situated at the vascular pole of the glomerulus. It comprises: (a) the macula densa; (b) the extraglomerular mesangium (described above); and (c) the terminal portion of the afferent arteriole with its renin-producing granular cells, as well as the beginning of the efferent arteriole (Fig. 3).

The macula densa is a plaque of specialized cells within the thick ascending limb at the site where the latter is affixed to the extraglomerular mesangium of the parent glomerulus. The most obvious structural features are the large, narrowly packed, cell nuclei, which account for the name 'macula densa' (Zimmermann 1933).

In contrast to other parts of the thick ascending limb, the cells of the macula densa do not interdigitate with each other but have a polygonal outline. The luminal cell membrane is densely studded by stubby microvilli and bears one cilium. At their bases, the cells display numerous infoldings and folds of the plasma membrane; the latter are anchored to the underlying basement membrane, blending with the matrix of the extraglomerular mesangium (Kriz and Kaissling 1992). The lateral membrane of macula densa cells bears folds and finger-like villi that are frequently connected to those of neighbouring cells by desmosomes. Near the apex, the cells are joined by tight junctions consisting of several parallel junctional strands similar to those in the thick ascending limb throughout. The cells contain the usual cytoplasmic organelles, comprising some small mitochondria, Golgi apparatus, and smooth endoplasmic reticulum; free ribosomes are abundant but rough endoplasmic reticulum is rare.

The lateral intercellular spaces are a prominent feature of the macula densa. Electron microscopic studies, and studies on isolated macula densa segments *in vitro*, have shown that the width of the lateral intercellular spaces varies under different functional conditions (Kaissling and Kriz 1982; Kirk *et al.* 1985). In agreement with the suggestion that water flow through the macula densa epithelium is secondary to active sodium reabsorption, compounds such as furosemide, that block sodium transport, as well as high osmolalities of impermeable solutes such as mannitol, are associated with narrowing of the intercellular spaces (Kaissling and Kriz 1982; Alcorn *et al.* 1986). The spaces are apparently dilated under most physiological conditions, usually regarded as normal control conditions. The most conspicuous immunocytochemical difference between macula densa cells and any other epithelial cell of the nephron is the high content of nitric oxide synthase I (Mundel *et al.* 1992; Persson and Bachmann 2000) and of cyclo-oxygenase-2 (Schnermann 2001) in the former.

The granular cells are assembled in clusters within the terminal portion of the afferent arteriole, replacing smooth muscle cells (Fig. 3). Their name refers to the cytoplasmic granules, which are dark, membrane-bound, and irregular in size and shape. Renin, the major secretion product, is stored in these granules. Small granules with crystalline substructure represent protogranules containing both renin prosegment and mature renin. Renin release occurs by exocytosis into the surrounding interstitium (Taugner and Hackenthal 1989).

Granular cells are modified smooth muscle cells. Under conditions requiring enhanced renin synthesis (e.g. volume depletion or stenosis of the renal artery) additional smooth muscle cells located upstream in the wall of the afferent arteriole transform into granular cells. Granular cells are connected to the extraglomerular mesangial cells, to adjacent smooth muscle cells, and to endothelial cells by gap junctions, and are densely innervated by sympathetic nerve terminals (Taugner and Hackenthal 1989).

The structural organization of the JGA suggests a regulatory function. Goormaghtigh in 1937 (Goormaghtigh 1937) was the first to propose that some component of the distal urine is sensed by the macula densa and this information is used to adjust the tonus of the glomerular arterioles, thereby producing a change in glomerular blood flow and filtration rate. Moreover, since the JGA is the major site of renin secretion, the function of the JGA is of great systemic relevance. There is wide agreement that the rate of Cl-transport through the macula densa cells is the sensing step and that adenosin is the decisive mediator that produces the effects on the granular cells and smooth muscle cells of the glomerular arterioles (Schnermann 2002).

References

Abrahamson, D. R. (1987). Structure and development of the glomerular capillary wall and basement membrane. *American Journal of Physiology* **253**, F783–F794.

Adler, S. and Eng, B. (1993). Integrin receptors and function on cultured glomerular endothelial cells. *Kidney International* **44**, 278–284.

Alcorn, D., Anderson, W. P., and Ryan, G. B. (1986). Morphological changes in the renal macula densa during natriuresis and diuresis. *Renal Physiology* **9**, 335–347.

Amizuka, N. *et al.* (1997). Cell-specific expression of the parathyroid hormone (PTH)/PTH-related peptide receptor gene in kidney from kidney-specific and ubiquitous promoters. *Endocrinology* **138**, 469–481.

Andrews, P. M. (1988). Morphological alterations of the glomerular (visceral) epithelium in response to pathological and experimental situations. *Journal of Electron Microscopy Technique* **9**, 115–144.

Bachmann, S., Kriz, W., Kuhn, C., and Franke, W. W. (1983). Differentiation of cell types of the mammalian kidney by immunofluorescence microscopy using antibodies to intermediate filament proteins and desmoplakins. *Histochemie. Histochemistry. Histochimie* **77**, 365–394.

Bagchus, W. M., Hoedemaeker, P. J., Rozing, J., and Bakker, W. W. (1986). Glomerulonephritis induced by monoclonal anti-Thy 1.1 antibodies.

A sequential histological and ultrastructural study in the rat. *Laboratory Investigation* **55**, 680–687.

Barajas, L. (1997). Cell-specific protein and gene expression in the juxtaglomerular apparatus. *Clinical and Experimental Pharmacology & Physiology* **24**, 520–526.

Barajas, L. *et al.* Pathology of the juxtaglomerular apparatus including Bartter's syndrome. In *Renal Pathology* (ed. C. C. Tisher and B. M. Brenner), pp. 877–912. Philadelphia: Lippincott, 1989.

Bek, M. *et al.* (1999). Characterization of prostanoid receptors in podocytes. *Journal of the American Society of Nephrology* **10**, 2084–2093.

Blantz, R. C., Gabbai, F. B., and Wilson, C. B. (1991). Glomerular hemodynamic (GH) response to changes in volume status after lysis of mesangial cells (MC). *Journal of the American Society of Nephrology* **1**, 661 (abstract).

Border, W. A., Okuda, S., and Nakamura, T. (1989). Extracellular matrix and glomerular disease. *Seminars in Nephrology* **9**, 307–317.

Brees, D. K., Ogle, R. C., and Williams, J. C., Jr. (1995). Laminin and fibronectin content of mouse glomerular and tubular basement membrane. *Renal Physiology and Biochemistry* **18**, 1–11.

Breier, G., Albrecht, U., Sterrer, S., and Risau, W. (1992). Expression of vascular endothelial growth factor during embryonic angiogenesis and endothelial cell differentiation. *Development* **114**, 521–532.

Breuss, J. M. *et al.* (1993). Restricted distribution of integrin $\beta 6$ mRNA in primate epithelial tissue. *Journal of Histochemistry and Cytochemistry* **41**, 1521–1527.

Bulger, R. E. and Hebert, S. C. Structural-functional relationships in the kidney. In *Diseases of the Kidney* (ed. R. W. Schrier and A. Gottschalk), pp. 3–63. Boston/Toronto: Little, Brown and Company, 1988.

Bulger, R. E., Eknoyan, G., Purcell, D. J., and Dobyan, D. C. (1983). Endothelial characteristics of glomerular capillaries in normal, mercuric chloride-induced, and gentamicin-induced acute renal failure in the rat. *Clinical Investigation* **72**, 128–141.

Burgeson, R. E. *et al.* (1994). A new nomenclature for laminins. *Matrix Biology* **14**, 209–211.

Burridge, K. *et al.* (1988). Focal adhesion: transmembrane junctions between the extracellular matrix and the cytoskeleton. *Annual Review of Cell Biology* **4**, 487–525.

Cockwell, P., Chakravorty, S., Girdlestone, J., and Savage, C. O. S. (2002). Fractalkine expression in human renal inflammation. *Journal of Pathology* **196**, 85–90.

Cosio, F. G., Sedmak, D. D., and Nahman, N. S. (1990). Cellular receptors for matrix proteins in normal human kidney and human mesangial cells. *Kidney International* **38**, 886–895.

Couchman, J. R., Beavan, L. A., and McCarthy, K. J. (1994). Glomerular matrix: synthesis, turnover and role in mesangial expansion. *Kidney International* **45**, 328–335.

Daniels, B. S. (1993). The role of the glomerular epithelial cell in the maintenance of the glomerular filtration barrier. *American Journal of Nephrology* **13**, 318–323.

Daniels, B. S. *et al.* (1993). Glomerular permeability barrier in the rat. *Clinical Investigation* **92**, 929–936.

Deen, W. M., Bohrer, M. P., and Brenner, B. M. (1979). Macromolecule transport across glomerular capillaries: application of pore theory. *Kidney International* **16**, 353–365.

Deen, W. M., Lazzara, M., and Myers, B. D. (2001). Structural determinants of glomerular permeability. *American Journal of Physiology. Renal Physiology* **281**, F579–F596.

De Vriese, A. S. *et al.* (2001). Antibodies against vascular endothelial growth factor improve early renal dysfunction in experimental diabetes. *Journal of the American Society of Nephrology* **12**, 993–1000.

Drenckhahn, D. and Franke, R. P. (1988). Ultrastructural organization of contractile and cytoskeletal proteins in glomerular podocytes of chicken, rat, and man. *Laboratory Investigation* **59**, 673–682.

Drumond, M. C. and Deen, W. M. (1994). Structural determinants of glomerular hydraulic permeability. *American Journal of Physiology* **266**, F1–F12.

Drumond, M. C., Kristal, B., Myers, B. D., and Deen, W. M. (1994). Structural basis for reduced glomerular filtration capacity in nephrotic humans. *Clinical Investigation* **94**, 1187–1195.

Durbeej, M., Henry, M. D., and Campbell, K. P. (1998). Dystroglycan in development and disease. *Current Opinion in Cell Biology* **10**, 594–601.

Dworkin, L. D., Ichikawa, I., and Brenner, B. M. (1983). Hormonal modulation of glomerular function. *American Journal of Physiology* **244**, F95–F104.

Elger, M., Sakai, T., Winkler, D., and Kriz, W. (1991). Structure of the outflow segment of the efferent arteriole in rat superficial glomeruli. *Contributions to Nephrology* **95**, 22–33.

Elger, M., Sakai, T., and Kriz, W. (1998). The vascular pole of the renal glomerulus of rat. *Advances in Anatomy Embryology and Cell Biology* **139**, 1–98.

Endlich, K., Kriz, W., and Witzgall, R. (2001a). Update in podocyte biology. *Current Opinion in Nephrology and Hypertension* **10**, 331–340.

Endlich, N., Nobiling, R., Kriz, W., and Endlich, K. (2001b). Expression and signaling of parathyroid hormone-related protein in cultured podocytes. *Experimental Nephrology* **9**, 436–443.

Farquhar, M. G. The glomerular basement membrane: a selective macromolecular filter. In *Cell Biology of Extracellular Matrix* (ed. E. D. Hay), pp. 365–418. New York: Plenum Press, 1991.

Farquhar, M. G. and Palade, G. E. (1962). Functional evidence for the existence of a third cell type in the renal glomerulus. Phagocytosis of filtration residues by a distinctive 'third' cell. *Journal of Cell Biology* **13**, 55–87.

Feng, D. *et al.* (2000). Ultrastructural localization of the vascular permeability factor/vascular endothelial growth factor (VPF/VEGF) receptor-2/FLK-1, KDR in normal mouse kidney and in the hyperpermeable vessels induced by VPF/VEGF-expressing tumors and adenoviral vectors. *Journal of Histochemistry and Cytochemistry* **48**, 545–555.

Fischer, K. *et al.* (2001). Extracellular nucleotides regulate cellular functions of podocytes in culture. *American Journal of Physiology. Renal Physiology* **281**, F1075–F1081.

Fong, A. *et al.* (1998). Fractalkine and CX3CR1 mediate a novel mechanism of leukocyte capture, firm adhesion, and activation under physiologic flow. *Journal of Experimental Medicine* **188**, 1413–1419.

Ford, M. D., Cauchi, J., Greferath, U., and Bertram, J. F. (1997). Expression of fibroblast growth factors and their receptors in rat glomeruli. *Kidney International* **51**, 1729–1738.

Fries, J. W., Sandstrom, D. J., Meyer, T. W., and Rennke, H. G. (1989). Glomerular hypertrophy and epithelial cell injury modulate progressive glomerulosclerosis in the rat. *Laboratory Investigation* **60**, 205–218.

Gibson, M. A., Kumaratilake, J. S., and Cleary, E. G. (1989). The protein components of the 12-nanometer microfibrils of elastic and nonelastic tissues. *Journal of Biological Chemistry* **264**, 4590–4598.

Goormaghtigh, N. (1937). L'appareil neuro-myo-artériel juxta-glomérulaire du rein: ses réactions en pathologie et ses rapports avec le tube urinifère. *Comptes rendus des seances de la Societe de biologie et de ses filiales* **124**, 293–296.

Guasch, A. and Myers, B. D. (1994). Determinants of glomerular hypofiltration in nephrotic patients with minimal change nephropathy. *Journal of the American Society of Nephrology* **4**, 1571–1581.

Halfter, W., Dong, S., Schurer, B., and Cole, G. (1998). Collagen XVIII is a basement membrane heparan sulfate proteoglycan. *Journal of Biological Chemistry* **273**, 25404–25412.

Hansen, K. and Abrass, C. K. (1999). Role of laminin isoforms in glomerular structure. *Pathology* **67**, 84–91.

Harvey, S. J. *et al.* (1998). Role of distinct type IV collagen networks in glomerular development and function. *Kidney International* **54**, 1857–1866.

Herman, W., Emancipator, S. N., Rhoten, R. I. P., and Simonson, M. S. (1998). Vascular and glomerular expression of endothelin-1 in normal human kidney. *American Journal of Physiology. Renal Physiology* **275**, F8–F17.

Hora, K. *et al.* (1990). Three-dimensional study of glomerular slit diaphragm by quick-freezing and deep-etching replica method. *European Journal of Cell Biology* **53**, 402–406.

Horvat, R. *et al.* (1986). Endothelial cell membranes contain podocalyxin—the major sialoprotein of visceral glomerular epithelial cells. *Journal of Cell Biology* **102**, 484–491.

Huang, T. W. and Langlois, J. C. (1985). Podoendin. A new cell surface protein of the podocyte and endothelium. *Journal of Experimental Medicine* **162**, 245–267.

Huber, T. B. *et al.* (1998). Catecholamines modulate podocyte function. *Journal of the American Society of Nephrology* **9**, 335–345.

Hudson, B. G., Kalluri, R., Gunwar, S., and Noelken, M. E. (1994). Structure and organization of type IV collagen of renal glomerular basement membrane. *Contributions to Nephrology* **107**, 163–167.

Hugo, C. *et al.* (1997). Extraglomerular origin of the mesangial cell after injury—a new role of the juxtaglomerular apparatus. *Clinical Investigation* **100**, 786–794.

Kaissling, B. and Kriz, W. (1982). Variability of intercellular spaces between macula densa cells: a transmission electron microscopic study in rabbits and rats. *Kidney International* **22** (Suppl. 12), 9–17.

Kanwar, Y. S. (1984). Biology of disease. Biophysiology of glomerular filtration and proteinuria. *Laboratory Investigation* **51**, 7–21.

Karkavelas, G. and Kefalides, N. A. (1988). Comparative ultrastructural localization of collagen types III, IV, VI and laminin in rat uterus and kidney. *Journal of Ultrastructure and Molecular Structure Research* **100**, 137–155.

Katz, A. *et al.* (1991). Renal entactin (nidogen): isolation, characterization and tissue distribution. *Kidney International* **40**, 643–652.

Kazatchkine, M. D. *et al.* (1982). Immunohistochemical study of the human glomerular C3b receptor in normal kidney and in seventy-five cases of renal diseases. *Clinical Investigation* **69**, 900–912.

Kerjaschki, D. and Farquhar, M. G. (1983). Immunocytochemical localization of the Heymann antigen (gp 330) in glomerular epithelial cells of normal Lewis rats. *Journal of Experimental Medicine* **157**, 667–686.

Kerjaschki, D., Sharkey, D. J., and Farquhar, M. G. (1984). Identification and characterization of podocalyxin-the major sialoprotein of the renal glomerular epithelial cell. *Journal of Cell Biology* **98**, 1591.

Kiberd, B. A. (1992). The functional and structural changes of the glomerulus throughout the course of murine lupus nephritis. *Journal of the American Society of Nephrology* **3**, 930–939.

Kirk, K. L., Bell, P. D., Barfuss, D. W., and Ribadeneira, M. (1985). Direct visualization of the isolated and perfused macula densa. *American Journal of Physiology* **248**, F890–F894.

Kobayashi, N. *et al.* (1998). Nonuniform microtubular polarity established by CHO1/MKLP1 motor protein is necessary for process formation of podocytes. *Journal of Cell Biology* **143**, 1961–1970.

Kreidberg, J. A. and Symons, J. M. (2000). Integrins in kidney development, function, and disease. *American Journal of Physiology. Renal Physiology* **279** (2), F233–F242.

Kreisberg, J. I., Venkatachalam, M., and Troyer, D. (1985). Contractile properties of cultured glomerular mesangial cells. *American Journal of Physiology* **249**, F457–F463.

Kriz, W. (2002). Podocyte is the mayor culprit accounting for the progression of chronic renal disease. *Microscopy Research and Technique* **57**, 189–195.

Kriz, W. and Kaissling, B. Structural organization of the mammalian kidney. In *The Kidney: Physiology and Pathophysiology* (ed. D. W. Seldin and G. Giebisch), pp. 707–777. New York: Raven Press, 1992.

Kriz, W., Elger, M., Lemley, K. V., and Sakai, T. (1990). Mesangial cell–glomerular basement membrane connections counteract glomerular capillary and mesangium expansion. *American Journal of Nephrology* **10** (Suppl. 1), 4–13.

Kriz, W., Elger, M., Mundel, P., and Lemley, K. V. (1995a). Structure-stabilizing forces in the glomerular tuft. *Journal of the American Society of Nephrology* **5**, 1731–1739.

Kriz, W., Hähnel, B., Rösener, S., and Elger, M. (1995b). Long-term treatment of rats with FGF-2 results in focal segmental glomerulosclerosis. *Kidney International* **48**, 1435–1450.

Larsson, L. and Maunsbach, A. B. (1980). The ultrastructural development of the glomerular filtration barrier in the rat kidney: a morphometric analysis. *Journal of Ultrastructure Research* **72**, 392–406.

Latta, H., Maunsbach, A. B., and Madden, S. C. (1960). The centrolobular region of the renal glomerulus studied by electron microscopy. *Journal of Ultrastructure Research* **4**, 455–472.

Lebrun, F., Morel, F., Vassent, G., and Marchetti, J. (1992). Cholinergic effects on intracellular free calcium concentration in renal corpuscle: role of parietal sheet. *American Journal of Physiology* **262**, F248–F255.

Lemley, K. V. *et al.* (1992). The glomerular mesangium: capillary support function and its failure under experimental conditions. *Clinical Investigation* **70**, 843–856.

Lethias, C. *et al.* (1994). Structure, molecular assembly and tissue distribution of facit collagen molecules. *Contributions to Nephrology* **107**, 57–63.

Madri, J. A., Roll, F. J., Furthmayr, H., and Foidart, J. M. (1980). Ultrastructural localization of fibronectin and laminin in the basement membranes of the murine kidney. *Journal of Cell Biology* **86**, G82–G87.

Mattot, V. *et al.* (2002). Loss of VEGF164 and VEGF188 isoforms impairs postnatal glomerular angiogenesis and renal arteriogenesis in mice. *Journal of the American Society of Nephrology* **13**, 1548–1560.

Mbassa, G., Elger, M., and Kriz, W. (1988). The ultrastructural organization of the basement membrane of Bowman's capsule in the rat renal corpuscle. *Cell and Tissue Research* **253**, 151–163.

Mendrick, D. L. and Rennke, H. G. (1988). Induction of proteinuria in the rat by a monoclonal antibody against SGP-115/107. *Kidney International* **33**, 818–830.

Miner, J. H. (1999). Renal basement membrane components. *Kidney International* **56**, 2016–2024.

Mohan, P. S. and Spiro, R. G. (1986). Macromolecular organization of basement membranes. *Journal of Biological Chemistry* **261**, 4328–4336.

Monnens, I. (2001). Thin glomerular basement membrane disease. *Kidney International* **60**, 799–800.

Morello, R. *et al.* (2001). Regulation of glomerular basement membrane collagen expression by LMX1B contributes to renal disease in nail patella syndrome. *Nature Genetics* **27**, 205–208.

Morita, M., White, R. H. R., and Raafat, F. (1988). Glomerular basement membrane thickness in children. *Pediatric Nephrology (Berlin, Germany)* **2**, 190–195.

Mundel, P. and Kriz, W. (1995). Structure and function of podocytes: an update. *Anatomy and Embryology* **192**, 385–397.

Mundel, P., Elger, M., Sakai, T., and Kriz, W. (1988). Microfibrils are a major component of the mesangial matrix in the glomerulus of the rat kidney. *Cell and Tissue Research* **254**, 183–187.

Mundel, P. *et al.* (1992). Expression of nitric oxide synthase in kidney macula densa cells. *Kidney International* **42**, 1017–1019.

Müller, E. *et al.* (1999). Possible involvement of heat shock protein 25 in the angiotensin II-induced glomerular mesangial cell contraction via p. 38 MAP kinase. *Journal of Cellular Physiology* **181**, 462–469.

Nagata, M. and Kriz, W. (1992). Glomerular damage after uninephrectomy in young rats. II. Mechanical stress on podocytes as a pathway to sclerosis. *Kidney International* **42**, 148–160.

Nagata, M., Yamaguchi, Y., and Ito, K. (1993). Loss of mitotic activity and the expression of vimentin in glomerular epithelial cells of developing human kidneys. *Anatomy and Embryology* **187**, 275–279.

Nitschke, R. *et al.* (2000). Angiotensin II increases the intracellular calcium activity in podocytes of the intact glomerulus. *Kidney International* **57**, 41–49.

Nitschke, R. *et al.* (2001). Acetylcholine increases the free intracellular calcium concentration in podocytes in intact rat glomeruli via muscarinic M(5) receptors. *Journal of the American Society of Nephrology* **12**, 678–687.

Noonan, D. M. *et al.* (1991). The complete sequence of perlecan, a basement membrane heparan sulfate proteoglycan, reveals extensive similarity with laminin a chain, low density lipoprotein-receptor, and the neural cell adhesion molecule. *Journal of Biological Chemistry* **266**, 22939–22947.

Ostendorf, T. *et al.* (1999). VEGF165 mediates glomerular endothelial repair. *Clinical Investigation* **104**, 913–923.

Ott, M. J., Olson, J. L., and Ballermann, B. J. (1993). Phenotypic differences between glomerular capillary (GE) and aortic (AE) endothelial cells in vitro. *Journal of the American Society of Nephrology* **4**, 564 (abstract).

Paul, L. C., Rennke, H. G., Milford, E. L., and Carpenter, C. B. (1984). Thy-1.1 in glomeruli of rat kidneys. *Kidney International* **25**, 771–777.

Pease, D. C. (1968). Myoid features of renal corpuscles and tubules. *Journal of Ultrastructure Research* **23**, 304–320.

Persson, A. E. G. and Bachmann, S. (2000). Constitutive nitric oxide synthesis in the kidney—functions at the juxtaglomerular apparatus. *Acta Physiologica Scandinavica* **169**, 317–324.

Petermann, A. *et al.* (1993). Polymerase chain reaction and focal contact formation indicate integrin expression in mesangial cells. *Kidney International* **44**, 997–1005.

Pihlajaniemi, T. (1996). Molecular properties of the glomerular basement membrane. *Contributions to Nephrology* **117**, 46–79.

Pricam, C., Humbert, F., Perrelet, A., and Orci, L. (1974). Gap junctions in mesangial and lacis cells. *Journal of Cell Biology* **63**, 349–354.

Raats, C. J. *et al.* (2000a). Expression of agrin, dystroglycan, and utrophin in normal renal tissue and in experimental glomerulopathies. *American Journal of Pathology* **156** (5), 1749–1765.

Raats, C. J., van den Born, J., and Berden, J. H. (2000b). Glomerular heparan sulfate alterations: mechanisms and relevance for proteinuria. *Kidney International* **57** (2), 385–400.

Rabb, H. *et al.* (1998). Leucocytes, cell adhesion molecules and ischemic acute renal failure. *Kidney International* **51**, 1463–1468.

Rasch, R. (1979). Prevention of diabetic glomerulopathy in streptozotocin diabetic rats by insulin treatment. Glomerular basement membrane thickness. *Diabetologia* **16**, 319–324.

Rebibou, J. M. *et al.* (1992). Functional endothelin 1 receptors on human glomerular podocytes and mesangial cells. *Nephrology, Dialysis, Transplantation* **7**, 288–292.

Regele, H. M. *et al.* (2000). Glomerular expression of dystroglycans is reduced in minimal change nephrosis but not in focal segmental glomerulosclerosis. *Journal of the American Society of Nephrology* **11** (3), 403–412.

Rodewald, R. and Karnovsky, M. J. (1974). Porous substructure of the glomerular slit diaphragm in the rat and mouse. *Journal of Cell Biology* **60**, 423–433.

Rostgaard, J. and Qvortrup, K. (2002). Sieve plugs in fenestrae of glomerular capillaries—site of the filtration barrier? *Cells, Tissues, Organs* **170**, 132–138.

Saito, A., Pietromonaco, S., Loo, A. K.-C., and Farquhar, M. G. (1994). Cloning and sequencing of gp330/megalin, the major Heymann nephritis antigen. *Journal of the American Society of Nephrology* **5**, 767 (abstract).

Sakai, T. and Kriz, W. (1987). The structural relationship between mesangial cells and basement membrane of the renal glomerulus. *Anatomy and Embryology* **176**, 373–386.

Sanes, J. R., Engvall, E., Butkowski, R., and Hunter, D. D. (1990). Molecular heterogeneity of basal laminae: isoforms of laminin and type IV collagen at the neuromuscular junction and elsewhere. *Journal of Cell Biology* **111**, 1685–1699.

Savage, C. O. S. (1994). The biology of the glomerulus: endothelial cells. *Kidney International* **45**, 314–319.

Savage, C. (1998). Injury mechanisms in vasculitis. *Kidney & Blood Pressure Research* **21**, 269–270.

Sawada, H., Stukenbrok, H., Kerjaschki, D., and Farquhar, M. G. (1986). Epithelial polyanion (podocalyxin) is found on the sides but not the soles of the foot processes of the glomerular epithelium. *American Journal of Pathology* **125**, 309–318.

Schlöndorff, D. (1987). The glomerular mesangial cell: an expanding role for a specialized pericyte. *The FASEB Journal* **1**, 272–281.

Schlöndorff, D., Nelson, P., and Luckow, B. (1997). Chemokines and renal disease. *Kidney International* **51**, 610–621.

Schnermann, J. (2001). Cyclooxygenase-2 and macula densa control of renin secretion. *Nephrology, Dialysis, Transplantation* **16**, 1735–1738.

Schnermann, J. (2002). Adenosine mediates tubuloglomerular feedback. *American Journal of Physiology. Renal Physiology* **283**, 276–277.

Schwartz, E., Goldfischer, S., Coltoff-Schiller, B., and Blumenfeld, O. O. (1985). Extracellular matrix microfibrils are composed of core proteins coated with fibronectin. *Journal of Histochemistry and Cytochemistry* **33**, 268–274.

Schwarzbauer, J. (1999). Basement membranes: putting up the barriers. *Current Biology* **9**, R242–R244.

Seiler, M. R., Rennke, H. G., Venkatachalam, M. A., and Cotran, R. S. (1977). Pathogenesis of polycation-induced alteration (fusion) of glomerular epithelium. *Laboratory Investigation* **36**, 48–61.

Sharma, R. *et al.* (2001). Both subtype 1 and 2 receptors of angiotensin II participate in regulation of intracellular calcium in glomerular epithelial cells. *Journal of Laboratory and Clinical Medicine* **138**, 40–49.

Spanidis, A. and Wunsch, H. (1979). Rekonstruktion einer Goormaghtigh'schen und einer Epitheloiden Zelle der Kaninchenniere. Dissertation edn, Dissertation, Heidelberg.

Spath, M. *et al.* (1995). Regulation of phosphoinositide hydrolysis and cytosolic free calcium induced by endothelin in human glomerular epithelial cells. *Nephrology, Dialysis, Transplantation* **10**, 1299–1304.

Sraer, J. D., Sraer, J., Ardaillou, R., and Mimoune, O. (1974). Evidence for renal glomerular receptors for angiotensin II. *Kidney International* **6**, 241–246.

Steffes, M. W. *et al.* (1983). Quantitative glomerular morphology of the normal human kidney. *Laboratory Investigation* **49**, 82–86.

Sterzel, R. B. *et al.* (2000). Elastic fiber proteins in the glomerular mesangium *in vivo* and in cell culture. *Kidney International* **58**, 1588–1602.

Stockand, J. and Sansom, S. (1998). Glomerular mesangial cells: electrophysiology and regulation of contraction. *Physiological Reviews* **78**, 723–744.

Striker, G. E. and Striker, L. J. (1985). Biology of disease. Glomerular cell culture. *Laboratory Investigation* **53**, 122–131.

Suga, S. *et al.* (2001). Vascular endothelial growth factor (VEGF 121) protects rats from renal infarction in thrombotic microangiopathy. *Kidney International* **60**, 1297–1308.

Taugner, R. and Hackenthal, E. *The Juxtaglomerular Apparatus*. Berlin: Springer-Verlag, 1989.

Taugner, R., Schiller, A., Kaissling, B., and Kriz, W. (1978). Gap junctional coupling between the JGA and the glomerular tuft. *Cell and Tissue Research* **186**, 279–285.

Thoenes, W. (1967). Endoplasmatisches Retikulum und 'Sekretkörper' im Glomerulumepithel der Säugerniere. Ein morphologischer Beitrag zum Problem der Basalmembranbildung. *Zeitschrift für Zellforschung und mikroskopische Anatomie* **78**, 561–582.

Timpl, R. and Dziadek, M. (1986). Structure, development, and molecular pathology of basement membranes. *International Review of Experimental Pathology* **29**, 1–112.

Tisher, C. C. and Brenner, B. M. Structure and function of the glomerulus. In *Renal Pathology* (ed. C. C. Tisher and B. M. Brenner), pp. 92–110. Philadelphia: Lippincott, 1989.

Trenchev, P., Dorling, J., Webb, J., and Holborrow, E. J. (1976). Localization of smooth muscle-like contractile proteins in kidney by immunoelectron microscopy. *Journal of Anatomy* **121**, 85–95.

Tryggvason, K. (1995). Molecular properties and diseases of collagens. *Kidney International* **47** (Suppl. 49), 24–28.

Van Den Berg, J. *et al.* (2000). Interleukin-4 and interleukin-13 act on glomerular visceral epithelial cells. *Journal of the American Society of Nephrology* **11**, 413–422.

Vasmant, D., Maurice, M., and Feldmann, G. (1984). Cytoskeleton ultrastructure of podocytes and glomerular endothelial cells in man and in the rat. *Anatomical Record* **210**, 17–24.

Wang, J. *et al.* (1993). Amelioration of antioxidant enzyme suppression and proteinuria in cyclosporin-treated puromycin nephrosis. *Nephron* **65**, 418–425.

Welling, L. W., Zupka, M. T., and Welling, D. J. (1995). Mechanical properties of basement membrane. *News in Physiological Sciences* **10** (1), 30–35.

Wiggins, R. C., Fantone, J., and Phan, S. H. Mechanisms of vascular injury. In *Renal Pathology* (ed. C. C. Tisher and B. M. Brenner), pp. 965–993. Philadelphia: Lippincott, 1989.

Winkler, D., Elger, M., Sakai, T., and Kriz, W. (1991). Branching and confluence pattern of glomerular arterioles in the rat. *Kidney International* **39** (Suppl. 32), S2–S8.

Woods, A. and Couchman, J. R. (1992). Protein kinase C involvement in focal adhesion formation. *Journal of Cell Science* **101**, 277–290.

Yamamoto, T. *et al.* (1998). Expression of types I, II, and III TGF-beta receptors in human glomerulonephritis. *Journal of the American Society of Nephrology* **9**, 2253–2261.

Yang, G. C. H. and Morrison, A. B. (1980). Three large dissectable rat glomerular models reconstructed from wide-field electron micrographs. *Anatomical Record* **196**, 431–440.

Yurchenco, P. D. and Ruben, G. C. (1987). Basement membrane structure in situ: evidence for lateral associations in the Type IV collagen network. *Journal of Cell Biology* **105**, 2559–2568.

Yurchenco, P. D. and Cheng, Y.-S. (1994). Laminin self-assembly: a three-arm interaction hypothesis for the formation of a network in basement membranes. *Contributions to Nephrology* **107**, 47–56.

Zhao, J. *et al.* (1994). Characterization of C-type natriuretic peptide receptors in human mesangial cells. *Kidney International* **46**, 717–725.

Zimmermann, K. W. (1929). Ueber den Bau des Glomerulus der menschlichen Niere. *Zeitschrift für mikroskopisch-anatomische Forschung* **18**, 520–552.

Zimmermann, K. W. (1933). Ueber den Bau des Glomerulus der Saeugerniere. *Zeitschrift für mikroskopisch-anatomische Forschung* **32**, 176–278.

3.2 Glomerular injury and glomerular response

John Feehally, Jürgen Floege, John Savill, and A. Neil Turner

Introduction

Most glomerular diseases are immune-mediated, and described by the generic term glomerulonephritis (GN). But other mechanisms of glomerular disease should be borne in mind, including important metabolic and deposition diseases, particularly diabetic nephropathy and amyloidosis, as well as inherited disruption of glomerular structure [e.g. Alport syndrome (AS)] and toxic endothelial injury that leads to thrombotic microangiopathy (TMA). Furthermore, although the glomerulus is the primary site of damage, subsequent injury to the tubulointerstitium plays a major role in the overall outcome of glomerular disease.

Many forms of GN are characterized by the deposition of immune reactants, particularly immunoglobulins and complements, in the glomerulus which is accompanied by varying degrees of glomerular inflammation and injury. However, both cellular and humoral immune mechanisms may provoke glomerular injury in the absence of such deposits.

Classification of glomerular disease

A classification of glomerular disease is presented in Table 1. The classification of non-immune glomerular disease is straightforward, reflecting distinct disease processes and clinical presentations—for example, diabetes, amyloid, and inherited glomerular damage. The classification of GN is, however, more challenging and reflects the evolving view of its pathogenesis over more than 40 years.

The clinical classification of GN has changed little since the widespread introduction of renal biopsy in the 1950s and 1960s when patterns of disease were defined from the combined observations made by light microscopy, electron microscopy (EM), and either immunoperoxidase or immunofluorescence microscopy. In some conditions, there is additional classification on the basis of serological markers and extrarenal disease. However, early optimism that immunopathogenesis for each histological pattern of disease would soon be clarified has not been fulfilled, except in a minority of conditions. Therefore, the classification of GN used in this book still reflects the predominance of morphological categorization, except where aetiological factors are clearly identified (e.g. HIV-associated nephropathy), an associated multisystem disease is defined (e.g. lupus nephritis), or the immunopathogenesis is well characterized [e.g. antiglomerular basement membrane (anti-GBM) disease]. In a number of the major categories of GN, we are still far from establishing the immunopathogenesis, and evidence increasingly suggests that more than one aetiology and more than one immunopathogenic pathway can produce a single morphological entity; membranous nephropathy and IgA nephropathy (IgAN) are good examples of this pathogenic heterogeneity.

Detailed descriptions of the pathogenesis of individual patterns of glomerular disease are given in subsequent chapters. In this chapter, we consider the genetic background to glomerular injury, the range of mechanisms which can initiate glomerular injury, and the glomerular response to such injury, including the recruitment of extraglomerular as well intrinsic cells and effector molecules. We will consider how such an injury may resolve either by healing or with irreversible glomerular scarring. Although the focus is on events in the glomerulus, it is also important to bear in mind that tubulointerstitial injury and scarring are also key features of glomerular disease that make a major contribution to the eventual degree of renal damage or recovery. For didactic reasons, we will discuss each of these sequentially, but recognizing that divisions between initiation of injury, adaptive response to injury, and regenerative events leading to resolution may in clinical practice be less clear, with multiple processes continuing in parallel. An overview of the known processes is presented in Fig. 1. This chapter emphasizes the enormous progress in the understanding of glomerular disease mechanisms over recent years, building on earlier insights from animal models with the increasingly powerful techniques of molecular genetics and cell biology.

Animal models of glomerular disease

Much progress has been made from the study of a wide range of animal models of glomerular disease mostly established in rodents or rabbits. These have been extremely informative about mechanisms by which immune injury is initiated, as well as the subsequent inflammatory events and their resolution either by healing or scarring. Some of these models appear to mimic both the morphology and immunopathogenesis of human disease very closely; for example, Heymann nephritis closely resembles human membranous nephropathy, and experimental allergic GN has much in common with Goodpasture's disease. Animal models for non-immune glomerular injury have also been developed. The commonly used experimental models are shown in Tables 2(a) and (b).

It is important, however, to bear in mind that these are only models providing insights that need to be evaluated in humans with glomerular disease before the proposed disease mechanisms can be accepted, or therapeutic strategies that are developed from such insights can be planned and tested in the clinical setting.

Table 1 Classification of glomerular disease

Category	Main site of injury	Presumed mechanism	Known aetiological factors	Associated extrarenal disease	Typical clinical presentation
Minimal change disease	Podocyte	Circulating T cell factor	Atopy Immunization	Hodgkin's disease Other lymphoma	Nephrotic syndrome
Focal segmental glomerulosclerosis	Podocyte	Circulating factor			Nephrotic syndrome
Membranous nephropathy	Podocyte and GBM	Autoimmune *In situ* immune complexes	Malignancy Gold, D-penicillamine	Malignancy	Nephrotic syndrome
IgA nephropathy	Mesangial	IgA glycosylation Immune complexes (?)		Henoch–Schönlein purpura	Haematuria
Mesangiocapillary (membranoproliferative)	Mesangial Capillary wall	Immune complexes	Nephritic factors Cryoglobulinaemia HCV + other chronic infection	Cryoglobulinaemia Chronic infection Lipodystrophy	Nephritic/nephrotic syndrome
Lupus nephritis	All sites	*In situ* immune complexes		Systemic lupus	Variable
Focal segmental necrotizing GN					ARF
Goodpasture's disease	Capillary wall	Autoimmune	Hydrocarbons	Lung haemorrhage	
Pauci-immune	Capillary wall	Autoimmune (?)	ANCA	Systemic vasculitis	
Thrombotic microangiopathy (TMA)	Endothelial	Endothelial cell injury—secondary platelet thrombi	*E. coli* O157, Shiga toxin Cyclosporin, tacrolimus, mitomycin C Pregnancy Genetic predisposition—factor H Altered vWF protease activity	Extrarenal TMA	ARF
Amyloid	Mesangial Capillary wall	Amyloid protein deposition	Plasma cell malignancy Chronic inflammation	Myeloma Rheumatoid, Crohn's, etc.	Nephrotic syndrome

Why does glomerular injury occur?

This section considers the known major mechanisms that initiate glomerular injury in man. The common mechanisms are shown in Table 3. There has been recent progress in the identification of a number of genetic mutations that lead to altered glomerular structure, mostly of the glomerular capillary wall, and predispose to subsequent glomerular injury; as well as genetic backgrounds that promote susceptibility to GN. There is increasing evidence that autoimmunity has a major role in the pathogenesis of GN; not only in Goodpasture's disease, but also in antineutrophil cytoplasmic antibodies (ANCA)-associated vasculitis, and perhaps in membranous nephropathy. Such autoimmunity may be mediated by both humoral and cellular immunity.

Immune complex deposition is usually considered the basis for patterns of GN characterized by granular immune deposits; however, the concept has evolved far from the early notion that the passive trapping of preformed circulating immune complexes (CIC) was the sole mechanism, and now includes *in situ* immune complex formation with either intrinsic glomerular antigens or planted extrinsic antigens. It is also recognized that direct infection of glomerular cells may provoke injury as well as infection resulting in GN through immune mechanisms. There is also a clearer appreciation of the range of endothelial insults that can provoke glomerular arteriolar and capillary injury, leading to TMA. Metabolic injury is common, particularly diabetes mellitus, and ischaemia and hypoxaemia may contribute to both acute and chronic glomerular injury.

Secondary glomerular injury, driven mainly by altered pressure within the glomerular capillary bed, as well as glomerular hypertrophy, may also occur following reduction in number of functioning nephrons, and contribute to progressive glomerular failure.

Genetic contributions to glomerular injury

Mutations in structural proteins of the glomerular capillary wall

Glomerular injury may develop as a consequence of genetic defects leading to structural abnormalities of cellular or extracellular glomerular proteins. Although the defect is present from birth, the

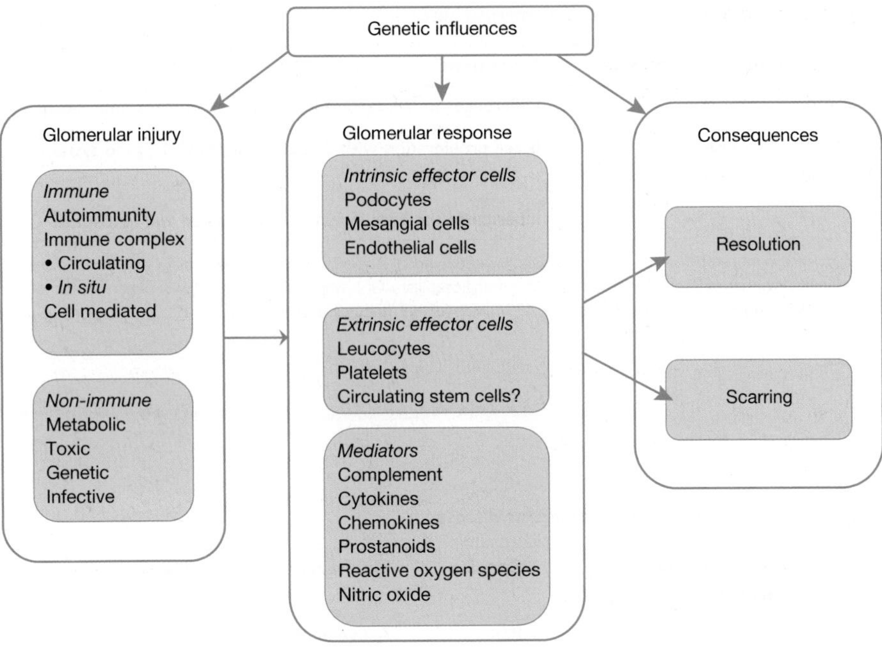

Fig. 1 Overview of mechanisms of glomerular injury.

clinical expression of glomerular injury may not be manifest until adult life. Mutations so far identified result in disordered structure and function of the glomerular capillary wall, either in the glomerular basement membrane (GBM) or in the podocyte. The commonest of these conditions are the structural defects in type IV collagen in the GBM which lead to AS and other closely related forms of hereditary nephritis. Recent evidence has also implicated genetic defects in podocyte and slit diaphragm proteins including podocin, alpha-adducin, and nephrin, which result in congenital and familial forms of nephrotic syndrome, and may also be associated with sporadic causes of nephrotic syndrome (Khoshnoodi and Tryggvason 2001).

Collagen IV

Type IV collagen in the GBM is a well-ordered glycoprotein in which three alpha chains are associated with a globular non-collagenous domain. The six different alpha chains are transcribed from genes expressed in pairs on different chromosomes—α-1 and α-2 on chromosome 13, α-3 and α-4 on chromosome 2, and α-5 and α-6 on the X chromosome. Known mutations leading to AS are predominant in the α-5 gene leading to an X-linked disorder; and on chromosome 2 in the α-3 gene leading to the less common autosomal recessive AS. A rare form of autosomal dominant AS is also described, but the underlying mutation remains uncertain (Kashtan 2000). The consequence of the COL4 mutations is the failure of the ordered structure of collagen IV. Mutated alpha chains and other alpha chains with which they normally assemble are missing from the structure completely in affected individuals; heterozygotes, including female carriers, have mosaic patterns. The GBM in the early phase of the disease has lost the microstructure demonstrable by EM—the lamina densa and the external and internal laminae rarae are poorly defined, the GBM may be variably thick and thin, and in due course the structure becomes more chaotic with 'basket weaving' and lamellation. The first clinical manifestation of this disordered GBM is haematuria, with proteinuria following as glomerular injury advances. Since collagen IV is also a major element in cochlear basement membrane, nerve deafness commonly occurs.

Although the collagen IV defect is well defined, the process by which this leads on to extensive glomerular injury and glomerulosclerosis is poorly understood. There is, however, no evidence for the involvement of another inherited defect, nor any predictable environmental factor. On available evidence, the collagen IV defect is sufficient to provoke progressive irreversible injury.

Slit diaphragm proteins

There has been recent rapid progress in our understanding of the podocyte slit diaphragm and the genetic defects in slit diaphragm proteins that contribute to inherited glomerular disease.

Nephrin Nephrin is an intrinsic component of the glomerular slit diaphragm. It has a crucial role in the maintenance of the integrity of the glomerular barrier. A mutation in NPHS1, the gene for nephrin, and failure of nephrin production is the fundamental abnormality in the congenital nephrotic syndrome of the Finnish type (Kestila *et al.* 1998). This is supported by an animal model in which administration of a monoclonal antibody against rat nephrin causes immediate but reversible heavy proteinuria (Topham *et al.* 1999). The rats lose nephrin expression and show severe foot process effacement, which recovers as proteinuria resolves.

It seems very probable that an analogous mutation on nephrin or another podocyte/slit diaphragm protein will prove to underlie diffuse mesangial sclerosis and other types of congenital nephritic syndrome, but none has yet been identified.

Podocin NPHS2 is the gene for podocin, a protein solely expressed in podocytes. An adult form of autosomal recessive focal segmental

Table 2a Animal models of glomerular disease: spontaneous glomerular disease

Human disease	Spontaneous disease in animal	Comment
IgA nephropathy	ddY mouse	Differences in IgA system in rodents cf. humans limit interpretation
Lupus nephritis	[NZBxNZW]F1 mouse MRL/lpr mouse	B cell proliferation with defects in fas/APO-1 ligand system
Alport syndrome	Dogs	Inheritance patterns include both X-linked and autosomal

Table shows spontaneous glomerular disease in inbred laboratory animals which has been widely studied. Note also that certain glomerular diseases are widespread in feral and domestic mammals, e.g. membranous nephropathy and mesangiocapillary GN; while others are virtually unknown, for example, anti-GBM disease. This has been most widely studied in dogs (Vilafranca *et al.* 1994). For further discussion, see Wilson (2001).

Table 2b Animal models of glomerular disease: induced glomerular disease

Human disease	Name of induced animal model	Species	Mechanism of induction	Comment
Membranous nephropathy	Heymann nephritis	Rat	Active immunization with Fx1A (renal tubular cell extract) Passive immunization with anti-Fx1A antibody	
Mesangial proliferative GN	Anti-Thy 1.1 nephritis	Rat	Passive immunization with anti-Thy 1.1 (rat mesangial antigen)	Usually acute, can be chronic
IgA nephropathy	—	Rat	DNP–anti-DNP immune complexes: infusion of CIC *or* IC formed *in situ*	Differences in IgA system in rodents, cf. humans limit interpretation
Anti-GBM disease	Experimental allergic GN (EAG) Nephrotoxic nephritis (Masugi nephritis)	Rat Rat	Active immunization with rat GBM or α3 chain of type IV collagen Passive immunization with heterologous anti-GBM antibody	
Pauci-immune necrotizing GN	ANCA mouse Mercuric chloride	Mouse Rat	Infusion of ANCA Polyclonal B cell activation with anti-MPO antibodies	
Lupus nephritis	—	Rat	Passive immunization with antibodies against DNA or phospholipid Active immunization with peptides from Sm antigen Graft-versus-host disease	Less widely studied than spontaneous models
Minimal change disease/FSGS FSGS	Puromycin aminonucleoside or adriamycin nephrosis Overload proteinuria	Rat Rat	Direct podocyte and tubular cell toxicity of puromycin or adriamycin Heterologous albumin overload leads to podocyte injury	Not steroid responsive
Congenital nephrotic syndrome	Nephrin 'knock-out' Mab-5-1-6	Mouse Rat	Genetic disruption of slit diaphragm Monoclonal antinephrin antibody disrupts slit diaphragm	
Diabetic nephropathy	Streptozotocin toxicity	Rat	Induces diabetes by islet cell toxicity followed by diabetic nephropathy	Usually non-progressive Kimmelstiel–Wilson lesions not seen
Alport syndrome	—	Mouse	COL4A3 and COL4A4 'knock outs'	

This table shows models which have been widely studied because they can be consistently reproduced and appear most closely related to human glomerular disease. There are many other models and variants which have been induced in laboratory animals. For further discussion, see Wilson (2001).

Table 3 Common categories of glomerular injury

Mechanism	Site of glomerular injury	Human disease
Immune mediated		
Autoimmune		
Intrinsic glomerular antigen		
α3 Chain of collagen IV	GBM	Goodpasture's disease
?	Podocyte	Membranous nephropathy
Planted antigen		
Bacterial components	GBM	Poststreptococcal GN
?DNA, ?nucleosome	Subendothelial, mesangial, subepithelial	Lupus nephritis
Drugs (gold, D-penicillamine)	Podocyte	Membranous nephropathy
Circulating immune complexes		
HBV infection	Mesangium	Mesangial proliferative GN
?Streptococcal components	GBM + mesangium	Poststreptoccal GN
In situ immune complexes	GBM	Membranous nephropathy
Physicochemical characteristics of antibody		
IgA1 glycosylation	Mesangial	IgA nephropathy
Cryoglobulins	GBM	Cryoglobulinaemia
Cellular immunity		
?T cell product	Podocyte	Minimal change disease
Metabolic		
Inherited	Podocyte	Fabry's disease (α-galactosidase deficiency)
Acquired	Endothelial cell, mesangial cell, and podocyte	Diabetic nephropathy
Deposition diseases		
Amyloid	Mesangium, GBM	AA and AL amyloid
Light chains	Mesangium, GBM disease	Light- and heavy-chain deposition
Thrombotic microangiopathy	Endothelial	HUS/TTP
Genetic mutation altering glomerular structure		
Nephrin [NPHS1 gene]	Podocyte	Finnish congenital nephrotic syndrome
Podocin [NPHS2 gene]	Podocyte	FSGS
α-Adducin	Podocyte	FSGS
Glomerular hypertension and hypertrophy	All	Secondary progression following nephron loss of any cause

glomerulosclerosis (FSGS) has been linked to NPHS2 mutations (Boute *et al.* 2000), and mutations are also found in some patients with sporadic FSGS, and appear to be associated with steroid resistance (Winn 2002).

α-Actinin-4 Mutation in the gene for the podocyte protein, α-actinin-4, has recently been described in some families with the uncommon autosomal dominant form of FSGS, which typically is manifest clinically in adult life (Kaplan *et al.* 2000). α-Actinin-4 is found in many tissues, but is highly expressed in podocytes, where it cross-links actin. The mutated protein appears to bind F-actin more tightly.

Why mutations in podocin and α-actinin-4, which affect every podocyte, should lead to a glomerular injury which is initially focal and segmental in FSGS is not clear. However, it has been argued that changes in oncotic pressure due to heavy proteinuria produces alterations in the ultrafiltration coefficient which are maximal at the glomerular hilum (Johnson 1997). Heavy proteinuria may itself result in tubulointerstitial injury with secondary glomerulosclerosis, but additional unidentified intraglomerular processes may also contribute.

Possible roles for these and other podocyte and slit diaphragm proteins in other sporadic human forms of GN as well as experimental models are the subjects of intensive investigation. For example, there is now evidence to link changes in the glomerular nephrin distribution to proteinuria in experimental models of nephrotic syndrome (Luimula *et al.* 2000), as well as early information on nephrin expression in human GN (Huh *et al.* 2002; Kim *et al.* 2002).

There is also a recent report that a transient neonatal nephrotic syndrome has occurred after passive transfer from the mother of antibodies against a podocyte enzyme, neutral endopeptidase (Debiec *et al.* 2002).

Genetic predisposition to glomerular disease

There has been widespread interest in the concept that genetic predisposition plays a significant role in susceptibility to glomerular disease (Phelps and Rees 2001). There is no doubt that first-degree relatives of those with many patterns of glomerular disease have an increased risk of disease. Candidate genes include those influencing the immune response (e.g. the highly polymorphic genes coding for HLA and the T cell receptor) and polymorphisms in genes for effector proteins such as those of the complement cascade and cytokines and growth factors. A number of associations have been identified, but studies have often been inconsistent, in particular showing significant racial variation in the power and specificity of such associations (Table 4). This may reflect the lack of power in many small reported studies. It also suggests that the susceptibility genes remain so far unidentified, but are in linkage disequilibrium with those genes being studied. It may also suggest that the genetic basis for susceptibility to these uncommon diseases play a minor role compared to environmental and other aetiological factors. The slow progress is best exemplified in IgAN, the commonest pattern of GN in many parts of the world. A very wide range of possible associations have been reported with few consistent patterns (Hsu *et al.* 2000). However, studies of kindreds susceptible to IgAN has now established a locus on chromosome 6, 6q22-23 (Gharavi *et al.* 2000) although the susceptibility gene itself has not yet been identified within that locus. Nor is it yet known whether such a locus is involved in the much more common sporadic cases of IgAN.

Mutations in factor H or other complement regulatory proteins also predispose to TMA, at least in familial cases (Taylor 2001).

Other genes are also implicated in promoting progression of chronic renal disease, including GN. These particularly include polymorphic genes coding for proteins of the renin–angiotensin system. These are discussed further in Chapter 11.1.

Immune-mediated glomerular injury

Deposition of immunoglobulin and complement in the glomerulus is a familiar feature of many patterns of glomerular disease. This does not always signal immune-mediated glomerular damage, for example, 'trapping' of circulating immunoglobulins is commonly observed in diabetic nephropathy and is not thought to be important in pathogenesis. However, in the majority of cases immunoglobulin deposition is pathogenic, and deposits through a range of immune and less commonly, non-immune mechanisms. Once deposited, it engages a number of key effector mechanisms including complement leucocytes (most often neutrophils, monocyte/macrophages, and T cells) and a number of soluble factors including cytokines, growth factors, proteases, and proteins of the coagulation cascade (see Section 'Immediate effector mechanisms').

Mechanisms of glomerular deposition of immunoglobulin

Most glomerular diseases develop as a result of immune dysregulation, either an inappropriate immune response to self-antigens occurring through a failure of tolerance, 'autoimmunity', or an ineffectual response to a foreign antigen. Since there is no direct evidence for involvement of antigens from exogenous microorganisms or other agents in most human GN, the mechanism is often presumed to be autoimmune: immune tolerance to a self-antigen has been broken and a pathological immune response results. The precise molecular identity of the autoantigen is known for very few glomerular diseases: Goodpasture's disease is the best defined exception; and an increasingly convincing case is also being made for the centrality of autoimmunity to neutrophil granule enzymes in small vessel vasculitis associated with ANCA.

Autoimmunity

In health, a tension exists between the normal immune response to foreign antigen and 'tolerance', which is the cellular process that prevents an immune response to self-antigen.

Tolerance develops because self-reactive T and B cells are clonally deleted during fetal and neonatal life, although small numbers survive outside the thymus. In the thymus, lymphocytes with very high affinity for autoantigens are deleted, and lymphocytes with negligible affinity for any self-antigen–MHC combinations are deleted—negative and positive selection, respectively. Since lymphocytes with specificity for self-antigens can be detected in normal individuals, autoimmune disease would be universal if there were not additional means of regulation. Regulatory T cells (CD4+ and some CD25+) control autoimmune responses to many peripheral antigens; regulatory cells with specificity for potential autoantigens are generated by 'thymic education'. The AIRE gene plays a key role in this process, and if that gene is deleted, multiple autoimmune conditions result both in a knockout mouse and in the human equivalent—autoimmune polyglandular syndrome, APS-1 (Anderson *et al.* 2002). However, these patients are not susceptible to all autoimmune diseases, and renal autoimmunity has been identified only very rarely in patients with homozygous AIRE mutations, despite the proven expression of at least one renal autoantigen in the thymus (Wong *et al.* 2001).

Peripheral self-reactive T and B cells can be stimulated to generate a cellular and humoral response to a 'self-antigen' if there are simultaneous 'danger signals', which are presented by signalling through the

Table 4 Genetic associations with human glomerular disease

Disorder	Caucasian		Asian (Japanese)	
	HLA specificity	**Relative risk**	**HLA specificity**	**Relative risk**
Goodpasture's disease	DR2[w15] DRB1*1501	10.5 8.5	Not studied	
Pauci-immune necrotizing GN	No consistent findings		Not studied	
IgA nephropathy	HLA Class II—no consistent findings 6q22-23 (gene not identified)		DR4 Not studied	2.6
Membranous nephropathy	DR3	5.6	DR2[w15]	6.8
Minimal change nephrotic syndrome	DR7	5.8	DR8	10.1

The best defined associations using serological and/or molecular techniques are shown, with information on racial variations where this is known.
For further review, see Phelps and Rees (2001).

innate immune system, triggered by pattern receptors evolved to recognize features of pathogens, or by cytokines generated by other triggered cells (Galluci and Matzinger 2001).

Three ways of breaking tolerance have been proposed. Only in a few examples are these proven to operate in a human disease, and it is possible for more than one of these mechanisms to act together. Firstly, *molecular mimicry*, in which a pathogen by chance generates peptide–MHC complexes that closely resemble autoantigen-derived peptide–MHC (Wucherpfennig 2001). When presented in a proinflammatory environment (with 'danger signals'), this results in an immune response that accidentally cross-reacts with self. Second, there may be *exposure* to a subtly altered antigen. Immunization with heterologous antigen (from a different species) with adjuvant (to provide 'danger signals') is the classic way of creating an experimental model. This happens rarely in life, though subtly altered antigens may be given inadvertently. The outbreak of erythropoietin autoimmunity in Europe 1999–2002 (Casadevall *et al.* 2002) may be an example of this. The slightly different molecular sequence or shape generates an immune response that is not subject to the usual degree of regulation because of the different peptide; however, it is similar enough to cross-react with the autoantigen. Third, *altered* antigen processing, in which inflammation or some other perturbation leads to the antigen being internalized in a different way (e.g. in a different multimolecular complex) or by a different cell type to that involved in 'thymic education', creating new peptide–MHC combinations that are not subject to regulation. The disease will only be self-perpetuating if the altered antigen presentation persists.

Infection or toxins may contribute to these processes by releasing antigens from sequestered sites so they have access to T cells, by altering host proteins to make them more immunogenic, or by molecular mimicry. Certain bacteria and viruses also express 'superantigens', which can activate T cells directly and may lead to polyclonal B cell expansion. Once there is an inflammatory response, the further release of antigens may result in the generation of additional autoantibodies, a process known as 'determinant spreading'. Activation of T cells may be further enhanced by the release of cytokines and lymphokines, and the conversion of normally innocuous cells into antigen-presenting cells via the upregulated or *de novo* expression of HLA class II molecules.

Immunoglobulin specific for glomerular components

Antiglomerular basement membrane autoantibodies

Anti-GBM antibodies initiate the 'classical' autoimmune mechanism in GN. Autoimmunity to the non-collagenous domain of α_3 Type IV collagen results in anti-GBM disease, Goodpasture's disease, with glomerular capillary wall deposition of circulating IgG, subsequent complement fixation, and severe glomerular injury. In smokers and others in whom antibody can gain access to the alveolar basement membrane, severe antibody-mediated lung haemorrhage may also occur. Although anti-GBM disease is rare, its immunopathogenesis has been extensively studied as a paradigm of autoimmunity. It is discussed in further detail in Chapter 3.11.

Autoantibodies reacting with other glomerular components

Evidence linking circulating autoantibodies to injury of glomerular cells is tantalizing, but much less well established than in anti-GBM disease. Autoantibodies to *glomerular epithelial cells* are widely postulated to be present in membranous nephropathy, resulting in *in situ* formation of immune complexes and podocyte injury (discussed below). Some patients with systemic lupus may have autoantibodies to components of *glomerular endothelial cells* (Perry *et al.* 1993). The importance of autoantibodies reacting with *mesangial cells* is, perhaps, least well established at present; a report of such autoimmunity in IgAN has not been confirmed (O'Donoghue *et al.* 1991).

Immune complexes

Granular deposits in the glomerulus are a feature of many types of human and experimental GN. These typically contain immunoglobulin of one or more isotype as well as complement components, appearing on EM as discrete electron dense deposits. They may occur in subepithelial, subendothelial, and mesangial locations within the glomerulus. They are usually referred to as 'immune complexes', and are often assumed to represent antigen–antibody complexes. This presumption derives from classical experiments of Germuth Dixon and others in the 1950s and 1960s (Wilson 2001) in which serum sickness induced in animals by injection of bovine serum albumin produced circulating antigen–antibody complexes and extensive subendothelial and mesangial granular deposits. The different patterns of glomerular injury seen in humans (mesangial proliferative, membranous, and crescentic) were produced by varying the experimental conditions in these serum sickness studies. Although this mechanism of injury undoubtedly applies to some types of GN, it is now clear that such granular deposits are not always derived from circulating antigen–antibody complexes but may arise through a range of immune and non-immune mechanisms. In the simplest exposition of this mechanism, the glomerulus is an innocent bystander, and CIC are passively trapped during their passage through the glomerulus. In this scenario, there is no intrinsic glomerular abnormality, but rather it is the composition of the CIC which predisposes to trapping. The unique features of the glomerular capillary bed favour such deposition, since it is a high-pressure, high-flow capillary system with a porous endothelium.

Animal studies performed in the 1970s, when passive trapping of CIC was thought to be the major mechanism for granular deposits in human GN, showed a range of factors that govern the extent of glomerular deposition and influence whether deposits were predominantly in mesangial, subendothelial, or subepithelial locations. These include antigen–antibody ratio, manipulation of the size and charge of CIC, as well as the antibody avidity, blood flow, complement, and the capacity of the reticulo-endothelial system to clear CIC. Subendothelial and mesangial deposits were frequently found; however, it proved difficult to provoke subepithelial deposition in a 'membranous' pattern with infusion of preformed immune complexes.

In human GN, the passive trapping of CIC with nephritogenic characteristics might arise from a number of mechanisms. First, exogenous antigen may provoke an antibody response with characteristics predisposing to CIC formation. This especially occurs in situations of antigen excess, which might occur during acute infection explaining the transient GN often associated with acute viral and bacterial infections. More likely, it would occur in chronic persistent infection with sustained viraemia or bacteraemia, especially if there is a vigorous humoral response to antigen, but impaired cell-mediated immunity prevents clearance of infection. Second, autoimmunity may result in a CIC response to an intrinsic antigen or neoantigen—systemic lupus being the archetype. Third, there may be failure of clearance of CIC from the circulation, normally achieved by engagement with the complement receptor, CR1, on erythrocytes followed by clearance by the monocyte–phagocyte system.

Although CIC may be present in many immune diseases associated with GN, it is important to emphasize that, with a few exceptions, there is virtually no direct evidence that passive trapping of CIC is a key pathogenic mechanism in human glomerular disease. Such evidence is hard to acquire, given that direct infusion experiments of the sort that established the paradigm in experimental animals are not justifiable in humans. Nevertheless, indirect evidence is also slight. Measurement of CIC has proved unhelpful in clinical practice—there is no consistent evidence in most types of GN that CIC levels equate to renal disease activity. CIC assays do not usually identify specific antigens, but rely on the binding of immunoglobulin or complement components—and may not always measure CIC as was once supposed. For example, the widely used C1q binding assay for CIC may measure free anti-C1q antibodies rather than C1q held within CIC. Even in lupus, often regarded as the archetypical immune complex disease, DNA–anti-DNA complexes are only found in circulation in small amounts (Adu *et al.* 1981) and although DNA and anti-DNA antibodies have been eluted from the kidney (Winfield *et al.* 1977) this does not amount to proof that trapped CIC are directly nephritogenic (Berden 1997; Berden *et al.* 2002).

In most human GN the antigen is unknown. Where it is known, evidence has been sought for specific antigens in both CIC and glomerular deposits. It should be recognized that, even if antigen is found in glomerular deposits, it does not necessarily mean it has deposited in trapped CIC.

The best evidence for the deposited CIC mechanism comes from GN associated with infective agents. In poststreptococcal GN (PSGN), CIC containing streptococcal antigen may be present (Friedman *et al.* 1984; Yoshizawa *et al.* 1992), although streptococcal antigens are not consistently found in glomerular deposits (Nordstrand *et al.* 1999). In chronic hepatitis B virus (HBV) infection, virus-containing CIC are also present and HBV is found in glomerular deposits (Johnson and Couser 1990). However, it is probable that other mechanisms are also involved in GN in these contexts (see below).

In situ immune complex formation

Heymann nephritis and membranous nephropathy

A retreat from the CIC paradigm began in the 1970s when it proved difficult to provoke subepithelial immune deposits by infusion of preformed IC, and continued when Couser and Salant showed that the subepithelial deposits in Heymann nephritis, which bears close morphological resemblance to human membranous nephropathy, could be reproduced by the infusion of antibody directed against the renal tubular antigenic preparation, Fx1A, with which the animals had previously been immunized (Couser and Salant 1980). Fx1A is a relatively crude renal tubular extract, and it is now clear that the glycoprotein antigen, gp330 or megalin, is irregularly expressed on visceral epithelial cells. Infusion of antibody leads to heterologous IgG deposition onto gp330, which is associated with clathrin-coated pits on the foot processes of podocytes, and following fixation of antibody the immune complexes thus formed are released, and accumulate on the subepithelial surface of the GBM leading to the formation of the characteristic electron dense deposits (Kerjaschki and Neale 1996). Thus, the granular deposits are not caused by trapping of CIC but are formed *in situ*. The remarkable similarity between the morphology of Heymann nephritis and human membranous nephropathy strongly suggests similar mechanisms operate in the human condition, but despite extensive searches no evidence of gp330 or another similar glomerular antigen has been found in human membranous nephropathy (Collins 1981). Nevertheless, the complete absence of subendothelial and mesangial deposits in idiopathic MN and the replication of the injury with antibodies directed against the podocyte support an autoimmune explanation. An alternative explanation for the membranous pattern of GN could be that small CIC deposits on the subendothelial surface, dissociate, traverse the GBM, and reform in the subepithelial space. This mechanism may be more likely in secondary forms of membranous nephropathy, for example, that associated with chronic hepatitis B infection.

Planted antigens

The possibility that molecules could deposit in the glomerulus for non-immune reasons and then be a target for circulating antibodies was first described by Mauer who showed that heat aggregated human IgG localized in the rat mesangium without renal injury. When the kidney was then transplanted into a syngeneic recipient immunized against human IgG, circulating antihuman IgG antibodies rapidly bound to the planted IgG resulting in mesangial deposits of rat and human immunoglobulins and a proliferative GN (Mauer *et al.* 1973). Numerous other molecules have been studied, particularly cationic molecules which preferentially bind to anionic sites on the GBM. These mechanisms lead to a variety of histological patterns of injury including membranous, as well as proliferative GN.

There is some evidence that such planted antigens may play a part in human GN. In PSGN, cationic streptococcal proteins can be eluted from the glomerulus, but are usually found in the mesangium early in the course of the disease rather than in the subepithelial 'humps' that are the characteristic immune deposits of the established disease. Planted antigens may also play a role in lupus nephritis, since DNA is highly cationic and could therefore be deposited at anionic sites, especially along the capillary wall. Here, they may act as a focus for *in situ* complex formation, although it now appears more likely that the nucleosome (DNA–histone complex) is a key to glomerular deposition rather than DNA itself (Berden 1997).

Explanations for lack of antigen in glomerular deposits

Specific antigens have been found infrequently in glomerular deposits in human GN despite extensive investigation. This has a number of possible aetiological and pathogenic implications.

First, it may indicate that there is a specific antigen involved, but the correct antigen has not been searched for. Given the uncertain aetiology of the much human glomerular disease, it is perfectly reasonable to suspect that more focused searches will increasingly identify the antigens associated with a growing number of human patterns of GN.

Second, the original aetiological agent may no longer be in the glomerulus. Given the lapse of time between initiation of disease and diagnostic renal biopsy in many types of GN, the original antigen provoking immune deposits may have disappeared from the glomerulus, and deposits continue to form by additional mechanisms such as the accretion of anti-idiotypic antibodies directed against the immunoglobulin first involved in the immune complexes.

Third, it may be that there never was an antigen involved in the pathogenesis. Mechanisms by which immune deposits form in the glomerulus without antigen involvement should always be considered.

Infection-associated glomerular injury

Glomerular disease may be a consequence of direct infection of glomerular cells (see below). More commonly, it is the consequence of deposition of antigen–antibody complexes formed in response to antigen from the infecting organism, often as a consequence of the inability to eliminate the foreign antigen. For example, HBV infection, in which infection, particularly in fetal or early life, results in tolerance and a chronic carrier state. Despite a strong humoral response, viral infection persists because the cell-mediated response required for elimination of HBV from the liver is impaired. The consequence is a state of persistent antigenaemia with circulating antigen–antibody complexes, which predisposes to glomerular injury.

It has also been proposed that injury may occur indirectly as a result of cross-reactivity of antibodies, which are a response to components of the infective agent contributing to an autoimmune response against intrinsic glomerular components. A further explanation is that bacterial components act as 'superantigens' stimulating polyclonal production of antibodies with broad reactivity promoting both immune complex formation and autoimmunity against glomerular components (Tomai *et al.* 1990).

Deposition of immune macromolecules other than immune complexes

There are a number of macromolecular assemblies in the circulation involving immunoglobulin which may be nephritogenic independent of classical antigen–antibody reactions. Rheumatoid factors are found in some forms of glomerular disease, including PSGN, and may lead to granular deposits. Cryoglobulins may also be deposited, local haemodynamic and concentration phenomena probably allowing them to be trapped in the glomerulus.

The sequence of pathogenic events in IgAN may be another example of an antigen-independent mechanism. Although the granular mesangial IgA and complement deposits might suggest CIC deposition, no antigen corresponding to a likely aetiological agent has been consistently found in the mesangial deposits, although many have been proposed. Dimers and larger polymers of IgA (pIgA) are increased in the circulation and some of these are rheumatoid factors. Electrical charge may be important since pIgA eluted from renal biopsies is markedly anionic compared to serum IgA; although how such anionicity would favour mesangial deposition is unclear. Altered IgA1 glycosylation also plays a role in mesangial deposition. There is abnormal *O*-glycosylation of the hinge region in serum IgA1 in IgAN (Hiki *et al.* 1998; Allen 1999); and the same defect is even more striking in IgA1 eluted from the kidneys of these patients (Allen 2001; Hiki *et al.* 2001). The altered glycosylation may itself directly promote interaction with cell surface and matrix proteins (Kokubo *et al.* 1998). But altered IgA1 glycosylation also promotes IgA1 self-aggregation *in vitro*, and therefore presumably encourages formation of macromolecular aggregates *in vivo* (Hiki *et al.* 1996). It also predisposes to the formation of IgA1–IgG complexes, thus creating the possibility of the deposition of circulating complexes which lack exogenous antigen (Tomana *et al.* 1999; Kokubo *et al.* 2000).

Immune-mediated glomerular injury without deposition of immune reactants

Pauci-immune necrotising GN

This pattern of acute severe glomerular injury is often associated with ANCA and extrarenal manifestations of small vessel vasculitis. Little or no immunoglobulin or complement deposition is found in the glomerulus ('pauci-immune') despite the presence of a focal segmental necrotizing GN, which may be very severe, causing rapidly progressive renal failure. There is now *in vivo* evidence that ANCA have a pathogenic role in the small vessel injury in the glomerulus and elsewhere in this condition (Xiao *et al.* 2002). In addition to ANCA, T cells play a critical role in the development of epithelial cell crescents in 'pauci-immune' necrotizing GN and other forms of severe GN (Atkins *et al.* 1996). This is discussed further in Chapter 4.5.3.

Immune-mediated injury without deposition of immune reactants and without overt glomerular inflammation

In minimal change nephrotic syndrome (MCNS) and primary FSGS, there is glomerular capillary wall dysfunction manifest as nephrotic syndrome, and evidence of associated podocyte injury, seen on renal histology chiefly as effacement of podocyte foot processes. There is a continuing debate whether MCNS and FSGS are two elements at each end of a spectrum of disease with the possibility of progression from MCNS to FSGS. An alternative view is that they have distinct mechanisms, which initiate podocyte injury, but share some common pathways, which lead to nephrotic syndrome.

There is substantial, albeit indirect, evidence for an immune pathogenesis in these conditions; particularly in the impressive response to a range of immunosuppressive therapies including corticosteroids, cyclosphosphamide, and cyclosporin. This response is much more clear-cut in MCNS than in FSGS. Yet, no immune deposits are seen and there is no active inflammatory process seen histologically. In MCNS, a reversible T cell abnormality leading to production of a factor creating glomerular capillary wall permeability was postulated 30 years ago (Shalhoub 1974). However, it still remains unidentified, although supernatants from T cell hybridomas generated from patients with MCNS provoke proteinuria and foot process effacement when infused into rats (Koyoma *et al.* 1991).

Circulating factor(s), not yet fully characterized, are also associated with recurrence of nephrotic syndrome after transplantation in primary FSGS (Dantal *et al.* 1994; Savin *et al.* 1995). The role of such factors in the pathogenesis of FSGS in native kidneys is not yet clear; nor is it known if the putative circulating factors in MCNS and FSGS are related.

Deposition of monoclonal immunoglobulins

Glomerular disease can be a consequence of extracellular deposition of circulating immunoglobulins or their derivative, proteins, whose innate properties predispose to glomerular deposition and lead to their subsequent pathogenicity. The commonest patients in this category are those with AA and AL amyloid, in whom disordered protein synthesis results in formation of amyloid fibrils. Less common are familial forms of amyloid, light and heavy chain deposition disease, and fibrillary and immunotactoid glomerulopathies (see Chapter 4.2.2). These deposits do not provoke any inflammatory or secondary immune response, but the mass of inert fibrillar protein increases unless the underlying disease process is interrupted, and these deposits relentlessly impair glomerular function.

Cell-mediated immune injury

Cellular mechanisms may be involved in the immune response which initiates glomerular injury, and also in the very early inflammatory events that are a consequence of the immune response.

While immune complex mechanisms are more common, certain glomerular diseases develop primarily through cell-mediated immunity. Studies in experimental models of crescentic nephritis have provided convincing evidence for a direct role for T cells in mediating proteinuria and crescent formation (Atkins *et al.* 1996). It is thought that T cells sensitized to endogenous or exogenous antigen present in the glomeruli recruit macrophages, which leads to a local delayed-type hypersensitivity reaction. In certain models, $CD8^+$ T cells have also been shown to mediate crescent formation via perforins (enzymes that act similarly to the complement membrane attack complex).

Immediate effector mechanisms

Once immunoglobulin has deposited by the range of mechanisms discussed above, it may engage a number of key effector mechanisms including complement, leucocytes (most often neutrophils, monocyte/macrophages, T cells, and natural killer cells), and a number of soluble factors including cytokines, growth factors, proteases, and proteins of the coagulation cascade.

Complement

The complement system (Fig. 2) is an amplifying cascade of proteins which evolved as part of the innate immune system (Morgan 2000; Hebert *et al.* 2001; Welch 2001). In some circumstances, complement protects against renal injury, for example, in promoting clearance of immune complexes, thus explaining why inherited complement component deficiencies are associated with lupus and other immune-complex-mediated diseases. Its protective role may, however, be superceded in immune injury by a sequence of events following immunoglobulin deposition that produces cell injury and promotes inflammation. The central event in the complement cascade is the cleavage of C3, which leads to the production of the membrane attack complex (C5b-9), and to C3 fragments, which are active in inflammation. Complement can be activated by immune complexes via the classical pathway, initiated by the binding of C1q to the Fc portion of the antibody. Classical pathway activation typically occurs in diffuse proliferative lupus nephritis, cryoglobulinaemia, and membranoproliferative GN type I. In this setting, both serum C3 and C4 are usually low. Complement can also be activated via the mannose-binding pathway initiated by a lectin (mannose-binding lectin, MBL), which has a similar structure to C1q. The role of the mannose-binding pathway in GN has not yet been clearly established.

Finally, the complement cascade can also be initiated via the alternative pathway, an amplification loop for C3 activation, which is independent of immune complexes, but is triggered by polysaccharide antigens, dimeric or polymeric IgA, injured cells, or endotoxins. This

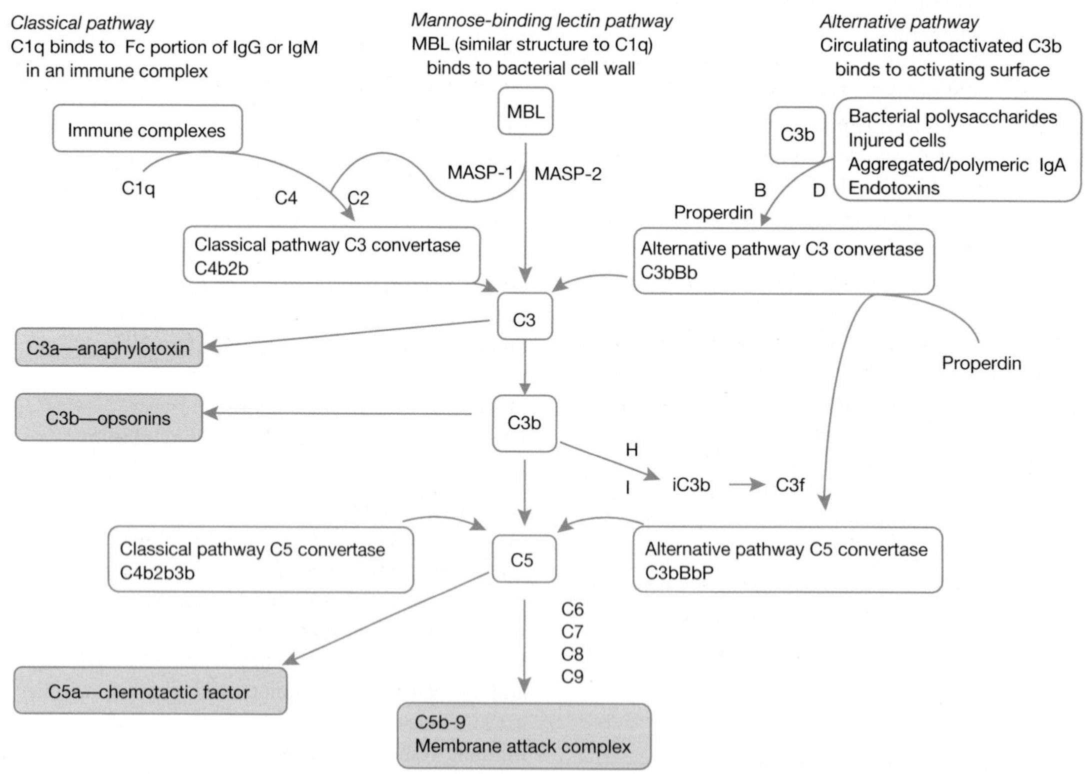

Fig. 2 *The complement cascade.* The complement system is a self-amplifying cascade of proteins that generates a membrane attack complex, which is cytolytic; the cascade promotes inflammation by the activity of the fragments it produces. The amplifying cascades occur because activated fragments of the components combine to make convertase enzymes that degrade C3 and C5. The complement cascade is controlled in part by the very short active life of many of its components. There are also inhibitory regulatory proteins, most notably factors H and I inhibiting C3b. Activated fragments of any component are designated b, for example, C3b; anaphylatoxic fragments are designated a, for example, C5a. Inflammatory functions of complement components are shown in shaded boxes.

pathway appears to be activated in mesangiocapillary GN type II, and in some cases of PSGN. Serum C3 is typically low, but C4 is normal. Nephritic factors are autoantibodies that stabilize various convertases in the complement pathway, and modify their action; they play a key role in the pathogenesis of mesangiocapillary GN (see Chapter 3.8).

Activation of the complement pathway has several consequences. First, leucocyte recruitment is facilitated by C3a and C5a. Second, formation of terminal opsonic complement fragments such as C3b on the surface of glomerular structures and cells may engage β_2 integrin receptors (i.e. $\alpha_m\beta_2$ also known as CR3 or Mac-1) on myeloid leucocytes, directing leucocyte attachment and spreading, and then trigger secretion of injurious granules into the tightly circumscribed space between the leucocyte and the glomerular cell. This phenomenon is termed 'frustrated phagocytosis' as granule contents that would normally be directed to a membrane-bound phagosome within the leucocyte reach the cell surface. Third, engagement of the terminal components of the complement cascade with the formation of the membrane attack complex, C5b-9, can literally 'punch holes' in target cells and trigger glomerular cell death by necrosis. C5b-9 can also produce sublytic injury that can activate rather than destroy cells contributing to ongoing tissue injury, for example, in Heymann nephritis and human membranous nephropathy (Nangaku *et al.* 2002).

Tissue injury is not an inevitable consequence of engagement of the complement cascade (Sheerin *et al.* 2001). An extensive system of complement regulatory proteins, both on cell membranes and in serum, provides checks and controls on the cascade (Nangaku 1998).

The liver is the major site of synthesis of complement components, and in glomerular injury most components of the cascade are recruited from the circulation. However, intrinsic glomerular cells and renal tubular cells can also synthesise C3, C4, factor H, and also complement regulatory proteins, providing an additional contribution to tissue injury and its control (Nangaku 1998; Sheerin *et al.* 2001; Welch 2001).

Recruitment of leucocytes

In many tissues, leucocytes are recruited from blood by traversing the wall of postcapillary venules. This occurs through the coordinated action of leucocyte chemoattractants acting to promote leucocyte spreading and movement (which may be prevented by extracellular matrix), adhesion molecules, and endothelial cell proteases that 'clip' attachments between endothelial cells (Fig. 3). Most of the general principles of this cascade of molecular and cellular interactions have been implicated in the recruitment of leucocytes to glomeruli, but there are important differences from this paradigm. First, glomerular capillaries are high-pressure, high-flow hemi-arterioles. Second, leucocytes can disrupt glomerular function merely by adhering to glomerular endothelial cells/basement membrane—they need not cross the vessel wall. This offers therapeutic opportunities based on promoting detachment from vessel walls.

In a typical acute inflammatory response there is a clear temporal sequence in recruitment of different leucocyte types. Thus, neutrophils are recruited within a few hours to reach a peak in numbers at ~24 h; monocytes are recruited rather more slowly, the maximum number typically being reached at 48 h when maturation into macrophages is already well advanced; and lymphocytes follow with an even slower rate. There is now strong evidence that such sequential recruitment reflects sequential expression of chemoattractant cytokines or chemokines (Nelson *et al.* 2001a) (Table 5). However, there are variations of this theme, an example being selective monocyte recruitment driven by activation of T cells in a tissue.

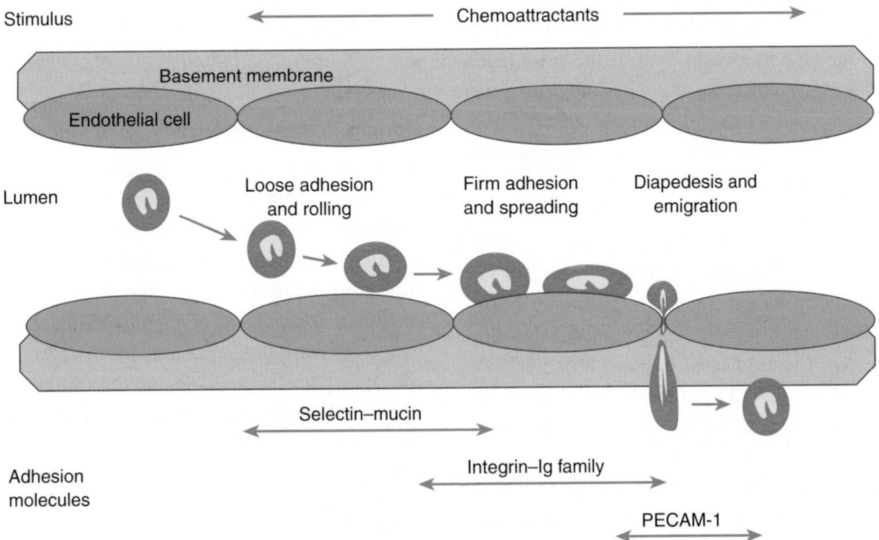

Fig. 3 Key events in leucocyte emigration from vessels. Generation of chemoattractants at sites of inflammation leads to activation of both endothelium and passing leucocytes. Initially selectin–mucin interactions mediate loose adhesion and 'rolling' of leucocytes along the endothelium at a rate considerably slower than blood flow. With activation of leucocyte integrins, firm leucocyte adhesion and spreading occur, mediated by integrin interaction with immunoglobulin superfamily counter–receptors. Endothelial cell proteases such as matrix metalloproteinase-7 'clip' sticky molecules such as syndecan-1 that otherwise bind leucocytes attached to chemokines on the basal aspect of endothelial cells. Finally, diapedesis of leucocytes occurs, an event in which PECAM-1 may be particularly important.

Table 5 Chemokines and their receptors likely to be important in glomerulonephritis

Family	Name	Source	Responding cells	Receptor
CXC	CXCL2 (MIP-2; GRO-β)	Leucocytes, tissue cells	Neutrophil	CXCR2
	CXCL5 (ENA78)	Epithelium	Neutrophil	CXCR2
	CXCL1 (GRO-α)	Leucocytes, fibroblasts	Neutrophil (fibroblast)	CXCR2
	CXCL7 (NAP-2)	Platelet basic protein	Neutrophil (fibroblast)	CXCR2
	CXCL8 (IL-8)	Leucocytes, tissue cells	Neutrophil (basophil, T cell)	CXCR1, CXCR2
CC	CL2 (MCP-1)	Leucocytes, tissue cells	Monocytes (basophil)	CCR2
	CCL3 (MIP-1α)	Leucocytes	Monocyte (other leucocytes)	CCR1, CCR5
	CCL4 (MIP-1β)	Leucocytes	Monocyte (other leucocytes)	CCR5
	CCL5 (RANTES)	T cells, platelets	Monocyte (T cell, eosinophil)	CCR1, CCR3, CCR5
Other chemokines	CX3CL1 (fractalkine)	Endothelial cells	Monocytes, natural killer cells, T cells	CX3CR1

There has been a recent rationalization of nomenclature for chemokines and their receptors. Previous terminology is also shown.
GRO, growth-related oncogene; IL-8, interleukin-8; MIP, macrophage inhibitory protein; MCP-1, monocyte chemoattractant protein-1; NAP-2, neutrophil activating peptide-2; RANTES, regulated upon activation normal T-cell expressed and secreted.

Capacity to induce injury

Neutrophils, the archetypal inflammatory leucocyte, exemplify the astonishing potential for injury of tissue consequent upon engagement of systems that have evolved to kill invading micro-organisms (Table 6). In turn, however, these injurious mechanisms are kept in check by an equally complex network of checks and balances (Table 6). Not all of these tissue-damaging systems are available to other leucocyte types. For example, as monocytes mature into macrophages they lose expression of myeloperoxidase, limiting their potential to damage tissue through the generation of halides. However, cytotoxic lymphocytes and natural killer cells possess other powerful mechanisms for injuring neighbouring cells such as the combination of granule enzymes plus Fas ligand.

The recruitment of leucocytes exposes resident cells at inflamed sites to injurious stimuli which in different microenvironments may produce different outcomes. Thus, high levels of noxious stimuli may 'murder' resident cells through induction of necrosis, lower levels may trigger altruistic 'suicide' by engaging the physiological death 'programme' of apoptosis (see below). Activated macrophages have particular potential to delete glomerular cells by engaging apoptosis. Activated cells of a macrophage line can induce 'cytolysis' of mesangial cells in co-culture (Mene *et al.* 1996), and macrophages are also known to direct developmental cell death (Lang and Bishop 1993; Diez Roux and Lang 1997). Furthermore, activated macrophages isolated from experimentally inflamed rat glomeruli and bone-marrow-derived macrophages activated by lipopolysaccharide and interferon-γ (but not quiescent macrophages) induced both suppression of mitosis and a dramatic increase in apoptosis of mesangial cells (Duffield *et al.* 2000). Experiments with inhibitors and macrophages from relevant 'knock-out' mice show that this reduction in mesangial cell numbers are mediated by products of macrophage-inducible nitric oxide synthase (iNOS or NOS2) in concert with another factor, probably tumour necrosis factor-α (TNF-α).

Table 6 Neutrophil products that may contribute to tissue injury and their antagonists

Injurious products	Antagonists
Oxygen radicals	*Radical 'scavengers'*
Superoxide anion (O_2^-)	Superoxide dismutase
Hydrogen peroxide (H_2O_2)	Catalase
Hydroxyl radical ($OH^\bullet$)	Uric acid
Singlet Oxygen ($^1O_2$)	*Anti-proteinases*
Hypochlorous acid (HoCl)	α_2 Macroglobin
N-chloramines	
Neutral proteinases	
Elastase	
Cathepsin G	
Collagenase	
Non-enzymatic cationic proteins	
Defensins	

Direct infection of glomerular cells

Immune-mediated GN is often a consequence of infection remote from the kidney, the immune response leading to deposition of immunoglobulin and complement as discussed above. However, it may also be the result of direct infection of glomerular cells.

Human immunodeficiency virus infection

The commonest pattern of glomerular disease described in association with human immunodeficiency virus (HIV) infection is a collapsing variant of FSGS, but other patterns reported include mesangial proliferative GN, with and without IgA deposits, and TMA. It was for some time controversial whether there was direct and continuing infection of glomerular cells in HIV, and whether this contributed to the pathogenesis of the glomerular lesion. However, there is now clear evidence that HIV particles are detected in podocytes in renal biopsies in HIV-associated nephropathies with evidence of active viral replication (Bruggeman *et al.* 2000). This may act as a reservoir to promote persistence of infection (Winston 2001). The presence of replicating virus does not necessarily prove that infection is directly contributing to glomerular injury. However, at least *in vitro* in murine cell systems, there is now evidence that podocyte behaviour is substantially altered by HIV infection (Nelson *et al.* 2001b).

Hepatitis B virus

The involvement of HBV is typically through its involvement in immune deposits in membranous and mesangiocapillary forms of HBV-associated GN. It is usually assumed to have been derived from the circulation. There is, however, evidence for direct infection for glomerular cells in patients with GN from an area where HBV is endemic (Lai *et al.* 1996). It has not, however, been established if glomerular cell infection contributes to the pathogenesis of GN.

Hepatitis C virus

There is some evidence that Hepatitis C virus (HCV) RNA is present in the kidney, although it has not been localized to the glomerulus (Sabry *et al.* 2002).

Endothelial cell injury—thrombotic microangiopathy

Direct injury to glomerular endothelial cells provokes a response usually manifest as TMA (Ruggenenti *et al.* 2001). While such insults are usually systemic, the consequences are particularly damaging to the glomerular capillaries, although other intrarenal vessels will often show similar damage. The endothelial injury is produced not only by a range of 'toxins' including bacterial products and drugs, but also by intrinsic injury in relation to pregnancy or hypertension. Such injury may be predisposed to by genetic variations in the complement regulatory protein, factor H, or by abnormal activity of proteases that cleave the von Willebrand factor. Whatever the precipitating factor, endothelial disruption follows a common process characterized by platelet activation and deposition, and microvascular thrombosis. This produces overwhelming glomerular injury, which is often irreversible.

The clinical syndrome associated with TMA is variously described as haemolytic–uraemic syndrome (HUS) and thrombotic thrombocytopenic purpura (TTP). These terms are poorly defined, but HUS is usually preferred when renal injury and acute renal failure dominate the clinical presentation.

Extrinsic toxins producing TMA include the verotoxin of *Escherichia coli* O157, and Shiga toxin, as well as a number of drugs, particularly cyclosporin, tacrolimus, and mitomycin C. A very similar series of pathogenic events will occasionally be associated with use of oral contraceptive agents, occur with pre-eclampsia, or develop in the postpartum period. TMA can also rarely complicate accelerated hypertension. These complications are uncommon and appear idiosyncratic. There is no clear evidence that dose exposure predicts the minority who develop overt TMA in response to these toxins or drugs. This may suggest that an additional predisposition, perhaps genetic, is also present in those who succumb. This is supported by growing evidence that TMA occurs in its uncommon familial forms because mutations in control proteins of the complement system produce susceptibility. Factor H mutations are the best described (Taylor 2001), but so far it has not been shown that these mutations are widespread in individuals with sporadic or toxin-induced TMA.

Metabolic injury

Diabetic nephropathy is one of the commonest causes of glomerular disease. It is conventionally considered to be a microvascular complication of diabetes mellitus, indicating that the glomerular capillary is the prime site of injury. However, the adverse effects of a hyperglycaemic milieu on glomerular structure and function are far more widespread. There is extensive experimental evidence that mesangial cells and podocytes as well as glomerular endothelial cells are injured by hyperglycaemia and its consequences, and that the subsequent responses of all three cell types contribute to progressive diabetic nephropathy.

Ischaemia

Ischaemia and hypoxaemia are significant contributors to glomerular injury. Atherosclerotic renal disease is the commonest cause, provoking ischaemia either through conduit artery stenosis/occlusion or through intrarenal arterial narrowing or subsequent cholesterol embolization. Sustained hypertension, even in the absence of atherosclerosis, will produce arteriolar injury and narrowing with secondary glomerular ischaemia. Medium and large vessel vasculitis (e.g. polyarteritis nodosa) also lead to patchy cortical ischaemia. The intrarenal vasoconstriction and blood flow diversion characteristic of acute tubular necrosis complicating glomerular disease will always produce a degree of glomerular ischaemia, although failure of the protective mechanisms which usually make such ischaemia reversible may lead to cortical necrosis with irreversible ischaemic glomerular damage.

Sustained hypoxaemia also results in glomerular hypertrophy and injury, as seen in the glomerular disease that may accompany congenital cyanotic heart disease, or sickle cell disease.

'Mechanical' injury

The glomerulus is susceptible to injury resulting from signification perturbations of its physical characteristics including perfusion pressure and size. Glomerular injury of this type is rarely primary, most often part of a continuing process of secondary injury which contributes to progression of renal failure even after primary immune mechanisms in GN have ceased. These changes occur when the primary GN has resulted in a significant reduction in the number of functioning nephrons, and there is failure of the usual autoregulatory processes that maintain pressure and filtration relationships in the glomerulus (Brenner 1997). Systemic hypertension is an almost universal feature of advancing glomerular disease in this setting and failure of afferent arteriolar autoregulation allows glomerular hypertension to develop. Secondary glomerular injury then exacerbates and accelerates further deterioration in renal function. These processes occur when systemic hypertension and reduced nephron number complicate any primary renal disease. This sequence of events is in contrast with the situation in essential hypertension in which the afferent glomerular arteriole takes the brunt of the injury but autoregulatory mechanisms usually protect the glomerulus.

A second characteristic promoting this type of injury is glomerular hypertrophy. This may be secondary to a reduction in functioning nephron number, but may also be congenital. This not only occurs in the rare congenital oligomeganephronia which predisposes to glomerulosclerosis, but also may have a racial basis: thus, a greater susceptibility of African-Caribbean children to glomerulosclerosis in the context of nephrotic syndrome has been attributed to their larger glomeruli (Fogo *et al.* 1990).

Sustained proteinuria is also a characteristic feature of such secondary glomerular injury and contributes to changes in the glomerular microcirculation through alterations in oncotic pressure and also by promoting tubulo-interstitial injury.

A characteristic feature of these predominantly haemodynamic forms of glomerular injury is that they manifest as focal, segmental glomerular sclerotic lesions. This presumably reflects local differences in the glomerular microcirculation that promote injury or restrict repair, although these are not well defined (Johnson 1997; Kriz *et al.* 2001).

What are the consequences of glomerular injury?

Changes in the mesangium

Given the relative ease with which mesangial cells can be cultured, much more information is available about their response to injury in comparison to other intrinsic glomerular cells. Located strategically in the centre of the glomerular tuft, mesangial cells and their surrounding matrix provide anatomical support and modulate various glomerular functions. Mesangial cells have many features of vascular smooth muscle cells, including a contractile apparatus that can alter glomerular microcirculation and ultrafiltration. Changes in the mesangial cell secretory and/or synthetic activity may result in acquisition by the mesangial cell of a proinflammatory and profibrotic phenotype.

In contrast to the intraglomerular mesangium, relatively little is known about the extraglomerular mesangial cells, a part of the juxtaglomerular apparatus. These cells may serve as a source of mesangial cell regeneration via migration into the mesangial stalk and local proliferation following severe mesangial disruption (Hugo *et al.* 1997).

Early consequences of mesangial injury

In the initial phase, injury to mesangial cells may result in mesangial apoptosis, necrosis, or activation of the cells.

In the case of mesangial apoptosis or necrosis and disruption of the surrounding extracellular matrix, the mesangial stabilizing capacity is lost. The resulting 'mesangiolysis' is a feature of various human and experimental glomerular diseases (Morita and Churg 1983). Whereas mesangiolysis represents the most severe type of mesangial injury, the majority of immunologic, metabolic, or haemodynamic insults to the mesangium will result in cell activation only. Alternatively, minor injury, which induces no more than very subtle cell changes, may result in their priming, that is, marked amplification of the response towards a second injurious stimulus (Floege *et al.* 1993a).

One of the earliest responses of activated mesangial cells to humoral or cell-mediated injury is their potential to produce and release a large number of pro- and/or anti-inflammatory products (Table 7) (Mene *et al.* 1989; Striker *et al.* 1991; Sterzel *et al.* 1993). These factors acting in an autocrine, paracrine, or even an endocrine fashion can greatly alter the proliferative, synthetic, or contractile mesangial cell phenotype. Some of the products, such as reactive

Table 7 Secretory products of activated mesangial cells

Mesangial cell secretory products	Examples
Low molecular weight mediators	Prostaglandins Platelet-activating factor (PAF) Reactive oxygen species Nitric oxide (NO)
Cytokines and growth factors	Connective tissue growth factor (CTGF) Fibroblast growth factor (FGF-1 and -2) Monocyte and granulocyte–monocyte colony stimulating factor (M-CSF, GM-CSF) Hepatocyte growth factor (HGF) Insulin-like growth factor-1 (IGF-1) Interleukins (1, 6, 8, 10, 12) Leukaemia inhibitory factor (LIF) Nerve growth factor (NGF) Platelet-derived growth factor (PDGF-A, -B, -C, -D) Transforming growth factor-β (TGF-β) Tumour necrosis factor (TNF-α) Vascular endothelial growth factor (VEGF)
Chemokines	CXCL1—Growth-related oncogene (GRO) CXCL8—IL-8 CXCL10—Interferon-γ-inducible protein 10 (IP10) CCL2—Monocyte chemoattractant protein-1 (MCP-1) CCL3, CCL4—Macrophage inflammatory protein (MIP-1α, -1β, -2) Macrophage migration inhibitory factor (MIF) CCL5—RANTES
Hormones	Endothelin Components of the renin–angiotensin system
Enzymes and inhibitors	Matrix degrading enzymes Aminopeptidase N Tissue plasminogen-activator (t-PA) and inhibitor (PAI-1) Tissue factor Complement C3

oxygen species, nitric oxide, or particular cytokines (e.g. FGF-2), may also act as endogenous pathways through which glomerular injury is initially amplified. Finally, many secretory products not only affect the behaviour of neighbouring mesangial cells but also of other intrinsic or infiltrating cells in the glomerulus.

Proliferation and accumulation of mesangial cells

Infiltration of the mesangium by inflammatory cells, in particular monocyte/macrophages, is a feature of many types of GN, and will result in mesangial hypercellularity. However, a second, often greater contributor to mesangial hypercellularity, is proliferation of the intrinsic mesangial cells. Whereas in health the proliferative turnover of mesangial cells is low (e.g. in a normal rat about 1 per cent of the glomerular cells are renewed daily, of which about 20 per cent are mesangial cells) (Pabst and Sterzel 1983), proliferation of these cells can increase dramatically in disease.

Of the various endogenous factors that affect mesangial cell behaviour (Table 8) (Mene *et al.* 1989; Striker *et al.* 1991; Sterzel *et al.* 1993), *in vitro* and animal data suggest that PDGF, in particular PDGF-B, has an especially important role (Floege and Johnson 1995): mesangial cells produce PDGF and PDGF B-chain and its receptor are overexpressed in glomerular diseases. Infusion of PDGF-BB or glomerular transfection with a PDGF B-chain cDNA induce mesangial proliferative changes *in vivo*. PDGF B-chain or β-receptor knock-out mice fail to develop a mesangium. Finally, specific antagonism of PDGF B-chain can reduce mesangial proliferative changes in an experimental model (Floege *et al.* 1999). Transient antagonism of PDGF B-chain during the active phase of a mesangial proliferative GN can prevent both functional and morphological progressive renal damage (Ostendorf *et al.* 2001). Since anti-PDGF treatment in tumour patients has shown little toxicity, suggesting that PDGF is not required in normal adult life, targeting growth factors such as PDGF may become an attractive therapeutic approach to mesangial proliferative diseases.

As well as a proliferative response mesangial cells may also be driven into cellular hypertrophy, which is particularly relevant for diabetic nephropathy. The molecular controls of the cell cycle that determine progression, that is, mitosis or exit from the cell cycle, that is, apoptosis or arrest, have been studied in great detail over recent years (Schocklmann 1999; Shankland 2000).

Table 8 Examples of regulators of mesangial cell proliferation in cell culture

Mitogenic	Antimitogenic
Arginine–vasopressin	ACE-inhibitors
Dinucleotides, adenosine triphosphate	C-type natriuretic peptide (CNP)
Endothelin-1	Heparan sulfate proteoglycans
Epidermal growth factor	Heparins (both anticoagulant and non-anticoagulant)
FGF-2	HMG-CoA-reductase inhibitors
IL-1	IL-4, IL-10
Insulin	Interferon-γ
Insulin-like growth factor-1	Mycophenolic acid
PDGF (-B, -C, -D)	Nitric oxide (NO)
Stretch	TGF-β (high concentrations)
TGF-β (low concentrations)	Trapidil
Thrombin	Verotoxin

Expansion of the mesangial extracellular matrix

Increased cell proliferation is usually accompanied by increased mesangial production and deposition of extracellular matrix (Eng *et al.* 1994). However, expansion of the mesangial matrix may become prominent, for example, in diabetic nephropathy, without major changes in mesangial cell number. The expanded mesangial matrix contains increased amounts of proteins present in the normal mesangium; but also contains proteins not normally expressed in the glomerulus, such as interstitial collagen types I and III (Table 9) (Floege *et al.* 1991; Lehmann and Schleicher 2000), which may be of importance in initiating mesangial sclerosis.

Apart from increased production of extracellular matrix proteins, mesangial cells also regulate the degradation of the matrix (Table 9) (Mene *et al.* 1989; Striker *et al.* 1991; Sterzel *et al.* 1993; Couchman *et al.* 1994; Davies 1994). Mesangial cells release matrix-degrading enzymes, and also their inhibitors such as plasminogen activator inhibitor-1 (PAI-1) and tissue inhibitor of metalloproteinases-1 (TIMP-1). For example, upregulation of PAI-1 synthesis by mesangial cells makes an important contribution to matrix accumulation, and since glomerular PAI-1 expression is regulated by the renin–angiotensin system, it represents one of the non-haemodynamic modes of action of ACE inhibitors and angiotensin receptor-1 antagonists (Oikawa *et al.* 1997).

A growth factor with a particularly well-established function in glomerular matrix accumulation is transforming growth factor-β (TGF-β). Like PDGF, it is produced by mesangial cells, induced in them by other growth factors, in particular angiotensin II, and over-expressed in various glomerular diseases (Peters *et al.* 1997). TGF-β contributes to mesangial cell matrix accumulation by both increasing the synthesis of matrix proteins and decreasing their proteolytic degradation (Border 1994). Transgenic overexpression of TGF-β in the kidney results in progressive fibrosis, and antagonism of TGF-β reduces glomerular matrix accumulation (Peters *et al.* 1997). However, apart

Table 9 Extracellular matrix proteins and matrix-degrading enzymes produced by mesangial cells

Extracellular matrix proteins	Matrix-degrading enzymes
Chrondroitin sulfate proteoglycans	Cathepsins
Collagens I, III, IV, V, VI, VIII	Endo-exoglycosidases
Dermatan sulfate proteoglycans	Metalloproteinases (MMP-1, -2, -3, -7, -9, -10)
Elastic fibre proteins	Plasminogen activators (u-PA, t-PA)
Fibronectin	
Heparan sulfate proteoglycans	
Laminin	
Nidogen/entactin	
Osteopontin	
Tenascin	
Thrombospondin	

from its profibrotic role, TGF-β also exerts potent anti-inflammatory and immunosuppressive effects (Shull *et al.* 1992). Nevertheless, recent data suggest that it may be safe to antagonize TGF-β for prolonged periods in adult life (Yang *et al.* 2002).

Late adaptive and regenerative responses

Mesangial cells may counteract intraglomerular hypertension through their contractile capacity. This, in turn, is influenced by various peptides (e.g. angiotensin II, endothelin-1), growth factors (PDGF, TNF-α), autacoids (e.g. prostaglandins, NO), as well as other small molecules (e.g. histamine, norepinephrine, dopamine). In addition to acute contraction, the mesangial cells also regulate their cytoskeleton in response to hypertension. For example, in angiotensin-II-induced hypertension in rats mesangial cells exhibit *de novo* expression of alpha-smooth muscle actin, which is likely to result in higher cell 'stiffness' and may therefore represent an adaptation to increased physical forces acting on the cells (Johnson *et al.* 1991).

Following a mesangial proliferative response to injury, mesangial cells have a tremendous capacity to reconstitute a normal mesangial morphology even after pronounced histological change. This occurs through mesangial cell apoptosis (see below) and the production of antimitogenic factors, the removal of excess matrix through the action of mesangial proteases and antifibrotic factors, and the production of factors that will counteract various proinflammatory products (Savill 1999; Kriz *et al.* 2003).

Excess extracellular matrix can be removed by various proteases, whose role is well established in the resolution phase of experimental mesangial proliferative GN (Davies *et al.* 1992). The importance of proteases in removing excess matrix is supported by evidence that an age-dependent decrease in glomerular metalloproteinase activity exists in parallel to the development of spontaneous glomerulosclerosis in the rat (Reckelhoff and Baylis 1993).

It is important to define when and how the capacity for mesangial regeneration is overriden. Experimentally, even severe mesangiolysis can be fully reversed and complete structural restoration usually occurs (Floege *et al.* 1991; Yamamoto *et al.* 1994; Kriz *et al.* 2003). However, under some experimental conditions, for example, following repetitive mesangial damage with mesangiolysis, segmental glomerular sclerosis and adhesions with Bowman's capsule can develop, which histologically resemble FSGS (Stahl *et al.* 1992). In human glomerular diseases, a pathogenetic role of mesangiolysis in the development of FSGS and other pathological lesions, such as nodular diabetic glomerulosclerosis, has also been suggested (Saito *et al.* 1988). Since the mesangium through its contractile apparatus counteracts the expanding force of the high intracapillary pressure within the glomerulus, mesangiolysis in the presence of intraglomerular hypertension will be deleterious and may result in 'mesangial failure' (Kriz *et al.* 2003). There is also experimental evidence that the extent of secondary podocyte damage following the primary mesangial injury is a crucial factor that determines whether mesangial injury resolves or progresses (Ostendorf *et al.* 2001; Kriz *et al.* 2003) (Fig. 4).

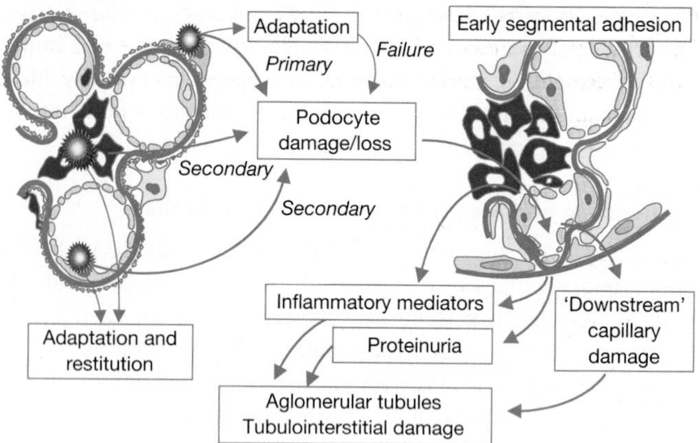

Fig. 4 *Mechanisms of podocyte injury and their consequences.* Primary damage to glomerular endothelial and mesangial cells as well as podocytes may induce adaptive changes. If these are insufficient, podocyte damage and/or loss may occur, resulting in the formation of an early segmental adhesion with attachment of the glomerular basement membrane to Bowman's capsule. Consequences of such early glomerular damage may include proteinuria, release of inflammatory mediators into the surrounding tissue, in particular, the adjacent renal interstitium, as well as downstream capillary damage. Finally, aglomerular tubules and tubulointerstitial damage may result.

Changes in glomerular epithelium/Bowman's space

Glomerular epithelial injury has two distinct consequences: (a) responses of the parietal glomerular epithelial cells, resulting in crescent formation; and (b) responses of the visceral glomerular epithelial cells, resulting in glomerular protein loss and/or scarring. Proteinuria is exclusively a function of visceral cell injury, but the contribution of visceral glomerular epithelial cells to crescent formation is still unresolved.

Crescent formation

The formation of a glomerular epithelial crescent is a common feature of many severe, acute forms of GN. Most typically it is associated with necrotizing GN which is often focal and segmental; which most often occurs in ANCA positive small vessel vasculitis, and less commonly with anti-GBM disease, IgAN, or other primary GN.

The formation of a crescent represents a final common pathway in acute, severe glomerular tuft injury. The cellular, humoral, and other mechanisms involved in crescent formation are discussed in detail in Chapter 3.10.

Podocyte injury disrupts the filtration barrier

The main clinical consequence of immunologic, toxic, metabolic, or haemodynamic damage to podocytes is proteinuria. If podocyte damage is extensive enough, the nephrotic syndrome will develop. The main structural abnormality that is associated with a leaky glomerular filter is effacement of the foot processes of the podocyte with a loss of the slit diaphragm between the foot processes. This process may involve all podocytes or may be localized to areas of pathology such as sites of accumulation of immune complexes. Common associated structural changes in the podocytes include pseudocyst formation, microvillus formation on the apical aspect of the cell, and either partial or complete detachment of the cell from the underlying GBM.

New understanding of individual molecules that constitute the slit diaphragm or molecules involved in the attachment of the foot processes to the GBM has led to major advances in identifying individual pathogenetic steps in the onset of proteinuria. A rapidly growing number of podocyte molecules have been identified, which when genetically deleted or functionally impaired by injection of antibodies, contributes to foot process effacement (Mundel *et al.* 2001) (see Section 'Genetic contributions to glomerular injury').

Adaptive and regenerative capacity of podocytes

Following primary mesangial and glomerular endothelial injury, secondary podocyte changes are a central determinant in the process of glomerular scarring. Following glomerular damage with ensuing glomerular hypertension and/or hypertrophy, podocytes can adapt to the expanding tuft or increased stretch by changes of their cytoskeleton (e.g. the *de novo* expression of desmin), and cellular hypertrophy. However, unlike mesangial and endothelial cells, secondary or primary podocyte loss in the course of glomerular disease cannot be easily replaced by podocyte replication. Injured podocytes have the capacity to replicate, as occasionally shown by podocyte DNA synthesis and mitoses in GN, but usually engage in a defective cell cycle with acytogenetic mitosis leading to bi-(multi) nucleation rather than increased cell numbers (Floege *et al.* 1993b; Kriz *et al.* 1995; Nagata *et al.* 1995; Kriz 1996; Petermann *et al.* 2002). This indicates that the podocyte is not in a state of terminal differentiation but rather that cell cycle progression and in particular cell division are being actively suppressed. For example, high levels of cyclin-dependent kinase inhibitors p21 and p27, key cell cycle regulators, are found in normal and injured podocytes (Shankland *et al.* 1997; Nagata *et al.* 1998; Shankland 1999). However, the potential for active interference with podocyte replication still remains poorly developed in contrast to current possibilities for mesangial and endothelial cells.

One disease entity, which may prove particularly useful in our understanding of podocyte differentiation, is collapsing glomerulosclerosis. This disease is associated with rapid renal failure and primarily occurs in African-American patients, often in association with HIV infection. In this disease, the podocytes lose several of their differentiation markers such as WT1 or GLEPP1, while reacquiring markers expressed early in podocyte development (Barisoni *et al.* 1999). Foot processes are lost and cells, presumably derived from the podocytes, accumulate in sclerotic areas and appear to multiply. It is assumed that these dedifferentiated podocytes are no longer able to provide support for the normal patency, structure, and function of the glomerular capillaries. Interestingly, this phenotype can be mimicked in mice by transgenically overexpressing parts of the HIV genome (Kopp *et al.* 1992).

Podocyte damage and loss—the final common pathway of glomerular scarring

In addition to residual disease-specific glomerular changes, advanced stages of many progressive glomerular diseases are characterized by the non-specific changes of FSGS and ultimately diffuse global glomerulosclerosis. FSGS is characterized histologically by adhesions between the glomerular tuft and Bowman's capsule, hyalinization and obliteration of capillary lumina, and endocapillary foam cell formation and/or deposition of macromolecules such as IgM or C3 in affected areas. Initially, these changes are focal (i.e. observed in only some glomeruli) and segmental (affecting only some parts of the glomerular tuft). The finding of FSGS late in the course of many types of GN suggests a final common pathway of glomerular damage.

Various glomerular events, particularly if combined, lead to an imbalance of intraglomerular forces resulting in podocyte stretch, damage and/or loss of podocytes in the urine (Hara *et al.* 1998; Kriz *et al.* 1998) (Fig. 4). The relative inability of differentiated podocytes to undergo regenerative growth, as discussed above, is believed to be of central importance in the development focal podocyte detachments from the GBM resulting in GBM denudation (Rennke and Klein 1989; Kriz *et al.* 1998). GBM denudations, that is, exposed extracellular matrix, are likely have a high capability to attach to other cells and matrices, in particular, parietal glomerular epithelial cells and their basement membrane, resulting in early adhesions between the glomerular tuft and Bowman's capsule. Early adhesions, in turn, will impose markedly altered physical forces upon the involved capillary loop and its covering podocytes and thus initiate further podocyte damage, ultimately resulting in the development of a segmental sclerotic lesion. Another consequence of adhesion formation between the glomerular tuft and Bowman's capsule is a process termed 'misdirected filtration', that is, flow of plasma ultrafiltrate into the periglomerular and peritubular interstitium (Kriz *et al.* 2001), the consequences of which are discussed below. In the course of podocyte damage, the described changes occur in a heterogenous fashion. Whereas the early onset of FSGS particularly in juxtamedullary glomeruli (Rich 1957) may be explained by local haemodynamic conditions and/or tissue oxygenation, it is less clear why in the renal cortex glomerulosclerosis develops in a focal and segmental manner.

Compelling clinical evidence for this concept is derived from observations in the diabetic Pima Indian population (Pagtalunan 1997). Members of this Native American group which is susceptible to type 2 diabetic nephropathy have a reduction in podocyte number, so that each podocyte serves a larger glomerular surface area. More importantly, progression of diabetes to overt nephropathy is associated with a further decrement in podocyte numbers. Further evidence is derived from the clinical observations that patients with extreme glomerulomegaly as an adaption to nephron loss, be it congenital in oligomeganephronia (Elfenbein *et al.* 1974), or due to surgical resection of more than two-thirds of renal mass (Novick *et al.* 1991), or as a consequence of excessive obesity (Kambham *et al.* 2001), are prone to develop FSGS and subsequent renal failure.

As well as this rather mechanical view of the pathogenesis of FSGS, it is very likely that damage to podocytes will also alter their biochemical functions. Due to the difficulties of maintaining podocytes in culture, the biochemical consequences of mechanical stress on podocytes have only recently been studied (Endlich *et al.* 2001; Petermann et al. 2003). Given the role of podocytes in producing extracellular matrix proteins of the GBM (Torbohm *et al.* 1989; Floege *et al.* 1992), it is conceivable that mechanical strain of the podocytes leads to alterations in GBM turnover and/or composition. Furthermore, podocytes are potent producers of various cytokines *in vitro* and *in vivo*, including various PDGF chains, FGF-2, VEGF, heparin-binding epidermal growth factor-like growth factor (HB-EGF) and TGF-β (Takeuchi *et al.* 1992; Floege *et al.* 1993b; Simon *et al.* 1995; Shankland *et al.* 1996). Although the pathophysiological role of most of these cytokines in podocyte injury remains to be established, at least some, such as FGF-2, appear to contribute to the development of glomerulosclerosis (Floege *et al.* 1995).

Changes in the glomerular endothelium

The glomerular endothelial lining is a unique cellular structure given its large pores, which allow free access of plasma to the mesangium and the GBM on the one hand, but on the other hand normally prevents intracapillary coagulation, and cell adhesion. In a normal rat, about 1 per cent of the glomerular cells are renewed daily, of which about 80 per cent are endothelial cells (Pabst and Sterzel 1983), that is, individual cells exhibit a long half-life. Because of this long half-life of glomerular endothelial cells, manifestations of structural injury may be delayed and thus difficult to be ascribed to a particular injurious event. The picture is complicated further by the fact that under physiological conditions endothelial cells modify the behaviour of neighbouring cells, for example, by inhibiting the migration and proliferation of mesangial or smooth muscle cells (Casscells 1992; Morigi *et al.* 1993).

Early events

Early glomerular endothelial injury is a feature of many human diseases, including pre-eclampsia, HUS, lupus nephritis, most types of vasculitides, and many glomerulonephritides as well as renal transplant rejection (Ballerman 1997). Glomerular endothelial damage also characterizes a variety of conditions associated with glomerular hypertension and hyperperfusion (Rennke 1988).

The most dramatic consequence of glomerular endothelial injury is capillary thrombosis such as occurs in TMA (see Chapters 10.6.3 and 10.6.4). While the role of endothelial damage in glomerular thrombosis is obvious, its role in the early pathogenesis of glomerulosclerosis is less well understood. In several experimental models of progressive renal damage, the endothelium is the initial site of injury (Jaenke *et al.* 1993; Lee *et al.* 1995). For example, biochemical alterations of glomerular endothelial cell function have been detected early after 5/6 nephrectomy in the rat, when hypertension is already established but no sclerotic changes are yet present (Lee *et al.* 1995). It is likely that in these instances the acute alteration of intracapillary pressure and shear forces affects the normal endothelial phenotype. The glomerular endothelium may also suffer 'collateral damage' in instances where the primary injury is confined to the mesangium. Thus, in anti-Thy 1.1 nephritis, immune-mediated primary mesangial cell damage is accompanied by secondary glomerular capillary ballooning, microaneurysm formation, and loss of endothelial cells (Iruela-Arispe *et al.* 1995). Both direct and 'collateral' damage to the endothelium may result in excess endothelial apoptosis and the necessity for growth factor-dependent endothelial repair.

Adaptive and regenerative events

Even extensive damage to glomerular endothelial cells can be completely reversible and may not result in progressive renal disease (human examples include PSGN and HUS). Experimentally, glomerular repair following severe mesangiolytic and secondary glomerular endothelial damage includes enhanced endothelial cell proliferation as well as features of angiogenesis (Iruela-Arispe *et al.* 1995). This proliferative and antiapoptotic endothelial response appears to be driven in large part by the 165-isoform of VEGF (Ostendorf *et al.* 1999; Masuda *et al.* 2001), which is overexpressed in neighbouring mesangial cells during mesangial proliferative GN (Noguchi *et al.* 1998). Besides $VEGF_{165}$, the 121-isoform is also able to promote endothelial regeneration in thrombotic glomerular microangiopathy (Kim *et al.* 2000).

If complete restoration of the glomerular endothelium cannot be achieved, the consequence for the glomerulus may be dramatic. For example, only 4 days of specific $VEGF_{165}$ antagonism or inhibition of glomerular angiogenesis through the administration of cyclooxygenase-2 (COX-2) inhibitors during the early phase of experimental mesangial proliferative disease were sufficient to result in progressive renal failure within a few weeks (Ostendorf *et al.* 1999; Kitahara *et al.* 2002). In agreement with these experimental data, some clinical observations show that in HUS the extent of glomerular endothelial injury predicts the likelihood of loss of renal function (Morel-Maroger *et al.* 1979; Matsumae *et al.* 1996). Similarly, in hypertensive chronic renal damage, progressive glomerulosclerosis was associated with an excess of glomerular endothelial cell apoptosis (Kitamura *et al.* 1998).

'Downstream events' following glomerular damage

The increase in intraglomerular pressure and the proteinuria that accompany most progressive glomerular diseases appear to mediate, in part, the accompanying tubular and interstitial cell injury (Remuzzi and Bertani 1998). Unlike the selective proteinuria that occurs in the reversible renal damage in MCNS, non-selective proteinuria as observed in virtually all progressive glomerular diseases contains numerous substances that can activate tubular cells, such as cytokines, growth factors, lipids, iron proteins that can generate reactive oxygen species, and complement proteins that can be activated in the tubule (Remuzzi and Bertani 1998; Eddy 2001; Nangaku *et al.* 2002). The consequence is the appearance in the urine of either cellular debris embedded in proteinaceous casts (i.e. granular casts) or even renal cells with maintained phenotypic characteristics such as podocytes (Hara *et al.* 1998). Whether these casts and cell debris are also sufficient to mechanically block the tubular system is currently unknown. Another consequence of proteinuria is the development of tubulointerstitial cellular infiltrates and possibly even the breakdown of immunologic protection of the renal tubular system (Kurts *et al.* 2001).

In addition to proteinuria as a universal mediator of progressive tubulointerstitial damage, inflammatory mediators generated within the glomerulus can also effect 'downstream' events by acting in and around the peritubular capillaries (Fine *et al.* 2000). Of possible greater importance is the exit of inflammatory mediators into the periglomerular and peritubular interstitium via filtration through the glomerular mesangial stalk or as a consequence of 'misdirected filtration' (see above) in areas of adhesions between the glomerular tuft and Bowman's capsule (Kriz *et al.* 2001). Finally, 'downstream' damage to the renal microvasculature, for example, induced by transmission of increased blood pressure into the peritubular compartment, and the resulting hypoxia, have recently received attention as a mechanism contributing to progressive renal failure (Fine *et al.* 2000). The loss of tubulointerstitial microvasculature that results from a disturbed balance of angiogenic (e.g. vascular endothelial growth factor—VEGF) and antiangiogenic factors (e.g. thrombospondin-1) in the course of inflammatory renal changes has led to new therapeutic approaches in progressive renal failure, namely the stimulation of angiogenesis in the tubulointerstitial compartment with angiogenic mediators such as VEGF (Kang *et al.* 2002).

Final outcome of glomerular injury

Once the processes of glomerular injury so far described have run their course, there are a wide range of possible eventual outcomes (Figs 1 and 4). On the one hand, there may be complete resolution of glomerular disease without demonstrable functional or morphological consequences. On the other hand, there may be severe glomerulosclerosis (and tubulointerstitial fibrosis) leading sooner or later to renal failure. But in almost all glomerular diseases there will also be a proportion of patients who recover. In PSGN, for example, this proportion is very high; while in crescentic GN, in the absence of treatment, it is very low. Whilst, in general, it is true that the more severe the initial injury the less the likelihood of recovery, PSGN is a notable exception since an apparently severe acute glomerular inflammation can resolve with remarkable efficiency. It is this striking clinical observation that has led to the recent emphasis on the study of glomerular repair mechanisms which is described below.

However, at the present time we remain very ill-informed about the processes that predict, in any individual patient, whether resolution or scarring will predominate. Such predictive information would be of enormous value in clinical practice, not only in improving the accuracy of prognostication for individual patients, but also in informing decisions about the justification for intensive, and often relatively toxic, treatment regimens.

Can we promote glomerular repair?

Most experimental work in GN has concentrated on molecular and cellular mechanisms implicated in initiation and amplification of glomerular injury. From time to time, particularly in the more severe and acute forms of GN, the patient may present in these early stages of the disease process, and therapy can be directed at this phase of injury. More commonly, however, glomerular disease presents once it is well established, so the clinician is much more concerned with promoting resolution of injury and repair. Ideally, repair requires a number of processes to proceed in an integrated fashion to achieve restitution without irreversible injury. Infiltrating inflammatory cells must be removed from the glomerulus, as must injured intrinsic cells. This must then be followed by regeneration of intrinsic cells at an appropriate tempo, and removal of excess matrix restoring the normal balance of matrix production and breakdown (see Section 'What are the consequences of glomerular injury?'). All these processes must proceed at a tempo and efficiency that minimizes the risk that secondary mechanical and haemodynamic changes supervene, which produce systemic and glomerular hypertension and promote glomerulosclerosis. These mechanisms are discussed further in Chapter 11.1. Here we focus on the earlier phases of repair.

The power of these repair mechanisms allowing resolution of glomerular injury is nowhere more obvious than in the majority of cases of PSGN. Here, florid acute inflammation of glomeruli appears to resolve completely, at least as assessed by resolution of clinical abnormalities. Recent work has highlighted the importance of deletion of 'unwanted' cells from glomeruli as a key mechanism in the resolution of the glomerular response to injury.

Cellular kinetics and cell death in glomerular injury

Infiltration with leucocytes and increases in glomerular cell numbers are stereotyped features of inflammatory glomerular injury. For example, in PSGN there is marked infiltration with inflammatory myeloid leucocytes, mainly neutrophils and monocyte/macrophages. The vast majority of these leucocytes are likely to have been recruited by generation of chemoattractant complement fragments and local secretion of chemokines (Wada *et al.* 1994; Oda *et al.* 1997). There is also glomerular cell proliferation (Oda *et al.* 1997) with marked increases in glomerular endothelial cell and mesangial cell numbers (Ludwigsen and Sorensen 1978). Cell kinetics can be studied with some accuracy in PSGN since the clinical onset is usually well defined; glomerular endothelial cell proliferation predominates in the first week (Oda *et al.* 1997), and mesangial cell proliferation in the second and third weeks (Ludwigsen and Sorensen 1978). There is a rapid reduction in cell numbers as PSGN resolves, glomerular endothelial cell and mesangial cell numbers returning to normal by approximately 8 and 24 weeks, respectively (Ludwigsen and Sorensen 1978). Cessation in cell birth by mitosis is not sufficient to explain this, and there must be potent mechanisms for clearance of both leucocytes and excess resident glomerular cells as PSGN resolves.

Apoptosis

Apoptosis (programmed cell death), the physiologic means for safe deletion of unwanted or excess cells (Kerr *et al.* 1972; Wyllie *et al.* 1980), is a candidate mechanism for returning the glomerular cell complement to normal as PSGN and other 'proliferative' forms of glomerular injury resolve. The molecular programme that results in apoptotic cell death is now well defined (Wyllie 1997). Morphological appearances of apoptosis include condensation of cytoplasm and nuclear heterochromatin, cellular shrinkage with preservation of organelles, and in some cell lineages, active blebbing of the dying cell leading to reduction in cell volume by the release of membrane-bound apoptotic bodies. A key event is activation of cysteine proteases termed 'caspases' (because they cleave a variety of target proteins at aspartate residues). Caspases dismantle the cell (Salvesen and Dixit 1997; Thornberry *et al.* 1997; Thornberry and Lazebnik 1998), and by cleaving an inhibitor (Enari *et al.* 1998), also activate an endonuclease that leads to typical internucleosomal fragmentation of chromatin (so-called caspase-activated DNAse). This event can be detected in tissues by the TUNEL technique (Gavrielli *et al.* 1992), which detects DNA cleaved by endonucleases. There is increased TUNEL labelling in glomeruli in PSGN (Oda *et al.* 1997).

Importantly, apoptosis is much more than programmed cell death—it is a programme for swift and safe cell clearance. By contrast with accidental cell death or necrosis, in which proinflammatory release of injurious cell contents is inevitable, apoptosis *in vivo* almost invariably leads to recognition and rapid uptake by phagocytes of intact, membrane-bound apoptotic cells or bodies (Wyllie *et al.* 1980; Savill 1997). The phagocytes involved may be either the professional scavengers of the body, macrophages, or healthy neighbours acting as 'semi-professional' phagocytes when large numbers of apoptotic cells must be removed. Phagocytic clearance of apoptotic cells *in vivo* is highly efficient and remarkably rapid (Savill 1997).

Clearance of glomerular leucocytes

Neutrophils

Neutrophils are programmed to die by apoptosis and animal models of immune-mediated glomerular injury supported a role for granulocyte apoptosis in the resolution of glomerular injury. In nephrotoxic nephritis in rats, there is clear evidence of neutrophil apoptosis leading to clearance both by glomerular inflammatory macrophages and mesangial cells acting as semi-professional phagocytes (Savill *et al.* 1992). In the Concanavalin-A/anti-Con-A model of immune complex nephritis, in which brief accumulation of neutrophils is almost exclusively limited to the lumen of glomerular capillaries and resolves in about 24 h, there is histological evidence of neutrophil apoptosis and phagocytosis of apoptotic neutrophils by intraluminal macrophages, especially where neutrophils are 'trapped' in thrombosed capillary loops (Hughes *et al.* 1997a).

Histological studies may underestimate the quantitative significance of neutrophil clearance from glomeruli by apoptosis (Hughes *et al.* 1997a). When the fate of infused radiolabelled syngeneic neutrophils was followed during resolution of glomerular injury, about two-thirds of recruited neutrophils meeting their fate locally were no longer histologically detectable at 24 h, presumably because they were rapidly degraded by phagocytes: 50 per cent of detectable autoradiographic foci representing neutrophils retained at 24 h were inside macrophages.

Neutrophil deletion by apoptosis is likely to promote resolution of inflammatory glomerular injury. Neither macrophages nor mesangial cells taking up apoptotic neutrophils release proinflammatory mediators, such as eicosanoids (Meagher *et al.* 1992) or chemokines (Hughes *et al.* 1997b). Furthermore, deliberately activated macrophages receive an important 'anti-inflammatory' signal from ingesting apoptotic cells, which results in marked inhibition of the release of proinflammatory cytokines such as TNF-α; this signal is mediated, in part, by autocrine/paracrine effects of the anti-inflammatory cytokine TGF-β1 (Voll *et al.* 1977; Fadok *et al.* 1998). Therefore, deletion of neutrophils undergoing apoptosis via uptake by activated macrophages could be a key proresolution event in self-limited glomerular inflammation such as PSGN.

Monocyte/macrophages

Although freshly isolated blood monocytes are susceptible to apoptosis, maturation into macrophages coincides with development of resistance to many proapoptotic stimuli. Nevertheless, studies in a rat model of crescentic GN not only emphasize the proliferative capacity of extravasated cells of the monocyte lineage (Lan *et al.* 1993), but also demonstrate that monocyte/macrophages can undergo apoptosis *in situ* (Lan *et al.* 1997). Studies of the fate of labelled macrophages also have emphasized that, unlike neutrophils, emigration via the lymphatic vessels is the major route for removal of macrophages from inflamed sites (Bellingan *et al.* 1996) perhaps to undergo apoptosis in draining lymph nodes.

Cells of the monocyte/macrophage lineage migrating from inflamed sites might carry with them intracellular 'parcels' of inflammatory cells undergoing degradation after recognition as apoptotic. For example, in ConA/anti-ConA nephritis, occasional macrophages bearing radiolabelled foci (compatible with earlier uptake of dying neutrophils) were observed in hilar lymph nodes (Hughes *et al.* 1997a). In the lymph node, macrophage-like immature myeloid dendritic cells can ingest apoptotic cells and present certain antigens derived from the apoptotic 'meal' via both MHC Class I and Class II to CD8+ and CD4+ T lymphocytes, respectively (Alberts *et al.* 1998a,b; Inaba *et al.* 1998). This antigen presentation might promote tolerance rather than incite ongoing immune responses (Steinman *et al.* 2000).

Clearance of resident glomerular cells

Mesangial cells

In glomerular injury, mesangial cells adopt a myofibroblast-like phenotype, expressing α-smooth muscle actin (Johnson *et al.* 1991). In experimental nephritis, these cells are deleted from glomeruli by undergoing apoptosis (Baker *et al.* 1994; Shimizu *et al.* 1995), and phagocytosis, mainly by healthy neighbours (Baker *et al.* 1994). Some of the TUNEL-positive apoptotic cells identified in PSGN (Oda *et al.* 1997) may, therefore, represent mesangial cells. It will be important to define mechanisms regulating mesangial cell survival versus deletion by apoptosis (Table 10) since there is growing evidence that unscheduled and excessive mesangial cell apoptosis may favour progression to hypocellular, functionless scars. There is a negative feedback control—macrophage capacity to direct mesangial cell apoptosis is suppressed by the uptake of apoptotic cells—which should provide important regulation of mesangial cell number (Duffield *et al.* 2000).

Glomerular endothelial cells

Similarly, apoptosis may be an important counterbalance to mitosis in the regulation of glomerular endothelial cell number. There is evidence of (undesirable) endothelial cell apoptosis in progression to scarring of glomerular injury experimentally induced by nephrotoxic globulin (Shimizu *et al.* 1996, 1997). There is already good evidence that macrophages can dock onto and induce apoptosis in unwanted microvascular endothelial cells in the developing rodent eye (Lang *et al.* 1993; Duffield *et al.* 2000).

Deranged cell clearance and failed resolution

If apoptosis of infiltrating leucocytes and excess resident cells plays an important role in resolution then derangements in cell clearance by apoptosis could be critical in promoting the persistence of glomerular injury (Ren *et al.* 1998).

First, failed clearance of leucocytes undergoing apoptosis will result in secondary necrosis of non-ingested apoptotic cells and lead to direct tissue injury by noxious cell contents as well as to indirect exacerbation

Table 10 Stimuli reported to trigger mesangial cell apoptosis

Non-specific
Serum starvation
Detachment
Shear stress
Hydrostatic pressure
DNA damage
Reactive oxygen species
Ionizing radiation
Cytotoxic drugs
Specific
Anti-Thy 1.1 antibodies
Anti-Fas antibodies
TNF-α
IL-1α
IL-1β
C1q
Anti-ds DNA antibodies
LDL
Lovastatin
Nitric oxide
Superoxide
Cyclic AMP

TNF, tumour necrosis factor; IL-1, interleukin-1; LDL, low density lipoprotein.
Reviewed in Savill (1999).

Table 11 Possible approaches to promoting resolution of glomerular injury

Problem	Therapeutic aim	Approach
Leucocyte infiltration	Block recruitment Diminish activation Promote deletion	Block adhesion molecules; block chemokines Inhibit 'master' cytokines (TNF-α, IFNγ) Trigger leucocyte apoptosis: ?targeted Fas ligand
Excess glomerular cell proliferation	Block proliferation Promote deletion excess cells	Block PDGF, etc. Trigger glomerular cell apoptosis: ?targeted Fas ligand
Excess matrix deposition	Block matrix accumulation Promote matrix resorption	TGF β1 inhibitors; TIMP inhibitors Stimulate/supplement matrix metalloproteinases
Endothelial cell loss	Promote survival/proliferation	Administer VEGF or other angiogenic factors
Podocyte loss	Repopulate podocytes	Tissue engineering
Nephron loss	Repopulate nephron	Tissue engineering

of inflammatory injury due to macrophage secretion of proinflammatory mediators (Ren *et al.* 1998). Additionally, failure of macrophage clearance of apoptotic leucocytes bearing ingested antigens might allow such cells to be taken up by dendritic cells so that antigen is presented to T cells, setting up a persistent and potentially damaging immune response (Steinman *et al.* 2000). Although a number of cell surface recognition mechanisms ensure that macrophages can safely ingest apoptotic cells (reviewed in Savill 1997, 1998), recent data suggest that lectin-like functions of C1q, the first component of complement, are particularly important in binding apoptotic cells in glomeruli and 'bridging' them to C1q receptors on glomerular phagocytes (Korb *et al.* 1997; Botto *et al.* 1998). C1q 'knockout' mice spontaneously develop a lupus-like disorder with GN (Botto *et al.* 1998), as observed in C1q-deficient humans. These mice exhibit an excess of apoptotic cells in glomeruli consistent with diminished clearance and diminished capacity to clear labelled apoptotic cells administered to the more accessible inflamed peritoneum (Taylor *et al.* 2000). Therefore, diminished C1q-mediated clearance of apoptotic cells in glomerular injury could lead to persistent inflammatory injury, as a consequence of leakage of leucocyte contents and also presentation by dendritic cells of antigens derived from ingested apoptotic cells. Both these processes increase the risk of progressive scarring.

Second, progression to hypocellular scarring could ensue if clearance of excess resident cells by apoptosis was undesirably prolonged, as in the case of glomerular endothelial cell loss in progressive nephrotoxic nephritis in rats (Shimizu *et al.* 1997). Many possible stimuli could increase the rate of unscheduled glomerular cell loss by apoptosis (reviewed in Savill 1999). However, a unifying hypothesis is that failed clearance of apoptotic cells denies activated macrophages a crucially important anti-inflammatory signal, so that they continue to trigger apoptosis in resident cells, with the result that excess glomerular endothelial and mesangial cells are lost, and hypocellular scarring follows. Given the strictly limited regenerative potential of glomerular epithelial cells and the important structural consequences of their deletion (see above), it will also be important to determine whether and how unscheduled podocyte apoptosis might be triggered.

Therapeutic approaches to glomerular injury

In this chapter, we have described our rapidly growing understanding of the cellular processes and mechanisms of glomerular injury and repair. In principle, these insights offer many therapeutic opportunities to minimize injury and promote repair, provided that interventions can be timed correctly and targeted precisely. Until now, such focused interventions have not been available in clinical practice. Clinicians have relied on long-established treatments that interrupt many aspects of immune and inflammatory pathways with broad specificity, for example, glucocorticoids, cyclophosphamide, and plasma exchange, as well as treatment targeting the consequences of superimposed haemodynamic or metabolic damage, for example, ACE inhibitors and normalization of blood glucose.

More specific molecular approaches are now being developed and tested in animal models, although not yet widely available in the clinic. These approaches are summarized in Table 11. They include blocking leucocyte infiltration, minimizing intrinsic glomerular cell proliferation, promoting clearance of unwanted cells, restoring the balance of extracellular matrix deposition and removal, and avoiding excessive glomerular endothelial cell and podocyte loss.

Promotion of resolution through increased cell clearance

There is good evidence that apoptosis promotes resolution of inflammation, and that deranged cell clearance can perturb safe resolution. Furthermore, some drugs used to promote resolution of glomerular injury may act by enhancing safe clearance of glomerular cells by apoptosis. At least one beneficial effect of glucocorticoids in severe inflammatory glomerular injury may be to promote safe, anti-inflammatory phagocyte clearance of apoptotic cells.

There is also intense effort focused on defining so-called 'endogenous anti-inflammatory agents', of which activated glucocorticoids may be but one. For example, lipoxins and eicosanoids formed at inflamed sites by metabolism of arachodonic acid appear not only to have endogenous anti-inflammatory effects, halting neutrophil recruitment to inflamed sites, but also appear to have endogenous proresolution effects since they can promote macrophage clearance of apoptotic cells. Such agents have high potential for development into useful proresolution drugs.

References

Adu, D., Dobson, J., and Williams, D. G. (1981). DNA–antiDNA circulating immune complexes in the nephritis of systemic lupus erythematosus. *Clinical and Experimental Immunology* **43**, 605–614.

Alberts, M. L., Sauter, B., and Bhardwaj, N. (1998a). Dendritic cells acquire antigen from apoptotic cells and induce class I-restricted CTLs. *Nature* **392**, 86–89.

Alberts, M. L. *et al.* (1998b). Immature dendritic cells phagocytose apoptotic cells via $\alpha_v\beta_5$ and CD36 and cross-present antigens to cytotoxic T lymphocytes. *Journal of Experimental Medicine* **188**, 1359–1368.

Allen, A. C. (1999). Analysis of IgA1 O-glycans in IgA nephropathy by fluorophore-assisted carbohydrate electrophoresis. *Journal of the American Society of Nephrology* **10**, 1763.

Allen, A. C. (2001). Mesangial IgA1 in IgA nephropathy exhibits aberrant O-glycosylation. *Kidney International* **60**, 969.

Anderson, M. S. *et al.* (2002). Projection of an immunological self shadow within the thymus by the Aire protein. *Science* **298**, 1395–1401.

Atkins, R. C. *et al.* (1996). Modulators of crescentic glomerulonephritis. *Journal of the American Society of Nephrology* **7**, 2271–2278.

Baker, A. J. *et al.* (1994). Mesangial cell apoptosis: the major mechanism for resolution of glomerular hypercellularity in experimental mesangial proliferative glomerulonephritis. *Journal of Clinical Investigation* **94**, 2105–2116.

Ballerman, B. J. Endothelial responses to immune injury. In *Immunologic Renal Disease* (ed. E. G. Neilson and W. G. Couser), pp. 627–654. Philadelphia: Lippincott-Raven, 1997.

Barisoni, L. *et al.* (1999). The dysregulated podocyte phenotype: a novel concept in the pathogenesis of collapsing idiopathic focal segmental glomerulosclerosis and HIV-associated nephropathy. *Journal of the American Society of Nephrology* **10**, 51–61.

Bellingan, G. J. *et al.* (1996). *In vivo* fate of the inflammatory macrophage during the resolution of inflammation: inflammatory macrophages do not die locally but emigrate to the draining lymph nodes. *Journal of Immunology* **157**, 2577–2585.

Berden, J. H. (1997). Lupus nephritis. *Kidney International* **52**, 538–558.

Berden, J. H., Grootscholten, C., Jurgen, W. C., and van der Vlag, J. (2002). Lupus nephritis: a nucleosome waste disposal defect? *Journal of Nephrology* **15** (Suppl. 6), S1–S10.

Border, W. A. (1994). Transforming growth factor-beta and the pathogenesis of glomerular diseases. *Current Opinion in Nephrology and Hypertension* **3**, 54–58.

Botto, M. *et al.* (1998). Homozygous C1q deficiency causes glomerulonephritis associated with multiple apoptotic bodies. *Nature Genetics* **19**, 56–59.

Boute, N. *et al.* (2000). NHPS2, encoding the glomerular protein, podocin, is mutated in autosomal recessive steroid-resistant nephrotic syndrome. *Nature Genetics* **24**, 349–354.

Brenner, B. M. and Mackenzie, H. S. (1997). Nephron mass as a risk factor for progression of renal disease. *Kidney International* **63** (Suppl.), S124–S127.

Bruggeman, L. A. *et al.* (2000). Renal epithelium is a previously unrecognised site of HIV-1 infection. *Journal of the American Society of Nephrology* **11**, 2079–2087.

Casadevall, N. *et al.* (2002). Pure red-cell aplasia and antierythropoietin antibodies in patients treated with recombinant erythropoietin. *New England Journal of Medicine* **346**, 469–475.

Casscells, W. (1992). Migration of smooth muscle and endothelial cells. Critical events in restenosis. *Circulation* **86**, 723–729.

Collins, A., Andres, G., and McCuskey, R. (1981). Lack of evidence for a role of renal tubular antigen in human membranous glomerulonephritis. *Nephron* **27**, 297–301.

Couchman, J. R., Beavan, L. A., and McCarthy, K. J. (1994). Glomerular matrix: synthesis, turnover and role in mesangial expansion. *Kidney International* **45**, 328–335.

Couser, W. G. and Salant, D. J. (1980). *In situ* immune complex formation and glomerular injury. *Kidney International* **17**, 1–13.

Dantal, J. *et al.* (1994). Effect of plasma protein adsorption on protein excretion in kidney-transplant recipients with recurrent nephrotic syndrome. *New England Journal of Medicine* **330**, 7–14.

Davies, M. (1994). The mesangial cell: a tissue culture view. *Kidney International* **45**, 320–327.

Davies, M. *et al.* (1992). Proteinases and glomerular matrix turnover. *Kidney International* **41**, 671–678.

Debiec, H. *et al.* (2002). Antenatal membranous glomerulonephritis due to anti-neutral endopeptidase (NEP) antibodies. *New England Journal of Medicine* **346**, 2053–2060.

Diez Roux, G. and Lang, R. A. (1997). Macrophages induce apoptosis in normal cells *in vivo*. *Development* **124**, 3633–3641.

Duffield, J. S. *et al.* (2000). Activated macrophages direct apoptosis and suppress mitosis of mesangial cells. *Journal of Immunology* **164**, 2110–2119.

Eddy, A. (2001). Role of cellular infiltrates in response to proteinuria. *American Journal of Kidney Diseases* **37** (1 Suppl. 2), S25–S29.

Elfenbein, I. B., Baluarte, H. J., and Gruskin, A. B. (1974). Renal hypoplasia with oligomeganephronia: light, electron, fluorescent microscopic and quantitative studies. *Archives of Pathology* **97**, 143–149.

Enari, M. *et al.* (1998). A caspase-activated DNase that degrades DNA during apoptosis and its inhibitor ICAD. *Nature* **39**, 43–50.

Endlich, N. *et al.* (2001). Podocytes respond to mechanical stress *in vitro*. *Journal of the American Society of Nephrology* **12**, 413–422.

Eng, E. *et al.* (1994). Does extracellular matrix expansion in glomerular disease require mesangial cell proliferation? *Kidney International* **45** (Suppl.), S45–S47.

Fadok, V. A. *et al.* (1997). Immunosuppressive effects of apoptotic cells. *Nature* **390**, 350–351.

Fine, L. G., Bandyopadhay, D., and Norman, J. T. (2000). Is there a common mechanism for the progression of different types of renal diseases other than proteinuria? Towards the unifying theme of chronic hypoxia. *Kidney International* **75** (Suppl.), S22–S26.

Floege, J. and Johnson, R. J. (1995). Multiple roles for platelet-derived growth factor in renal disease. *Mineral and Electrolyte Metabolism* **21**, 271–282.

Floege, J. *et al.* (1991). Increased synthesis of extracellular matrix in mesangial proliferative nephritis. *Kidney International* **40**, 477–488.

Floege, J. *et al.* (1992). Altered glomerular extracellular matrix synthesis in experimental membranous nephropathy. *Kidney International* **42**, 573–585.

Floege, J. *et al.* (1993a). Infusion of platelet-derived growth factor or basic fibroblast growth factor induces selective glomerular mesangial cell proliferation and matrix accumulation in rats. *Journal of Clinical Investigation* **92**, 2952–2962.

Floege, J. *et al.* (1993b). Visceral glomerular epithelial cells can proliferate *in vivo* and synthesize platelet-derived growth factor B-chain. *American Journal of Pathology* **142**, 637–650.

Floege, J. *et al.* (1995). Basic fibroblast growth factor augments podocyte injury and induces glomerulosclerosis in rats with experimental membranous nephropathy. *Journal of Clinical Investigation* **96**, 2809–2819.

Floege, J. *et al.* (1999). A novel approach to specific growth factor inhibition *in vivo*: antagonism of PDGF in glomerulonephritis by aptamers. *American Journal of Pathology* **154**, 169–179.

Fogo, A. *et al.* (1990). Glomerular hypertrophy in minimal change disease predicts subsequent progression to focal segmental glomerulosclerosis. *Kidney International* **38**, 115–123.

Friedman, J. *et al.* (1984). Immunological studies of post-streptococcal sequelae: evidence for the presence of streptococcal antigens in circulating immune complexes. *Journal of Clinical Investigation* **74**, 1027–1034.

Gallucci, S. and Matzinger, P. (2001). Danger signals: SOS to the immune system. *Current Opinion in Immunology* **13**, 114–119.

Gavrielli, Y., Sherman, Y., and Ben-Sasson, S. A. (1992). Identification of programmed cell death *in situ* via specific labelling of nuclear DNA fragmentation. *Journal of Cell Biology* **119**, 493–501.

Gharavi, A. G. *et al.* (2000). IgA nephropathy, the most common cause of glomerulonephritis, is linked to 6q22-23. *Nature Genetics* **26**, 354–357.

Hara, M. *et al.* (1998). Urinary excretion of podocytes reflects disease activity in children with glomerulonephritis. *American Journal of Nephrology* **18** (1), 35–41.

Hebert, L. A. *et al.* Complement and complement regulatory proteins in renal disease. In *Immunologic Renal Disease* (ed. W. G. Couser and E. G. Neilson), pp. 367–394. Philadelphia: Lippincott, Williams & Wilkins, 2001.

Hiki, Y. *et al.* (1996). Association of asialo-galactosylβ1-3*N*-acetylgalactosamine on the hinge with a conformational instability of jacalin-reactive immunoglobulin A1 in immunoglobulin A nephropathy. *Journal of the American Society of Nephrology* **7**, 955.

Hiki, Y. *et al.* (1998). Analyses of IgA1 hinge glycopeptides in IgA nephropathy by matrix-assisted laser desorption/ionization time-of-flight mass spectrometry. *Journal of the American Society of Nephrology* **9**, 577.

Hiki, Y. *et al.* (2001). Mass spectrometry proves underglycosylation of glomerular IgA1 in IgA nephropathy. *Kidney International* **59**, 1077.

Hsu, S. I. *et al.* (2000). Evidence for genetic factors in the development and progression of IgA nephropathy. *Kidney International* **57**, 1818–1835.

Hughes, J. *et al.* (1997a). Neutrophil fate in experimental glomerular capillary injury in the rat: emigration exceeds *in situ* clearance by apoptosis. *American Journal of Pathology* **150**, 223–234.

Hughes, J. *et al.* (1997b). Human glomerular mesangial cell phagocytosis of apoptotic cells is mediated by a CD36-independent vitronectin receptor/thrombospondin recognition mechanism. *Journal of Immunology* **158**, 4389–4397.

Hugo, C. *et al.* (1997). Extraglomerular origin of the mesangial cell after injury. A new role of the juxtaglomerular apparatus. *Journal of Clinical Investigation* **100** (4), 786–794.

Huh, W. *et al.* (2002). Expression of nephrin in acquired human glomerular disease. *Nephrology, Dialysis, Transplantation* **17**, 478–484.

Inaba, K. S. *et al.* (1998). Efficient presentation of phagocytosed cellular fragments on the major histocompatibility complex class II products of dendritic cells. *Journal of Experimental Medicine* **188**, 2163–2173.

Iruela-Arispe, L. *et al.* (1995). Participation of glomerular endothelial cells in the capillary repair of glomerulonephritis. *American Journal of Pathology* **147**, 1715–1727.

Jaenke, R. S. *et al.* (1993). Capillary endothelium. Target site of renal radiation injury. *Laboratory Investigation* **68**, 396–405.

Johnson, R. J. (1997). Have we ignored the role of oncotic pressure in the pathogenesis of glomerulosclerosis? *American Journal of Kidney Diseases* **29**, 147–152.

Johnson, R. J. and Couser, W. G. (1990). Hepatitis B infection and renal disease: clinical, imunopathogenetic and therapeutic considerations. *Kidney International* **37**, 663–676.

Johnson, R. J. *et al.* (1991). Expression of smooth muscle cell phenotype by rat mesangial cells in immune complex nephritis. *Journal of Clinical Investigation* **87**, 847–858.

Kambham, N. *et al.* (2001). Obesity-related glomerulopathy: an emerging epidemic. *Kidney International* **59**, 1498–1509.

Kang, D. H. *et al.* (2002). Role of the microvascular endothelium in progressive renal disease. *Journal of the American Society of Nephrology* **13**, 806–816.

Kaplan, J. M. *et al.* (2000). Mutations in ACTN4, encoding alpha-actinin-4, cause familial focal segmental glomerulosclerosis. *Nature Genetics* **24**, 251–256.

Kashtan, C. E. (2000). Alport syndrome: renal transplantation and donor selection. *Renal Failure* **22**, 765–768.

Kerjaschki, D. and Neale, T. J. (1996). Molecular mechanisms of glomerular injury in in rat experimental membranous nephropathy (Heymann nephritis). *Journal of the American Society of Nephrology* **7**, 2518–2526.

Kerr, J. F. R., Wyllie, A. H., and Currie, A. R. (1972). Apoptosis: a basic biological phenomenon with widespread implications in tissue kinetics. *British Journal of Cancer* **26**, 239–257.

Kestila, M. *et al.* (1998). Positionally cloned gene for a novel glomerular protein-nephrin is mutated in congenital nephrotic syndrome. *Molecular Cell Biology* **1**, 575–582.

Khoshnoodi, J. and Tryggvason, K. (2001). Unraveling the molecular make-up of the glomerular podocyte slit diaphragm. *Experimental Nephrology* **9**, 355–359.

Kim, B. K. *et al.* (2002). Differential expression of nephrin in acquired human proteinuric diseases. *American Journal of Kidney Diseases* **40**, 964.

Kim, Y. G. *et al.* (2000). Vascular endothelial growth factor accelerates renal recovery in experimental thrombotic microangiopathy. *Kidney International* **58**, 2390–2399.

Kitahara, M. *et al.* (2002). Selective cyclooxygenase-2 inhibition impairs glomerular capillary healing in experimental glomerulonephritis. *Journal of the American Society of Nephrology* **13** (5), 1473–1480.

Kitamura, H. *et al.* (1998). Apoptosis in glomerular endothelial cells during the development of glomerulosclerosis in the remnant-kidney model. *Experimental Nephrology* **6**, 328–336.

Kokubo, T. *et al.* (1998). Protective role of IgA1 glycans against IgA1 self-aggregation and adhesion to extracellular matrix proteins. *Journal of the American Society of Nephrology* **9**, 2048.

Kokubo, T. *et al.* (2000). Humoral immunity against the proline-rich peptide epitope of the IgA1 hinge region in IgA nephropathy. *Nephrology, Dialysis, Transplantation* **15**, 28.

Kopp, J. B. *et al.* (1992). Progressive glomerulosclerosis and enhanced renal accumulation of basement membrane components in mice transgenic for human immunodeficiency virus type 1 genes. *Proceedings of the National Academy of Sciences of the USA* **89**, 1577–1581.

Korb, L. C. and Ahearn, J. M. (1997). C1q binds directly and specifically to surface blebs of apoptotic human keratinocytes. *Journal of Immunology* **158**, 4525–4528.

Koyama, A. *et al.* (1991). A glomerular permeability factor produced by human T cell hybridomas. *Kidney International* **40**, 453–460.

Kriz, W. R. (1996). Progressive renal failure—inability of podocytes to replicate and the consequences for development of glomerulosclerosis. *Nephrology, Dialysis, Transplantation* **11**, 1738–1742.

Kriz, W., Gretz, N., and Lemley, K. V. (1998). Progression of glomerular diseases: is the podocyte the culprit? *Kidney International* **54** (3), 687–697.

Kriz, W. *et al.* (1995). Long-term treatment of rats with FGF-2 results in focal segmental glomerulosclerosis. *Kidney International* **48**, 1435–1450.

Kriz, W. *et al.* (2001). Tracer studies in the rat demonstrate misdirected filtration and peritubular filtrate spreading in nephrons with segmental glomerulosclerosis. *Journal of the American Society of Nephrology* **12**, 496–506.

Kriz, W. *et al.* (2003). Pathways to recovery and nephron loss in anti-Thy-1 nephritis. *Journal of the American Society of Nephrology* **14** (7), 1904–1926.

Kurts, C. *et al.* (2001). Kidney protection against autoreactive CD8(+) T cells distinct from immunoprivilege and sequestration. *Kidney International* **60**, 664–671.

Lai, K. N. *et al.* (1996). Detection of hepatitis B virus DNA and RNA in kidneys of HBV related glomerulonephritis. *Kidney International* **50**, 1965–1977.

Lan, H. Y., Nikolic-Paterson, D. J., and Atkins, R. C. (1993). Trafficking of inflammatory macrophages from the kidney to draining lymph nodes during experimental glomerulonephritis. *Clinical and Experimental Immunology* **92**, 336–341.

Lan, H. Y. *et al.* (1997). Macrophage apoptosis in rat crescentic glomerulonephritis. *American Journal of Pathology* **151**, 531–538.

Lang, R. A. and Bishop, J. M. (1993). Macrophages are required for cell death and tissue remodeling in the developing mouse eye. *Cell* **74**, 453–462.

Lee, L. K. *et al.* (1995). Endothelial cell injury initiates glomerular sclerosis in the rat remnant kidney. *Journal of Clinical Investigation* **96**, 953–964.

Lehmann, R. and Schleicher, E. D. (2000). Molecular mechanism of diabetic nephropathy. *Clinica Chimica Acta* **297**, 135–144.

Ludwigsen, E. and Sorensen, F. H. (1978). Post-streptococcal glomerulonephritis: a quantitative glomerular investigation. *Acta Pathologica Microbiologica Scandinavica* **86**, 319–324.

Luimula, P. *et al.* (2000). Nephrin in experimental glomerular disease. *Kidney International* **58**, 1461–1468.

Masuda, Y. *et al.* (2001). Vascular endothelial growth factor enhances glomerular capillary repair and accelerates resolution of experimentally induced glomerulonephritis. *American Journal of Pathology* **159**, 599–608.

Matsumae, T., Takebayashi, S., and Naito, S. (1996). The clinico-pathological characteristics and outcome in hemolytic–uremic syndrome of adults. *Clinical Nephrology* **45**, 153–162.

Mauer, S. M. *et al.* (1973). The glomerular mesangium III: acute mesangial injury: a new model of glomerulonephritis. *Journal of Experimental Medicine* **137**, 553–570.

Meagher, L. C. *et al.* (1992). Phagocytosis of apoptotic neutrophils does not induce macrophage release of thromboxane B2. *Journal of Leukocyte Biology* **52**, 269–273.

Mene, P., Pugliese, F., and Cinotti, G. A. (1996). Adhesion of U-937 monocytes induces cytotoxic damage and subsequent proliferation of cultured human mesangial cells. *Kidney International* **50**, 417–423.

Mene, P., Simonson, M. S., and Dunn, M. J. (1989). Physiology of the mesangial cell. *Physiological Reviews* **69** (4), 1347–1424.

Morel-Maroger, L. *et al.* (1979). Prognostic importance of vascular lesions in acute renal failure with microangiopathic hemolytic anemia (hemolytic–uremic syndrome): clinicopathologic study in 20 adults. *Kidney International* **15**, 548–558.

Morgan, B. P. (2000). The complement system: an overview. *Methods in Molecular Biology* **150**, 1–13.

Morigi, M. *et al.* (1993). Supernatant of endothelial cells exposed to laminar flow inhibits mesangial cell proliferation. *American Journal of Physiology* **264**, C1080–C1083.

Morita, T. and Churg, J. (1983). Mesangiolysis. *Kidney International* **24**, 1–9.

Mundel, P., Schwarz, K., and Reiser, J. (2001). Podocyte biology: a footstep further. *Advances in Nephrology, Necker Hospital* **31**, 235–241.

Nagata, M. *et al.* (1995). Mitosis and the presence of binucleate cells among glomerular podocytes in diseased human kidneys. *Nephron* **70**, 68–71.

Nagata, M. *et al.* (1998). Cell cycle regulation and differentiation in the human podocyte lineage. *American Journal of Pathology* **153**, 1511–1520.

Nangaku, M. (1998). Complement regulatory proteins in glomerular diseases. *Kidney International* **54**, 1419–1428.

Nangaku, M., Pippin, J., and Couser, W. G. (2002). C6 mediates chronic progression of tubulointerstitial damage in rats with remnant kidneys. *Journal of the American Society of Nephrology* **13**, 928–936.

Nelson, P. J., Segerer, S., and Schlondorff, D. Chemoattractants and chemokines in renal disease. In *Immunologic Renal Disease* (ed. W. G. Couser and E. G. Neilson), pp. 521–550. Philadelphia: Lippincott, Williams & Wilkins, 2001a.

Nelson, P. J., Gelman, I. H., and Klotman, P. E. (2001b). Suppression of HIV-1 expression by cyclin-dependent kinases promotes differentiation of infected podocytes. *Journal of the American Society of Nephrology* **12**, 2827–2831.

Noguchi, K. *et al.* (1998). Activated mesangial cells produce vascular permeability factor in early-stage mesangial proliferative glomerulonephritis. *Journal of the American Society of Nephrology* **9**, 1815–1825.

Nordstrand, A., Norgren, M., and Holm, S. E. (1999). Pathogenic mechanism of acute post-streptococcal glomerulonephritis. *Scandinavian Journal of Infectious Diseases* **31**, 523–537.

Novick, A. C. *et al.* (1991). Long-term follow-up after partial removal of a solitary kidney. *New England Journal of Medicine* **325**, 1058–1062.

Oda, T. *et al.* (1997). Glomerular proliferating cell kinetics in acute post-streptococcal glomerulonephritis (APSGN). *Journal of Pathology* **183**, 359–368.

O'Donoghue, D. J., Darvill, A., and Ballardie, F. W. (1991). Mesangial cell autoantigens in immunoglobulin A nephropathy and Henoch–Schönlein purpura. *Journal of Clinical Investigation* **88**, 1522–1530.

Oikawa, T. *et al.* (1997). Modulation of plasminogen activator inhibitor-1 *in vivo*: a new mechanism for the anti-fibrotic effect of renin–angiotensin inhibition. *Kidney International* **5**, 164–172.

Ostendorf, T. *et al.* (1999). Vascular endothelial growth factor (VEGF165) mediates glomerular endothelial repair. *Journal of Clinical Investigation* **104** (7), 913–923.

Ostendorf, T. *et al.* (2001). Specific antagonism of PDGF prevents renal scarring in experimental glomerulonephritis. *Journal of the American Society of Nephrology* **12**, 909–918.

Pabst, R. and Sterzel, R. B. (1983). Cell renewal of glomerular cell types in normal rats. An autoradiographic analysis. *Kidney International* **24**, 626–631.

Pagtalunan, M. E. (1997). Podocyte loss and progressive glomerular injury in type II diabetes. *Journal of Clinical Investigation* **99**, 342–348.

Perry, G. J. *et al.* (1993). Antiendothelial cell antibodies in lupus: correlations with renal injury and circulating markers of endothelial damage. *Quarterly Journal of Medicine* **86**, 727–734.

Petermann, A. T. (2002). Mechanical stress reduces podocyte proliferation *in vitro*. *Kidney International* **61**, 40–50.

Petermann, A. T. *et al.* (2003). Mitotic cell cycle proteins increase in podocytes despite lack of proliferation. *Kidney International* **63**, 113–122.

Peters, H., Noble, N. A., and Border, W. A. (1997). Transforming growth factor-beta in human glomerular injury. *Current Opinion in Nephrology and Hypertension* **6**, 389–393.

Phelps, R. G. and Rees, A. J. Immunogenetics of renal disease. In *Immunologic Renal Disease* (ed. W. G. Couser and E. G. Neilson), pp. 105–138. Philadelphia: Lippincott, Williams & Wilkins, 2001.

Reckelhoff, J. F. and Baylis, C. (1993). Glomerular metalloprotease activity in the aging rat kidney: inverse correlation with injury. *Journal of the American Society of Nephrology* **3**, 1835–1838.

Remuzzi, G. and Bertani, T. (1998). Pathophysiology of progressive nephropathies. *New England Journal of Medicine* **339**, 1448–1456.

Ren, Y. and Savill, J. (1998). Apoptosis: the importance of being eaten. *Cell Death & Differentiation* **5**, 563–568.

Rennke, H. G. (1988). Glomerular adaptations to renal injury or ablation. Role of capillary hypertension in the pathogenesis of progressive glomerulosclerosis. *Blood Purification* **6**, 230–239.

Rennke, H. G. and Klein, P. S. (1989). Pathogenesis and significance of non-primary focal and segmental glomerulosclerosis. *American Journal of Kidney Diseases* **13**, 443–456.

Rich, A. R. (1957). A hitherto undescribed vulnerability of the juxtamedullary glomeruli in lipoid nephrosis. *Bulletins of the Johns Hopkins Hospital* **100**, 173–186.

Ruggenenti, P., Noris, M., and Remuzzi, G. (2001). Thrombotic microangiopathy, haemolytic uremic syndrome, and thrombotic thrombocytopenic purpura. *Kidney International* **60**, 831–846.

Sabry, A. A. *et al.* (2002). A comprehensive study of the association between hepatitis C virus and glomerulopathy. *Nephrology, Dialysis, Transplantation* **17**, 239–245.

Saito, Y. *et al.* (1988). Mesangiolysis in diabetic glomeruli: its role in the formation of nodular lesions. *Kidney International* **34**, 389–396.

Salvesen, G. S. and Dixit, V. M. (1977). Caspases: intracellular signalling by proteolysis. *Cell* **91**, 443–446.

Savill, J. (1997). Recognition and phagocytosis of cells undergoing apoptosis. *British Medical Bulletin* **53**, 1–18.

Savill, J. (1998). Apoptosis: phagocytic docking without shocking. *Nature* **392**, 442–443.

Savill, J. (1999). Regulation of glomerular cell number by apoptosis. *Kidney International* **56**, 1216–1222.

Savill, J. S. *et al.* (1992). Glomerular mesangial cells and inflammatory macrophages ingest neutrophils undergoing apoptosis. *Kidney International* **42**, 924–936.

Savin, V. J. *et al.* (1995). Circulating factor associated with increased glomerular permeability to albumin in recurrent focal segmental glomerulosclerosis. *New England Journal of Medicine* **334**, 878–883.

Schocklmann, H. O., Lang, S., and Sterzel, R. B. (1999). Regulation of mesangial cell proliferation. *Kidney International* **56**, 1199–1207.

Shalhoub, R. J. (1974). Pathogenesis of lipoid nephrosis: a disorder of T-cell function. *Lancet* **2**, 556–560.

Shankland, S. J. (1999). Cell cycle regulatory proteins in glomerular disease. *Kidney International* **56**, 1208–1215.

Shankland, S. J. and Wolf, G. (2000). Cell cycle regulatory proteins in renal disease: role in hypertrophy, proliferation, and apoptosis. *American Journal of Physiology. Renal Physiology* **278**, F515–F529.

Shankland, S. J. *et al.* (1996). Differential expression of transforming growth factor-beta isoforms and receptors in experimental membranous nephropathy. *Kidney International* **50**, 116–124.

Shankland, S. J. *et al.* (1997). Cyclin kinase inhibitors are increased during experimental membranous nephropathy: potential role in limiting glomerular epithelial cell proliferation *in vivo*. *Kidney International* **52**, 404–413.

Sheerin, N. S. *et al.* (2001). Protection and injury: the differing roles of complement in the development of glomerular injury. *European Journal of Immunology* **31**, 1255–1260.

Shimizu, A. *et al.* (1995). Apoptosis in the repair process of experimental proliferative glomerulonephritis. *Kidney International* **47**, 114–121.

Shimizu, A. *et al.* (1996). Apoptosis in progressive crescentic glomerulonephritis. *Laboratory Investigation* **74**, 941–951.

Shimizu, A. *et al.* (1997). Rare glomerular capillary regeneration and subsequent capillary regression with endothelial cell apoptosis in progressive glomerulonephritis. *American Journal of Pathology* **151**, 1231–1239.

Shull, M. M. *et al.* (1992). Targeted disruption of the mouse transforming growth factor-beta 1 gene results in multifocal inflammatory disease. *Nature* **359**, 693–699.

Simon, M. *et al.* (1995). Expression of vascular endothelial growth factor and its receptors in human renal ontogenesis and in adult kidney. *American Journal of Physiology* **268**, F240–F250.

Stahl, R. A. *et al.* (1992). A rat model of progressive chronic glomerular sclerosis: the role of thromboxane inhibition. *Journal of the American Society of Nephrology* **2**, 1568–1577.

Steinman, R. M. *et al.* (2000). The induction of tolerance by dendritic cells that have captured apoptotic cells. *Journal of Experimental Medicine* **191**, 411–416.

Sterzel, R. B., Schulze-Lohoff, E., and Marx, M. (1993). Cytokines and mesangial cells. *Kidney International* **39** (Suppl.), S26–S31.

Striker, L. J. *et al.* (1991). Mesangial cell turnover: effect of heparin and peptide growth factors. *Laboratory Investigation* **64**, 446–456.

Takeuchi, A. *et al.* (1992). Basic fibroblast growth factor promotes proliferation of rat glomerular visceral epithelial cells *in vitro*. *American Journal of Pathology* **141**, 107–116.

Taylor, C. M. (2001). Complement factor H and the haemolytic uraemic syndrome. *Lancet* **358**, 1200–1202.

Taylor, P. R. *et al.* (2000). A hierarchial role for classical pathway complement proteins in the clearance of apoptotic cells *in vivo*: a mechanism for protection against autoimmunity. *Journal of Experimental Medicine* **19**, 359–366.

Thornberry, N. A. and Lazebnik, Y. (1998). Caspases: enemies within. *Science* **281**, 1312–1316.

Thornberry, N. A., Rosen, A., and Nicholson, D. W. (1997). Control of apoptosis by proteases. *Advances in Pharmacology* **41**, 155–177.

Tomai, M. *et al.* (1990). Superantigenicity of streptococcal M protein. *Journal of Experimental Medicine* **172**, 359–362.

Tomana, M. *et al.* (1999). Circulating immune complexes in IgA nephropathy consist of IgA1 with galactose-deficient hinge region and antiglycan antibodies. *Journal of Clinical Investigation* **104**, 73.

Topham, P. S. *et al.* (1999). Nephritogenic mAb 5-1-6 is directed at the extracellular domain of rat nephrin. *Journal of Clinical Investigation* **104**, 1559–1566.

Torbohm, I. *et al.* (1989). Modulation of collagen synthesis in human glomerular epithelial cells by interleukin 1. *Clinical Experimental Immunology* **75**, 427–431.

Vilafranca, M. *et al.* (1994). Histological and immunohistological classification of canine glomerular disease. *Zentralbl Veterinarmed A* **41**, 599–610.

Voll, R. E. *et al.* (1977). Immunosuppressive effects of apoptotic cells. *Nature* **390**, 350–351.

Wada, T. *et al.* (1994). Detection of urinary interleukin-8 in glomerular diseases. *Kidney International* **46**, 455–460.

Welch, T. R. (2001). The complement system in renal diseases. *Nephron* **88**, 199–204.

Winfield, J. F., Faiferman, I., and Koffler, D. (1977). Avidity of anti-DNA antibodies in serum and glomerular eluates from patients with systemic lupus erythematosus. *Journal of Clinical Investigation* **59**, 90–96.

Winn, M. P. (2002). Not all in the family: mutations of podocin in sporadic steroid-resistant nephritic syndrome. *Journal of the American Society of Nephrology* **13**, 577–579.

Wilson, C. B. Immune models of glomerular injury. In *Immunologic Renal Disease* (ed. W. G. Couser and E. G. Neilson), pp. 711–778. Philadelphia: Lippincott, Williams & Wilkins, 2001.

Winston, J. A. *et al.* (2001). Nephropathy and establishment of a renal reservoir of HIV type 1 during primary infection. *New England Journal of Medicine* **344**, 1979–1984.

Wong, D., Phelps, R. G., and Turner, A. N. (2001). The Goodpasture antigen is expressed in the human thymus. *Kidney International* **60**, 1777–1783.

Wucherpfennig, K. W. (2001). Mechanisms for the induction of autoimmunity by infectious agents. *Journal of Clinical Investigation* **108**, 1097–1104.

Wyllie, A. H. (1997). Apoptosis: an overview. *British Medical Bulletin* **53**, 451–465.

Wyllie, A. H., Kerr, J. F. R., and Currie, A. R. (1980). Cell death: the significance of apoptosis. *International Reviews in Cytology* **68**, 251–306.

Xiao, H. *et al.* (2002). Antineutrophil cytoplasmic autoantibodies specific for myeloperoxidase cause glomerulonephritis and vasculitis in mice. *Journal of Clinical Investigation* **110**, 955–963.

Yamamoto, T. *et al.* (1994). Sustained expression of TGF-beta 1 underlies development of progressive kidney fibrosis. *Kidney International* **45**, 916–927.

Yang, Y. A. *et al.* (2002). Lifetime exposure to a soluble TGF-beta antagonist protects mice against metastasis without adverse side effects. *Journal of Clinical Investigation* **109**, 1607–1615.

Yoshizawa, N. *et al.* (1992). Role of a streptococcal antigen in the pathogenesis of acute poststreptococcal glomerulonephritis. *Journal of Immunology* **148**, 3110–3116.

3.3 The patient with proteinuria and/or haematuria

J. Stewart Cameron

Haematuria and/or proteinuria *without symptoms* have become a common presentation for renal diseases since simple and rapid 'stix' testing became widely available. Urine is tested routinely during medical consultations for any complaint, during pregnancy, during insurance examinations, and on entry into many forms of employment such as the armed forces. In some countries such as Japan, Korea, and Taiwan there is routine urine testing of all schoolchildren, although the utility of this practice is questionable.

Proteinuria and haematuria, either alone or together, form one of the primary presenting symptoms of renal disease but the quality of the evidence base is very poor: strategies for who should have their urine tested, how someone found to have a positive test should be further investigated and managed, and what to do with those whose further investigations are negative in the presence of continued urinary abnormality have almost never been subjected to prospective, comparative studies. Guidelines, such as those for haematuria of the American Urological Association (Grossfeld *et al.* 2001a,b) and the Scottish Intercollegiate Guideline Network (SIGN) (1997) on both haematuria and proteinuria are based entirely on grade B evidence and consensus statements.

The patient with proteinuria

There are no signs of proteinuria unless the excretion is greater than several grams per 24 h: in that case the urine may become frothy, because protein lowers the surface tension of the urine and permits a relatively stable foam to form—an observation first made by Hippocrates—and this may be a valuable way of dating the onset of profuse proteinuria.

The physiological and pathological basis of proteinuria

Glomerular retention and leakage of protein molecules

Proteins are excluded from glomerular filtrate by a mechanism only partly understood (Myers and Guasch 1994; Schurek 1994; Oikama and Fogo 1995; D'Amico and Bazzi 2003). The glomerular filter (see Chapter 3.1) acts as a high capacity ultrafiltration membrane. It is made up of highly modified vascular endothelial cells, with only a thin cytoplasm and large pores allowing almost direct access of filtrate to the basement membrane, which has on its outside a unique pericyte—the glomerular epithelial cell or podocyte. This structure permits a high flux of solvent (water) and does not retard the passage of molecules up to an Einstein–Stokes radius (r_s) of about 1.5 nm. Solutes gain access to Bowman's space by convection and diffusion down concentration gradients. In the case of small solutes, such as sodium, transfer is almost entirely convective, but for larger solutes such as proteins both convection and diffusion are important. The glomerular barrier acts to minimize the diffusion, which would otherwise occur across the capillary wall from the high concentration of protein in the plasma to the very low concentration in the filtrate, and thus helps to maintain that concentration gradient.

The complex podocyte provides a barrier to the penetration of large molecules (Daniels 1993; Wickelgren 1999). How this may be achieved is not yet fully understood, but molecular analysis of some inherited conditions has led to progress. Single molecules may be mutated or missing, such as nephrin (Tryggvason 1999; Wang *et al.* 2002) and podocin (Caridi *et al.* 2001) on the podocyte cell surface, or with α-actinin-4 (Kaplan *et al.* 2000) within the cell. In the Finnish congenital nephrotic syndrome, nephrin, an essential constituent of the slit diaphragm 'zipper' structure (Rodewald and Karnovsky 1974) is absent whilst *p*-cadherin and CD2AP probably anchor the podocyte cytoskeleton to the slit diaphragm (see Chapters 3.1 and 16.4.4 for details). Electron microscopic tracer studies show that even proteins of large r_s and molecular mass can traverse the basement membrane with relative freedom, although the fixed negative charge on the membrane does inhibit penetration of anionic molecules (Figs 2 and 3) (Daniels 1993).

Size selectivity

At a molecular size greater than 1.5 nm begins a cut-off of glomerular filtration of proteins with increasing molecular radius (Fig. 1). The urinary clearance (sieving coefficent) of albumin is normally less than 0.01 per cent of water, whilst the clearance of proteins such as smaller immunoglobulin light chains approaches that of the glomerular filtration rate (GFR). Using polydisperse dextran clearance as a probe (Deen *et al.* 1985), a model suggesting the presence of water-filled cylindrical pores of about 4.7 nm diameter occupying about 10 per cent of the glomerular filtration area was evolved. It must be emphasized that the physical existence of these 'pores' remains a mathematical construct (Simpson 1986) although there are claims (Hironaka *et al.* 1993) that they can be visualized using ultra-high resolution scanning electron microscopy. Models of the distribution of these pores yield results that fit different sets of experimental data, and it is not clear yet which model is best (Myers and Guasch 1994).

That *charge selectivity* also operates (Comper and Glasgow 1995) is suggested by data from experimental animals using charged dextrans (Bohrer *et al.* 1978) (Fig. 2), and by comparing uncharged polyvinylpyrroloidone (Hulme and Hardwicke 1968) or neutral dextran (Robson *et al.* 1974) clearances with those of charged proteins of similar

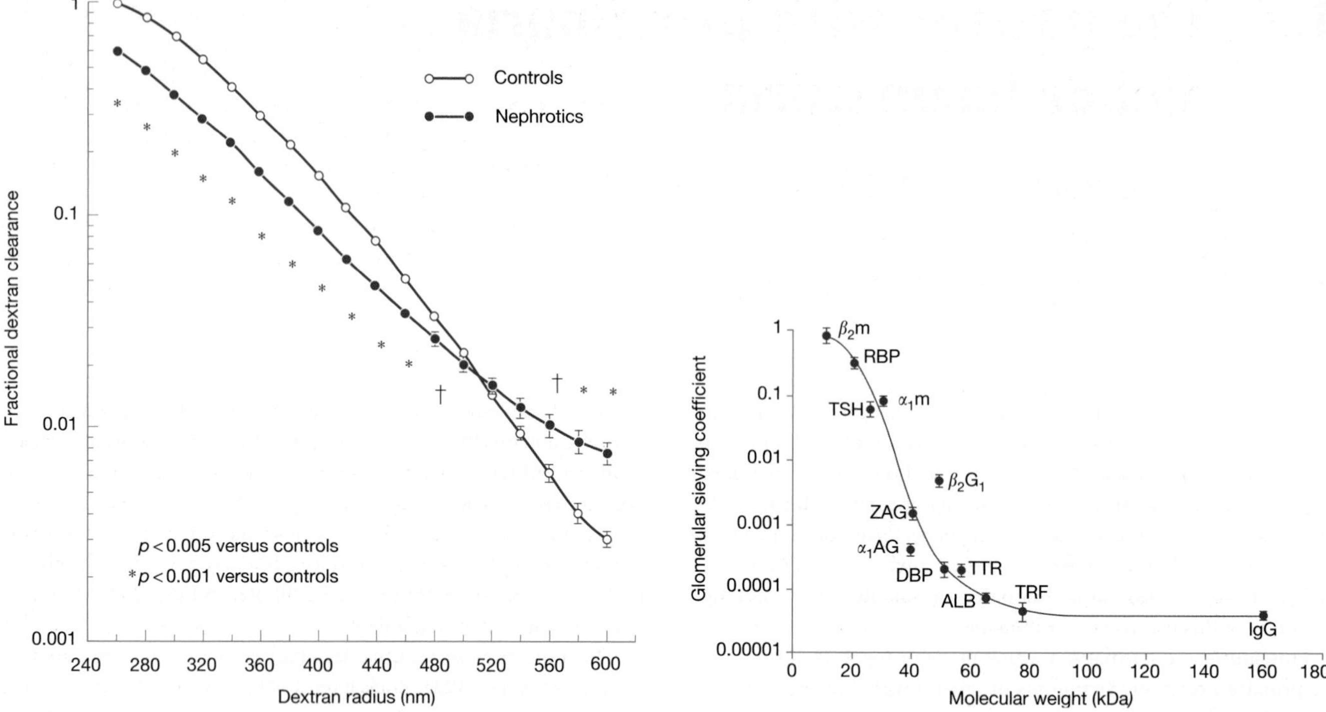

Fig. 1 Left: glomerular permselectivity determined by excretion of neutral dextrans in normal individuals and in nephrotic subjects with either minimal change nephropathy or membranous nephropathy. Note that small molecules are restricted from entry into the urine despite considerable proteinuria, whilst larger molecules are filtered into the urine more readily in the nephrotic subjects. Note also that there is no difference between the sieving profiles of the two groups of nephrotics despite their differing pathogenesis and histological appearances. [From Myers and Guasch (1994) with permission.] Right: the human glomerular sieving profile in patients with 'knockout' of tubular reabsoprtion as a result of inherited tubulopathies, mainly Dent's disease and Lowe's syndrome. See text for discussion. [From Norden *et al.* (2001), with permission.]

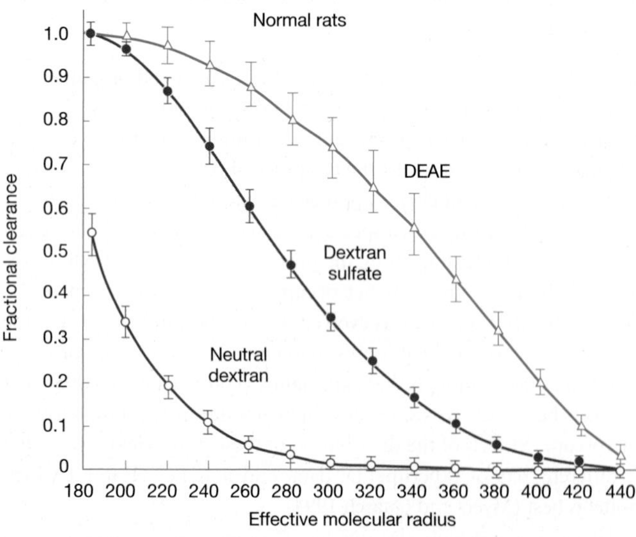

Fig. 2 Charge selectivity in the rat. The entry into the urine of similarly sized dextrans is affected by charge, negatively charged molecules being excluded and positively charged molecules facilitated for any given molecular size [from Bohrer *et al.* (1978) with permission].

molecular weight. Clearance data are available also from native molecules with a wide range of p*I* in humans: these include IgG (Deckert *et al.* 1988; Tencer *et al.* 1999), albumin (Ghiggeri *et al.* 1987; Candiano *et al.* 1990; Taylor *et al.* 1997), and amylase (Fox *et al.* 1994) (Fig. 3). Unfortunately, the effect of tubular reabsorption cannot be assessed in these studies [see Fig. 1 (right) and below]. In experimental animals using electron microscopy cationic molecules with an r_s of 5–6 nm such as IgG and ferritin can be seen penetrating the endothelial cell and entering the basement membrane, because these bear a negative surface charge; whereas anionic molecules of the same size are excluded completely.

This charge selectivity almost certainly arises from the high density of negative charges present on the structures of the glomerular capillary wall, principally heparin sulfate (Kanwar and Farquhar 1979; Raats *et al.* 2000). Thus the glomerular wall can be pictured as having two filtration barriers in series; an inner, charge-dependent electrostatic barrier on the surface of endothelial cells and the inner basement membrane; and a more external, mainly size-selective barrier in the outer basement membrane and slit diaphragms of the foot processes.

In humans, the proteinuria which develops with disease shows a gradual loss of glomerular discrimination for proteins of 60–1000 kDa (r_s = 3.5–20 nm). Loss of glomerular anionic sites is found even without structural alterations in the glomeruli, such as in minimal change proteinuria (Washizawa *et al.* 1993). However, in minimal change disease, the clearance of smaller molecules of dextran ($r_s < 4.8$ nm) is actually *decreased* compared with normal (Robson *et al.* 1974), whilst

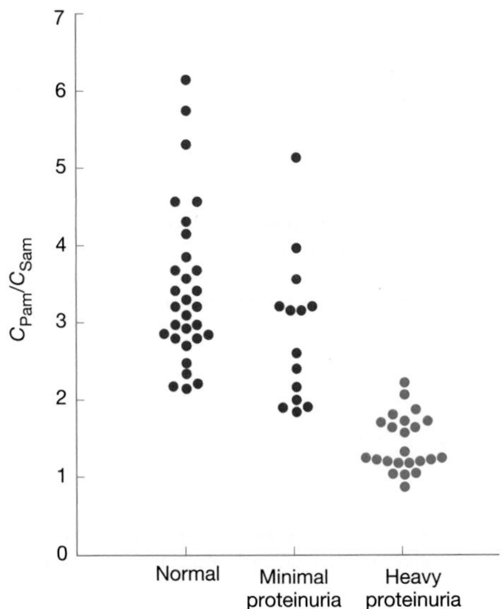

Fig. 3 Charge selectivity in human nephrotic subjects. The ratio in the urine of more cationic pancreatic isoamylase (p*I* 7.0) to more anionic salivary isoamylase (p*I* 5.9–6.4) is shown. In patients with profuse proteinuria, the ratio approaches 1.0, suggesting loss of charge selectivity in the glomerulus (from Fox *et al.* 1994 with permission).

that of larger dextrans is normal or increased (Fig. 2). This is present also in diabetes mellitus, lupus, and membranous nephropathy (Hulme and Hardwicke 1968; Myers and Guasch 1994). Again, these data have been interpreted in terms of a heteroporous model. A practical consequence of the partially preserved size selectivity even in disease is that glomerular proteinuria consists overwhelmingly of the predominant plasma protein, albumin.

Tubular reabsorption of proteins

This occurs predominantly—if not exclusively—into proximal tubular cells by endocytosis, with digestion of the absorbed protein within intracellular vesicles (Maack 2000). Anionic molecules do not compete for reabsorption (Bernard *et al.* 1988) but cationic or small molecules may do so (Park and Maack 1984). In the rabbit the uptake of albumin is a low-affinity–high-capacity process (Park and Maack 1984), which accounts for some albumin in normal urine even though the amount filtered is very small; presumably the same is true in humans. The large multispecific receptor megalin is involved in uptake into tubular cells (Leheste *et al.* 1999) together with cubulin (Birn *et al.* 2000; Christensen and Birn 2001), and many protein molecules have ligand epitopes for these molecules. Comper and colleagues (Eppel *et al.* 1999) have suggested controversially (Christensen and Birn 2000) that in addition considerable amounts of *intact* albumin may be reabsorbed by a transcellular route in rodents but the role of this in humans, if any, is unknown.

In the rat micropuncture can determine the concentration of protein in the proximal tubular fluid directly (Oken *et al.* 1981; Tojo and Endou 1992), which normally is between 1 and 10 mg/l. In man such direct measurement of tubular fluid is not feasible and there has been a long dispute about how much filtration and tubular reabsorption of various proteins occurs in health or disease. Norden *et al.* (2001) point out that the Fanconi syndrome arising from inherited disorders such as Dent's disease and Lowe's syndrome represents essentially a 'knockout' model of tubular protein reabsorption in man, allowing a description of a sieving profile for the human glomerulus (Fig. 1, right). The tubulopathy in Dent's disease arises from a mutation in the CLCN-5 gene whose product is probably concerned with the acidification of intracellular vesicles involved in protein endocytosis. A likely concentration for albumin in human glomerular filtrate of 3.5 ± 0.4 mg/l was derived, in agreement with data in rodents and implying a filtration of 500–700 mg of albumin daily. Of this, at least one-tenth normally appears in the urine, that is rather less than 90 per cent of filtered albumin is usually reabsorbed.

Lower molecular weight proteins of 10–45 kDa (r_s 1.5–3.0 nm) are filtered at rates from 1 to 80 per cent of the GFR, the latter figure being reached for lysozyme, β_2-microglobulin, and fragments of IgG light chains (Fig. 1, right). There is extensive reabsorption of these low molecular weight proteins in the proximal tubule (about 98 per cent of the filtered load) so that only about 100 mg/24 h are normally excreted in humans, along with some 15–20 mg of albumin. A consequence of the extensive filtration and major reabsorption of small molecular weight proteins is that in proximal tubular damage of any kind, low molecular weight protein will predominate in the urine (Norden *et al.* 2001 and Chapter 5.1). Because of their ready filtration and extensive reabsorption, the plasma concentrations of low molecular weight proteins are in health very low, their turnover by renal catabolism is very rapid and they accumulate in the plasma during uraemia. Thus the kidney is a major site of disposal for many small molecular weight proteins, including peptide hormones such as insulin growth hormone and parathyroid hormone (PTH), and also many cytokines and chemokines.

Clinical proteinuria

Methods of detecting and measuring proteinuria

Table 1 summarizes some of the tests used in clinical practice for the detection and measurement of proteinuria (Pesce and First 1979).

A visible cloudiness or even a solid coagulum on heating is rarely used today having been all but replaced by various 'stix' tests. These depend on the fact that titration curves of certain dyes is shifted in the presence of protein, especially albumin; light chains and some low molecular weight proteins are *not* detected by stix tests. They are buffered to keep the pH constant and leaving the stix in the urine will wash out the buffer and give a false reading—they should be read immediately. Some people with colour blindness have difficulty in reading the colour changes. Commercial stix such as Albustix® are very sensitive, giving a trace or positive reading with many normal urine samples containing only about 100 mg/l of protein. There is only a crude relationship between the urinary concentration of protein and the stix reading.

Sulfosalicylic acid (SSA) precipitation (0.5 ml of 3 per cent solution to 0.5 ml urine), which can be read in a densitometer has been used to give a rough quantitative reading but this again has been superseded almost everywhere by the stix tests. The reference methods for quantitation are the Kjeldahl measurement of precipitated nitrogen or the biuret method which measures peptide bonds. However, dye-binding methods which are reliable, accurate, and easy to perform, such as those applied to the measurement of serum albumin, are widely applied to urine, for example Coomassie brilliant blue (McElderry *et al.* 1982), as well as

Table 1 Different methods of detecting and measuring urine protein

Method	Description	Detection limit	Comments
Kjeldahl	Remove non-protein nitrogen, digest protein, measure protein nitrogen	10–20 mg/l	Reference and research method
Biuret	Copper reagent, measures peptide bonds	50 mg/l	Requires precipitation of proteins, used for 24-h measurement in some laboratories
Turbidimetric	Addition of trichloracetic or sulfosalicylic acids alters colloid properties and produces turbidity to be read in densitometer. Benzethomecin also used	50–100 mg/l	Imprecise, different readings for albumin and globulin
Dye-binding	Indicator changes colour in presence of protein (e.g. Coomassie brilliant blue)	50–100 mg/l	Different proteins bind differently; several different dyes in use; used in many laboratories for 24-h excretion
Nephelometric	Specific antialbumin antibody used		Measures albumin excretion not total protein. Does not detect globulins
Stick tests	Impregnated with indicator dye (bromocresol green) which changes colour in the presence of protein	100 mg/l	Reacts poorly with globulins. Usual clinical screening test

nephelometric tests—which rely on measuring albumin only—using specific antibodies, for example in the Beckman 'Array 360'® analyser.

The concentration and excretion of protein in the urine varies with both posture and exercise through changes in glomerular haemodynamics, and overnight collections may not reflect the 24-h output of protein. However, the difficulties of obtaining accurate 24-h urine collections in clinical practice also apply to proteinuria. Given the relative constancy of creatinine excretion, the urine creatinine can be used to correct the protein concentration in 'spot', untimed samples of urine. In normal children (Barratt 1983; Elises *et al.* 1988) the urinary albumin–creatinine ratio is less than 10 mg/mmol creatinine and in adults (Ginsberg *et al.* 1983) less than 21 mg/mmol (0.2 mg/mg). Both these suggested limits are probably too high, since by using nephelometry rarely do normal people exhibit more than 1–2 mg/mmol creatinine (Norden *et al.* 2001). An advantage of using the mg/mg ratio is that by coincidence, the resultant figure is almost exactly the same as the corresponding figure for grams per 24 h. The correlation between 24-h protein excretion and the protein creatinine ratio is 0.95 or better across the whole range of proteinuria and regardless of renal function (although the 95 per cent confidence limits are wide), so that 'spot' urines can be recommended for routine practice in preference to 24-h collections (Chitalia *et al.* 2001).

Normal proteinuria

The 24-h excretion of protein is 80 ± 24 mg (mean ± SD) in normal individuals, so that 128 mg/24 h (Berggård 1970) represents the mean + 2SD, a rate of excretion of 103 μg/min total protein. More than half of this consists of small molecular weight proteins or protein fragments, although albumin is the largest single component (40 mg/24 h or 28 μg/min). This represents less than 0.1 mg/mg creatinine (11 mg/mmol) in spot urine samples.

Pathological proteinuria

Proteinuria in excess of this modest limit can come about by:

1. The glomerular filter becoming more permeable to proteins of large molecular size in addition to those of low molecular weight ('glomerular' proteinuria). This is by far the most common cause of proteinuria in clinical practice.
2. The proximal tubule being damaged so that normally reabsorbed proteins, principally of low molecular weight, pass into the urine ('tubular' proteinuria). This usually occurs as part of the Fanconi syndrome of multiple proximal tubular dysfunction (see Chapter 5.3) and is much less common in isolation but may occur in combination with 'glomerular' proteinuria.
3. A marked increase in the plasma concentration of protein in the circulation, so that the amount filtered exceeds the reabsorptive capacity of the proximal tubule ('overflow' proteinuria): IgG light chains and light chain fragments in myeloma, and of lysozyme in monomyelocytic leukaemia are the only clinical examples.

'Glomerular' proteinuria

Glomerular proteinuria thus is 85–99 per cent albumin accompanied by other relatively low molecular weight proteins. In less selective proteinurias, however, other higher molecular weight components such as immunoglobulins and even macroglobulins are visible using electrophoresis on cellulose acetate or acrylamide gel. Glomerular proteinuria may be only a few hundred mg/24 h; on rare occasions however, it can be as much as 100 g/24 h. Only glomerular leakage can account for the presence of more than about 1.5 g protein/24 h. Because it is mostly albumin, glomerular proteinuria is readily assessed by stix or nephelometric methods.

How the glomerular barrier leaks excess protein in disease remains unclear (Savin 1993; D'Amico and Bazzi 2003). Loss of fixed anionic charge is a tempting hypothesis (Washizawa *et al.* 1993; Raats *et al.* 2000) particularly in minimal change nephropathy (Carrie *et al.* 1981). Although there appears to be loss of negative charge in the Finnish congenital nephrotic syndrome (Vernier *et al.* 1983) the proteinuria in this condition is known to result from loss of nephrin from the podocytes (see Chapter 16.4.4). A confusing factor is that the surface area of the podocyte bearing anionic heparan sulfate decreases with the simplification ('fusion') of the podocyte foot processes over the basement membrane, in proportion to the amount of proteinuria (Powell 1976) and this simplification may well be one of its causes (Daniels 1993).

Other experimental studies suggest focal areas of increased permeability from detatchment of the epithelial podocytes (Daniels 1993), or focally over immunological lesions such as immune aggregates. Interestingly, micropuncture data in animals with focally sclerosed glomeruli showed that most of the proteinuria originated from glomeruli that appeared relatively normal on histological examination. Agents known to increase glomerular protein permeability are the C5b-9 active complex of complement in models of membranous nephropathy, and leucocyte and monocyte products in proliferative glomerulonephritides, particularly proteases, eicosanoids, and cytokines such as tumour necrosis factor-α (TNF-α) and interleukin-1β (see Chapter 3.1).

It is also clear that glomerular haemodynamics can alter glomerular permeability profoundly but reversibly, an increase in intraglomerular capillary pressure being associated with the induction of proteinuria, with increases in both convective and conductive diffusion of protein into the glomerular space (Weening and van der Val 1987). The clinical importance of these observations is that measures to reduce glomerular hypertension by afferent arteriolar constriction (cyclosporin, low protein diets, and non-steroidal anti-inflammatory drugs) or by relaxing the efferent arteriole [angiotensin-converting enzyme (ACE) inhibitors, AT1 anatagonists, and dipyridamole] can reduce clinical proteinuria substantially, in a synergistic fashion. One can predict (see Chapter 1.3) that all these manoeuvres will lead to a concomitant reduction in GFR and in addition that agents which increase intraglomerular pressure such as angiotensin will induce proteinuria, which is again the case (Yoshioka *et al.* 1986). One example of this may be the reversible but sometimes profuse proteinuria associated with some cases of renal artery stenosis (Eiser *et al.* 1982).

'Tubular' proteinuria

Tubular proteinuria often accompanies—and is masked by—glomerular proteinuria in glomerular diseases ('mixed proteinuria'), but may occur also in isolation, such as in the Fanconi syndrome from any of its many causes (see Chapter 5.3). An important pointer is the *quantity of protein in the urine*; in tubular proteinuria. There is almost never excretion of more than 1.5 g/24 h (100 mg/mmol creatinine in spot urines); whereas in glomerular proteinuria excretion commonly exceeds 3–5 g/24 h. All except the most specific chemical tests will miss most low molecular weight proteins if present in isolation, because they are poorly precipitated in the sulfosalicylic acid test, are not denatured reliably on heating, and do not react with stix or antibodies designed to be principally sensitive to albumin. These statements particularly apply to immunoglobulin light chains. Cellulose acetate or sodium dodecyl sulfate polyacrylamide gel electrophoresis (SDS–PAGE) remains the easiest way to assess the pattern of proteinuria, and both are valuable in the diagnosis and assessment of tubular proteinuria.

Specific radioimmunoassays and enzyme-linked immunosorbent assays (ELISAs) have long been available for β_2-microglobulin (MW 12 kDa), one of the many microglobulins that make up most tubular proteinuria. Unfortunately although a very sensitive indicator of tubular damage, this protein is unstable in urine of normal pH (5–6.5) and even alkalinization of urine to pH 7 or above immediately on voiding may not stop degradation. Normally, less than 0.4 μg/l of β_2-microglobulin is present in urine. Lysozyme (MW 15 kDa) can also be used (Barratt 1983): normally excretion is less than 1 mg/mmol creatinine (10 μg/mg); α_1-microglobulin (MW 30 kDa) and retinol-binding protein (MW 21 kDa) have been studied also (Tomlinson *et al.* 1997), and have advantages in screening both for isolated tubular damage (such as in inherited tubulopathies and heavy metal exposure) or to detect tubulointerstitial damage in glomerular diseases such as nephrotic syndromes.

'Overflow' proteinuria: immunoglobulin light chains in the urine

The only important example of 'overflow' proteinuria in clinical practice is plasma cell dyscrasias. Assays for γ, α, and μ immunoglobulin chains by immunoelectrophoresis are, of course, an essential part of the diagnosis of myeloma, and may be found also in the urine of patients with primary amyloidosis, light chain nephropathy, and in some patients with immunotactoid glomerulopathy (see Chapter 4.2.2). Monoclonal 'spikes' are found also in the serum of a proportion of initially normal elderly individuals. The most accurate and sensitive method for detection of monoclonal proteinuria in urine is immunofixation using specific antisera to probe blots of electrophoresed urine. Often in the presence of good renal function, concentrations of light chain fragments in the plasma are negligible whilst abundant in urine. The only study available (Chew *et al.* 1999) to guide clinical policy is inconclusive. One can suggest arbitrarily that all nephrotic (or proteinuric) patients aged over 45 years should have immunoelectrophoresis performed on their urine, otherwise only suspicious cases should be investigated.

Secreted proteins; urinary casts (Scherberich 1990)

Some 20–30 mg/24 h of non-plasma protein is contributed by the renal tubules and the lower urinary tract. Much of this is Tamm–Horsfall protein (Hoyer and Seiler 1979), an easily polymerized 200-kDa glycoprotein that appears to be identical with uromodulin (Hession *et al.* 1987). Tamm–Horsfall protein is secreted into the tubular fluid only by the ascending thick limb and early distal convoluted tubule. It is a major constituent of renal tubular casts (McQueen 1966), along with albumin and traces of many plasma proteins, including immunoglobulins (Rustecki *et al.* 1971). Secretory IgA is added by the lower urinary tract including the urethral glands (Bienenstock and Tomasi 1968) together with trace quantities of proteins of prostatic or seminal vesicular origin (Rosenmann and Boss 1979). Bohle *et al.* (1988) have suggested that some of the secretory IgA found in the urine has its origin in the renal tubules in disease as well as in health, together with some IgM. Finally, tubular cell brush-border proteins and cytosolic enzymes are shed into the urine in small quantities, and increases in their urinary concentration may be a useful sign of tubular damage (see Chapter 1.2).

The finding of proteinuria on stick testing of a casual urine sample

Many entirely healthy individuals will have their urine examined and protein is found, often 'trace' or '+' (Table 2). Some positive results will be the result of recent exercise (see below, 'Jogger's nephritis'). Two to five per cent of children (Vehaskari and Rapola 1982), 5 per cent of young adults, and up to 16 per cent of the elderly will show proteinuria on testing of a single sample. However, the yield of significant treatable disease is very small and the general view is that it is not cost-effective to perform routine tests on the population as a whole, whether adult or paediatric (Anonymous 1988). Nevertheless urinary screening has been routine in Japanese schoolchildren since 1974, and also in Taiwan (Lin *et al.* 2000). This analysis of over 10 million urinary screenings in Taiwanese schoolchildren from 1992 to 1996 revealed that 119 children progressed towards or into renal failure (1 : 100,000); similar data have been reported from Japan, usually again without any cost analyses.

Table 2 Prevalence of dipstick/SSA proteinuria in apparently healthy individuals

Study and reference	Prevalence (%)
Schoolchildren	
10 studies from 1950	
(Vehaskari and Rapola 1982)	0.6–6.4
1000–50,000 children	(weighted mean 2.2)
Young adults	
Male armed forces recruits	
McLean (1919)	5.6
Murphy (1944)	3.0
Sinniah (1977)	0.9
College students, both sexes	
Diehl and McKinney (1944)	5.3
Burden (1933)	26.0
Lee (1920)	5.0
Adults, both sexes	
Blatherwick (1942) (>20 mg/dl)	1.7
Alwall (1973)	1.7
Yudkin (1988) (microalbuminuria)	9.4
Bigazzi (1992) (microalbuminuria)[a]	10.0
UK Diabetes Study (1993) (>50 mg/l)[a]	4.0
Ritz (1994) (>20 mg/l)[a]	3.0
Elderly (>60 years)	
Sawyer (1988)	6.6
Casiglia (1993)	10.0
>80 years	
Casiglia (1993)	16.1

[a] Hypertensive subjects excluded [for full details of references see Ritz *et al.* (1994) and Vehaskari and Rapola (1982)].

Microalbuminuria >20–50 mg/l.

Obviously in some groups at risk—for example, patients with diabetes mellitus (Viberti 1988) and/or hypertension (Ritz *et al.* 1994)—urine testing is essential. In addition to affecting prognosis in patients with diabetes mellitus, it has been suggested that proteinuria is a predictor of poor survival from vascular disease in the general population (Yudkin *et al.* 1988), and when the presence of vascular disease is allowed for (Kannel *et al.* 1984) also in the elderly (Damsgard *et al.* 1990) and in patients with hypertension (Ritz *et al.* 1994) or malignant disease (Sawyer *et al.* 1988). In the author's opinion, screening for proteinuria should be limited to these 'at risk' groups. Microalbuminuria is discussed below.

Occasionally, proteinuria may be factitious (Tojo *et al.* 1990), egg albumin or other protein being added to the urine; even more rarely parents may add protein to their child's urine, as a variety of the Munchausen syndrome by proxy (Meadow 1977). Electrophoresis of the urine will easily demonstrate foreign proteins such as ovalbumin. Pseudoproteinuria may be noted in patients receiving infusions of gelatin (MW 30 kDa)-based volume expanders such as 'gelofusine', which are readily filtered at the glomerulus (Jones *et al.* 1999), if the molybdate pyrogallol or possibly other dye-binding methods are used.

Postural proteinuria (orthostatic proteinuria) and persistent symptomless isolated proteinuria

In a proportion of those with protein found in a casual daytime specimen, often adolescents and especially young males, proteinuria is found in excess of the normal limits but is normal during recumbency. The usual way of testing this is to check the first urine passed on rising in the morning. There are no red cells even in the proteinuric daytime urine, or casts other than occasional hyaline casts. Blood pressure, renal function and renal imaging are normal.

This *postural or orthostatic proteinuria* has been recognized for more than a century, but its exact pathogenesis is unknown; almost certainly it represents an exaggerated intraglomerular haemodynamic response to change with posture (Robinson 1980). However, in the past decade arterial entrapment of renal veins, particularly the left (the 'nutcracker' phenomenon, Fig. 6), has been suggested as a plausible alternative explanation, at least in some patients (Devarajan 1993; Lee *et al.* 1996; Eksim *et al.* 1999). However, it is not clear why some patients with this vascular anomaly suffer haematuria or even severe bleeding (see below), and others proteinuria. Reasonably, however, in proteinuric patients surgical relief has not been tried to see if it results in improvement of the proteinuria. Data on renal biopsies in patients with postural proteinuria are confusing, because not all the patients studied in this way actually had true orthostatic proteinuria, and thus some showed minor glomerular changes (Robinson 1980) as found in isolated persistent proteinuria (see below).

The long-term prognosis of orthostatic proteinuria is benign in virtually all cases over many decades (Rytand and Spreiter 1981; Springberg *et al.* 1982), although it frequently persists for this long. It should also not be forgotten that there is an orthostatic component to almost all proteinuria (Wan *et al.* 1995). The absence of haematuria and return of the proteinuria to normal values (not simply diminution) during recumbency is required before it can be labelled 'orthostatic', and a benign prognosis given. Similarly *isolated persistent proteinuria* of modest dimensions (0.5–1.5 g/24 h) in all samples with preserved renal function no red cells and normal renal imaging is almost always benign, as long-term follow-ups of children (McLaine and Drummond 1970), university students (Levitt 1967), and adults (Antoine *et al.* 1968) demonstrate.

Proteinuria together with persistent microscopic haematuria

This finding if persistent should alert to the possibility of structurally damaged kidneys. A careful search for urinary casts should be made, and will often indicate by their presence that activity or scarring is present, or by their absence that the outlook may be good. In some cases only benign glomerular disease will be found, such as resolving acute nephritis, or a milder form of IgA-associated nephropathy; but focal segmental glomerulosclerosis, crescentic nephritis, membranous nephropathy, or mesangiocapillary glomerulonephritis may be present. Non-glomerular diseases may present in this fashion also, including atheroembolic disease, papillary necrosis and other toxic nephropathies, sickle-cell disease, tuberculosis, and reflux nephropathy. In the middle-aged or older patient amyloid or even diabetes mellitus may be found; one-third of diabetic nephropathy patients have microscopic haematuria. Thus renal biopsy will often be necessary in these circumstances, especially if reduced renal function, hypertension, or both are present. Renal function should be checked ideally by measuring the GFR (or cystatin C plasma concentrations if available) if the plasma creatinine is normal or near normal. In addition, some form of renal imaging (usually a renal and urinary tract ultrasound) will be needed, not just to localize the kidneys for the biopsy but because reflux nephropathy, polycystic kidneys, atheroembolic disease, and renal tuberculosis may present as haematuria with proteinuria. Finally, serology should be done (see next section). If renal function is within normal limits for age, it may be justified to wait for a year or two, observing renal function by further measurements of GFR or cystatin C concentrations, because assessment of plasma creatinine is inadequate at or near normal function (see Chapter 1.3).

The diagnostic approach to proteinuria (Fig. 4)

The test should be repeated two or three times, again on casual samples, which most adult patients or parents can do themselves: in many, results will be negative. This repetitive testing will also allow further assessment of whether haematuria is also consistently present. An early morning specimen of urine should be included to assess whether the proteinuria, even if regularly present in daytime urine, is postural. If it is, the patient may be reassured. Usually, no renal investigations should be required,

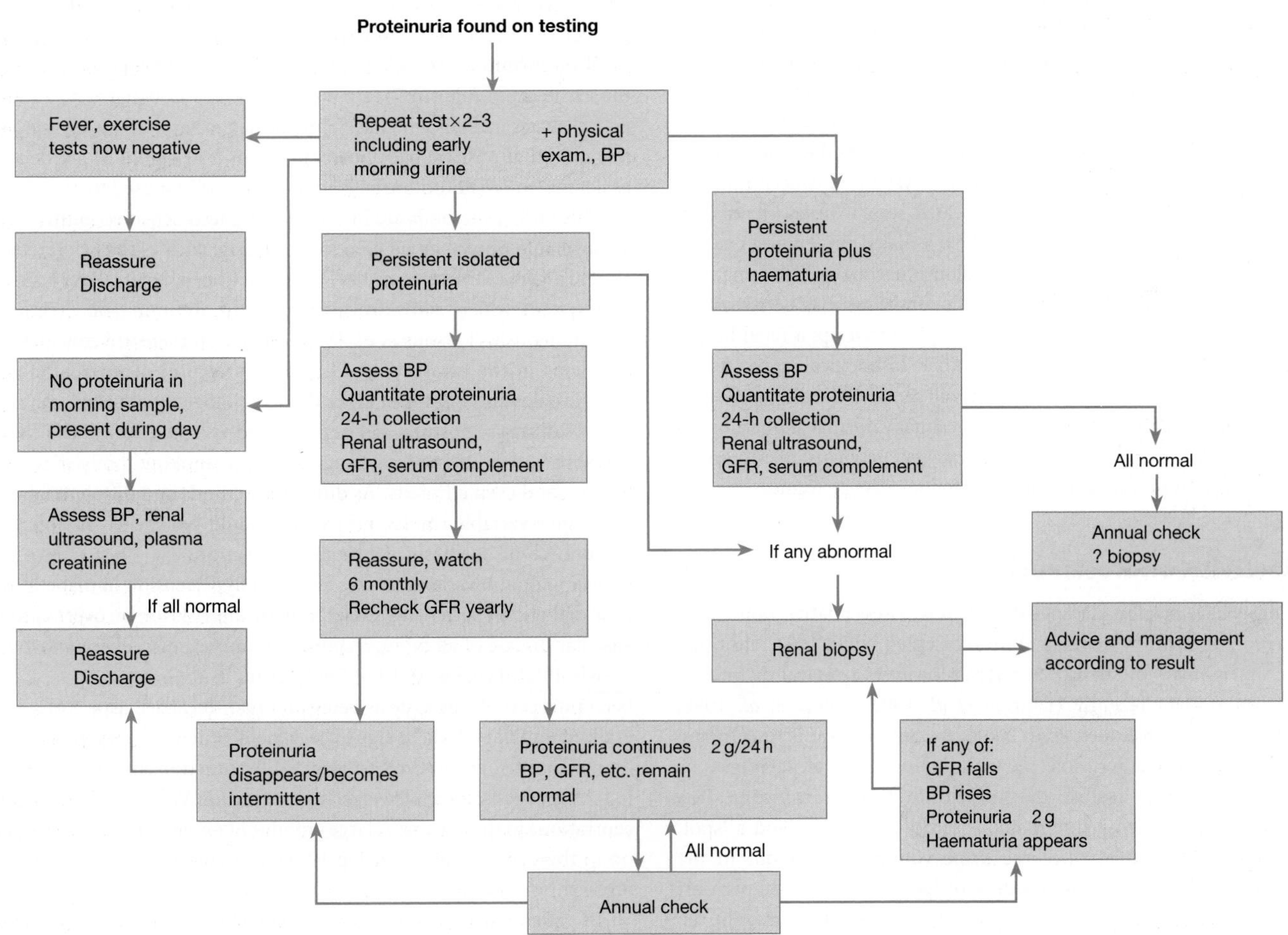

Fig. 4 An algorithm describing suggested management of a patient with symptomless proteinuria.

although in many cases the additional reassurance of a normal renal ultrasound and plasma creatinine is helpful to both doctor and patient. Follow-up is not necessary, but the individual will need to be warned that future samples passed (as an example) for employment or insurance purposes may again contain protein.

If, however, proteinuria is persistent and present day and night, a history should be taken including medicines or drugs ingested, for example, gold or penicillamine (see Chapter 4.9); and an examination performed to exclude associated disease. The persistent but transient proteinuria of fever (Marks *et al.* 1970), recent exercise—so called 'jogger's nephritis' (see below)—and of cardiac failure (Albright *et al.* 1983) need exclusion. Mild proteinuria associated with hypertension and reversed by treatment may be also seen (Ritz *et al.* 1994). However, in patients showing only hypertensive nephrosclerosis on biopsy, it has been realized recently that proteinuria may be more profuse—up to nephrotic dimensions in some patients (Mujais *et al.* 1987; Innes *et al.* 1993). Proteinuria together with hypertension and haematuria will almost always be associated with some form of underlying renal scarring, often from nephritis. A spot urine sample should be used to assess how much protein is being passed (for a full 24-h urine sample—see above) and a blood sample taken for plasma creatinine and serum albumin estimations. A renal and urinary tract ultrasound should be arranged. In some cases tests for hepatitis B and C and for syphilis, should be done, together with serum complement concentrations. Patients over the age of 45 years should have a serum protein electrophoresis test to check for the presence of paraproteins.

If two normal-sized and normally shaped kidneys are found on ultrasound, the renal function and serum C3 complement are normal, the blood pressure is normal, and no haematuria is present (i.e. persistent isolated proteinuria), a renal biopsy is not necessary, at least in the first instance. Ideally, an isotope-based assessment of GFR is best if renal function is relatively normal, but a serum cystatin C concentration if available, or a creatinine clearance repeated several times, may be an acceptable substitute (see Chapter 1.3). If isolated proteinuria exceeds 2 g/24 h, even in the absence of hypoalbuminaemia and oedema, it is possible that a minimal change nephrotic syndrome may be present or appear later, and such patients need to be followed up; a renal biopsy would usually be done to exclude other histological appearances. However, if a biopsy is performed it will (unlike the situation with postural proteinuria) not always show a virtually normal glomerulus: as well as minimal change lesions, mild mesangial nephritis, membranous nephropathy, or occasionally sclerosing lesions may be found.

Selectivity of proteinuria

Attempts have been made since the 1950s to assess relative glomerular discrimination for proteins in clinical disease (White 1981) although little use is made of such tests today. However, a revival of interest has been evident recently (Laurent *et al.* 1993; Tencer *et al.* 1998; Bazzi et al. 2000; Bakouch *et al.* 2001). A common test is to compare the clearance of a larger molecule with that of a smaller: IgG, IgM, or α_2-macroglobulin, against that of albumin or transferrin. This requires only a roughly simultaneous sample of plasma and a 'spot' untimed urine sample, since the urine volume cancels out in the relationship C_{large}/C_{small}. A clearance of IgG greater than 20 per cent (0.20) of transferrin or albumin represents 'non-selective' proteinuria; less than 0.10 is 'highly selective' (and suggests that a minimal change lesion may be present), whilst the range beween 0.10 and 0.20 is of little discriminatory value. The proteins can be measured conveniently in urine and plasma by radial immunodiffusion (Cameron and Blandford 1966) or by laser nephelometry. These tests of relative glomerular permeability are of limited value in predicting histology, except to distinguish minimal change nephrotic syndrome from other forms of nephritis or glomerular disease (see Chapters 1.7 and 3.4). An alternative approach is to perform SDS–PAGE on the urine followed by silver staining and/or Western blotting, and examine the result qualitatively by inspection (Brocklebank *et al.* 1991) or by scanning of individual protein peaks. This gives a general pattern of all the protein species present, including whether tubular proteinuria is present in addition to glomerular proteinuria in those with glomerular disease—an indicator of tubulointerstitial involvement, as noted above (Bazzi *et al.* 1997).

Microalbuminuria

Excretion of albumin in apparently healthy patients with diabetes mellitus which exceeds normal amounts, but is less than that detectable on Albustix® or similar tests, was first described using radioimmunoassay by Keen and Chlouverakis in 1963. It is common, prevalent in about one-third of Type I diabetics (see Chapter 4.1). This appears to be a reliable early predictor of the later appearance of overt, stix-positive proteinuria and diabetic nephropathy (Mogensen and Christensen 1984; Viberti 1988) and thus permits targetted renoprotective intervention. Normal individuals excrete less than 30 μg of albumin/min (~30 mg/l or 43 mg/24 h) (Metcalf *et al.* 1992), whilst the sensitivity of Albustix® is about 100 mg/l (150–250 mg/24 h). Patients with diabetes mellitus who have proteinuria greater than 20 μg/min, but less than that positive by Albustix® (i.e. 30–250 mg/24 h) are defined as having 'microalbuminuria'. Nephelometry is best used to assay albumin, but other methods are in use, and stix tests sensitive in this range are available which can be used for screening, such as the Micral-Test® (Boehringer) (Minetti *et al.* 1997) and the Clinitek® 50 (Bayer), a two-pad system which allows measurement of albumin and creatinine simultaneously (Parsons *et al.* 1999). However, there are considerable problems in the measurement and interpretation of microalbuminuria (Lydakis and Lip 1998), since there is biological variation with time of day, diuresis, posture and activity, and in some series also blood pressure within the normal range and age, smoking, body mass (see below), and even ethnicity. As different methods and different laboratories give variable results, no patient should be labelled as 'microalbuminuric' on the basis of a single observation.

Microalbuminuria correlates also with hypertension in diabetic and non-diabetic hypertensive subjects, with the risk for or overt cardiovascular disease of all types, response to trauma, and general mortality (Lewis 1998; Lydakis and Lip 1998; Evans and Greaves 1999). It has been interpreted variously as being an organ-localized aspect of a generalized capillary leak, a sign of a general inflammatory process, or an indicator of generalized endothelial dysfunction. In support of the latter hypothesis, there are correlations with von Willebrand factor concentrations in the plasma. A large amount of research is currently going on in this area (Lydakis and Lip 1998) particularly in relation to early intervention studies.

In patients with systemic lupus erythematosus showing apparently normal urine and renal function, microalbuminuria is present in the majority, some of whom subsequently develop overt clinical proteinuria and nephritis (Terai *et al.* 1987; Valente de Almeida *et al.* 1999). This agrees with the observation (see Chapter 4.7.2) that such patients usually do have minor changes of nephritis on biopsy even in the presence of clinically normal urine. In minimal change nephrotic patients after remission, however, normal albumin excretion rates are present.

Proteinuria and progression of renal diseases

For a quarter of a century it has been known that greater proteinuria is associated with poorer outcome in glomerular disease (Cameron 1979), and for almost as long that progression in some normally non-proteinuric diseases such as reflux nephropathy (Kincaid-Smith and Becker 1979) is associated with appearance of an increasing proteinuria. In parallel came the realization that even in what appeared to be primarily glomerular diseases, events in the tubules and interstitium correlated better with renal function (Schainuk *et al.* 1970) and poor outcome than glomerular appearances. During the 1980s, speculation that both these might represent more than an epiphenomenon of more severe renal injury increased (Williams *et al.* 1988; Cameron 1990; D'Amico 1991). In the past decade, the hypothesis has been proposed that traffic of protein through the glomerulus and back though the tubules might be a toxic event in the kidney and a cause of interstitial nephritis. Some of the most convincing evidence that this was so, emerged from studies of overload proteinuria following infusions of protein into normal animals (Lawrence and Brewer 1981; Eddy *et al.* 1989).

Recently, evidence has accumulated to show that pathological quantities of proteinuria leaking through damaged glomeruli are indeed toxic to the renal tubules, with release of inflammatory mediators and chemoattractants, as well as complement activation and expression of adhesion molecules and profibrotic cytokines (Burton and Harris 1996; Abbate *et al.* 1999; Kairaitis and Harris 2001). However, the exact component of pathological proteinuria which is responsible for this activation remains obscure, as pure albumin seems incapable of inducing this inflammation. Current candidate molecules include chemically altered or lipid-bearing albumin, filtered complement and cytokines, transferrin-iron, IgG, and lipoproteins. Despite this important gap in our knowledge, the reduction of the amount of filtered protein and its uptake by the tubules has become a major therapeutic goal, and has proved to be capable of slowing progression of renal injury in almost all proteinuric states. The most powerful and best-studied antiproteinuric agents so far are the ACE inhibitors, which reduce proteinuria and slow progression in both diabetic (Weidmann *et al.* 1993) and non-diabetic nephropathies (Gansevoort *et al.* 1995; de Jong *et al.* 1997; Jafar *et al.* 2001) by lowering intraglomerular pressures through efferent arteriolar vasodilatation. AT1 receptor inhibitors seem equally capable, and may be synergistic with ACE inhibitors.

The patient with haematuria

Visible blood in the urine (macroscopic haematuria), or blood detected on microscopy (microscopic haematuria) or the finding of haemoglobin in the urine are cardinal symptoms of renal disease. In *macroscopic haematuria* the urine may be bright red, but more often after a dwell time in the bladder is brownish and may be likened to tea or Coca Cola especially in acid urine. Usually, the amount of blood lost is trivial but in some patients (almost always with bleeding lesions of the urinary tract but also in medullary 'sponge' kindey) major bleeding with clot colic can be seen with anaemia if prolonged. The significance and seriousness of the finding of *microscopic haematuria* is independent of the number of red cells (Messing *et al.* 1989), although there is an increase in significant and life-threatening findings in relation to the quantity of blood in the urine if macroscopic haematuria is included in the analysis (Mariani *et al.* 1989) (see below).

Testing for blood in the urine

This presents practical problems both in methodology and interpretation. In health and at rest less than 1 μl of blood containing less than 10^7 red blood cells is excreted per day in 2 l of urine; thus, the concentration of erythrocytes is less than 5 per μl and usually only 1 per μl of unspun urine. Unfortunately, the upper limit for the number of red cells in normal urine is not clearly defined, perhaps because of normal individuals with thin glomerular capillary basement membranes: 90 per cent of normal individuals will have less than 1 erythrocyte/μl of urine, that is about 10^5 cells/h, but a few will have up to 10 times this number. Only 5 ml of blood (containing 25×10^9 red cells) are needed to give pink macroscopic haematuria in a litre of urine (25,000 cells/μl); twice this will give easily visible haematuria. A number of substances such as drugs and foods may give a pink-red colour to the urine (phenindione, phenolphthalein, beetroot (Thompson 1996), rifampicin, occasionally chloroquine, desferrioxamine, and sulfasalazine) and thus may be confused with haematuria. Urate crystals may be mistaken for blood on the diaper of babies, and phosphates are on occasion red enough to cause confusion. Haemoglobin and myoglobin may be excreted as free compounds when intravascular haemolysis or rhabdomyolysis occur, and will need to be differentiated from haematuria by examination and/or sepectroscopy of the supernatant of spun fresh urine. Porphyrins may also discolour urine and be mistaken for haematuria.

How do red cells get into the urine?

Minute leaks from ruptured small vessels in lesions in the renal papilla or the lower urinary tract are relatively easy to understand. However, renal bleeding is more obscure (Schurek 1994). Even if all the red cells came through the kidney, probably only one and at most 10 red cells normally pass through each nephron in 24 h. Thus, it is not surprising that illustrations of red cells traversing the GBM are unusual, even in haematuric illnesses (Collar *et al.* 2001). Most of these cells are 'dysmorphic' (Loh *et al.* 1990) and are hence presumably of renal origin (see below). At least some originate from the lower urinary tract. Why some forms of nephritis apparently confined to the mesangium such as IgA nephropathy cause microscopic or even macroscopic haematuria is completely obscure. Red cells are seen free in the tubular lumens in biopsies from patients with IgA and other haematuric nephropathies, and an additional origin from the peritubular capillaries cannot be excluded.

Dipstick tests for haematuria

The reaction in dipstick tests for haematuria is between the haemoglobin or myoglobin and compounds such as *o*-toluidine and detects the haemoglobin from lysed red cells only; these break up more quickly in dilute and alkaline urine. The sticks react also with filtered haemoglobin from intravascular haemolysis, haemoglobinuria, and with free filtered myoglobin in rhabdomyolysis with myoglobinuria. False positive tests may be noted also in the presence of some bacteria containing peroxidase (Lam 1995).

A practical problem is that the sensitivity of the sticks is close to the normal range of red cell excretion (1–5 cells/μl) (Daum *et al.* 1988), so that some normal individuals will show positive reactions from time to time, especially after vigorous exercise, ('jogger's nephritis'—see below), both from red cells and free myoglobin. Compared with microscopy of fresh urine, dipstick tests show 100 per cent sensitivity, but only 62 per cent specificity; the latter figure is low mainly because the tests are so sensitive. Nevertheless, the test is cost-effective (Mariani *et al.* 1984). Negative results may be obtained using stix testing in urines containing ascorbic acid as a result of mega doses of vitamin C (Brigden 1992).

Urine microscopy for haematuria

Microscopy of unspun normal urine usually shows about one red blood cell/μl, and is best done in *fresh* concentrated acid urine (such as early morning urine) to avoid break-up of the cells. Haemoglobinuria or myoglobinuria can only be excluded, of course, by doing both tests, and a positive stix text should always be followed by microscopy of fresh urine to confirm haematuria. Counts of red cells are best done in a Fuchs–Rosenthal counting chamber on unspun unstained urine; the use of phase contrast rather than bright field illumination greatly improves the precision of the count. Concentration of the urine by centrifugation is particularly useful for *qualitative* analysis—to look for the presence and the type of casts, or of white cells (Fogazzi *et al.* 1999); but 'quantitation' 'per high power field' done in this way is hopelessly unreliable in spun urines done casually (Corwin and Silverstein 1988) and should be consigned to history, although still widely practised. If this technique *is* to be used, then the centrifugation and volume of resuspension should be optimized, for example 10 ml of urine at 2000–2500 rpm in a 16-cm rotor centrifuge (~1250*g*) for 5 min, with 9.5 ml supernatant decanted and the sediment gently resuspended in the remaining 0.5 ml, and examination of 50 μl under a 24 × 32 mm coverslip (Fogazzi *et al.* 1999). Casts are often found around the outside margins of the preparation, the much smaller red cells throughout the field.

Exercise-related haematuria: 'jogger's nephritis'

Vigorous exercise leads to a temporary microscopic haematuria (Kincaid-Smith 1982; Kallmeyer and Miller 1993; Jones and Newhouse 1997) as well as proteinuria. Weight-bearing exercise (running) more readily leads to haematuria than non-weight-bearing exercise (cycling or swimming) (McInnis *et al.* 1998). The red cells are dysmorphic (see next section) (Fassett *et al.* 1982) and may be accompanied by a few red cell casts, which suggests a renal origin, but in the past others have suggested they arise mainly from the bladder (see Kincaid-Smith 1982 for discussion). On occasion, the haematuria can be macroscopic (Ubels *et al.* 1999) and needs to be distinguished from the rarer 'march' haemoglobinuria, and myoglobinuria following rhabdomyolysis of severe exercise, which however, can occur with only trivial exercise in some inherited muscle enzyme disorders. Haematuria is present during and for 1–2 h after exercise, but can persist on occasion for as long as 72 h. There is some evidence that adequate hydration minimizes or avoids the problem.

Where in the urinary tract do the red cells come from?

It is obviously valuable to be able to distinguish renal bleeding from mainly 'medical' causes from that arising mainly from 'urological' lesions of the lower urinary tract. The presence of other than trivial concomitant proteinuria almost always indicates a renal—usually but not always glomerular—origin of the haematuria. This is because, except in major bleeding (more than 50 ml/24 h), there is simply not enough protein lost in the blood to give a positive result on stix testing (Tapp and Copley 1988). The presence of red cell casts similarly confirms glomerular (or at least renal) haematuria (Rath *et al.* 1990) and in the presence of either cystourethroscopy is unnecessary.

Dysmorphic red cells

Birch and Fairley reintroduced this century-old idea (Birch and Fairley 1979; Fairley and Birch 1982) (see Chapter 1.2 for details). Glomerular haematuria usually contains a high proportion of bizarrely shaped cells, including acanthocytes with considerable anisocytosis, whilst the red cells resulting from bleeding into the urinary tract are usually smooth disks (see Chapter 1.2 for illustrations). Acanthocytes (G1 cells), with their knob-like protrusions (sometimes also called 'Mickey Mouse' cells from the resemblance of the projections to round ears), appear to be more specific for glomerular as opposed to renal bleeding (Loh *et al.* 1990; Köhler *et al.* 1991; see also Fogazzi *et al.* 1999 and Chapter 1.2 for illustrations). However, a number of observers have been unable to reproduce accurately the distinction of glomerular from non-glomerular haematuria using either percentage of dysmorphic cells or acanthocytes alone, and Zaman and Proesmans (2000) suggest that both indices must be used to achieve useful accuracy (>90 per cent sensitivity and specificity). Others find that the degree of urine concentration and time from passage of the urine had major effects on the appearance of the red cells (Schramek *et al.* 1989; Briner and Reinhart 1990; Rath *et al.* 1990).

Phase-contrast microscopy of unspun urine (Birch *et al.* 1983) was the standard method to begin with, but is routine in only a few clinics in part because it is strongly observer-dependent. Automated red cell analysers designed for flow cytometry of blood (Shichiri *et al.* 1986, 1988) have also been used to make the distinction. However, analysis of red cell size does not accurately divide glomerular from non-glomerular haematuria unless the haematuria is profuse. More recently, several dedicated urine flow cytometric machines have been described which have sensitivities of about 85 per cent and specificities of 95 per cent for glomerular versus other haematurias (e.g. Angulo *et al.* 1999; Apeland *et al.* 2001), comparable to expert urine microscopy. Again, performance is in general better, the more red cells are present in the specimen. In view of the steady fall-off in the performance of urine microscopy even in renal units, access to such a machine should now be part of the armamentarium; although urine microscopy by an experienced observer using phase-contrast microscopy remains the 'gold standard' in this area. Other techniques have been used, such as scanning electron microscopy, confocal microscopy, flow cytometry using antihaemoglobin antibody, and staining for Tamm–Horsfall protein, but at the moment none of these techniques is in general use.

Causes of haematuria

Unlike proteinuria, which almost always arises from the kidney, haematuria may arise from anywhere in the urinary tract. The list of conditions which may cause haematuria is long (Table 3); some may give rise to

Table 3 Principal causes of haematuria

Disorders of coagulation	*Infections*
Bleeding disorders (haemophilia, etc.)[a]	Acute bacterial pyelonephritis/cystitis[a]
Vascular diseases	Tuberculous cystitis[a]
Aortic aneurysm[b]	Schistosomiasis[a]
Atheroembolism of renal artery[b]	Prostatitis[a]
Renal artery stenosis[a]	*Stone disease*
Renal vein thrombosis[c]	Anywhere in the urinary tract[a]
Glomerular diseases	Ca oxalate crystalluria[a]
Haematuria (almost) invariable	Uric acid crystalluria[a]
IgA nephropathy and other mesangial disorders[a]	*Trauma*
Thin membrane disease	To kidney, bladder, ureter, urethra[c]
Alport's syndrome	*Miscellaneous*
Mesangiocapillary glomerulonephritis	Relief of obstruction
Active/healing endocapillary nephritis	Loin pain–haematuria syndrome[a]
Vasculitis and lupus nephritis[a,c]	Bladder and urethral 'polyps'
Focal segmental glomerulosclerosis[a]	Prostatic calculus
Haematuria variably present	Urethral caruncle
Membranous nephropathy[c]	Familial telangectasia
Amyloidosis	Arteriovenous malformation[c]
Diabetes mellitus[a]	Endometriosis[a]
Miscellaneous disorders: Fabry's disease, etc.[c]	Chemical and interstital cystitis[a]
Renal interstitial diseases	Meatal ulcers
Interstitial nephritis[a]	Foreign body[c]
Polycystic disease of various types	Trapped renal vein[c] ('Nutcracker' phenomenon)
Renal medullary diseases	Exercise (temporary)
Papillary necrosis from analgesics, diabetes, sickle-cell disease[c]	Factitious (added human/animal blood)
Medullary 'sponge' kidney	Djenkol bean, canatharides, etc. ingestion
Renal tuberculosis[a]	
Reflux nephropathy[c]	
Pelviureteric junction obstruction[c]	
Tumours of the urinary tract	
Wilms' tumour[b]	
Renal cell carcinoma[b]	
Transitional cell carcinomas[b]	
Carcinoma of the prostate[b]	
Carcinoma of the urethra[b]	

[a] Require treatment.

[b] Life-threatening.

[c] May require treatment.

Almost every condition on this list may present on occasion as macroscopic haematuria, although in some conditions, particularly some glomerular pathology (e.g. membranous nephropathy) this may be rare.

either macroscopic or microscopic haematuria, others, mostly 'medical' causes, only ever present with microscopic haematuria. Unreported trauma (Anonymous 1979) must not be forgotten. The most important point to remember in the diagnosis of haematuria is that *the likelihood of finding any one of these conditions varies with age*: the principal causes of haematuria in an infant, a child or young adult, and a middle-aged or elderly subject are quite different, and consequently the most effective strategies of investigation will be different at various ages.

Persistent symptomless isolated microscopic haematuria: the strategy of investigation

This, first described by Vigla and Rayer in 1837 is common in apparently healthy individuals. The problem is that the stix in use are sensitive to amounts of haematuria within the normal range and there is no clear definition of 'abnormal' haematuria. There are, in addition, far fewer data for the prevalence of haematuria in general populations than exist for proteinuria (Table 4; see Grossfeld *et al.* 2001a). In children, about 1 per cent have repeatedly detectable haematuria (Vehaskari *et al.* 1979), a much smaller proportion than that showing proteinuria in girls, but greater in boys (Table 2). In adults, haematuria is more common with increasing age; perhaps 12 per cent of young adults have a positive stick test (Froom *et al.* 1984) whilst in those over the age of 50 years 10–16 per cent show positive results (Britton *et al.* 1989). In tropical and developing countries, the prevalence of schistosomiasis or sickle-cell trait at any age, and bladder stones in children, alters the incidence and probable causes (see below).

These large proportions of symptomless individuals with positive stix tests or microscopy render it necessary to plan and evaluate the investigation of haematuria with care. Obviously invasive and/or expensive

Table 4 Prevalence of haematuria at various ages in healthy populations

Study and reference	Prevalence (%)
Children	
Dodge *et al.* (1976)	0.7 (girls), 0.5
	0.1 (boys)
Vehaskari *et al.* (1979)	1.0–4.0
Young male armed forces recruits 18–33 years	
Froom *et al.* (1984)	5.2
Older adults (>50 years)	
Mariani *et al.* (1989)	13 (males and females)
Mohr *et al.* (1986)	13 (males)
	14 (females)
Ritchie *et al.* (1986)	2.5 (males, age not stated)
Thompson (1987)	4 (males, aged 40–90 years)
Messing *et al.* (1989)	13 (males)
Britton *et al.* (1989)	18 (males)
Elderly (>75 years)	
Mohr *et al.* (1986)	13 (males)
	9 (females)

Different criteria were used to define the upper limit of 'normal' and hence the lower limit of 'microhaematuria' in all of these studies. The original papers should be consulted for details, which illustrate the difficulties of defining and diagnosing microhaematuria.

investigations must be used with precision on selected patients, but clear and complete data to guide their use do not exist as yet. A further problem has been that the detection of haematuria naturally lies with primary care physicians, but its subsequent evaluation is undertaken by both urologists and nephrologists, none of whom have communicated well with each other hitherto, and who approach the whole problem with attitudes formed from studying only subgroups of haematuria. The main difference in causes and approach relates to the *age of the individual.* A final point is that non-medical pressures to (over-) investigate may be present, such as employment or medicolegal issues.

Numerous algorithms to direct the investigation of haematuria in developed countries have been produced (e.g. Jaffe *et al.* 2001), including a recent recommendation from the American Urological Association (Grossfeld *et al.* 2001a,b); although few have been prospectively evaluated, and none on large populations. The (often unstated) target of these algorithms is usually the older patient, although strategies for children have been described also (e.g. Diven and Travis 2000). Given the importance of the age of the subject, an *age-dependent* algorithm for investigation of isolated haematuria is suggested in Fig. 5. A family history is important, and other family members may need their urine tested on occasion. Industrial exposure to toxic dyes and chemicals, cyclophosphamide administration, abuse of analgesics (Chapter 6.2) or so-called 'Chinese' herbs (Chapter 6.9) should be sought, and a smoking history should be taken in view of the relation of these to bladder and other urothelial cancers.

In every case, the first thing to do is to *repeat the test several times* over a period of 1–2 weeks. Mariani *et al.* (1984, 1989) required two or three tests to be positive before diagnosing haematuria to be present, but one must not forget that in many potentially life-threatening conditions, haematuria may be intermittent. In addition, active infections in the urinary tract should be sought and if found, treated; haematuria will often disappear after eradication.

Major points of continuing debate (Fig. 5) include the nature of any initial imaging: the traditional intravenous urography (IVU) has largely been replaced by an ultrasound, with IVU reserved for later use in selected patients (Jaffe *et al.* 2001). However, Khadra *et al.* (2000) point out that a considerable proportion of patients with tumours will remain undiagnosed unless both techniques are employed, as suggested in Fig. 5. The utility (or lack of it) of performing urinary cytology has been debated also. When to do flexible cystoscopy on subjects with persisting haematuria has been the subject of controversy also, and again must be viewed in relation to age.

Haematuria in children and younger (<40 years) adults (Cilento *et al.* 1995)

In patients with isolated symptomless haematuria *under the age of 40 years*, the chances of finding significant urological disease are very low—only about 2 per cent in the study of Froom *et al.* (1984), and no tumours were identified under this age in the large series of 982 patients with microscopic haematuria of Khadra *et al.* (2000). Thus investigation of this group centres largely around evaluation of potential 'medical' sources of the blood in the urine. Significant disease in less than 2 per cent of a young haematuric population has been reported, with good medium-term prognosis (Vehaskari *et al.* 1979; Túri *et al.* 1989; Hisano *et al.* 1991). Nevertheless neoplasms can be found even in 30-year-olds (Sharfi and Hassan 1994; Reynard 2000) and some individualization of management will be needed.

It is important in children and young adults with haematuria to obtain and test specimens from other members of the family, because the presence of a familial haematuria completely alters the picture (see Chapters 16.4.1–16.4.4). Either Alport's syndrome or the so-called 'benign' familial haematuria with thin basement membranes may be present, or polycystic or other cystic kidney diseases. Crystalluria-associated familial haematuria has been described also (Praga *et al.* 2000). If no red cell casts or dysmorphic cells are present and a clotting screen is normal, it is often forgotten that infection of the urinary tract, including the prostate in males, and the urethra in both sexes are the most common cause of haematuria at all ages, but additional symptoms such as dysuria are usually present. *Urine culture* should be one of the first investigations, although fastidious organisms may not be evident immediately.

Usually a *renal ultrasound* will be done, but very few cases will require a *cystourethroscopy*. Significant morphological findings in the kidney and urinary tract are uncommon under the age of 45 years (0–2 per cent) (Froom *et al.* 1984; Grossfeld *et al.* 2001a), although Ritchie *et al.* (1986) detected a single carcinoma of the bladder in a 37-year-old during their survey of 10,000 'normal' men, and Reynard (2000) one in a 31-year-old. In screening of 55,000 adults who worked for the Hitachi company (Yamagata *et al.* 1996) 478 patients with isolated haematuria on repeated testing were investigated and followed up: in half, the haematuria disappeared, and no patient developed renal insufficiency. In black patients and others at risk [not all patients with sickle-cell trait appear obviously of African or Middle-Eastern origin! (Oksenhendler *et al.*1984)], the possibility of sickle-cell heterozygosity as a cause of minor papillary necrosis must be remembered (see Chapter 4.11) and haemoglobin electrophoresis should be done.

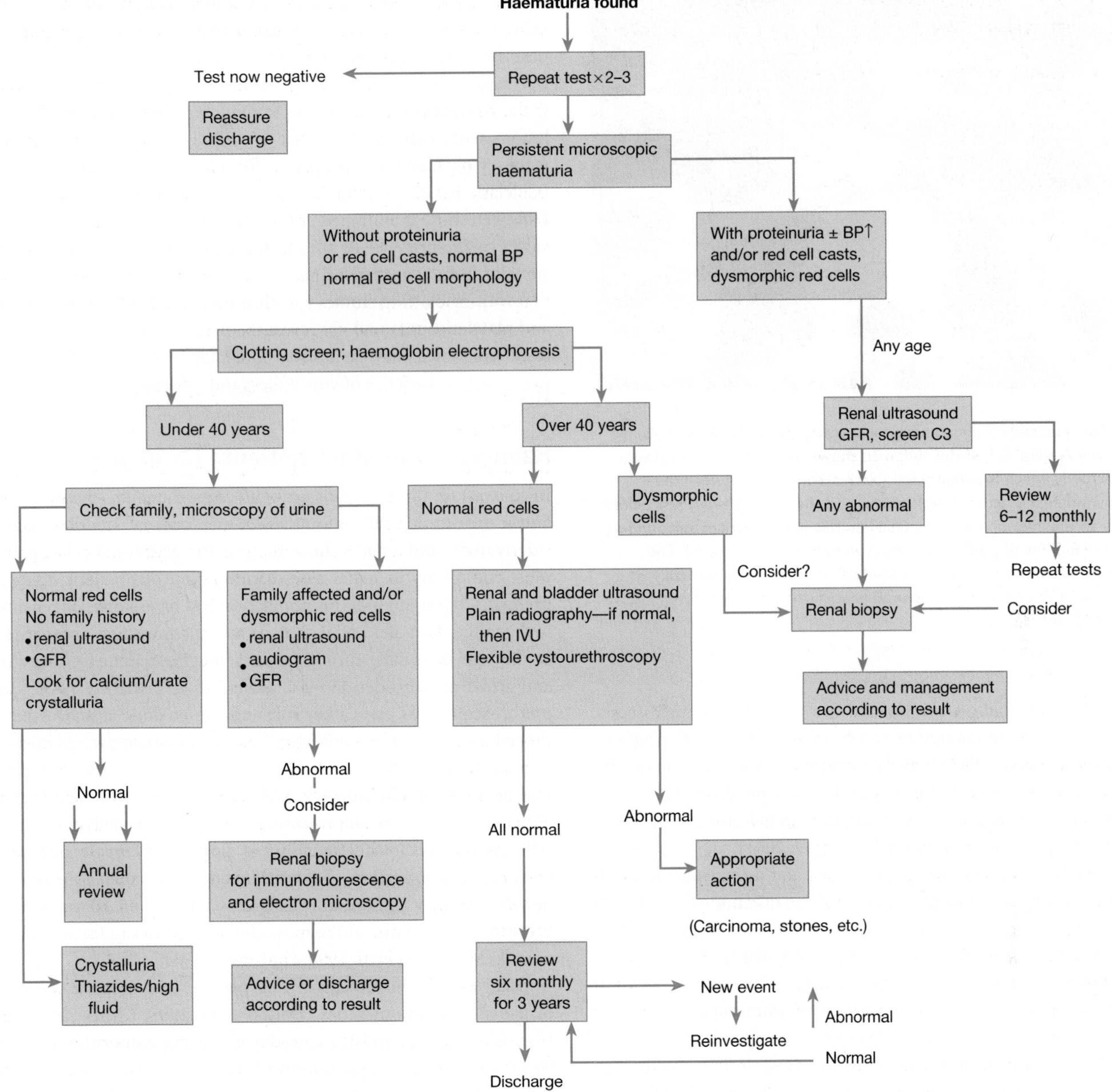

Fig. 5 An algorithm describing suggested management of a patient with symptomless haematuria.

Experienced observers can detect sickled red cells in the urine (Fogazzi *et al.* 1996). Males and the left kidney (see below) are more commonly the source of the haematuria in sickle-cell disease. On the renal ultrasound examination, minor degrees of medullary 'sponge' kidney may be revealed (see Chapter 17.5) or hydronephrosis is present; this is a cause of sudden gross macroscopic haematuria after trivial trauma. Renal calculi are a rare cause of symptomless haematuria in children from developed countries, but common in the developing world (Chapters 8.1–8.3), but many Caucasian children show a high calcium oxalate or uric acid excretion without lithiasis, which appears to be the cause of the haematuria, probably through microcrystalluria (Perrone *et al.* 1991; Stapleton 1994). Polycystic kidney disease may be revealed in the absence of a family history, but proteinuria is often present as well in these patients (see below). Renal haemangiomas are a rare but well-documented cause, and in infants and children up to about 5 years of age, Wilms' tumour must not be forgotten; about one-fourth of the patients with Wilms' tumours show microscopic haematuria although this is poorly documented in the literature.

The 'nutcracker' phenomenon of left renal vein entrapment between the aorta and the superior mesenteric artery although known since 1972 (De Schepper 1972) has only received attention recently. It can lead to microscopic or even profuse macroscopic haematuria relieved by surgery (Shaper *et al.* 1994; Chuang *et al.* 1997; Lidove *et al.* 2001). As imaging and angiographic techniques have improved (Wolfish *et al.* 1986), and with this ease of diagnosis (Fig. 6), it has been identified more frequently, although it remains a rare phenomenon.

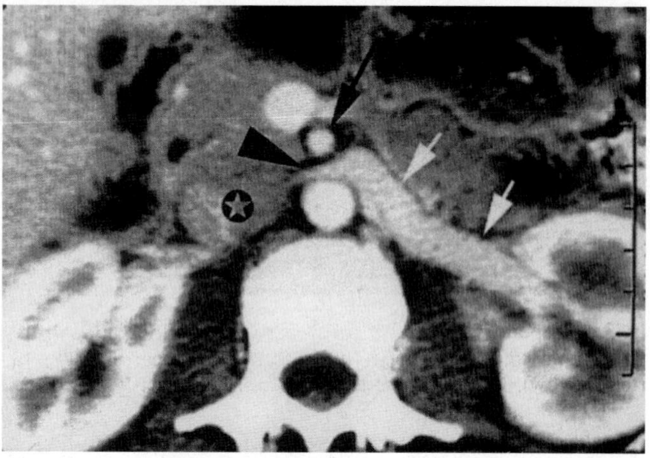

Fig. 6 The 'nutcracker' phenomenon in a young woman with unexplained haematuria. A spiral CT of the abdomen shows the dilated left renal vein (white arrows) which is compressed (black arrowhead) between the superior mesenteric artery (black arrow) and the aorta (below) just before its entry to the inferior vena cava (star). In this patient varices surrounding the pelvis (and out of plane, the ureter) were not demonstrated. The 'nutcracker' phenomenon has been invoked also, but more debatably, as a possible cause of orthostatic (postural) proteinuria (see text). From Lidove *et al.* (2001) with permission.

Arteriovenous malformations may also present with microscopic haematuria, and again awareness and imaging are the key to diagnosis (Subramanyam *et al.* 1983). Finally, one must beware the patient who has an obvious 'cause' for episodes of macroscopic haematuria, such as polycystic kidneys, but has in addition renal stones—or worse a bladder or uroepithelial tumour (Dedi *et al.* 2001).

If, in addition to red cells, red cell casts and dysmorphic red cells are found and renal ultrasound is normal, the question of whether to perform a *renal biopsy* will arise and has been much debated for both adults (Copley *et al.* 1987; De Caestecker and Ballardie 1990; Topham *et al.* 1994; McGregor *et al.* 1998) and children (Piqueras *et al.* 1998). If done, this will often show minor patterns of glomerular change, but may reveal thin membrane nephropathy or mesangial IgA deposition, and thus in immunofluorescence-negative cases, electron microscopy should be performed. Alport's syndrome (Chapter 16.4.1) will often present as isolated haematuria before any deafness or associated proteinuria occurs, usually between 5 and 15 years of age, and will present also as immunofluorescence-negative microscopic haematuria; the finding of deafness or eye changes in other members of the family may render a renal biopsy unnecessary, but if one is performed, electron microscopy to examine basement membrane morphology is crucial. Renal biopsy findings in children and young adults with microscopic haematuria rarely alter treatment, and their value should not be exaggerated; their main aim is to provide a definite diagnosis which may have important implications for prognosis and genentic counselling, such as in Alport's syndrome (Topham *et al.* 1994; Piqueras *et al.* 1998).

Factitious haematuria may be induced by adding blood obtained by fingerprick or from animal or avian (chicken) sources; these red cells may show nuclei which gives the game away, but factitious haematuria using human blood can be very difficult to detect. Rarely, parents will even add blood to their child's urine, another variety of Munchausen syndrome by proxy (Meadow 1977).

Use of warfarin should not be forgotten, which in the past was the cause in isolation of both microscopic and even macroscopic haematuria; but with modern levels of anticoagulation [INR (international normalized ratio) of two to three times normal], in almost every case if the haematuria is macroscopic there will prove to be a lesion or lesions within the urinary tract as well. Therefore imaging perhaps cytology plus, where appropriate, flexible cystoscopy should be done (Culclasure *et al.* 1994; Van Savage and Fried 1995; Avidor *et al.* 2000). However, those maintained at higher INR (3–4) for mechanical heart valves or the presence of antiphospholipid antibody may bleed occasionally from a normal urinary tract. Finally, one should not forget that routine clotting studies (prothrombin and kaolin–cephalin times and platelet count) will *not* reveal the presence of some rarer clotting disorders which may be an occasional cause of microscopic haematuria, such as varieties of von Willebrand's disease.

Haematuria in older patients (>40 years)

In contrast, in those *over the age of 40 years*, the main causes of haematuria are 'urological'. About 10–20 per cent of middle-aged and elderly males and females show microscopic symptomless haematuria, most commonly in males as a manifestation of prostatic disease or urethritis, but up to half this population will have stones or renal tract malignancy (Grossfeld *et al.* 2001b) and the investigation of patients at this age is initially urological and imaging-based, seeking stones and growths (Schröder, 1994; Grossfeld *et al.* 2001b). Flexible cysto-urethroscopy thus plays a key role and can be done as an out-patient procedure as part of a 'single stop' evaluation of haematuria including also ultrasound examination. Nevertheless, various forms of nephritis may be found even in the very elderly (see Chapter 14.2) and the presence of more than trivial proteinuria, red cell casts, or dysmorphic red cells should alert to the possibility of glomerular disease, and a *renal biopsy* should be performed if renal imaging is normal. Polycystic kidney disease may present also as late as 70 or even 80 years of age. Infections remain one of the most common causes in the older group as well (Murakami *et al.* 1990; Paul *et al.* 1993).

Malignant disease presents in 1–25 per cent (commonly 2–5 per cent) of patients in various series (Britton *et al.* 1989; Khadra *et al.* 2000; Grossfeld *et al.* 2001a) with a steadily increasing proportion from 40 to 90 years of age (12–34 per cent in Khadra *et al.*'s series). In Murakami's study of more than 1000 middle-aged Japanese haematurics, 3 per cent had urinary tract malignancies, 5 per cent stones, and 11 per cent parenchymal renal disease. Similarly in Mariani's survey (1989) of 1000 individuals with haematuria, 77 (8 per cent) had cancers and an additional 23 per cent had conditions for which at least observation was required; only 12 patients had glomerulonephritis.

An ideal strategy of *imaging* has not been defined at this age either, and ultrasonography, computed tomography (CT) scanning, and IVU all have advantages in certain situations (Grossfeld *et al.* 2001b). CT has the highest sensitivity for both renal masses and urinary tract stones, ultrasound best defines cystic lesions, and IVU urothelial lesions (Chapter 1.6). In practice today renal and bladder ultrasound examination are the usual first step, together with a plain abdominal radiograph (Corwin and Silverstein 1988; Spencer *et al.* 1990; Grossfeld *et al.* 2001b). If negative, an IVU should be performed if the haematuria persists for 3 months or more (Jaffe *et al.* 2001), as this still remains the best imaging method to diagnose transitional cell lesions of the upper urinary tract. CT will be preferred by many in addition to either, but is more expensive. *Flexible cystourethroscopy* usually will be needed to diagnose or exclude bladder tumours, since *urine cytology*, although highly specific (94 per cent), has a very low sensitivity—only 42 per cent in one study (Chahal *et al.* 2001). Thus, a negative result should not be reassuring, cystoscopy is likely to be needed in positive cases in any case and thus this test has only a minor role to play, principally in patients *not* submitted to flexible cystoscopy, or during follow-up in negative cases. *Voided tumour markers* have been used also (Grossfeld and Carroll 1998) but although under extensive investigation, none as yet are sensitive and specific enough to avoid cystoscopy if negative (Grossfeld *et al.* 2001b).

Haematuria in tropical and developing countries

Few data are available from parts of the world where *Schistosoma haematobium* and sickle-cell trait are common to determine local optimum strategies of investigation (Sharfi and Hassan 1994; Muraguri *et al.* 1997; Hall and Fentiman 1999; Dawam *et al.* 2001) but in general throughout areas affected by *S. haematobium* this is the major cause of microscopic haematuria, to the point where it forms a useful screening test for this infection alone, with high specificity but understandably a rather low sensitivity (Hammad *et al.* 1997; Anosike *et al.* 2001). The precocious bladder tumours in infected patients aged less than 40 years of age must be remembered also in evaluating younger haematuric patients in or from endemic areas (Sharfi and Hassan 1994). In contrast, the overall impact of sickle cell trait in Africa seems to be small as a cause of haematuria (Muraguri *et al.* 1997; Hall and Fentiman 1999; Dawam *et al.* 2001) although still important to recognize. In children, urinary tract stones are common specially in the bladder.

The patient whose investigations are negative

In a proportion of patients, greater in the young (perhaps as many as 80 per cent) and less in the older patients (ca 20 per cent), no cause may be found even after exhaustive investigation (which may or may not include a renal biopsy); many of those patients not submitted to biopsy probably have thin glomerular basement membranes, but even biopsy and full urological evaluation may reveal nothing. These patients with negative investigations require follow-up, particularly those over 40 years of age since, for example, a few will have undiagnosed bladder tumours. If a lesion is present but has not been identified by the first screening, however, it will almost always present within 3 years (Murakami *et al.* 1990; Khadra *et al.* 2000) and longer study is unproductive. Yet again, no clear strategy of management can be outlined which is based on good evidence, and the incidence of new findings is low—about 3 per cent. Follow-up for urine testing and cytology at 6-monthly intervals up to 3 years have been advocated by the American Urological Association (Grossfeld *et al.* 2001b), unless of course some new event appears, such as macroscopic haematuria, or persistent dysuria in the absence of infection, which require immediate reinvestigation.

Routine screening for microscopic haematuria?

Should population screening for haematuria be performed in those *without* an increased risk factor being present (i.e. family history, exposure to dyes, chemicals or analgesics, or smoking)? Certainly routine screening does not seem useful in the young, such as in schoolchildren (Benbassat *et al.* 1996) unless a family history is present, but nevertheless since 1974 all schoolchildren in Japan, Korea, and Taiwan have had their urine screened for both proteinuria and haematuria but with only minimal return in identification of patients with chronic treatable disorders. Given the frequency of significant findings in older males (25 per cent in some series) half of whom showed urological disease and 0.8 per cent undiagnosed bladder tumours, whether the elderly should have urinary screening for haematuria has been much debated (Anonymous 1988; Grossfeld *et al.* 2001b). Britton *et al.* (1989) screened 68 per cent of 855 men over 60 in a general practice, and found 13 per cent to have microscopic haematuria. Of these, 45 per cent had urological abnormalities, including four bladder tumours and one prostate cancer. Messing *et al.* (1989) had 235 apparently well men over the age of 50 test their urine weekly for haematuria over a year: 44 of them showed at least one positive test at some time, and 31 had a full urological evaluation. Fifteen of these had serious disease, eight of them cancers. A further study on 856 men (Messing *et al.* 1995) showed that because of the rapidity of growth of the tumours, annual screening would be needed to be effective. Thus even here the cost-effectiveness is relatively low (Froom *et al.* 1997) and despite these findings, at the moment no Western government and no professional organization recommends routine screening of even the middle-aged or elderly for haematuria, and several have recommended against the practice (Grossfeld *et al.* 2001a).

Macroscopic haematuria

The differing underlying causes in various age groups found for microscopic haematuria are present also in macroscopic haematuria, with 'nephrological' conditions predominating under the age of 40 and 'urological' conditions becoming steadily predominant over that age. In an important study of 948 patients with macroscopic haematuria, Khadra *et al.* (2000) noted a lower proportion of patients with macroscopic haematuria in whom no diagnosis was reached after investigation (52.5 per cent) compared with microscopic haematuria (68.5 per cent). Of 199 patients in their study who had macroscopic haematuria and neoplasms (183 being bladder tumours), six were under 40 years of age at the time of diagnosis, and two under 30. This proportion rose, however, to 15 per cent in 40–50 year olds and up to 35 per cent in 70–80 year olds and for macroscopic haematuria the divide should perhaps be at 30 or even 20 years of age. On occasions it will be justified in a high-risk patient even younger than this. Other than that, the diagnostic approach to the diagnosis of macroscopic haematuria can be the same as for microscopic haematuria (Fig. 5) and is well established. Nevertheless, in 53 per cent of 948 patients with macroscopic haematuria (Khadra *et al.* 2000), no lesion was found and at follow-up only half still had haematuria; no new tumours were identified from 2.5 to 4.2 years later. In 146 patients with macroscopic haematuria in whom no diagnosis emerged from initial investigation (Sells and Cox 2001) followed for 2.5 years or more, only one developed a transitional cell tumour, and he had recurrent macroscpic bleeding. Thus routine follow-up is not justified in patients in whom no cause is identified, even those with macroscopic haematuria.

Pain and haematuria

In some patients, haematuria, either macroscopic or microscopic, may be associated with loin pain (Fox and Saunders 1978). This can be associated with IgA nephropathy (Macdonald *et al.* 1975), and we have seen this also in patients with thin membrane disease as emphasized by Hebert *et al.* (1996). The renal colic of ureteric or renal lithiasis is well known. In addition, however, there is a poorly defined group of patients, usually young women, who may be diagnosed by exclusion as the loin pain–haematuria syndrome (see below). The dominant feature is the pain, and the haematuria may be intermittent.

Persistent microscopic haematuria with associated proteinuria

This has been discussed above (see Hisano and Ueda 1991).

Acute macroscopic haematuria with proteinuria: the 'acute nephritic syndrome'

This has also been called 'acute glomerulonephritis', but because this term carries implications of histology, pathogenesis, and outcome, which apply to only some patients, the term 'acute nephritic syndrome' is preferable (see Chapters 3.9–3.12); the underlying causes are listed in Table 3.

Recurrent macroscopic haematuria, with or without proteinuria

This may result from glomerulonephritis in younger patients, but also as recurrent bleeding from urinary tract lesions; again the difference in likely causes between younger and older patients needs emphasis. In some patients with glomerular disease and macroscopic haematuria the volume overload and hypertension are absent, the haematuria appears at the same time as the infection, and the syndrome may then be called 'recurrent haematuria'. In a few of these patients, the haematuria may be accompanied by loin pain, fever, and adenopathy, or be precipitated by exercise. Some patients' urine may be reddish almost all the time, and this is almost the only state in which glomerular bleeding can be so profuse as to cause anaemia. Usually, renal biopsy in such patients will show IgA nephropathy, mesangial nephritia negative immunofluorescence or C3 alone, but some patients with thin membrane nephropathy or Alport's syndrome may present in this fashion also. In a minority, usually with IgA nephropathy (Fogazzi *et al.* 1992) but also in thin membrane disease (Abt *et al.* 2000) or Henoch–Schönlein purpura (Kobayashi *et al.* 2001), acute renal failure supervenes. There is speculation that this may result from tubular erythrophagocytosis during the acute haematuric episode (Sheerin *et al.* 1999). Erythrophagocytosis by macrophages may be observed also in the urinary sediment (Anders and Schlondorff 1998), and is diagnostic of inflammatory disease withn the kidney, almost certainly glomerulonephritis.

Special forms of haematuria and proteinuria

Loin pain–haematuria syndrome

Loin pain is an important symptom of renal disease (see Chapter 1.1; Eastwood 1978; and Fox and Saunders 1978) and often presents together with haematuria such as in renal or ureteric stones, gravel or crystalluria, and those with urinary tract infections. Acute glomerulonephritis or IgA nephropathy may also present variable loin pain, especially during attacks of macroscopic haematuria (Macdonald *et al.* 1975); a proportion of such patients go into acute renal failure (see above). Some patients have pain in the loin which is referred from the spine.

Definition

However, patients have been described apparently distinct from all these groups, who have come to be called the 'loin pain–haematuria syndrome' (Anonymous 1992; Weisberg *et al.* 1993; Winearls and Bass 1994; Burke and Hardie 1996). This term was first used by Little *et al.* (1967) and its definition remains imprecise and one of exclusion: a patient with intermittent or persistent severe loin pain, and intermittent or persistent haematuria (usually microscopic but ocasionally sufficient to produce even clot colic), in the presence of a normal cystoscopy and intravenous urogram, no or minor proteinuria, sterile urine, and (if performed) a renal biopsy which does not show any form of primary or secondary glomerulonephritis. Not all patients included under this heading have had haematuria, or it is present only intermittently, or disappears. We have reviewed 22 patients who appear to satisfy these criteria in an unpublished study which is referred to throughout this section, and others have reported their experience (Burden *et al.* 1975, 1979; Leaker *et al.* 1990; Lucas *et al.* 1995). Cases have been described worldwide, from the United States, France, Canada, Australia, Italy, and Finland as well as from the United Kingdom, although most experience has accumulated in this country.

Patients are usually young women, and attacks become less frequent and gradually remit in middle age; it has not been described in patients older than 50 years, although children as young as 6 have been seen (Burke and Hardie 1996)—our youngest patient was aged 14. Three of our patients have been males, and this has been noted by others (Habte *et al.* 1981). Little *et al.* (1967) described these patients as 'anxious, introspective, demanding of medical attention; occasionally fabricating evidence' and this remains true, to the point where some observers believe that in all cases there is evidence of 'malingering' or at least somatization.

On the other hand, the effect of chronic severe pain, especially pain which the medical profession persistently denies (and with this denial of effective analgesia), must lead to abnormalities of attitude and behaviour. Very often before being referred to a nephrologist or a urologist, the patient will have been seen by a psychiatrist. These young women are often medical workers, although never in our experience or in the published literature, doctors: that is, nurses, medical aides, medical receptionists, laboratory staff, medical secretaries, and even in children or relatives of the above. Psychiatrists have studied a number of patients and have emphasized the resemblance to other somatoform disorders (Kelly 1992, 1994; Lucas *et al.* 1992, 1995), that is, bodily symptoms without physical cause but the result of somatization of psychiatric events. Lucas *et al.* (1995) compared 15 patients with the loin pain–haematuria syndrome with 10 patients with complicated painful stone disease, and noted a greater prevalence of other unexplained symptoms, more frequently the onset of loin pain following a major life event, feelings of responsibility for parental distress, and more frequent experience of family illness or death during childhood; both groups were equally anxious or depressed. Thus, the condition may be primarily a psychiatric disorder (Hall *et al.* 1997), and this is supported by the fact that although a variety of histological, radiological, and haemostatic abnormalities have been described, none of these is common or consistently present. Blood pressure is normal, the pain is often unilateral (at least to begin with) and examination reveals nothing except sometimes loin tenderness.

Clinical investigations

Renal function (unless nephrectomy has been performed) is normal, the urinary red cells are dysmorphic on phase contrast microscopy suggesting a renal, probably glomerular, origin (Leaker *et al.* 1990) but red cell casts are absent. Occasionally patients have an excretion of protein greater than normal, but never more than 1 g/24 h. By definition there are no stones present, but in some patients there is a history (which may be doubtful) of having passed a stone previously. Urine is sterile and on culture the ESR is normal even during attacks and haematology and routine plasma biochemistry are unremarkable. CRP appears not to have been measured.

Radiological findings

Little *et al.* (1967) and Burden *et al.* (1975, 1979) described tortuosity, beading, and obliteration of intrarenal medium-sized vessels, present in the majority of (but not all) patients. In some patients with unilateral pain, the changes were observed only on the painful side. Occasionally quite large areas of underperfusion were noted within the kidney (Burden *et al.* 1979) (Fig. 7), and Bergroth *et al.* (1987) reported reversible intrarenal arterial spasm. However, in almost all of our patients arteriography revealed nothing abnormal. Woolfson *et al.* (1993) examined ureteric peristalsis, but this appeared normal.

Histological findings

Histological changes have in general been mild or absent, apart from the intrarenal vessels. Mild mesangial hypertrophy and patchy interstitial fibrosis and tubular atrophy have been described (Burden *et al.* 1975), but a number of renal biopsies in our own series were completely normal and all in the series of Leaker *et al.* (1990). The renal vessels, however, often show marked abnormalities (Fletcher *et al.* 1979) for age, with hyalinosis (Fig. 8), lesions resembling atheroma, intimal hyperplasia, or an 'onion skin' appearance, and in one patient microaneurysms, affecting arcuate to segmental arteries. There was prominent deposition of C3 in the affected vessels (Naish *et al.* 1975; Fletcher *et al.* 1979) whilst C4 was reported by Burden *et al.* (1979). The deposition of C3 in vessel walls is, of course, a non-specific finding in many arteriopathies, and immunoglobulins have never been recorded. Miller *et al.* (1994) reported a single patient in whom obvious radiological vascular changes were evident, and in whom deposition of properdin and C5b-9 could be demonstrated as well as C3 in the arterioles. Hebert *et al.* (1996) described 7 patients with the syndrome of loin-pain–haematuria who had thin basement membranes in their glomerular capillaries.

Pathogenesis

If this syndrome has a physical basis in the kidney, the radiological and histological evidence suggests that it may result from disease affecting the intrarenal vessels, the only structure within the parenchyma of the kidney bearing pain-sensitive nerve fibres. However, patients with other severe diseases of the intrarenal vasculature such as the haemolytic–uraemic syndrome, accelerated hypertension and cholesterol atheroembolism never experience similar pain. Nor is there any explanation as to why it is usually unilateral, at least to begin with, or why it may move subsequently to a remaining or an autotransplanted kidney.

Since it is a condition predominantly affecting young women, many of whom have been taking an oestrogen-containing contraceptive, these have been implicated by some. Burden *et al.* (1975) present a convincing anecdote of a patient whose attacks were temporally related to oestrogen substitution after oophorectomy, which is supported by its

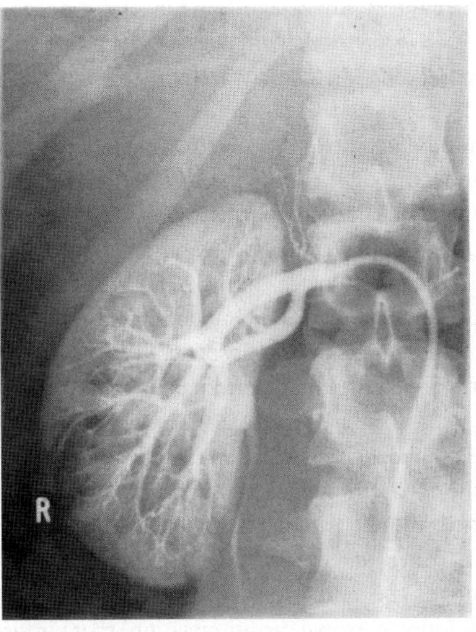

(a)

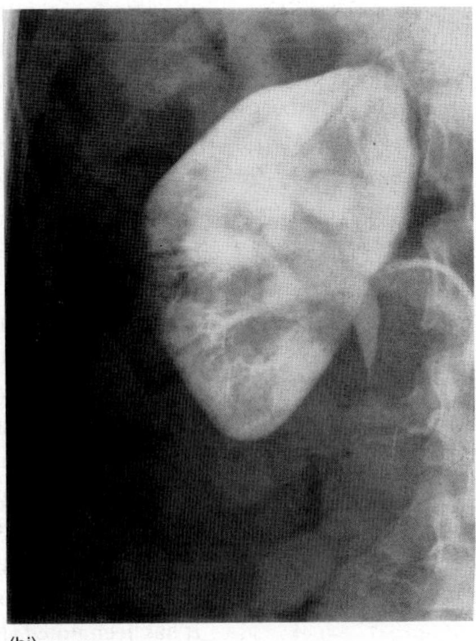
(bi)

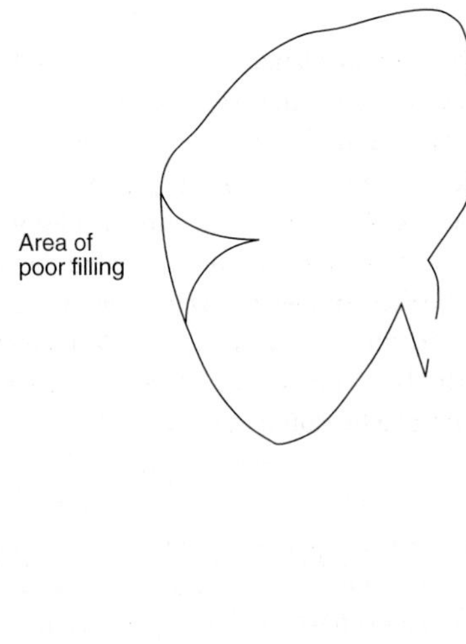

(bii)

Fig. 7 Arteriogram of right kidney of a patient with loin pain–haematuria syndrome. (a) Initial flush showing diminished perfusion in the lower lateral area; (b) nephrogram indicating poor concentration of dye in the area of abnormal perfusion (reproduced by kind permission of Dr Richard Burden, Nottingham City Hospital, UK).

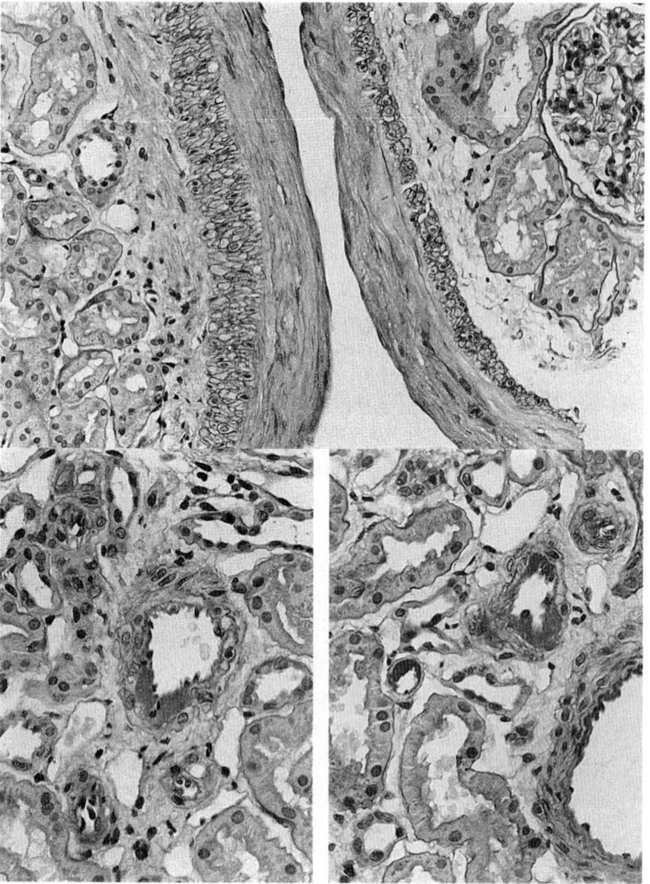

Fig. 8 Vessels from a 32-year-old normotensive male with the loin pain–haematuria syndrome. At the top, extensive endothelial hyperplasia is demonstrated in a medium-sized vessel. In the two lower panels, widespread hyaline changes in small arterioles are shown, which resemble those seen in patients with cyclosporin-induced vasospasm (by courtesy of Professor G. H. Neild).

age and sex incidence. In contrast temporary remission has been reported during pregnancy in three patients (Aber and Higgins 1982; Burke and Hardie 1996).

The nature of this vascular pathology, if it exists, remains obscure. Several lines of evidence support the idea of intravascular coagulation being a primary or a secondary event: the details of the vessel pathology (Burden *et al.* 1975), and evidence of platelet activation (Parbtani and Cameron 1979; Leaker *et al.* 1990), fibrin deposition and evidence of fibrinolysis (Leaker *et al.* 1990), failure of plasma to support prostacyclin production by endothelial cells (Siegler *et al.* 1988), or factor XII deficiency (Smellie *et al.* 1987) all support this suggestion. Leaker *et al.* (1990) draw attention also to the similarities between their histological findings in 13 of 20 biopsies (Fig. 7) and those seen in patients taking cyclosporin (see Chapter 11.5), again suggesting that vasospasm may be the primary event (Bergroth *et al.* 1987).

Clinical course

The condition runs a relapsing intermittent course over periods of several years, but eventually the attacks of severe pain become less common, until they finally cease in many cases by middle age (Aber and Higgins 1982). Renal function remains normal throughout, and the microscopic haematuria may wax and wane. The severe pain, not surprisingly, disrupts the life of the patients considerably, to the point of suicide attempts in a few. By the time patients get to a nephrologist, many are seriously disturbed, and reassurance that the clinician has seen similar cases before, is aware of the condition and may be able to help, may produce immediate relief in someone who has become hostile and bruised by prolonged contact with sceptical doctors. On the other hand, their continued support presents many challenges to the physician.

Treatment

The management of this syndrome is completely unsatisfactory. No treatment is of proven value in the long-term for the majority of patients. Prednisolone or antiplatelet agents do not usually meet with much success. I am not aware of any substantial data on the use of hydralazine, α-blockers, ACE inhibitors, AT1 anatgonists, or calcium channel blockers to relieve the vasospasm. Usually conventional analgesics are the mainstay of treatment, and often opioids or equivalent drugs are required, sometimes in fairly large doses; but it is striking that in the majority of patients the dosage needed is stable, and the drugs are not required between attacks if they are intermittent. Neild (personal communication) recommends tricyclic antidepressives, which are also platelet membrane stabilizing agents, administered at night to avoid sedation. Other approaches in intractable cases have been the use of long-term intrathecal morphine (Prager *et al.* 1995), and capsaicin (Bultitude 1995; Armstrong *et al.* 2000). Transcutaneous nerve stimulation (TENS) has been used, by ourselves and others (Chin 1992; Dimski *et al.* 1992) but without lasting relief.

Given that the principal problem is pain, interruption of the pain fibres running along the renal vessels, either by stripping under direct vision (Little *et al.* 1967), injection of temporary anaesthetic agents, or destruction of the renal nerves by alcohol or similar substances, has attractions. In some cases injections give prolonged relief lasting weeks or months, but usually the pain recurs. Nerve stripping operations have the disadvantage that reinnervation occurs within about 6 months (Gazdar and Dammin 1970) although this reinnervation is usually incomplete (Hansen *et al.* 1994). This may account for the return of pain (see below).

Nephrectomy should be avoided (although a number of sufferers from this condition find a urologist willing to perform the operation), because it has the obvious penalty of nephron loss and rarely leads to complete relief from pain, which recurs (usually immediately) in the opposite loin. In occasional cases, doctors have been driven by requests from patients themselves to perform bilateral nephrectomy after all else has failed, putting the patient on dialysis (Gibson *et al.* 1994; Talic *et al.* 1994). This is not a course many patients or doctors would be willing to accept in a patient with normal renal function (Winearls and Bass 1994). This extreme state may be achieved accidentally also by technical problems during autotransplantation. This operation conserves renal function and denervates the kidney, at least temporarily (see above) and has been publicized by Sheil *et al.* (1985, 1987, 1998) although it had been done previously (Aber and Higgins 1982; Turini *et al.* 1995). It has been noted (N. F. Jones, personal communication) that perfusion of the kidney *ex vivo* after excision has been a problem in some autografts, supporting the idea of vasospasm as the primary pathological event, and leading in some to vascular thrombosis (Burke and Hardie 1996). Autotransplantation, which can be done through laparoscopy

(Gill *et al.* 2000), has since been studied by a number of groups (Chin 1992; Dimski *et al.* 1992; Harney *et al.* 1994; Burke and Hardie 1996; Chin *et al.* 1998). Despite some encouraging reports on long-term follow-up (Sheil *et al.* 1987, 1998; Chin 1992; Turini *et al.* 1995; Spitz 1997; Chin *et al.* 1998), return of pain at the site of the autotransplanted kidney is common (Hutchinson *et al.* 1987; Dimski *et al.* 1992; Harney *et al.* 1994), and is probably underestimated by the published reports (see Weisberg *et al.* 1993 and Burke and Hardie 1996 for review), although it is often less intense than before and more easily controlled by analgesics.

Clearly the management of these unfortunate patients is a matter of decades rather than months or years, and requires the cooperation of experts in psychiatry, pain relief, and urology or transplantation, as well as nephrology.

Proteinuria and nephrotic syndrome in massive obesity

Apart from the well-recognized associations of obesity [usually defined as a body mass index (BMI) of >30] such as hypertension, insulin resistance, and diabetes mellitus, proteinuria is common in those attending morbid obesity (body weight > 120 kg) clinics (Cohen 1975; Dornfeld 1989) being present in 40 per cent of patients, with 5 per cent showing an abnormal urinary sediment. In those patients in whom weight loss could be achieved, proteinuria usually disappeared. Metcalf *et al.* (1992) noted a strong relationship between generally subclinical levels of proteinuria and BMI in a population study of nearly 6000 subjects aged more than 45 years, and microalbuminuria is associated with obesity (see above).

In some a full nephrotic syndrome appears, as first noted by José Weisinger and colleagues in 1974: Praga *et al.* (2001) review the 15 or so patients published previously, although there are others (Lim *et al.* 1974; Velosa *et al.* 1975; Shimamura *et al.* 1990). They add a series of 15 such patients studied by themselves. In the United States, Kambham *et al.* (2001) described an even larger series of 71 proteinuric obese patients, 31 with a nephrotic syndrome and/or renal insufficiency and pointed out that this association seems to become more common, perhaps as levels of obesity in the general population increase. Oedema is usually mild in these patients, or even absent for long periods despite nephrotic-range proteinuria (Praga *et al.* 2001) and the serum albumin remains nearer normal when compared with nephrotic controls with focal segmental glomerulosclerosis. Males are in a slight excess over females, 75 per cent of Kambham's and 100 per cent of Praga's patients were Caucasian and the condition may be seen from older children to the elderly. Hypertension is not prominent, but sleep apnoea is common (Jennette *et al.* 1987; Bailey *et al.* 1989; Praga *et al.* 2001). Conversely Sklar and Chaudhary (1988) reported proteinuria in obese sleep apnoeic patients, which diminished on giving oxygen, although Casserly *et al.* (2002) in a series of 148 sleep apnoeic patients found only eight with increased proteinuria. Not surprisingly perhaps, diabetes mellitus may develop later in these obese patients. Equally all were markedly hyperlipidaemic, but surprisingly less so than the idiopathic focal segmental glomerulosclerosis (FSGS) controls, in both the series of Praga *et al.* (2001) and Kambham *et al.* (2001).

Even nephrotic range proteinuria may diminish or disappear with weight loss (Shimamura *et al.* 1990), suggesting that at least in the early stages it may be functional in nature, perhaps depending upon the increased concentrations of renin and angiotensin present in obese subjects (Tuck *et al.* 1981) which diminish on fasting. This is supported by the effect of ACE inhibition on proteinuria in obese subjects, which diminishes in parallel with that achieved by weight loss (Praga *et al.* 1995) and by the finding of juxtaglomerular apparatus (JGA) hyperplasia by Kambham *et al.* (2001). However, Praga *et al.* (2001) reported poor results with ACE inhibitors and negligible achievement of weight loss.

Renal histology has been studied in only a few cases other than the large series of Kambham *et al.* (2001), but nephrotic patients have shown minimal change lesions (usually with glomerulomegaly) reported in six sporadic cases, and in one patient with membranous nephropathy renal venous thrombosis has been reported. However, in the majority of patients, including 57/71 in Kambham *et al.*'s (2001) series, lesions resembling those of idiopathic FSGS were seen. This is of some general interest in view of theories of nutrition and hyperfiltration in the genesis of such lesions, and some of these patients were Afro-Americans, who have relative glomerulopenia and relative glomerulomegaly when compared with Caucasians, and thus are particularly susceptible to segmental sclerosing glomerular lesions. Praga *et al.* (2001) report that the mean diameter of the glomeruli in their (Caucasian) patients with FSGS exceeded that of control nephrotic patients with FSGS by 25 per cent (mean 256 versus 199 μm), which implies double the glomerular volume, a finding replicatd by Kambham *et al.* (2001) (226 versus 168 μm) in a population 75 per cent Caucasian.

Outcome in obese proteinuric patients has been little studied, but the patients of Kambham *et al.* (2001) and Praga *et al.* (2001) both survived better than control patients with FSGS, 5-year survival without renal failure being 86 per cent versus 48 per cent in Kambham's series. Most had been treated with ACE inhibitors and some with corticosteroids, but without any evident effect as in the seven of Praga *et al.*'s 15 patients, who went into chronic renal failure with steadily increasing proteinuria—although more slowly than FSGS controls. However, four of these patients already had diminished renal mass on one side at diagnosis.

Congenital cyanotic heart disease, polycythaemia, and proteinuria

Apart from possible subacute endocarditis, thrombosis, and embolism, it has been known since Weber's first description in 1909 that patients with persistent cyanosis, hypoxaemia, and high haematocrit may develop proteinuria, which can reach nephrotic dimensions (Drummond *et al.* 1963; Spear 1964; Spear 1977) and even result in decline in renal function (Hagley *et al.* 1992; Krull *et al.* 1992; Dittrich *et al.* 1998). The magnitude of the proteinuria correlates with the degree and duration of the polycythaemia (Rennie 1966; Krull *et al.* 1992), as do the depression of inulin and *p*-aminohippurate clearances, and rise in the filtration fraction (Table 5). Concentrating ability and urinary acidification are in contrast not affected.

Now that many cyanotic heart conditions can be corrected surgically in infancy or childhood, this problem has diminished in importance, and Flanagan *et al.* (1991) noted only five nephrotic patients amongst 83 such patients over the age of 21 years. A greater proportion than usual of patients with cyanotic heart disease show urinary tract abnormalities on IVU [7/45 (15 per cent) in Rennie's series], particularly Fallot's tetralogy, and one patient in his series had papillary necrosis.

Table 5 Renal clearances in 20 patients with congenital cyanotic heart disease

Haematocrit 71.3 + 10.6
Haemoglobin 24.1 + 3.5
C_{inulin} 70.3 + 22.0 ml/min/1.73 m^2
$C_{creatinine}$ 80.5 + 26 ml/min/1.73 m^2
C_{PAH} 224.8 + 67.6 ml/min/1.73 m^2
Filtration fraction 0.32 + 0.075
Renal blood flow 836 + 238 ml/min/1.78 m^2
Proteinuria 1.87 + 0.78 g/24 h

Unpublished data of IBD Rernie (1966).

Renal plasma flow is diminished but GFR is partially maintained in these extreme degrees of polycythaemia by a considerable increase in the filtration fraction (Table 5; De Jong *et al.* 1983; Krull *et al.* 1992). This reverses promptly as the haematocrit is lowered (De Jong *et al.* 1983), with a concomitant reduction in the level of proteinuria. Hyperuricaemia is often present also. Hida *et al.* (2002) describe a nephrotic patient with FSGS and glomerulomegaly whose proteinuria diminished to less than 1g/24h during treatment with an ACE inhibitor.

The renal histology is striking, with enormous enlargement of the glomeruli and a relative increase in mesangial area. Ultrastructural studies of three patients (Burke *et al.* 1977) showed basement membrane thickening in addition to the mesangial expansion. In Hida's (2002) patient FSGS was a striking finding. Proteinuria has been described also in polycythaemic individuals with chronic lung disease (Rosenmann *et al.* 1972; Wilcox *et al.* 1982) and those living at altitudes (Naeye 1965). Again in these patients filtration fraction was greatly increased with a reduced renal plasma flow, which reversed after venesection (Wilcox *et al.* 1982).

References

Abbate, M., Benigni, M., Bertani, T., and Remuzzi, G. (1999). Nephrotoxicity of increased glomerular protein traffic. *Nephrology, Dialysis, Transplantation* **14**, 304–312.

Aber, G. M. and Higgins P. M. (1982). The natural history and management of the loin pain–haematuria syndrome. *British Journal of Urology* **54**, 613–615.

Abt, A. B., Carroll, L. E., and Mohler, J. H. (2000). Thin basement membrane disease and acute renal failure secondary to gross hematuria and tubular necrosis. *American Journal of Kidney Diseases* **35**, 533–536.

Albright, P., Brensilver, J., and Cortell, S. (1983). Proteinuria in congestive heart failure. *American Journal of Medicine* **3**, 272–275.

Anders, H. J. and Schlondorff, D. (1998). Urinary erythrophagocytosis in proliferative glomerulonephritis. *New England Journal of Medicine* **339**, 925–926.

Angulo, J. C., Lopez-Rubio, M., Guil, M., Burgaleta, C., and Sanchez-Chapado, M. (1999). The value of comparative volumetric analysis of urinary and blood erythrocytes to localize the source of hematuria. *Journal of Urology* **162**, 119–126.

Anonymous (1979). Haematuria after closed trauma. *British Medical Journal* **i**, 841–842 (editorial).

Anonymous (1988). Is routine urinalysis worthwhile? *Lancet* **i**, 747 (editorial).

Anonymous (1992). Loin pain/haematuria syndrome. *Lancet* **340**, 701–702 (editorial).

Anosike, J. C., Nwoke, B. E., and Njoku, A. J. (2001). The validity of haematuria in the community diagnosis of urinary schistosomiasis. *Journal of Helminthology* **75**, 223–225.

Antoine, B., Symvoulidis, A., and Dardenne, M. (1968). La stabilité évolutive des états de proteinurie permanente isolée. *Nephron* **6**, 526–536.

Apeland, T., Mestad, O., and Hetland, Ø (2001). Assessment of haematuria: automated flow cytometry *vs* microscopy. *Nephrology, Dialysis, Transplantation* **16**, 1615–1619.

Armstrong, T., Maclean, A. D., Hayes, M., Morgans, B. T., and Tulloch, D. N. (2000). Early experience of intra-ureteric capsaicin infusion in loin-pain haematuria syndrome. *BJU International* **85**, 233–237.

Avidor, Y., Nadu, A., and Matzkin, H. (2000). Clinical significance of gross hematuria and its evaluation in patients receiving anticoagulant and aspirin treatment. *Urology* **55**, 22–24.

Bailey, R. R., Lynn, K. L., Burry, A. F., and Drennan, C. (1987). Proteinuria, glomerulomegaly and focal segmental scerosis in a grossly obese man with obstructive sleep apnea syndrome. *Australian and New Zealand Journal of Medicine* **19**, 473–474.

Barratt, T. M. (1983). Proteinuria. *British Medical Journal* **287**, 1489–1490.

Bakouch, O., Torffvit, O., Rippe, B., and Tencer, J. (2001). High proteinuria selectivity index based upon IgM is a stong predictor of poor renal survival in glomerular diseases. *Nephrology, Dialysis, Transplantation* **16**, 1357–1363.

Bazzi, C., Petrini, C., Rizza, V., Arrigo, G., Beltrame, A., and D'Amico, G. (1997). Characterization of proteinuria in primary glomerulonephritides. SDS–PAGE patterns: clinical significance and prognostic value of low molecular weight ('tubular') proteins. *American Journal of Kidney Diseases* **29**, 27–35.

Bazzi, C., Petrini, C., Rizza, V., Arrigo, G., and D'Amico, G. (2000). A modern approach to selectivity of proteinuria and tubulointerstitial damage in nephrotic syndrome. *Kidney International* **58**, 1732–1741.

Benbassat, J., Gergawi, M., Offringa, M., and Drukker, A. (1996). Symptomless microhaematuria in schoolchildren: causes for variable management strategies. *Quarterly Journal of Medicine* **89**, 845–854.

Berggård, I. Plasma proteins in normal urine. In *Proteins in Normal and Pathological Urine* (ed. H. Manuel, H. Bétuel, and J.-P. Revillard), p. 719, Basel: Karger, 1970.

Bergroth, V., Konttinen, Y., Nordstrom, D., and Laasonen, L. (1987). Loin pain and haematuria syndrome: possible association with intrarenal arterial spasms. *British Medical Journal* **294**, 1657.

Bernard, A., Amor, A. O., Viau, C., and Lauwerys, R. (1988). The renal uptake of proteins: a nonselective process in conscious rats. *Kidney International* **34**, 175–185.

Bienenstock, J. and Tomasi, T. B., Jr. (1968). Secretory gamma-A in normal urine. *Journal of Clinical Investigation* **47**, 1162–1171.

Birch, D. F. and Fairley, K. F. (1979). Haematuria: glomerular or non-glomerular? *Lancet* **ii**, 845–846.

Birch, D. *et al.* (1983). Urinary erythrocyte morphology in the diagnosis of glomerular hematuria. *Clinical Nephrology* **20**, 78–84.

Birn, H. *et al.* (2000). Cubulin is an albumin binding protein important for renal tubular albumin absorption. *Journal of Clinical Investigation* **105**, 1353–1361.

Bohle, A., Olivera de Cavalcanti, V., and Laberke, H.-G. (1988). Is there any tubular secretion of protein? *Clinical Nephrology* **29**, 28–34.

Bohrer, M. P., Baylis, C., Humes, H. D., Glassock, R. J., Robertson, C. R., and Brenner, B. R. (1978). Permselectivity of the capillary wall. Facilitated filtration of circulating polycations. *Journal of Clinical Investigation* **61**, 72–78.

Brigden, M. L. (1992). High incidence of significant urinary ascorbic acid in a West coast population. Implication for routine analysis. *Clinical Chemistry* **38**, 426–431.

Briner, V. A. and Reinhart, W. H. (1990). *In vitro* production of glomerular red cells: role of pH and osmolality. *Nephron* **56**, 13–18.

Britton, J. P., Dowell, A. C., and Whelan, P. O. (1989). Dipstick haematuria and bladder cancer in men over 60: results of a community study. *British Medical Journal* **299**, 1010–1012.

Brocklebank, T., Cooper, E. H., and Richmond, K. (1991). Sodium dodecyl sulphate polyacrylamide gel electrophoresis patterns of proteinuria in various renal diseases of childhood. *Pediatric Nephrology* **5**, 371–375.

Bultitude, M. I. (1995). Capsaicin in treatment of loin pain–haematuria syndrome. Lancet **345**, 921–922.

Burden, R. P., Booth, L. J., Ockenden, B. G., Boyd, W. N., Higgins, P. McR., and Aber, G. M. (1975). Intrarenal vascular changes in adult patients with recurrent haematuria and loin pain—a clinical, histological, and angiographic study. *Quarterly Journal of Medicine* **44**, 433–447.

Burden, R. P., Dathan, J. R., Etherington, M. D., Guyer, P. B., and McIver, A. G. (1979). The loin pain/haematuria syndrome. *Lancet* **i**, 897–900.

Burke, J. R. and Hardie I. R. (1996). Loin pain hematuria syndrome. *Pediatric Nephrology* **10**, 216–220.

Burke, J. R., Glasgow, E. F., McCredie, S. A., and Powell, H. R. (1977). Nephropathy in cyanotic congenital heart disease. *Clinical Nephrology* 7, 38–42.

Burton, C. and Harris, K. G. P. (1996). The role of proteinuria in progression of chronic renal failure. *American Journal of Kidney Diseases* **27**, 765–775.

Cameron, J. S. Clinicopathologic correlations in glomerular disease. In *Kidney Disease—Present Status. IAP Mongraph* (ed. W. Sommers), pp. 76–97. Baltimore, MD: Williams & Wilkins, 1979.

Cameron, J. S. (1990). Proteinuria and progression in human glomerular diseases. *American Journal of Nephrology* **10** (Suppl. 1), 81–87.

Cameron, J. S. and Blandford, G. (1966). The simple assessment of of selectivity in heavy proteinuria. *Lancet* **ii**, 242–247.

Candiano, G., Ginevri, F., Acerbo, S., Garberi, A., Gusmano, R., and Ghiggeri, G. M. (1990). Analysis of albumin charge by direct immunofixation in ultrathin gels. *Kidney International* **37**, 1002–1005.

Caridi, G. *et al.* (2001). Prevalence, genetics and clinical features of patients carrying podocin mutations in steroid-resistant nonfamilial focal segmental glomerulosclerosis. *Journal of the American Society of Nephrology* **12**, 2742–2746.

Carrie, B. J., Salyer, W. R., and Myers, B. D. (1981). Minimal change nephropathy: an electrochemical disorder of the glomerular membrane. *American Journal of Medicine* **70**, 262–268.

Casserly, L. F. *et al.* (2002). Proteiuria in sleep apnea. *Kidney International* **60**, 1484–1489.

Chahal, R., Gogoi, N. K., and Sundaram, S. K. (2001). Is it necessary to perform urine cytology in screening patients with hematuria ? *European Urology* **39**, 283–286.

Chew, S. T. H., Fitzwilliam, J., Indridason, O. S., and Kovalik, E. C. (1999). Role of urine and serum protein electrophoresis in the evaluation of nephrotic-range proteinuria. *American Journal of Kidney Diseases* **34**, 135–139.

Chin J. L. (1992). Loin pain–hematuria syndrome: role for renal transplantation. *Journal of Urology* **147**, 987–989.

Chin, J. L., Kloth, D., Pautler, S. E., and Mulligan, M. (1998). Renal autotransplantation for the loin pain–hematuria syndrome: long-term follow-up of 26 cases. *Journal of Urology* **160**, 1232–1235 (discussion pp. 1235–1236).

Chitalia, V. C., Kothari, J., Wells, E. J., Livesey, J. H., Robson, R. A., Searle, M. and Lynn, K. L. (2001). Cost–benefit analysis and prediction of 24-hour proteinuria from the spot urine protein–creatinine ratio. *Clinical Nephrology* **55**, 436–447.

Christensen, E. and Birn, H. (2000). Renal handling of albumin in the normal rat. *Kidney International* **57**, 1207–1208; (reply in Comper, W., Eppel, G., Osicka. T., Glasgow, E. F., and Jablonski, P. *ibid* 1208–1209).

Christensen, E. and Birn, H. (2001). Megalin and cubulin: synergistic endocytic receptors in renal proximal tubule. *American Journal of Physiology* **280**, F1208–F1209.

Chuang, C. K., Chu, S. H., and Lai, P. C. (1997). The nutcracker syndrome managed by autotransplantation. *Journal of Urology* **157**, 1833–1834.

Cilento, B. G., Jr., Stock, J. A., and Kaplan, B. W. (1995). Hematuria in children: a practical approach. *Urological Clinics of North America* **22**, 43–55.

Cohen, A. H. (1975). Massive obesity and the kidney. *American Journal of Pathology* **81**, 117–127.

Collar J. E., Lavda, S., Cairns, T. D. H., and Cattell, V. (2001). Red cell traverse through thin glomerular basement membranes. *Kidney International* **59**, 2069–2072.

Comper, W. D. and Glasgow, E. F. (1995). Charge selectivity in kidney ultrafiltration. *Kidney International* **47**, 1242–1251.

Copley, J. B., James, M. A. J., and Hasbargen, J. A. (1987). 'Idiopathic' hematuria. A prospective evaluation. *Archives of Internal Medicine* **147**, 434–437.

Corwin, H. L. and Silverstein, M. D. (1988). The diagnosis of neoplasia in patients with asymptomatic microscopic hematuria: a decision analysis. *Journal of Urology* **139**, 1002–1006.

Culclasure, T. F., Brady, V. J., and Hasbargen, J. A. (1994). The significance of hematuria in the anticoagulated patient. *Archives of Internal Medicine* **154**, 649–652.

D'Amico, G. (1991). The clinical role of proteinuria. *American Journal of Kidney Diseases* **17**, 48–52.

D'Amico, G. and Bazzi, C. (2003). Pathophysiology of proteinuria. *Kidney International* **64**, 809–825.

Daniels, B. S. (1993). The role of the glomerular epithelial cell in the maintenance of the glomerular filtration barrier. *American Journal of Nephrology* **13**, 318–323.

Daum, G. S., Krolikowski, F. J., Reuter, K. L., Colby, J. M., and Silva, W. M. (1988). Dipstick evaluation of hematuria in abdominal trauma. *American Journal of Clinical Pathology* **89**, 538–542.

Dawam, D., Kalayi, G. D., Osuide, J. A., Muhammad, I., and Garg, S. K. (2001). Haematuria in Africa: is the pattern changing? *BJU International* **87**, 326–330.

De Caestecker, M. P. and Ballardie, F. W. (1990). Unexplained haematuria may be due to slowly progressive glomerular disease. *British Medical Journal* **301**, 1171–1172.

Deckert, T., Feldt-Rasmussen, B., Dhurup, R., and Deckert, M. (1988). Glomerular size and charge selectivity in insulin-dependent diabetes mellitus. *Kidney International* **33**, 100–106.

Dedi, R., Bhandari, S., Turney, J. H., Borwnjohn, A. M., and Earley, I. (2001). Causes of haematuria in adult polycystic kidney disease. *British Medical Journal* **323**, 386–388.

Deen, W. M., Bridges, C. R., Brenner, B. R., and Myers, B. D. (1985). Heteroporous model of glomerular size selectivity: application to normal and nephrotic humans. *American Journal of Physiology* **249**, F374–F389.

De Jong, P. E., Weening, J. J., Donker, A. J. M., and van der Hem, G. K. (1983). The effect of phlebotomy on renal function and proteinuria in a patients with congenital cyanotic heart disease. *Nephron* **33**, 225–226.

De Jong, P. E., de Zeeuw, D., and Mogensen, C. E., ed. (1997). Proteinuria and progressive renal disease. *Nephrology, Dialysis, Transplantation* **12** (Suppl. 2), 1–85.

De Schepper, A. (1972). 'Nutcracker' fenomeen van de vena renalis en veneuze pathologie van der linker niere. *Journal Belge de Radiologie* **55**, 507–511.

Devarajan, P. (1993). Mechanisms of orthostatic proteinuria: lessons from a transplant donor. *Journal of the American Society of Nephrology* **4**, 36–39.

Dimski, D. S. *et al.* (1992). Renal autotransplantation in the loin pain–hematuria syndrome: a cautionary note. *American Journal of Kidney Diseases* **20**, 180–184.

Dittrich, S., Haas, N. A., Buhrer, C., Muller, C., Dahnert, I., and Lange, C. E. (1998). Renal impairment in patients with long-standing cyanotic congenital heart disease. *Acta Paediatrica* **87**, 949–954.

Diven, S. C. and Travis, L. B. (2000). A practical primary care approach to hematuria in children. *Pediatric Nephrology* **14**, 65–72.

Dodge, W. F., West, C. D., Smith, E. H., and Bunce, H. B., III. (1976). Proteinuria and hematuria in schoolchildren: epidemiology and early natural history. *Journal of Pediatrics* **88**, 327–347.

Dornfeld, L. P. Obesity. In *Textbook of Nephrology* 2nd edn. (ed. R. J. Glassock and S. G. Massry), pp. 989–995. Baltimore, MD: Williams and Wilkins, 1989.

Drummond, K. N., Vernier, R. L., Worthen, H. G., and Good, R. A. (1963). The associated occurrence of the nephrotic syndrome and congenital heart disease. *Pediatrics* **31**, 103–114.

Eastwood, N. B. (1978). Loin pain—renal or parietal? *Lancet* **i**, 318.

Eddy, A. A., McCulloch, L., Adams, J., and Liu, E. J. (1989). Interstitial nephritis induced by homologous protein load. *Laboratory Investigation* **135**, 719–733.

Eiser, A. R., Katz, S. M., and Swatz, C. (1982). Reversible nephrotic range proteinuria with renal artery stenosis: a clinical example of renin-associated proteinuria. *Nephron* **30**, 374–377.

Eksim, M., Bakkaloglu, S. A., Tümer, N., Sanlidilek, U., and Salih, M. (1999). Orthostatic proteinuria as a result of venous compression (nutcracker pheonomenon)—a hypothesis testable with modern imaging techniques. *Nephrology, Dialysis, Transplantation* **14**, 826–827.

Elises, J. S., Griffiths, P. D., Hocking, M. D., Taylor, C. M., and White, R. H. R. (1988). Simplified quantification of urinary protein excretion in children. *Clinical Nephrology* **30**, 225–229.

Eppel, G., Osicka, T., Pratt, L., Jablonski, P., Howden, B. O., Glasgow, E. F., and Comper, W. D. (1999). The return of glomerular-filtered albumin to the rat renal vein. *Kidney International* **56**, 1861–1870.

Evans, G. and Greaves, I. (1999). Microalbuminuria as a predictor of outcome. *British Medical Journal* **318**, 27–28.

Fairley, K. F. and Birch, D. F. (1982). Hematuria: a simple method for identifying glomerular bleeding. *Kidney International* **21**, 105–108.

Fassett, R. G., Owen, J. E., Fairley, J., Birch, D. F., and Fairley, K. F. (1982). Urinary red cell morphology during exercise. *British Medical Journal* **285**, 1455–1457.

Flanagan, M. F., Hourihan, M., and Keane, J. F. (1991). Incidence of renal dysfunction in adults with congenital cyanotic heart disease. *American Journal of Cardiology* **68**, 403–406.

Fletcher, P., Al-Khader, A. A., Parsons, V., and Aber, G. M. (1979). The pathology of intrarenal vascular lesions associated with the loin-pain–haematuria syndrome. *Nephron* **24**, 150–154.

Fogazzi, G. B., Banfi, G., and Ponticelli, C. (1992). Acute tubular necrosis caused by gross haematuria in a patient with focal and segmental necrotizing glomerulonephritis. *Nephron* **61**, 102–105.

Fogazzi, G. B., Leong, S. O., and Cameron, J. S. (1996). Don't forget sickle cells in the urine in investigating a patient for haematuria. *Nephrology, Dialysis, Transplantation* **11**, 723–725.

Fogazzi, G. B., Ponticelli, C., and Ritz, E.. *The Urinary Sediment* 2nd edn., pp. 16–17. Oxford: Oxford University Press, 1999.

Fox, J., Quin, J. D., O'Reilly, D. St. J., and Boulton-Jones, J. M. (1994). Glomerular charge selectivity in primary glomerulopathies. *Clinical Science* **87**, 421–425.

Fox, M. and Saunders, N. R. (1978). Significance of loin pain in women. A study of 100 consecutive cases referred to a urological clinic. *Lancet* **i**, 115–117.

Froom, P., Ribak, J., and Benbassat, J. (1984). Significance of microhaematuria in young adults. *British Medical Journal* **288**, 20–21.

Froom, P., Froom, J., and Ribak, J. (1997). Asymptomatic microscopic hematuria—is investigation necessary? *Journal of Clinical Epidemiology* **50**, 1197–1200.

Gansevoort, R. T., Sluiter, W. J., Hemmelder, M. H., de Zeeuw, D., and de Jong, P. E. (1995). Antiproteinuric effect of blood-pressure-lowering agents: a meta-analysis of comparative trials. *Nephrology, Dialysis, Transplantation* **10**, 1963–1974.

Gazdar, A. F. and Dammin, G. J. (1970). Neural degeneration and regeneration in human renal transplants. *New England Journal of Medicine* **283**, 22–24.

Ghiggeri, G. M. *et al.* (1987). Renal selectivity properties towards endogenous albumin in minimal change nephropathy. *Kidney International* **32**, 69–77.

Gibson, P., Winney, R. J., Masterson, G., and Fowles, R. G. (1994). Bilateral nephrectomy and haemodialysis for the treatment of severe loin-pain haematuria syndrome. *Nephrology, Dialysis, Transplantation* **9**, 1640–1641.

Gill, I. S., Uzzo, R. G., Hobart, M. G., Streem, S. B., Goldfarb, D. A., and Noble, M. J. (2000). Laparoscopic retroperitoneal live donor right nephrectomy for purposes of allotransplantation and autotransplantation. *Journal of Urology* **164**, 1500–1504.

Ginsberg, J. M., Chang, B. S., Matarese, R. A., and Garella, S. (1983). Use of single voided urine samples to estimate quantitative proteinuria. *New England Journal of Medicine* **309**, 1543–1546.

Grossfeld, G. D. and Carroll, P. R. (1998). Evaluation of asymptomatic microscopic hematuria. *Urologic Clinics of North America* **25**, 661–676.

Grossfeld, G. D., Litwin, M. S., Wolf, J. S., Jr., Hricak, H., Shuler, C. L., Agerter, D. C., and Carroll, P. R. (2001a). Evaluation of asymptomatic microscopic hematuria in adults: the American Urological Association best practice policy—Part I: Definition, detection, prevalence, and etiology. *Urology* **57**, 599–603.

Grossfeld, G. D., Litwin, M. S., Wolf, J. S., Jr., Hricak, H., Shuler, C. L., Agerter, D. C., and Carroll, P. R. (2001b). Evaluation of asymtomatic microscopic hematuria in adults: the American Urological Association best practice policy—Part II: patient evaluation, cytology, voided markers, imaging, cystoscopy, nephrology evaluation and follow-up. *Urology* **57**, 604–610.

Habte, B., Dobbie, J. W., and Boulton-Jones, M. (1981). The loin pain–haematuria syndrome in males. *Scottish Medical Journal* **26**, 118–120.

Hagley, M. T., Murphy, D. P., Mullins, D., and Zarconi, J. (1992). Decline in creatinine clearance in a patient with glomerulomegaly associated with congenital cyanotic heart disease. *American Journal of Kidney Diseases* **20**, 177–179.

Hall, A. and Fentiman, A. (1999). Blood in the urine of girls in an area of Ghana with a low prevalence of infections with Schistosoma haematobium. *Transactions of the Royal Society of Tropical Hygiene and Medicine* **93**, 411–412.

Hall, R., Mailis, A., and Rapoport, A. (1997). Hematuria-loin pain syndrome: its existence as a discrete clinicopathological entity cannot be supported. *Clinical Journal of Pain* **13**, 171–177.

Hammad, T. A., Gabr, N. S., Talaat, M. M., Orieby, A., Shawky, E., and Strickland, G. T. (1997). Hematuria and proteinuria as predictors of Schistomsoma hamatobium infection. *American Journal of Tropical Medicine and Hygiene* **57**, 363–367.

Hansen, J. M. *et al.* (1994). The transplanted human kidney does not achieve functional innervation. *Clinical Science* **87**, 13–20.

Harney, J., Rodgers, E., Campbell, E., and Hickey, D. P. (1994). Loin pain–haematuria syndrome: how effective is renal autotransplantation in its treatment ? *Urology* **44**, 493–496.

Hebert, L. A. *et al.* (1996). Loin-pain hematuria syndrome associated with thin glomerular basement membrane disease and haemorrhage into renal tubules. *Kidney International* **49**, 168–173.

Hession, C. *et al.* (1987). Uromodulin (Tamm–Horsfall glycoprotein): a renal ligand for lymphokines. *Science* **237**, 1479–1484.

Hida, K., Wada, J., Yamasaki, H., Nagake, Y., Zhang, H., Sugiyama, H., Shitaka, K., and Makino, H. (2002). Cyanotic congenital heart disease associated with glomerulomegaly and focal segmental glomerulosclerosis: remission of nephrotic syndrome with angiotensin converting enzyme inhibitor. *Nephrology, Dialysis, Transplantation* **17**, 144–147.

Hironaka, K., Makino, H., Yamasaki, Y., and Ota, Z. (1993). Pores in the glomerular basement membrane revealed by ultrahigh-resolution scanning electron microscopy. *Nephron* **64**, 647–649.

Hisano, S. and Ueda, K. (1991). Asymptomatic haematuria and proteinuria: renal pathology and clinical outcome in 54 children. *Pediatric Nephrology* **3**, 229–234.

Hisano, S. *et al.* (1991). Asymptomatic isolated microhematuria: natural history of 136 children. *Pediatric Nephrology* **5**, 578–581.

Hoyer, J. and Seiler, M. W. (1979). Pathophysiology of Tamm–Horsfall protein. *Kidney International* **16**, 279–289.

Hulme, B. and Hardwicke, J. (1968). Human glomerular permeability to macromolecules in health and disease. *Clinical Science* **34**, 515–529.

Hutchison, S. M. W., Doig, A., and Jenkins, A. M. (1987). Recurrence of the loin pain haematuria syndrome after renal transplantation. *Lancet* **i**, 1501–1502.

Innes, A., Johnston, P. A., Morgan, A. G., Davison, A. M., and Burden, R. P. (1993). Clinical features of benign hypertensive nephrosclerosis at time of renal biopsy. *Quarterly Journal of Medicine* **86**, 271–275.

Jafar, T. H., Stark, P. C., Schmid, C. H., Landa, M., Maschio, G., Marcantonio, C. *et al.* (2001). Proteinuria as risk factor for the progression of non-diabetic renal disease. *Kidney International* **60**, 1131–1140.

Jaffe, J. S., Ginsberg, P. C., Gill, R., and Harkaway, R. C. (2001). A new diagnostic algorithm for the evaluation of microscopic hematuria. *Urology* **57**, 889–894.

Jennette, J. C., Charles, L., and Grubb, W. (1987). Glomerulomegaly and focal segmental glomerulosclerosis associated with obesity and the sleep-apnea syndrome. *American Journal of Kidney Diseases* **10**, 470–472.

Jones, G. R. and Newhouse, I. (1997). Sport-related hematuria: a review. *Clinical Journal of Sport Medicine* **7**, 119–125.

Jones, C. R., Sumeray, M., Heys, A., and Woolfson, R. G. (1999). Pseudo-proteinuria following *gelofusine* infusion. *Nephrology, Dialysis, Transplantation* **14**, 944–945.

Kallmeyer, G. and Miller, N. M. (1993). Urinary changes in ultra-long distance marathon runners. *Nephron* **64**, 119–121.

Kanwar, Y. S. and Farquhar, M. S. (1979). Anionic sites in the glomerular basement membrane *in vivo* and *in vitro* localization in the lamina densae rarae by cationic probes. *Journal of Cell Biology* **81**, 137–153.

Kaplan, J. M. *et al.* (2000). Mutations of ACTN4, encoding alpha-actinin-4, cause familial focal segmental glomerulosclerosis. *Nature Genetics* **24**, 251–256.

Kairaitis, L. K. and Harris, D. C. H. (2001). Tubular-interstitial interactions in proteinuric renal diseases. *Nephrology* **6**, 198–207.

Kelly, B. (1992). Psychological aspects of loin pain/haematuria syndrome. *Lancet* **340**, 1294 (letter).

Kelly, B. (1994). Psychiatric issues in the 'loin pain and haematuria syndrome'. *Australian and New Zealand Journal of Psychiatry* **28**, 302–306.

Khadra, M. H., Pickard, R. S., Charlton, M., Powell, P. H., and Neal, D. E. (2000). A prospective analysis of 1930 patients with hematuria to evaluate current practice. *Journal of Urology* **163**, 524–527. *See also:* Messing, E. M. Editorial comment *ibid* 527; Mariani, A. J., Chahal, R., and Sundaram, S. K. (letters) *ibid* **164**, 545.

Kambham, N., Markowitz, G. S., Valeri, A. M., Lin, J., and D'Agati, V. (2001). Obesity-related glomerulopathy: an emerging epidemic. *Kidney International* **59**, 1498–1509.

Kincaid-Smith, P. (1982). Haematuria and exercise-related haematuria. *British Medical Journal* **285**, 1595–1597.

Kincaid-Smith, P. and Becker, G. (1979). Reflux nephropathy and chronic atrophic pyelonephritis. *Journal of Infectious Diseases* **138**, 774–780.

Kobayashi, Y., Omori, S., Kamimaki, I., Ikeda, M., Akaoaka, K., Honda, M., Ogata, K., and Morikawa, Y. (2001). Acute reversible renal failure with macroscopic hematuria in Henoch–Schönlein purpura. *Pediatric Nephrology* **16**, 742–744.

Köhler, H., Wandel, E., and Brunck, B. (1991). Acanthocyturia—a characteristic marker for glomerular bleeding. *Kidney International* **40**, 115–120.

Krull, F., Ehrich, J. H., Wurster, W., Toel, U., and Rothganger, S. (1992). Renal involvement in patients with congenital cyanotic heart disease. *Acta Paediatrica Scandinavica* **80**, 1214–1219.

Lam, M. H. (1995). False 'hematuria' due to bacteriuria. *Archives of Pathology and Laboratory Medicine* **119**, 717–721.

Laurent, J., Phillipon, C., Lagrue, G., Laurent, G., Weil, B., and Rostocker, G. (1993). Proteinuria selectivity index—prognostic value in lipoid nephrosis and related diseases. *Nephron* **65**, 185–189.

Lawrence, G. M. and Brewer, D. B. (1981). Effect of strain and sex on the induction of hyperalbuminuric proteinuria in the rat. *Clinical Science* **61**, 751–756.

Leaker, B. R., Gordge, M. P., Patel, A., and Neild, G. H. (1990). Haemostatic changes in the loin pain haematuria syndrome: secondary to renal vasospasm? *Quarterly Journal of Medicine* **76**, 969–979.

Lee, S. J., You, E. S., Lee, J. E., and Chung, E. C. (1996). Left renal vein entrapment syndrome in two girls with orthostatic proteinuria. *Pediatric Nephrology* **11**, 218–220.

Leheste, J. R. *et al.* (1999). Megalin knockout mice as an animal model of low molecular weight proteinuria. *American Journal of Pathology* **155**, 1361–1370.

Levitt, J. I. (1967). The prognostic significance of proteinuria in young college students. *Annals of Internal Medicine* **66**, 685–696.

Lewis, J. B. (1998). Microalbuminuria: accuracy and economics. *American Journal of Kidney Diseases* **32**, 524–528.

Lidove, O., Orizco, R., Guéry, B., Correas, J.-M., Robino, C., and Méjean, A. (2001). A young woman with intermittent macroscopic haematuria. *Nephrology, Dialysis, Trasnplantation* **16**, 853–855.

Lim, V. S., Sibley, R., and Spargo, B. (1974). Adult lipoid nephrosis: clinico-pathologic correlations. *Annals of Internal Medicine* **81**, 1314–1320.

Lin, C.-H., Sheng, C.-C, Chen, C.-H., Lin, C.-C., and Chou, P. (2000). The prevalence of heavy proteinuria and progression risk factors in children undergoing urinary screening. *Pediatric Nephrology* **14**, 953–959.

Little, P. J., Sloper, J. S., and de Wardener, H. E. (1967). A syndrome of loin pain and haematuria associated with disease of peripheral renal arteries. *Quarterly Journal of Medicine* **36**, 253–259.

Loh, E. H., Keng, V. W., and Ward, P. B. (1990). Blood cells and red cell morphology in the urine of healthy children. *Nephron* **34**, 185–187.

Lucas, P. A., Leaker, B. R., and Neild, G. H. (1992). Psychiatric aspects of the loin pain/haematuria syndrome. *Lancet* **340**, 1038 (letter).

Lucas, P. A., Leaker, B. R., Murphy, M., and Neild G. H. (1995). Loin pain and haematuria syndrome: a somatoform disorder. *Quarterly Journal of Medicine* **88**, 703–709.

Lydakis, C. and Lip, G. Y. H. (1998). Micoalbuminuria and cardiovascular risk. *Quarterly Journal of Medicine* **91**, 381–391.

Maack, T. Renal filtration, transport, and metabolism of protein. In *The Kidney* 3rd edn. (ed. D. W. Seldin and G. Giebisch), pp. 2235–2267. Philadelphia: Lippincott, Williams and Wilkins, 2000.

Macdonald, I. M., Fairley, K. F., Hobbs, J. B., and Kincaid-Smith, P. (1975). Loin pain as a presenting symptom of idiopathic glomerulonephritis. *Clinical Nephrology* **3**, 129–133.

Mariani, A. J., Luangphinith, S., Loo, S, Scottolini, A., and Hodges, C. V. (1984). Dipstick chemical urinalysis: an accurate cost-effective screening test. *Journal of Urology* **132**, 64–66.

Mariani, A. J., Mariani, M. C., Macchioni, C., Stams, U. K., Hariharan, A., and Moriera, A. (1989). The significance of adult haematuria: 1000 haematuria evaluations including a risk–benefit and cost effectiveness analysis. *Journal of Urology* **141**, 350–355.

Marks, M. L., McLaine, P. N., and Drummond, K. N. (1970). Proteinuria in children with febrile illnesses. *Archives of Disease in Childhood* **45**, 250–253.

McElderry, L. A., Tarbit, I. F., and Cassells-Smith, A. J. (1982). Six methods for urinary protein compared. *Clinical Chemistry* **28**, 356–360.

McGregor, D. O., Lynn, K. I., Bailey R. R., Robson, R. A., and Gardner, J. (1998). Clinical audit of the use of renal biopsy in the management of isolated microscopic hematuria. *Clinical Nephrology* **49**, 345–348.

McInnis, M. D., Newhouse, I. J., von Duvillard, S. P., and Thayer, R. (1998). The effect of exercise intensity on hematuria in healthy male runners. *European Journal of Applied Physiology and Occupational Physiology* **79**, 99–105.

McLaine, P. N. and Drummond, K. N. (1970). Benign persistent asymptomatic proteinuria in childhood. *Pediatrics* **46**, 548–552.

McQueen, E. G. (1966). Composition of urinary casts. *Lancet* **i**, 397–398.

Meadow, R. (1977). Munchausen syndrome by proxy. The hinterland of child abuse. *Lancet* **ii**, 343–345.

Messing, E. M., Young, T. B., Hunt, V. B., Webbie, J. M., and Rust, P. (1989). Urinary tract cancer found by home screening with haematuria dipstick in healthy men over 50 years of age. *Cancer* **64**, 2361–2367.

Messing, E. M. *et al.* (1995). Hematuria home screening: repeat test results. *Journal of Urology* **154**, 57–61.

Metcalf, P., Baker, J., Scott, A., Wild, C., Scragg, R., and Dyson, E. (1992). Albuminuria in people at least 40 years old: effect of obesity, hypertension and hyperlipidemia. *Clinical Chemistry* **38**, 1802–1808.

Miller, F., Lane, B. P., Kirsch, M., Ilamathi, E., Moore, B., and Finger, M. (1994). Loin pain–hematuria syndrome with a distinctive vascular lesion and alternative pathway complement activation. *Archives of Pathology and Laboratory Medicine* **118**, 1016–1019.

Minetti, E. E., Cozzi, M. G., Granata, S., and Guidi, E. (1997). Accuracy of the urinary albumin titrator stick 'Micral-Test' in kidney disease patients. *Nephrology, Dialysis, Transplantation* **12**, 78–80.

Mogensen, C. E. and Christensen, C. K. (1984). Predicting diabetic nephropathy in insulin-dependent patients. *New England Journal of Medicine* **311**, 89–93.

Mohr, D. N., Offord, K. P., Owen, R. A., and Melton, J. III. (1986). Asymptomatic microhematuria and urologic disease: a population-based study. *Archives of Internal Medicine* **256**, 224–229.

Mujais, S. K., Emmanouel, D. S., Kasinath, B. S., and Spargo, B. H. (1987). Marked proteinuria in hypertensive nephrosclerosis. *American Journal of Nephrology* **5**, 190–195.

Muraguri, P. W., McLigeyo, S. O., and Kayima, J. K. (1997). Proteinuria other selected abnormalities and hypertension among teenage secondary school students in Nairobi, Kenya. *East African Medical Journal* **74**, 467–473.

Murakami, S., Igarashi, T., Hara, S., and Shimazaki, J. (1990). Strategies for asymptomatic microscopic hematuria: a prospective study of 1034 patients. *Journal of Urology* **144**, 99–101.

Myers, B. D. and Guasch, A. (1994). Mechanisms of proteinuria in nephrotic humans. *Nephrology, Dialysis, Transplantation* **8**, 107–112.

Naeye, R. L. (1965). Children at high altitude. Pulmonary and renal abnormalities. *Circulation Research* **16**, 33–38.

Naish, P. F., Aber, G. M., and Boyd, W. N. (1975). C3 deposition in renal arterioles in the loin pain and haematuria syndrome. *British Medical Journal* **3**, 746.

Norden, A. G. W. *et al.* (2001). Glomerular protein sieving and implications for renal failure in Fanconi syndrome. *Kidney International* **60**, 1885–1892.

Oikawa, T. and Fogo, A. (1995). Mechanisms and significance of proteinuria. *Nephrology* **1**, 95–103.

Oken, D., Kirschbaum, B. B., and Landwehr, D. M. (1981). Micropuncture studies of the mechanism of normal and pathological proteinuria. *Contributions to Nephrology* **24**, 1.

Oksenhendler, E., Bourbigot, B., Desbazeille F., Droz, D., Choquenet, C., Girot, R., and Jungers, P. (1984). Recurrent haematuria in 4 white patients with sickle cell trait. *Journal of Urology* **132**, 1201–1203.

Parbtani, A. and Cameron, J. S. (1979). Platelet involvement in the loin pain/haematuria syndrome. *Lancet* **ii**, 1330.

Park, C. H. and Maack, T. (1984). Albumin absorption and catabolism by isolated perfused convoluted tubules of the rabbit. *Journal of Clinical Investigation* **73**, 767–777.

Parsons, M., Newman, D. J., Pugia, M., Newall, R. G., and Price, C. P. (1999). Performance of a reagent strip device for quantitation of the urine albumin: creatinine ratio in a point of care setting. *Clinical Nephrology* **51**, 220–227.

Paul, A. B., Collie, D. A., Wild, S. R., and Chisholm, G. F. (1993). An integrated haematuria clinic. *British Journal of Clinical Practice* **47**, 128–130.

Perrone, H. C., Aizen, H., Torporvski, J., and Schor, N. (1991). Metabolic disturbance as a cause of recurrent hematuria in children. *Kidney International* **39**, 807–811.

Pesce, A. and First, R. M. *Proteinuria. An integrated Review.* New York, NY: Marcel Dekker, 1979.

Piqueras, A. I., White, R. H. R., Raafat, F., Moghal, N., and Milford, D. V. (1998). Renal biopsy diagnosis in children presenting with hematuria. *Pediatric Nephrology* **12**, 386–391.

Powell, H. R. (1976). Relationship between proteinuria and epithelial cell changes in minimal change glomerulopathy. *Nephron* **16**, 310–317.

Praga, M., Hernández, E., Andres A., Leon, M., Ruilope, L. M., and Rodicio, J. L. (1995). Effects of bodyweight loss and captopril treatment on proteinuria associated with obesity. *Nephron* **70**, 35–41.

Praga, M., Alegre, R., Hernández, E., Morales, E., Domínguez-Gil, B., Careño, A., and Andrés, A. (2000). Familial hematuria caused by hypercalciuria and hyperuricosuria. *American Journal of Kidney Diseases* **35**, 141–145.

Praga, M., Hernández, E., Morales, E., Campos, A. P., Valero, M. A., Martínez, M. A., and León, M. (2001). Clinical features and long-term outcome of obesity-associated focal segmental glomerulosclerosis. *Nephrology, Dialysis, Transplantation* **16**, 1790–1798.

Prager, J. P., DeSalles, A., Wilkinson, A., Jacobs, M., and Csete, M. (1995). Loin pain hematuria syndrome: pain relief with intrathecal morphine. *American Journal of Kidney Diseases* **25**, 629–631.

Raats, C. J. I., van den Borne, J., and Berden, J. H. M. (2000). Glomerular heparan sulfate alterations: mechanisms and relevance for proteinuria. *Kidney International* **57**, 385–400.

Rath, B., Turner, C., Hartley, B., and Chantler, C. (1990). Evaluation of light microscopy to localise the site of haematuria. *Archives of Disease in Chidhood* **65**, 338–340.

Rennie, I. D. B. MD Thesis, University of London, 1966.

Reynard, J. (2000). All patients with haematuria should undergo cystoscopy. *British Medical Journal* **320**, 1598.

Ritchie, C. D., Bevan, E. A., and Collier, St. J. (1986). The importance of occult haematuria found at screening. *British Medical Journal* **292**, 681–683.

Ritz, E., Nowicki, M., Fliser, D., Hörner, D., and Klimm, H.-P. (1994). Proteinuria and hypertension. *Kidney International* **47** (Suppl. 47), s-76–s-80.

Robinson, R. R. (1980). Isolated proteinuria in asymptomatic patients. *Kidney International* **18**, 395–406.

Robson, A. M., Giangiacomo, J., Kienstra, R. A., Naqvi, S. T., and Ingelfinger, J. R. (1974). Normal glomerular permeability and its modification by minimal change nephrotic syndrome. *Journal of Clinical Investigation* **54**, 1190–1199.

Rodewald, R. and Karnovsky, M. J. (1974). Porous substructure of the glomerular slit diaphragm in the rat and mouse. *Journal of Cell Biology* **60**, 423–433.

Rosenmann, E. and Boss, J. H. (1979). Tissue antigens in normal and pathologic urines: a review. *Kidney International* **16**, 337–344.

Rosenmann, E., Dwarka, L., and Boss J. H. (1972). Proliferative glomerulopathy in rheumatic heart disease and chronic lung disease. *American Journal of Medical Science* **264**, 213–223.

Rustecki, G. J., Goldsmith, C., and Schreiner, G. E. (1971). Characterization of proteins in urinary casts. Fluorescent antibody identification of Tamm–Horsfall protein in matrix and serum proteins in granules. *New England Journal of Medicine* **284**, 1049–1052.

Rytand, D. A. and Spreiter, S. (1981). Prognosis in postural (orthostatic) proteinuria. Forty to forty five year follow-up of six patients after diagnosis by Thomas Addis. *New England Journal of Medicine* **305**, 618–621.

Savin, V. J. (1993). Mechanisms of proteinuria in noninflammatory glomerular diseases. *American Journal of Kidney Diseases* **21**, 347–362.

Sawyer, N., Wadsworth, J., Wijnen, M., and Gabriel, R. (1988). Prevalence, concentration, and prognostic importance of proteinuria in patients with malignancies. *British Medical Journal* **296**, 1295–1298.

Schainuk, L. I., Benditt, F. P., Striker, G. E., and Cutler, R. E. (1970). Structural–functional correlations in renal disease. II. The correlations. *Human Pathology* **1**, 631–643.

Scherberich, J. E. (1990). Urinary proteins of tubular origin: basic immunological and clinical aspects. *American Journal of Nephrology* **10** (Suppl. 1), 43–51.

Schramek, P., Moristch, A., Haschkowitz, H., Binder, B. R., and Maier, M. (1989). *In vitro* generation of dysmorphic erythrocytes. *Kidney International* **36**, 72–77.

Schröder, F. H. (1994). Microscopic haematuria requires investigation. *British Medical Journal* **309**, 70–72.

Schurek, H. J. (1994). Mechanisms of glomerular proteinuria and hematuria. *Kidney International* (Suppl. 47), s12–s16.

Scottish Intercollegiate Guidelines Network (1997). *Investigation of Asymptomatic Microscopic Haematuria in Adults.* SIGN publication no. 17, Edinburgh. *Investigation of Proteinuria in Adults.* SIGN publication no. 18, Edinburgh.

Sells, H. and Cox, R. (2001). Undiagnosed macroscopic haematuria revisited: a follow-up of 146 patients. *BJU International* **88**, 6–8.

Shaper, P. R. L., Jackson, J. F., and Williams, G. (1994). The nutcracker syndrome: an uncommon cause of haematuria. *British Journal of Urology* **74**, 144–146.

Sharfi, A. R. and Hassan, O. (1994). Investigation of haematuria in Khartoum. *East African Medical Journal* **71**, 29–31.

Sheerin, N. S., Sacks, S. H., and Fogazzi, G. B. (1999). *In vitro* erythrophagocytosis by renal tubular cells and tubular toxicity by haemoglobin and iron. *Nephrology, Dialysis, Transplantation* **14**, 1391–1397.

Sheil, A. G. R., Ibels, L. S., and Thomas, M. A. B. (1985). Renal autotransplantation for severe loin-pain/haematuria syndrome. *Lancet* **ii**, 1216–1217.

Sheil, A. G. R., Ibels, L. S., Pollock, C., Graham, J. C., and Short, J. (1987). Treatment of loin pain haematuria syndrome by renal transplantation. *Lancet* **ii**, 907–908.

Sheil, A. G., Chui, A. K., Verran, D. J., Boulas, J., and Ibels, L. S. (1998). Evaluation of the loin pain/hematuria syndrome treated by autotransplantation or radical renal neurectomy. *American Journal of Kidney Diseases* **32**, 215–220.

Shichiri, M., Oowada, A., Nishio, Y., Tomita, K., and Shigai, T. (1986). Use of autoanalyser to examine urinary red cell morphology in the diagnosis of glomerular haematuria. *Lancet* **ii**, 781–782.

Shichiri, M. *et al.* (1988). Red cell volume distribution curves in diagnosis of glomerular and non-glomerular haematuria. *Lancet* **i**, 908–910.

Shimamura, Y. *et al.* (1990). Improvement of nephrotic syndrome in an obese patient after weight loss and treatment with an anti-allergic drug. *Journal of Medicine* **21**, 337–347.

Siegler, R. L., Brewer, E. D., and Hammond, E. (1988). Platelet activation and prostacyclin supporting capacity in the loin pain hematuria syndrome. *American Journal of Kidney Diseases* **12**, 156–160.

Simpson, F. O. (1986). Is current research into basement membrane chemistry and ultrastructure providing any new insights into the way the glomerular basement membrane functions ? *Nephron* **43**, 1–4.

Sklar, A. H. and Chaudhary, B. A. (1988). Reversible proteinuria in obstructive sleep apnea syndrome. *Archives of Internal Medicine* **148**, 87–89.

Smellie, S. W., Lambert, M., Lavenne, E., and van Cangh, P. J. (1987). Factor XII deficiency associated with loin pain/haematuria syndrome. *Lancet* **ii**, 1330.

Spear, G. S. (1964). The glomerulus in cyanotic congenital heart disease and pulmonary hypertension: a review. *Nephron* **1**, 238–248.

Spear, G. S. (1977). The glomerular lesion of cyanotic congenital heart disease. *Johns Hopkins Medical Journal* **140**, 185–188.

Spencer, J., Lindsell, D., and Matorakou I. (1990). Ultrasonography compared with intravenous urography in the investigation of adults with haematuria. *British Medical Journal* **301**, 1074–1076. (But see also discussion of this paper: Stenlake, P. S., Wallace, D. M. A., Cattell, W. R., Webb, J. A. W., and Whitfield, H. G. Investigation of adults with haematuria. *British Medical Journal* **301**, 1396–1397, and the authors' reply.)

Springberg, P. D. *et al.* (1982). Fixed and reproducible orthostatic proteinuria: results of a 20 year follow-up study. *Annals of Internal Medicine* **97**, 516–519.

Spitz, A., Huffman, J. L., and Mendez, R. (1997). Autotransplantation as an effective therapy for the loin-pain hematuria syndrome: case report and a review of the literature. *Journal of Urology* **157**, 1554–1559.

Stapleton, F. B. (1994). Hematuria associated with hypercalciuria and hyperuricosuria: a practical approach. *Pediatric Nephrology* **8**, 756–761.

Subramanyam, B. R., Lefleur, R. S., and Bosniak, M. A. (1983). Renal arteriovenous fistulas and aneurysm: sonographic findings. *Radiology* **149**, 261–263.

Talic, R. F., Parr, N., and Hargreave, T. B. (1994). Anephric state after graft nephrectomy in a patient treated with autotransplantation for bilateral metachronous loin/pain haematuria syndrome. *Journal of Urology* **152**, 1194–1195.

Tapp, D. C. and Copley, J. B. (1988). Effect of red blood cell lysis on protein quantitation in hematuric states. *American Journal of Nephrology* **8**, 190–193.

Taylor, C. M., Neuhaus, T. J., Shah, V., Dillon, S., and Barratt, T. M. (1997). Charge and size selectivity of proteinuria in children with idiopathic nephrotic syndrome. *Pediatric Nephrology* **11**, 404–410.

Tencer, J., Torffvit, O., Thysell, H., Rippe, B., and Grubb, A. (1998). Proteinuria selectivity index based upon α_2-macroglobulin or IgM is superior to the IgG based index in differentiating glomerular diseases. *Kidney International* **54**, 1098–1105.

Tencer, J., Torffvit, O., Thysell, H., Rippe, B., and Grubb, A. (1999). Urine IgG2/IgG4-ratio indicates the significance of the charge selective properties of the glomerular capillary wall for the macromolecular transport in glomerular diseases. *Nephrology, Dialysis and Transplantation* **14**, 1425–1429.

Terai, C., Nojima, Y., Takano, K., Yamada, A., and Takaku, F. (1987). Determination of urinary albumin excretion by radioimmunoassay in patients with subclinical lupus nephritis. *Clinical Nephrology* **27**, 79–83.

Thompson, I. M. (1987). The evaluation of microscopic hematuria: a population-based study. *Journal of Urology* **138**, 1189–1190.

Thompson, W. G. (1996). Things that go red in the urine and others that don't. *Lancet* **347**, 5.

Tojo, A. and Endou, H. (1992). Intrarenal handling of proteins in rats using fractional micropuncture technique. *American Journal of Physiology* **263**, F601–F606.

Tojo, A. *et al.* (1990). Factitious proteinuria in a young girl. *Clinical Nephrology* **33**, 299–302.

Tomlinson, P. A., Dalton, R. N., Hartley, B., Haycock, G. B., and Chantler, C. (1997). Low molecular weight protein excretion in glomerular disease: a comparative analysis. *Pediatric Nephrology* **11**, 285–290.

Topham, P. S., Harper, S. J., Furness, P., Harris, K. P. G., Walls, J., and Feehally, J. (1994). Glomerular disease as a cause of isolated microscopic haematuria. *Quarterly Journal of Medicine* **87**, 329–335.

Tryggvason, K. (1999). Unraveling the mechanisms of glomerular ultrafiltration: nephrin, a key component of the slit diaphragm. *Journal of the American Society of Nephrology* **10**, 2440–2445.

Tuck, M. L., Sowers, J. R., Dornfeld, L. P., Kledzick, G., and Maxwell, M. H. (1981). The effect of weight reduction on blood pressure, plasma renin activity, and plasma aldosterone levels in obese patients. *New England Journal of Medicine* **304**, 930–933.

Túri, S. *et al.* (1989). Long-term follow-up of patients with persistent/recurrent, isolated haematuria: a Hungarian multi-center study. *Pediatric Nephrology* **3**, 235–239. [See also the editorial and discussion of this paper: Vehaskari, V. M. (1989). Asymptomatic hematuria—a cause for concern? *Pediatric Nephrology* **3**, 240–241; Gauthier, B. and Trachtman, H. (1989). Asymptomatic hematuria. *Pediatric Nephrology* **4**, 296–297.]

Turini, D., Barbanti, G., Beneforti, P., and Lazzeri, M. (1995). Autotransplantation for intractable loin pain: report of a case with long-term follow up. *Journal of Urology* **153**, 389–391.

Ubels, F. J., van Essen, G. G., de Jong, P. E., and Stegman, C. E. (1999). Exercise induced macroscopic hematuria: run for a diagnosis? *Nephrology, Dialysis, Transplantation* **14**, 2030–2031.

Valente de Almeida, R., Rocha de Carvalho, J. G., de Azevedo, A. F., Mulinari, R. A., Ioshhi S. O., da Rosa Utiyama, S., and Nisihara, R. (1999). Microalbuminuria and renal morphology in the evaluation of subclinical lupus nephritis. *Clinical Nephrology* **52**, 218–229.

Van Savage, J. G. and Fried, F. A. (1995). Anticoagulant-associated haematuria: a prospective study. *Journal of Urology* **153**, 1594–1596.

Vehaskari V. M. and Rapola, J. (1982). Isolated proteinuria: analysis of a school age population. *Journal of Pediatrics* **101**, 661.

Vehaskari, V. M., Rapola, J., Koskimies, O., Savilahti, E., Vilska, J., and Hallman, N. (1979). Microscopic hematuria in schoolchildren: epidemiology and clinicopathologic evaluation. *Journal of Pediatrics* **95**, 676–684.

Velosa, J. A., Donadio, J. V., and Holley K. E. (1975). Focal segmental glomerulopathy. A clinicopathological study. *Mayo Clinic Proceedings* **50**, 121–133.

Vernier, R. W., Klein, D. J., Sisson, S. P., Mahan, J. D., Ogema, T. R., and Brown, D. B. (1983). Heparan-sulfate rich anionic sites in the human glomerular basement membrane. Decreased concentration in congential nephrotic syndrome. *New England Journal of Medicine* **309**, 1001–1009.

Viberti, G. F. (1988). Etiology and prognostic importance of proteinuria in diabetes. *Diabetes Care* **11**, 840–845.

Wan, L. L., Yano, S., Hiromura, K., Tsukada, Y., Tomono, S., and Kawazu, S. (1995). Effects of posture on creatinine clearance and protein excretion in patients with various renal diseases. *Clinical Nephrology* **43**, 312–317.

Wang, S.-X., Rastaldi, M. P., Pätäri A., Ahola, H., Hekkilä, E., and Holthöfer, H. (2002). Patterns of nephrin and a new- proteinuria-associated protein expression in human renal diseases. *Kidney International* **61**, 141–147.

Washizawa, K., Kansai, S., Mori, T., Komiyama, A., and Shigematsu, H. (1993). Ultrastructural alteration of glomerular anionic sites in nephrotic patients. *Pediatric Nephrology* **7**, 1–5.

Weening, J. J. and Van der Val, A. (1987). Effect of decreased perfusion pressure on glomerular permeability in the rat. *Laboratory Investigation* **47**, 144–149.

Weidmann, P., Boehlen, L. M., and de Courten, M. (1993). Effects of different antihypertensive drugs on human diabetic proteinuria. *Nephrology, Dialysis, Transplantation* **8**, 582–584.

Weisberg, L. S., Bloom, P. B., Simmons, R. L., and Viner, E. D. (1993). Loin pain hematuria syndrome. *American Journal of Nephrology* **13**, 229–237.

White, R. H. R. (1981). The clinical applications of selectivity of proteinuria. *Contributions to Nephrology* **24**, 63–71.

Wickelgren, I. (1999). First components found for kidney filter. *Science* **286**, 225–226.

Wilcox, C. S., Payne, J., and Harrison B. D. W. (1982). Renal function in patients with chronic hypoxaemia and cor pulmonale following reversal of polycythaemia. *Nephron* **30**, 173–177.

Williams, P. S., Fass, G., and Bone, J. M. (1988). Renal pathology and proteinuria determine progression in untreated mild/moderate renal failure. *Quarterly Journal of Medicine* **67**, 343–354.

Winearls, C. G. and Bass, C. (1994). The loin pain–haematuria syndrome. *Nephrology, Dialysis, Transplantation* **9**, 1537–1539.

Wolfish, N. M., McLaine, P. N., and Martin, D. (1986). Renal vein entrapment syndrome: frequency and diagnosis. *Clinical Nephrology* **26**, 96–100.

Woolfson, R. G., Lewis, C. A., Hill, P. D., Hilson, A. J., and Neild, G. H. (1993). Ureteric peristalsis studies in loin pain–haematuria syndrome: another diagnostic disappointment. *British Journal of Urology* **72**, 291–292.

Yamagata, K., Yamgata, Y., Kobayashi, M., and Koyama, A. (1996). A long-term follow-up of asymptomatic hematuria and/or proteinuria in adults. *Clinical Nephrology* **45**, 281–288.

Yoshioka, T., Mitarai, T., Kon, V., Deen, W. M., and Ichikawa, I. (1986). Role for angiotensin II in an overt functional proteinuria. *Kidney International* **30**, 538–545.

Yudkin, J. S., Forrest, R. D., and Jackson, C. A. (1988). Microalbuminuria as predictor of vascular disease in non-diabetic subjects. *Lancet* **ii**, 530–533.

Zaman, Z. and Proesmans, W. (2000). Dysmorphic erythrocytes and G1 cells as markers of glomerular haematuria. *Pediatric Nephrology* **14**, 980–984.

3.4 The nephrotic syndrome: management, complications, and pathophysiology

Raymond A.M.G. Donckerwolcke and J. Stewart Cameron

The nephrotic syndrome (NS), recognized as an entity for over half a century (Cameron and Hicks 2002) is defined by massive continued urinary protein losses resulting in hypoalbuminaemia and oedema formation. These are associated with modifications in kidney function, and with complications such as increased susceptibility to infections, thromboembolism, altered lipid and carbohydrate metabolism, and losses of binding proteins in the urine.

Oedema, the usual presenting complaint, is the consequence of abnormal accumulation of interstitial fluid, and becomes obvious if in excess of 10 per cent of body weight. This is usually associated with proteinuria greater than 40 mg/m^2 BSA/h (>3.5 g/24 h in a 70 kg adult) leading to hypoalbuminaemia of less than 25 g/l. However in slowly developing nephrotic syndromes significant proteinuria and hypoalbuminaemia may persist for prolonged periods without evident oedema, while in children with minimal changes and NS in relapse, oedema may appear even before a low serum albumin appears. Thus, there is only an approximate boundary between the NS and persisting proteinuria, with borderline patients. The older the patient, the lesser the degree of proteinuria and hypoalbuminaemia at which oedema may be observed.

Clinical features and investigation

The oedema

Nephrotic oedema is noticeable first only around the eyes in the morning, and the ankles in the evening, but with increasing retention there is permanent swelling of ankles and face (Fig. 1), with a sacral pad and oedematous elbows. The effects of gravity are less evident in children than adults, in whom oedema is generally dependent: young children with NS may suffer considerable ascites and facial oedema without ankle oedema.

In adults retention of up to 4 l of salt and water remains undetectable, revealed only by weighing. With increasing oedema, ascites may appear followed by pleural effusions, which are usually bilateral, occasionally unilateral, and usually limpid, but sometimes opaque and chylous. Genital oedema may be distressing, especially in males. The oedema remains soft and pitting even when profound, but if it remains untreated for long periods it may become indurated and pit only with difficulty especially around the ankles. Ankle swelling may be asymmetrical if deep venous thrombosis supervenes. Striae may appear even if no corticosteroids are being given, and the skin may actually split and weep spontaneously. Needlestick punctures may also weep profusely. The liver is often painlessly enlarged, especially in children.

The jugular venous pressure is usually normal or low, but if raised in association with a low or normal blood pressure in an older adult with NS this raises suspicion of cardiac amyloidosis as a cause (see Chapters 4.2.1 and 14.2). The nails may show white bands corresponding to periods of hypoalbuminaemia (Fig. 2a).

If extreme hyperlipidaemia is present (see below) xanthomas may form periorbitally and elsewhere (Fig. 2b). In patients with progressive forms of nephritis underlying the syndrome, symptoms and signs of uraemia and hypertension may appear. The NS is often chronic, and the psychological effects of a condition which (together with its treatment) distorts the patient's body image must not be forgotten. Prolonged hospital admissions and fear of renal failure take their toll of morale.

In the medical history, the ingestion of medicines (prescribed or 'over the counter'), prior acute or chronic infections, allergies, or any features suggestive of a systemic disorder such as lupus erythematosus should be noted. A history of macroscopic haematuria may be obtained, but this is unusual except in postinfectious or mesangiocapillary glomerulonephritis. The possibility of an associated tumour, usually in the lung or large bowel should be kept in mind in older patients (see Chapter 3.14). Finally, the family history may be revealing on occasion, as in Alport's syndrome or the Finnish form of congenital nephrotic syndrome.

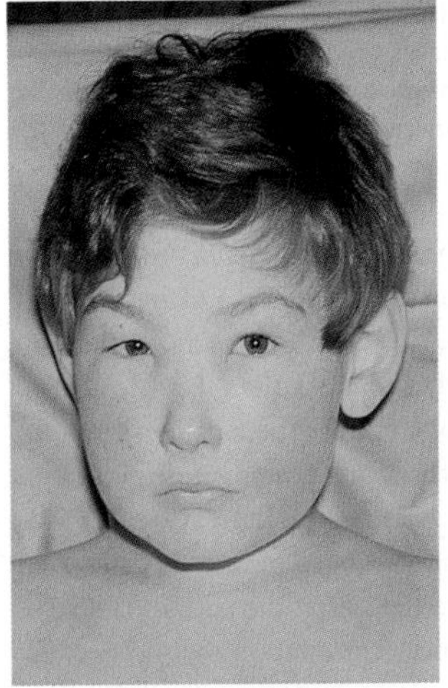
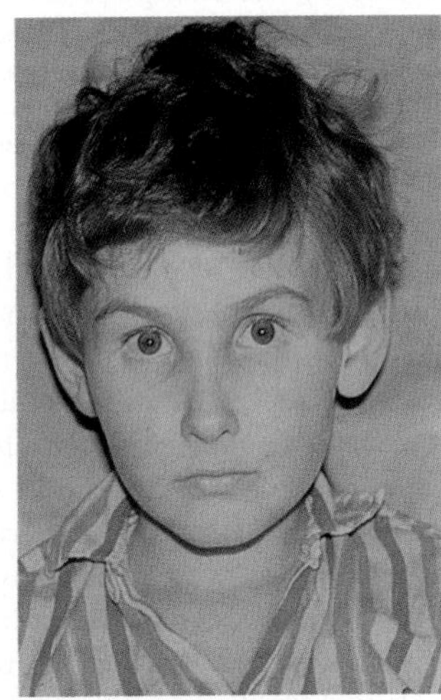

Fig. 1 Facial oedema in the nephrotic syndrome (left). Note that after diuresis (right) the face is thin, reflecting the tissue protein losses suffered by most patients with an active nephrotic syndrome of long duration.

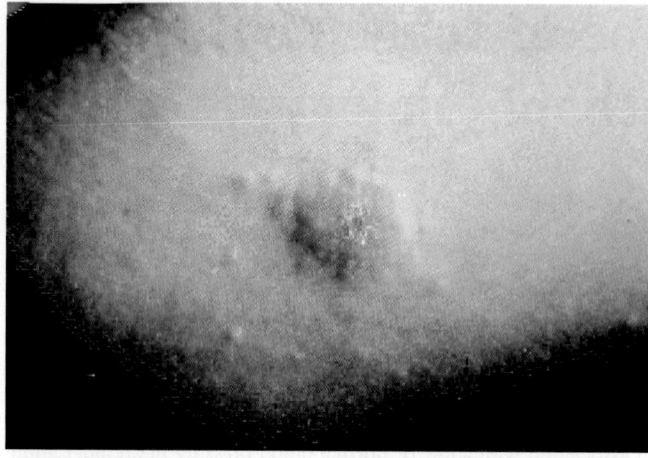

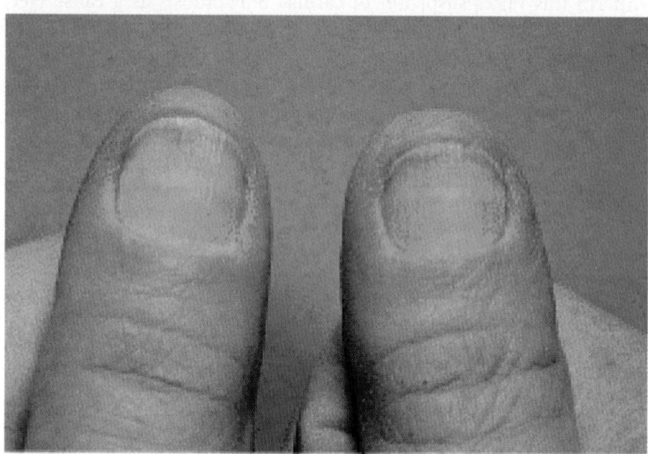

Fig. 2 (a) Left: a xanthoma on the elbow of a child with a persistent nephrotic syndrome from focal segmental glomerulosclerosis who had extreme hyperlipidaemia. As he went into endstage renal failure and his proteinuria diminished somewhat, the hyperlipidaemia remitted in part and the xanthomas disappeared spontaneously. (This patient was observed in the period before effective hypolipidaemic therapy was available.) (b) The white-banded nail of an adult nephrotic patient with membranous nephropathy, representing a period of relapse when there was a severe nephrotic syndrome and profound hypoalbuminaemia. The exact pathogenesis of this type of nail appearance is not known; in some patients the nail becomes diffusely white from the lunula outwards as the disease continues (sometimes called a 'half and half' nail).

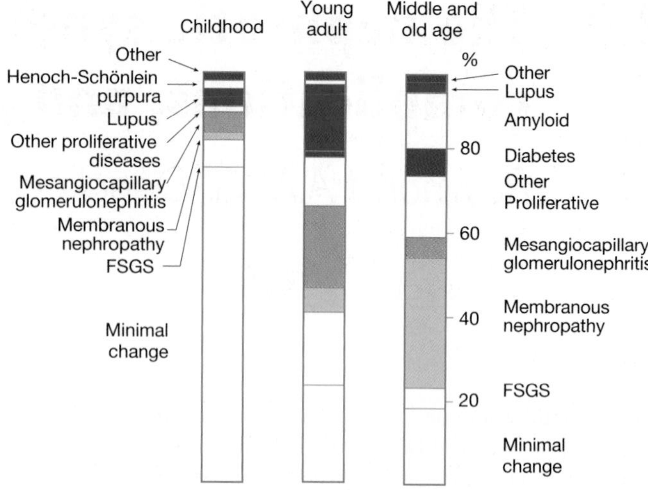

Fig. 3 Underlying histological appearances found in renal biopsies from more than 1000 nephrotic patients of all ages seen at Guy's Hospital 1963–1990. Note that the majority of children under the age of 15 years have minimal change disease, the proportion falling steadily from 2 to 15 years of age. However minimal changes remains an important cause of the nephrotic syndrome in adult nephrotics, and overall is the commonest form. Membranous nephropathy, in contrast, becomes steadily more common with age and is the commonest form of nephrotic syndrome in elderly patients.

Investigation of patients with the nephrotic syndrome follows closely on that of those with persistent proteinuria and haematuria discussed in Chapter 3.3. The majority opinion today is that all nephrotic adults and all nephrotic children less than 1 and over 10 years of age should have a renal biopsy, even if their urine shows no casts or red cells. If no unusual features are present and persistent microscopic haematuria and red cell casts are absent, treatment can be started with corticosteroids (see Chapter 3.5). The underlying renal biopsy appearances differ according to the age of the patient (Fig. 3).

Renal imaging usually by ultrasound examination will be needed. A glomerular filtration rate (GFR) measurement using a single injection of radioactive tracer or contrast is desirable, in addition to the obligatory measurement of plasma creatinine (see Chapter 1.3); in some very oedematous patients it may be better to wait until oedema has been minimized because of problems with equilibration of the isotope. Almost all patients show some reduction in GFR when the data are corrected for ideal weight for height, for reasons discussed below, and an initially reduced GFR is not necessarily an indicator of structural renal damage. The proteinuria must be quantitated on several 24 h urines as a baseline. Serological measurements should include a slide test for antinuclear factors, together with a specific assay for ds-DNA antibody, hepatitis B and C serology, complement concentrations; in patients over 45 years of age a chest radiograph and protein electrophoresis searching for paraproteins should be carried out. A VDRL or equivalent investigation may be needed to exclude syphilis, remembering that low titres of antibody against treponemes are induced by previous yaws. ANCA tests will rarely be needed since patients with vasculitis very rarely develop a nephrotic state, unless they have recovered function after severe renal damage. A routine anti-GBM antibody is likewise unnecessary because of the rarity of this type of presentation, but should of course be done if the immunohistology suggests linear capillary wall IgG deposits (see Chapter 3.11).

Proteinuria and urinary findings

The pathogenesis, diagnosis, detection, and quantitation of proteinuria are discussed in Chapter 3.3. The only symptom of profuse proteinuria itself is urinary frothing, which some patients may notice, and which may provide a valuable clue as to when major proteinuria began. Findings on urine microscopy or testing for haematuria depend upon the underlying cause of the proteinuria, and range from a bland sediment and no or only intermittent red cells and only fatty casts in the case of minimal changes, to an 'angry' sediment with abundant red cells, red cell and granular casts (see Chapter 1.2), or even visible blood in the urine, in cases of severe mesangiocapillary or crescentic nephritis.

Hypoalbuminaemia

Urinary losses of albumin are the major factor in the development of hypoalbuminaemia, but the possible role of catabolism of reabsorbed albumin in the tubule remains controversial. Thus, severe hypoalbuminaemia may be seen in the presence of only moderate albuminuria. Turnover studies have shown that the fractional catabolic rate of albumin is increased, but the absolute catabolic rate is decreased (Kaysen and Al Bander 1990). Losses of protein into the intestine as part of a generalized increase in capillary permeability often have been proposed (Schulze *et al.* 1980) but not confirmed.

Pathogenesis of nephrotic oedema

The pathogenesis of oedema formation in nephrotics is still not entirely understood (Schrier and Fassett 1988; Palmer and Alpern 1997; Vande Walle and Donckerwolcke 2001). The two major systems involved in oedema formation are the capillaries and the kidneys.

The capillaries

The extracellular compartment of body water is made up of plasma water and interstitial fluid. These are in dynamic equilibrium and fluid movement across the capillaries is the result of the balance between filtration and reabsorption due to changes in capillary and tissue hydraulic and oncotic pressure, and changes in capillary permeability. The Starling equation describes the contribution of these factors to fluid movement:

$$(\mathrm{Jv}) = \mathrm{Kf} \times S \times \mathrm{EFP},$$

where EFP (effective filtration pressure) is calculated as $(P_c - P_i) - (\pi_c - \pi_i)$; Kf is the ultrafiltration coefficient, and S is capillary surface area.

Fluid movement is different along the length of the capillary vessel, related in turn to changes in pressure (Fig. 4). Along the capillary the hydrostatic pressure (P_c) decreases, whilst the colloid osmotic pressure (π_c) increases slightly as water is filtered into the interstitium. The positive EFP at the arterial side (±4 mmHg) results in a high filtration rate (= 60 l/24 h), while the negative EFP value (−2.8 mmHg) promotes fluid reabsorption at the venous side. Net fluid filtered (filtered minus reabsorbed fluid = 4–6 l/24 h) is removed by lymph flow back into the circulation. This is associated with a slightly negative hydrostatic pressure (P_i) in the interstitium (−2 mmHg) (Taylor 1981).

Although the capillary permeability to albumin is low, the interstitial concentration is about 40 per cent of that of plasma, resulting in a π_i of 12 mmHg (Fig. 4a). In nephrotic patients, this normal fluid balance is disrupted. When π_c decreases because of urinary losses of albumin, there will be increased loss of fluid into the interstitium from the capillaries, resulting in oedema. However, important changes in the interstitium will limit oedema formation. The accumulation of interstitial fluid increases P_i and when P_i reaches zero, interstitial tissue resistance increases and limits filtration.

The filtered fluid from the capillaries has a lower protein content, leading to dilution of the interstitial fluid and this will reduce interstitial oncotic pressure. Thereby the interstitial fluid oncotic pressure will decrease in parallel with plasma colloid osmotic pressure (COP). Also, increased interstitial hydrostatic pressure accelerates lymph flow. The return of interstitial fluid to the vascular space is enhanced and the washout of the interstitium leads to further reduction of the concentration of albumin in the interstitial fluid. Koomans *et al.* (1985) have shown that in nephrotics a decrease of plasma COP from 23 to 10 mmHg will decrease the transcapillary COP gradient by only 2–3 mmHg. Thus, a new balance is achieved consisting of a higher tissue pressure, increased lymph flow and a decrease in both interstitial fluid and plasma albumin concentration (Fig. 4b).

However, in some situations this equilibrium will not be achieved. This is the case in patients with extremely low plasma albumin concentrations, such as in children with a congenital nephrotic syndrome. In these patients, plasma COP is so low that even a decrease of interstitial COP to values near zero will not allow achievement of a new equilibrium. Also in minimal change nephrotic syndrome during a rapidly developing relapse, the decrease in plasma COP may be too fast

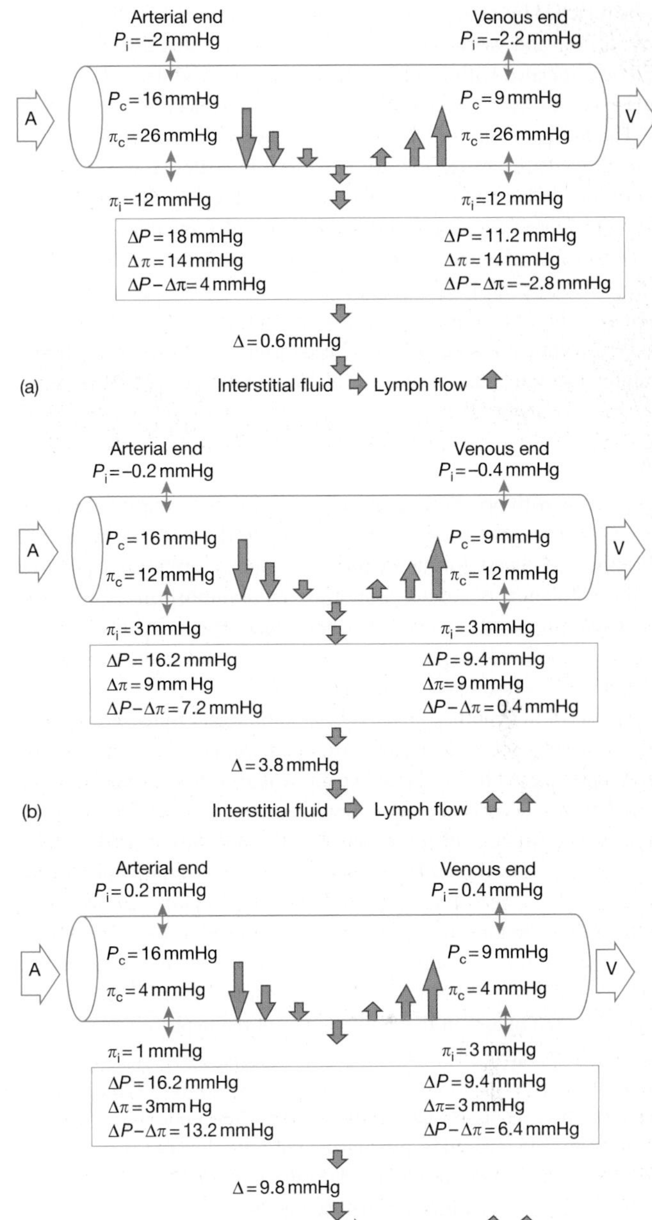

Fig. 4 Starling forces in and around the capillary in normal individuals and nephrotic syndrome (Vande Walle and Donckerwolcke 2001). Reproduced wih permission from Springer-Verlag. See the text for explanation.

to be matched by an appropriate decrease of interstitial COP, increased lymph flow and vascular refill. During this stage this disequilibrium will be associated with insufficient vascular refill and decreased circulating blood volume (Vande Walle and Donckerwolcke 2001) (Fig. 4c).

The presence and contribution of changes in general capillary permeability coefficient (Kf) is still a matter of debate. However, under conditions of hypoalbuminaemia the permeability of the capillary to protein seems to decrease and this will also contribute to maintenance of the oncotic gradient between capillaries and interstitium (Fadnes 1975; Golden *et al.* 1990). Based on all these considerations, oedema formation in the nephrotic syndrome cannot be related only to reduced plasma oncotic pressure inducing hypovolaemia with secondary renal sodium retention, but a primary renal defect in sodium and water excretion must be involved.

The kidneys

All patients with NS show renal sodium and water retention, but this may show important differences according to the stage of the NS. At onset of the NS and during the phase of oedema formation a positive sodium balance is found, but after an equilibrium is reached renal sodium excretion again matches intake. However, this is not a stable situation, and sodium retention may occur occasionally in long-standing NS (Vande Walle *et al.* 1996).

The classical hypothesis related renal sodium and water retention to hypovolaemia (underfill theory). Loss of albumin by the kidneys is not fully compensated by increased hepatic synthesis, the plasma albumin concentration decreases, and the resulting reduction of COP increases fluid movements out of the vessels into the interstitium and thereby decreases plasma volume. The reduction of plasma volume will activate the sympathetic nervous system, and the renin–angiotensin axis, promote AVP secretion and suppress atrial natriuretic peptide (ANP). Interaction of these systems stimulates renal sodium and water retention. Arguments have been provided that at least in some patients and during limited phases in the development of the nephrotic syndrome, renal sodium retention is stimulated by hypovolaemia (Usberti *et al.* 1984; Kumugai *et al.* 1985). In children with NS, clinical symptoms of hypovolaemia are occasionally noticed but in these patients, even when blood volume is assessed by plasma and red cell volume measurements, a decrease was seldom found (Vande Walle *et al.* 1995).

In adult patients with minimal change NS, an exaggerated fall in plasma volume has been observed when patients go from recumbent to standing position (Joles *et al.* 1993) suggesting the presence of hypovolaemia. However, several other studies failed to show a consistent reduction in blood and plasma volume in nephrotic patients (Dorhout Mees *et al.* 1979).

Elevated concentrations of plasma renin and aldosterone have been found in nephrotics, and in some patients sodium and water excretion increases by manoeuvres known to expand blood volume (such as intravenous albumin infusion and head-out water immersion), and is associated with a decrease in concentrations of vasoactive hormones (Rasher *et al.* 1986). Blockage of endogenous aldosterone by large doses of spironolactone resulted in enhanced natriuresis only in nephrotics and not in controls while on a high sodium intake (Shapiro *et al.* 1990). Both are arguments for involvement of increased RAAS activity, probably related to hypovolaemia. Other findings pointing to hypovolaemia are the non-osmotic related increased production of antidiuretic hormone in patients with the NS and increased plasma catecholamine concentrations and urinary clearances found in patients with NS (Usberti *et al.* 1984).

In nephrotic patients, increased proximal as well as distal tubular sodium reabsorption are present, and this also points to extrarenal stimulation of sodium retention (Grausz *et al.* 1972; Vande Walle *et al.* 1996). All these data are arguments in favour of water and sodium retention mediated by hypovolaemia. However, such abnormalities were only found in patients with rapid progression to the nephrotic syndrome and in others with extremely low serum albumin values (Vande Walle *et al.* 1996).

While all these observations are arguments in favour of a contracted plasma volume as the initiating factor for water and sodium retention, there is ample evidence that this is not the case in the majority of patients with the nephrotic syndrome. One study has shown that renal sodium retention already starts in the incipient nephrotic syndrome when plasma albumin is only slightly decreased (Vande Walle *et al.* 1995). In these patients, no difference in blood volume was found when measurements made during this phase and when in remission were compared. In other studies of patients with incipient remission of oedema, natriuresis was shown to precede an increase in plasma albumin (Brown *et al.* 1982; Koomans *et al.* 1987). Both observations are arguments against reduced plasma oncotic pressure being the primary mechanism for sodium retention. Several reports have indicated the lack of increased renin and aldosterone concentrations during the phase of oedema formation in NS, or found only modest increases in renal sodium excretion in response to blood volume expansion by head out water immersion or albumin infusion (Geers *et al.* 1984; Rabelink *et al.* 1993). While manoeuvres to achieve blood volume expansion in nephrotic patients resulted in appropriate elevations of plasma ANP concentrations, such increase in endogenous production of ANP was associated with a blunted natriuresis (Perico and Remuzzi 1993).

The most convincing evidence against hypovolaemia as the primary cause of sodium retention in the nephrotic syndrome are studies in experimental animals. In a rat model of unilateral proteinuric renal disease induced by puromycin amoninucleoside infusion, impaired urinary sodium excretion was limited to the proteinuric kidney despite the fact that both kidneys were affected by similar changes in blood volume and plasma COP (Chandra *et al.* 1981; Ichikawa *et al.* 1983).

Thus, these data from the literature and our own observations (Koomans *et al.* 1987; Palmer and Alpern 1997; Schrier and Fassett 1998) allow us to reformulate the sequence of events leading to renal water and sodium retention in NS. The basic abnormality seems to be a primary renal disturbance and exists in all cases of NS. Sodium retention occurs at an early stage when no significant decrease in serum albumin is noticed. Sodium retention continues through the stage of oedema formation. By sodium and water retention and redistribution of albumin stores most patients are able to maintain plasma COP above a critical minimum and conserve their blood volume. In these patients, sodium retention is not related to increased vasoactive hormones but the primary renal defect has yet to be identified.

Some patients, especially minimal change NS in early relapse, experience temporary hypovolaemia due to a disequilibrium in albumin redistribution. If progression to the nephrotic stage is too fast and compensatory mechanisms are insufficient, blood volume can only be maintained by secondary stimulation of vasoactive hormones maximizing renal sodium retention. The majority of these patients eventually achieve a new equilibrium, characterized by oedema, low plasma albumin concentrations and stable blood volume. A persistently unstable circulation is found only if the plasma COP decrease below a critical level (± 8 mmHg). The relative roles of sodium retention due to hypovolaemia, and primary sodium retention by intrarenal defects, probably vary during the different stages in the development of the NS (Vande Walle and Donckerwolcke 2001).

Changes in kidney function

In nephrotics, conflicting observations on GFR have been made (Berg and Bohlin1982; Löwenborg and Berg 1999), although in the majority a decreased GFR was found (Geers *et al.* 1984; Shapiro *et al.* 1986). If GFR and renal plasma flow (RPF) were only volume dependent, they would be increased in hypervolaemic patients and during hypovolaemia the decrease of RPF would be more important than the decrease in GFR, resulting in increased filtration fraction (FF). In addition, a decrease in plasma oncotic pressure would also result in an increased GFR and RPF, but changes in GFR will be larger than changes in RPF and result also in increased FF. However an inverse correlation between FF and oncotic pressure was found in patients with the NS. Therefore, the decrease in FF commonly found in nephrotic patients implicates a decrease of the permeability of the glomerular basement membrane (Kf) (Berg and Bohlin 1982; Myers and Guasch 1993).

Different nephron segments are involved in sodium retention in the NS. One study attributed impaired sodium excretion to decreased GFR and showed correction of both sodium excretion and GFR by volume expansion (Shapiro *et al.* 1986). Several tubular segments may be involved in renal sodium retention. In incipient nephrotic syndrome and during hypovolaemia increased tubular sodium retention was found at both proximal and distal tubules. In the distal tubule, at least part of increased sodium reabsorption is related to increased sodium/potassium exchange and is stimulated by aldosterone (Vande Walle and Donckerwolcke 2001). In patients with stable circulatory volume, sodium retention is not related to increased vasoactive hormones and seems to be localized in the most distal nephron segments. The molecular mechanism of renal sodium avidity has been attributed in PAN nephrotic rats to stimulation of Na, K-ATPase and increased expression of epithelial sodium channels of cortical collecting duct cells (Deschenes et al. 2002). Increased distal tubular sodium reabsorption has been attributed to resistance to ANP (Perico and Remuzzi 1993) and experience in nephrotic animals and patients are in accordance with this assumption. The abnormality was related to a specific cellular alteration in the ANP signalling pathway. Evidence has been provided that increased cGMP phosphodiesterase activity blunts the cellular actions of cyclic guanosine monophosphate, the second messenger of ANP normally produced in response to ANP's interaction with its biologically active receptor (Valentin *et al.* 1992).

A defect in urinary concentration capacity was found in humans with NS and similarly in adriamycin-induced NS in rats (Fernandez-Llama *et al.* 1998). The abnormality was associated with a decreased expression of Na^+ transporters (Na–K–2Cl, Na^+/H^+ exchanger NHE-3 and Na, K-ATPase, $\alpha 1$) in the thick ascending limb, and of renal medullary aquaporin-1 water channels in the thin descending limb of Henle's loop and of aquaporin 2 and 3 in the collecting duct. The concentrating defect was related to the failure to generate a high osmolality in the renal medulla and osmotic equilibrium in the collecting duct. The defect found in experimental studies, however, may follow a toxic effect of adriamycin (Apostol *et al.* 1997; Fernandez-Llama 1998). We and others observed a defect in urinary diluting capacity following a water load in patients with the NS (Vande Walle *et al.* 1996). This abnormality maybe related to decreased Na–K–2Cl transport and thereby failure to generate a hypotonic luminal fluid by the cortical thick ascending limb of Henle's loop. However, we found the abnormality only in patients with hypovolaemia and suggest that decreased Na^+ absorption in Henle's loop maybe related to low distal nephron sodium delivery. It is not clear how the reduced Na^+ reabsorption in Henle's loop fits with the decreased sodium excretion in patients with NS.

Symptomatic treatment of nephrotic oedema

When oedema formation is severe, symptomatic treatment is required, independent of any specific measures that may be available to treat the underlying condition. The first step is to ensure a reasonably low intake of sodium compatible with a relatively normal diet, but in patients with hypovolaemia who require maximal sodium retention to maintain circulatory volume, particularly children, this policy can be dangerous. In patients with hypervolaemia, and in those requiring diuretics a low sodium intake (50–70 mmol/24 h in adults) should be given. An additional goal of sodium restriction is potentiation of the antiproteinuric effects of ACE inhibitors, discussed below.

Patients with the NS often show relative resistance to diuretic (Kirschner *et al.* 1992), which has been attributed to a multifactorial decreased delivery of the drug to the active sites in the tubular brush border of the kidney (Wilcox 2002). Diuretics are protein-bound, which limits the diuretic to the vascular space and maximizes its delivery to the kidney. Hypoalbuminaemia will result in a larger extravascular distribution and reduce its availability (Keller *et al.* 1982), as well as increasing its inactivation to the glucuronide within the kidney (Pichette *et al.* 1996). In addition, it has been shown that binding of free filtered frusemide to urinary proteins decreases the inhibitory effect on loop Cl^- reabsorption (Kirschner *et al.* 1990); although Agarwal *et al.* (2000) found that displacement of frusemide from urinary albumin using sulfasoxazole made little difference to its diuretic activity. Experimental studies have shown that the active drug is less effective in inhibiting Cl^- reabsorption in the loop of Henle of nephrotic rats than in control rats (Keller *et al.* 1982). The tubuli of analbuminaemic rats are resistant to frusemide, but of practical importance this can be overcome by intravenous administration of the frusemide bound to albumin (Inoue *et al.* 1987). While the extent of absorption of frusemide in healthy individuals and nephrotics may be identical, a delayed delivery to the active sites may diminish the response to oral therapy. Other drugs may have a better bioavailability such as bumetanide (1–10 mg) or torsemide (10–50 mg), because of their hepatic rather than renal metabolism (Brater *et al.* 1984; Krämer *et al.* 1999).

Frusemide is most often used in doses of 40 mg up to 200 mg/24 h, doses higher than used in other diseases. When the efficiency of oral diuretics is impaired, a continuous intravenous administration should be considered. Constant infusion is preferred to bolus administration, because it prevents a rebound in postdiuretic sodium reabsorption. This effect has been documented by several studies (Krämer *et al.* 1999). Addition of other distal-acting diuretics may be necessary to obtain an effect, but in patients with low plasma aldosterone concentrations, the effect of added spironolactone is often disappointing unless given in very high dosages (600 mg/24 h), which often induce nausea. Additional metolazone 5–20 mg on alternate days has been used also, with success reported by some authors.

Intravenous albumin administration would seem at first sight to be the treatment of choice in patients with hypoalbuminaemia and hypovolaemia, but is rapidly excreted into the urine, and may lead to circulatory overload and hypertension in patients with hypervolaemia. Therefore the detection of hypovolaemia is of particular importance. Clinical symptoms alone are often unreliable for evaluation of blood volume and plasma albumin and oncotic pressure do not allow assessment of the blood volume status. Intrinsic renal diseases may be more often associated with sodium retention independent of volume status.

Thus it would be useful to have clinical measures of blood volume status to guide treatment. Concentrations of vasoactive hormones are not available for a quick diagnosis. We have shown that the association of low FE_{Na^+} and increased $[U_{K^+}/(U_{K^+} + U_{Na^+})]$ ratio correlated best with clinical symptoms of hypovolaemia and significantly elevated levels of plasma renin, aldosterone, noradrenaline, and vasopressin. If $[U_{(K^+)}/(U_{K^+} + U_{Na^+})] \times 100$ is higher than 60 per cent, salt-free albumin infusion (1.5 ml/kg BW of a 20 per cent solution) can safely be administered (Donckerwolcke *et al.* 2003). The diameter and collapsibility of the inferior vena cava and the left atrial volume measured by ultrasonography have been advocated as an index of central filling in nephrotic children (Dönmez *et al.* 2001) and deserve more exploration.

Intravenous salt-free albumin has been used also rather sparingly—and controversially (Dorhout Mees 1996) by some authors in adults, but more commonly in children with severe hypovolaemia, which is uncommon in adult nephrotics. A dose of 100 ml of 20 per cent solution, combined with a high dose (usually 250–500 mg) of oral or 250 mg per 1.72 m^2 BSA intravenous frusemide was recommended in adults (Davison *et al.* 1974) and in children (Haws and Baum 1993). However, intravenous albumin alone has little effect in inducing a diuresis in patients with NS (Rabelink *et al.* 1993) or in hypoalbuminaemic cirrhotic patients (Chalasani *et al.* 2001). Direct comparison of diuretic alone versus a diuretic plus intravenous albumin showed no advantage for the latter regime in one study (Akcicek *et al.* 1995), but a modest benefit in another (Fliser *et al.* 1999). In cirrhotics (in whom the confounding variable of proteinuric binding of frusemide was absent) albumin alone or in combination did not enhance the diuresis (Chalasani *et al.* 2001). Each of these manoeuvres can be dangerous if employed alone, since IV albumin may induce severe or even fatal pulmonary oedema if a diuresis is not induced, and high-dose frusemide can induce severe volume depletion and hypotension. If employed, it is best to use the double regime on alternate days, to allow re-equilibration of interstitial and plasma albumin and saline. Despite the fact that the albumin passes quite quickly into the urine and the lack of evidence of an effect of albumin alone, this regime does seem to permit rapid removal of up to 35–40 l over 2 weeks in severely oedematous nephrotic adults.

Finally, gentle ultrafiltration using either a haemodialysis machine or (less commonly) peritoneal dialysis has been used in such resistant patients ever since the introduction of dialysis (Fauchald *et al.* 1985). This may lead to acute renal failure if pursued too vigorously, however, and perhaps albumin could be used in combination with ultrafiltration, but this has not been adequately tested.

Reduction of proteinuria

Apart from symptomatic relief of oedema, much evidence has accumulated (Burton and Harris 1996; Abbate *et al.* 1999; Jafar *et al.* 2001) that suggests proteinuria is directly toxic to the renal tubules and leads eventually to an interstitial infiltrate and renal fibrosis (see Chapter 11.1). Additionally, reduction in proteinuria leads to improvement in plasma albumin concentrations and consequent improvement in lipid and coagulation parameters (see below). Thus, reduction of proteinuria has become a major goal in the management of patients with persisting proteinuria from chronic conditions leading to renal failure (see Chapters 11.1 and 11.2).

Since the first descriptions (Michielsen *et al.* 1973; Arisz *et al.* 1976), a number of manoeuvres (Table 1) have been outlined that can reduce nephrotic-range proteinuria arising from any type of histological change, when specific treatment to reduce or eliminate proteinuria is not available. All of these seem to act through reversible haemodynamic changes, and are accompanied by a greater or smaller reduction in the GFR, important in patients with either structural glomerular damage and/or reversible reduction in GFR. This therapeutic ratio is more favourable using ACE inhibitors than with any other agent except perhaps dipyridamole. Whilst any reduction in the mean arterial blood pressure will reduce proteinuria, the effect of ACE inhibitors is present even when the reduction in proteinuria is corrected for that achieved by lowering the blood pressure to an equivalent extent using other agents (Gansevoort *et al.* 1995a). The effect of these manoeuvres in reducing proteinuria is additive (Table 1) and all may have a final common action in reducing intraglomerular capillary hydraulic pressure, P_c (de Jong *et al.* 1992). On the one hand, non-steroidal anti-inflammatory drugs (NSAIDs), protein restriction, and cyclosporin most likely exert their antiproteinuric effect by increasing afferent glomerular arteriolar tone; whilst ACE inhibitors, AT1 antagonists (Kurokawa 1999) and possibly dipyridamole, act through decreasing efferent glomerular arteriolar tone (de Jong *et al.* 1992). The combination of ACE inhibitor and AT1 antagonist is additive (Russo *et al.* 2001). Improvements in glomerular permeability seiving profiles during treatment with indomethacin (Golbetz *et al.* 1989) or ACE inhibitors (de Zeeuw *et al.* 1990) are almost certainly the result of these haemodynamic changes.

A number of controlled trials of the renoprotective effects of ACE inhibitors in proteinuric patients with various underlying renal conditions have been performed (see Gansevoort *et al.* 1995a and Chapters 11.1 and 11.2), which suggest that the strategy of using a long-acting ACE inhibitor such as enalapril, ramipril, or lisinopril to reduce protein excretion in long-term nephrotic patients should form a part of the long-term

Table 1 Inhibition of proteinuria in (non-diabetic) nephrotic patients by different agents

Preglomerular vasoconstriction	
NSAIDs	
Indomethacin	Arisz *et al.* (1976)
Naproxen	Vriesendorp (1985)
Low protein diet	Kaysen *et al.* (1991)
Cyclosporin	Tejani *et al.* (1987)
Postglomerular vasodilatation	
ACE inhibitors[a]	Gansevoort *et al.* (1995a)
AT1 receptor antagonists	Kurokawa (1999)
Dipyridamole	Kan *et al.* (1974), de Jong *et al.* (1988)
Combined therapy	
Indomethcin + lisinopril	Heeg *et al.* (1991)
Enalapril + low protein diet	Ruilope *et al.* (1992), Gansevoort *et al.* (1995b)
Captopril + ibuprofen	Allon *et al.* (1990)
ACE inhibitor + AT1 antagonist	Russo *et al.* (2001)[b], Laverman *et al.* 2002

[a] Mainly lisinopril and elalapril have been studied, but captopril, fosinopril (Keilani *et al.* 1993), ramipril, and benazapril have similar effects.

[b] Note that patients in this study all had IgA nephropathy, with a mean proteinuria of only 1.9 g/24 h.

management of all such patients today. AT1 receptor antagonists also are under trial, as are combinations of both. It is important to restrict sodium at the same time to 50–60 mmol/24 h, since the inhibitory effect on proteinuria is much greater in sodium-depleted than sodium-replete patients (Heeg *et al.* 1989), and the effect can be completely abrogated by a sodium intake of 200 mmol/24 h of sodium. Also, the maximum effect will not be achieved for several weeks with ACE inhibitors, in contrast to NSAIDs, with which a reduction in proteinuria is evident within a week or two. Lisinopril 5 mg is usually effective in reducing proteinuria by one third, and today is probably the recommended treatment; 10 mg/24 h will halve the proteinuria, but with a 25 per cent reduction in GFR. Addition of a small dose and an NSAID into the regime can be considered in both adults (Allon *et al.* 1990; Heeg *et al.* 1991) and children (Trachtman and Gauthier 1988), but the further reduction in GFR will carry with it a greater risk of acute renal failure.

Nephrectomy to eliminate proteinuria

In a few unfortunate individuals, proteinuria remains torrential despite aggressive treatment, postural hypotension is prominent, oedema persists, the plasma creatinine increases, and protein malnutrition becomes increasingly severe. These are usually young and show severe ('malignant') focal and segmental glomerulosclerosis (see Chapter 3.5); if elderly, amyloidosis. In this situation, it may be useful to contemplate nephrectomy, dialysis, and intensive nutrition, an approach now standard in the Finnish congenital NS (see Chapter 16.4.4) before the infants have become too malnourished (Kim *et al.* 1992). Unilateral nephrectomy has been used also in neonatal nephrotics (Mattoo *et al.* 1992) and also in focal segmental glomerulosclerosis, with decrease in proteinuria and an increase in albumin in some cases, but no change in others.

Bilateral surgical nephrectomy through a midline incision is the standard procedure (Bienz *et al.* 1994), but other means have been employed to achieve a 'medical' nephrectomy. These include the administration of mercurial diuretics or NSAIDs in very high doses (Bamelou and Legrain 1982), cyclosporin and angiotensin (Rieu *et al.* 1994), or the injection of polymers, autologous thrombus (Olivero *et al.* 1993), coils, gelfoam, or fat into the renal artery. Both approaches have advantages and disadvantages; we have used only surgery and NSAIDs under these circumstances.

Complications of the nephrotic syndrome

The NS, mainly through alterations in concentration of plasma proteins, affects every cell and every tissue in the body. There is selective loss of low molecular weight protein in the urine as discussed in Chapter 3.3, together with a general overproduction of all hepatically synthesized proteins (Fig. 5). Thus, low molecular weight proteins tend to be depleted in the plasma, with accumulation of the higher molecular weight species. Proteins smaller than 180–200 kDa show lower plasma concentrations, and above this size increased levels. Proteins with fast turnovers in health are more resistant to depletion than those with slower normal synthetic rates.

The abnormalities found in NS result from the effects of these alterations in the protein environment, directly as a result of altered concentrations (e.g. in coagulation) or as a secondary result of induced alterations in cellular function (e.g. binding of increased LDL to platelets or endothelium).

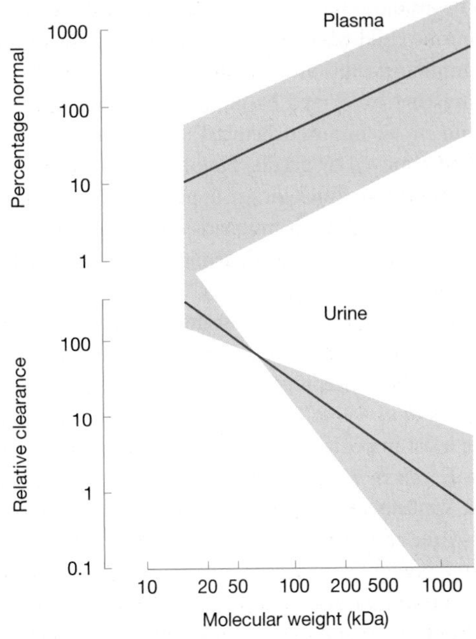

Fig. 5 The relationship between (lower panel) the loss of proteins into the urine in relation to molecular weight in nephrotic patients, and (upper panel) the concentrations of proteins in the plasma in relationship to molecular weight. It can be seen that there is a reciprocal relationship between the two sets of measurements. One hypothesis which would explain this relationship is that all proteins are synthesized in excess in the nephrotic syndrome, and those of low molecular weight are lost predominantly in the urine. Thus, those of low molecular weight are depleted, and those of high molecular weight accumulate in the plasma.

Infections in nephrotic patients

Incidence and clinical features

Although no longer a major problem in developed countries, infections remain a formidable challenge in nephrotics throughout the developing world (Elidrissy 1982; Gulati *et al.* 1997). Early papers from developed countries described a similar situation (Arneil 1961) but such reports are rare today (Rusthoven and Kabins 1978). However, sepsis remains an important cause of deaths in children with NS even today: 6/10 deaths in 389 children with minimal change NS were from sepsis (International Study of Kidney Disease in Children 1984) and Gorensek *et al.* (1988) also showed that peritonitis remains a threat.

Although minimal changes underlies the NS in most cases, this may reflect only the fact that it is the most common form in childhood; we have seen pneumococcal peritonitis also in children with mesangiocapillary glomerulonephritis and in Henoch–Schönlein purpura. Most organisms implicated are encapsulated, and the predominance of pneumococcal infections is striking; others, such as *staphylococcus*, are notable for their almost complete absence. The clinical infections rate is higher in children treated with cytotoxic drugs than in those treated with prednisone alone, being highest in those treated with chlorambucil (6.5 per cent) compared with cyclophosphamide (1.5 per cent) (Latta *et al.* 2001).

Primary peritonitis

This is a particular feature of children with NS. Our oldest case was aged 21, but even older patients have been noted (Chuang *et al.* 1999).

Onset may be insidious but is usually sudden, and should be suspected in any nephrotic child who develops abdominal pain. Unfortunately, this is a common symptom associated with hypovolaemia, and the diagnosis must be confirmed by direct microscopic examination of a Gram stain or an immunochemical search for bacterial antigens in ascitic fluid removed by needle. Blood cultures are usually positive also, but of course take much longer to perform. Hypotension, shock, and even acute renal failure (Cavagnaro and Lagomarsino 2000) may follow rapidly, sometimes with disseminated intravascular coagulation (see below).

In the past, the organism was almost always *Streptococcus pneumoniae*, but other organisms have become relatively more common; these include β-haemolytic streptococci, *Haemophilus* and Gram-negative bacteria (Speck *et al.* 1974; Tain *et al.* 1999). Even so, *S. pneumoniae* remains the most important organism: half in Krensky *et al.*'s (1982) series, with *E. coli* in 25 per cent and Gorensek *et al.* (1988) noted 11/37 cases. *S. pneumoniae* peritonitis also may be more common in Black than White children (O'Regan *et al.* 1980). Although now treatable, primary pneumococcal peritonitis is still a major illness, and remains an important cause of death in nephrotics in both the developing (Elidrissy 1982) and developed worlds (Gorensek *et al.* 1988). Penicillin-resistant strains of *S. pneumoniae* are now emerging (Giebink 2001).

Cellulitis

This may arise from skin lesions, either spontaneous or as a result of venepuncture, and are usually the result of β-haemolytic streptococci or a variety of Gram-negative bacteria. Usually the clinical diagnosis is clear with obvious demarcation of the infected area; the patient may be toxic, febrile, or even become hypotensive. Other patients run a more indolent course with an area of infection, which remains localized. It is difficult to stain or culture organisms from fluid aspirated from the area, but as in primary peritonitis, blood cultures are usually positive.

Miscellaneous infections

Viral infections Relapses of the minimal change NS often follow not only viral upper respiratory infections, but also viral infections, especially measles, which may induce remission of the minimal change NS, and the disease was even used as a treatment for the condition before the advent of corticosteroids (Janeway *et al.* 1948). The major threat is either varicella (see below) or measles, especially to children receiving either corticosteroid or cytotoxic agents.

Other organisms Particularly in the developing world, infections (including peritonitis) may arise from a variety of other organisms, such as *Bacterium alkaligenes*, *Bacteroides*, *Aerobacter*, and *Streptococcus viridans* (Choudhry and Gai 1977). Tuberculosis, common in developing areas, affected almost 10 per cent of all nephrotic children in one large series from India (Gulati *et al.* 1997).

Pathogenesis of infections in nephrotics

Although physical factors such as fluid collections in cavities, ruptured fragile skin, and dilution of local humoral defences by oedema are important, it seems likely that immunological factors play the major role in the susceptibility of nephrotic patients to infection.

Low serum IgG concentrations are characteristic of nephrotic patients (Giangiacomo *et al.* 1975) for unclear reasons (see Chapter 3.5). However, low IgG does not seem to play an important role in infections in NS, since in patients with inherited common hypogammaglobulinaemia concentrations less than 2 g/l are needed to provoke serious infections, a level rarely seen in nephrotics. Also in deficiencies of IgG, infections tend to be staphylococcal, chronic, and sinopulmonary in site.

Factor B is crucial in the primitive, antigen non-specific alternative pathway of the complement system. Its molecular weight is only 55 kDa and thus is lost in the urine in the NS with lowered plasma concentrations (McLean *et al.* 1977; Anderson *et al.* 1979). The alternative pathway is of particular significance to the opsonization of encapsulated organisms, such as *S. pneumoniae*, and whilst the addition of IgG had no effect on opsonization by nephrotic sera, addition of purified factor B resulted in improvement. Matsell and Wyatt (1993) have pointed also to the importance of urinary losses of another alternative pathway component, *factor I*. By 20 years of age, most individuals have acquired specific antibodies against a variety of pneumococcal capsular antigens. Thus, it is only during childhood that there is this peculiar vulnerability to *S. pneumoniae*.

Transferrin is essential for normal lymphocyte function, and acts as a carrier for a number of metals, including *zinc*. Warshaw *et al.* (1984) suggested that, *in vitro*, added transferrin could restore defective function in lymphocytes from nephrotics to normal, and Bensman *et al.* (1984) suggest that urinary losses of zinc result in diminished production of the zinc-dependent thymic hormone thymulin.

There is abundant—but confusing—evidence that lymphocyte function is depressed in nephrotic patients, especially those with minimal change disease (see Chapter 3.5). This depression of T-cell function appears to arise from serum factor(s) which may persist in remission and which may or may not be specific for minimal change disease, independent of treatment. There are fewer data on polymorph function, but Yetgkin *et al.* (1980) and Sillix *et al.* (1983) demonstrated impaired phagocytosis of *Staphylococcus aureus* and *E. coli* by polymorphonuclear leucocytes from nephrotics, even when the assays were performed in normal serum.

Treatment and prophylaxis

Obviously, prompt induction of remission of oedema or proteinuria are the most important goals and the decline in death rate from infection in nephrotic children is probably the result of this. Meticulous care must be taken over asepsis concerning breaches in skin.

In children who have already experienced pneumococcal infection, there is a good case for using prophylactic penicillin at least whilst the child is oedematous since recurrences are well known (Anderson *et al.* 1979; Moore *et al.* 1980). For some time pneumococcal vaccines against capsular antigens have been available, and their use in nephrotic children seems logical (Tejani *et al.* 1985) as the response when given in remission is sufficient. During relapse, however, when treated with high doses of prednisone (~20 mg/kg/day) or with cytotoxic therapy, vaccination may not give protection. We recommend delaying vaccination up to 14 days after discontinuation of these treatments. However, recurrent pneumococcal sepsis has been reported in children immunized after a first attack (Primack *et al.* 1979; Moore *et al.* 1980). Persistence of the antibody is low in relapsing cases (Spika *et al.* 1986), and protection should not be trusted too far (Güven *et al.* 2004). The emergence of non-vaccine serotypes in immunized individuals, and antibiotic resistance, are increasing problems (Giebink 2001).

The most important feature of treatment for established sepsis in a nephrotic patient is that it should begin quickly. This, in turn, rests with anticipation, suspicion, and rapid diagnosis. The ESR is useless in nephrotic children, the white cell count may be misleading in those taking corticosteroids or immunosuppressants and the C-reactive protein is not always available, or too late to be of use.

Parenteral antibiotics should always be used, even when the infection appears to be localized, because septicaemia is almost always present. Antibiotics should be begun as soon as cultures have been taken; results of sensitivity tests should not be awaited. In children, benzylpenicillin should always be a component of the antibiotic therapy; conversely when pneumococcus is observed, backup broad-spectrum therapy is needed, because it may not be the only organism present. A broad-spectrum cephalosporin, perhaps with an aminoglycoside, may be used as initial 'blind' treatment in adults. Blood pressure, peripheral temperature, and venous pressure should be watched carefully, colloid given as necessary and heparin given for anticoagulation because of the danger of secondary thrombosis (Futrakul 1978, and see next section). Finally, the need for supplementary corticosteroids in those taking these drugs, or in those who have just stopped them, should be remembered. Any severe infection should prompt discontinuation of cytotoxic therapy.

In nephrotic children with active disease, varicella/chicken pox is a threat. Those taking high-dose corticosteroids or other immunosuppressive agents within the previous 3 months are at risk of severe progressive disseminated disease. Following contact with infected persons, zoster immune globulin should be administered within 72 h. Active varicella zoster infection should be treated with intravenous acyclovir, and cyclophosphamide or chlorambucil should be discontinued. In several countries, an effective varicella vaccine is available. Low to moderate doses of prednisone do not contraindicate administration of the live virus vaccine. In these patients, seroconversion is similar to healthy children, but relapses of the NS following vaccination have been noticed (Alpay *et al.* 2002).

Thromboembolic complications

Introduction

Thrombosis in both the arterial and the venous circulations is a relatively frequent and serious complication of NS (Cameron 1984; Cameron *et al.* 1988) being associated with clinical symptoms in about 10 per cent of nephrotic adults and 2–3 per cent of children (Andrew and Brooker 1996; Lilova *et al.* 2000). Subclinical thrombotic complications hve been reported to occur in up to 50 per cent of adults and 28 per cent of children with NS (Hoyer *et al.* 1986).

Abnormalities of coagulation

It remains unclear what causes the increased tendency to thromboembolism in nephrotic patients. No single protein factor appears overwhelmingly important, although most changes in NS might be expected to lead to enhanced coagulability (Table 2) (see Cameron 1984; Cameron *et al.* 1988; Kanfer 1990; Rabelink *et al.* 1994 for details).

Physical factors

Nephrotic patients are relatively immobile and may have haemoconcentration from hypovolaemia, especially in childhood. Whole blood viscosity is increased by both the increase in haematocrit with changes in red cell deformability, and increased plasma viscosity arising from high fibrinogen concentrations (Zwaginga *et al.* 1994). These conditions also favour margination of platelets and increased platelet aggregability (Rabelink *et al.* 1994).

Table 2 Concentrations of proteins important in coagulation in the nephrotic syndrome in relation to molecular weight

Protein	MW (Da)	Concentration in nephrotic plasma
Zymogens and cofactors		
Von Willebrand factor	840,000	Raised
Factor V	350,000	Raised
Factor I (fibrinogen)	330,000	Raised
Factor VII	200,000	Raised–normal
Factor XI	160,000	Normal–reduced
Factor XII	79,000	Normal–reduced
Factor II (prothrombin)	72,000	Normal–reduced
Factor X	56,000	Normal–reduced
Factor IX	55,400	Normal–reduced
Regulator proteins		
α_1-Macroglobulin	840,000	Raised
Plasminogen	81,000	Normal–reduced
Protein S	75,000	Normal–reduced
α_2-Antiplasmin	70,000	Normal–reduced
Antithrombin III	68,000	Normal–reduced
Protein C	65,000	Raised–normal
α_1-Antitrypsin	54,000	Reduced

Alterations in zymogens and cofactors

Numerous studies of adults (Cameron *et al.* 1988) and children (Kanfer 1990; Elidrissy *et al.* 1991; Andrew and Brooker 1996) survey concentrations and/or activities of procoagulant zymogens and their cofactors in NS. In general, plasma concentrations of factors of the intrinsic pathway of coagulation are reduced, and occasional patients with a bleeding tendency from this have been reported (Handley and Lawrence 1967); but all other zymogens or cofactors are either present in normal—or more usually raised—concentrations, particularly von Willebrand factor, fibrinogen, and factors V, X, and VII. Concentrations of prothrombin (factor II) are in general normal. Whether increases in zymogen concentrations, over and above the great excess in which all are present in normal circumstances will induce a 'prethrombotic' state is not clear; none is rate-limiting at the concentrations found in normal plasma. However, it is worth noting that in normal individuals, fibrinogen and factor VIIc concentrations are independent variables predicting vascular disease. Zwaginga *et al.* (1994) and Rabelink *et al.* (1994) point to a crucial role of raised fibrinogen concentrations, particularly under flow conditions.

Alterations in fibrinolytic and regulator proteins

Some of this group of proteins are concerned both with inhibiting fibrinolysis (which limits thrombosis) but also thrombin generation (which promotes thrombosis), complicating prediction of likely effects. Also, activity of the several modulators of plasmin and thrombin summate; concentrations of some may go down and some up. Thus, even though concentrations of antithrombin III are very low in NS (10–20 per cent normal) (Kauffmann *et al.* 1978), total functional antithrombin activity is normal (Kanfer 1990) because of the increase in α_2-macroglobulin concentration (Boneu *et al.* 1981). Rydzewski *et al.* (1986) also noted low concentrations of α_1-antitrypsin, but felt that the increases in α_2-macroglobulin did not compensate for losses of antithrombin III. Consistently, plasminogen concentrations have been found to be low in nephrotics, but the role of plasmin inhibitors (Du *et al.* 1985) is not yet clear.

The vitamin K-dependent natural anticoagulant protein C, and its cofactor protein S (Clouse and Comp 1986; Preissner 1990), are activated by the thrombin–thrombomodulin complex and inherited deficiencies are associated with venous thromboses. They antagonize the action of activated factors V and VIII and stimulate release of plasminogen activator from endothelial cells. Protein S is in addition responsible for binding of protein C to platelets and endothelial cells, where anticoagulant activity is expressed. Protein S exists in the plasma in a free active form, and also in an inactive form bound to C4b-binding protein. Despite a molecular weight of 62 kDa, which leads to the expected urinary losses (Cosio *et al.* 1985), concentrations of protein C remain normal or even increased in nephrotic plasma (Rostoker *et al.* 1987; Gouault-Heilmann *et al.* 1988); while there are conflicting reports concerning the functional activity of the molecule (Vaziri *et al.* 1988). Only the free protein S is active, but there is disagreement about even total concentrations of protein S in nephrotic plasma (Gouault-Heilman *et al.* 1988; Vaziri *et al.* 1988; Citak *et al.* 2000), although functional levels are usually low, which might play a part in nephrotic hypercoagulability (Vigano-Angelo *et al.* 1987).

Factor V, previously thought of as a purely procoagulant zymogen, is also a cofactor of protein C (Svensson and Dahlbäck 1994). Mutations of factor V that permit its procoagulant action but eliminate its anticoagulant cofactor function have been described in as many as 30–40 per cent of otherwise normal patients who suffer deep vein thromboses (Factor V_{Leiden}) (Voorberg *et al.* 1994). However, study of small number of nephrotic patients with thrombosis did not suggest an increased frequency of potentially thrombogenic factor V mutations (Irish 1997).

Thus, the immensely complex balance of coagulant, fibrinolytic, and regulator proteins is much disturbed by the dysproteinaemia of the nephrotic state. It seems unlikely that the increases in zymogens and other promoters of coagulation will enhance coagulation in view of the excess normally present in plasma, except perhaps fibrinogen. Urinary losses of regulator proteins may be important; there is no convincing evidence that total antithrombin activity is reduced in nephrotics when all the changes are summed up. Fibrinolysis has been less studied in nephrotics, and it may be here that the effects of dysproteinaemia, if any, are to be found. Conventional tests of coagulation such as the prothrombin time are usually normal in NS (Andrassy *et al.* 1980). The partial thromboplastin time may be prolonged in the few patients with low intrinsic pathway activities (factors XII, XI, and IX). However, it is safe to biopsy these patients without fresh frozen plasma, as it is in those with a lupus 'anticoagulant' (antiphospholipid antibody) (Kant *et al.* 1981).

Alterations in platelet function

Three possible mechanisms by which platelet hyperaggregability may arise in NS have been explored (Cameron 1991): effects of lowered serum albumin on platelet prostaglandin metabolism, effects of hyperlipidaemia on platelet membrane lipids, and effects of increased von Willebrand factor concentrations.

The platelet count in nephrotic patients has been reported as either normal or mildly raised (Cameron 1984). Abnormalities of platelet aggregation and thromboxane production in platelets from nephrotic patients studied *ex vivo* are well recognized. To what extent these data reflect events *in vivo* is not clear, but the data of Zwaginga *et al.* (1994), who studied whole nephrotic blood under flow conditions, throw doubt on their relevance. *In vitro*, hyperaggregability of stirred nephrotic platelet-rich plasma to ADP stimulation, with occasional spontaneous aggregation, is seen. This can be reversed by addition of concentrated urine protein (Bang *et al.* 1973) or of purified albumin both *in vitro* and *in vivo* by infusion (Remuzzi *et al.* 1979). This is unlikely to depend upon increased availability of arachidonic acid for thromboxane synthesis as proposed by Jackson *et al.* (1982) and Schiepatti *et al.* (1984), at least *in vivo*.

Hyperlipidaemia is a prominent feature of the NS. Lipoproteins bind to platelets, LDL-enhancing and HDL-inhibiting aggregation; these effects may be mediated through effects on adenylate cyclase. Hyperlipidaemia is associated in NS with spontaneous aggregation (Jackson *et al.* 1982) and dietary lipids will alter the composition of platelet membrane lipid. There are also opposing effects of LDL and HDL on endothelial cell production of prostacyclin (see below), which is a powerful modulator of platelet activity. LDL from nephrotic plasma is enriched in lysolecithin (Joles *et al.* 1994), and lysolecithin-containing LDL are toxic to endothelial cells, diminishing nitric oxide production (Kugiyama *et al.* 1990), which is an inhibitor of platelet adhesion under flow conditions.

Hyperaggregability to ristocetin (a cationic compound) is present in *in vitro* inplatelets from nephrotic adults, which appeared to be independent of the depletion of albumin, or the availability of arachidonate but is probably related to the greatly increased concentrations of von Willebrand factor in nephrotic plasma (Bennett and Cameron 1987), to which ristocetin binds in a triple complex with the platelet. Suggestions of altered charge on platelets from nephrotic patients based on indirect methodology (Levin *et al.* 1985) have not been sustained by direct measurement (Cohen *et al.* 1988; Böhler *et al.* 1992).

Alterations in endothelial cell function

Endothelial cells are known to play a very active role in maintaining the free flow of blood *in vivo*. Their function has been studied little in nephrotic patients, but Stroes *et al.* (1995) showed impaired response to endothelium-dependent vasodilatation, possibly as the result of the alterations in circulating lipids (Kugiyama *et al.* 1990; Joles *et al.* 1994). Alterations in endothelial function could be important in nephrotic hypercoagulability.

Role of drugs

Corticosteroids The description of thromboses in nephrotic patients coincided with the introduction of corticosteroids in their treatment (Calcagno and Rubin 1961); in Egli's (1974) paediatric survey, 26 of 59 patients who developed thrombosis were taking steroids at the time. Corticosteroids increase the concentration of some zymogens (Ozsolylu *et al.* 1962), and prothrombin times and APTT may be shortened under steroid treatment (Ueda *et al.* 1987). The action of warfarin is also antagonized by corticosteroids (Menczel and Dreyfuss 1960). On the positive side, steroids tend to increase concentrations of antithrombin III (Thaler and Lechner 1978) and inhibit platelet aggregation (Glass *et al.* 1981), at least in large doses.

Diuretics Most patients who develop thrombosis are receiving diuretics, since almost all are oedematous; some develop thrombosis during diuresis (Lilova *et al.* 2000) possibly from the increased haematocrit induced by diuretics. The already increased blood viscosity in nephrotics as a result of high fibrinogen concentrations increases steeply with increasing haematocrit. It may be that the more judicious use of diuretics during the 1970s and 1980s has led to a decrease in the frequency of thromboses, for example, of the pulmonary artery in children (Egli *et al.* 1973; Egli 1974), which we no longer observe. Another factor may be the common practice of giving albumin infusions at the same time as powerful diuretics, especially when the latter are given intravenously.

Peripheral venous thrombosis and pulmonary embolism

Deep vein thrombosis

Thrombosis of the deep calf veins is common in NS, overt in 3–12 per cent of adults (Llach 1982; Cameron 1984), whilst occult thrombi may be detectable in as many as 25 per cent by Doppler ultrasonography (Andrassy *et al.* 1980). It is not clear how common deep vein thrombosis is in childhood; less than 1 per cent of the 4158 paediatric patients identified through a MEDLINE search by Andrew and Brooker (1996) showed clinically-evident deep vein thrombosis, and Mehls *et al.* (1987) reported only two cases amongst 204 nephrotic children. However, the study of Hoyer *et al.* (1986) discussed below on pulmonary emboli in children with the nephrotic syndrome, suggests that thrombi must be more common than this at a subclinical level, and 8/16 thrombotic episodes in the series of NS patients in Bulgaria (Lilova *et al.* 2000) were in the leg.

Pulmonary emboli

Not surprisingly in view of these data, pulmonary emboli are also common: at a clinical level about 0–15 (median 7) per cent of adult nephrotics have embolism (Cameron *et al.* 1988), and in our series of those with minimal changes, 8 per cent. However, if ventilation–perfusion (*V*/*Q*) isotope scanning is done routinely, 9–26 (median 12) per cent of adult nephrotics show evidence of pulmonary emboli, often symptomless (Cameron 1984). Nevertheless only a single patient in our own adult series up to 1982, followed for a total of 2100 patient-years, had actually died from pulmonary embolism. As for DVT, children seem to be less affected: Egli's data (1974) discovered only a single child of 3377 with clinical embolism. But, in contrast, 2 of 204 cases of Mehls *et al.* (1987) had pulmonary emboli, and Jones and Hébert (1991) reported a major pulmonary vein embolus in a child, and Lilova *et al.* (2000) another. As in adults, a systematic study of pulmonary *V*/*Q* scans in 26 nephrotic children (Hoyer *et al.* 1986) showed evidence of emboli in a much higher proportion—7 (35 per cent).

Other venous thrombi

Other venous thrombi are much less common, with the exception of renal vein thrombosis, discussed below. However subclavian or axillary, jugular, iliac, portal, splenic, hepatic, and mesenteric vein thrombosis have all been described (see Cameron 1984 and Cameron *et al.* 1988 for references). Sagittal sinus thrombosis has been described both in children and adults, and we have seen a fatal case in which the thrombus extended to include superficial cortical veins. We have also seen a nephrotic child with priapism.

Arterial thrombosis

In all series reported in adults, arterial thrombosis is much less common than venous thrombosis (Cameron 1984). Also, in children the proportion of thromboses at a venous site (73–81 per cent) was greater than in arteries (19–27 per cent) (Andrew and Brooker 1996; Lilova *et al.* 2000). Thrombosis of almost every artery has been recorded, and is summarized in detail in Cameron (1984) and Cameron *et al.* (1988). Multiple arterial thrombi in the same patient have been recorded also (Lye and Tan 1991) as well as both venous and arterial thrombi in the renal vessels (Kennedy *et al.* 1991).

One of the most common sites is the femoral artery, found usually in children (10 cases in Egli's survey of 1973) often in association with attempts at femoral vein puncture in hypovolaemic subjects, and also in adults (Kanfer *et al.* 1970). A femoral artery thrombosis was the only instance amongst our 90 nephrotic adults with minimal change. Pulmonary artery thrombosis was common in the past, being the single most common site in the paediatric study of Egli (1974), and has been in an adult (Kanfer *et al.* 1970). Now, it seems almost to have disappeared. It is not clear how many of these cases may have in fact have originated as pulmonary emboli (Jones and Hébert 1991). Haemoconcentration seems the likely factor, since the only other condition in which pulmonary artery thrombosis may be seen is polycythaemic congenital cyanotic heart disease.

Renal venous thrombosis in nephrotic patients

This controversial topic has been reviewed extensively in the past (Llach 1982, 1985). Controversy exists not only about its incidence, but also how energetically it should be sought, and how it should best be managed especially when symptomless. All agree that it is most commonly found in association with membranous nephropathy, usually idiopathic but also in secondary forms such as in lupus (Appel *et al.* 1976), after gold therapy (Nelson and Birchmore 1979), and after transplantation (Liaño *et al.* 1988), as well as in the Heymann model of membranous nephropathy in rats. The reason for this predilection for membranous nephropathy has so far eluded explanation.

Prevalence

The apparent prevalence of renal vein thrombosis varies according to whether a clinical or a venographic diagnosis in symptomless patients is considered. Also, since renal vein thrombosis and membranous nephropathy are associated, those series with a high proportion of patients with membranous nephropathy (as in several American series) will show a higher incidence of renal vein thrombosis. Rather consistent clinical prevalences from 4 to 8 per cent have been reported in membranous nephropathy (Trew *et al.* 1978; Noel *et al.* 1979; Cameron *et al.* 1988), whilst in several American series using *venography*, up to 50 per cent have been reported (Llach 1982; Wagoner *et al.* 1983). In contrast, in Europe the prevalence is much lower, from 13 to 18 per cent (Andrassy *et al.* 1980; Cameron *et al.* 1988; Rostoker *et al.* 1992). In another American series, it was only 9 per cent (Pohl *et al.* 1984). In other forms of NS, the incidence of renal venous thrombosis is much lower, clinically 0–5 per cent (Andrassy *et al.* 1980; Llach 1982); of 322 such nephrotics in our own series only five (1.5 per cent) were affected (Cameron *et al.* 1988). Venography demonstrated subclinical thrombi, but only in 0–16 per cent of cases (Llach 1982).

Clinical diagnosis and evaluation

Renal venous thrombosis may present acutely with loin pain, haematuria, renal enlargement, pain and swelling in the ispilateral testicle in males, and deterioration in renal function; or as a slower decline in renal function without dramatic signs or symptoms. Leg oedema increases if the vena cava is involved, although caval thrombosis can be surprisingly silent. Thrombosis of renal veins may be unilateral, and men are more commonly affected than women. About 35 per cent of patients with renal venous thrombosis will have pulmonary emboli which are clinically evident or show up on scanning (see Cameron *et al.* 1988 for detailed discussion).

It has yet to be established that seeking symptomless renal venous thrombi is useful (Rostocker *et al.* 1992), since their prognosis appears to be benign (see below), or how frequently or at what intervals rescreening must be undertaken. Nor is it clear what diagnostic strategy should be adopted: until recently, renal venography was the standard investigation, but being expensive and invasive was little employed for screening symptomless patients with NS, even those with membranous nephropathy. However, colour duplex Doppler ultrasonography (Avasthi *et al.* 1983) is easy and safe to perform, and although it has never been evaluated against MRI scanning (Tempany *et al.* 1992) or spiral CT, both of which have advocates, it probably remains the best diagnostic approach today. Surprisingly in view of the divergence of opinion in the past, no recent studies using Doppler duplex ultrasound have beeen published in nephrotic patients.

Prognosis

The prognosis of untreated renal venous thrombosis, whether clinically evident or silent, is no longer clear since virtually all patients now receive heparin and/or warfarin as soon as a diagnosis is made. In particular, the prognosis of radiographically diagnosed, symptomless renal venous thrombosis in the absence of anticoagulation is not known. Functional renal impairment is an adverse prognostic sign (Laville *et al.* 1988) but in many instances recovery of renal function is possible and recanalization of the veins usually occurs.

Treatment and prophylaxis of thrombosis in nephrotics

Thromboses in children, being more frequently arterial, will on average be more serious clinically than in adults.

Treatment of evident thrombosis

Patients should be mobilized, sepsis avoided or treated promptly, dehydration from incidental causes (e.g. diarrhoea) treated, diuretics used with care, and haemoconcentration minimized. Anticoagulation carries the usual risks and presents additional difficulties in nephrotic patients. *Heparin* acts mainly through activation of antithrombin III, whose concentration may be diminished in nephrotics (Kauffman *et al.* 1978). Thus, higher doses of heparin are required in NS to achieve anticoagulation, although there are probably additional explanations (Vermylen *et al.* 1987b) and Sie *et al.* (1988) describe normal plasma concentrations of heparin cofactor II (molecular weight 66 kDa) in nephrotics. Heparin binds also to α_2-macroglobulin and to endothelial cell surfaces, as well as promoting platelet aggregation in some patients. *Warfarin* similarly presents problems in nephrotics (Ganeval *et al.* 1986), mainly because it is bound to albumin whose concentration may change therapeutically or spontaneously; however, it increases antithrombin III concentrations (Andrassy *et al.* 1980).

Whether nephrotic patients with symptomless deep venous thrombosis should receive anticoagulation treatment has never been studied adequately; probably if they also have symptomless pulmonary emboli, most physicians would anticoagulate. If the physician *does* wish to anticoagulate every nephrotic with a symptomless deep vein thromboses, then he or she will have to anticoagulate one quarter.

Patients with symptomatic thromboses should receive anticoagulation using warfarin with an INR maintained at 2–4, with similar treatment for children (Andrew and Brooker 1996). Special consideration needs to be given to nephrotics with renal venous thrombosis (Kanfer 1994), irrespective of how the diagnosis was reached. In the face of an incidence of overt or occult pulmonary emboli of 35 per cent, it is difficult to argue against anticoagulating all of them, although evidence of benefit from doing this is not available in symptomless patients. There appears to be no advantage either to thrombectomy or local fibrinolytic therapy (Laville *et al.* 1988). In most cases in which warfarin has been used and subsequent venography performed, the renal vein had recanalized (Kassirer 1979; Llach 1982), but in some it did not (Laville *et al.* 1988). Five of 27 patients in Laville's series had bleeding complications from anticoagulation (see above).

When—and on what grounds—anticoagulation can be stopped also remains unclear. Data from the general population with deep vein thrombosis (Petiti *et al.* 1986) suggests a minimum of 3 months, with some extra benefit from 6 months. However, stopping the warfarin at any time in the continuing presence of NS may lead to rethrombosis (Briefel *et al.* 1978), and a reasonable policy is to continue warfarin until the oedema remits, or at least until the serum albumin is greater than 25 g/l. This may result in anticoagulation being required for some years.

Patients with diagnosed thrombi and an antiphospholipid antibody should have a higher level of anticoagulation, with an INR of 3–4 (Piette 1994), which needs to be maintained as long as the antiphospholipid antibody persists. At the moment there are no clear indications for prophylactic anticoagulation in patients with antiphospholipid antibodies; high titres of IgG antibody carry the greatest risk of subsequent thrombosis, but at the moment data do not justify treatment—although others have expressed the opposite point of view (see next paragraph).

Prophylactic anticoagulation in nephrotic patients?

Given the very high incidence of thrombotic complications (10 per cent of adults and 3 per cent of children), should all nephrotics—or at least all those with membranous nephropathy—receive prophylactic anticoagulation? Bellomo and Atkins (1993) and Sarasin and Schifferli (1994) conclude that warfarin anticoagulation *is* justified in all patients with membranous nephropathy, and should lead to lowered morbidity. Sarasin and Schifferli (1994) argue further that anticoagulation for every nephrotic may be justified. The problem lies with the quality of the data fed into the decision models used in these analyses, and it will be interesting to see if these reviews have altered clinical practice. After all, patients at risk of thrombosis from familial antithrombin III, protein C, or protein S deficiencies are *not* recommended for prophylactic anticoagulation (Pabinger *et al.* 1994). The benefit of prophylactic anticoagulation with warfarin in children with NS remains even more unclear, alhough some recommend treatment in patients with unstable steroid-resistant NS.

Other possible approaches to prophylaxis are subcutaneous low molecular weight or synthetic heparins but there are no reports of this in nephrotics. Also, there is a case for giving at-risk subgroups (e.g. those with membranous nephropathy or antiphospholipid antibody) low-dose aspirin (75 mg daily, which is safe with steroids) and dipyridamole (100–200 mg three times a day), as suggested by Andrassy (1980). This has the advantage of being safe, and might also be justified on the grounds of the extra risk of vascular disease (see next section).

Lipid abnormalities in the nephrotic syndrome

Hyperlipidaemia is the most common complication of the NS, to the point where some authors have considered it a part of the definition of the syndrome: hypercholesterolaemia is present in 90 per cent of patients with a urinary protein excretion of over 3 g/24 h (Kasiske 1998). The importance of hyperlipidaemia lies in its contribution to the development of atherosclerosis, and possibly also to the progression or induction of renal damage leading to or aggravating chronic renal failure (Samuelsson *et al.* 1997). Abnormalities occur in all aspects of lipid metabolism in nephrotic patients.

Nephrotic hyperlipidaemia (Kasisike 1998; Wheeler 2001) is characterized by an increased plasma concentration of cholesterol, both free and cholesterol esters (total plasma cholesterol > 5.2 mmol/l). The hyperlipidaemia correlates inversely and strongly with serum albumin concentration [although dyslipidaemia has been reported in patients with nephrotic-range proteinuria without hypoalbuminaemia, and in remission (Zilleruelo *et al.* 1984)]. It is independent, however, of the underlying cause of the NS including lupus (Jovén *et al.* 1993). Increases in fasting triglyceride (TG) concentration are less common, and more often found in patients with severe NSs. The profile of lipoproteins, mixtures of apolipoprotein and lipids, is characterized by increases in TG-rich very low-density lipoprotein (VLDL), and in parallel of intermediate density lipoprotein (IDL) and of low-density lipoprotein (LDL) particles. Kashyap *et al.* (1980) showed reduced apolipoprotein C-II in VLDL from nephrotics, which may be important since Apo C II is an activator of lipoprotein lipase (see below). Deighan *et al.* (1998) demonstrated that LDL from nephrotics are rich in the smaller, denser, more atherogenic LDL III than normal. In contrast, high density lipoprotein (HDL) concentrations are usually normal, although an important reduction of the HDL-2 fraction is found (Short *et al.* 1986), and some studies have reported low total HDL concentrations in very severe NSs (Appel *et al.* 1985). The composition of the HDL is also altered from normal (Jovén *et al.* 1987).

Lipoprotein (a) [Lp(a)] concentrations are also increased (Stenvinkel *et al.* 1993; Doucet *et al.* 2000) and it has been demonstrated that increased plasma concentrations of apolipoprotein (a) (>300 mg/l) are a strong independent predictor of adverse vascular events in the general population. Plasma concentrations in the normal population vary 100-fold, on the basis of genetic heterogeneity and molecular polymorphism.

Lipiduria is well recognized in the NS, and fatty urinary casts are a characteristic feature (see Chapter 1.2). Cholesterol, phospholipid, free fatty acids, and TG are all present in nephrotic urine. HDL is also present (Short *et al.* 1986) and Gitlin *et al.* (1958) showed that labelled HDL appeared in the urine when injected into nephrotics, whereas VLDL did not, presumably on the basis of molecular size.

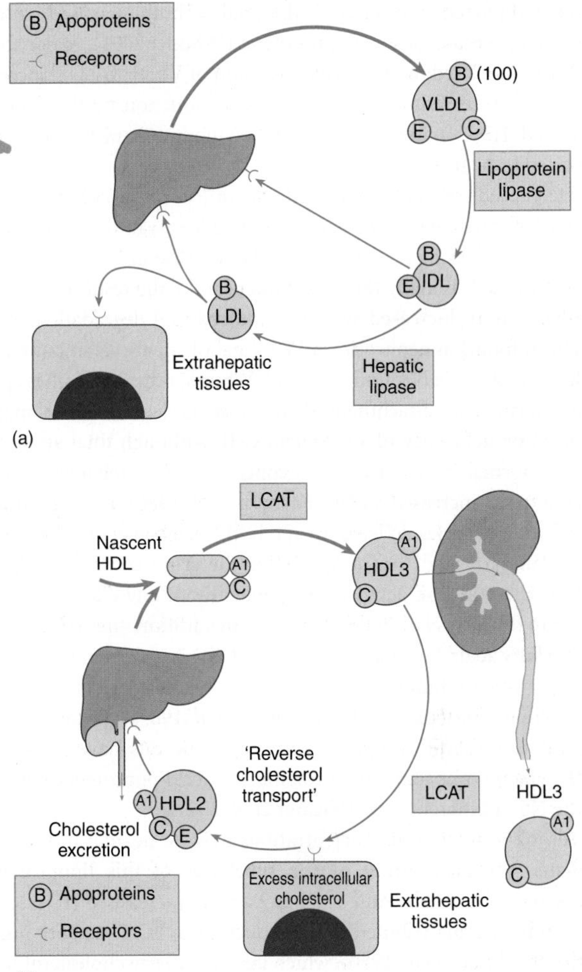

Fig. 6 (a) Abnormalities of very low-density lipoprotein (VLDL), IDL, and LDL in the nephrotic syndrome. Hepatic overproduction of VLDL leads to an increase in plasma concentration of this lipoprotein and its products, intermediate (IDL) and low (LDL) density lipoprotein. In addition the activity of endothelial lipoprotein lipase is reduced, so that catabolism of VLDL is retarded. Excess VLDL may deposit in vascular structures (see the text for details). (b) Abnormalities of high density lipoprotein (HDL) in the nephrotic syndrome. Secretion of nascent HDL by the liver is increased. HLD-3 tends to be lost in the urine since its molecular weight is higher than that of HDL-2. LCAT activity is reduced, which also inhibits conversion of HDL-3 to HDL-2. Removal of cholesterol from tissues to the liver is inhibited by this defective maturation of HDL (see text for additional details). Modified from Wheeler D.C., Varghese, Z., and Moorhead, J.F. (1989). Hyperlipidaemia in the nephrotic syndrome. *American Journal of Nephrology* **9** (Suppl. 1), 78–84, with permission of the authors and publishers.

Pathogenesis of the hyperlipidaemia of the nephrotic syndrome

This is complex and understood only in part (Fig. 6). Lipoproteins transport TGs in plasma. They may be categorized according to apolipoprotein composition and density into high density (which contain apolipoprotein AI) and VLDL, IDL, and LDL (containing apolipoprotein B) (Vaziri 2003). The plasma concentration of the various lipoproteins is dependent on the balance between synthesis and catabolism. The liver synthesizes and secretes VLDL into the circulation. The determinants of VLDL catabolism are endothelial-bound lipoprotein lipase (LpL) which requires the availability of apoprotein C-II (apo CII). Lipoprotein lipase tethers triglyceride-rich lipoprotein to the vascular endothelium, where it is hydrolyzed. Normal VLDL metabolism is also dependent on HDL by recirculation of apo CII from HDL-3 to VLDL. Nascent HDL is formed by surface constituents of VLDL, free cholesterol and phospholipids and matures in the circulation. During maturation HDL particles accumulate cholesterol, which is esterified by lecithin cholesterol acyltransferase (LCAT) to form cholesterol esters. These sink into the core as nascent HDL is converted to HDL-3 and subsequently to HDL-2. The TG-depleted VLDL is taken up by the liver or interacts with cholesterol ester-rich HDL-2. HDL-2 is processed by lipase to HDL-3. The end-product of hydrolysis of VLDL, low density lipoprotein (LDL), is also directly synthesized by the liver.

Hyperlipidaemia in the NS is the result of both increased synthesis and decreased catabolism of lipoproteins (Wheeler 2001). Major abnormalities are related to impaired conversion of VLDL to LDL, increased hepatic LDL secretion, increased Lp(a) production by the liver, and impaired HDL maturation. The following mechanisms have been reported to be involved:

Decreased receptor-mediated clearance of circulating VLDL (Warwick *et al.* 1990, 1992; Kaysen and de Sain-van der Velden 1999) now seems crucially responsible for the increase in VLDL concentrations, although initially this was thought to be the result of increased synthesis. Both increased synthesis and reduced degradation of TGs has been found in nephrotics. VLDL catabolism also is impaired by a reduced endothelial-bound LpL pool. While synthesis of LpL is apparently normal, its attachment to the vascular endothelium may be reduced by deficiency of apoprotein C-II. Although total apoprotein C-II is normal in nephrotics, its concentration is relatively reduced related to the increased VLDL (Kashyap *et al.* 1980). Patients with NS have VLDL particles deficient in apo C-II (Deighan *et al.* 2000). Thus, proteinuria, through loss of ApoC-II in the urine, contributes directly to the defect in LpL activity, independently of any effect on plasma albumin (Shearer *et al.* 2001). However, in addition, the concentration of free fatty acids (normally albumin-bound) is increased in nephrotic plasma, which inhibits LpL (Nikkilä and Pykäpistö 1968) and nephrotic sera inhibit LpL *in vitro* (Vermylen *et al.* 1987a). Detailed studies in analbuminaemic compared with nephrotic rats have shown that both hypoalbuminaemia and proteinuria affect lipoprotein catabolism in the NS in different ways (Shearer *et al.* 2001).

Although total HDL concentrations may be normal in nephrotic patients, the distribution of the subclasses of this lipoprotein is abnormal, with a reduction of HDL-2 and an increase in HDL-3. This pattern has been attributed to the reduction in LCAT activity present in the NS (Cohen *et al.* 1980), which inhibits reverse cholesterol transport and thus impairs VLDL lipolysis by reducing the availability of apoprotein C-II. This loss of LCAT activity is probably multifactorial, since it is small enough to be lost in the urine, and also is potentiated by albumin which is reduced.

There is increased hepatic synthesis of all the lipid and protein moieties of VLDL and LDL which have been studied, in both human and in experimental NS (Kaysen 1991; Wheeler *et al.* 1991; Warwick and Packard 1993), an abnormality which in most cases returns to normal on remission. Probably an increase in apolipoprotein synthesis is the prime mover, and the accumulation of lipid a secondary event. Thus while conversion of VLDL to LDL is impaired, the principal pathway promoting the increase in LDL concentrations is through increased synthesis of LDL apoB100 by the liver (de Sain-van der Velden *et al.* 1998a); it is not clear yet what signal stimulates this (see below). The activity of cholesterol ester transfer protein (CETP), an enzyme that catalyzes the exchange of the cholesterol ester-rich core of HDL-2 for the TG-rich core of VLDL remnant particles, yielding LDL, is increased also in nephrotics, stimulating the normal pathway for LDL production (Kaysen 1992).

Elevated plasma Lp(a) concentrations result also from increased hepatic synthesis (De Sain-van der Velden *et al.* 1998a). Lp(a) consists of a molecule of LDL to which one molecule of the apolipoprotein apo(a) has been covalently attached to apoB100. Its molecular weight varies from 60 to 230 kDa according to the number of kringle repeats in the molecule, and both Lp(a) and its fragments are excreted in the urine in increased quantities in nephrotics (Doucet *et al.* 2000), the kidney also being an important site of metabolism of the molecule.

Chylomicra have been little studied in the NS (Levy *et al.* 1990; Warwick *et al.* 1992a), but surprisingly in view of the data on impaired VLDL clearance, there seem to be no differences in the timing or height of chylomicron response to a fat meal in nephrotic subjects.

The primary stimulus responsible for triggering all these abnormalities of lipid metabolism in the NS has not been elucidated. The apparent coregulation of production of different proteins supports the hypothesis that reduced oncotic pressure or albumin concentration increases transcription of a group of liver-regulated proteins (Davis *et al.* 1980; Appel *et al.* 1985). Plasma viscosity has been suggested as the important factor, but this has also been denied (Appel *et al.* 1985). Infusion of albumin alone, or dextran, will acutely lower cholesterol and triglyceride in nephrotic patients or in nephrotic rats, but this effect may not operate in the long-term.

Consequences of hyperlipidaemia in nephrotic syndrome

Similar lipid abnormalities to those associated with NS have been shown to be major risk factors for atherosclerosis in the general population. However, the evidence to support the idea that this operates also within nephrotic patients, although plausible, remains scanty. The hyperlipidaemia of the NS was shown to increase the relative risk for myocardial infarction 5.5-fold and the relative risk of coronary death 2.8-fold compared to controls in a Californian population (Ordoñez *et al.* 1993). However, the only previous epidemiologic data, from the population in the South East of England (Wass *et al.* 1979) found no differences in incidence or outcomes compared to matched local controls. Numerous other small studies are inadequate and/or anecdotal, although the rapid appearance of aortic atheroma in some chronic nephrotics is striking, especially in children (Kallen *et al.* 1977; Hopp *et al.* 1994). The duration of the nephrotic hyperlipidaemia appears to be critical in inducing vascular damage, and it is patients with unremitting proteinuria and hypoalbuminaemia who are most at risk. Conversely, in remitting or minor NS vacular risk appears less. It must not be forgotten either that other risk factors, such as smoking (Chapter 4.12.2), obesity, hypertension (Section 9), and hyperuricaemia (Chapter 6.4) must contribute strongly to vascular disease in nephrotic patients, as they do in the general population, and require management also.

The principal mechanisms of vascular damage appear to be associated with circulating LDL. Increased levels of LDL lead to increased scavenger-mediated LDL uptake by monocytes, inducing formation of foam cells within the vascular walls. Oxidized LDL is more rapidly taken up than normal LDL. Rupture of foam cells releases oxidized LDL and free radicals. Oxidized LDL causes apoptosis of endothelial cells, associated with endothelial dysfunction. The significance of the increased Lp(a) as a risk factor for atherosclerosis in the setting of NS is not yet known.

Elevated plasma TG concentrations are associated with a faster rate of deterioration of renal function in patients with glomerular disease (Hunsicker *et al.* 1997; Samuelson *et al.* 1997). Hyperlipidaemia may be associated also with the development of glomerular and interstitial renal disease in animal studies, but evidence remains persistently lacking of this in humans (Yang *et al.* 1999; Wheeler 2001). Endothelial damage may favour influx of lipoprotein into the mesangium, leading to proliferation and sclerosis. Also, filtered lipoproteins may accumulate in the tubular interstitium leading to a chronic inflammatory reaction. Interstitial foam cells are of macrophage origin, and accumulate in relation to duration but not intensity of the proteinuria (Neugarten and Schlondorff 1991).

Confounding factors such as proteinuria and hypertension made the assessment of any beneficial effect of treating hyperlipidaemia on progression of renal disease difficult in humans, although amply demonstrated in animal models (Harris *et al.* 1990). However, a recent meta-analysis of 13, generally small, controlled trials involving a total of 362 patients with diverse progressive renal diseases (but over two thirds diabetic), demonstrated that the rate of progression of renal disease to renal failure was slowed using various types of lipid-lowering therapy (statins, gemfibrozil, probucol). The rate of decline in GFR decreased by 0.16 (CI 0.03–0.27) ml/min/month [1.9 (CI 0.3–3.4) ml/min/year], comparable to the effect of reducing proteinuria using ACE inhibitors, and four times that achieved using protein restriction (Fried *et al.* 2001). The treatment of transient NS of less than some months' duration, however, does not at present seem justified (Keane *et al.* 1992; Olbricht and Koch 1992).

Treatment of hyperlipidaemia in the nephrotic syndrome

General measures

Although dietary fat restriction is usually recommended in hyperlipidaemic states, only severe fat restriction is associated with significant reduction in plasma lipids in NS. Dietary supplementation with fish oil has some lipid-lowering effect, but the effect on progression of renal disease has been found mainly in patients with IgA nephropathy (see Chapter 3.9). D'Amico and Gentile (1991) showed that a low-fat, low cholesterol diet in membranous nephropathy with NS, although it had no effect on proteinuria, reduced plasma total and LDL cholesterol concentrations by 24 and 27 per cent, respectively. Similar figures (28 and 32 per cent) were obtained using a vegetarian soy-protein, polyunsaturated fat diet; HDL cholesterol declined also, but by only 14 per cent.

Obviously, if major reduction of proteinuria or remission can be obtained, abnormalities of lipid metabolism will regress towards normal (Kaysen 1991). Gansevoort *et al.* (1994) reported that apolipoprotein(a) concentrations were reduced in nephrotic patients by giving lisinopril 10 mg/24 h together with indomethacin 150 mg/24 h, and Keilani *et al.* (1993) found that fosinopril 10–20 mg alone reduced proteinuria and also total cholesterol, LDL cholesterol, and Lp(a) concentrations. Several studies have documented the lipid-lowering effects of agents such as statins, bile acid sequestrants, fibric acids, fish oil, and probucol in patients with NS.

Statins (HMG CoA reductase inhibitors)

Lipid-lowering interventions, in order to decrease progression of renal disease should be directed towards lowering of TG-rich lipoproteins (Attman *et al.* 1999). While several drugs can achieve lowering of plasma lipids in nephrotics, HMG CoA reductase inhibitors (statins) have been shown to be the most effective agents (Massy *et al.* 1995). These drugs are inhibitors of the enzyme 3-hydroxy-3-methyl coenzyme A (HMG CoA), reducing cholesterol synthesis. They lead also to upregulation of hepatic LDL receptors, and thus to increased clearance of LDL from plasma in addition. They reduce both LDL and triglyceride levels, the latter through activation of lipoprotein lipase. Finally, these versatile drugs correct endothelial dysfunction through up-regulation of endothelial NO-synthase and decreasing endothelial superoxide production, as well as inhibiting proliferation of smooth muscle cells within the vascular wall (Dogra *et al.* 2002). They also have anti-inflammatory effects and inhibit cell proliferation, and thereby may decrease progression of renal disease (O'Donnell 2001).

Several statins have been shown to reduce LDL cholesterol in nephrotic patients by 35–40 per cent and TGs by 15–30 per cent in short-term studies. Simvastatin dosages ranging from 10 to 40 mg/24 h are required to lower cholesterol below 120 mg/l (3.1 mmol/l) (Rabelink *et al.* 1988; Warwick *et al.* 1992); there is no effect on Lp(a) concentrations. However, an effect on albuminuria and progression of renal disease has still to be shown in long-term studies (Samuelson 1998; Attman *et al.* 1999; Olbricht *et al.* 1999), although the recent meta-analysis of Fried *et al.* (2001) discussed above is encouraging. Other agents such as pravastatin (Toto *et al.* 1992) and lovastatin (Chan *et al.* 1992) have been used also in nephrotic patients with similar results, but simvastatin has been most studied in nephrotics. Olbricht *et al.* (1999) described 56 adults treated for 2 years, and noted a reduction in LDL cholesterol of 47 per cent with no change in HDL cholesterol. In general, statins are safe: however, both lovastatin and simvastatin rarely lead to rhabdomyolysis (Corpier *et al.* 1988) occasionally with acute renal failure, in the majority of cases the result of interactions with concomitant cyclosporin or gemfibrozil. Symptomless increases in muscle enzymes are often noted (Israeli *et al.* 1989; Olbricht *et al.* 1999), and the drug should be stopped if creatine kinase increases to greater than 500 i.u./l. Simvastatin has been reported to adversely affect growth in rats also, and has thus generally been avoided in children; pravastatin does not appear to have this disadvantage (Querfeld 1999).

Other treatments

Cholesterol is lowered less by fibrates than by statins, although they have a powerful effect on TGs in nephrotics as in other subjects (Groggel *et al.* 1989) since they stimulate lipoprotein lipase activity, and hence reduce VLDL cholesterol. However, since in nephrotics (unlike in renal failure) the main need is to reduce LDL cholesterol concentrations, it does not seem that fibrates are the best drugs to use—unless hypertriglyceridaemia is present as well. Fibrates induce muscle necrosis more frequently than statins, and fenofibrate produces a confusing increase in plasma creatinine which may be interpreted as a fall-off in renal function. Finally, the risk of gallstones is increased by both clofibrate and benzafibrate.

Probucol does not affect TG concentrations at all, but is effective in lowering cholesterol. Unfortunately, it may reduce HDL cholesterol concentrations as well as LDL cholesterol in many subjects. Its exact mode of action remains uncertain, and moreover no large population studies in cardiovascular disease are available. Its main attraction is that it reduces concentrations of the strongly atherogenic oxidized LDL by its antioxidant effect. Probucol has been used in nephrotic patients (Valeri *et al.* 1986; Iida *et al.* 1987), including children because of doubts about statins mentioned above (Querfeld *et al.* 1999), with a reduction in cholesterol concentrations; but it was taken off the market in 1999, and may not be reintroduced.

Nicotinic acid (1–6 g/24 h) and its derivatives, and bile acid binding resins (cholestyramine and colestipol) have both been used wth successful reduction of cholesterol concentrations in nephrotic patients, but have severe and frequent side-effects which lead to poor compliance, and they are little used today.

Lipopheresis

In patients with FSGS, statin treatment associated with lipopheresis resulted in a prolonged reduction of LDL cholesterol. Reduction of LDL by 60–70 per cent was achieved which persisted following discontinuation of lipopheresis. The effect on protein excretion and serum albumin levels was not consistent in all treated patients, although some achieved remission of the NS (Brunton *et al.* 1999; Muso *et al.* 1999).

Protein wasting and protein intake

Many nephrotic patients become seriously wasted during the course of their illness (Fig. 1), presumably the result not only of protein losses, but also catabolism of much larger amounts of protein in the renal tubules. The optimal dietary protein intake for patients with a persisting NS remains controversial. Although recommended in the past, it has long been known that a high protein intake (>1.5 g/kg/24 h) leads to an increase in urinary protein excretion but without any increase in serum albumin or total plasma protein concentrations. In contrast, reduction in protein intake to 0.8 g/kg/24 h reduces proteinuria, although with controversial effects on serum albumin concentration (Mansy *et al.* 1989; Kaysen 1991) and a risk of protein malnutrition (Guarneiri *et al.* 1989). Therefore, a dietary protein intake of 0.8 g of protein of high biological value/kg/24 h, plus 1 g protein per gram of proteinuria, has been advocated widely in adults with the NS. In fact 0.8 g/kg/24 h represents an average protein intake in Europe, although less than American norms.

Alterations in carbohydrate metabolism in nephrotics

Unlike lipid metabolism, there appear to be no direct clinical consequences of the changes in carbohydrate metabolism in the NS (Bridgman *et al.* 1975; Loschiavo *et al.* 1983). Accelerated glycogenolysis, elevated resting insulin and impaired response to oral glucose loading with a diabetic-like plasma glucose curve have all been reported.

Loss of binding and transport proteins and hormones in the urine

A number of plasma proteins important in the transport of metals, hormones, and drugs are of relatively small molecular weight and thus are lost easily into the urine of nephrotic patients (Table 3). Free protein hormones, especially of low molecular weight, are also lost. These findings, however, although interesting, are usually of little clinical significance.

Metal-binding proteins

Low serum iron and losses of transferrin (molecular weight 87 kDa) and associated iron into the urine are features of NS (Brown *et al.* 1984). Transferrin turnovers show increased synthesis and degradation, presumably in renal tubules after reabsorption, and Prinsen *et al.* (2001) point to a failure of increased synthesis to replace the losses as the cause of the low plasma concentrations. True iron deficiency (Brown *et al.* 1984) is, however, rare since urinary losses of iron are at most 0.5–1.0 mg/24 h. In addition, the transferrin–iron complex binds to many proliferating cells, and the effects of transferrin depletion on immunity may not depend entirely upon zinc deficiency (Warshaw *et al.* 1984).

Table 3 Loss of binding proteins in urine in the nephrotic syndrome

Diagnostic technique	Authors	*n*	Total	Percentage
Doppler	Andrassay *et al.* (1980)	21	84	25
Clinical	Combined series[a]	12	191	6
	Llach (1982)	3	118	2.5
	Pohl *et al.* (1984)	3	59	5.5
	Cameron *et al.* (1988)[b]	11	90	12
Total		29	458	6

[a] Kanfer *et al.* (1970); Kendall *et al.* (1971); Thompson *et al.* (1974); Bernard *et al.* (1977); Kauffman *et al.* (1978). All these papers reported concentrations of coagulation factors in nephrotics.

[b] All minimum changes.

Caeruloplasmin has a molecular weight of 151 kDa is lost in the urine and its plasma concentration is low (Brown *et al.* 1984). Low red-cell and plasma copper concentrations heve been reported by some authors in nephrotic children (Štec *et al.* 1990) and rats (Pedraza-Chaverri *et al.* 1994), but no clinical consequences of these losses of copper have been found.

Zinc circulates bound mainly to albumin and also to transferrin, and zinc is reduced in plasma, hair, and white cells in NS (Reimold 1980; Štec *et al.* 1990) and in plasma in nephrotic rats (Pedraza-Chaverri *et al.* 1994). Increased synthesis of α_2-macroglobulin and its tight binding of zinc lower the biological availability of the metal (de Sain-van der Velden *et al.* 1998b). Hypogeusia may be found in nephrotics (Mahajan *et al.* 1982), and the possible effects in reducing cell-mediated immunity have been discussed above (Bensman *et al.* 1984; Warshaw *et al.* 1984).

Loss of vitamins and hormones in the urine

A number of abnormalities of calcium and vitamin D metabolism have been described, in part the result of losses of vitamin D binding protein (molecular weight 59 kDa) and its associated vitamin in the urine (Vaziri 1993; Harris and Ismail 1994). Bone biopsies are usually normal, although some may show osteomalacia and/or hyperparathyroidism (Mittal *et al.* 1999) but without symptoms, and vitamin D and/or calcium supplementation is not necessary (Mehls 1990). However, nephrotics with reduced renal function do more readily develop bone disease (Tessitore *et al.* 1984), and earlier treatment than usual with vitamin D may have a place in those evolving into uraemia.

Despite losses of thyroid-binding globulin (molecular weight 85 kDa) in the urine (Vaziri 1993) accompanied by bound T_3 and T_4, plasma concentrations of T_3, T_4, and TSH are usually normal in nephrotic patients, although the T_3 may be rather low and the T_4 raised with increased reverse T_3. In general, this is of no clinical significance, although cases of hypothyroidism remitting once proteinuria ceased have been reported (Fonseca *et al.* 1991) and hypothyroidism is a regular feature of the Finnish congential NS (Mattoo 1994).

Cortisol-binding protein (molecular weight 52 kDa) is lost in nephrotic urine and in one study (Musa *et al.* 1967) plasma concentration was reduced, but not in another (Loschiavo *et al.* 1983). More important is binding of prednisolone to albumin (see below).

Erythropoietin has a molecular weight of 33 kDa and is thus readily lost in the urine, in both health and in proteinuric patients (Vaziri *et al.* 1992). A number of nephrotic patients, both children and adults, suffering anaemia disproportionate to their renal function have been described, whose anaemia responded to epoetin administration (Feinstein *et al.* 2001).

Despite the large number of drugs normally bound in part to albumin, the gross reductions in serum albumin in nephrotics give rise to remarkably few problems (Gugler and Arzanoff 1976). Those concerning warfarin (Ganeval *et al.* 1986) have been discussed above. Prednisolone is normally bound to albumin, but despite this even severe hypoalbuminaemia doses of prednisolone are not modified either in nephrotic adults (Frey and Frey 1984) or children (Miller *et al.* 1990; Rostin *et al.* 1990), since the levels of free drug equilibrate rapidly to nearly normal concentrations. However, Miller *et al.* (1990) suggest that differential pharmacokinetics may account for differing profiles of toxicity, as in the Boston drug surveillance programme.

Renal effects of the nephrotic syndrome

Acute renal failure in nephrotic patients (Smith and Hayslett 1992)

Apparently 'idiopathic' acute renal failure is an occasional but important complication of NS, and can be distinguished from acute renal failure from identifiable causes such as interstitial nephritis, thrombosis, sepsis, or contrast media. About 100 such cases have been published (Koomans *et al.* 1992; Smith and Hayslett 1992) mostly in previous decades; it may be that this complication has become less common in recent years, but under-reporting is also possible.

This complication occurs mostly in older patients of either gender, overwhelmingly (81 per cent) in those with minimal change/FSGS histology, despite the overall preponderance of young children in the latter group. In such children, acute renal failure is, in contrast, very rare, and usually follows either sepsis or thrombosis (Cameron *et al.* 1988; Cavangnaro and Lagomarsino 2000). Most adult patients present already in acute renal failure; few develop it subsequent to diagnosis, or in relapse. One-sixth were judged to be seriously hypovolaemic or in shock, and all had a very low serum albumin. Urine volume is low, containing less than 5 mmol/l Na^+ and unresponsive to diuretics and/or volume repletion, loaded with protein, and containing red cells and often red cell casts. Thus, renal biopsy is almost always necessary to establish a diagnosis, as this pattern of sediment suggests a proliferative nephritis rather than minimal changes.

The role of hypovolaemia and reduced renal perfusion is not clear; in many patients the circulation was full or overfull and hypertension was common. In six childhood patients during relapse of the NS, we observed a decrease in GFR below 20 ml/min/1.73 m^2 associated with normal RPF and a significant decrease of FF, inversely correlated with vasoactive hormones (renin, noradrenaline) and positively correlated with plasma oncotic pressure. Following intravenous albumin infusion, in none of these patients did the FF increase. These data are in agreement with a severely reduced Kf as the cause of acute renal failure in patients with the NS (Vande Walle *et al.* 2004).

Moderate to severe tubular changes were present in the majority of reported cases, amounting to frank tubular necrosis in about one-fourth. Proteinaceous casts are an important feature in only a minority (Chamberlain *et al.* 1966; Venkataseshan *et al.* 1993). Interstitial oedema is usually present, perhaps indicating increased interstitial pressure (Lowenstein *et al.* 1970). Blood vessel changes are frequent, and have been thought by some to be important in the pathogenesis (Jennette and Falk 1990), but these may be the result of the age of the patients (see Chapter 1.5).

Management of these often elderly and severely ill patients is difficult. They continue to pass large amounts of protein in tiny amounts of urine, have very low serum albumin and sometimes unstable circulation, and are of course uraemic. If not already malnourished, they rapidly become so. Obviously, they require dialysis by some form of blood purification with gentle ultrafiltration and salt-free albumin infusions given cautiously to avoid pulmonary oedema. Supplementary intravenous nutrition may be required, with an obligation to filter large enough volumes to make this possible. Should they receive concomitant treatment with corticosteroids and/or cyclophosphamide? Clearly, the risks are high, but some authors have suggested that treatment in this fashion led to a diuresis, and it may help eliminate or reduce the proteinuria. Others have seen no benefit, and there is no clear answer to this question. Outcome is serious, with a mortality in published cases of 18 per cent, and another 20 per cent survive but never recover renal function. Recovery of renal function often takes several months rather than weeks. A few patients have gone on to have further relapses of their NS, but without renal failure in these episodes.

In nephrotic children, acute renal failure is very rare (Cameron *et al.* 1988; Cavagnaro and Lagomarsino 2000). In the majority of these few cases some other factor—major sepsis or thrombosis—was present. Recovery has been usual, although one of our patients lost both her legs as a result of associated aortic thrombosis, and was still relapsing 10 years later.

Renal tubular dysfunction in nephrotics

A Fanconi syndrome has been described in a small number of nephrotic patients. Some of these had reversible tubular defects dependent upon tubular damage from proteinuria (Shioji *et al.* 1974) but in most, the tubular defect arises from tubular damage as part of the underlying disease (Praga *et al.* 1991), and do worse than those without glycosuria/aminoaciduria. In children, this finding (Boissou *et al.* 1980; McVicar *et al.* 1980) or β_2-microglobulinuria (Portman *et al.* 1986) can help differentiate children with focal segmental glomerulosclerosis from those with only minimal change lesions.

Proteinuria and progression of renal failure

This topic is dealt with in Chapters 11.1 and 3.3, and above.

References

General articles

Bernard, D. B. (1988). Extrarenal complications of the nephrotic syndrome. (Nephrology Forum). *Kidney International* **33**, 1184–1202.

Cameron, J. S., Ogg, C. S., and Wass, V. J. Complications of the nephrotic syndrome. In *The Nephrotic Syndrome* (ed. J. S. Cameron and R. J. Glassock), pp. 849–920. New York: Marcel Dekker, 1988.

Kaysen, G. A., ed. (1993). The nephrotic syndrome: pathogenesis and consequences. *American Journal of Nephrology* **13**, 309–428.

Orth, S. R. and Ritz, E. (1998). The nephrotic syndrome. *New England Journal of Medicine* **38**, 1202–1211.

Bibliography

Abbate, M. *et al.* (1999). Nephrotoxicity of increased glomerular protein traffic. *Nephrology, Dialysis, Transplantation* **14**, 304–312.

Agarwal, R. *et al.* (2000). Urinary protein binding does not affect response to furosemide in patients with nephrotic syndrome. *Journal of the American Society of Nephrology* **11**, 1100–1105.

Akcicek, F. *et al.* (1995). Diuretic effect of frusemide in patients with nephrotic syndrome: is it potentiated by intravenous albumin? *British Medical Journal* **310**, 162–163.

Allon, M., Pasque, C. B., and Rodriguez, M. (1990). Acute effects of captopril and ibuprofen on proteinuria in patients with nephrosis. *Journal of Laboratory and Clinical Medicine* **116**, 462–468.

Alpay, H. *et al.* (2002). Varicella vaccination in children with steroid-sensitive nephrotic syndrome. *Pediatric Nephrology* **17**, 181–183.

Anderson, D. C. *et al.* (1979). Assessment of factor B, serum opsonins, granulocyte chemotaxis and infection in nephrotic syndrome of children. *Journal of Infectious Diseases* **140**, 1–11.

Andrassy, K., Ritz., E., and Bommer, J. (1980). Hypercoagulability in the nephrotic syndrome. *Klinische Wochenschrift* **58**, 1029–1036.

Andrew, M. and Brooker, L. A. (1996). Hemostatic complications in renal disorders of the young. *Pediatric Nephrology* **10**, 88–99.

Apostol, E. *et al.* (1997). Reduced renal medullary water channel expression in puromycin aminonucleoside—induced nephrotic syndrome. *Journal of the American Society of Nephrology* **8**, 15–24.

Appel, G. B. *et al.* (1976). Renal vein thrombosis, nephrotic syndrome and systemic lupus erythematosus. An association in four cases. *Annals of Internal Medicine* **85**, 310–317.

Appel, G. B. *et al.* (1985). The hyperlipidemia of the nephrotic syndrome. Relation to plasma albumin concentration, oncotic pressure and viscosity. *New England Journal of Medicine* **312**, 1544–1548.

Arisz, L. *et al.* (1976). The effect of indomethacin on proteinuria and kidney function in the nephrotic syndrome. *Acta Medica Scandinavica* **199**, 121–125.

Arneil, G. C. (1961). 164 children with nephrosis. *Lancet* **ii**, 1103–1110.

Attman, P. O., Alanpovic, P., and Samuelson, O. (1999). Lipoprotein abnormalities as a risk factor for progressive nondiabetic renal disease. *Kidney International* **56** (S71), 14–17.

Avasthi, P. S. *et al.* (1983). Noninvasive diagnosis of renal vein thrombosis by ultrasonic echo-Doppler flowmetry. *Kidney International* **23**, 882–887.

Bamelou, A. and Legrain, M. (1982). Medical nephrectomy with anti-inflammatory non-steroidal drugs. *British Medical Journal* **284**, 234.

Bang, N. U. *et al.* (1973). Enhanced platelet function in glomerular renal disease. *Journal of Laboratory and Clinical Medicine* **81**, 651–655.

Bellomo, R. and Atkins, R. C. (1993). Membranous nephropathy and thromboembolism: is prophylactic anticoagulation warranted? *Nephron* **63**, 249–254.

Bennett, A. and Cameron, J. S. (1987). Hyperaggregability of platelets to ristocetin in the nephrotic syndrome not dependent upon thromboxane production or serum albumin concentration. *Clinical Nephrology* **27**, 182–188.

Bensman, A. *et al.* (1984). Decreased biological activity of serum thymic hormone (thymulin) in children with nephrotic syndrome. *International Journal of Pediatric Nephrology* **5**, 201–204.

Berg, U. and Bohlin, A. B. (1982). Renal hemodynamics in minimal change nephrotic syndrome of childhood. *International Journal of Pediatric Nephrology* **3**, 187–192.

Bienz, N. *et al.* (1994). Bilateral nephrectomy for uncontrollable nephrotic syndrome in primary amyloidosis with subsequent improvement in hepatic function. *Clinical and Laboratory Haematology* **16**, 85–88.

Bohler, T. *et al.* (1992). Increased aggregation with normal surface charge and deformability of red blood cells in children with nephrotic syndrome. *Clinical Nephrology* **38**, 119–124.

Boissou, F., Barthe, F. L., and Pierragi, M. Th. (1980). Severe idiopathic nephrotic syndrome with tubular dysfunction (report of nine pediatric cases). *Clinical Nephrology* **14**, 135–141.

Boneu, B. *et al.* (1981). Comparison of progressive antithrombin activity and concentration of three thrombin inhibitors in nephrotic syndrome. *Thrombosis and Haemostasis* **46**, 623–625.

Brater, D. C. *et al.* (1984). Bumetamide and furosemide in heart failure. *Kidney International* **26**, 183–189.

Bridgman, J. F. *et al.* (1975). Insulin and growth hormone secretion in the nephrotic syndrome. *Quarterly Journal of Medicine* **44**, 115–123.

Briefel, G. R. *et al.* (1978). Recurrent renal vein thrombosis consequent to membranous glomerulonephritis. *Clinical Nephrology* **10**, 32–37.

Brown, E. A. *et al.* (1982). Sodium retention in nephrotic syndrome is due to an intrarenal defect: evidence from steroid induced remission. *Nephron* **39**, 290–295.

Brown, E. A. *et al.* (1984). Urinary iron loss in the nephrotic syndrome—an unusual case of iron deficiency with a note on the excretion of copper. *Postgraduate Medical Journal* **160**, 125–128.

Brunton, C., Varghese, Z., and Moorhead, J. (1999). Lipopheresis in the nephrotic syndrome. *Kidney International* **56** (S71), 6–90.

Burton, C. and Harris, K. P. G. (1996). The role of proteinuria in the progression of chronic renal failure. *American Journal of Kidney Diseases* **27**, 765–775.

Calcagno, P. L. and Rubin, M. I. (1961). Physiologic considerations concerning corticosteroid therapy and complications in the nephrotic syndrome. *Journal of Pediatrics* **58**, 686–706.

Cameron, J. S. (1984). Thromboembolic complications of the nephrotic syndrome. *Advances in Nephrology* **13**, 75–114.

Cameron, J. S. Platelets in renal disease. In *Platelets in Health and Disease* (ed. C. P. Page), pp. 228–260. Oxford: Blackwell, 1991.

Cameron, J. S. and Hicks, J. A. (2002). The origins and development of the concept of a Nephrotic Syndrome. *American Journal of Nephrology* **22**, 240–247.

Cameron, J. S., Ogg, C. S., and Wass, V. J. Complications of the nephrotic syndrome. In *The Nephrotic Syndrome* (ed. J. S. Cameron and R. J. Glassock), pp. 849–920. New York: Marcel Dekker, 1988.

Cavagnaro, F. and Lagomarsino, E. (2000). Peritonitis as a risk factor of acute renal failure in nephrotic children. *Pediatric Nephrology* **15**, 248–251.

Chalasani, N. *et al.* (2001). Effects of albumin/furosemide mistures on responses to furosemide in hypoalbuminemic patients. *Journal of the American Society of Nephrology* **12**, 1010–1016.

Chamberlain, M. J., Pringle, A., and Wrong, O. M. (1966). Oliguric renal failure in the nephrotic syndrome. *Quarterly Journal of Medicine* **35**, 215–235.

Chan, P. C. K. *et al.* (1992). Lovastatin in glomerulonephritis patients with hyperlipidaemia and heavy proteinuria. *Nephrology, Dialysis, Transplantation* **7**, 93–99.

Chandra, M., Hoyer, J. L., and Lewy, J. E. (1981). Renal function in rats with unilateral proteinuria produced by renal perfusion with aminonucleoside. *Pediatric Research* **15**, 340–344.

Choudhry, V. P. and Gai, D. P. (1977). Peritonitis in the nephrotic syndrome. *Indian Pediatrics* **14**, 405–408.

Chuang, T. F. *et al.* (1999). Spontaneous bacterial peritonitis as the presenting feature in an adult with nephrotic syndrome. *Nephrology, Dialysis, Transplantation* **14**, 181–182.

Citak, A. *et al.* (2000). Hemostatic problems and thromboembolic complications in nephrotic children. *Pediatric Nephrology* **14**, 138–142.

Clouse, L. H. and Comp, P. C. (1986). The regulation of hemostasis: the protein C system. *New England Journal of Medicine* **314**, 1298–1304.

Cohen, H. T. *et al.* (1988). Red-cell surface charge in patients with nephrotic syndrome. *Lancet* **i**, 1459 (letter).

Cohen, S. L. *et al.* (1980). The mechanism of hyperlipidaemia in nephrotic syndrome—role of low albumin and the LCAT reaction. *Clinica Chimica Acta* **104**, 393–400.

Corpier, C. L. *et al.* (1988). Rhabdomyolysis and renal injury with lovastatin use. Report of two cases in cardiac allograft recipients. *Journal of the American Medical Association* **260**, 239–241.

Cosio, F. G. *et al.* (1985). Plasma concentrations of the natural anticoagulants protein C and protein S in patients with proteinuria. *Journal of Laboratory and Clinical Medicine* **106**, 218–222.

D'Amico, G. and Gentile, M. G. (1991). Pharmacological and dietary treatment of lipid abnormalities in nephrotic patients. *Kidney International* **39**, (Suppl. 31), S65–S69.

Davis, R. A. *et al.* (1980). Very low density lipoprotein secretion by cultured rat hepatocytes: inhibition by albumin and other macromolecules. *Journal of Biological Chemistry* **255**, 2039–2045.

Davison, A. M. *et al.* (1974). Salt-poor human albumin in managment of nephrotic syndrome. *British Medical Journal* **i**, 481–484.

Deighan, C. *et al.* (2000). Patients with nephrotic range proteinuria have apolipoprotein C and E deficient VLDL1. *Kidney International* **58**, 1238–1246.

Deighan, C. J. *et al.* (1998). Increased atherogenicity of low-density lipoprotein in heavy proteinuria. *Nephrology, Dialysis, Transplantation* **13**, 1183–1188.

de Jong, P. E., Anderson, S., and de Zeeuw, D. (1992). Glomerular preload and afterload reduction as a tool to lower urinary protein leakage: will such treatments also help to improve renal function outcome? *Journal of the American Society of Nephrology* **3**, 1333–1341.

de Jong, P. E. *et al.* (1988). Is the antiproteinuric effect of dipyridamole hemodynamically mediated? *Nephron* **50**, 292–294.

de Sain-van der Velden, M. G. *et al.* (1998a). Evidence for increased synthesis of lipoprotein (a) in the nephrotic syndrome. *Journal of the American Society of Nephrology* **9**, 1474–1481.

de Sain-van der Velden, M. G. *et al.* (1998b). Plasma α_2 macroglobulin is increased in nephrotic patients as a result of increased synthesis alone. *Kidney International* **54**, 530–535.

Deschenes, D., Feraille, E., and Doucet, A. (2003). Mechanism of oedema in the nephrotic syndrome. Old theories and new ideas. *Nephrology, Dialysis, Transplantation* **18**, 454–456.

de Zeeuw, D. *et al.* (1990). Mechanism of the antiproteinuric effect of angiotensin converting enzyme inhibition. *Contributions to Nephrology* **83**, 160–165.

Dogra, G. K., Watts, G. F., Hermann, S., Thomas, M. A. B., and Irish, A. B. (2002). Statin therapy improves brachial artery endothelial function in nephrotic syndrome. *Kidney International* **62**, 550–557.

Donckerwolcke, R. A. M. G. *et al.* (2003). Distal nephron sodium-potassium exchange in children with nephrotic syndrome. *Clinical Nephrology* **59**, 259–266.

Dönmez, O. *et al.* (2001). Inferior vena cava indices determine volume load in minimal lesion nephrotic syndrome. *Pediatric Nephrology* **16**, 251–255.

Dorhout Mees, E. J. (1996). Does it make sense to administer albumin to the patient with nephrotic oedema? *Nephrology, Dialysis, Transplantation* **11**, 1224–1226.

Dorhout Mees, E. J. *et al.* (1979). Observations on edema formation in the nephrotic syndrome in adults with minimal lesions. *American Journal of Medicine* **67**, 378–384.

Doucet, C. *et al.* (2000). Lipoprotein(a) in the nephrotic syndrome: molecular analysis of lipoprotein(a) and apolipoprotein(a) fragments in plasma and urine. *Journal of the American Society of Nephrology* **11**, 507–513.

Du, X. H. *et al.* (1985). Nephrotic syndrome with renal vein thrombosis: pathogenic importance of plasmin inhibitor (alpha-2-antiplasmin). *Clinical Nephrology* **24**, 186–191.

Egli, F. (1974). *Thromboembolism beim nephrotischer Syndrom in Kindesalter.* Thesis, University of Basel.

Egli, F., Eimiger, P., and Stalder, G. (1973). Thromboembolism in the nephrotic syndrome. *Pediatric Research* **8**, 803 (abstract).

Elidrissy, A. T. H. (1982). Primary peritonitis and meningitis in nephrotic syndrome in Riyadh. *International Journal of Pediatric Nephrology* **3**, 9–12.

Elidrissy, A. T. H. *et al.* (1991). Haemostatic measurements in childhood nephrotic syndrome. *European Journal of Pediatrics* **150**, 374–378.

Fadnes, H. O. (1975). Protein concentration and hydrostatic pressure insubcutaneous tissue of rats in hpoproteinemia. *Scandinavian Journal of Clinical and Laboratory Investigation* **35**, 441–446.

Fauchald, P., Noddeland, H., and Norseth, J. (1985). An evaluation of ultrafiltration as treatment for diuretic-resistent oedema in nephrotic syndrome. *Acta Medica Scandinavica* **17**, 127–131.

Feinstein, S. *et al.* (2001). Erythropoietin deficiency causes anemia in nephrotic children with normal renal function. *American Journal of Kidney Diseases* **37**, 736–742.

Fernandez-Llama, P. *et al.* (1998). Concentrating defect in experimental nephrotic syndrome. Altered expression of aquaporins and thick ascending limb Na+ transporters. *Kidney International* **54**, 170–179.

Fliser, D. *et al.* (1999). Co-administration of albumin and furosemide in patients with the nephrotic syndrome. *Kidney International* **55**, 629–634.

Fonseca, V., Thomas, M., and Sweny, P. (1991). Can urinary thyroid loss cause hypothyroidism? *Lancet* **338**, 475–476.

Frey, F. J. and Frey, B. M. (1984). Altered plasma protein-binding of prednisolone in patients with the nephrotic syndrome. *American Journal of Kidney Diseases* **3**, 339–348.

Fried, L. P., Orchard, T. J., and Kasiske, B. L. (2001). For the lipids and renal disease progression meta analysis study group. Effect of lipid reduction on the progression of renal disease: a meta analysis. *Kidney International* **59**, 260–269.

Futrakul, P. (1978). Primary peritonitis syndrome: a state of hypercoagulability in the nephrotic syndrome. *Journal of the Medical Association of Thailand* **61**, 268–273.

Ganeval, D. *et al.* (1986). Pharmacokinetics of warfarin in the nephrotic syndrome and effect on vitamin K dependent clotting factors. *Clinical Nephrology* **25**, 75–80.

Gansevoort, R. T. *et al.* (1994). Symptomatic antiproteinuric treatment decreases serum lipoprotein(a) concentration in patients with glomerular proteinuria. *Nephrology, Dialysis, Transplantation* **9**, 244–250.

Gansevoort, R. T. *et al.* (1995a). Antiproteinuric affect of blood-pressure-lowering agents: a meta-analysis of comparative trials. *Nephrology, Dialysis, Transplantation* **10**, 1963–1974.

Gansevoort, R. T., de Zeeuw, D., and de Jong, P. E. (1995b). Additive antiproteinuric effect of ACE inhibition and a low-protein diet in human renal disease. *Nephrology, Dialysis, Transplantation* **10**, 497–504.

Geers, A. B. *et al.* (1984). Functional relationships in the nephrotic syndrome. *Kidney International* **26**, 324–330.

Giangiacomo, J. *et al.* (1975). Serum immunoglobulins in the nephrotic syndrome. *New England Journal of Medicine* **293**, 8–12.

Giebink, G. S. (2001). The prevention of pneumococcal disease in children. *New England Journal of Medicine* **345**, 1177–1183.

Gitlin, D. *et al.* (1958). Studies on the metabolism of plasma proteins in the nephrotic syndrome. II The lipoproteins. *Journal of Clinical Investigation* **37**, 172–184.

Glass, F., Lippton, H., and Kadowitz, P. J. (1981). Effects of methylprednisolone and hydrocortisone on aggregation of rabbit platelets induced by arachidonic acid and other aggregating substances. *Thrombosis and Haemostasis* **46**, 676–679.

Golbetz, H. *et al.* (1989). Mechanism of the antiproteinuric effect of indomethacin in nephrotic humans. *American Journal of Physiology* **25**, F44–F51.

Golden, M. H. *et al.* (1990). Effacement of glomerular foot processes in kwashiorkor. *Lancet* **336**, 1472–1474.

Gorensek, M. J., Lebel, M. H., and Nelson, J. D. (1988). Peritonitis in children with nephrotic syndrome. *Pediatrics* **81**, 849–856.

Gouault-Heilmann, M. *et al.* (1988). Total and free protein S in nephrotic syndrome. *Thrombosis Research* **49**, 37–42.

Grausz, H., Lieberman, R., and Earley, L. E. (1972). Effect of plasma albumin and sodium reabsorption in patients with the nephrotic syndrome. *Kidney International* **1**, 47–54.

Groggel, G. C. *et al.* (1989). Treatment of nephrotic hyperlipoproteinemia with gemfibrozil. *Kidney International* **36**, 266–271.

Guarneiri, G. F. *et al.* (1989). Nutritional status in patients on long-term low-protein diet or with nephrotic syndrome. *Kidney International* **36** (Suppl. 27), S195–S200.

Gugler, R. and Azarnoff, D. L. (1976). Drug protein binding and the nephrotic syndrome. *Clinical Pharmacokinetics* **1**, 25–35.

Gulati, S. *et al.* (1997). Tuberculosis in childhood nephrotic syndrome in India. *Pediatric Nephrology* **11**, 695–698.

Güven, A. G., Akman, S., Bahat, E., Senyurt, M., Yüzbey, S., Uguz, A., and Yegin, O. (2004). Rapid decline of anti-pneumococcal antibody levels in nephrotic children. *Pediatric Nephrology* **19**, 61–65.

Handley, D. A. and Lawrence, J. R. (1967). Factor IX deficiency in the nephrotic syndrome. *Lancet* **i**, 1079–1081.

Harris, R. C. and Ismail, N. (1994). Extra renal complications of the nephrotic syndrome. *American Journal of Kidney Diseases* **23**, 477–497.

Harris, K. P. *et al.* (1990). Lovastatin ameliorates the development of glomerulosclerosis and uraemia in experimental nephrotic syndrome. *American Journal of Kidney Diseases* **15**, 16–23.

Haws, R. M. and Baum, M. (1993). Efficacy of albumin and diuretic therapy in children with nephrotic syndrome. *Pediatrics* **91**, 1142–1146.

Heeg, J. E., de Jong, P. E., and de Zeeuw, D. (1991). Additive antiproteinuric effect of angiotensin-converting enzyme inhibition and non-steroidal anti-inflammatory drug therapy: a clue to the mechanism of action. *Clinical Science* **81**, 367–372.

Heeg, J. E. *et al.* (1989). Efficacy and variability of the antiproteinuric effect of ACE inhibition by lisinopril. *Kidney International* **36**, 272–279.

Hopp, L. *et al.* (1994). Acute myocardial infarction in a young boy with nephrotic syndrome: a case report and review of the literature. *Pediatric Nephrology* **8**, 290–294.

Hoyer, P. F. *et al.* (1986). Thromboembolic complications in children with nephrotic syndrome. *Acta Paediatrica Scandinavica* **75**, 804–810.

Hunsicker, L. G. *et al.* (1997). Predictors of the progression of renal disease in the modification of diet in renal disease study. *Kidney International* **51**, 1908–1919.

Ichikawa, J. *et al.* (1983). Role of intrarenal mechanism in the impaired salt excretion of experimental nephrotic syndrome. *Journal of Clinical Investigation* **71**, 91–103.

Iida, H. *et al.* (1987). Effect of probucol on hyperlipidemia in patients with nephrotic syndrome. *Nephron* **47**, 280–283.

Inoue, M., Okagima, K., and Itoh, K. (1987). Mechanism of furosemide resistance in albuminemic rats and hypoalbuminemic patients. *Kidney International* **32**, 198–202.

International Study of Kidney Disease in Children (1984). Minimal change nephrotic syndrome in children: deaths occurring during the first five to fifteen years. *Pediatrics* **73**, 497–501.

Irish, A. B. (1997). The factor V Leiden mutation and risk of thrombosis in the nephrotic syndrome. *Nephrology, Dialysis, Transplantation* **12**, 1680–1683.

Israeli, A. *et al.* (1989). Lovastatin and elevated creatine kinase: results of rechallenge. *Lancet* **i**, 725.

Jackson, C. A. *et al.* (1982). Relationship between platelet aggregation, thromboxane synthesis and albumin concentration in nephrotic syndrome. *British Journal of Haematology* **52**, 69–77.

Jafar, T. H. *et al.* (2001). Proteinuria as a modifiable risk factor for the progression of non-diabteic renal disease. *Kidney International* **60**, 1131–1140.

Janeway, C. A. *et al.* (1948). Diuresis in children with nephrosis. Comparison of response to injection of normal human serum albumin and to infection, particularly measles. *Transactions of the Association of American Physicians* **61**, 108–111.

Jennette, J. C. and Falk, R. J. (1990). Adult minimal change glomerulopathy with acute renal failure. *American Journal of Kidney Diseases* **16**, 432–437.

Joles, J. A. *et al.* (1993). Plasma volume regulation: defences against edema formation (with special emphasis on hypoproteinemia). *American Journal of Nephrology* **13**, 399–412.

Joles, J. A. *et al.* (1994). Lipoprotein phospholipid composition and LCAT activity in nephrotic and analbuminemic rats. *Kidney International* **46**, 97–104.

Jones, C. L. and Hébert, D. (1991). Pulmonary thrombo-embolism in the nephrotic syndrome. *Pediatric Nephrology* **5**, 56–58.

Joven, J., Villabona, C., and Vilella, E. (1993). Pattern of hyperlipoproteinemia in human nephrotic syndrome: influence of renal failure and diabetes. *Nephron* **64**, 565–569.

Joven, J. *et al.* (1987). High density lipoproteins in untreated nephrotic syndrome without renal failure. *Nephrology, Dialysis, Transplantation* **2**, 149–153.

Kallen, R. J. *et al.* (1977). Premature coronary atherosclerosis in a 5-year old with corticosteroid-refractory nephrotic syndrome. *American Journal of Diseases in Children* **131**, 976–980.

Kan, K. *et al.* (1974). Dipyridamole for protein suppression. *Journal of the American Medical Association* **229**, 557–558.

Kanfer, A. (1990). Coagulation factors in the nephrotic syndrome. *American Journal of Nephrology* **10** (Suppl. 1), 63–68.

Kanfer, A. (1994). Prophylactic anticoagulation for renal vein thromosis. *Journal of Nephrology* **7**, 251–253.

Kanfer, A. *et al.* (1970). Coagulation studies in 45 cases of nephrotic syndrome without uremia. *Thrombosis Diathesis Haemorrhagica* **24**, 562–571.

Kant, S. K. *et al.* (1981). Glomerular thrombosis in systemic lupus erythematosus: prevalence and significance. *Medicine (Baltimore)* **60**, 71–86.

Kashyap, H. L. *et al.* (1980). Apolipoprotein CII and lipoprotein lipase in human nephrotic syndrome. *Atherosclerosis* **35**, 29–40.

Kasiske, B. (1998). Hyperlipidemia in patients with chronic renal disease. *American Journal of Kidney Diseases* **32S**, 142–156.

Kassirer, J. P. Thrombosis and embolism of the renal vessels. In *Strauss and Welt's Diseases of the Kidney* (ed. L. E. Earley and C. W. Gottschalk), pp. 1385–1402. Boston: Little Brown, 1979.

Kauffmann, R. H. *et al.* (1978). Acquired antithrombin III deficiency and thrombosis in the nephrotic syndrome. *American Journal of Medicine* **65**, 607–613.

Kaysen, G. A. (1991). Hyperlipidemia of the nephrotic syndrome. *Kidney International* **39** (Suppl. 31), S8–S15.

Kaysen, G. A. (1992). Nephrotic hyperlipidemia: primary abnormalities in both lipoprotein catabolism and synthesis. *Mineral and Electrolyte Metabolism* **18**, 212–216.

Kaysen, G. A. and Al Bander, H. (1990). Metabolism of albumin and immunoglobulins in the nephrotic syndrome. *American Journal of Nephrology* **10** (Suppl. 1), 36–42.

Kaysen, G. A. and de Sain-van der Velden, M. (1999). New insights in the nephrotic syndrome. *Kidney International* **S71**, 18–21.

Keane, W. F., St Peter, J. V., and Kasiske, B. L. (1992). In the aggressive management of hyperlipidemia in nephrotic patients mandatory? *Kidney International* **42** (Suppl. 38), S134–S141.

Keilani, T. *et al.* (1993). Improvement of lipid abnormalities associated with proteinuria using fosinopril, and angiotensin-converting enzyme inhibitor. *Annals of Internal Medicine* **118**, 246–254.

Keller, E., Hoppe-Seyler, G., and Schollmeyer, P. (1982). Disposition and diuretic effect of furosemide in the nephrotic syndrome. *Clinical Pharmacology and Therapeutics* **32**, 442–449.

Kennedy, J. S. *et al.* (1991). Simultaneous renal arterial and venous thrombosis in the nephrotic syndrome: treatment with intra-arterial urokinase. *American Journal of Medicine* **90**, 124–127.

Kim, M. S., Primack, W., and Harmon W.E. (1992). Congenital nephrotic syndrome: pre-emptive bilateral nephrectomy and dialysis before renal transplantation. *Journal of the American Society of Nephrology* **3**, 260–263.

Kirschner, K. A., Voelker, J. R., and Brater, D. C. (1990). Intratubular albumin blunts the response to furosemide. *Journal of Pharmacology and Experimental Therapeutics* **252**, 1097–1101.

Kirschner, K. A., Voelker, J. R., and Brater, D. C. (1992). Tubular resistance to furosemide contributes to the attenuated diuretic response in nephrotic rats. *Journal of the American Society of Nephrology* **2**, 1201–1207.

Koomans, H. A., Boer, W. H., and Dorhout Mees, E. J. (1987). Renal function during recovery from minimal lesion nephrotic syndrome. *Nephron* **47**, 173–178.

Koomans, H. A., Hené, R. J., and Dorhout Mees, E. J. Acute renal failure complicating nephrotic syndrome. In *Oxford Textbook of Clinical Nephrology* 1st edn. (ed. J. S. Cameron, A. M. Davison, J.-P. Grünfeld, D. N. S. Kerr, and E. Ritz), pp. 1034–1040. London: Oxford University Press, 1992.

Koomans, H. A. *et al.* (1985). Lowered plasma protein content of tissue fluid in patients with the nephrotic syndrome: observations during disease and recovery. *Nephron* **40**, 391–395.

Krämer, B. K., Schweda, F., and Riegger, G. (1999). Diuretic treatment and diuretic resistance in heart failure. *American Journal of Medicine* **106**, 90–96.

Krensky, A. M., Ingelfinger, J. M., and Grupe, W. E. (1982). Peritonitis in childhood nephrotic syndrome. *American Journal of Diseases of Children* **136**, 732–736.

Kugiyama, K. *et al.* (1990). Impairment of endothelium-dependent arterial relaxation by lysolecithin-modified low-density lipoproteins. *Nature* **344**, 160–162.

Kumugai, H. *et al.* (1985). Role of renin angiotensin aldosterone on minimal change nephrotic syndrome. *Clinical Nephrology* **23**, 229–235.

Kurokawa, K. (1999). Effects of candesartan on the proteinuria of chronic glomerulonephritis. *Journal of Human Hypertension* **13** (Suppl. 1), s57–s60.

Latta, K., vom Schnakenburg, C., and Ehrich, J. H. H. (2001). A meta-analysis of cytotoxic treatment for frequently relapsing nephrotic syndrome in children. *Pediatric Nephrology* **16**, 271–282.

Laverman, G. D., Navins, G., Henning, R. G., de Jong, P. E., and de Zeeuw, D. (2002). Dual renin angiotensin system blockade at optimal doses for proteinuria **62**, 1020–1025.

Laville, M. *et al.* (1988). The prognosis of renal vein thrombosis: a re-evaluation of 27 cases. *Nephrology, Dialysis, Transplantation* **3**, 247–256.

Levin M. *et al.* (1985). Steroid-responsive nephrotic syndrome: a generalised disorder of membrane negative charge. *Lancet* **ii**, 239–242.

Levy, E. *et al.* (1990). Experimental nephrotic syndrome: removal and tissue distribution of chylomicrons and very low density lipoproteins of normal and nephrotic origin. *Biochimica Biophysica Acta* **1043**, 259–266.

Liaño, F. *et al.* (1988). Allograft membranous glomerulonephritis and renal-vein thrombosis in a patient with a lupus anticoagulant factor. *Nephrology, Dialysis, Transplantation* **3**, 684–689.

Lilova, M. I., Velkovski, I. G., and Topalov, I. B. (2000). Thromboembolic complications in children with nephrotic syndrome in Bulgaria. *Pediatric Nephrology* **15**, 74–78.

Llach, F. Nephrotic syndrome: hypercoagulability, renal vein thrombosis and other thromboembolic complications. In *The Nephrotic Syndrome* (ed. B. M. Brenner and J. H. Stein), pp. 121–144. New York: Churchill-Livingstone, 1982.

Llach, F. (1985). Hypercoagulability, renal vein thrombosis, and other thrombotic complications of nephrotic syndrome (Nephrology Forum). *Kidney International* **28**, 429–439.

Loschiavo, C. *et al.* (1983). Carbohydrate metabolism in patients with nephrotic syndrome and normal renal function. *Nephron* **33**, 257–261.

Löwenborg, E. K. M. and Berg U. (1999). Influence of albumin on renal function in nephrotic syndrome. *Pediatric Nephrology* **16**, 251–255.

Lowenstein, J., Schacht, R. G., and Baldwin, D. S. (1970). Renal failure in minimal change nephrotic syndrome. *American Journal of Medicine* **70**, 227–233.

Lye, W.-C. and Tan, C.-C. (1991). Multiple arterial thromboses in nephrotic syndrome. *Nephrology, Dialysis, Transplantation* **6**, 55–56.

Mahajan, S. *et al.* (1982). Zinc metabolism in nephrotic syndrome. *Kidney International* **23**, 129 (abstract).

Mansy, H. *et al.* (1989). Effect of a high protein diet in patients with the nephrotic syndrome. *Clinical Science* **77**, 445–451.

Massy, Z. A., Ma, J. Z., Louis, T. A., and Kasiske, B. L. (1995). Lipid lowering therapy in patients with renal disease. *Kidney International* **48**, 188–198.

Matsell, D. G. and Wyatt, R. J. (1993). The role of I and B in peritonitis associated with nephrotic syndrome of children. *Pediatric Research* **34**, 84–88.

Mattoo, T. K. (1994). Hypothyroidism in infants with nephrotic syndrome. *Pediatric Nephrology* **8**, 657–659.

Mattoo, T. K. *et al.* (1992). Nephrotic syndrome in the first year of life and the role of unilateral nephrectomy. *Pediatric Nephrology* **6**, 16–18.

McLean, R. H. *et al.* (1977). Decreased serum factor B concentration associated with decreased opsonisation of *Escherichia coli* in the nephrotic syndrome. *Pediatric Research* **11**, 910–916.

McVicar, M., Exeni, R., and Susin, M. (1980). Nephrotic syndrome and multiple tubular defects in children; an early sign of focal glomerulosclerosis. *Journal of Pediatrics* **87**, 918–922.

Mehls, O. (1990). Ask the expert: is it correct to supplement patients with nephrotic syndrome with vitamin D and calcium? *Pediatric Nephrology* **4**, 519.

Mehls, O. *et al.* (1987). Hemostasis and thromboembolism in children with nephrotic syndrome: differences from adults. *Journal of Pediatrics* **110**, 862–867.

Menczel, J. and Dreyfuss, F. (1960). Effect of prednisone on blood coagulation time in patients on dicoumarol therapy. *Journal of Laboratory and Clinical Medicine* **56**, 14–20.

Michielsen, P. *et al.* Indomethacin treatment of membranoproliferative glomerulonephritis. In *Glomerulonephritis* Vol. I (ed. P. Kincaid-Smith, T. H. Mathew, and E. L. Becker), p. 611. New York: John Wiley, 1973.

Miller, P. F. W. *et al.* (1990). Pharmacokinetics of prednisolone in children with nephrosis. *Archives of Disease in Childhood* **65**, 196–200.

Mittal, S. K. *et al.* (1999). Bone histology in patients with nephrotic syndrome and normal renal function. *Kidney International* **55**, 1912–1919.

Moore, D. H. *et al.* (1980). Recurrent pneumococcal sepsis and defective opsonisation after pneumococcal polysaccaride vaccine in a child with nephrotic syndrome. *Journal of Pediatrics* **96**, 882–885.

Musa, B. J., Seal, U. S., and Doe, R. P. (1967). Excretion of corticosteroid binding globulin, thyroxine binding globulin and total protein in adult males with nephrosis. Effect of sex hormone. *Journal of Clinical Endocrinology* **27**, 768–774.

Muso, E. *et al.* (1999). Low density lipoprotein apheresis therapy for steroid resistant nephrotic syndrome. *Kidney International* **56** (S71), 122–125.

Myers, B. D. and Guasch, A. (1993). Selectivity of the glomerular filtration barrier in healthy and nephrotic humans. *American Journal of Nephrology* **13**, 311–317.

Nelson, D. C. and Birchmore, D. A. (1979). Renal vein thrombosis associated with nephrotic syndrome and gold therapy in rheumatoid arthritis. *Southern Medical Journal* **72**, 1616–1618.

Neugarten, J. and Schlondorff, D. (1991). Lipoprotein interactions with glomerular cell and matrix. *Contemporary Issues Nephrology* **24**, 173–206.

Nikkilä, E. A. and Pykäpistö, O. (1968). Regulation of adipose tissue lipoprotein lipase synthesis by intracellular free fatty acid. *Life Sciences* **7**, 1303–1309.

Noel, L. H. *et al.* (1979). Long term prognosis of idiopathic membranous glomerulonephritis: study of 116 untreated patients. *American Journal of Medicine* **66**, 82–90.

O'Donnell, M. P. (2001). Mechanisms and clinical importance of hypertriglyceridemia in the nephrotic syndrome. *Kidney International* **59**, 380–382.

Olbricht, C. J. and Koch, K. M. (1992). Treatment of hyperlipidemia in nephrotic syndrome: time for a change? *Nephron* **62**, 125–129.

Olbricht, C. *et al.* **(for the Simvastatin in Nephrotic Syndrome Study Group)** (1999). Simvastatin in nephrotic syndrome. *Kidney International* **56** (S71), S113–S116.

Olivero, J. J., Frommer, J. P., and Gonzalez, J. M. (1993). Medical nephrectomy: the last resort for intractable complications of the nephrotic syndrome. *American Journal of Kidney Diseases* **21**, 260–263.

Ordoñez, J. D. *et al.* (1993). The increased risk of coronary heart disease associated with nephrotic syndrome. *Kidney International* **44**, 638–642.

O'Regan, S., Mongeau, J., and Robitaille, P. (1980). Primary peritonitis in the nephrotic syndrome. *International Journal of Pediatric Nephrology* **1**, 216–217.

Ozsosylu, S., Strauss, H. S., and Diamond, L. K. (1962). Effects of corticosteroids on coagulation of the blood. *Nature* **195**, 1214–1215.

Pabinger, I. *et al.* (1994). The risk of thromboembolism in asymptomatic patients with protein C and protein S deficiency: a prospective cohort study. *Thrombosis and Haemostasis* **71**, 441–445.

Palmer, B. and Alpern, R. (1997). Pathogenesis of edema formation in the nephrotic syndrome. *Kidney International* **59**, 21–27.

Pedraza-Chaverri, J. *et al.* (1994). Copper and zinc metablism in aminonucleoside-induced nephrotic syndrome. *Nephron* **66**, 87–92.

Perico, N. and Remuzzi, G. (1993). Edema of the nephrotic syndrome: the role of the atrial peptide system. *American Journal of Kidney Diseases* **22**, 355–366.

Petiti, D. B., Strom, B. L., and Melmon, K. L. (1986). Duration of warfarin anticoagulant therapy and the probabilities of recurrent thromboembolism and haemorrhage. *American Journal of Medicine* **81**, 255–259.

Pichette, V., Geadah, D., and de Souich, P. (1996). The influence of moderate hypoalbuminemia on the renal metabolism and dynamics of furosemide in the rabbit. *British Journal of Pharmacology* **119**, 885–890.

Piette, J.-C. (1994). Prevention of recurrent thrombosis in the antiphospholipid syndrome. *Lupus* **3**, 73–74.

Pohl, M. A. *et al.* (1984). Renal vein thrombosis in membranous and membranoproliferative glomerulonephritis. *IXth Congress of the International Society of Nephrology*. Los Angeles. p. 119A (abstracts).

Portman, R. J., Kissane, J. M., and Robson, A. M. (1986). Use of β-microglobulin to diagnose tubulo-interstitial lesions in children. *Kidney International* **30**, 91–98.

Praga, M. *et al.* (1991). Tubular dysfunction in nephrotic syndrome: incidence and prognostic implications. *Nephrology, Dialysis, Trasnplantation* **6**, 683–688.

Preissner, K. T. (1990). Biological relevance of the protein C system and laboratory diagnosis of protein C and protein S deficiencies. *Clinical Science* **78**, 351–364.

Primack, W. A. *et al.* (1979). Failure of pneumococcal vaccine to prevent *Streptococcus pneumoniae* sepsis in nephrotic children. *Lancet* **ii**, 1192.

Prinsen, B. H. C. M. T. *et al.* (2001). Transferrin synthesis is increased in nephrotic patients insufficiently to replace urinary losses. *Kidney International* **12**, 1017–1025.

Querfeld, U. (1999). Should hyperlipidemia in children with the nephrotic syndrome be treated? *Pediatric Nephrology* **13**, 77–84.

Querfeld, U. *et al.* (1999). Probucol for treatment of hyperlipidemia in persistent nephrotic syndrome. Report of a prospective uncontrolled multicenter study. *Pediatric Nephrology* **13**, 7–12.

Rabelink, A. J. *et al.* (1988). Effects of simvastatin and cholestyramine on lipoprotein profile in hyperlipidaemia of nephrotic syndrome. *Lancet* **ii**, 1335–1338.

Rabelink, T. J., Bijlsma, J. A., and Koomans, H. A. (1993). Isooncotic volume expansion in the nephrotic syndrome. *Clinical Science* **84**, 627–632.

Rabelink, T. J. *et al.* (1994). Thrombosis and hemostasis in renal disease. *Kidney International* **46**, 287–296.

Rasher, W., Tulassay, T., and Seyberth, H. W. (1986). Diuretic and hormonal response to head-out water immersion in nephrotic syndrome. *Journal of Pediatrics* **109**, 609–614.

Reimold, E. W. (1980). Changes in zinc metabolism during the course of the nephrotic syndrome. *American Journal of Diseases of Children* **134**, 46–50.

Remuzzi, G. *et al.* (1979). Platelet hyperaggregability and the nephrotic syndrome. *Thrombosis Research* **16**, 345–354.

Rieu, P. *et al.* (1994). Medical nephrectomy with CsA and angiotensin II in a case of life-threatening membranous glomerulonephritis. *Nephrology, Dialysis, Transplantation* **9**, 83–84.

Rostin, M. *et al.* (1990). Pharmacokinetics of prednisolone in children with the nephrotic syndrome. *Pediatric Nephrology* **4**, 470–473.

Rostoker, G. *et al.* (1987). High level of protein C and S in nephrotic syndrome. *Nephron* **46**, 20–21.

Rostoker, G. *et al.* (1992). Asymptomatic renal-vein thrombosis in adult nephrotic syndrome. Ultrasonography and urinary fibrin–fibrinogen degradation products: a prospective study. *European Journal of Medicine* **1**, 19–22.

Ruilope, L. M. *et al.* (1992). Additive antiproteinuric affect of converting enzyme inhibition and a low protein intake. *Journal of the American Society of Nephrology* **3**, 1307–1311.

Russo, D. *et al.* (2001). Coadministration of losartan and enalapril exerts additive antiproteinuric effect in IgA nephropathy. *American Journal of Kidney Diseases* **38**, 18–25 (see also editorial comment *ibid.* 182–185).

Rusthoven, J. and Kabins, S. A. (1978). Hemophilus influenzae cellulitis with bacteremia, peritonitis and pleuritis in an adult with the nephrotic syndrome. *Southern Medical Journal* **71**, 1433–1435.

Rydzewski, A., Mysilwiec, M., and Soszka, J. (1986). Concentration of three thrombin inhibitors in the nephrotic syndrome in adults. *Nephron* **42**, 200–203.

Samuelson, O., Mulec, H., and Knight-Gibson, C. (1997). Lipoprotein abnormalities are associated with increased rate of progression of human chronic renal insufficiency. *Nephrology, Dialysis, Transplantation* **12**, 1908–1915.

Samuelson, O. *et al.* (1998). Flustatin reduce both cholesterol rich and triglyceride-rich apo-containing lipoproteins in patients with renal dyslipidemia. *70th European Atherosclerosis Society Congress* (abstract).

Sarasin, F. P. and Schifferli, J. A. (1994). Prophylactic oral anticoagulation in nephrotic patients with idiopathic membranous nephropathy. *Kidney International* **45**, 578–585.

Schiepatti, A. *et al.* (1984). The metabolism of arachidonic acid by platelets in the nephrotic syndrome. *Kidney International* **25**, 671–676.

Schrier, R. and Fassett, R. (1998). A critique of the overfill hypothesis of sodium and water retention in the nephrotic syndrome. *Kidney International* **53**, 1111–1117.

Schulze, G. *et al.* (1980). Gastointestinal protein loss in the nephrotic syndrome studied with ^{51}Cr albumin. *Nephron* **25**, 227–230.

Shapiro, M. D. *et al.* (1986). Role of glomerular filtration rate in the impaired sodium and water excretion of patients with the nephrotic syndrome. *American Journal of Kidney Diseases* **8**, 81–87.

Shapiro, M. D. *et al.* (1990). Role of aldosterone in the sodium retention of patients with the nephrotic syndrome. *American Journal of Nephrology* **10**, 44–48.

Shearer, G. C. *et al.* (2001). Hypoalbuminemia and proteinuria contribute separately to reduced lipoprotein catabolism in the nephrotic syndrome. *Kidney International* **59**, 179–189.

Shioji, R. *et al.* (1974). Reversible tubular dysfunction associated with chronic renal failure in an adult patient with the nephrotic syndrome. *Clinical Nephrology* **2**, 76–80.

Short, C. D. *et al.* (1986). Serum and urinary high density lipoproteins in glomerular disease with proteinuria. *Kidney International* **29**, 1224–1228.

Sié, P. *et al.* (1988). Plasma levels of plasma co-factor II in nephrotic syndrome of children. *Nephron* **48**, 175–176.

Sillix, D. *et al.* (1983). Impaired granulocyte function in the nephrotic syndrome. *Kidney International* **23**, 135 (abstract).

Smith, J. D. and Hayslett, J. P. (1992). Reversible renal failure in the nephrotic syndrome. *American Journal of Kidney Diseases* **19**, 201–203.

Speck, W. T., Dresdale, S. S., and McMillan, R. W. (1974). Primary peritonitis and the nephrotic syndrome. *American Journal of Surgery* **127**, 267–269.

Spika, J. S. *et al.* (1986). Decline of vaccine-induced antipneumococcal antibody in children with nephrotic syndrome. *American Journal of Kidney Diseases* **7**, 466–470.

Štec, J. *et al.* (1990). Zinc and copper metabolism in nephrotic syndrome. *Nephron* **56**, 186–187.

Stenvinkel, P. *et al.* (1993). Lipoprotein(a) in nephrotic syndrome. *Kidney International* **44**, 1116–1123.

Stroes, E. S. G. *et al.* (1995). Impaired endothelial function in patients with nephrotic range proteinuria. *Kidney International* **48**, 544–550.

Svensson, P. J. and Dahlbäck, B. (1994). Resistance to activated protein C as a basis for venous thrombosis. *New England Journal of Medicine* **330**, 517–522.

Tain, Y.-L., Lin, G.-J., and Cher, T.-W. (1999). Microbiological spectrum of septicemia and peritonitis in nephrotic children. *Pediatric Nephrology* **13**, 835–837.

Taylor, A. E. (1981). Capillary fluid filtration, Starling forces and lymph flow. *Circulation Research* **49**, 557–575.

Tejani, A. *et al.* (1985). Persistence of protective pneumococcal antibody following vaccination in patients with a nephrotic syndrome. *American Journal of Nephrology* **4**, 32–37.

Tejani, A. *et al.* (1987). Cyclopsorine-induced remission of relapsing nephrotic syndrome in children. *Journal of Pediatrics* **111**, 1056–1062.

Tempany, C., Morton, R. A., and Marshall, F. F. (1992). MRI of the renal veins: assessment of non-malignant venous thrombosis. *Journal of Computer Assisted Tomography* **16**, 929–934.

Tessitore, N. *et al.* (1984). Bone histology and calcium metabolism in patients with nephrotic syndrome and normal or reduced renal function. *Nephron* **37**, 153–159.

Thaler, E. and Lechner, K. Thrombophilie bei erworbenem Antithrombin III-Mangel von Patienten mit nephrotischem Syndrom. In *Niere und Hämostase* Vol. 5 (ed. R. Marx and H. Thiess), pp. 123–129. Stuttgart: Schattauer, 1978.

Toto, R. D., Vega, G. L., and Grundy, S. M. (1992). Pravastatin improves hypercholesterolemia of the nephrotic syndrome by enhancing clearance of apolipoprotein B. *Journal of the American Society of Nephrology* **3**, 321 (abstract).

Trachtman, H. and Gauthier, B. (1988). Effect of angiotensin-converting enzyme inhibitor therapy on proteinuria in children with renal disease. *Journal of Pediatrics* **112**, 295–298.

Trew, P. A. *et al.* (1978). Renal vein thrombosis in membranous glomerulonephritis: incidence and association. *Medicine (Baltimore)* **57**, 69–82.

Ueda, N. *et al.* (1987). Effect of corticosteroids on coagulation factors in children with nephrotic syndrome. *Pediatric Nephrology* **1**, 286–289.

Usberti, M. *et al.* (1984). Role of plasma vasopressin in the impairment of water excretion in nephrotic syndrome. *Kidney International* **25**, 422–429.

Valentin, J. P. *et al.* (1992). Cellular basis for blunted volume expansion natriuresis in experimental nephrotic syndrome. *Journal of Clinical Investigation* **90**, 1302–1312.

Valeri, A. *et al.* (1986). Treatment of hyperlipidemia of the nephrotic syndrome: a controlled trial. *American Journal of Kidney Diseases* **8**, 388–396.

Vande Walle, J. G. and Donckerwolcke, R. A. (2001). Pathogenesis of edema formation in the nephrotic syndrome. *Pediatric Nephrology* **16**, 283–293.

Vande Walle, J. G. *et al.* (1995). Volume regulation in children with early relapse of minimal-change nephrosis with or without hypovolemic symptoms. *Lancet* **346**, 148–152.

Vande Walle, J. G. *et al.* (1996). Renal sodium handling in children with nephrotic relapse: relation to hypovolemic symptoms. *Nephrology, Dialysis, Transplantation* **11**, 2202–2208.

Vande Walle, J. G. *et al.* (2004). ARF in children with minimal change nephrotic syndrome may be related to functional changes of the glomerular basal membrane. *American Journal of Kidney Diseases* (accepted for publication).

Vaziri, N. D. (1993). Endocrinological consequences of the nephrotic syndrome. *American Journal of Nephrology* **13**, 360–364.

Vaziri, N. D. (2003). Molecular mechanisms of lipid disorders in nephrotic syndrome. *Kidney International* **63**, 1964–1976.

Vaziri, N. D. *et al.* (1988). Increased levels of protein C activity, protein C concentration, total and free protein S in nephrotic syndrome. *Nephron* **49**, 20–23.

Vaziri, N. D. *et al.* (1992). Plasma concentration and urinary excretion of erythropoietin in adult nephrotic syndrome. *American Journal of Medicine* **92**, 35–40.

Venkataseshan, V. S. *et al.* (1993). Renal failure due to tubular obstruction by large protein casts in patients with massive proteinuria. *Clinical Nephrology* **39**, 321–326.

Vermylen, C. G. *et al.* (1987a). Inhibition of lipoprotein lipase by plasma from children with the steroid responsive nephrotic syndrome. *Pediatric Research* **22**, 197–200.

Vermylen, C. G. *et al.* (1987b). Decreased sensitivity to heparin *in vitro* in steroid-responsive nephrotic syndrome. *Kidney International* **31**, 1396–1401.

Vigano-D'Angelo, S. *et al.* (1987). Protein S deficiency occurs in the nephrotic syndrome. *Annals of Internal Medicine* **107**, 42–47.

Voorberg, J. *et al.* (1994). Association of idiopathic venous thromboembolism with a single point-mutation at Arg^{506} of factor V. *Lancet* **343**, 1535–1536.

Vriesendorp, R. *et al.* (1985). Antiproteinuric effect of naproxen and indomethacin. A double-blind crossover study. *American Journal of Nephrology* **5**, 236–242.

Wagoner, R. D. *et al.* (1983). Renal vein thrombosis in idiopathic membranous glomerulopathy and nephrotic syndrome: incidence and significance. *Kidney International* **23**, 368–374.

Warshaw, B. L. *et al.* (1984). Decreased serum transferrin concentrations in children with nephrotic syndrome: effect on lymphocyte proliferation and correlation with serum transferrin levels. *Clinical Immunology and Immunopathology* **33**, 210–219.

Warwick, G. L. and Packard, C. J. (1993). Lipoprotein metabolism in the nephrotic syndrome. *Nephrology, Dialysis, Transplantation* **8**, 385–396.

Warwick, G. L. *et al.* (1990). Low density lipoprotein (LDL) apoprotein metabolism in the nephrotic syndrome. *Metabolism* **39**, 187–192.

Warwick, G. L. *et al.* (1992). Effect of simvastatin on plasma lipid and lipoprotein concentrations and low-density lipropotein metabolism in the nephrotic syndrome. *Clinical Science* **82**, 701–708.

Wass, V. J. *et al.* (1979). Does the nephrotic syndrome increase the risk of cardiovascular disease? *Lancet* **ii**, 664–667.

Wheeler, D. C. (2001). Lipid abnormalities in the nephrotic syndrome: the therapeutic role of statins. *Journal of Nephrology* **14** (Suppl. 4), 70–75.

Wheeler, D. C. *et al.* (1991). Characterisation of the binding of low-density lipoproteins to cultured rat mesangial cells. *Nephrology, Dialysis, Transplantation* **6**, 701–708.

Wilcox, C. (2002). New insights into diuretic use in patients with chronic renal disease. *Journal of the American Society of Nephrology* **13**, 798–805.

Yang, W. Q. *et al.* (1999). Serum lipid concentration correlate with the progression of chronic renal failure. *Clinical Laboratory Science* **12**, 104–108.

Yetgkin, S., Guy, Y., and Saatçi, U. (1980). Non-specific immunity in nephrotic syndrome. *Acta Paediatrica Scandinavica* **69**, 21–24.

Zilleruelo, G. *et al.* (1984). Persistence of serum lipid abnormalities in children with idiopathic nephrotic syndrome. *Journal of Pediatrics* **104**, 61–64.

Zwaginga, J. J. *et al.* (1994). Thrombus formation and platelet vessel wall interaction in the nephrotic syndrome under flow conditions. *Journal of Clinical Investigation* **93**, 204–211.

3.5 Minimal change and focal–segmental glomerular sclerosis

Alain Meyrier and Patrick Niaudet

History and definition

The term 'lipoid nephrosis' was coined by Munk (1913) to describe patients with oedema, heavy proteinuria, hypoproteinaemia, and hyperlipidaemia, in whom renal microscopy showed normal glomeruli and lipid droplets in the tubular cells. When the same was shown to be a consequence of abundant proteinuria, whatever its cause, 'nephrotic syndrome' was considered preferable. Light microscopy and immunofluorescence were helpful in recognizing the underlying pathology. Many patients—mainly children—had minimal changes on light microscopy and were referred to as having 'minimal-change' nephrotic syndrome, or 'idiopathic nephrotic syndrome' (INS) or 'nephrosis', a denomination still widely used. However, Rich (1957) had already noted that children with nephrosis may display focal and segmental lesions on juxtamedullary glomeruli.

INS is characterized by massive proteinuria, hypoalbuminaemia, hyperlipidaemia, oedema, and, by light microscopy, minimal-glomerular changes, focal–segmental glomerulonephritis (FSGS) and diffuse mesangial proliferation. These features are associated with visceral epithelial cell foot process effacement on electron microscopy and insignificant deposition of immunoglobulins or complement by immunofluorescence. A question remains: do minimal-change nephrosis and FSGS represent two facets of the same disease, or distinct pathophysiologic entities?

The unitary view

The unitary view is the most appropriate regarding treatment options. It is compatible with varied causes and/or pathophysiological mechanisms. Rather than distinguishing FSGS from minimal changes, the best guide to prognosis and to subsequent response to other drugs is the initial response to glucocorticoids. Patients with FSGS generally suffer a more severe disease, are often resistant to corticosteroids, and are prone to progressing to renal failure. In the early stages, however, FSGS and minimal-change disease are indistinguishable (Kashgarian *et al.* 1974). Several facts favour the single-disease concept: a number of patients with FSGS respond to steroids whilst some steroid-resistant patients have no sclerotic changes on adequate biopsies (Habib 1973). The best illustration of this is the appearance of renal biopsy carried out shortly after relapse of nephrotic syndrome following transplantation in a patient whose primary renal disease was FSGS. Despite heavy proteinuria, the glomeruli initially show minimal changes. Several studies (Rumpelt and Thoenes 1974; Velosa *et al.* 1975; Newman *et al.* 1976), are consistent with common pathophysiological factors operating at different intensity in minimal-change nephrosis and FSGS.

The pluralistic view

More recent data have comforted the belief of many nephrologists, especially those caring for adults, that minimal-change disease and FSGS are different entities. The latter clearly appears to be a podocyte disease (Kriz *et al.* 1994) that develops to the cell and the scar variants of the glomerular lesion and less frequently to the so called 'collapsing' subset of FSGS. The notion of 'podocyte dysregulation' (Bariéty *et al.* 1998, 2001; Barisoni *et al.* 1999), the different expression of cyclin-dependent kinase inhibitors in minimal-change disease and in FSGS, the role of these cell cycle disturbances leading to podocyte proliferation and maturation (Shankland *et al.* 2000), and identification of Parvovirus B 19 in glomeruli of patients suffering from FSGS (Tanawattanachaoren *et al.* 2000; Moudgil *et al.* 2001) and similarly of SV 40 in patients with FSGS (Li *et al.* 2002) are in favour of distinct entities. The detractors of the unitary view consider that the finding that intrarenal transcription of CTL-effectors and TGF-β1 in a majority of children with FSGS, contrasting with the rare occurrence of this phenomenon in children with minimal-change disease (Strehlau *et al.* 2002) is in favour of the pluralistic view. Moreover, that this intrarenal gene expression anticipates development to FSGS in steroid resistant cases may be considered a valuable argument for sorting out one histologic pattern from the other.

Demography

The incidence of INS varies with age, race, and geography. The annual incidence in children in three areas of the United States has been estimated to be 2–2.7 per 100,000 (McEnery and Strife 1982), with a cumulative prevalence of 16 per 100,000. Whereas INS accounts for only 25 per cent of adult cases (Cameron *et al.* 1974), it is by far the most common cause of nephrotic syndrome in children (see Chapter 3.3). Almost all nephrotic children under 6 years of age in Western countries suffer from 'nephrosis'.

In the United Kingdom, its incidence is sixfold greater in Asian than in White European children (Sharples *et al.* 1985). This is also true for Indians (Srivastava *et al.* 1975) and in Asia. INS is rare in Africa (Coovadia *et al.* 1979).

There is a male/female ratio of 2/1 in children (International Study of Kidney Disease in children 1978). Male preponderance is also observed in adults (Korbet 1995).

In the United States, the incidence of FSGS in children with nephrosis has increased from 23 per cent before 1990 to 47 per cent afterwards. This was observed in all ethnic groups, including Caucasians, Black

Americans, and Hispanics (Bonilla-Felix *et al.* 1999). The authors reviewed the clinical charts of 152 children with nephrosis seen between 1978 and 1997, including 105 with a renal biopsy. Minimal-change nephropathy was present in 35 per cent and FSGS in 31 per cent of all biopsies. Even considering the assumption that all patients without histological examination had minimal changes, the total incidence of minimal change disease in this population was only 55 per cent. The same increased incidence has been observed in adults, but especially in Blacks and Hispanics, at least in the United States (Braden *et al.* 2000). To our knowledge, there have been no report outside the United States indicating a similar increase in the incidence FSGS in children or adults with nephrosis.

The nephrotic syndrome tends to be more severe in blacks (Korbet 1995). White South African children with minimal-change disease seem to have a long-term outcome similar to that reported in Europe, whereas Black children are generally corticosteroid resistant (Coovadia and Adhikari 1989) (see Chapter 3.14).

Conditions with a possible aetiologic role in nephrosis

Many factors are commonly cited as possible 'causes' or temporally associated conditions for INS. They include infectious diseases, drugs, allergies, vaccinations, and some malignancies. It is not at all clear what final common pathway permits these differing factors to result in the common clinical and pathological outcome of minimal-change disease, or less commonly FSGS, or how this relates to ideas on pathogenesis outlined below.

Allergy

Allergy is associated with up to 30 per cent of cases (Lagrue and Laurent 1984), which suggests some involvement of type IV reactions in the pathogenesis of minimal-change disease. Among a list of anecdotal cases, the allergens reported include fungi, poison ivy, ragweed and timothy grass pollen, house dust, medusa stings, bee stings, and cat fur.

A food allergen may be responsible for relapsing episodes of steroid-sensitive nephrosis, such as cow's milk and egg. Laurent *et al.* (1987) evaluated the effect of an oligoantigenic diet given for 10–15 days to 13 patients with an unsatisfactory response to corticosteroids. This diet coincided with improvement of proteinuria in nine, including complete remission in five.

Drugs

A number of drugs may induce a nephrotic syndrome with the histopathological appearance of minimal-change disease. The list comprises apparently unrelated drugs such as non-steroidal anti-inflammatory agents, including salazopyrine and mesalasine, D-penicillamine, lithium, rifampicin, heavy metals (gold, mercury), and trimethadione (see Chapter 19.1).

Malignancy

The association with malignancies mainly concerns lymphomatous disorders and solid tumours. Detailed description is to be found in Chapter 3.13.

Viral infections

The knowledge that HIV carriage may elicit a severe form of FSGS (HIVAN) (see Chapter 3.12) shed a new light on possible other viral aetiologies of nephrosis. The description of Parvovirus B 19 associated FSGS drew attention to the fact that a common, benign viral illness in childhood may later be complicated with nephrotic syndrome which can no longer be termed 'idiopathic'.

Tanawattanacharoen *et al.* (2000) studied renal biopsies from 40 children with various glomerulopathies, including classic FSGS, collapsing glomerulopathy, minimal-change disease and membranous glomerulopathy. The prevalence of Parvovirus B 19 DNA identified by polymerase chain reaction (PCR) was greater ($p < 0.05$) among patients with classic and collapsing FSGS compared with patients with other diagnoses. Considering that they failed to localize Parvovirus B 19 nucleic acid within kidney tissue, the authors suggested that past infection might have triggered the process leading to podocyte injury and further development to FSGS.

Moudgil *et al.* (2001) detected Parvovirus B 19 by *in situ* hybridization in glomerular visceral and parietal glomerular cells and in tubular cells from 18/23 patients with 'collapsing glomerulopathy', 6/27 patients with classic FSGS, 3/19 patients with HIVAN, and 7/27 controls. The significantly higher prevalence of Parvovirus B 19 in renal biopsies of patients with collapsing glomerulopathy suggested that in susceptible individuals this virus may induce collapsing glomerulopathy following podocyte infection.

Li *et al.* (2002) detected DNA sequences homologous to the simian virus SV 40 regulatory genome by PCR in urinary cells from 15 (41 per cent) of 36 patients with FSGS, 2 (10 per cent) of 20 patients with other kidney diseases, and 1 (4 per cent) of 22 healthy volunteers. SV 40 regulatory region genome was detected from peripheral blood mononuclear cells at similar frequencies in patients with FSGS (35 per cent), other glomerular diseases (20 per cent), and healthy volunteers (22 per cent). SV 40 genome was detected by PCR in kidney tissues from 17 (56 per cent) of 30 of patients with FSGS and 4 (20 per cent) of 20 patients with minimal-change disease and membranous nephropathy ($p < 0.01$). These preliminary data seem to adduce further evidence that viruses other than HIV may cause the podocyte disease which characterizes FSGS.

Inheritance

The familial occurrence of INS is well known. White (1973) found that 3.3 per cent of 1877 patients with INS had affected family members, mainly siblings.

In the past few years, there have been several reports on the molecular genetic basis of some familial cases of INS with FSGS. The discovery of molecular defects leading to FSGS has provided important insight in the critical role of newly identified podocyte proteins of the glomerular filtration barrier to proteins (Pollak 2002).

Linkage analysis was carried out in a large family in which the disease followed an autosomal dominant mode of inheritance (Mathis *et al.* 1998). The severity was variable. Some patients developed severe proteinuria or endstage renal disease (ESRD) by the fourth decade whilst others had only mild proteinuria. The responsible gene was located on chromosome 19q13. Mutations in the gene encoding α-actinin-4, an actin-filament cross-linking protein, were found in affected patients (Kaplan *et al.* 2000). This gene was known to be up-regulated in experimental nephrotic syndrome. *In vitro*, mutant α-actinin-4 binds filamentous actin more strongly than does wild-type α-actinin-4. Regulation of the actin cytoskeleton of glomerular podocytes may be altered in these patients.

Another family with autosomal dominant FSGS was studied for linkage analysis (Winn *et al.* 1999a,b). The disease was diagnosed during the third decade of life with high-grade proteinuria progressing to ESRD in a relatively high percentage of cases. The authors found a linkage to chromosome 11q21–q22 with a maximum lod score of 9.89. In the same report, Winn *et al.* (1999b) described another large family with autosomal dominant FSGS but no linkage to chromosome 11q21 or to chromosome 19q13.

Fuchshuber *et al.* (1995) mapped a locus to chromosome 1q25–q31 for autosomal recessive nephrotic syndrome characterized by an early onset, steroid resistance, rapid progression to renal failure and no recurrence after transplantation. Using a positional cloning approach, Boute *et al.* (2000) identified the causative gene, NPHS2, which is only expressed on podocytes and encodes podocin. By immunoelectron microscopy, podocin is located at the foot processes, opposite the slit diaphragm (Roselli *et al.* 2002). This 42 kDa protein is structurally related to human stomatin, an adapter protein which links mechanosensitive channels to the cytoskeleton on the cell surface. Podocin may link membrane proteins, such as nephrin, to the cytoskeleton. Thirty different NPHS2 mutations, comprising non-sense, frameshift, and missense mutations, were found to segregate with the disease. Podocin mutations have been identified also in 15–30 per cent of patients with the sporadic form of steroid resistant INS (Frishberg *et al.* 2002; Karle *et al.* 2002).

CD2-associated protein (CD2AP) that anchors CD2 receptors of T lymphocytes to the cytoskeleton is also expressed on the podocyte. Shih *et al.* (1999) observed that mutant mice lacking CD2AP develop proteinuria and renal failure. They showed that CD2AP and nephrin interact directly suggesting an important role of this protein in the anchoring of nephrin to the slit diaphragm or into the signalling pathways (Shih *et al.* 2001). No mutation in the CD2AP gene has been reported in the human.

The Wilms' tumour suppressor gene WT-1 encodes a transcription factor presumed to regulate the expression of numerous target genes through DNA binding. It plays a key role in kidney and gonad maturation and, when mutated, in the occurrence of nephroblastoma and/or glomerular diseases (Denys–Drash syndrome and Frasier syndrome). The WT-1 gene contains 10 exons covering approximately 50 kb of genomic DNA. Exons 1–6 encode a proline/glutamine rich transcriptional regulatory region, whereas exons 7–10 encode the four zinc fingers of the DNA-binding domain. Two alternative splicing regions, one corresponding to the 17 amino acids encoded by exon 5 and the other to three amino acids [lysine–threonine–serine (KTS)] encoded by the 3′ end of exon 9, lead to the synthesis of four isoforms with definite and stable proportions and different functions. The target genes potentially regulated, most often negatively, by WT-1 include genes coding for transcription factors such as PAX2, PAX8, NovH, and WT-1, and for growth factors or their receptors: IGF-II, IGFR, PDGF-A, TGF-β, EGFR (Reddy and Licht 1996). WT-1 is strongly expressed during embryofetal life (Pritchard-Jones *et al.* 1990). In the mature kidney, WT-1 expression persists only in podocytes and epithelial cells of Bowman's capsule. WT-1 gene disruption in mice results in the absence of kidneys and gonads suggesting a key role of WT-1 in the maturation of the genitourinary tract.

Frasier syndrome is characterized by male pseudohermaphroditism and progressive glomerulopathy (Frasier *et al.* 1964). Proteinuria is discovered during childhood, usually between 2 and 6 years of age, or later. It increases progressively with time and does not respond to corticosteroids or to immunosuppressive agents. The disease runs a slow progressive course to ESRD. Renal biopsy shows FSGS. No recurrence is observed after transplantation. Patients have female external genitalia and it is often the evaluation of primary amenorrhoea in nephrotic females that leads to diagnosing 46, XY gonadal dysgenesis, frequently complicated by gonadoblastoma.

Barbaux *et al.* (1997) detected point mutations in the donor splice site in intron 9 of the WT-1 gene. These mutations were heterozygotous, and appeared *de novo* in the two patients whose parents were studied. The mutations result in loss of the +KTS isoform. Similar intronic mutations have also been described by Kikuchi *et al.* (1998) and by Klamt *et al.* (1998). This indicates that donor splice-site mutations in WT-1 intron 9 are constant in Frasier syndrome. The former definition of Frasier syndrome included only 46, XY patients with a female phenotype. However, Frasier syndrome mutations may be responsible for isolated persistent glomerulopathy, with focal sclerosis, in genetically female patients and in patients with the Denys–Drash syndrome (Demmer *et al.* 1999; Denamur *et al.* 1999).

Nephrotic syndrome with FSGS has been reported in patients with mitochondrial cytopathies (Kurogouchi *et al.* 1998; Doleris *et al.* 2000; Hotta *et al.* 2001) (see Chapter 16.7). An A–G transition at position 3243 in mitochondrial DNA was reported in some of these patients who presented with isolated nephrotic syndrome or with nephrotic syndrome in association with mitochondrial myopathy, encephalopathy, lactic acidosis and stroke-like episodes (MELAS), or progressive external ophtalmoplegia (PEO). Other patients develop diabetes mellitus or hearing loss.

Some familial cases of minimal-change nephrotic syndrome are associated with other abnormalities, such as microcephaly and hiatus hernia, as in the syndrome of Galloway and Mowat (1968). Spondyloepiphyseal dysplasia was found in association with FSGS (Ehrich *et al.* 1990). Other conditions, including myelodysplastic syndromes, have also been reported in association with early-onset nephrotic syndrome (Bogdanovic *et al.* 2001).

Histocompatibility antigens and idiopathic nephrotic syndrome

A three- to fourfold increased incidence of HLA-DR7 in nephrotic children has been reported (Alfiler *et al.* 1980; de Mouzon-Cambon *et al.* 1981). Clark *et al.* (1990) found a strong association between HLA-DR7 and the *DQB1* gene of *HLA-DQW2* and steroid-sensitive nephrosis, and suggested that the β-chains of DR7 and DQW2 contribute to disease susceptibility.

HLA-DR3 has been associated with steroid-resistant nephrosis in children, with a relative risk of 3. The incidence of HLA-DR3-DR7 is increased in steroid-resistant patients with a relative risk of 9.3. An association between HLA-DR4 and idiopathic nephrotic FSGS leading to ESRD was found in 57 adult patients by Glicklich *et al.* (1988).

An association with HLA-B8 was reported in Europe. Children with atopy and HLA-B12 have a 13-fold increased risk of developing nephrosis.

Clinical features

Children

The disease may be discovered on routine urine analysis, but oedema is the most frequent presenting symptom (see Chapter 3.4). The onset is usually rapid. Oedema increases gradually and becomes clinically detectable when fluid retention exceeds 3–5 per cent of body weight. It is often initially apparent around the eyes and misdiagnosed as allergy. Oedema is gravity-dependent. During the day, periorbital oedema decreases whilst it localizes at the lower extremities. In the reclining position, it localizes on the back. It is white, soft, and pitting. Oedema of the scrotum and penis, or labia, may also be observed. Anasarca may develop. The abdomen may bulge with umbilical or inguinal hernias. When ascites builds up rapidly, the child complains of abdominal pain and malaise. Abdominal pain may also result from severe hypovolaemia, peritonitis, pancreatitis, thrombosis, or steroid-induced gastritis. Shock is not unusual, following sudden fall of plasma albumin, with abdominal pain and peripheral circulatory failure. Emergency treatment is mandatory. Blood pressure is usually normal, but sometimes elevated. Nephrosis may also be revealed by a complication. Peritonitis due to *Streptococcus pneumoniae* is a classical mode of onset. Other infections include meningitis, cellulitis, and pneumonia. Deep-vein or arterial thromboses and pulmonary embolism may also occur during the first attack or during a relapse (see Chapter 3.4).

Adults

The clinical picture in adults is similarly characterized by generalized oedema. However, especially in FSGS the onset may be insidious. Also, hypovolaemic shock and abdominal pain are quite unusual. Blood pressure is normal or moderately elevated.

Laboratory abnormalities

Urine analysis

Nephrotic-range proteinuria is defined as greater than 50 mg/kg per day or 40 mg/h per m^2 in children and 3.5 g/24 h in adults, but the mean value during the first days of an attack may be higher. Proteinuria is also dependent on the plasma protein concentration, and may decrease as serum albumin concentrations decline.

In young children the urinary protein/creatinine ratio or $U_{albumin}/U_{creatinine}$ ratio are useful. For these two indices, the nephrotic range is 200–400 mg/mmol.

The nature of proteinuria depends on the severity of the lesions. In minimal-change, steroid-sensitive nephrotic syndrome, proteinuria consists mainly of albumin and low molecular weight proteins, whilst in severe nephrotic syndrome with glomerular lesions and steroid resistance the urine also contains globulins. This can be seen on polyacrylamide gel electrophoresis and can also be quantified by means of the selectivity index, that is, the ratio of IgG to albumin or transferrin clearance (see Chapter 3.4). A favourable index would be below 0.10, or better below 0.05; a poor index is above 0.15–0.20. There is a considerable overlap in results and the test has limited value, especially in adults. Some children with severe steroid-resistant nephrotic syndrome have both glomerular and tubular proteinuria.

Macroscopic haematuria is rare, occurring in 1 per cent of steroid responders and in 3 per cent of non-responders. Persistent microscopic haematuria is more common, and may be observed up to 30 per cent of patients.

Blood chemistry

Serum proteins are markedly reduced, to less than 50 g/l. Albumin concentration is usually less than 20 g/l and may be less than 10 g/l. Electrophoresis of plasma proteins shows a typical pattern with low albumin, increased α_2-globulins and, to a lesser extent, β-globulins whilst gammaglobulins are decreased. IgG is considerably decreased, IgA slightly, and IgM is increased. Among other proteins, fibrinogen, and β-lipoproteins are increased, whilst small molecules such as antithrombin III are lost in the urine and decreased. A detailed analysis of the hyperlipidaemia of nephrotic syndrome and its related complications is to be found in Chapter 3.4.

Serum electrolytes are usually within the normal range. Low plasma sodium may be related to dilution from inappropriate renal water retention. Mild hyponatraemia may be an artefact related to hyperlipidaemia. Serum calcium is consistently low as a result of hypoalbuminaemia. Ionized calcium may be decreased in persistent nephrotic syndrome, due to urinary loss of 25-hydroxyvitamin D_3. Blood urea and plasma creatinine are often within the normal range, or increased in relation to functional renal insufficiency.

Haematology

Haemoglobin and the haematocrit may be increased in patients with a reduced plasma volume, which is sometimes associated with the first attack or a relapse, with sudden and heavy urinary loss of albumin. Microcytic anaemia may be observed in chronic, steroid-resistant nephrotic syndrome, in some cases following urinary loss of transferrin (see Chapter 3.4). Thrombocytosis is common.

Renal function

Renal function is usually normal, but some patients have a reduction of the glomerular filtration rate (GFR) attributed to hypovolaemia, with complete return to normal after remission. A reduced GFR may also be found despite normal effective plasma flow (Dorhout Mees *et al.* 1979; Bohlin 1984). Bohman *et al.* (1984) showed a close relationship between the degree of foot-process effacement and both the GFR and the filtration fraction, suggesting that foot process effacement leads to a reduction of the glomerular filtering area and/or of permeability to water and small solutes. This reduction is transitory, with a rapid return to normal after remission. Tubular functions are occasionally altered with glycosuria, aminoaciduria, hypokalaemia, and acidosis (see Chapter 3.4).

Acute renal failure complicating nephrosis (see also Chapter 3.4)

Marked oliguria occurs mainly in adults, particularly in middle-aged or older patients (Cameron *et al.* 1974). It may also occur in children (Sakarlan *et al.* 1994). Oliguric renal failure may be the presenting symptom. A role for hypovolaemia with poor renal perfusion is unlikely, since plasma volume is not significantly decreased. Bilateral renal-vein thrombosis is easily recognized by sonography. Interstitial nephritis has been reported, especially following the use of frusemide. Skin rash and eosinophilia are suggestive of this diagnosis (see Chapter 19.1).

Acute renal failure is usually reversible, often with high dose furosemide induced diuresis, especially with intravenous infusion of albumin (Fliser *et al.* 1999). In some cases—where glomerular structure is close to normal on initial histology, renal failure may last for as long as a year (Sakarlan *et al.* 1994) and sometimes be irreversible (Raij *et al.* 1976).

Renal biopsy in idiopathic nephrotic syndrome

Indications

Renal biopsy is not indicated at onset in a child 1–8 years old with typical symptoms. Complete remission obtained by corticosteroids is a major support for the diagnosis. Biopsy is, however, indicated at onset in circumstances suggesting another type of glomerular disease, including moderate nephrotic syndrome or a long previous course of minor proteinuria, macroscopic haematuria, marked hypertension, and/or persistent renal insufficiency. A decreased plasma C3 fraction is also an indication for performing a biopsy. Age under 12 months and over 11 years is another indication, even in patients with a typical picture. However, the main indication is failure to respond to a 4-week course of prednisone given and taken in adequate dosage. Renal biopsy is sometimes indicated in steroid-dependent patients, but in general therapeutic interventions do not depend on histology. A biopsy is necessary before starting cyclosporin treatment, to allow assessment of nephrotoxicity on a later biopsy. Since INS is much less common in adults, a renal biopsy is usually performed before any treatment.

Histopathology

Light microscopy shows three patterns: minimal changes, diffuse mesangial proliferation, and FSGS. Their relative incidence is difficult to determine. Minimal changes are found in the majority of children, and FSGS in only 5–7 per cent (Southwest Paediatric Nephrology Study Group 1985). Mesangial proliferation is reported in a small number (3–5 per cent) of patients. These proportions are different in adults, half of whom have minimal-change disease, and half focal–segmental sclerosis. Immunofluorescence reveals no immune material. Mesangial deposits of IgM, and, more rarely, of IgA, IgG, and C3 have, however, been reported.

Minimal-change disease

Under light microscopy the glomeruli are mostly normal. Mild changes, including podocyte swelling and vacuolation, a slight increase in mesangial matrix and mild, focal–mesangial hypercellularity may be seen (Churg *et al.* 1970; Cameron *et al.* 1974). Lipid vacuoles and degenerative changes of proximal tubules are rare. Scattered foci of tubular lesions and interstitial fibrosis may be observed, such as obstruction by hyaline casts, dilatation with epithelial cell thinning, tubular basement membrane thickening, interstitial foam cells, and calcium deposits. Vascular changes are absent in children. In adults they are age-related (Cameron *et al.* 1974).

Ultrastructural changes are constant, mainly involving podocytes and mesangial stalks. Podocyte foot-process effacement is generalized (Fig. 1) and closely related to the degree of proteinuria. Immunoelectron microscopy has shown that the expression of nephrin is lower than normal in regions where the foot processes are effaced (Huh *et al.* 2002). Other epithelial changes consist of microvilli formation and numerous protein reabsorption droplets. The glomerular basement membranes (GBMs) are normal. The endothelial cells are often swollen.

Diffuse mesangial proliferation

It is not always easy to draw the line between 'mild' and 'marked' mesangial hypercellularity. A subset of patients shows a marked increase in mesangial matrix associated with hypercellularity (Churg *et al.* 1970; Waldherr *et al.* 1978). However, peripheral capillary walls are normal, and immunofluorescence does not show humps. Electron microscopy shows foot-process effacement (Fig. 2).

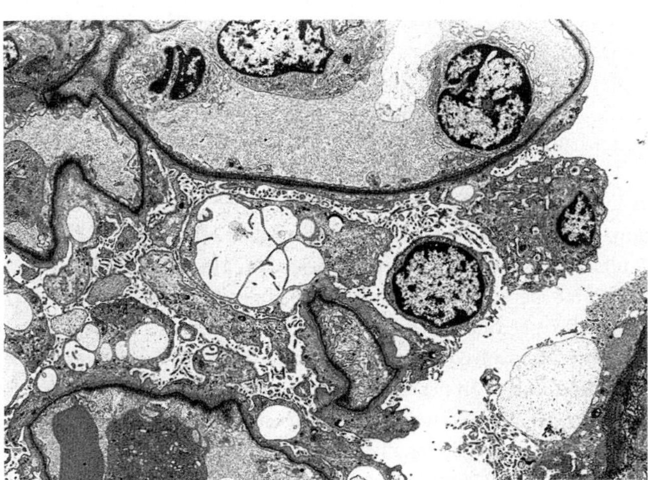

Fig. 1 Minimal-change disease (electron microscopy). The glomerular basement membrane is normal; the cytoplasm of the podocytes is vacuolated, with effacement of foot processes and microvilli. Methenamine silver, 2800×.

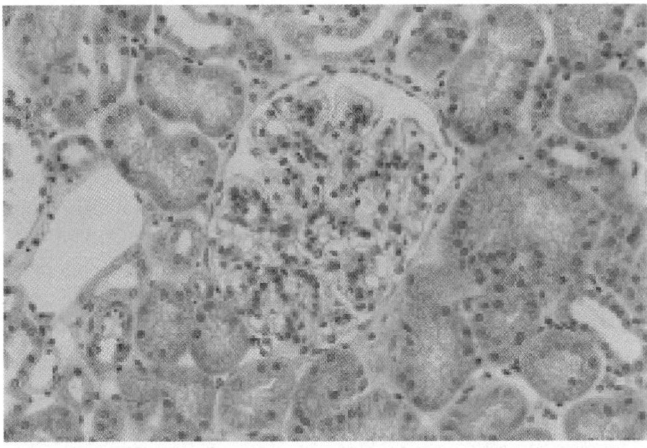

Fig. 2 Diffuse mesangial proliferation: the glomerular basement membrane is normal but there is an increased number of mesangial cells and amount of mesangial matrix. Masson's trichrome, 250×.

Mesangial hypercellularity has been attributed a prognostic significance (Schwartz and Lewis 1985). Waldherr *et al.* (1978) found a higher rate of initial steroid resistance and of progression to renal failure. Other studies failed to confirm these findings (Southwest Pediatric Nephrology Study Group 1985). Diffuse mesangial proliferation may be associated with FSGS.

Primary focal–segmental glomerulosclerosis

General description of 'classic' focal–segmental glomerulosclerosis

FSGS is characterized by focal lesions affecting a variable proportion of glomeruli at any time during the course of the disease (Churg *et al.* 1970; Habib 1973). They predominate in the deeper cortex and juxtamedullary glomeruli are mainly affected (Rich 1957). Focal changes are frequently limited to part of the tuft. Fogo *et al.* (1990) and Muda *et al.* (1994) have shown that glomerular hypertrophy is common in FSGS, and that such hypertrophy found in minimal-change disease is somewhat predictive of further development to FSGS.

By serial three-dimensional (3D) ultrathin sections the distribution of focal sclerosis is more widespread than that observed by conventional microscopy. Fogo *et al.* (1995) studied renal biopsies from 15 adults and six children. Sclerosis assessed on a single section involved 31.5 ± 6.8 per cent of glomeruli in adults, contrasting with only 11.7 ± 5.7 per cent in children. After 3D screening, the percentage of glomeruli involved by sclerosis increased to 48.0 ± 6.6 per cent in adults and 23.2 ± 7.4 per cent in children. The greater increase in sclerosis after 3D analysis in children versus adults reflected the predominance of small peripheral, that is, more segmental, lesions in children than adults. Similar findings were described by Fuiano *et al.* (1996). They concur to indicate that FSGS is less segmental and probably less focal than previously thought.

The lesion of FSGS affects a few capillary loops, which stick together either at the hilum or at the periphery of the tuft, often at both. Howie and Brewer (1984) and Ito *et al.* (1984) considered that the location of lesions has a prognostic significance: the clinical course is considered more benign when they are peripheral (the so-called tip lesion; Fig. 3), although this opinion is not shared by all (Morita *et al.* 1990; Schwartz *et al.* 1995). Hyaline material is often present within sclerotic areas, appearing as a peripheral rim or as round deposits obstructing lumens (Fig. 4). Foamy endothelial cells and lipid inclusions may be found. At the periphery of sclerotic segments there is, in most cases, a clear 'halo' (Fig. 5). The segmental lesion has a different appearance depending on whether it affects a group of capillary loops free in Bowman's space or is adherent to Bowman's capsule. The 'free' sclerotic segments are surrounded by a layer of cuboid podocytes ('cobblestones') in close apposition to the clear 'halo'. When the sclerotic lesion adheres to Bowman's capsule, podocytes are no longer identifiable and a synechia links the collapsed capillary loops covered by the 'halo' to Bowman's capsule basement membrane. The rest of the tuft and the non-sclerotic glomeruli show either 'minimal changes' or 'mesangial proliferation' with foot-process effacement.

In some areas, the tuft is separated from Bowman's capsule by a continuous layer of parietal epithelial cells progressing along the outer aspect of the tuft, thereby circumscribing an empty slit and assuming the appearance of a pseudotubule. This pseudotubule persists in obsolescent glomeruli, which allows retrospective diagnosis of terminal forms of FSGS.

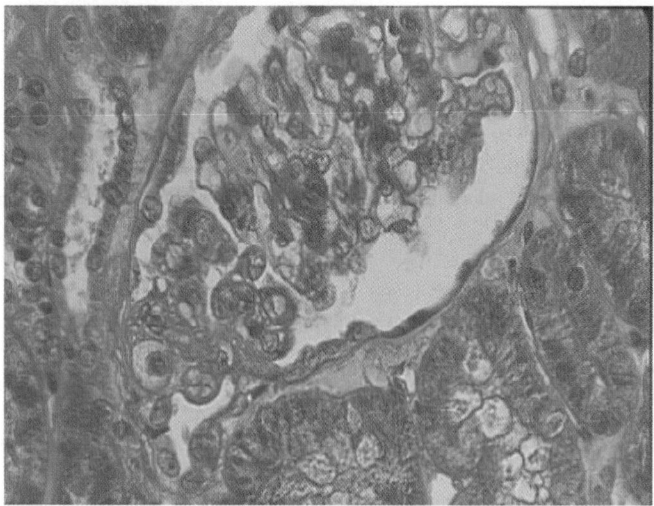

Fig. 3 Typical tip lesion. The photomicrograph is focused on the 'glomerular outlet'. Note the 'cell-type' of this form of focal–segmental glomerulonephritis, with abundant, swollen macrophages in the capillary lumens. Masson's trichrome, 600×. Courtesy: Prof. Jean Bariéty, Paris VI University, Broussais-Hôtel Dieu Medical School and INSERM U 430, Paris.

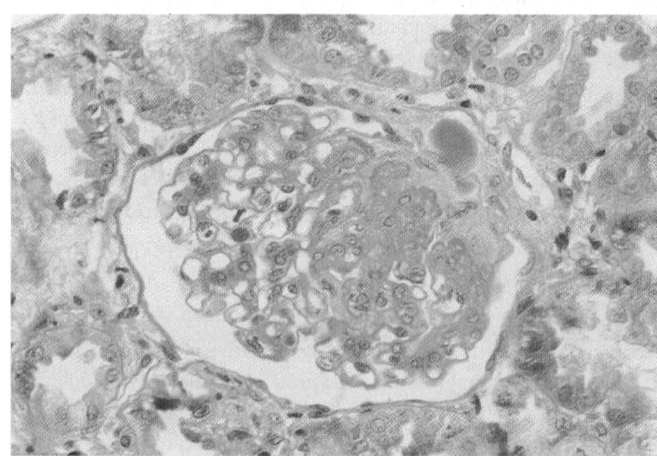

Fig. 4 Focal–segmental sclerosis/hyalinosis: obliteration of capillary lumens at the vascular pole of the glomerulus by a combination of sclerosis and hyalinosis. Masson's trichrome, 320×.

Histological variants

A recent consensus conference proposed a new classification for FSGS. Five patterns have been defined: FSGS not otherwise specified (NOS), perihilar variant, cellular variant, tip variant, and collapsing variant. (D'Agati 2003). However, it has become clear that despite its histological diversity FSGS begins as a podocyte disease, which progresses from a cellular to a scar lesion. (Schwartz and Korbet 1993; Kriz *et al.* 1994, 1998; Rydel *et al.* 1995; Schwartz *et al.* 1995; Bariéty *et al.* 1998; Schwartz 2000). Relapse of nephrotic primary FSGS on a renal

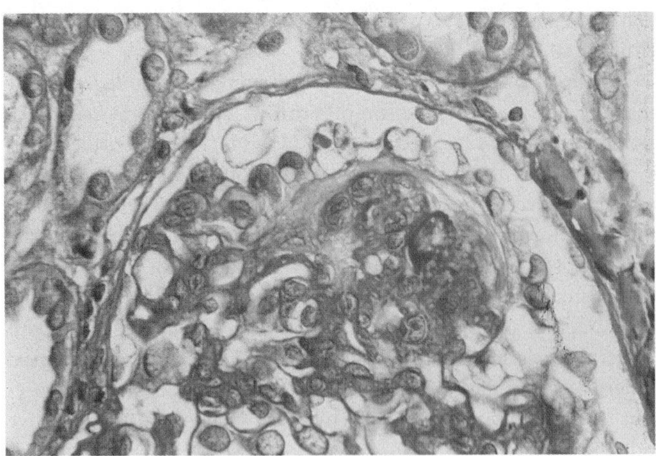

Fig. 5 Focal–segmental sclerosis/hyalinosis: segmental lesion of the tuft characterized by the deposition of hyaline material in the inner side of glomerular basement membrane, and a ring of detached podocytes separated from the glomerular basement membrane by a clear 'halo'. Masson's trichrome, 520×.

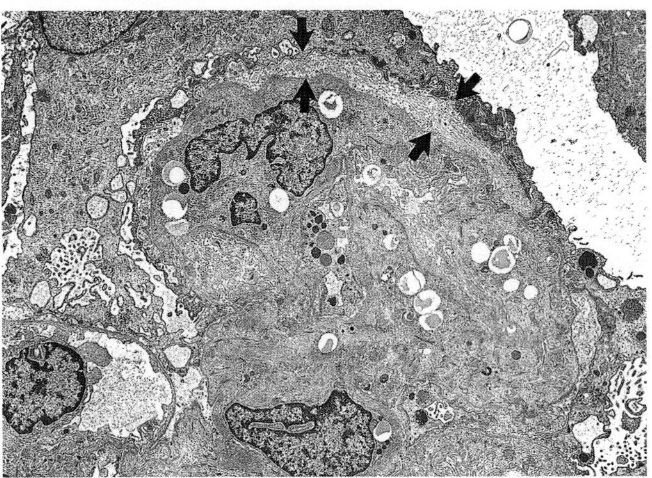

Fig. 6 Focal–segmental sclerosis/hyalinosis (electron microscopy): note the presence around the collapsed capillary loops of multilayered basement-membrane material in a subepithelial location (arrows). Uranyl acetate–lead citrate, 2380×.

transplant offers a privileged model to study the incipient lesion in man and to follow its progression (Verani 1986; Korbet *et al.* 1988; Bariéty *et al.* 2001). Within weeks following recurrence of proteinuria podocytes observed by electron microscopy appear swollen and vacuolated. Some vacuoles are round and by immunofluorescence appear to contain IgA. The podocytes exhibit strong mitotic activity, with multinucleation and expression of the PCNA and Ki-67 proliferation markers. The number of visceral epithelial cells seems to be increased, although it has not been clearly established whether these podocytes undergo replication or just gather in clusters. Podocytes detached from the glomerular basement membranes assume a round shape and form grape-like clusters of cells on the outer aspect of the tuft. Their number may be such that they assume the appearance of a pseudocrescent. Some appear to drift free in the urinary chamber, and migrate into the tubular lumen, a phenomenon first noted by Oda *et al.* (1998). Other dysmorphic podocytes assume a 'cobblestone' pattern covering the outer aspect of the tuft. The parietal epithelial cells of Bowman's capsule facing this line of cuboid cells usually proliferate and form a pluricellular stratum. Underlying endocapillary lesions comprise foam cells, macrophages, and mesangial cell proliferation along with capillary loop collapse. This subset of FSGS is the 'cellular lesion' (Schwartz and Lewis 1985). Further stages are characterized by extracellular matrix build-up, comprising ubiquitous collagen, leading to the 'scar lesion', variably hilar, peripheral, or central (Schwartz and Korbet 1993; Schwartz *et al.* 1995).

Glomerular obsolescence follows. FSGS is an irreversible scarring process, as demonstrated by repeat biopsies (Velosa *et al.* 1975; Nash *et al.* 1976). The whole tuft is sclerotic, often in association with conspicuous interstitial and tubular damage. In children, focal global sclerosis should be differentiated from 'congenital glomerulosclerosis', which is a developmental anomaly frequently found in kidneys of infants and young children (Kohaut *et al.* 1976) and is not associated with tubulointerstitial changes. In normal adults, the number of sclerotic glomeruli increases with age (Kaplan *et al.* 1975) and their interpretation on biopsies from patients older than 40 is difficult. (Cameron *et al.* 1974).

Tubular atrophy and interstitial fibrosis are common and proportional to the glomerular damage (Hyman and Burkholder 1973; Newman *et al.* 1976). Overlooked FSGS should therefore be suspected when tubular and interstitial changes are associated with minimal-glomerular changes. In rare instances, tubular lesions predominate (Hayslett *et al.* 1969). Foam cells may be seen in the interstitium and occasionally in the glomeruli. Vascular changes are rare in children, although subendothelial hyalinosis of afferent arterioles may be observed (Hyman and Burkholder 1974). In adults, they increase with age (Cameron *et al.* 1974). By immunofluorescence there are conspicuous deposits of IgM and C3 on the segmental lesions.

Electron microscopy shows that capillary obliteration is mainly due to paramesangial and subendothelial, finely granular deposits (Velosa *et al.* 1975) with endothelial cell disappearance or swelling, and increased mesangial matrix. Fatty vacuoles may be seen, among the abnormal deposits or in the cytoplasm of endothelial and mesangial cells. Synechiae are formed by apposition of a cloudy, acellular material containing thin and irregular layers of newly formed basement membrane (Fig. 6). Sclerotic lesions result from a marked increase in GBM-like material with capillary wall wrinkling and capillary collapse (Rumpelt and Thoenes 1974). Collagen fibres are seen within some segmental areas. Studies in animals (Couser and Stilmant 1975) and in nephrotic patients have shown that proteinuria precedes the development to focal sclerotic lesions. The same sequence was reported in patients with recurrence after transplantation.

Collapsing glomerulopathy

Collapsing glomerulopathy is regarded by some observers as an autonomous condition, although others consider it as no more than a severe form of cellular FSGS (Meyrier 1999b). In 1986, Weiss *et al.* published a paper on '*A new clinicopathologic entity*' observed in a small group of patients with glomerular 'collapse' and nephrotic syndrome rapidly progressing to renal failure, (Weiss *et al.* 1986). These features closely resembled those of the newly described HIV-associated nephropathy, and in fact some of their patients were HIV-1 infected.

Eight years later, Detwiler *et al.* (1994) reported on 16 HIV negative patients with idiopathic FSGS, a rapid course and collapsing glomerular features characterized by segmental or global wrinkling and collapse of the glomerular capillary walls with prominent hypertrophy and hyperplasia of the overlying podocytes. Biopsies containing any glomeruli with global collapse and/or over 20 per cent of glomeruli with segmental collapse were considered to be 'collapsing glomerulopathy'. In fact, earlier descriptions of FSGS all comprised a collapsing component of some capillary loops (Velosa *et al.* 1975; Schwartz and Lewis 1985). Korbet *et al.* (1988) studied two cases of recurrent FSGS on renal allografts. Focal glomerular abnormalities were found by 1 month in one patient and by 11 months in the other. They consisted of segmental epithelial cell proliferation with mitotic figures and collapse of glomerular capillaries. This cellular and collapsing lesion was later (5 months and 4.5 years, respectively) followed by a scar lesion. [The same was later found by Bariéty *et al.* (2001) after relapse of non-collapsing forms of FSGS on renal transplants.] Despite such precedents, Valeri *et al.* (1996) defended the view of a new entity and concluded that idiopathic collapsing glomerulopathy is a variant of FSGS with increasing incidence, distinct clinicopathological features, Black racial predominance, a rapidly progressive course and relative steroid resistance (Fig. 7).

Since then, numerous articles have appeared which all consider 'collapsing glomerulopathy' as a distinct form of FSGS, that may be 'idiopathic' (Nagata *et al.* 1998; Toth *et al.* 1998; Barisoni *et al.* 1999, 2000), recur on a renal transplant (Clarkson *et al.* 1998), represent a variety of *de novo* glomerular disease after renal transplantation (Meehan *et al.* 1998; Nadasdy *et al.* 2002), or be associated with Loa Loa (Pakasa *et al.* 1997), Parvovirus B 19 (Moudgil *et al.* 2001), or Simian virus SV 40 (Li *et al.* 2002) infection.

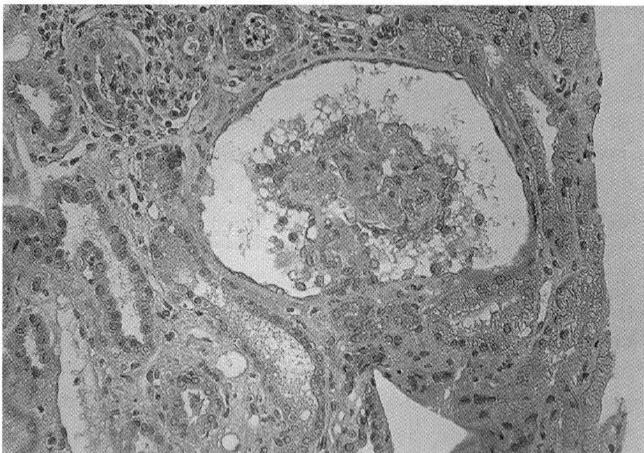

Fig. 7 Collapsing form of cell-FSGS. The glomerular tuft is shrunken within Bowman's capsule. Most capillary loops are obliterated. Build-up of excess extracellular matrix appears in green. The tuft is surrounded with a crown of podocytes with several layers suggesting proliferation and formation of a 'pseudocrescent'. Numerous podocytes (identified as such by immunohistochemistry and confocal laser microscopy as described in Bariéty *et al.* 1998) are drifting free in the urinary chamber. The detached podocytes lose most of their specific markers and acquire macrophagic and cytokeratin specific epitopes, indicating a process of cell dedifferentiation and transdifferentiation (see Bariéty *et al.* 2001) Masson's trichrome, 400×. Courtesy: Prof. Jean Bariéty, Paris VI University, Broussais-Hôtel Dieu Medical School and INSERM U 430, Paris

Whether 'collapsing glomerulopathy' should be regarded as a new entity or just the extreme form of 'primary' cellular focal–segmental glomerulonephritis has been debated (Meyrier 1999b). Furthermore, it appears that the 'collapsing' variant of FSGS might just be the non-specific consequence of glomerular ischaemia. The cellular and collapsing forms of FSGS have been associated with conspicuous vascular lesions in renal allografts (Meehan *et al.* 1998). Nadasdy *et al.* (2002) studied three cases of collapsing glomerular changes in renal allografts that showed a zonal distribution of lesions associated with obliterative vascular changes. They suggested that the morphological pattern of collapsing glomerulopathy in renal allografts may not represent the same disease process as collapsing glomerulopathy in native kidneys.

In any event, this particular variant of FSGS has elicited a host of remarkable papers which have shed a new light on the phenomena of podocyte dedifferentiation and transdifferentiation observed in the cellular variant of FSGS.

Cell dedifferentiation and transdifferentiation in cellular focal–segmental glomerulonephritis

Since 1998, a number of studies, especially, but not exclusively regarding collapsing forms of FSGS, have shown that the process inducing the podocyte disease that characterizes this condition is accompanied by striking changes occurring in these visceral epithelial cells. These changes have been attributed to a profound cell cycle derangement.

The normal mature podocyte is unable to replicate and does not express the proliferation markers PCNA and Ki-67. It is characterized by the expression of numerous epitopes comprising Wilms' tumour protein-1 (WT-1), common acute lymphoblastic leukaemia antigen (CALLA), C3b receptor (CR1), glomerular epithelial protein-1 (GLEPP-1), podocalyxin, synaptopodin, and vimentin. The first stages of FSGS, as observed when the lesions relapse on a renal transplant (Bariéty *et al.* 2001) and in 'collapsing glomerulopathy' (Bariéty *et al.* 1998; Barisoni *et al.* 1999, 2000) are characterized by loss of normal podocyte epitopes, and acquisition of macrophagic and cytokeratin markers. Nuclear proliferation markers PCNA and Ki-67 are expressed indicating strong mitotic activity. Such 'podocyte dysregulation' is accompanied by podocyte detachment from the basement membranes, and migration into the urinary chamber and the tubular lumens where they assume a round shape and occasionally coexpress macrophagic and cytokeratin epitopes. By laser confocal microscopy some of these round cells coexpress CD 68 or cytokeratin markers and original podocyte markers such as podocalyxin. Shankland *et al.* (2000) showed that the expression of cyclins and cyclin inhibitors of the Cip/Kip family differ among patients with minimal-change disease or idiopathic membranous glomerulopathy and those with cellular focal–segmental glomerulonephritis. These remarkable findings are summarized in Table 1.

IgM-associated nephropathy and other immunofluorescence patterns

Cohen *et al.* (1978) proposed that mesangial IgM be considered a separate entity 'IgM-associated nephropathy'. They contended that

Table 1 Differential expression of cyclin-dependent kinase inhibitors in human glomerular disease

	p57	p27	p21	Ki-67
Controls	+	+	−	−
Minimal-change disease	+	+	−	−
Membranous glomerulopathy	+	+	−	−
FSGS, cellular variant	−	−	+	+
FSGS, collapsing variant	−	−	+	+
HIV-associated FSGS	−	−	+	+

The expression by podocytes of the cyclin-dependent kinase inhibitors p57, p27, and p21 and the proliferation marker Ki-67 differs among control renal tissue and glomerular disease tissue. Notably, the cellular and collapsing variants of idiopathic FSGS and HIV-associated FSGS share a similar podocyte phenotype. Data summarizing Shankland *et al.* (2000).

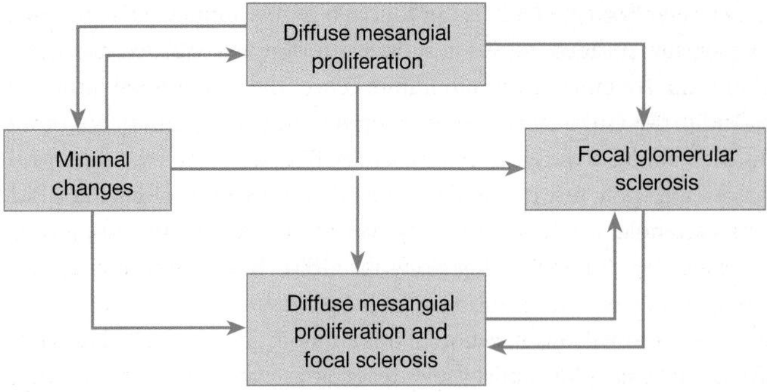

Fig. 8 The different histological patterns of idiopathic nephrotic syndrome and their possible sequential evolution.

IgM mesangial deposits portend either poor response to corticosteroids or progression to renal failure. Other studies have not confirmed this view (Bhuyan and Srivastava 1987; Andal *et al.* 1989). Immunofluorescence confirmed that even though IgM was the immunoglobulin most frequently found in the glomeruli, there was no correlation between these deposits and initial response to therapy or final outcome (Habib *et al.* 1988). IgM deposits have also been described in association with diffuse mesangial proliferation and with focal–mesangial sclerosis. In fact, IgM is a large molecule that can be non-specifically trapped in an injured glomerulus, and it is likely that mesangial IgM deposits represent an epiphenomenon. The same applies to IgG mesangial deposits (Habib *et al.* 1988).

A number of patients with nephrosis display mesangial deposits of IgA. They are classified by some as Berger's disease, especially when they experience macroscopic haematuria (Southwest Pediatric Nephrology Study Group 1985; Lai *et al.* 1989). Others consider that mesangial IgA in patients with minimal changes, that is, without cellular proliferation is merely coincidental. (Barbiano di Belgiojoso *et al.* 1986; Habib *et al.* 1988). This probably applies to nephrosis associated with mesangial IgA deposits occurring in Asians, and would explain a favourable response to steroids, which would not be the case in true Berger's disease.

Relation between the different histological patterns

All published series include cases with morphological transition among the main histological patterns (Fig. 8) on repeat biopsies. A number of patients with minimal changes on a first biopsy have FSGS on a later biopsy. They usually have a more severe disease, either steroid-resistant or highly steroid-dependent. FSGS develops along with an aggravation of the disease (Tejani 1985).

Conversely, some patients with diffuse mesangial proliferation, whether or not associated with focal sclerosis on a first biopsy, may show minimal change or FSGS on a later biopsy (Southwest Pediatric Nephrology Study Group 1985).

In conclusion, it may be considered that, at least in children, minimal-change disease, FSGS, and diffuse mesangial proliferation represent histological variants of nephrosis that may be found alone or in any combination on sequential biopsies in the same patient.

Pathophysiology

Mechanisms of proteinuria

Every clinician faced with a patient having nephrosis and generalized oedema, from puffy face to swollen feet, has suspected that this condition differs from other oedematous states, in that fluid seems to ooze from every capillary in the body. The concept of a generalized disorder was supported when Levin *et al.* (1985) and Boulton-Jones *et al.* (1986) presented indirect data indicating that loss of negative charges was not restricted to the glomeruli, but was also found on blood cell membranes. However, other investigators have failed to reproduce Levin's findings on red cells (Feehally *et al.* 1986; Sewell and Brenchley 1986) or on platelets (Cohen *et al.* 1988) by direct measurement of charge.

The anionic glomerular basement membrane

The barrier to serum albumin rests in part upon the presence of anionic (negative) charges on the endothelium, the GBM, and the foot processes. Negative charges repulse the anionic serum albumin molecules, whose isoelectric point is 4.6. Albuminuria of nephrosis might then be due to loss of the glomerular polyanion elicited by a circulating factor.

In minimal-change disease, the contrast between absence of lesions on light microscopy and massive proteinuria has long suggested an electrochemical disorder of the GBM. This hypothesis was substantiated by demonstration that the glomerular K_f is diminished despite increased permeability to serum albumin. Pore-size studies using polyvinylpyrrolidone (Robson *et al.* 1974) or dextrans with Einstein–Stokes radii between 2.0 and 4.8 nm (Carrie *et al.* 1981) as test macromolecules have adduced evidence to a reduction of the 'pore' size of the barrier contrasting with massive albuminuria, suggesting a loss of glomerular negative charges. Kitano *et al.* (1993), using polyethylamine as a cationic probe, reported a decrease in the anionic charges of the GBM in minimal-change disease. Carrie *et al.* (1981), studied renal biopsy sections stained by colloidal iron and showed that its glomerular uptake was markedly reduced. They envisaged a reduced sialic acid content in the GBM, as sialic acid residues are the major chemical group responsible for glomerular negative charges (Blau and Haaz 1973). Guasch *et al.* (1993), using dextran sulfate to evaluate the charge selectivity of the barrier, confirmed that impairment of this barrier contributes to the abundant albuminuria of nephrotic syndrome.

Van den Born *et al.* (1992) produced a mouse monoclonal antibody to partially purified heparan sulfate proteoglycan isolated from rat glomeruli. By indirect immunofluorescence, the monoclonal antibody bound to the GBM on rat kidney sections. Using electron microscopy a diffuse staining of the whole width of the GBM was observed. After intravenous injection, the monoclonal antibody was localized along the GBM with a granular staining, and 1 day later in the mesangium with a concomitant decrease in staining along the GBM. By electron microscopy, 1 h after injection, the antibody was bound mainly to the inner side of the GBM. Intravenous injection of this antibody in rats resulted in selective proteinuria. This model shows that neutralization of heparan sulfate anionic charges may contribute to increasing albuminuria.

The slit diaphragm proteins

Recent knowledge regarding the paramount role of the slit diaphragm and of the numerous proteins forming its 'raft' framework, which prevents serum albumin from transiting through the GBM have shed a new light on the mechanisms of proteinuria in nephrosis. Figure 9 in Chapter 3.1 shows the complex molecular architecture of the three membrane domains that form the apical cell membrane above the slit diaphragm, the slit diaphragm domain and the 'sole' of the foot processes.

Novel podocyte proteins such as podocin, nephrin, and many others have been identified. Each may be genetically abnormal and thus induce massive proteinuria, as described above (Antignac 2002). This forcibly leads us to conceive that the acquired factor, or factors, eliciting nephrosis and the relapse of FSGS on renal transplants may also affect some of these key albumin-restraining proteins (Furness 1999).

Immunofluorescence microscopy, PCR, and Western blot analysis have shown that nephrin is redistributed on podocytes of nephrotic patients, especially, but not exclusively those with minimal-change disease and FSGS (Doublier *et al.* 2001). Kerjaschki (2001) produced a comprehensive review of the molecular bases of focal glomerulosclerosis. It is likely that these findings apply to at least some forms of minimal-change disease.

To quote Kerjaschki (2001): 'At the molecular level, FSGS and presumably also minimal change nephrosis are not definite entities, but rather syndromes, as isolated or combined damage to any of the listed podocyte proteins could result in identical clinical and histopathological features'.

At the time of writing this it seems likely that molecular genetics will help in discovering new mutations in the proteins that form the complex framework of the slit diaphragm. In turn, some, if not each of these inborn molecular distortions might conceivably have an acquired counterpart, not necessarily due to a single factor (Devarajan and Spitzer 2002). This would nicely explain the variety of histological glomerular lesions observed in INS, the differing responses of the same lesion to corticosteroids, cyclosporin, and other therapeutic agents, as well as the discrepancy between forms that do, versus those that do not, relapse in renal transplants.

The immune system in idiopathic nephrotic syndrome

Cellular immunity

Shalhoub (1974) postulated that nephrosis might be secondary to a disorder of T-lymphocyte function. He hypothesized that expansion of a T-lymphocyte clone results in the production of a lymphokine, which increases the permeability of the glomerular filtration barrier to proteins. The arguments supporting this hypothesis were the response of the disease to corticosteroids and to alkylating agents, the remission occurring in association with measles, which depresses cell-mediated immunity, the susceptibility of patients to pneumococcal infections, and the occurrence of minimal-change nephrotic syndrome in patients with Hodgkin's disease.

Peripheral blood T-lymphocyte subpopulations have actually been shown to be altered in children during a relapse, with an increase in memory T-cell subsets (CD45RO+CD4+T cells and CD45RO+CD8 T cells) (Yan *et al.* 1998). Increased expression of the IL-2 receptor on the T-lymphocyte surface is found in patients with minimal-change disease during the proteinuric phase, but not during remission (Topaloglu *et al.* 1994).

Cell-mediated immunity is depressed in patients with INS, and returns to normal with remission. Their lymphocytes have an impaired responses to mitogens (Sasdelli *et al.* 1981; Taube *et al.* 1984). This decreased response is partly reversible when normal human serum is added to the culture medium instead of autologous serum, suggesting both an intrinsic defect of the cells and presence of inhibitory factors in the serum (Al-Azzawi *et al.* 1994). Macrophages may be responsible for the impaired response of mononuclear cells to mitogens. The proliferative response of these cells returns to normal at the time of remission. Therefore, a soluble factor may inhibit the proliferative response of T lymphocytes. Other abnormalities of cell-mediated immunity have been described in minimal-change nephrosis. Skin reactivity to common antigens and recall response to common antigens are decreased during relapses, with a return to normal during remission (Fodor *et al.* 1982).

Sahali *et al.* (2001) used a subtracted cDNA library screening to identify genes that might be differentially expressed in patients in relapse compared to those in remission. They found several upregulated genes, some of which are closely involved in T-cell activation. Relapsing patients display persistently high levels of nuclear factor-κB (NF-κB) DNA binding activity and downregulation of IκBα mRNA, which may account for increased production of several cytokines. In contrast, NF-κB binding activity returns to normal during remission with concomitant upregulation of IκBα and downregulation of most of the cytokines. An upregulation of c-maf expression and a downregulation of IL-12Rb2 during relapse may suggest that T-cell activation in patients with minimal-change disease evolves towards a T-helper-2 phenotype (Sahali *et al.* 2002).

Humoral immunity

Patients with minimal-change disease have depressed serum IgG levels. This is more pronounced during relapses, but persists during remission (Giangiacomo *et al.* 1975). Conversely, serum IgM is elevated. Altered serum levels of IgG and IgM may be secondary to abnormal T-cell regulation of immunoglobulin synthesis (Yokoyama *et al.* 1987). Factors B and D are decreased during relapses, but return to normal during remission. Specific antibodies to pneumococcal or streptococcal antigens are reduced in patients up to 20 years after remission. This suggests that patients with minimal-change nephrotic syndrome have a defect of the immune response that is not directly related to the nephrotic state. However, it does not imply that it is pathogenic.

Schnaper and Aune (1985, 1987, 1990) reported the presence of a lymphokine, the soluble immune-response suppressor (SIRS), in the urine and serum from patients with steroid-responsive nephrotic syndrome, including minimal-change nephrotic syndrome and other histopathological forms of nephrotic syndrome. SIRS is produced by regulatory T lymphocytes, and inhibits both delayed hypersensitivity reactions and antibody responses. SIRS may contribute to the decreased immune responsiveness of patients with minimal-change disease (Schnaper 1990).

Circulating factors

Increased production of several lymphokines by activated T lymphocytes may alter glomerular permeability to albumin. Lagrue *et al.* (1975) described a 'vascular permeability factor', or VPF, a lymphokine found in the supernatant of concanavalin A-activated lymphocytes from patients with minimal-change disease that enhances vascular permeability when injected in guinea pigs (Sobel *et al.* 1977). The VPF, distinct from IL-2, is produced by T lymphocytes. Cyclosporin suppresses *in vitro* VPF production (Heslan *et al.* 1986, 1991). Tanaka *et al.* (1992) found that supernatants of peripheral mononuclear cells stimulated with concanavalin injected in the renal artery of rats induce proteinuria along with reduction of the GBM anionic charges.

Koyama *et al.* (1991) found a glomerular permeability factor in the supernatant of a T-cell hybridoma derived from peripheral T lymphocytes from a patient with minimal-change disease. The supernatant induced proteinuria when injected in the rat. Histology showed partial fusion of glomerular epithelial cell foot processes without immune deposits.

Several studies have shown increased *in vitro* production of IL-2, IL-4, and interferon-γ by lymphocytes and high plasma and urine concentrations of the soluble IL-2 receptor in patients in relapse. The soluble IL-2r suppresses lymphocyte proliferation. Patients in relapse have increased CD4+ and CD8+ IL-13 mRNA expression as compared to patients in remission or controls (Yap *et al.* 1999). The IL-13 and IL-4 cytokines are produced by stimulated TH2 lymphocytes. Activation of TH2 lymphocytes is known to play a key role in atopy. Glomerular epithelial cells express IL-4 and IL-13 receptors and both cytokines increase transcellular ion transport in cultured cells as well as basolateral secretion of lysosomial proteinases (Van den Berg *et al.* 2000, 2002). Such effects of IL-4 and IL-13 may explain an alteration of glomerular permeability.

Increased IL-2 concentrations have been found in supernatants of lymphocyte culture from patients with idiopathic nephrosis (Lagrue *et al.* 1988), and IL-2 can induce proteinuria and a reduction of the anionic sites of the GBM when injected in the rat kidney (Kawaguchi *et al.* 1987; Heslan *et al.* 1988). Nephrotic syndrome has been observed in patients treated with recombinant IL-2 and α-interferon (Rosenberg *et al.* 1987; Hisanaga *et al.* 1990; Traynor *et al.* 1994). Garin *et al.* (1994) reported an increased serum concentration of IL-8 and the presence of its mRNA in mononuclear cells from patients with minimal-change disease during relapses. They also found that IL-8 may affect the metabolism of the GBM and postulated that it might alter glomerular permeability. Serum concentrations of tumour necrosis factor-α and its mRNA in peripheral mononuclear cells from patients with INS are increased in comparison with controls or patients in remission (Bustos *et al.* 1994).

One of the most convincing arguments for a role of circulating factors in the pathogenesis of the disease is the possible recurrence of nephrotic syndrome after renal transplantation in patients with steroid-resistant FSGS. Savin *et al.* (1996) found in some patients with FSGS a serum factor which increases the permeability to albumin of isolated rat glomeruli. This factor was strongly predictive of recurrence of proteinuria after renal transplantation. A vascular permeability factor, which induces proteinuria when injected into the renal artery of rats, was found in the serum from transplanted patients who had recurrence of the nephrotic syndrome (Zimmerman 1984; Sharma *et al.* 2002), but attempts to isolate the factor(s) have failed. Dantal *et al.* (1994) treated patients with recurrent FSGS with plasma protein A adsorption. The administration to rats of material eluted from the protein A columns increased urinary albumin excretion. The factor, or factors that may be responsible for immediate nephrotic syndrome after transplantation seem to be bound to an immunoglobulin (Dantal *et al.* 1998).

The Buffalo/Mna strain of rats spontaneously develops proteinuria with FSGS at two months of age. Le Berre *et al.* (2002) found that the nephrotic syndrome recurs when Buffalo/Mna rats receive a kidney from a healthy LEW.1W rat. Conversely, proteinuria and renal lesions regress when kidneys from a Buffalo/Mna rat are transplanted into normal LEW.1W rats. Although recurrence of proteinuria is not immediate after transplantation in these rats, this model may be helpful to clarify the pathogenesis of the disease and the mechanisms of recurrence after transplantation in man.

Two other observations indicate that the kidneys are not primarily affected, but rather circulating factors render the GBM more permeable to proteins. Lagrue *et al.* (1991) reported the case of a woman with steroid-resistant FSGS, who twice delivered children who were proteinuric and hypoalbuminaemic at birth. In each infant, proteinuria and nephrotic syndrome disappeared within 2 and 3 weeks respectively. The second observation concerns a 20-year-old male with minimal-change disease who died of cerebral haemorrhage, and whose kidneys were transplanted into two recipients whose primary renal disease was not nephrosis. In both cases, proteinuria subsided and then disappeared within 6 weeks, along with disappearing features of minimal-change disease (Ali *et al.* 1994).

Pathogenesis of glomerular sclerosis

Focal–segmental glomerulosclerosis—a podocyte disease

It can be safely admitted that the podocyte is the major player in the genesis of FSGS (Kriz 1994; Kihara 1997; Kriz and Lemley 1999). It is tempting to believe that in human FSGS a factor, or factors, that injure the glomerular visceral epithelial cell are responsible for both GBM hyperpermeability and a 'podocyte disease' preceding focal sclerosis. These factors may be humoral, mechanical, or both.

In rats, puromycin- and adriamycin-induced early lesions comprise podocyte detachment from the glomerular basement membrane, effacement of foot processes, and an increased in organelle content, followed by the typical lesion of focal sclerosis (Fries 1989). This recalls the electron microscopic observations of Grishman *et al.* (1976) showing in the human that a toxic substance, heroin, induces nephrotic syndrome with FSGS in which the initial lesions affect glomerular podocytes.

The visceral epithelial cell is the first victim of the process that leads to focal scarring in cases of relapse after renal transplantation (Verani and Hawkins 1986; Korbet *et al.* 1988; Bariéty *et al.* 2001).

Serial histological observations, confirmed earlier findings in patients with focal sclerosis (Grishman and Churg 1975; Schwartz and Lewis 1985).

Kriz (1996) stressed the inability of podocytes to replicate, the loss of even a single podocyte possibly initiating the degeneration of the whole glomerulus. The same team showed that mechanical stress *per se* affects this particular cell, a cell that is essential in maintaining the glomerular structure (Kriz *et al.* 1994; Endlich *et al.* 2001). This could bear a relationship with the increased glomerular diameter observed in FSGS (Fogo *et al.* 1990; Savin 1993; D'Agati 1994; Muda *et al.* 1994) and partly be in keeping with a haemodynamic 'Brennerian' interpretation of secondary FSGS (Rennke and Klein 1989).

Growth factors in the development of focal–segmental glomerulosclerosis

FSGS is basically composed of excess matrix and sclerosis. The pathophysiology of a lesion so destructive for the glomerular tuft is still a matter of speculation. Conversely, there is a host of arguments for the role of growth factors in promoting excess synthesis of extracellular matrix comprising ubiquitous collagen, proteoglycans, and glycoproteins. Among the many likely candidates for eliciting collagen secretion, angiotensin 2, platelet-derived growth factor, thromboxane A_2, deposition of macromolecules, coagulation factors, lipids, and transforming growth factor-β could possibly be at work (Ichikawa *et al.* 1991; Border *et al.* 1995; Floege *et al.* 1995; Tanaka *et al.* 1995; Sasaki *et al.* 1999).

Treatment and outcome in children

Symptomatic treatment

Diet

Diet should include a protein intake of around 130–140 per cent of the normal daily allowance according to statural age. Salt restriction is mandatory for the prevention and treatment of oedema, and a very low salt diet is necessary in case of massive oedema. Fluid restriction is recommended for moderate to severe hyponatraemia (plasma sodium concentration < 125 mmol/l). A reduction of saturated fat is advisable. Carbohydrates are given preferentially as starch or dextrin–maltose, avoiding sucrose which increases lipid disturbances.

Hypovolaemia

Hypovolaemia, a consequence of rapid loss of serum albumin may be aggravated by diuretics. This complication requires emergency treatment by rapid infusion of plasma (20 ml/kg) or albumin 20 per cent (1 g/kg) administrated with monitoring of heart rate, respiratory rate, and blood pressure (see Chapter 3.4).

Diuretics

Diuretics should only be used in cases of severe oedema, after hypovolaemia has been corrected. Patients with anasarca may be treated with furosemide (1–2 mg/kg) or, if necessary, furosemide and salt-poor albumin (1 g/kg infused over 4 h) to increase the rate of diuretic delivery to the kidney (Fliser *et al.* 1999). This approach is immediately effective, but not longlasting. Moreover, respiratory distress with congestive heart failure have been observed in some patients (Haws and Baum 1993). Spironolactone (5–10 mg/kg) may be prescribed provided serum creatinine is normal. Diuretics must be used with caution. They may induce intravascular volume depletion with a risk of thromboembolism and of acute renal failure. Refractory oedema with serous effusions may require drainage of ascites and/or pleural effusions. Head-out immersion has been reported to be helpful in these cases (Rasher *et al.* 1986).

Thromboembolism (see also Chapter 3.4)

All nephrotic patients with severe hypoalbuminaemia are at risk for thromboembolic complications. Prevention includes mobilization, avoiding haemoconcentration and treating early sepsis or volume depletion. Prophylactic warfarin must be given to patients with a plasma albumin concentration below 20 g/l, a fibrinogen level greater than 6 g/l, or an antithrombin III level less than 70 per cent of normal. Patients at risk may alternatively be treated with low-dose aspirin and dipyridamole, although no controlled trials have been performed to demonstrate their efficacy for preventing thrombosis (McBryde 2001).

Heparin is given initially if thrombosis occurs, alone or with thrombolytic agents. Heparin dosage obtaining therapeutic efficacy is often greater than normally, due to decreased antithrombin III levels.

Antihypertensive drugs

Hypertension must be treated, using a β-blocker or a calcium channel blocker during acute episodes. In cases of persisting hypertension, an angiotensin-converting enzyme (ACE) inhibitor or an inhibitor of angiotensin 2 receptors are preferred.

Infections and immunizations

Prophylaxis of *S. pneumoniae* with oral penicillin is often prescribed in children during initial corticosteroid treatment. Although antibody response to pneumonococcal vaccine is blunted in children with steroid responsive nephrotic syndrome (Spika 1982), vaccination with the conjugated pneumococcal vaccine (7vPCV) is recommended (Overturf 2000). In cases of peritonitis, antibiotics against both *S. pneumoniae* and Gram-negative organisms are started after peritoneal fluid sampling. Varicella is a serious disease in patients receiving immunosuppressive treatment or daily corticosteroids. Varicella immunity status should therefore be assessed. In case of exposure, early prevention by acyclovir must be instituted. Immunization with a live virus is contraindicated in immunosuppressed patients.

Hyperlipidaemia (see also Chapter 3.4)

Hyperlipidaemia is a risk factor for atherosclerosis and may play a role in the progression of chronic renal failure. Experience with hypolipidaemic drugs in nephrotics is still limited but HMG-Co reductase inhibitors seem effective in decreasing hypercholesterolaemia (Coleman *et al.* 1996; Sanjad *et al.* 1997). Creatine phosphokinase levels must be monitored at regular intervals. Although long-term side-effects of these drugs are not known, it is reasonable to consider a lipid-lowering regimen in children with a persistent nephrotic syndrome.

Miscellaneous (see also Chapter 3.4)

Calcium metabolism may be altered by urinary loss of 25-hydroxycholecalciferol and its carrier protein. Preventive treatment with vitamin D supplements is advisable. Thyroxine substitution may be indicated, but only in patients with documented hypothyroidism due to urinary loss of iodinated proteins.

Specific treatment

The prognosis of INS is directly related to the response to corticosteroids. This treatment must be applied in all cases of INS whatever the histopathology, even in FSGS, both in children and in adults (Agarwal *et al.* 1994).

The majority of patients are steroid-responsive: 89 per cent of children studied by White *et al.* (1970) and 98 per cent of the patients with minimal changes on histology. Steroid responders may relapse, but the majority still responds over the subsequent course (Habib and Kleinknecht 1971). Only 1–3 per cent of patients initially steroid-sensitive subsequently become steroid-resistant and are defined as 'late non-responders' (Habib and Kleinknecht 1971; Siegel *et al.* 1974; Trainin *et al.* 1975). Conversely, patients who do not respond to an initial steroid regimen given at an adequate dosage usually remain non-responders. Response to corticosteroids is therefore the best prognostic index, not only since non-responders are more exposed to complications of persistent nephrotic syndrome, but also (and mainly) because they may develop ESRD after several years.

Initial treatment

Steroids should not be started too early as spontaneous remission may occur in 5 per cent of cases within the first 8–15 days (Habib and Kleinknecht 1971; Cameron *et al.* 1974). Some of these early spontaneous remissions are definitive, others are not. Infection must be sought and treated before starting steroids, not only to prevent the risk of overwhelming sepsis during treatment, but also because occult infection may be responsible for steroid resistance (McEnery and Strife 1982). Metronidazole must not be forgotten for preventing malignant *Strongyloides stercoralis* infestation in patients from countries where carriage of this worm is endemic.

Corticosteroids

Steroid therapy is started when the diagnosis of INS is most likely in a child or after renal biopsy has been performed. Prednisone remains the reference drug. Prednisolone has the advantage of being soluble in water, making treatment easier in young children, but it may fail to induce remission in some patients who respond quickly to the same dosage of prednisone. The vagaries of its intestinal absorption and drug interactions, for instance with aluminium gels, may explain resistance to this form of corticosteroid regimen.

The International Study of Kidney Disease in Children regimen consists of prednisone, 60 mg/m^2/day with a maximum of 80 mg/day, in divided doses for 4 weeks followed by 40 mg/m^2/day with a maximum of 60 mg/day in divided doses, on three consecutive days per week for 4 weeks. The Arbeitsgemeinschaft für pädiatrische Nephrologie (1979) showed that an alternate-day regimen (40 mg/m^2 every other day for 4 weeks) resulted in a significantly lower number of patients with relapses and fewer relapses per patient. It also showed that on alternate days prednisone can be given in a single dose rather than in divided doses.

A response occurs in most cases within 10–15 days (median 11 days). According to the International Study of Kidney Disease in Children (1981), approximately 90 per cent of responders enjoy remission 4 weeks after starting steroids, less than 10 per cent are pushed to remission after 2–4 more weeks of a daily regimen. A few more patients go into remission after 8–12 weeks of daily steroids (Schlesinger *et al.* 1968; International Study of Kidney Disease in Children 1978), but prolongation of daily steroid treatment beyond 4 or 5 weeks dramatically increases the risk of side-effects. An alternative for patients who are not in remission after 4 weeks is to inject three to four pulses of methylprednisolone (1 g/1.73 m^2). This additional regimen seems to be associated with fewer side-effects than prolongation of daily high-dose steroids and probably produces remission more rapidly in the few patients who would have entered the second month of daily therapy (Murnaghan *et al.* 1984).

Duration of initial steroid therapy bears on the risk of relapse. The APN compared a standard regimen of 4-week daily prednisone and 4 weeks of alternate-day prednisone with a shorter course comprising prednisone given at a dose of 60 mg/m^2/day until the urine was protein free, followed by alternate day prednisone until serum albumin returned to normal (Arbeitsgemeinschaft für pädiatrische Nephrologie 1979). Treatment lasted approximately 1 month in children receiving the short course. However, these children had a relapse rate that was doubled so that, at the end of the trial, they had received an amount of prednisone substantially greater than in the standard treatment group.

Following an 8-week steroid regimen, 50–70 per cent of children experience relapses. Several controlled studies have compared the 8-week regimen with longer duration of steroid regimen (3–7 months) including 4–8 weeks of daily prednisone followed by alternate-day prednisone (Ueda *et al.* 1988; Ehrich *et al.* 1993; Ksiazek *et al.* 1995; Norero *et al.* 1996; Bagga *et al.* 1999). With a follow-up of 2 years, a significant reduction of 25–30 per cent in the relapse rate was observed with a prednisone regimen of 3 months or more.

The number of children with frequent relapses is also decreased with a longer course of prednisone. A longer duration is more important than the cumulative dose of prednisone in reducing the risk of relapse. This relative risk decreases by 0.133 (13 per cent) for every additional month of treatment up to 7 months (Hodson *et al.* 2000). There are no data showing that treating for more than 7 months is beneficial. However, an alternate-day regimen over a year did not reduce the rate of relapse compared to a 5-month alternate-day regimen (Kleinknecht *et al.* 1982). Although the studies were not designed to analyse the side-effects of glucocorticoids, the authors did not report increased toxicity with longer duration of treatment.

Corticosteroid-responsive nephrosis in children

Nephrosis is steroid responsive in most cases, at least in children. About 30 per cent of patients experience only one attack and are definitively cured after a single course of steroids. Persistent remission for 18–24 months after stopping adequate treatment is likely to reflect definitive cure, and the risk of later relapses is low. About 10–20 per cent of patients relapse several months after stopping treatment and are apparently free of disease after three or four episodes which respond to a standard course of corticosteroids. The remaining 50–60 per cent experience frequent relapses as soon as steroid therapy is stopped or when dosage is decreased. In some cases, exacerbations of proteinuria are only transient, and spontaneous remissions are observed (Wingen *et al.* 1985). The risk of relapse is greater in children aged less than 5 years at onset and in males. These steroid dependent patients often raise difficult therapeutic problems.

Steroid-dependent nephrotics may be treated with repeated courses of prednisone, 60 mg/m^2/day, continued 3 days after the urine has become protein free, followed by alternate-day prednisone, 40 mg/m^2, for 4 weeks as proposed by the International Study of Kidney Disease in Children (1981). Another option is based on treating relapses with daily prednisone, 40–60 mg/m^2, until proteinuria has disappeared for 4–5 days. Thereafter, prednisone is switched to alternate days and the dosage is tapered to 15–20 mg/m^2 every other day, according to the steroid threshold, that is, the dosage at which the relapse has occurred. Treatment is then continued for 12–18 months. The first approach allows better definition in terms of relapses but is associated with more relapses. The latter regimen is associated with less steroid side effects as the cumulative dosage is lower. Prolonged courses of alternate-day steroid therapy are often well tolerated by young children and growth velocity is not affected. However, prednisone dosage must be as low as possible for reducing side-effects. In adolescents, steroid therapy is often accompanied by decreased growth velocity.

A controlled trial has shown that deflazacort reduces the risk of relapse in comparison with equivalent doses of prednisone, without additional side-effects (Broyer *et al.* 1997).

The role of upper respiratory tract infections in exacerbating nephrotic syndrome has been highlighted in all series: 71 per cent of relapses were preceded by such an event in a prospective study, although only 45 per cent of respiratory infections were followed by an exacerbation of proteinuria (McDonald *et al.* 1986). Mattoo *et al.* (2000) found that the risk of relapse was decreased during upper respiratory tract infections when prednisone was given daily for 5 days rather than on alternate days.

Leisti *et al.* (1977) suggested a role for postcorticosteroid adrenal suppression in triggering relapses, and some clinicians have suggested a possible prevention by low-dose maintenance hydrocortisone (Leisti *et al.* 1978).

Alternative treatments

An alternative treatment is required in children who relapse on alternate-day prednisone therapy and suffer severe side-effects such as growth retardation, behaviour disturbances, Cushingoid features, hypertension, cataract, or osteopenia. Such treatment is also indicated in children at risk of toxicity such as diabetes or during puberty, in children with severe relapses accompanied by thrombotic complications or severe hypovolaemia and in those with poor compliance (Anonymous, 1994).

Alternative treatments include levamisole which has a weak steroid sparing effect, alkylating agents such as cyclophosphamide or chlorambucil and cyclosporin.

Levamisole

The beneficial effect of levamisole was first described by Tanphaichitr *et al.* (1980), and was subsequently reported to reduce the risk of relapse in steroid-dependent patients (Niaudet *et al.* 1984; Mehta *et al.* 1986; Drachman *et al.* 1988; Mongeau *et al.* 1988). A significant steroid-sparing effect at a dose of 2.5 mg/kg every other day was demonstrated in a prospective controlled trial (British Association for Paediatric Nephrology 1991). Another controlled study confirmed the efficacy of levamisole for preventing relapses (Dayal 1994). However, the beneficial effect of levamisole is not sustained after stopping treatment.

Levamisole given for 6 months was compared with cyclophosphamide given for 8–12 weeks in a retrospective study involving 51 children with steroid dependent nephrotic syndrome (Alsaran *et al.* 2001). The relapse rate and the cumulative dose of prednisone were reduced to the same extent with both drugs.

Side-effects occasionally include neutropenia, agranulocytosis, vomiting, cutaneous rash, neurological symptoms including insomnia, hyperactivity, and seizures (Palcoux 1994). In fact, levamisole is well tolerated in most children.

Alkylating agents

Alkylating agents have been used for more than 50 years to achieve long-lasting remission. Three drugs have been used: cyclophosphamide, chlorambucil, and mechlorethamine.

Cyclophosphamide

The efficacy of cyclophosphamide for preventing relapses of INS was reported almost 40 years ago, and was proven in a prospective study by Barratt and Soothill (1970), who compared an 8-week course of cyclophosphamide to prednisone alone. A trial found a 48 per cent relapse rate after a mean follow-up of 22 months in children treated with a combination of cyclophosphamide and prednisone compared to a 88 per cent relapse rate in patients on prednisone alone.

Several studies have addressed the relation between dose and duration of treatment and therapeutic efficacy. Treatment for 12 weeks at a daily dose of 2 mg/kg was found more effective than an 8-week course, with 67 per cent as compared to 22 per cent remaining in remission after 2 years (Arbeitsgemeinschaft für pädiatrische Nephrologie 1987). However, a randomised trial showed that prolonging the course of cyclophosphamide from 8 to 12 weeks did not further reduce the proportion of children experiencing relapses (Ueda *et al.* 1990).

Cyclophosphamide is less effective in patients with steroid dependency compared to patients with frequent relapses (Arbeitsgemeinschaft für pädiatrische Nephrologie 1982).

The incidence of relapse after cyclophosphamide is significantly higher in patients with FSGS (73 per cent) or mesangial proliferation, compared to 22 per cent in children with minimal changes (Siegel *et al.* 1981).

Cyclophosphamide toxicity includes bone marrow depression, haemorrhagic cystitis, gastrointestinal disturbances, alopecia, and infection. Leucopenia is frequently observed, but weekly haematological monitoring may limit its severity and concomitant steroids help blunt marrow depression. Haemorrhagic cystitis rarely occurs. Alopecia, which is variably pronounced, remits a few weeks after stopping treatment. Viral infections can be overwhelming if cyclophosphamide is not stopped in due time.

Long-term toxiciy includes malignancy, pulmonary fibrosis, ovarian fibrosis, and sterility. Gonadal toxicity is well established and the risk of sterility is greater in boys than in girls. The cumulative threshold dose above which oligo/azoospermia may be feared lies between 150 and 250 mg/kg (Hsu *et al.* 1979; Trompeter *et al.* 1981). Azoospermia is reversible in some patients (Buchanan *et al.* 1975). In females, the cumulative dose associated with sterility is greater, but not well defined. Pregnancies have been reported after treatments longer than 18 months (Watson *et al.* 1986).

Chlorambucil

Beneficial results have also been achieved with chlorambucil in steroid-responsive nephrosis. Grupe (1973) demonstrated the efficacy of chlorambucil given for 2.5–12 weeks, with a relapse rate of only 13 per cent. Grupe *et al.* (1976), in a controlled trial of chlorambucil for 6–12 weeks, observed prolonged remissions of 1–3 years. Baluarte *et al.* (1978) obtained similar results in relapsing, steroid-responsive nephrosis. Williams *et al.* (1980) showed that low daily doses are preferable: 91 per cent of patients on a dose of 0.3 mg/kg and 80 per cent of those on 3 mg/kg were still in remission 4 years later.

Acute toxic effects are less frequent with chlorambucil than with cyclophosphamide. Leucopenia and thrombocytopenia may occur, and are reversible within 1–3 weeks. Severe microbial and viral infections have been reported, including malignant hepatitis and measles encephalitis.

Long-term toxic effects include the risk of developing cancer or leukaemia, which has only been reported in patients who had prolonged courses of treatment (Kleinknecht *et al.* 1977; Müller and Brandis 1981). Gonadal toxicity, as with cyclophosphamide, essentially affects boys. Azoospermia is total and probably irreversible at cumulative doses above 10–20 mg/kg. No case of azoospermia was reported in patients given less than 8 mg/kg.

Cyclosporin

Cyclosporin has been shown in a number of uncontrolled studies to reduce the incidence of relapses in 75–90 per cent of patients with steroid-dependent nephrotic syndrome. However, most patients experience relapses when the dosage is tapered, or when cyclosporin is withdrawn. The patients thus behave with cyclosporin as they did with steroids; that is, they become cyclosporin dependent. The relapse rate usually returns to the pretreatment rate. Hulton *et al.* (1993) found that patients in whom cyclosporin had been discontinued and later restarted had more relapses, requiring steroids in addition to cyclosporin in order to maintain remission.

The effects of cyclosporin have been evaluated in two comparative trials in steroid-sensitive patients. Cyclosporin at a dosage of 6 mg/kg/day for 3 months, then tapered over 3 months was compared with chlorambucil given for 2 months. At 12 months, 30 per cent of patients who had received chlorambucil and only 5 per cent of those who were still in remission on cyclosporin (Niaudet 1992). A multicentre randomized controlled trial compared cyclosporin for 9 months then tapered over 3 months, with oral cyclophosphamide for 2 months (Ponticelli *et al.* 1993a). After 2 years, 25 per cent of the patients (50 per cent of adults and 20 per cent of children) who had received cyclosporin had not relapsed, whilst 63 per cent of those treated with cyclophosphamide (40 per cent of adults and 68 per cent of children) were still in remission. During the year following treatment, the relapse rate (1.8 versus 0.7) and the steroid dosage required (109 versus 23 mg/kg/year) were significantly higher in children who had received cyclosporin.

Tejani *et al.* (1991) led a randomized controlled trial comparing low-dose prednisone and cyclosporin versus high-dose prednisone for 8 weeks as first line treatment in 28 children. Thirteen of the 14 children receiving the combined treatment went into remission compared to only 8/14 receiving prednisone alone ($p < 0.05$). The duration of remission after ending treatment was comparable in both groups. Ingulli and Tejani (1992) reported that severe hypercholesterolaemia may inhibit cyclosporin efficacy, and require higher dosages for similar results.

Considering cyclosporin dependency, this treatment must be pursued to prevent new relapses. Thus, some consider that steroid-dependent patients should first be treated with alkylating agents before resorting to cyclosporin, given its potential nephrotoxicity (British Association for Paediatric Nephrology 1994; Niaudet and Habib 1994).

Cyclosporin use carries a risk of nephrotoxicity. It is often difficult to determine if the decrease of renal function is merely functional, or due to the natural progression of the disease or to the nephrotoxic effect of the drug, in particular in patients who do not respond to treatment. In these cases, it is advisable to reduce dosage or even stop the treatment. Renal function improvement of is in favour of functional renal insufficiency or drug nephrotoxicity. Nevertheless, lesions of chronic nephrotoxicity can develop without any appreciable decline of the GFR (Habib and Niaudet 1994; Meyrier *et al.* 1994). It is often necessary to continue treatment for a long time and repeat renal biopsies are highly advisable to detect these lesions. They most often consist of tubulointerstitial injury, characterized by stripes of interstitial fibrosis containing clusters of atrophic tubules and by vascular lesions.

Other side-effects are of less concern: hypertension, hyperkalaemia, hypertrichosis, gum hypertrophy, and hypomagnesaemia are common but easily manageable.

Azathioprine, mycophenolate mofetil

Abramowicz *et al.* (1970) performed a controlled, multicentre trial in children showing that azathioprine had no effect in preventing relapses, but preliminary data suggest that empirical treatment with mycophenolate mofetil has a beneficial effect in inducing remission (Choi *et al.* 2002). The possible role of this agent in INS is under study, but not clear yet.

Steroid-resistant idiopathic nephrotic syndrome in children

In children, steroid resistance may be defined as failure to respond to at least 4 weeks of daily prednisone, 60 mg/m^2. Some clinicians continue the treatment for one or two weeks whilst others favour a series of three methylprednisolone pulses. In an International Study of Kidney Disease in Children prospective study (1978), 94 per cent of the patients who responded after 8 weeks had already responded after 4 weeks. According to this definition, less than 10 per cent of children are non-responders.

Alkylating agents

Although alkylating agents have limited efficacy in steroid-resistant patients, they are still widely used, alone or in combination with corticosteroids, cyclophosphamide more often than chlorambucil. The rate of full or partial remission is higher in patients with partial steroid resistance, those with late steroid resistance, or those in whom initial renal biopsy has shown minimal changes, by comparison with those showing initial resistance to corticosteroids and/or those with FSGS. The International Study of Kidney Disease in Children performed a controlled randomized trial and concluded on the lack of beneficial effect of oral cyclophosphamide in children with steroid resistant FSGS (Tarshish *et al.* 1996). In a controlled trial including 13 children with steroid resistant minimal-change disease, intravenous pulses of cyclophosphamide were shown to be beneficial when compared to oral cyclophosphamide (Ehlence *et al.* 1994).

Chlorambucil has been used with some success in small uncontrolled studies. Baluarte *et al.* (1980) described remissions in 10 of 17 cases. Williams *et al.* (1980) treated six children who all went into remission with a follow-up of 1.3–9.4 years.

Pulse methylprednisolone plus alkylating agents

A protocol consisting of methylprednisolone pulses, and oral prednisone with or without alkylating agents was shown to induce complete remission in 21/32 children (Tune *et al.* 1995). Despite the high cumulative dose of steroids side-effects were reported to be minimal. Although these results are encouraging, a multicentre study did not confirm the efficacy of pulse methylprednisolone (Guillot *et al.* 1993). Among 15 children with FSGS who received a mean of 15 pulses, only four maintained complete remission whilst five had a poor outcome with progression to ESRD or death. Waldo *et al.* (1992) did not observe remission in 10 children who were so treated whilst Hari *et al.* (2001) reported a 65 per cent response rate.

Combined immunosuppression including vincristine

Trompeter (1987) proposed aggressive immunosuppression including vincristine, cyclophosphamide, and prednisolone for patients with FSGS, refractory nephrotic syndrome, and/or rapid progression to renal failure. Lasting remission was observed in 7/21 children. Almeida *et al.* (1994) observed a complete and stable remission in only 2/7 children who were treated in this fashion.

Azathioprine

Azathioprine was considered ineffective in steroid-resistant patients after the report of Abramowicz *et al.* (1970), who found no difference between a 3-month course of azathioprine and a placebo.

Cyclosporin

Initial reports on the use of cyclosporin in steroid-resistant INS showed poor results (Niaudet and Habib 1994). These were uncontrolled studies, each involving a limited number of patients. A prospective protocol of the French Society of Pediatric Nephrology included 65 children who were treated by an association of cyclosporin and prednisone (Niaudet and the French Society of Pediatric Nephrology 1994). Complete remission was observed in 42 per cent of the children (48 per cent of those with minimal change disease and 30 per cent of those with FSGS), whilst 6 per cent entered in partial remission and 52 per cent did not respond. The remission rate was higher in patients who had initially responded to steroids but had developed steroid resistance (71 per cent) compared with initially steroid non-responders (33 per cent). Progression to chronic or terminal renal failure was observed only in patients who had had a partial remission (one patient) or in those who did not respond to the treatment (12 patients including five with minimal-change disease and seven with FSGS).

Gregory *et al.* (1996) treated 15 children with steroid resistant INS with an association of moderate doses of cyclosporine and prednisone. They observed a remission in 13 children after a mean duration of treatment of two months.

Ingulli *et al.* (1995) observed interesting results in Black American and Hispanic children with steroid resistant FSGS treated with a long course of cyclosporin. Dosage was adjusted according to serum cholesterol levels. Five of the 21 children progressed to terminal renal insufficiency, which represents a significantly lower percentage than was observed in a comparable previous series of 54 children of whom 42 (78 per cent) had progressed to ESRD.

Ponticelli *et al.* (1993b) compared the effect of a course of cyclosporin with a symptomatic treatment. Seven of the 22 patients treated with cyclosporin entered into remission, six in partial remission and nine did not respond. Remission was long-lasting in only 38 per cent of the patients who responded. In the control group, only 3/19 patients had a partial remission. Tejani and Liberman (1993) also performed a randomized double blind trial comparing cyclosporin to a placebo during a 6-month period. Proteinuria decreased in 12 treated patients and in only 2/12 patients receiving the placebo. The decrease of the GFR was comparable in both groups.

Singh *et al.* (1999) reported the effect of cyclosporin in 42 children with steroid resistant FSGS. Mean proteinuria decreased from 7.1 to 1.8 g/day whilst serum albumin increased from 2.1 g/dl to 3.5 g/dl. Mean serum creatinine increased from 0.85 to 1.26 mg/dl. Twenty-five patients responded with complete remission.

In sum, cyclosporin is effective in approximately 40 per cent of steroid-resistant patients. It should be used in combination with corticosteroids. The dose of cyclosporin may have to be increased in patients with high serum cholesterol levels. Close monitoring of serum creatinine levels is mandatory.

Tacrolimus (FK 506)

A few patients have been treated with this immunophillin modulator (McCauley *et al.* 1993). The results were not very convincing.

Non-steroidal anti-inflammatory drugs

Non-steroidal anti-inflammatory drugs decrease proteinuria. Donker *et al.* (1978) found a reduction of proteinuria in patients with focal sclerosis as a result of simultaneous reduction of the GFR. This effect was enhanced by a sodium-restricted diet, but was immediately reversible when the drug was discontinued. A clear reduction in proteinuria, with an increase in plasma albumin, was also reported in patients treated with meclofenamate in an uncontrolled study (Velosa *et al.* 1985). Apart from these seemingly encouraging reports, a high incidence of irreversible renal failure was observed in a prospective randomized study (Kleinknecht *et al.* 1980). Thus, non-steroidal anti-inflammatory drugs may help reduce proteinuria in some patients with steroid-resistant INS. However, these drugs must be administered with extreme caution. Their efficacy, along with the reversibility of renal insufficiency induced by these rather dangerous agents must be assessed at regular intervals by stopping treatment for several days.

Angiotensin-converting enzyme inhibitors

A decrease of proteinuria by 50 per cent without a concomitant decrease in GFR was reported in children with steroid-resistant nephrotic syndrome following treatment with ACE inhibitors (Milliner and Morgensten 1991). The role of ACE inhibitors in preventing deterioration of renal function that has been reported in experimental animals with reduced renal mass (see Section 9) is another reason to consider this prescription in patients with refractory INS.

The combination of an ACE inhibitor such as captopril and a non-steroidal anti-inflammatory drug such as indomethacin was reported to decrease proteinuria still more effectively, but the patient must be carefully followed (Allon *et al.* 1990).

Pefloxacin

Pruna *et al.* (1992) reported that pefloxacin was effective in both steroid-resistant and -dependent patients. However, a disappointing experience was reported in a series of six steroid-resistant patients (Geffriaud-Ricouard *et al.* 1993).

Long-term outcome in children with idiopathic nephrotic syndrome

Initially steroid-responsive patients

About one-third of patients have only one attack and are definitively cured after the course of corticosteroids. About 10–20 per cent of patients relapse several months after stopping the treatment and a cure takes place after three or four episodes, which respond to a standard course of corticosteroids. The remaining 40–50 per cent of patients experience frequent relapses either as soon as steroid therapy is stopped or when the dosage is decreased. These patients are steroid dependent and the disease may have a prolonged course. However, if the patient continues to respond to steroids, the risk of progression to chronic renal failure is minimal.

Schärer and Minges (1973) found that 22 per cent of patients had only one attack and 35 per cent of the relapsing patients continued to relapse after 10 years. Trompeter *et al.* (1985) reported the late outcome of 152 children steroid-responsive nephrotic syndrome after a follow-up of 14–19 years: 127 (83 per cent) were in remission, four had hypertension, 10 were still relapsing, and 11 had died. The duration of the disease was longer in children who had started before the age of 6 years. Wynn *et al.* (1988) found that 15 per cent of 132 patients had a persistent relapsing course with a mean follow-up of 27.5 year. Lewis *et al.* (1989) reported on 26 patients over the age of 20 years at last follow-up, of whom 5 (19.2 per cent) were still relapsing in adulthood.

Koskimies *et al.* (1982), analysed all patients with INS in Finland from 1967 to 1976: 94 of 114 cases responded to corticosteroids—24 per cent of these had no relapse, 22 per cent infrequent relapses, and 54 per cent frequent relapses, more than two-thirds being in long remission at time of report. None of these patients developed renal insufficiency and none died from the disease.

It is noteworthy that this generally good long-term prognosis is also observed in patients with steroid-responsive focal and segmental glomerular sclerosis: the 19 children reported by Arbus *et al.* (1982) remained responders, and none had renal insufficiency after a mean follow-up of 10 years.

Late non-responders

Some patients who initially respond to steroids become unresponsive after a few months to more than 10 years. This course was noted in 2–5 per cent of patients with steroid-sensitive nephrotic syndrome (Trainin *et al.* 1975; Srivastava *et al.* 1985). These patients may later achieve remission either after another course of steroid treatment or, more often, after cyclophosphamide or cyclosporin. However, they may also progress to end-stage renal failure.

In summary, the long-term outcome of steroid-sensitive nephrotic syndrome may be considered as excellent for the majority of patients, in spite of the fact that approximately 50 per cent experience multiple relapses, the duration of the disease being longer with younger age at onset. After 10–15 years, 10–20 per cent of patients continue to relapse. Very few patients become late non-responders, and even fewer, probably less than 1 per cent, go into endstage renal failure, with the exception of some groups that include a majority of African-American children.

Primary non-responders

The main difference between responders and non-responders is the tendency of the latter to develop endstage renal failure, which is seen in less than 3 per cent of responders, even in the highly selected series. This complication occurs in 50 per cent or more of the steroid resistant patients after a follow-up of 10 years. The only 'benefit' of the decrease of GFR is the improvement of the nephrotic syndrome due to a decrease of proteinuria.

We have retrospectively analysed in the Enfants Malades series the outcome of 181 children with steroid-resistant idiopathic nephrotic syndrome who have been followed for at least 5 years. Eighty-five per cent were primary non-responders, 15 per cent late non responders, and 13 had a sibling affected by the same disease. Initial renal biopsy had shown MCD in 62 cases and FSGS in 119 cases. Renal survival rates were 65 per cent at 5 years, 50 per cent at 10 years, and 34 per cent at 15 years. Interestingly, the rate of progression to endstage renal failure was similar in patients with minimal changes or with FSGS on initial biopsy.

The data reported in other series are difficult to compare, as most of them deal with patients with FSGS. The Southwest Pediatric Nephrology Study Group (1985) reported 75 children with FSGS followed for periods of 7–217 months. Twenty-one per cent had progressed to endstage renal failure, 23 per cent had decreased GFR, 37 per cent had a persistent nephrotic syndrome and 11 per cent were in remission.

Progression to endstage renal failure has been reported to be more rapid in patients of African or Hispanic descent when compared with Caucasians. Ingulli and Tejani (1991) found that among 57 African American and Hispanic children, 50 per cent of them had reached endstage renal failure in 3 years and 95 per cent reached this stage after six years. In addition, among the children with INS, the proportion of those with steroid resistant FSGS tends to be more important in African-American and Hispanic children.

Treatment and outcome in adults

There are hints that adult nephrosis is not the same disease as in children. This is true in terms of glomerular lesions of FSGS (Fogo *et al.* 1995) and especially in terms of progression and treatment. Evolution and treatment in adults and children must then be discussed separately. However, the reader must forgive us for some repetitions between the foregoing section and this one, as some series include children and adults.

Response to corticosteroid therapy

Considerable differences in treatment schedules between adults and children have been reported in the literature (Korbet *et al.* 1988a; Meyrier and Simon 1988; Fujimoto *et al.* 1991; Mak *et al.* 1996; Nakayama *et al.* 2002) making comparisons of treatment results difficult. Definitions of steroid sensitivity, dependence, resistance, and multiple relapses vary among papers dealing with adult nephrosis, owing to lack of unified agreement regarding treatment protocol. Despite these shortcomings, an analysis of the literature (Meyrier and Simon 1988) showed that response to corticosteroids does not seem to differ greatly according to age, although it appears to be somewhat lower in adults (Fig. 9).

Minimal-change disease

The response of nephrosis to corticosteroids in adults is much slower than in children (Nolasco *et al.* 1986; Fujimoto *et al.* 1991; Korbet *et al.* 1994; Korbet 1995, 1999; Rydel *et al.* 1995; Mak *et al.* 1996; Nakayama *et al.* 2002). Fujimoto *et al.* (1991) treated 33 patients having adult-onset minimal-change disease with prednisolone at 1 mg/kg/day for 4–8 weeks, followed by slow tailing off, for a total duration of over 6 months. Seventy-six per cent of patients were pushed into remission within 8 weeks, but in the extant cases the longest time to remission was 4 months. Five patients went into remission whilst the steroid dosage was being tapered. Mak *et al.* (1996) treated 40 patients with adult-onset minimal-change nephropathy. The remission rate was 46 per cent by the fourth week, 69 per cent by the eighth week, 85 per cent by the sixteenth week, and 87 per cent by the twenty-first week. These figures clearly show that corticosteroid resistance in adult nephrosis should not be pronounced before 4 months, and probably even 6 months of treatment. However, it is clear that such long, full-dose treatment courses entail a proportionally increased risk of iatrogenic complications.

Another difference stems from the trend toward a diminished frequency of relapses with increasing age, provided nephrosis did not start during childhood.

Nolasco *et al.* (1986) followed 89 patients with adult-onset minimal change, 58 of whom responded to corticosteroid treatment: 24 per cent never relapsed, 56 per cent relapsed on a single occasion or infrequently, and only 21 per cent were frequent relapsers. Korbet *et al.* (1988b) followed 40 adults with minimal-change disease: 34 were treated with prednisone, and 31 (91 per cent) achieved remission, of whom only three suffered multiple relapses. Relapses were infrequent in 99 adult nephrotics with minimal-change disease followed by Wang *et al.* (1982) for 3–102 months. In 85 patients whose urine was protein-free for at least 6 months, four relapsed; of 46 who were protein-free for 24 months, three relapsed; of 37 followed for 36–96 months, only three relapsed. Nair *et al.* (1987) treated 54 adults with minimal-change disease. Only 17 had relapses, a rate of 31 per cent at 3 years of follow-up. Fujimoto *et al.* (1991) also found an incidence of relapse significantly lower in patients older than 30 years. Nakayama *et al.* (2002) analysed retrospectively 62 Japanese adult cases of minimal-change nephrotic syndrome. Five experienced remission spontaneously. Fifty-three entered complete remission, three partial remission, and one patient showed no response to corticosteroids. Fifty-three patients with complete remission were divided into two groups: 38 early responders who experienced remission completely within 8 weeks after starting treatment and 15 late responders who experienced remission after 8 weeks. Thirty-three patients experienced a relapse; 13 experienced multiple relapses. Fifty-three patients with remission were divided into three groups: 16 patients who experienced relapse within 6 months after the initial response (early relapsers), 17 who experienced relapse after 6 months (late relapsers), and 20 non-relapsers. Mean age at onset was younger in early relapsers than in late or non-relapsers. Age at onset correlated inversely with relapse rate in 53 patients with remission and correlated positively with timing of the first relapse in 33 relapsers.

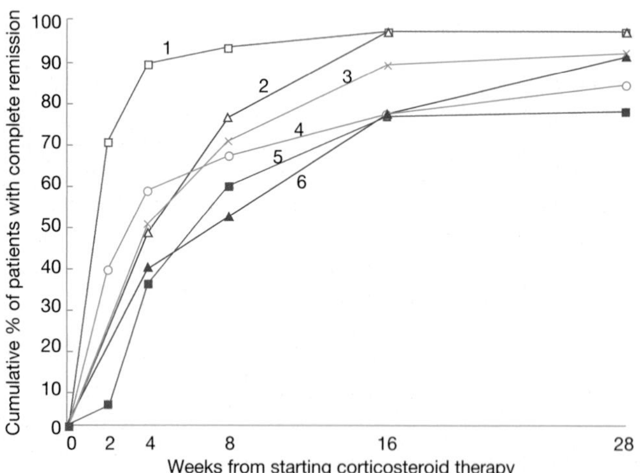

Fig. 9 Comparing the time of response to corticosteroid treatment in children (1) shows that the definition of corticosteroid resistance in adults (2–6) is in the order of 4 months. Many articles in the literature on the treatment of adult nephrosis are biased, as they adopt the same definition of 'steroid resistance' as for children, that is, 6–8 weeks of this regimen without remission. (1) International Study of Kidney Disease in Children (1981); (2) Fujimoto *et al.* (1991); (3) Mak *et al.* (1996); (4) Nakayama *et al.* (2002); (5) Nolasco *et al.* (1986); (6) Korbet *et al.* (1981). Source: Nakayama *et al.* (2002), with permission.

Thus, the experience of nephrologists treating adult nephrosis is comparable in Europe, America, and the Far East, with a multiple relapse rate in the order of 10–20 per cent, as opposed to a greater percentage in children.

Apart from age, insufficient treatment might also explain some of the relapses observed in adults. In four of six reports published between 1971 and 1988, patients were treated with a long course of steroids; in the other two a short regimen was used. The remission rate was comparable with the two treatment modes, but duration of remission was superior when patients received more than 8 months of prednisone. On comparing two groups of adult nephrotics of the same age, Simon and Meyrier (1989) showed that a long initial alternate-day corticosteroid regimen followed by slow tapering is effective in obtaining sustained remission in adult minimal-change disease.

Focal–segmental glomerulosclerosis

The prognosis of FSGS in adults depends on abundance of proteinuria and response to corticosteroids. Figure 10 indicates the prognostic value of 24-hr protein excretion in FSGS. Non-nephrotic proteinuria entails a good prognosis, and does not represent an indication for corticosteroid treatment. Nephrotic proteinuria portends an evolution to renal insufficiency that represent an indication for treatment. Proteinuria in excess of 14 g/24 h at presentation is ominous and predicts a precipitous course to ESRD.

Three points must be made. First, nephrotic FSGS in adults must always be allowed to benefit from a course of corticosteroid treatment, followed by other drugs when ineffective. Second, high-dose prednisone is clearly more effective than dosages less than 1 mg/kg/day. Third, as analysed above, response of FSGS to corticosteroids is much slower in adults than in children and that steroid resistance cannot be

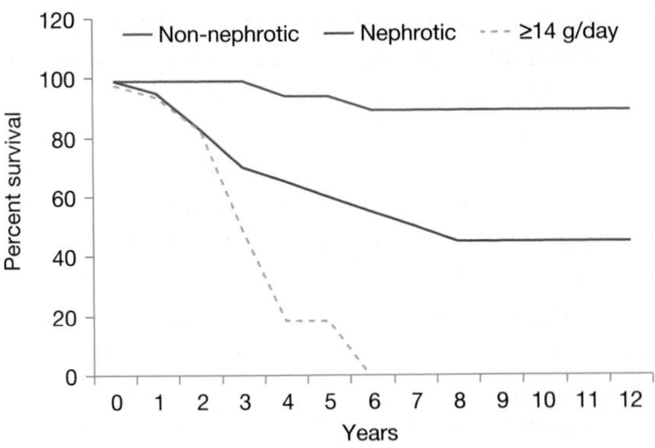

Fig. 10 The amount of 24 h proteinuria is the best predictor of outcome in FSGS. Source: Korbet (1999), with permission.

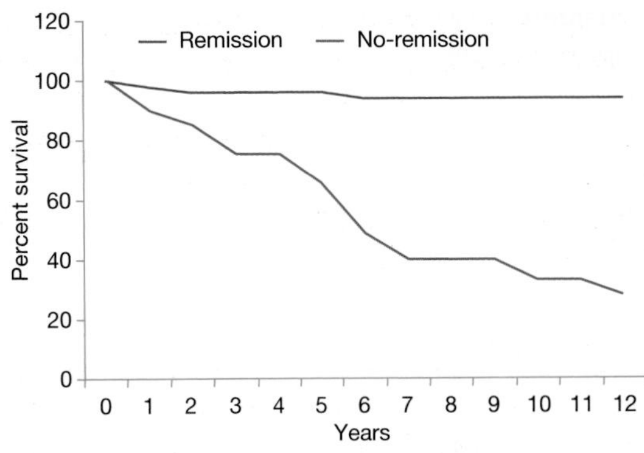

Fig. 11 Cumulative renal survival in patients achieving a complete remission as compared with those not achieving remission. Source: Korbet (1999), with permission.

Table 2 Response to corticosteroids in adult patients with idiopathic nephrotic syndrome (1961–1986)

	Patients (*n*)	Complete remissions (%)	Partial remissions (%)	Failures (%)
Minimal changes	301	226 (75.8)	21 (7)	55 (18.2)
Focal sclerosis	153	24 (15.6)	31 (20.2)	98 (64.2)
Biopsy not done	48	31 (64.6)	0 (0)	17 (35.4)
Total	502	281 (55.8)	52 (10.3)	170 (33.9)

pronounced before a minimum of 4 months of full-dose corticosteroid treatment Korbet (2002) (Table 2).

The necessity to treat adults with corticosteroids suffering from nephrotic FSGS has been a late concept. Until recently, nephrotic FSGS was considered a steroid-resistant disease. Then Pei *et al.* (1987), Banfi *et al.* (1991), Korbet (1994), and Meyrier (1999b) pointed out that, given its reputation for steroid resistance, many nephrologists caring for adults did not even try to treat them. The same authors showed that, in fact, this subset of nephrosis should always be treated with a long course of full-dose steroids, and that partial or even complete remission can be obtained, albeit less frequently than in minimal-change disease. Such findings are of practical importance, as steroid sensitivity of FSGS is a strong predictor of stable renal function up to 10 years of follow-up, whereas steroid resistance is predictive of development to ESRD in about 57 per cent of cases within an average of 6.5 years (Fig. 11). Whether corticosteroids prevent the further progression of focal sclerosis or just select a subset of patients whose evolution would have been favourable in any case is an academic debate and not an argument to eschew affirmative treatment.

That full dosage is more effective than timid low-dose prednisone regimens has now been established. Several publications dating back to the seventies dealt with prednisone dosages ranging from 0.2 to 0.5 mg/kg/day (Velosa *et al.* 1975; Newman *et al.* 1976; Beaufils *et al.* 1978). The rate of complete remission was at best 15 per cent, of partial remission 40 per cent and none of the patients was pushed to complete remission. Using full dose treatment, that is in the order of 1 mg/kg/day, complete remission was achieved in 35–45 per cent and partial remission in 15–25 per cent of the cases (Rydel *et al.* 1995; Cattran and Rao 1998; Ponticelli *et al.* 1999).

Time to remission is the third issue at stake that bears on treatment duration. Ponticelli *et al.* (1999) analysed the majority of published series and determined that in case of treatment duration shorter than 16 weeks the complete plus partial remission rate is in the order of 15 per cent, whilst treatments longer than 16 weeks are credited with a remission rate of 61 per cent. Such figures are essential to interpret treatment trials comparing the results of alternative drugs with those of corticosteroids, trials in which the definition of steroid resistance in adults is the same as that applied in paediatrics, that is absence of remission after a 1-month course of glucocorticoids.

Response to conventional immunosuppressive therapy

A review of the experience with various immunosuppressive regimens using cyclophosphamide, chlorambucil, and mechlorethamine published between 1966 and 1986 (Meyrier and Simon 1988) is summarized in Table 3. The indications were the same as in children, namely steroid-resistant, steroid-dependent, or relapsing INS. There were no significant differences in response rates between adults and children. The passage of time has not modified these figures. However, newer drugs have since been marketed for preventing renal graft rejection. They were subsequently tried for treating steroid-resistant or -dependent INS.

Azathioprine deserves special mention, since it has occasionally been administered to adult nephrotics, with a few anecdotal successful results (Meyrier and Simon 1988). Cade *et al.* (1986) studied the effect of azathioprine in 13 adult patients, including 11 in whom nephrosis appeared after the age of 14. The diagnosis was FSGS in four and minimal change disease in nine. Six were steroid-resistant from the outset; the others had multirelapsing nephrotic syndrome, and four eventually developed resistance. The results of prolonged treatment with azathioprine were favourable: the 12 patients who complied with follow-up progressively attained complete remission. Such observations should be an incentive to undertake large-scale, prospective controlled studies on the effect of 18 months of azathioprine in adult nephrosis.

Table 3 Response of adult patients with INS to conventional immunosuppressive drugs

	Patients (*n*)	Complete remissions (%)	Partial remissions (%)	Failures (%)
Minimal change disease	152	123 (80.9)	13 (8.5)	16 (10.5)
Focal sclerosis	63	16 (25.4)	8 (12.7)	36 (61.9)
Total	215	139 (64.6)	21 (9.8)	52 (25.6)

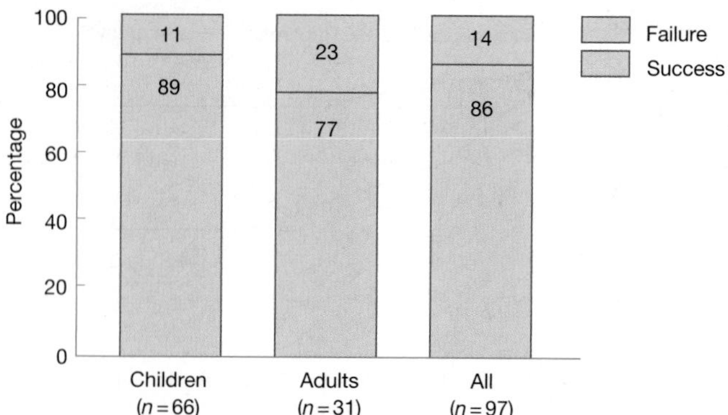

Fig. 12 Results of cyclosporin treatment in corticosteroid-sensitive nephrosis (minimal-change disease and FSGS). 'Success' regarded as complete remission or patterns of remission after dose reduction or withdrawal of steroids. [From Meyrier and Collaborative Group of the Société de Néphrologie (1989), with permission of the publisher.]

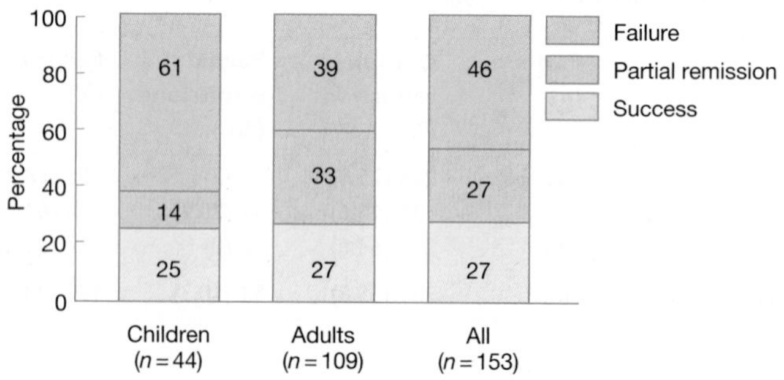

Fig. 13 Results of cyclosporin treatment in corticosteroid-resistant INS (minimal-change disease and FSGS). 'Success' regarded as complete remission or maintenance of remission after dose reduction or withdrawal of steroids. [From Meyrier and Collaborative Group of the Société de Néphrologie (1989), with permission of the publisher.]

Response to treatment with cyclosporin

Treatment of adult INS with cyclosporin was undertaken in 1986 (Meyrier and Collaborative Group of the Société de Néphrologie 1989; Meyrier *et al.* 1992, 1994; Ponticelli *et al.* 1993a,b; Cattran *et al.* 1999). Only minor differences were observed between children and adults treated with this drug.

In adults who respond to corticosteroids but suffer multiple relapses, cyclosporin-induced complete remission or maintained remission after dose reduction or withdrawal of steroids slightly less frequently in adults (77 per cent) than in children (89 per cent) (Meyrier and Collaborative Group of the Société de Néphrologie 1989). The success rate was lower in steroid-resistant patients, whether adults or children (Figs 12 and 13). The main difference stemmed from the interpretation of 'partial remission'. Apparently, more adults than children achieved such partial remission. The addition of low doses of corticosteroids produced slightly better results than with cyclosporin alone. As in children, cyclosporin had the major advantage of reducing the threshold of corticosteroid sensitivity and allowing a reduction in steroid dosage, or withdrawal.

Few controlled studies have been undertaken. Cattran *et al.* (1999) undertook a randomized trial in 49 adults, with two arms: cyclosporin plus prednisone versus placebo plus prednisone. The study was pursued for 104 weeks. The remission rate in the placebo subset was no better than 10 per cent. In the cyclosporin group, partial remission was slightly less than 60 per cent at 12 and 26 weeks and complete remission was in the order of, at best, 20 per cent. The results concerning renal function came as a surprise since, contrary to the majority of published series (especially that of Meyrier *et al.* 1994), renal function improved, rather than declined in the group with FSGS treated with cyclosporin.

Cyclosporin dependence: renal tolerance

A major concern in the treatment of adult nephrosis with cyclosporin is cyclosporin dependency. It has been published repeatedly that the drug exerts a suspensive, not a curative, effect on nephrotic syndrome, with a majority of cases relapsing when it is tapered to a stop. This in turn led to the prospect of using indefinitely a potentially nephrotoxic drug to maintain remission. The issue was reconsidered in the light of long-term surveillance of a series of adult patients treated with cyclosporin (Meyrier *et al.* 1994). This study showed that in one-third of cases, comprising a majority of patients with steroid-dependent, cyclosporin-responsive, minimal-change disease, treatment pursued for longer than 2 years followed by slow tailing off ended in persistent remission. The investigators suggested that in some instances the suspensive effect of cyclosporin on the ill-identified immunological process with induces massive proteinuria provides the time to reach a phase of extinction of the disease, which had already been observed in papers on the natural history of lipoid nephrosis published before corticosteroids were available, as specified above in the section dealing with children.

Concerning tolerance, Meyrier *et al.* (1994) established that in adults the cut-off dosage above which the drug in its previous presentation (Sandimmune®) becomes dangerously nephrotoxic in nephrosis is 5.5 mg/kg per day. Finally, in the light of repeat renal biopsies, renal tolerance appeared to differ according to the type of primary glomerular disease. Renal function and renal histology remained remarkably stable in patients with minimal-change disease. Conversely, in most cases renal function continued to deteriorate in patients with FSGS. Follow-up biopsies found a significant increase in glomeruli with segmental scars, obsolescent glomeruli, and interstitial fibrosis. The severity of tubulointerstitial lesions and fibrosis correlated positively with the percentage of glomeruli with segmental scars on the precyclosporin biopsy and with the serum creatinine at the time of beginning treatment. Thus, cyclosporin can be detrimental for patients with FSGS, especially those with pre-existing renal insufficiency and tubulointerstitial damage, and should be used with extreme caution in such patients (Korbet 1995). This caveat should probably apply with increased conviction regarding Neoral®, considering its better bioavailability. It is likely that the maximum safe dosage of this form of cyclosporin should be much lower than 5.5 mg/kg/day, although no data of the literature has yet determined the cut-off dosage beyond which toxicity should be feared.

Other immunosuppressive agents

Tacrolimus (FK 506)

As noted above, few children with INS have been treated with FK 506 (McCauley *et al.* 1993). The drug was nephrotoxic, dependency was observed and overall results were not superior to cyclosporin. Schweda *et al.* (1997) reported the case of a young woman with minimal-change disease, steroid dependency, and subsequent steroid resistance in whom remission was achieved with 4 mg/kg/day of FK 506. Follow-up was 20 months. The largest series dealing with a combination of tacrolimus and corticosteroids was published by Segarra *et al.* (2002). Twenty-five heavily proteinuric patients with proven resistance or dependency to cyclosporin were treated with tacrolimus and steroids for 6 months. Proteinuria decreased in 68 per cent, including 40 per cent complete remission and 8 per cent partial remission within 112 ±24 days. After tacrolimus discontinuation, 13/17 patients relapsed. Resuming treatment achieved complete remission in five, partial remission in four and reduction of proteinuria in four. After 2 years of follow-up 12 patients were in sustained remission. Acute, reversible toxicity was observed in 40 per cent.

Mycophenolate mofetil

Choi *et al.* (2002) treated empirically 46 patients with various glomerulopathies, including 11 with FSGS. Not all were nephrotic. The drug yielded short-term reduction in proteinuria. Renal function was stable in seven and worsened in four patients.

Recurrence of focal–segmental glomerulosclerosis in transplanted kidneys

Recurrence of nephrotic syndrome with FSGS was first reported by Hoyer *et al.* (1972). As the occurrence of nephrotic syndrome following transplantation (see Chapter 13.5) may be related to several causes, including *de novo* membranous nephropathy, allograft nephropathy, and chronic rejection, strict criteria have to be fulfilled before the diagnosis of recurrence is made in a transplanted patient with heavy proteinuria: past history of INS in the recipient associated with any of the morphological variants of this entity; demonstration in the graft of one of three patterns observed in patients with INS, and especially FSGS on late kidney graft biopsy. The rapid development of nephrotic syndrome after transplantation is an additional criterion, but not essential.

The overall risk of recurrence is estimated to be around 25 per cent, but it differs in children and in adult patients, as was shown in a single-centre study reporting eight recurrences in 16 children against three in 27 adults (Senggutuvan *et al.* 1990). In children, recurrence is more frequent when the disease started after rather than before 6 years of age (Habib *et al.* 1982).

Rapid development of endstage renal failure seems to be a major factor associated with recurrence. In most of the series a duration of disease shorter than 3 years was associated with a 50 per cent risk of recurrence (Leumann *et al.* 1980; Pinto *et al.* 1981; Habib *et al.* 1982).

The histopathological pattern observed on the first biopsy performed during the initial course of the disease is probably the most important predictive factor (Leumann *et al.* 1980; Maizel *et al.* 1981; Habib *et al.* 1982; Senggutuvan *et al.* 1990). Nephrosis recurred in 50–80 per cent of patients in whom mesangial proliferation was present on initial biopsy, whilst patients with minimal changes on the first biopsy had a recurrence rate of 20–25 per cent.

Risk factors for graft loss and graft loss resulting from recurrent FSGS of 101,808 renal transplant recipients were analysed by Abbott *et al.* (2001) from the 1999 data of the United States Renal Data System. Of these, 3861 recipients of renal transplants who had ESRD resulting from FSGS met inclusion criteria. The respective roles played by living donor donation and other factors was less straightforward than previously thought. As a percentage of all graft loss, recurrent FSGS accounted for 18.7 per cent in living donor recipients and 7.8 per cent in cadaveric recipients. In White recipients, the corresponding figures were 27 per cent and 13 per cent respectively. However, by multivariate analysis, factors associated with graft loss resulting from recurrent FSGS were white recipient, donor kidney Afro-American in White recipient, younger recipient age, and treatment for rejection. Black American recipients had higher rates of graft loss overall. A living donor was associated with superior overall graft survival. Among renal transplant, recipients with FSGS, White recipients had a higher risk of graft loss resulting from recurrent FSGS, disproportionately seen in recipients of Afro-American kidneys. The authors stressed that the role of donor–recipient race pairing on graft loss resulting from recurrent FSGS should be validated, considering that living donor had no association with graft loss from recurrent FSGS after correction for other factors.

Recurrence is usually marked by massive proteinuria as soon as urine is produced by the transplant (Maizel *et al.* 1981). Proteinuria and nephrotic syndrome may occur after several months or years, with a histological pattern suggesting recurrence.

Early graft biopsy shows typical electron microscopic changes, with fusion of epithelial-cell foot processes as early as 12 days following transplantation (Maizel *et al.* 1981). Focal sclerosis is invariably observed in patients who had immediate or early recurrence, at least on repeat biopsy. Bariéty *et al.* (2001) studied by immunohistochemistry and confocal laser microscopy six cases of FSGS that relapsed on a renal transplant. They observed that some 'dysregulated' podocytes, occasionally some parietal epithelial cells, and possibly some tubular epithelial cells underwent a process of transdifferentiation. This process of transdifferentiation was especially striking in podocytes that acquired macrophagic and cytokeratin epitopes that are absent from normal adult and fetal podocytes.

Recurrence is associated with an increased incidence of delayed graft function and acute rejection. Sixty per cent of patients with recurrence lost their graft, as compared with 23 per cent of those without recurrence in the Enfants Malades series. Similar failure rates were reported in other series (Pinto *et al.* 1981; Artero *et al.* 1992). Other patients show good renal function for many years despite proteinuria and nephrotic syndrome (Leumann *et al.* 1980; Pinto *et al.* 1981).

Plasma exchange have been used in several studies. The rate of persisting complete remission has varied from 8 to 67 per cent. The best results are observed when the treatment is started early after recurrence (Munoz *et al.* 1985; Dantal *et al.* 1991; Artero *et al.* 1992; Ohta *et al.* 2001). Immunoadsorption on a protein-A column was reported to be followed by more or less transient remission (Dantal *et al.* 1994).

Other treatments have been reported to reverse proteinuria, such as cyclophosphamide (Cochat *et al.* 1993; Cheong *et al.* 2000) and ACE inhibitors. Conflicting results have been observed with the use of cyclosporin in patients with recurrence. Banfi *et al.* (1991) found that 10 of 19 adult patients receiving cyclosporin as part of their immunosuppressive treatment showed recurrence. Moreover, cyclosporin did not improve the outcome of the disease compared to patients receiving azathioprine. Other studies have shown that cyclosporin given as part of the initial immunosuppressive regimen at conventional dosage does not modify the rate of recurrence. However, increased dose of cyclosporin may be beneficial in patients with recurrent nephrotic syndrome. Ingulli *et al.* (1990) reported two children with recurrent nephrotic syndrome following renal transplantation in whom proteinuria was controlled after high dose oral cyclosporin. Similarly, Srivastava *et al.* (1994) reported a rapid and sustained remission following high-dose oral cyclosporin in a child with recurrent nephrotic syndrome after renal transplantation. In the Enfants Malades group, 17 children with recurrence were treated with intravenous cyclosporin at an initial dose of 3 mg/kg per day which was afterwards adapted in order to maintain whole blood levels between 250 and 350 ng/ml. In 14 of the 17 cases (82 per cent), proteinuria completely disappeared after 20.8 ± 8.4 days (range: 12–40 days). The treatment was ineffective in the remaining three patients. Plasma exchanges were performed in four patients during the first 2 months and proteinuria regressed in three cases and persisted in one. Persistent remission was observed in 11 patients with a follow-up of 3.7 ± 3 years. Actuarial graft survival was 92 and 70 per cent at 1 and 5 years.

Management of patients who lose their graft due to recurrence is difficult. An incidence of 75 per cent multiple recurrences in successive allografts has been reported (Chandra *et al.* 1981; Senggutuvan *et al.* 1990) and the tendency to recur may persist for a long time, as shown by Senggutuvan *et al.* (1990) in a patient whose disease recurred on the fifth graft, 9 years after he was first started on dialysis.

References

Abbott, K. C. *et al.* (2001). Graft loss due to recurrent focal segmental glomerulosclerosis in renal transplant recipients in the United States. *American Journal of Kidney Diseases* **37**, 366–373.

Abramowicz, M. *et al.* (1970). Controlled trial of azathioprine in children with nephrotic syndrome. A report for the International Study of Kidney Disease in Children. *Lancet* **1**, 959–961.

Agarwal, S. K., Dash, S. C., Tiwari, S. C., and Bhuyan, U. N. (1993). Idiopathic adult focal segmental glomerulosclerosis: a clinicopathological study and response to steroid. *Nephron* **63**, 168–171.

Al-Azzawi, Y. H. M., Altawil, N. G., and Alshamaa, I. A. (1994). Lymphocyte transformation test in adult patients with minimal change nephrotic syndrome. *Scandinavian Journal of Immunology* **40**, 277–280.

Alfiler, C. A., Roy, L. P., Doran, T., Sheldon, A., and Bashir, H. (1980). HLA-DRW7 and steroid responsive nephrotic syndrome of childhood. *Clinical Nephrology* **14**, 71–74.

Ali, A. A. *et al.* (1994). Minimal-change glomerular nephritis. Normal kidneys in an abnormal environment? *Transplantation* **58**, 849–852.

Allon, M., Pasque, C., and Rodriguez, M. (1990). Acute effects of captopril and ibuprofen on proteinuria in patients with nephrosis. *Journal of Laboratory and Clinical Medicine* **116**, 462–468.

Almeida, M. P., Almeida, H. A., and Rosa, F. C. (1994). Vincristine in steroid-resistant nephrotic syndrome. *Pediatric Nephrology* **8**, 79–80.

Alsaran, K., Grisaru, S., Stephens, D., and Arbus, G. (2001). Levamisole *vs.* cyclophosphamide for frequently-relapsing steroid-dependent nephrotic syndrome. *Clinical Nephrology* **56**, 289–294.

Anonymous (1994). Consensus statement on management and audit potential for steroid responsive nephrotic syndrome. Report of a Workshop by the British Association for Paediatric Nephrology and Research Unit, Royal College of Physicians. *Archives of Disease in Childhood* **70**, 151–157.

Antignac, C. (2002). Genetic models: clues for understanding the pathogenesis of idiopathic nephrotic syndrome. *Journal of Clinical Investigation* **109**, 447–449.

Arbeitsgemeinschaft für pädiatrische Nephrologie (1979). Alternate-day *vs.* intermittent prednisone in frequently relapsing nephrotic syndrome. *Lancet* **i**, 401–403.

Arbeitsgemeinschaft für pädiatrische Nephrologie (1982). Effect of cytotoxic drugs in frequently relapsing nephrotic syndrome with or without steroid dependence. *New England Journal of Medicine* **306**, 451–454.

Arbeitsgemeinschaft für pädiatrische Nephrologie (1987). Cyclophosphamide treatment of steroid dependant nephrotic syndrome: comparison of eight week with 12 week course. *Archives of Diseases in Childhood* **62**, 1102–1106.

Arbus, G. S., Poucell, S., Bacheyie, G. S., and Baumal, R. (1982). Focal segmental glomerulosclerosis with idiopathic nephrotic syndrome: three types of clinical response. *Journal of Pediatrics* **101**, 40–45.

Artero, M., Biava, C., Amend, W., Tomlanovich, S., and Vincenti, F. (1992). Recurrent focal glomerulosclerosis: natural history and response to therapy. *American Journal of Medicine* **92**, 375–383.

Bagga, A., Hari, P., and Srivastava, R. N. (1999). Prolonged versus standard prednisolone therapy for initial episode of nephrotic syndrome. *Pediatric Nephrology* **13**, 824–827.

Baluarte, H. J., Hiner, L., and Gruskin, A. B. (1978). Chlorambucil dosage in frequently relapsing nephrotic syndrome: a controlled clinical trial. *Journal of Pediatrics* **92**, 295–298.

Baluarte, H. J., Gruskin, A. B., Polinski, M. S., Prebis, J. W., and Rosenblum, H. Chlorambucil therapy in the nephrotic syndrome. In *Pediatric Nephrology: Proceedings of the 5th International Pediatric Nephrology Symposium* (ed. A. B. Gruskin and H. E. Norman), pp. 423–429. The Hague: Martinus Nijhoff, 1980.

Banfi, G., Moriggi, M., Sabadini, E., Fellin, G., D'Amico, G., and Ponticelli, C. (1991). The impact of prolonged immunosuppression on the outcome of idiopathic focal–segmental glomerulosclerosis with nephrotic syndrome in adults. A collaborative retrospective study. *Clinical Nephrology* **36**, 53–59.

Barbaux, S. *et al.* (1997). Donor splice-site mutations in WT1 are responsible for Frasier syndrome. *Nature Genetics* **17**, 467–470.

Barbiano di Belgiojoso, G., Mazzucco, G., Casanova, S., Radaelli, L., Monga, G., and Minetti, L. (1986). Steroid-sensitive nephrotic syndrome with mesangial IgA deposits: a separate entity? *American Journal of Nephrology* **6**, 141–145.

Bariéty, J., Nochy, D., Mandet, C., Jacquot, C., Glotz, D., and Meyrier, A. (1998). Podocytes undergo phenotypic changes and express macrophagic-associated markers in idiopathic collapsing glomerulopathy. *Kidney International* **53**, 918–925.

Bariéty, J., Bruneval, P., Hill, G., Irinopoulou, T., Mandet, C., and Meyrier, A. (2001). Posttransplantation relapse of FSGS is characterized by glomerular epithelial cell transdifferentiation. *Journal of the American Society of Nephrology* **12**, 261–274.

Barisoni, L., Kriz, W., Mundel, P., and D'Agati, V. (1999). The dysregulated podocyte phenotype: a novel concept in the pathogenesis of collapsing idiopathic focal segmental glomerulosclerosis and HIV-associated nephropathy. *Journal of the American Society of Nephrology* **10**, 51–61.

Barisoni, L., Mokrzycki, M., Sablay, L., Nagata, M., Yamase, H., and Mundel, P. (2000). Podocyte cell cycle regulation and proliferation in collapsing glomerulopathies. *Kidney International* **58**, 137–143.

Barratt, T. M. and Soothill, J. F. (1970). Controlled trial of cyclophosphamide in steroid sensitive relapsing nephrotic syndrome of childhood. *Lancet* **ii**, 479–482.

Beaufils, H., Alphonse, J. C., Guedon, J., and Legrain, M. (1978). Focal glomerulosclerosis: natural history and treatment. A report of 70 cases. *Nephron* **21**, 75–85.

Bhuyan, U. N. and Srivastava, R. N. (1987). Incidence and significance of IgM mesangial deposits in relapsing idiopathic nephrotic syndrome of childhood. *Indian Journal of Medical Research* **86**, 53–60.

Blau, E. B. and Haaz, J. E. (1973). Glomerular sialic acid and proteinuria in human renal disease. *Laboratory Investigation* **28**, 477–481.

Bogdanovic, R. *et al.* (2001). Glomerular involvement in myelodysplastic syndromes. *Pediatric Nephrology* **16**, 1053–1057.

Bohlin, A. B. (1984). Clinical course and renal function in minimal change nephrotic syndrome. *Acta Paediatrica Scandinavica* **73**, 631–636.

Bohman, S. O., Jaremko, G., Bohlin, A. B., and Berg, U. (1984). Foot process fusion and glomerular filtration rate in minimal change nephrotic syndrome. *Kidney International* **25**, 696–700.

Bonilla-Felix, M. *et al.* (1999). Changing patterns in the histopathology of idiopathic nephrotic syndrome in children. *Kidney International* **55**, 1885–1890.

Border, W. A., Noble, N. A., and Ketteler, M. (1995). TGF-β: a cytokine mediator of glomerulosclerosis and a target for therapeutic intervention. *Kidney International* **47**, S59–S61.

Boulton-Jones, J. M., McWilliams, G., and Chandrachud, L. (1986). Variation in charge on red cells of patients with different glomerulopathies. *Lancet* **ii**, 186–189.

Boute, N. *et al.* (2000). NPHS2, encoding the glomerular protein podocin, is mutated in autosomal recessive steroid-resistant nephrotic syndrome. *Nature Genetics* **24**, 349–354.

Braden, G. L., Mulhern, J. G., O'Shea, M. H., Nash, S. V., Ucci, A. A., Jr., and Germain, M. J. (2000). Changing incidence of glomerular diseases in adults. *American Journal of Kidney Diseases* **35**, 878–883.

British Association for Pediatric Nephrology (1991). Levamisole for corticosteroid dependent nephrotic syndrome in childhood. *Lancet* **337**, 1555–1557.

Broyer, M., Terzi, F., Lehnert, A., Gagnadoux, M. F., Guest, G., and Niaudet, P. (1997). A controlled study of deflazacort in the treatment of idiopathic nephrotic syndrome. *Pediatric Nephrology* **11**, 418–422.

Buchanan, J. D., Fairley, K. F., and Barris, J. U. (1975). Return of spermatogenesis after stopping cyclophosphamide therapy. *Lancet* **ii**, 156–157.

Bustos, C., Gonzalez, E., Muley, R., Alonso, J. L., and Egido, J. (1994). Increase of tumour necrosis factor alpha synthesis and gene expression in peripheral blood mononuclear cells of children with idiopathic nephrotic syndrome. *European Journal of Clinical Investigation* **24**, 799–805.

Cade, R. *et al.* (1986). Effect of long-term azathioprine administration in adults with minimal-change glomerulonephritis and nephrotic syndrome resistant to corticosteroids. *Archives of Internal Medicine* **146**, 737–741.

Cameron, J. S., Turner, D. R., Ogg, C. S., Sharpstone, R., and Brown, C. B. (1974). The nephrotic syndrome in adults with minimal change glomerular lesions. *Quarterly Journal of Medicine* **43**, 461–488.

Carrie, B. J., Salyer, W. R., and Myers, B. D. (1981). Minimal change nephropathy: an electrochemical disorder of the glomerular membrane. *American Journal of Medicine* **70**, 262–268.

Cattran, D. C. and Rao, P. (1998). Long-term outcome in children and adults with classic focal segmental glomerulosclerosis. *American Journal of Kidney Diseases* **32**, 72–79.

Cattran, D. C. *et al.* (1999). A randomized trial of cyclosporine in patients with steroid-resistant focal segmental glomerulosclerosis. North America Nephrotic Syndrome Study Group. *Kidney International* **56**, 2220–2226.

Chandra, M., Lewy, J. E., Mouradian, J., Susin, M., and Hoyer, J. R. (1981). Recurrent nephrotic syndrome with three successive renal allografts. *American Journal of Nephrology* **1**, 110–114.

Cheong, H. I. *et al.* (2000). Early recurrent nephrotic syndrome after renal transplantation in children with focal segmental glomerulosclerosis. *Nephrology, Dialysis, Transplantation* **15**, 80–81.

Choi, M. J. *et al.* (2002). Mycophenolate mofetil treatment for primary glomerular diseases. *Kidney International* **61**, 1098–1114.

Churg, J., Habib, R., and White, R. H. R. (1970). Pathology of the nephrotic syndrome in children. *Lancet* **i**, 1299–1302.

Clark, A. G. B., Vaughan, R. W., Stephens, H. A. F., Chantler, C., Williams, D. G., and Welsh, K. I. (1990). Genes encoding the β-chains of HLA-DR7 and HLA-DQW2 define major susceptibility determinants for idiopathic nephrotic syndrome. *Clinical Science* **78**, 391–397.

Clarkson, M. R., O'Meara, Y. M., Murphy, B., Rennke, H. G., and Brady, H. R. (1998). Collapsing glomerulopathy—recurrence in a renal allograft. *Nephrology, Dialysis, Transplantation* **13**, 503–506.

Cochat, P. *et al.* (1993). Recurrent nephrotic syndrome after transplantation: early treatment with plasmapheresis and cyclophosphamide. *Pediatric Nephrology* **7**, 50–54.

Cohen, A. H., Border, W. A., and Glassock, R. J. (1978). Nephrotic syndrome with glomerular mesangial IgM deposits. *Laboratory Investigation* **38**, 610–619.

Coleman, J. E. and Watson, A. R. (1996). Hyperlipidaemia, diet and simvastatin therapy in steroid-resistant nephrotic syndrome of childhood. *Pediatric Nephrology* **10**, 171–174.

Coovadia, H. M. and Adhikari, M. (1989). Outcome of childhood minimal change disease. *Lancet* **i**, 1199–1200.

Coovadia, H. M., Adhikari, M., and Morel-Maroger, L. (1979). Clinicopathological features of the nephrotic syndrome in South African children. *Quarterly Journal of Medicine* **48**, 77–91.

Couser, W. G. and Stilmant, M. M. (1975). Mesangial lesion and focal glomerular sclerosis in the aging rat. *Laboratory Investigation* **33**, 491–501.

D'Agati, V. (1994). The many masks of focal segmental glomerulosclerosis. *Kidney International* **46**, 1233–1241.

D'Agati, V. (2003). Pathologic classification of focal-segmental glomerulosclerosis. *Seminars in Nephrology* **23**, 117–134.

Dantal, J. *et al.* (1991). Recurrent nephrotic syndrome following renal transplantation in patients with focal glomerulosclerosis: a one-center study of plasma exchange effects. *Transplantation* **52**, 827–831.

Dantal, J. *et al.* (1994). Effect of plasma protein adsorption on protein excretion in kidney-transplant recipients with recurrent nephrotic syndrome. *New England Journal of Medicine* **330**, 7–14.

Dantal, J. *et al.* (1998). Antihuman immunoglobulin affinity immunoadsorption strongly decreases proteinuria in patients with relapsing nephrotic syndrome. *Journal of the American Society of Nephrology* **9**, 1709–1715.

Dayal, U., Dayal, A. K., Shastry, J. C., and Raghupathy, P. (1994). Use of levamisole in maintaining remission in steroid-sensitive nephrotic syndrome in children. *Nephron* **66**, 408–412.

de Mouzon-Cambon, A. *et al.* (1981). HLA-DR7 in children with idiopathic nephrotic syndrome. Correlation with atopy. *Tissue Antigens* **17**, 518–524.

Demmer, L., Primack, W., Loik, V., Brown, R., Therville, N., and McElreavey, K. (1999). Frasier syndrome: a cause of focal segmental glomerulosclerosis in a 46,XX female. *Journal of the American Society of Nephrology* **10**, 2215–2218.

Denamur, E. *et al.* (1999). Mother-to-child transmitted WT1 splice-site mutation is responsible for distinct glomerular diseases. *Journal of the American Society of Nephrology* **10**, 2219–2223.

Detwiler, R. K., Falk, R. J., Hogan, S. L., and Jennette, J. C. (1994). Collapsing glomerulopathy: a clinically and pathologically distinct variant of focal segmental glomerulosclerosis. *Kidney International* **45**, 1416–1424.

Devarajan, P. and Spitzer, A. (2002). Towards a biological characterization of focal segmental glomerulosclerosis. *American Journal of Kidney Diseases* **39**, 625–636.

Doleris, L. M. *et al.* (2000). Focal segmental glomerulosclerosis associated with mitochondrial cytopathy. *Kidney International* **58**, 1851–1858.

Donker, A. J. M., Brentjens, J. R. H., and Van der Hem, G. K. (1978). Treatment of the nephrotic syndrome with indomethacin. *Nephron* **22**, 374–381.

Dorhout Mees, E. J., Roos, J. C., and Boer, P. (1979). Observations on edema formation in the nephrotic syndromes in adults with minimal lesion. *American Journal of Medicine* **67**, 378–384.

Doublier, S. *et al.* (2001). Nephrin redistribution on podocytes is a potential mechanism for proteinuria in patients with primary acquired nephrotic syndrome. *American Journal of Pathology* **158**, 1723–1731.

Drachman, R. *et al.* (1988). Immunoregulation with levamisole in children with frequently relapsing steroid responsive nephrotic syndrome. *Acta Paediatrica Scandinavica* **77**, 721–726.

Ehrich, J. H. H. and Brodehl, J. (1993). Long versus standard prednisone therapy for initial treatment of idiopathic nephrotic syndrome in children. Arbeitsgemeinschaft fur Padiatrische Nephrologie. *European Journal of Pediatrics* **152**, 357–361.

Ehrich, J. H. H., Offner, G., Shirg, E., Hoyer, P. F., Helmchen, U., and Brodehl, J. (1990). Association of spondylo-epiphyseal dysplasia with nephrotic syndrome. *Pediatric Nephrology* **4**, 117–212.

Elhence, R., Gulati, S., Kher, V., Gupta, A., and Sharma, R. K. (1994). Intravenous pulse cyclophosphamide—a new regime for steroid-resistant minimal change nephrotic syndrome. *Pediatric Nephrology* **8**, 1–3.

Endlich, N. *et al.* (2001). Podocytes respond to mechanical stress in vitro. *Journal of the American Society of Nephrology* **12**, 413–422.

Feehally, J., Samanta, A., Kinghom, H., Burden, A. C., and Walls, J. (1986). Red-cell surface charge in glomerular disease. *Lancet* **ii**, 635.

Fliser, D. *et al.* (1999). Coadministration of albumin and furosemide in patients with the nephrotic syndrome. *Kidney International* **55**, 629–634.

Floege, J. *et al.* (1995). Basic fibroblast growth factor augments podocyte injury and induces glomerulosclerosis in rats with experimental membranous nephropathy. *Journal of Clinical Investigation* **96**, 2809–2819.

Fodor, P., Saitua, M. T., Rodriguez, E., Gonzalez, B., and Schlesinger, L. (1982). T-cell dysfunction in minimal-change nephrotic syndrome of childhood. *American Journal of Diseases of Children* **136**, 713–717.

Fogo, A. *et al.* (1990). Glomerular hypertrophy in minimal change disease predicts subsequent progression to focal glomerular sclerosis. *Kidney International* **38**, 115–123.

Fogo, A., Glick, A. D., Horn, S. L., and Horn, R. G. (1995). Is focal segmental glomerulosclerosis really focal? Distribution of lesions in adults and children. *Kidney International* **47**, 1690–1696.

Frasier, S., Bashore, R. A., and Mosier, H. D. (1964). Gonadoblastoma associated with pure gonadal dysgenesis in monozygotic twins. *Journal of Pediatrics* **64**, 740–745.

Fries, J. W., Sandstrom, D. J., Meyer, T. W., and Rennke, H. G. (1989). Glomerular hypertrophy and epithelial cell injury modulate progressive glomerulosclerosis in the rat. *Laboratory Investigation* **60**, 205–218.

Frishberg, Y., Rinat, C., Megged, O., Shapira, E., Feinstein, S., and Raas-Rothschild, A. (2002). Mutations in NPHS2 encoding podocin are a prevalent cause of steroid-resistant nephrotic syndrome among Israeli-Arab children. *Journal of the American Society of Nephrology* **13**, 400–405.

Fuchshuber, A. *et al.* (1995). Mapping a gene (SRN1) to chromosome 1q25–1q31 in idiopathic nephrotic syndrome confirms a distinct entity of autosomal recessive nephrosis. *Human Molecular Genetics* **4**, 2155–2158.

Fuiano, G. *et al.* (1996). Serial morphometric analysis of sclerotic lesions in primary 'focal' segmental glomerulosclerosis. *Journal of the American Society of Nephrology* **7**, 49–55.

Fujimoto, S., Yamamoto, Y., Hisanaga, S., Morita, S., Eto, T., and Tanaka, K. (1991). Minimal change nephrotic syndrome in adults: response to corticosteroid therapy and frequency of relapse. *American Journal of Kidney Diseases* **17**, 687–692.

Furness, P. N., Hall, L. L., Shaw, J. A., and Pringle, J. H. (1999). Glomerular expression of nephrin is decreased in acquired human nephrotic syndrome. *Nephrology, Dialysis, Transplantation* **14**, 1234–1237.

Galloway, W. H. and Mowat, A. P. (1968). Congenital microcephaly and nephrotic syndrome in two sibs. *Journal of Medical Genetics* **5**, 319–321.

Garin, E. H., Blanchard, D. K., Matsushima, K., and Djeu, J. Y. (1994). IL-8 production by peripheral blood mononuclear cells in nephrotic patients. *Kidney International* **45**, 1311–1317.

Geffriaud-Ricouard, C., Jungers, P., Chauveau, D., and Grünfeld, J. P. (1993). Inefficacy and toxicity of perfloxacin in focal and segmental glomerulosclerosis with steroid resistant nephrotic syndrome. *Lancet* **341**, 1475.

Giangiacomo, J., Cleary, T. G., Cole, B. R., Hoffsten, P., and Robson, A. M. (1975). Serum immunoglobulins in the nephrotic syndrome. A possible cause of minimal change nephrotic syndrome. *New England Journal of Medicine* **293**, 8–12.

Glicklich, D., Haskell, L., Senitzer, D., and Weiss, R. A. (1988). Possible genetic predisposition to idiopathic focal segmental glomerulosclerosis. *American Journal of Kidney Diseases* **12**, 26–30.

Gregory, M. J. *et al.* (1996). Long-term cyclosporine therapy for pediatric nephrotic syndrome—a clinical and histologic analysis. *Journal of the American Society of Nephrology* **7**, 543–549.

Grishman, E. and Churg, J. (1975). Focal glomerular sclerosis in nephrotic patients: an electron microscopy study of glomerular podocytes. *Kidney International* **7**, 111–122.

Grishman, E., Churg, J., and Porush, J. G. (1976). Glomerular morphology in nephrotic heroin addicts. *Laboratory Investigation* **35**, 415–424.

Grupe, W. E. (1973). Chlorambucil in steroid dependent nephrotic syndrome. *Journal of Pediatrics* **82**, 598–606.

Grupe, W. E., Makker, S. P., and Ingelfinger, J. R. (1976). Chlorambucil treatment of frequently relapsing nephrotic syndrome. *New England Journal of Medicine* **295**, 746–749.

Guasch, A., Deen, W. M., and Myers, B. D. (1993). Charge selectivity of the glomerular filtration barrier in healthy and nephrotic humans. *Journal of Clinical Investigation* **92**, 2274–2282.

Guillot, A. P. and Kim, M. S. (1993) Pulse steroid therapy does not alter the course of focal segmental glomerulosclerosis. *Journal of the American Society of Nephrology* **4**, 276 (abstract).

Habib, R. (1973). Focal glomerulosclerosis. *Kidney International* **4**, 355–361.

Habib, R. and Niaudet, P. (1994). Comparison between pre- and posttreatment renal biopsies in children receiving cyclosporine for idiopathic nephrosis. *Clinical Nephrology* **42**, 141–146.

Habib, R., Hebert, D., Gagnadoux, M. F., and Broyer, M. (1982). Transplantation in idiopathic nephrosis. *Transplantation Proceedings* **14**, 489–495.

Habib, R., Girardin, E., Gagnadoux, M. F., Hinglais, N., Levy, M., and Broyer, M. (1988). Immunopathological findings in idiopathic nephrosis: clinical significance of glomerular 'immune deposits'. *Pediatric Nephrology* **2**, 402–408.

Hari, P., Bagga, A., Jindal, N., and Srivastava, R. N. (2001). Treatment of focal glomerulosclerosis with pulse steroids and oral cyclophosphamide. *Pediatric Nephrology* **16**, 901–905.

Haws, R. and Baum, M. (1993). Efficacy of albumin and diuretic therapy in children with nephrotic syndrome. *Pediatrics* **91**, 1142–1146.

Hayslett, J. P., Krassner, L. S., Klausse, G., Bensch, M. D., Kashgarian, M., and Epstein, F. H. (1969). Progression of lipoid nephrosis to renal insufficiency. *New England Journal of Medicine* **281**, 181–187.

Heslan, J. M., Branellec, A. I., Laurent, J., and Lagrue, G. (1986). The vascular permeability factor is a T lymphocyte produce. *Nephron* **42**, 187–188.

Heslan, J. M. J., Branellec, A. I., Pilatte, Y., Lang, P., and Lagrue, G. (1991). Differentiation between vascular permeability factor and IL-2 in lymphocyte supernatants from patients with minimal-change nephrotic syndrome. *Clinical and Experimental Immunology* **86**, 157–162.

Hisanaga, S. *et al.* (1990). Nephrotic syndrome associated with recombinant interleukin-2. *Nephron* **54**, 277–278.

Hodson, E. M., Knight, J. F., Willis, N. S., and Craig, J. C. (2000). Corticosteroid therapy in nephrotic syndrome: a meta-analysis of randomised controlled trials. *Archives of Disease in Childhood* **83**, 45–51.

Hotta, O., Inoue, C. N., Miyabayashi, S., Furuta, T., Takeuchi, A., and Taguma, Y. (2001). Clinical and pathologic features of focal segmental glomerulosclerosis with mitochondrial tRNALeu(UUR) gene mutation. *Kidney International* **59**, 1236–1243.

Howie, A. J. and Brewer, D. B. (1984). The glomerular tip lesion: a previously undescribed type of segmental glomerular abnormality. *Journal of Pathology* **142**, 205–220.

Hoyer, J. R., Raij, L., Vernier, R. L., Simmons, R. L., Najarian, J. S., and Michael, A. F. (1972). Recurrence of idiopathic nephrotic syndrome after renal transplantation. *Lancet* **ii**, 343–348.

Hsu, A. C., Folami, A. O., Bain, J., and Rance, C. P. (1979). Gonadal functions in males treated with cyclophosphamide for nephrotic syndrome. *Fertility and Sterility* **31**, 173–177.

Huh, W. *et al.* (2002). Expression of nephrin in acquired human glomerular disease. *Nephrology, Dialysis, Transplantation* **17**, 478–484.

Hulton, S. A., Neuhaus, T. J., Dillon, M. J., and Barratt, T. M. (1994). Long-term cyclosporin A treatment of minimal-change nephrotic syndrome of childhood. *Pediatric Nephrology* **8**, 401–403.

Hyman, L. R. and Burkholder, P. M. (1973). Focal sclerosing glomerulonephropathy with segmental hyalinosis. A clinicopathologic analysis. *Laboratory Investigation* **28**, 533–544.

Hyman, L. R. and Burkholder, P. M. (1974). Focal sclerosing glomerulonephropathy with hyalinosis. *Journal of Pediatrics* **84**, 217–225.

Ichikawa, I., Ikoma, M., and Fogo, A. (1991). Glomerular growth promoters, the common key mediator for progressive glomerular sclerosis in chronic renal diseases. *Advances in Nephrology* **20**, 127–148.

Ingulli, E. and Tejani, A. (1991). Racial differences in the incidence and renal outcome of idiopathic focal segmental glomerulosclerosis in children. *Pediatric Nephrology* **5**, 393–397.

Ingulli, E. and Tejani, A. (1992). Severe hypercholesterolemia inhibits cyclosporin A efficacy in a dose-dependent manner in children with nephrotic syndrome. *Journal of the American Society of Nephrology* **3**, 254–259.

Ingulli, E. *et al.* (1990). High-dose cyclosporine therapy in recurrent nephrotic syndrome following renal transplantation. *Transplantation* **49**, 219–221.

Ingulli, E., Singh, A., Baqi, N., Ahmad, S., Moazami, S., and Tejani, A. (1995). Aggressive, long-term cyclosporine therapy for steroid-resistant focal segmental glomerulosclerosis. *Journal of the American Society of Nephrology* **5**, 1820–1825.

International Study of Kidney Disease in Children (1978). Nephrotic syndrome: prediction of histopathology from clinical and laboratory characteristics at time of diagnosis. *Kidney International* **13**, 159–165.

International Study of Kidney Disease in Children (1981). The primary nephrotic syndrome in children. Identification of patients with minimal change nephrotic syndrome from initial response to prednisone. *Journal of Pediatrics* **98**, 561–564.

Ito, H. *et al.* (1984). Twenty-seven children with focal segmental glomerulosclerosis: correlation between the segmental location of the glomerular lesions and prognosis. *Clinical Nephrology* **22**, 9–14.

Kaplan, C., Pasternak, B., Shah, H., and Gallo, G. (1975). Age related incidence of sclerotic glomeruli in human kidneys. *American Journal of Pathology* **80**, 227–234.

Kaplan, J. M. *et al.* (2000). Mutations in ACTN4, encoding alpha-actinin-4, cause familial focal segmental glomerulosclerosis. *Nature Genetics* **24**, 251–256.

Karle, S. M., Uetz, B., Ronner, V., Glaeser, L., Hildebrandt, F., and Fuchshuber, A. (2002). Novel mutations in $NPHS_2$ detected in both familial and sporadic steroid-resistant nephrotic syndrome. *Journal of the American Society of Nephrology* **13**, 388–393.

Kashgarian, M., Hayslett, J. P., and Seigel, N. J. (1974). Lipoid nephrosis and focal sclerosis: distinct entities or spectrum of disease. *Nephron* **13**, 105–108.

Kawaguchi, H., Yamaguchi, Y., Nagata, M., and Itoh, K. (1987). The effects of human recombinant interleukin-2 on the permeability of glomerular basement membranes in rats. *Japanese Journal of Nephrology* **29**, 1–11.

Kerjaschki, D. (2001). Caught flat-footed: podocyte damage and the molecular bases of focal glomerulosclerosis. *Journal of Clinical Investigation* **108**, 1583–1587.

Kihara, I. *et al.* (1997). Podocyte detachment and epithelial cell reaction in focal segmental glomerulosclerosis with cellular variants. *Kidney International* **63** (Suppl.), S171–S176.

Kikuchi, H. *et al.* (1998). Do intronic mutations affecting splicing of WT1 exon 9 cause Frasier syndrome? *Journal of Medical Genetics* **35**, 45–48.

Kitano, Y., Yoshikawa, N., and Nakamura, H. (1993). Glomerular anionic sites in minimal change nephrotic syndrome and focal segmental glomerulosclerosis. *Clinical Nephrology* **40**, 199–204.

Klamt, B. *et al.* (1998). Frasier syndrome is caused by defective alternative splicing of WT1 leading to an altered ratio of WT1 +/−KTS splice isoforms. *Human Molecular Genetics* **7**, 709–714.

Kleinknecht, C., Guesry, P., Lenoir, G., and Broyer, M. (1977). High cost benefit of chlorambucil in frequent relapsing neprhosis. *New England Journal of Medicine* **296**, 48–49.

Kleinknecht, C., Broyer, M., and Gubler, M. C. (1980). Irreversible renal failure after indomethacin in steroid-resistant nephrosis. *New England Journal of Medicine* **302**, 691.

Kleinknecht, C., Broyer, M., Loirat, C., Nivet, H., Palcoux, J. B., and Parchoux, B. (1982). Comparison of short and long term treatment at onset of steroid sensitive nephrosis. Preliminary results of a multicentric controlled trial from the French Society of Pediatric Nephrology. *International Journal of Pediatric Nephrology* **3**, 45 (abstract).

Kohaut, E. C., Singer, B., and Leighton, H. (1976). The significance of focal glomerular sclerosis in children who have nephrotic syndrome. *American Journal of Clinical Pathology* **66**, 545–550.

Korbet, S. M. (1995). Management of idiopathic nephrosis in adults, including steroid-resistant nephrosis. *Current Opinion in Nephrology and Hypertension* **4**, 169–176.

Korbet, S. M. (1999). Clinical picture and outcome of primary focal segmental glomerulosclerosis. *Nephrology, Dialysis, Transplantation* **14** (Suppl. 3), 68–73.

Korbet, S. M. (2002). Treatment of primary focal segmental glomerulosclerosis. *Kidney International* **62**, 2301–2310.

Korbet, S. M., Schwartz, M. M., and Lewis, E. J. (1988a). Minimal-change glomerulopathy of adulthood. *American Journal of Nephrology* **8**, 291–297.

Korbet, S. M., Schwartz, M. M., and Lewis, E. J. (1988b). Recurrent nephrotic syndrome in renal allografts. *American Journal of Kidney Diseases* **11**, 270–276.

Korbet, S., Schwartz, M., and Lewis, E. (1994). Primary focal segmental glomerulosclerosis: clinical course and response to therapy. *American Journal of Kidney Diseases* **23**, 773–783.

Koskimies, O., Vilska, J., Rapola, J., and Hallman, N. (1982). Long-term outcome of primary nephrotic syndrome. *Archives of Disease in Childhood* **57**, 544–548.

Koyama, A., Fujisaki, M., Kobayashi, M., Igarashi, M., and Narita, M. (1991). A glomerular permeability factor produced by human T cell hybridoma. *Kidney International* **40**, 453–460.

Kriz, W. (1996). Progressive renal failure—inability of podocytes to replicate and the consequences for development of glomerulosclerosis. *Nephrology, Dialysis, Transplantation* **11**, 1738–1742.

Kriz, W. and Lemley, K. V. (1999). The role of the podocyte in glomerulosclerosis. *Current Opinion in Nephrology and Hypertension* **8**, 489–497.

Kriz, W., Hackenthal, E., Nobiling, R., Sakai, T., Elger, M., and Hahnel, B. (1994). A role for podocytes to counteract capillary wall distension. *Kidney International* **45**, 369–376.

Ksiazek, J. and Wyszynska, T. (1995). Short versus long initial prednisone treatment in steroid-sensitive nephrotic syndrome in children. *Acta Paediatrica* **84**, 889–893.

Kurogouchi, F. *et al.* (1998). A case of mitochondrial cytopathy with a typical point mutation for MELAS, presenting with severe focal–segmental glomerulosclerosis as main clinical manifestation. *American Journal of Nephrology* **18**, 551–556.

Lagrue, G., and Laurent, J. (1984). Role de l'allergie dans la néphrose lipoïdique. *Nouvelle Presse Médicale* **11**, 1465–1466.

Lagrue, G., Branellec, A., and Blanc, C. (1975). A vascular permeability factor in lymphocyte culture supernatants from patients with nephrotic syndrome. *Biomédecine* **23**, 73–75.

Lagrue, G., Branellec, A., Niaudet, P., Heslan, J. M., Guillot, F., and Lang, P. (1991). Transmission d'un syndrome nephrotique à deux nouveau-nés. Regression spontanée. *La Presse Médicale* **20**, 255–257.

Lai, K. N., Lai, F. M., Chan, K. W., Ho, C. P., Leung, A. C., and Vallance-Owen, J. (1989). An overlapping syndrome of IgA nephropathy and lipoid nephrosis. *American Journal of Clinical Pathology* **86**, 716–723.

Laurent, J., Rostoker, G., Robeva, R., Bruneau, C., and Martin-Govantes, J. (1987). Is adult idiopathic nephrotic syndrome food allergy? *Nephron* **47**, 7–11.

Le Berre, L. *et al.* (2002). Extrarenal effects on the pathogenesis and relapse of idiopathic nephrotic syndrome in Buffalo/Mna rats. *Journal of Clinical Investigation* **109**, 491–498.

Leisti, S., Koskimies, O., Rapola, J., Hallman, H., Perheentupa, J., and Vilska, J. (1977). Association of post-medication hypocortisolism with early first relapse of idiopathic nephrotic syndrome. *Lancet* **ii**, 795–796.

Leisti, S., Koskimies, O., Perheentupa, J., Vilska, J., and Hallman, N. (1978). Idiopathic nephrotic syndrome: prevention of early relapse. *British Medical Journal* **1**, 892.

Leumann, E. P., Briner, J., Donckerwolcke, R. A., Kuijten, R., and Largiader, F. (1980). Recurrence of focal segmental glomerulosclerosis in the transplant kidney. *Nephron* **25**, 65–71.

Levin, M., Walters, M. D. S., Smith, C., Gascoine, P., and Barratt, T. M. (1985). Steroid-responsive nephrotic syndrome: a generalized disorder of membrane negative charge. *Lancet* **ii**, 239–242.

Lewis, M. A., Davis, N., Baildom, E., Houston, I. B., and Postlethwaite, R. J. (1989). Nephrotic syndrome from toddlers to twenties. *Lancet* **i**, 255–259.

Li, R. M., Branton, M., Tanawattanacharoen, S., Falk, R. J., Jennette, J. C., and Kopp, J. B. (2002). Molecular identification of SV 40 infection in human subjects and possible association with kidney disease. *Journal of the American Society of Nephrology* **13**, 2320–2330.

Lieberman, K. and Tejani, A. (1996) A randomized placebo controlled double blind trial of cyclosporine in steroid resistant idiopathic focal segmental glomerulosclerosis in children. A report of the New York, New Jersey pediatric nephrology collaborative study group. *Journal of the American Society of Nephrology* **7**, 56–63.

Maizel, S. E., Sibley, R. K., Horstman, J. P., Kjellstrand, C. M., and Simmons, R. L. (1981). Incidence and significance of recurrent focal segmental glomerulosclerosis in renal allograft recipients. *Transplantation* **32**, 512–516.

Mak, S. K., Short, C. D., and Mallick, N. P. (1996). Long term outcome of adult-onset minimal change nephropathy. *Nephrology, Dialysis, Transplantation* **11**, 2192–2201.

Mathis, B. J. *et al.* (1998). A locus for inherited focal segmental glomerulosclerosis maps to chromosome 19q13. *Kidney International* **53**, 282–286.

Mattoo, T. K. and Mahmoud, M. A. (2000). Increased maintenance corticosteroids during upper respiratory infection decrease the risk of relapse in nephrotic syndrome. *Nephron* **85**, 343–345.

McBryde, K. D., Kershaw, D. B., and Smoyer, W. E. (2001). Pediatric steroid-resistant nephrotic syndrome. *Current Problems in Pediatric Adolescence Health Care* **31**, 280–307.

McCauley, J., Shapiro, R., Ellis, D., Igdal, H., Tzakis, A., and Starzl, T. (1993). Pilot trial of FK 506 in the management of steroid resistant nephrotic syndrome. *Nephrology, Dialysis, Transplantation* **8**, 1286–1290.

McDonald, N. E., Wolfish, N., McLaine, P., Phipps, P., and Rossier, E. (1986). Role of respiratory viruses in exacerbation of primary nephrotic syndrome. *Journal of Pediatrics* **108**, 378–382.

McEnery, P. T. and Strife, C. F. (1982). Nephrotic syndrome in childhood. Management and treatment in patients with minimal change disease, mesangial proliferation, or focal glomerulosclerosis. *Pediatric Clinics of North America* **29**, 875–894.

Meehan, S. M., Pascual, M., and Williams, W. W. (1998). *De novo* collapsing glomerulopathy in renal allografts. *Transplantation* **65**, 1192–1197.

Mehta, K. P., Ali, U., Kutty, M., and Kolhatkar, U. (1986). Immunoregulatory treatment for minimal change nephrotic syndrome. *Archives of Diseases in Childhood* **61**, 153–158.

Meyrier, A. (1992). Antiproteinuric and immunologic effects of cyclosporine A in the treatment of glomerular diseases. *Nephrology, Dialysis, Transplantation* **7** (Suppl. 1), 80–84.

Meyrier, A. (1999a). Treatment of primary focal segmental glomerulosclerosis. *Nephrology, Dialysis, Transplantation* **14** (Suppl. 3), 74–78.

Meyrier, A. Y. (1999b). Collapsing glomerulopathy: expanding interest in a shrinking tuft. *American Journal of Kidney Diseases* **3**, 801–803.

Meyrier, A. and Simon, P. Treatment of corticoresistant idiopathic nephrotic syndrome in the adult: minimal change disease and focal segmental glomerulosclerosis. In *Advances in Nephrology* (ed. J. P. Grünfeld *et al.*), pp. 127–150. Chicago: Year Book, 1988.

Meyrier, A. and Collaborative Group of the Société de Néphrologie (1989). Cyclosporine in the treatment of nephrosis. *American Journal of Nephrology* **9** (Suppl. 1), 65–71.

Meyrier, A., Noel, L. H., Auriche, P., and Callard, P. (1994). Long-term renal tolerance of cyclosporine A treatment in adult idiopathic nephrotic syndrome. *Kidney International* **45**, 1446–1456.

Milliner, D. and Morgensten, B. Z. (1991). Angiotensin converting enzyme inhibitor for reduction of proteinuria in children with steroid resistant nephrotic syndrome. *Pediatric Nephrology* **5**, 587–590.

Mongeau, J. G., Robitaille, P. O., and Roy, F. (1988). Clinical efficacy of levamisole in the treatment of primary nephrosis in children. *Pediatric Nephrology* **2**, 398–401.

Morita, M., White, R. H. R., Coad, N. A. G., and Faafat, F. (1990). The clinical significance of the glomerular location of segmental lesions in focal segmental glomerulonephrosclerosis. *Clinical Nephrology* **33**, 211–219.

Moudgil, A. *et al.* (2001). Association of parvovirus B19 infection with idiopathic collapsing glomerulopathy. *Kidney International* **59**, 2126–2133.

Muda, A. O., Feriozzi, S., Cinotti, G., and Faraggiana, T. (1994). Glomerular hypertrophy and chronic renal failure in focal segmental glomerulosclerosis. *American Journal of Kidney Diseases* **23**, 237–241.

Müller, W. and Brandis, M. (1981). Acute leukemia after cytotoxic treatment for non malignant disease in childhood. *European Journal of Pediatrics* **136**, 105–108.

Munk, F. (1913). Klinische Diagnostik der degenerativen Nierenkrankungen. *Klinische Medizin* **78**, 1–52.

Munoz, J., Sanchez, R., Perez-Garcia, R., Anaya, F., and Valderrabana, F. (1985). Recurrent focal segmental glomerulosclerosis in renal transplants. Proteinuria relapsing following plasma exchange. *Clinical Nephrology* **24**, 213–214.

Murnaghan, W. M., Vasmant, D., and Bensman, A. (1984). Pulse methylprednisolone therapy in severe idiopathic childhood nephrotic syndrome. *Acta Paediatrica Scandinavica* **73**, 733–739.

Nadasdy T., Allen C., and Zand, M. S. (2002). Zonal distribution of glomerular collapse in renal allografts: possible role of vascular changes. *Human Pathology* **33**, 437–441.

Nagata, M., Hattori, M., Hamano, Y., Ito, K., Saitoh, K., and Watanabe, T. (1998). Origin and phenotypic features of hyperplastic epithelial cells in collapsing glomerulopathy. *American Journal of Kidney Diseases* **32**, 962–969.

Nair, R. B., Date, A., Kirubakaran, M. G., and Shastry, J. C. M. (1987). Minimal change nephrotic syndrome in adults treated with alternate-day steroids. *Nephron* **47**, 209–210.

Nakayama, M., Katafuchi, R., Yanase, T., Ikeda, K., Tanaka, H., and Fujimi, S. (2002). Steroid responsiveness and frequency of relapse in adult-onset minimal change nephrotic syndrome. *American Journal of Kidney Diseases* **39**, 503–512.

Nash, M. A., Greifer, I., Olbing, H., Bernstein, J., Bennett, B., and Spitzer, A. (1976). The significance of focal sclerotic lesions of glomeruli in children. *Journal of Pediatrics* **88**, 806–813.

Newman, W. J. *et al.* (1976). Focal glomerular sclerosis: contrasting clinical patterns in children and adults. *Medicine (Baltimore)* **55**, 67–87.

Niaudet, P. (1992). Comparison of cyclosporin and chlorambucil in the treatment of steroid-dependent idiopathic nephrotic syndrome: a multicentre randomized controlled trial. The French Society of Paediatric Nephrology. *Pediatric Nephrology* **6**, 1–3.

Niaudet, P. and Habib, R. (1994). Cyclosporine in the treatment of idiopathic nephrosis. *Journal of the American Society of Nephrology* **5**, 1049–1056.

Niaudet, P., Drachman, R., Gagnadoux, M. F., and Broyer, M. (1984). Treatment of idiopathic nephrotic syndrome with levamisole. *Acta Paediatrica Scandinavica* **73**, 637–641.

Niaudet, P. and the French Society of Pediatric Nephrology (1994). Treatment of childhood steroid resistant idiopathic nephrosis with a combination of cyclosporine and prednisone. *Journal of Pediatrics* **125**, 981–985.

Nolasco, F., Cameron, J. S., Heywood, E. F., Hicks, J., Ogg C., and Williams, D. G. (1986). Adult-onset minimal change nephrotic syndrome: a long-term follow-up. *Kidney International* **29**, 1215–1223.

Norero, C., Delucchi, A., Lagos, E., and Rosati, P. (1996). Initial therapy of primary nephrotic syndrome in children: evaluation in a period of 18 months of two prednisone treatment schedules. Chilean Co-operative Group of Study of Nephrotic Syndrome in Children. *Revista Medica de Chile* **124**, 567–572.

Oda, T. *et al.* (1998). Clinicopathological significance of intratubular giant macrophages in progressive glomerulonephritis. *Kidney International* **53**, 1190–1200.

Ohta, T. *et al.* (2001). Effect of pre- and postoperative plasmapheresis on post-transplant recurrence of focal segmental glomerulosclerosis in children. *Transplantation* **71**, 628–633.

Overturf, G. D. (2000). American Academy of Pediatrics. Committee on Infectious Diseases. Technical report: prevention of pneumococcal infections, including the use of pneumococcal conjugate and polysaccharide vaccines and antibiotic prophylaxis. *Pediatrics* **106**, 367–376.

Pakasa, N. M., Nseka, N. M., and Nyimi, L. M. (1997). Secondary collapsing glomerulopathy associated with Loa loa filariasis. *American Journal of Kidney Diseases* **30**, 836–839.

Palcoux, J. B., Niaudet, P., and Goumy, P. (1994). Side effects of levamisole in children with nephrosis letter. *Pediatric Nephrology* **8**, 263–264.

Pei, Y., Cattran, D., Delmore, T., Katz, A, Lang, A., and Rance, P. (1987). Evidence suggesting under-treatment in adults with idiopathic focal segmental glomerulosclerosis. *American Journal of Medicine* **82**, 938–944.

Pinto, J., Lacerda, G., Cameron, J. S., Turner, D. R., Bewick, M., and Ogg, C. S. (1981). Recurrence of focal segmental glomerulosclerosis in renal allografts. *Transplantation* **32**, 83–89.

Pollak, M. R. (2002). Inherited podocytopathies: FSGS and nephrotic syndrome from a genetic point of view. *Journal of the American Society of Nephrology* **13**, 3016–3023.

Ponticelli, C. *et al.* (1993a). Cyclosporin versus cyclophosphamide for patients with steroid-dependent and frequently relapsing idiopathic nephrotic syndrome: a multicentre randomized controlled trial. *Nephrology, Dialysis, Transplantation* **8**, 1326–1332.

Ponticelli, C. *et al.* (1993b). A randomized trial of cyclosporine in steroid-resistant idiopathic nephrotic syndrome. *Kidney International* **43**, 1377–1384.

Ponticelli, C. *et al.* (1999). Can prolonged treatment improve the prognosis in adults with focal segmental glomerulosclerosis? *American Journal of Kidney Diseases* **34**, 618–625.

Pritchard-Jones, K. *et al.* (1990). The candidate Wilms' tumour gene is involved in genitourinary development. *Nature* **346**, 194–197.

Pruna, A. *et al.* (1992). Pefloxacin as first-line treatment in nephrotic syndrome. *Lancet* **340**, 728–729.

Raij, L., Keane, W. F., Leonard, A., and Shapiro, F. L. (1976). Irreversible acute renal failure in idiopathic nephrotic syndrome. *American Journal of Medicine* **61**, 207–214.

Rascher, W., Tulassay, T., Seyberth, H. W., Himbert, U., Lang, U., and Schärer, K. (1986). Diuretic and hormonal responses to head out water immersion in nephrotic syndrome. *Journal of Pediatrics* **109**, 609–614.

Reddy, J. C. and Licht, J. D. (1996). The WT1 Wilms' tumor suppressor gene: how much do we really know? *Biochimica et biophysica atca* **1287**, 1–28.

Rennke, H. G. and Klein, P. S. (1989). Pathogenesis and significance of non-primary focal and segmental glomerulosclerosis. *American Journal of Kidney Diseases* **13**, 443–456.

Rich, A. R. (1957). A hitherto undescribed vulnerability of the juxta medullary glomeruli in the lipoid nephrosis. *Bulletin of the Johns Hopkins Hospital* **100**, 173–179.

Robson, A. M., Giangiacomo, J., Kienstra, R. A., Naqui, S. T., and Ingelfinger, J. R. (1974). Normal glomerular permeability and its modification by minimal change nephrotic syndrome. *Journal of Clinical Investigation* **54**, 1190–1199.

Roselli, S. *et al.* (2002). Podocin localizes in the kidney to the slit diaphragm area. *American Journal of Pathology* **160**, 131–139.

Rosenberg, S. A. *et al.* (1987). A progress report on the treatment of 157 patients with advanced cancer using lymphokine activated killer cells and interleukin-2 alone. *New England Journal of Medicine* **316**, 889–897.

Rumpelt, H. J. and Thoenes, W. (1974). Focal and segmental sclerosing glomerulopathy: a pathomorphological study. *Virchow's Archives A: Pathology, Anatomy and Histology* **362**, 265–282.

Rydel, J. J., Korbet, S. M., Borok, R. Z., and Schwartz, M. M. (1995). Focal segmental glomerular sclerosis in adults: presentation, course, and response to treatment. *American Journal of Kidney Diseases* **25**, 534–542.

Sahali, D. *et al.* (2001). Transcriptional and post-transcriptional alterations of IkappaBalpha in active minimal-change nephrotic syndrome. *Journal of the American Society of Nephrology* **12**, 1648–1658.

Sahali, D. *et al.* (2002). A novel approach to investigation of the pathogenesis of active minimal-change nephrotic syndrome using subtracted cDNA library screening. *Journal of the American Society of Nephrology* **13**, 1238–1247.

Sakarlan, A., Timmons, C., and Seikaly, M. (1994). Reversible idiopathic acute renal failure in children with primary nephrotic syndrome. *Journal of Pediatrics* **125**, 723–727.

Sanjad, S. A., al-Abbad, A., and al-Shorafa, S. (1997). Management of hyperlipidemia in children with refractory nephrotic syndrome: the effect of statin therapy. *Journal of Pediatrics* **130**, 470–474.

Sasaki, T., Hatta, H., and Osawa, G. (1999). Cytokines and podocyte injury: the mechanism of fibroblast growth factor 2-induced podocyte injury. *Nephrology, Dialysis, Transplantation* **14** (Suppl. 1), 33–34.

Sasdelli, M., Cagnoli, L., Candi, P., Mandreoli, M., Bettrandi, E., and Zuchelli, P. (1981). Cell mediated immunity in idiopathic glomerulonephritis. *Clinical and Experimental Immunology* **46**, 27–34.

Savin, V. J. (1993). Mechanisms of proteinuria in noninflammatory glomerular diseases. *American Journal of Kidney Diseases* **21**, 347–362.

Savin, V. J. *et al.* (1996). Circulating factor associated with increased glomerular permeability to albumin in recurrent focal and segmental glomerulosclerosis. *New England Journal of Medicine* **334**, 878–883.

Schärer, K. and Minges, U. (1973). Long term prognosis of the nephrotic syndrome in childhood. *Clinical Nephrology* **1**, 182–187.

Schlesinger, E. R., Sultz, H. A., Mosher, W. E., and Feldman, J. G. (1968). The nephrotic syndrome. Its incidence and implications for the community. *American Journal of Diseases of Children* **116**, 623–632.

Schnaper, H. W. (1990). A regulatory system for soluble immune response suppressor production in steroid-responsive nephrotic syndrome. *Kidney International* **38**, 151–159.

Schnaper, H. W. and Aune, T. M. (1985). Identification of the lymphokine soluble immune response suppressor in urine of nephrotic children. *Journal of Clinical Investigation* **76**, 341–349.

Schnaper, J. W. and Aune, T. M. (1987). Steroid-sensitive mechanism of soluble immune response suppressor production in steroid-responsive nephrotic syndrome. *Journal of Clinical Investigation* **79**, 257–264.

Schwartz, M. W. and Lewis, E. J. (1985). Focal segmental glomerular sclerosis: the cellular lesion. *Kidney International* **28**, 968–974.

Schwartz, M. M. and Korbet, S. M. (1993). Primary focal segmental glomerulosclerosis: pathology, histological variants, and pathogenesis. *American Journal of Kidney Diseases* **22**, 874–883.

Schwartz, M. M., Korbet, S. M., Rydell, J., Borok, R., and Genchi, R. (1995). Primary focal segmental glomerular sclerosis in adults: prognostic value of histologic variants. *American Journal of Kidney Diseases* **25**, 845–852.

Schwartz, M. M. (2000). The role of podocyte injury in the pathogenesis of focal segmental glomerulosclerosis. *Renal Failure* **22**, 663–684.

Schweda, F., Liebl, R., Riegger, G. A., and Kramer, B. K. (1997). Tacrolimus treatment for steroid- and cyclosporin-resistant minimal-change nephrotic syndrome. *Nephrology, Dialysis, Transplantation* **12**, 2433–2435.

Segarra, A. *et al.* (2002). Combined therapy of tacrolimus and corticosteroids in cyclosporin-resistant or -dependent idiopathic focal glomerulosclerosis: a preliminary uncontrolled study with prospective follow-up. *Nephrology, Dialysis, Transplantation* **17**, 655–662.

Senggutuvan, P. *et al.* (1990). Recurrence of focal segmental glomerulosclerosis in transplanted kidneys: analysis of incidence and risk factors in 59 allografts. *Pediatric Nephrology* **4**, 21–28.

Sewell, R. F. and Brenchley, P. E. (1986). Red-cell surface charge in glomerular disease. *Lancet* **ii**, 635–636.

Shalhoub, R. J. (1974). Pathogenesis of lipoid nephrosis: a disorder of T cell function. *Lancet* **ii**, 556–559.

Shankland, S. J., Eitner, F., Hudkins, K. L., Goodpaster, T., D'Agati, V., and Alpers, C. E. (2000). Differential expression of cyclin-dependent kinase inhibitors in human glomerular disease: role in podocyte proliferation and maturation. *Kidney International* **58**, 674–683.

Sharma, M., Sharma, R., Reddy, S. R., McCarthy, E. T., and Savin, V. J. (2002). Proteinuria after injection of human focal segmental glomerulosclerosis factor. *Transplantation* **73**, 366–372.

Sharples, P. M., Poulton, J., and White, R. H. R. (1985). Steroid responsive nephrotic syndrome is more common in Asians. *Archives of Diseases in Childhood* **60**, 1014–1017.

Shih, N. Y. *et al.* (1999). Congenital nephrotic syndrome in mice lacking CD2-associated protein. *Science* **286**, 312–315.

Shih, N. Y., Li, J., Cotran, R., Mundel, P., Miner, J. H., and Shaw, A. S. (2001). CD2AP localizes to the slit diaphragm and binds to nephrin via a novel *C*-terminal domain. *American Journal of Pathology* **159**, 2303–2308.

Siegel, N. J., Gaudio, K. M., Krassner, L. S., MacDonald, B., Anderson, F. P., and Kashgarian, M. (1981). Steroid dependent nephrotic syndrome in children: histopathology and relapses after cyclophosphamide treatment. *Kidney International* **19**, 454–459.

Simon, P. and Meyrier, A. (1989). One-year, alternate day dosage, corticosteroid Rx reduces rate of further relapses in adult minimal change nephrosis. *Kidney International* **35**, 201 (abstract).

Singh, A., Tejani, C., and Tejani, A. (1999). One-center experience with cyclosporine in refractory nephrotic syndrome in children. *Pediatric Nephrology* **13**, 26–32.

Sobel, A. T., Branellec, A. L., Blanc, C. J., and Lagrue, G. A. (1977). Physiochemical characterization of a vascular permeability factor, produced by Con A stimulated human lymphocytes. *Journal of Immunology* **119**, 1230–1234.

Southwest Pediatric Nephrology Study Group (1985). Focal segmental glomerulosclerosis in children with idiopathic nephrotic syndrome. *Kidney International* **27**, 442–449.

Spika, J. S. *et al.* (1982). Serum antibody response to pneumococcal vaccine in children with nephrotic syndrome. *Pediatrics* **69**, 219–223.

Srivastava, R. N., Mayekar, G., Anand, R., Choudhry, V. P., Gnaî, O. P., and Tandon, H. D. (1975). Nephrotic syndrome in Indian children. *Archives of Diseases in Childhood* **50**, 626–680.

Srivastava, R. N., Agarwal, R. K., Moudgil, A., and Bhuyan, U. N. (1985). Late resistance to corticosteroids in nephrotic syndrome. *Journal of Pediatrics* **107**, 66–70.

Srivastava, R. N., Kalia, A., Travis, L. B., Diven, S. C., Gugliuzza, K. K., and Rajaraman, S. (1994). Prompt remission of post-renal transplant nephrotic syndrome with high-dose cyclosporine. *Pediatric Nephrology* **8**, 94–95.

Strehlau, J., Schachter, A. D., Pavlakis, M., Singh, A., Tejani, A., and Strom, T. B. (2002). Activated intrarenal transcription of CTL-effectors and TGF-beta1 in children with focal segmental glomerulosclerosis. *Kidney International* **61**, 90–95.

Tanaka, R., Yoshikawa, N., Nakamura, H., and Ito, H. (1992). Infusion of peripheral blood mononuclear cell products from nephrotic children increases albuminuria in rats. *Nephron* **60**, 35–41.

Tanaka, R., Sugihara, K., Tatematsu, A., and Fogo, A. (1995). Internephron heterogeneity of growth factors and sclerosis—modulation of platelet-derived growth factor by angiotensin II. *Kidney International* **47**, 131–139.

Tanawattanacharoen, S., Falk, R. J., Jennette, J. C., and Kopp, J. B. (2000). Parvovirus B19 DNA in kidney tissue of patients with focal segmental glomerulosclerosis. *American Journal of Kidney Diseases* **35**, 1166–1174.

Tanphaichitr, P., Tanphaichitr, D., Sureetanan, J., and Chatasigh, S. (1980). Treatment of nephrotic syndrome with levamisole. *Journal of Pediatrics* **96**, 490–493.

Tarshish, P., Tobin, J. N., Bernstein, J., and Edelmann, C. M., Jr. (1996). Cyclophosphamide does not benefit patients with focal segmental glomerulosclerosis. A report of the International Study of Kidney Disease in Children. *Pediatric Nephrology* **10**, 590–593.

Taube, D., Brown, Z., and Williams, D. G. (1984). Impaired lymphocyte and suppressor cell function in minimal change nephropathy membranous nephropathy and focal glomerulosclerosis. *Clinical Nephrology* **22**, 176–182.

Tejani, A. (1985). Morphological transitions in minimal change nephrotic syndrome. *Nephron* **39**, 157–159.

Tejani, A., Suthanthiran, M., and Pomerantz, A. (1991). A randomized controlled trial of low-dose prednisone and cyclosporin versus high-dose prednisone in nephrotic syndrome of children. *Nephron* **59**, 96–99.

Topaloglu, R., Saatci, U., Arikan, M., Canpinar, H., Bakkaloglu, A., and Kansu, E. (1994). T-cell subsets, interleukin-2 receptor expression and production of interleukin-2 in minimal change nephrotic syndrome. *Pediatric Nephrology* **8**, 649–652.

Toth, C. M. *et al.* (1998). Recurrent collapsing glomerulopathy. *Transplantation* **65**, 1009–1010.

Trainin, E. B., Boichis, H., Spitzer, A., Edelmann, C. M., and Greifer, I. (1975). Late non responsiveness to steroids in children with the nephrotic syndrome. *Journal of Pediatrics* **87**, 519–523.

Traynor, A., Kuzel, T., Samuelson, E., and Kanwar, Y. (1994). Minimal change glomerulopathy and glomerular visceral epithelial hyperplasia associated with alpha-interferon therapy for cutaneous T-cell lymphoma. *Nephron* **67**, 94–100.

Trompeter, R. S. Steroid resistant nephrotic syndrome: a review of the treatment of focal segmental glomerulosclerosis in children. In *Recent Advances in Pediatric Nephrology* (ed. K. Murakami, T. Kitagawa, K. Yabuta, and T. Sakai), pp. 363–371. Amsterdam: Excerpta Medica, 1987.

Trompeter, R. S., Evans, P. R., and Barratt, T. M. (1981). Gonadal function in boys with steroid responsive nephrotic syndrome treated with cyclophosphamide for short periods. *Lancet* **i**, 1177–1180.

Trompeter, R. S., Hicks, J., Lloyd, B. W., White, R. H. R., and Cameron, J. S. (1985). Long term outcome for children with minimal change nephrotic syndrome. *Lancet* **i**, 368–370.

Tune, B. M., Kirpekar, R. K., Reznik, V. M., Grisfold, W. R., and Mendoza, S. A. (1995). Intravenous methylprednisolone and oral alkylating agent therapy of prednisone-resistant pediatric focal segmental glomerulosclerosis: a long-term follow-up. *Clinical Nephrology* **43**, 84–88.

Ueda, N. *et al.* (1988). Intermittent versus long-term tapering prednisolone for initial therapy in children with idiopathic nephrotic syndrome. *Journal of Pediatrics* **112**, 122–126.

Ueda, N., Kuno, K., and Ito, S. (1990). Eight and 12 week courses of cyclophosphamide in nephrotic syndrome. *Archives of Disease in Childhood* **65**, 1147–1150.

Valeri, A., Barisoni, L., Appel, G. B., Seigle, R., and D'Agati, V. (1996). Idiopathic collapsing focal segmental glomerulosclerosis: a clinicopathologic study. *Kidney International* **50**, 1734–1746.

Van den Berg, J. G. *et al.* (2000). Interleukin-4 and interleukin-13 act on glomerular visceral epithelial cells. *Journal of the American Society of Nephrology* **11**, 413–422.

Van den Berg, J. G., Aten, J., Annink, C., Ravesloot, J. H., Weber, E., and Weening, J. J. (2002). Interleukin-4 and -13 promote basolateral secretion of H(+) and cathepsin L by glomerular epithelial cells. *American Journal of Physiology. Renal Physiology* **282**, F26–F33.

Van den Born, J., Van den Heuvel, L. P. W. J., Bakker, M. A. H., Veerkamp, J. H., Assmann, K. J. M., and Berden, J. H. M. (1992). A monoclonal antibody against GBM heparan sulfate induces an acute selective proteinuria in rats. *Kidney International* **41**, 115–123.

Velosa, J. A., Donadio, J. V., and Holley, K. E. (1975). Focal sclerosing glomerulopathy. *Mayo Clinic Proceedings* **50**, 121–132.

Velosa, J. A., Torres, V. E., Donadio, J. V., Jr., Wagoner, R. D., Holley, K. E., and Offord, K. P. (1985). Treatment of severe nephrotic syndrome with meclofenamate: an uncontrolled pilot study. *Mayo Clinic Proceedings* **60**, 586–592.

Verani, R. R. and Hawkins, E. P. (1986). Recurrent focal segmental glomerulosclerosis: a pathological study of the early lesion. *American Journal of Nephrology* **6**, 263–270.

Waldherr, R., Gubler, M., Levy, M., Broyer, M., and Habib, R. (1978). The significance of pure mesangial proliferation in idiopathic nephrotic syndrome. *Clinical Nephrology* **10**, 171–179.

Waldo, F. B., Benfield, M. R., and Kohaut, E. C. (1992). Methylprednisolone treatment of patients with steroid-resistant nephrotic syndrome. *Pediatric Nephrology* **6**, 503–505.

Wang, F., Loo, L. M., and Chua, C. T. (1982). Minimal change glomerular disease in Malaysian adults and use of alternate day steroid therapy. *Quarterly Journal of Medicine* **51**, 312–328.

Watson, A. R., Taylor, J., Rance, C. P., and Bain, J. (1986). Gonadal function in women treated with cyclophosphamide for childhood nephrotic syndrome: a long term follow-up study. *Fertility and Sterility* **46**, 331–333.

Weiss, M. A., Daquioag, E., Margolin, G., and Pollak, V. E. (1986). Nephrotic syndrome, progressive irreversible renal failure and glomerular 'collapse'. A new clinicopathologic entity? *American Journal of Kidney Diseases* **7**, 20–28.

White, R. H. R. (1973). The familial nephrotic syndrome. A European survey. *Clinical Nephrology* **1**, 215–219.

Williams, S. A., Makker, S. P., Ingelfinger, J. R., and Grupe, W. E. (1980). Long term evaluation of chlorambucil plus prednisone in idiopathic nephrotic syndrome of childhood. *New England Journal of Medicine* **302**, 929–933.

Wingen, A. M., Muller-Wiefel, D. E., and Scharer, K. (1985). Spontaneous remissions in frequently relapsing and steroid dependent idiopathic nephrotic syndrome. *Clinical Nephrology* **23**, 35–40.

Winn, M. P. *et al.* (1999a). Clinical and genetic heterogeneity in familial focal segmental glomerulosclerosis. International Collaborative Group for the Study of Familial Focal Segmental Glomerulosclerosis. *Kidney International* **55**, 1241–1246.

Winn, M. P. *et al.* (1999b). Linkage of a gene causing familial focal segmental glomerulosclerosis to chromosome 11 and further evidence of genetic heterogeneity. *Genomics* **58**, 113–120.

Wynn, S. R., Stickler, G. B., and Burke, E. C. (1988). Long term prognosis for children with nephrotic syndrome. *Clinical Pediatrics* **27**, 63–68.

Yan, K. *et al.* (1998). The increase of memory T cell subsets in children with idiopathic nephrotic syndrome. *Nephron* **79**, 274–278.

Yap, H. K., Cheung, W., Murugasu, B., Sim, S. K., Seah, C. C., and Jordan, S. C. (1999). Th1 and Th2 cytokine mRNA profiles in childhood nephrotic syndrome: evidence for increased IL-13 mRNA expression in relapse. *Journal of the American Society of Nephrology* **10**, 529–537.

Yokoyama, H., Kida, H., Abe, T., Koshino, Y., Yoshimura, M., and Hattori, N. (1987). Impaired immunoglobulin G production in minimal change nephrotic syndrome in adults. *Clinical and Experimental Immunology* **70**, 110–115.

Zimmerman, S. W. (1984). Increased urinary protein excretion in the rat produced by serum from patient with recurrent focal glomerular sclerosis after renal transplantation. *Clinical Nephrology* **22**, 32–38.

3.6 IgA nephropathies

Francesco Paolo Schena and Rosanna Coppo

Definition of IgA nephropathies

IgA nephropathies are characterized by the presence of diffuse mesangial deposits of IgA in the glomeruli which occur in selected pathological entities such as Berger's disease, Henoch–Schönlein purpura (Chapter 4.5.2), systemic lupus erythematosus (Chapters 4.7.1 and 4.7.2), and in liver diseases. Several systemic diseases in which an abnormal response of the IgA system is present may also be associated with IgA nephropathy. The renal disease may occur before and during the clinical course of the disease, and a wide variety of glomerular lesions may be present.

Primary IgA nephropathy (Berger's disease)

Primary IgA nephropathy, or Berger's disease, is mostly characterized by recurrent episodes of gross haematuria concomitant with upper respiratory tract infections or other mucosal inflammatory processes. In other patients, microscopic haematuria and/or proteinuria are the only symptoms. There is absence of any recognizable systemic disease (lupus erythematosus, Henoch–Schönlein purpura, cryoglobulinaemia), liver disease, or lower urinary tract diseases.

Clinical manifestations

At apparent onset

Haematuria

The first episode of macroscopic haematuria occurs generally between 15 and 30 years of age, which is often 7–10 years earlier than when a biopsy diagnosis is made. Since it is conceivable that the pathogenetic process leading to IgA deposit formation and clinical symptoms lasts several years, the true onset of primary IgA nephropathy is thus usually in the teens or even earlier. Affected children do not present symptoms and/or urinary signs before the age of 3 years; thereafter the frequency increases with age.

In many patients, the first sign is the abrupt appearance of macroscopic haematuria concomitant with inflammation, usually mucosal. Episodes of *macroscopic haematuria* can be associated with any of the events reported in Table 1, but the majority occur after mucosal infections, usually of the upper respiratory tract and less often of other sites (Fig. 1); rarely they occur after vaccination or heavy physical exercise. The interval between the precipitating event and the appearance of macrohaematuria is very short (12–72 h), compared with 1–3 weeks in postinfectious acute glomerulonephritis. The macrohaematuria persists for less than 3 days and is sometimes accompanied by flank and loin pain and, occasionally, fever. The colour of the urine is red or brown (coke-coloured); blood casts are common, rarely blood clots can be found. The number of recurrent episodes of gross haematuria is variable in adults, declining in frequency with increasing age in both

Table 1 Precipitating factors for haematuria in IgA nephropathy

Upper respiratory tract infections
  Tonsillitis
  Pharyngitis
  Bronchitis

Acute gastroenteritis
Hepatitis A/B
Periostitis
Staphylococcal osteomyelitis
Septic arthritis
Peritonitis
Lobar pneumonia
Erysipelas
Erythema polymorphus
Staphylococcal sepsis
Typhoid fever
Brucellosis
Infectious mononucleosis
Influenza-like syndromes
Rubella
Mumps
Herpes zoster
Tonsillectomy
Tooth extraction
Appendicectomy
Heavy physical exercise
Vaccine
BCG overdose

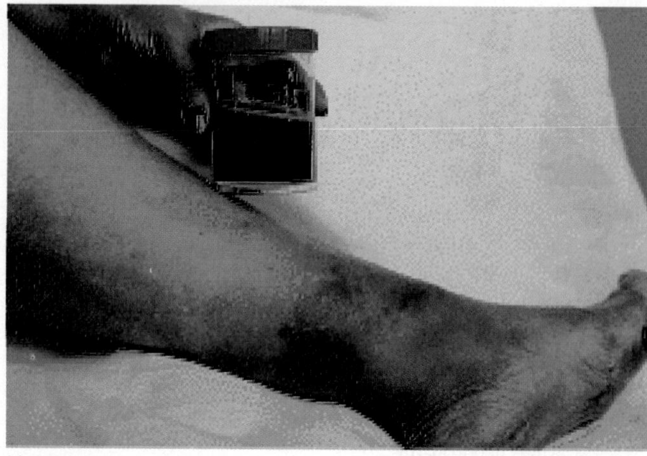

(a)

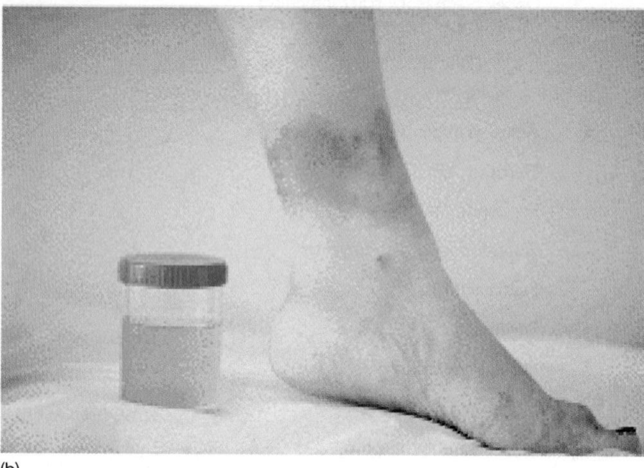

(b)

Fig. 1 'Coke'©-coloured urine in a patient with previously diagnosed primary IgA nephropathy during an episode of erysipelas (a). The urine shows a variation in colour a few days after the infectious episode (b) (see text).

sexes, whereas this is a characteristic feature of the clinical picture of the disease in 30–40 per cent of children.

The apparent onset in other cases is asymptomatic persistent microscopic haematuria and/or mild proteinuria. More than 5000 red blood cells/ml in the urine may be assumed as a possible presentation of the disease. In many cases microhaematuria is detected by chance as a result of pre-employment or blood donor screening in adults, or of investigation for sport or school screening programmes, particularly in Japan.

Due to the different attitude towards the performance of screening tests, the frequency of IgA nephropathy detected through persistent microscopic haematuria is higher in patients in Asia (67.4 per cent) than in Europe (39.4 per cent), North America (38.1 per cent), and Australia (30.2 per cent). Similar variations are reported in children, and a mean of 30–50 per cent of childhood patients are biopsied because of persistent microscopic haematuria with or without proteinuria. Macroscopic haematuria is more frequent in North American (56 per cent), Australian (46.5 per cent), and European (39.7 per cent) patients than those from Asia (11.5 per cent). In all patients, the presence of glomerular IgA immune deposits is concomitant with the clinical signs, except for a few cases in which IgA deposition appears months or years after the clinical onset of the disease.

Proteinuria

In asymptomatic patients, detected at routine medical examinations, chance proteinuria may be found in 3–13 per cent of cases. The degree of proteinuria tends to remain fairly stable. A transient increase in proteinuria occurs coinciding with episodes of gross haematuria or in subjects with a history of fever, sore throat, pain in the lumbar or loin region, dysuria, and transient suborbital or ankle oedema.

In some children (6 per cent), the clinical onset can be in full nephrotic syndrome, and only the renal biopsy allows a correct diagnosis of IgA nephropathy.

Other presentations

In a low percentage of patients the disease appears as acute renal failure (9 per cent), nephrotic syndrome (2.8–7.5 per cent), and/or hypertension (1.7–14.8 per cent). In a few cases, there is an acute nephritic syndrome, similar to poststreptococcal glomerulonephritis, at the onset of the disease. In these patients, macrohaematuria is associated with increased serum creatinine and urea, and also hypertension. In rare cases, the onset may be severe nephritic syndrome progressing to chronic renal failure due to crescentic lesions. Furthermore, in a few patients, acute oliguric failure, usually spontaneously reversible, accompanies the episodes of macrohaematuria, attributed to tubular obstruction by red blood cells. Other clinicians have observed the superimposition of poststreptococcal acute glomerulonephritis on the course of the IgA nephropathy. Finally, primary IgA nephropathy may recur after transplantation, with the appearance of microhaematuria and mild proteinuria.

At the time of renal biopsy

Haematuria

The episodes of macrohaematuria are more frequent during the first few years of the disease and then tend to disappear. The relative incidence of this symptom is greater in adolescents and young adults than in small children and older patients. This difference varies greatly in various geographical areas because of differences in the policy of submitting patients with this symptom for renal biopsy.

In some countries of the Asian Pacific area (Japan, Hong Kong, Singapore), microscopic haematuria together with asymptomatic proteinuria is the main clinical finding at the time of renal biopsy in children and in young adults undergoing school screening programmes or during the routine or regular medical examinations of male army recruits. By contrast, in Asia macroscopic haematuria is an unusual presenting symptom either at presentation or at renal biopsy. The prevalence of micro- and macrohaematuria in different areas of the world is shown in Fig. 2 (Schena 1990).

In a small number of patients presentation of the disease is characterized clinically by macrohaematuria, proteinuria, and rapid deterioration of renal function. In these cases, the histological examination of renal biopsy samples reveals prominent crescent formation that usually involve more than 30–50 per cent of the glomeruli. This condition has been called 'rapidly progressive glomerulonephritis' or 'malignant IgA nephropathy'.

Proteinuria

Proteinuria may be mild (<1 g/day), moderate (1–3 g/day), or severe (>3 g/day). Proteinuria of less than 3 g/day, as a clinical presentation, has been observed more frequently in Europeans (13.6 per cent) than

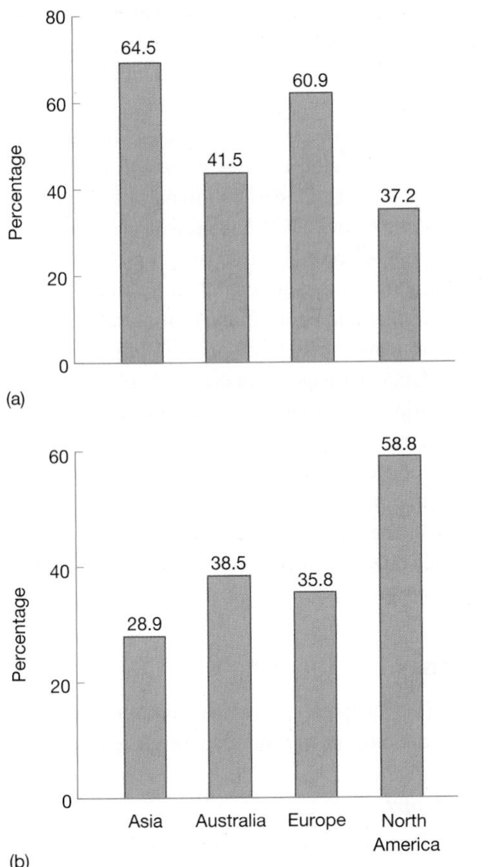

Fig. 2 Percentage of microhaematuria (a) and macrohaematuria (b) observed at clinical presentation and renal biopsy in patients with primary IgA nephropathy.

in North Americans (6.6 per cent), Asians (4.8 per cent), and Australians (3 per cent) (Schena 1990). At the time of renal biopsy, mild or moderate proteinuria is present in approximately 15 per cent of patients worldwide.

Nephrotic syndrome

The nephrotic syndrome rarely appears at the onset of the disease. Its occurrence is more prevalent later in the natural course of the disease and is greater in Asians and North Americans than in Australians and Europeans. The renal lesions may be minimal or severe.

Spontaneous remission of the nephrotic syndrome has been reported in a few patients with primary IgA nephropathy, mainly children, in whom the renal biopsy revealed a minimal change disease together with mesangial deposits of IgA. The occurrence of mild or minimal glomerular lesions, normal renal function, good response to corticosteroids, and a tendency to relapse clearly recalls minimal change disease, and it is possible that, in some cases, primary IgA nephropathy is superimposed upon a preceding, undiagnosed minimal change disease. This suggestion is supported by the finding of nephrotic children whose first renal biopsies failed to reveal IgA deposits, which were detected in a subsequent biopsy (Southwest Pediatric Nephrology Study Group 1985). Alternative explanations for this particular form of primary IgA nephropathy may be the possible intermittent appearance of mesangial IgA deposits, the failure to identify IgA at the initial biopsy, or the presence of the disease with IgA deposits in a focal distribution, affecting only some glomeruli.

Renal insufficiency

Acute renal failure, occurring in 3 per cent patients, is more common in the presence of macrohaematuria and red blood cell casts in tubules, and may occur on more than one occasion in the same patient. The long-term prognosis for these patients is excellent, while patients with more than 40 per cent of sclerosed glomeruli show irreversible renal failure. Acute renal failure occurs rarely in older patients.

Acute renal failure with rapid progression to endstage renal failure is frequent also in IgA nephropathy patients with necrotizing lesions in the segmental areas of the glomeruli, extracapillary lesions, and interstitial accumulation of monocytes and T lymphocytes. Some of these patients may have serum positivity for antineutrophil cytoplasmic antoantibodies (ANCA), mainly IgA antibodies. This novel subset of crescentic IgA nephropathy associated with high-titre of antimyeloperoxidase antibodies constitute an overlap group between IgAN and microscopic polyangitis (Allmaras *et al.* 1997).

The frequency of chronic renal insufficiency at the time of renal biopsy is greater in Australian (32.2 per cent), European (22.8 per cent), and North American patients (22.5 per cent) than in Asian patients (16 per cent). The difference may be accounted for by the different policies adopted towards renal biopsy in eastern and western areas of the world.

Hypertension

The frequency of hypertension in patients without renal insufficiency is greater than that found in the healthy population, matched for gender and age, and living in the same geographical area. At the clinical onset, hypertension is more frequent in Australian patients (14.8 per cent) than in Europeans (9.8 per cent), North Americans (7.5 per cent), and Asians (1.7 per cent). It commonly develops during the course of the disease, sometimes before serum creatinine is appreciably increased. At the time of renal biopsy, hypertension is more frequent in Australians (52.5 per cent) than in Europeans (24.7 per cent), North-Americans (24.2 per cent), and Asians (18.6 per cent). It is less common in children (5 per cent) and occurs more frequently in patients who present the disease after the age of 35 and in those with decreased renal function. In some subjects, hypertension accelerates the impairment of renal function. Malignant hypertension occurs in 7–15 per cent of patients and is associated with a rapid decline in renal function. In these cases, the renal biopsy reveals epithelial crescents in the majority of glomeruli.

Laboratory findings

Serum IgA

An elevated serum IgA is found in 35–50 per cent of patients. This marker may suggest the possible presence of the disease. The initial high values persist in some patients, and decline to normal in others. The IgA1 subclass is largely predominant, although in Afro-American patients the serum concentration of IgA2 is also elevated. This finding is in accordance with the deposition of IgA2 in the mesangium of 56 per cent of Afro-American patients.

IgA is unique amongst immunoglobulins for its ability to form multimers. High serum concentrations of polymeric IgA have been observed in one-fourth of patients; they may have an anti-IgG activity (rheumatoid factor) or an anti-IgA activity.

Immune complexes

In 30–70 per cent of patients, either adults or children, high titres of IgA immune complexes and a low frequency of IgG immune complexes have been found consistently in the blood of patients with primary IgA nephropathy (Coppo *et al.* 1995). The former are present both in the acute phase of the disease (fever, upper respiratory tract infection, and macrohaematuria) and in remission, the latter appear only in relapses (Schena *et al.* 1989b). The complexes may contain antibodies against bacterial, viral, and food antigens.

Proteinuria

The presence of proteinuria is closely correlated to an impairment of renal function. When proteinuria exceeds 2 g/day, there is an increased incidence of renal failure as well as an increased incidence of crescents in the renal biopsy. As heavy proteinuria often precedes the appearance of hypertension in progressive patients, its identification may be a useful marker of active nephritis. Patients with poorly selective proteinuria have worse clinical features, such as renal impairment, hypertension, and severe glomerulosclerosis (Woo *et al.* 1989). In contrast, selective proteinuria is associated with mild histological changes. In addition, selective proteinuria tends to be steroid responsive, whereas non-selective proteinuria is not.

Other laboratory features

Antistreptolysin O titres are elevated in a small number of patients. The presence of cryoglobulins and cryofibrinogen in serum and plasma has been observed in a few cases. High serum alpha-1 antitrypsin, haptoglobin, and orosomucoid may be found.

In a few cases of primary IgA nephropathy, ANCA, rarely of IgA class, have been detected. The disease is characterized by haematuria, proteinuria (sometimes in nephrotic range), and acute progressive renal insufficiency. Renal histological lesions may be those of a necrotizing and crescentic glomerulonephritis (Haas *et al.* 2000).

In 20–30 per cent of patients, IgA specific for alimentary antigens have been detected, but the serum levels of such antibodies did not correlate with IgA immune complexes or disease activity (Coppo *et al.* 1995). High serum IgA antibodies against *Haemophilus parainfluenzae* antigen, CMV, and EBV capsid antigen have been found in some patients.

Routine tests have indicated that serum complement (C3, C4, and factor B) is normal. Nevertheless, sensitive techniques able to detect small amounts of some neoantigens of C3, such as iC3b and C3b, provide evidence of complement activation in patients with primary IgA nephropathy, both adults and children (Coppo *et al.* 1982; Wyatt *et al.* 1987). Increased activated plasma C3 levels is present in 30 per cent of patients, frequently in patients with proteinuria and haematuria. Elevated levels at presentation correlate with subsequent deterioration of renal function and, thus, may be used as predictor of the subsequent course of IgA nephropathy (Zwirner *et al.* 1997).

Individual complement protein deficiencies have been observed in some IgA nephropathy patients. A partial deficiency of a complement component, such as factor H which controls the C3b amplification loop, has been found in some patients and in their relatives (Wyatt *et al.* 1982). Congenital C9 deficiency has been reported in three young Japanese males with primary IgA nephropathy (Yoshioka *et al.* 1992). Immunohistochemical staining of renal biopsy tissues showed IgA and C3 in association with C5, C8, and S-protein, while C5b-9 neoantigen was completely negative. These data demonstrate that the formation of the C5b-9 complex is not essential for the induction of glomerular disease.

Increased urinary excretion of cytokines (IL-6) and chemokines (MCP-1 and IL-8) have been observed in IgA nephropathy patients with severe renal damage. IL-6 excretion may be influenced by mesangial cell proliferation and MCP-1 is present when interstitial infiltration of macrophages occur (Grandaliano *et al.* 1996). IL-8 is elevated in urine of patients with acute renal damage and its excretion correlates with glomerular and endocapillary proliferation (Yokoyama *et al.* 1998). Reduced urinary EGF levels occur in IgA nephropathy patients with severe tubular damage (Ranieri *et al.* 1996). Recently, urinary EGF/MCP-1 ratio was proposed as a prognostic marker for evaluating progression of renal damage in the presence of mild proteinuria (Schena and Gesualdo 2001).

Other urinary markers of activity and glomerular damage have been signalled as the excretion of podocytes (Hara *et al.* 1998) and the excretion of activated macrophages (Hotta *et al.* 1999), but are not in regular use.

Renal biopsy

Renal biopsy (see Chapter 1.7) remains the most important tool for diagnosis and the most powerful predictor for renal outcome in IgAN.

Light microscopy

The first histological lesions that appear in the glomeruli are represented by increased extracellular matrix and hypercellularity of the mesangium. Subsequently, the spectrum of glomerular abnormalities may enlarge and virtually all morphological manifestations of glomerular damage, such as floculo-capsular adhesions, segmental sclerosis, and crescents may be observed. For this reason, different classifications have been used by renal pathologists. The grading of histological damage is based principally on the severity of cellular proliferation and glomerulosclerosis, on the number of crescents, and on the presence or absence of tubular atrophy and interstitial cellular infiltration or fibrosis. On the basis of similar renal pathological and immunohistological findings in Berger's disease and in Henoch–Schönlein nephritis, Lee *et al.* (1982) and Sinniah *et al.* (1985) used the classification of Meadow *et al.* (1972) for morphological distinction. Although only 20 IgAN patients were assessed in Lee's classification, it has been applied in a number of studies, including many patients, which have confirmed its utility. There are problems in using this classification: for example, Hass (1997) demonstrated that the tubulointerstitial damage was underscored and a new classification was proposed. After that, a number of other histological systems have been put forward (Southwest Pediatric Nephrology Study Group 1982; Kobayashi *et al.* 1983; Mina and Murphy 1985; Alamartine *et al.* 1991). All these systems may be divided into two groups: 'lumped' and 'split' (Wyatt *et al.* 1997). 'Lumped' systems are those introduced by Lee *et al.* (1982) and Mina and Murphy (1985). 'Split' systems include those of Kobayashi *et al.* (1983), Andreoli and Bergstein (1989), Alamartine *et al.* (1990), and Waldo *et al.* (1993). The lumped system is used for its simplicity and easy application in large multicentre studies. The scoring system as mild, moderate, or severe is valuable in the analysis of a large clinical database. The weakness of a lumped system is the lack of flexibility in interpretation and the chance that important isolated pathological changes be missed. The split system gives a detailed analysis of each lesion by introducing a global score which provides more information on the evaluation of glomeruli, tubules, interstitium, and vessels. This system has more flexibility and minimal intercentre variability. According to our experience, the use of a lumped system is useful for diagnosis and grading of IgAN, and the application of a split system for comparing two or more renal biopsies performed on the same patient. The use of a glomerular, tubular, interstitial, and vascular scores could be more informative on the progression of renal lesions.

To describe the renal lesion, we use the classification of Churg and Sobin (1982), accepted by the World Health Organization and recently updated (Churg *et al.* 1995). This classification has been in part revised by us (Table 2). The grading of histological damage is based principally on the severity of cellular proliferation and glomerulosclerosis, on the number of crescents, and on the presence or absence of tubular atrophy and interstitial cellular infiltration or fibrosis (Fig. 3). Thus, in order of severity of renal damage, we distinguish three grades (G): G1 (mild) includes IgAN patients with minor or minimal lesions; G2 (moderate) includes patients with focal–segmental or diffuse proliferative glomerulonephritis; G3 (severe) includes patients with sclerotic lesions in advanced chronic glomerulonephritis or end-stage renal disease. Table 3 shows our scoring system represented by a slightly modified Pirani and Salinas-Marrigal classification (1968). Renal biopsy containing at least six glomeruli is considered adequate for scoring of the renal biopsy specimens performed on the same patient.

Biopsies performed during or within episodes of macrohaematuria show a remarkable amount of polymorphs, macrophages, fibrin, and small crescents which later disappear. For this reason, renal biopsy is recommended after 30 days from the episode of macroscopic haematuria.

Biopsy specimens taken within the first year from the onset of disease usually show minor changes. In contrast, focal lesions, diffuse mesangial cell proliferation, and diffuse sclerosing glomerulonephritis are more frequent in patients examined 3 or more years after the clinical onset of disease. A renal biopsy study performed in patients in relationship to the appearance of haematuria and proteinuria at clinical onset in the presence of normal renal function (serum creatinine < 1.2 mg/dl or Ccr > 80 ml/min) revealed that the glomerular damage was more evident when the interval between clinical onset and renal biopsy was

Table 2 Histological classification of IgA nephropathy

Grade	Class	Glomerular changes	Tubulointerstitial changes
I[a] (mild)	A	Normal glomeruli	
	B	Slight mesangial cellularity	
	C	Slight mesangial matrix	
II[b] (moderate)	A	<25% of the glomeruli with moderate focal and segmental mesangial proliferation and rare sclerosis Rare small crescents	Occasional focal interstitial infiltrate
	B	Up to 50% of the glomeruli with moderate focal and segmental mesangial proliferation and/or sclerosis Capillary obstruction by endocapillary cell proliferation Adhesions and cellular crescents less than 25% of glomeruli	Focal interstitial infiltrate less than 25% of cortical area
	C	>50% of the glomeruli with segmental proliferation and/or sclerosis Adhesions and cellular crescents up to 50% of glomeruli	Tubular atrophy and interstitial infiltrate up to 50% of the cortical area
III[c] (severe)	A	<25% of the glomeruli with focal and segmental or global sclerosis Adhesions and fibrous crescents less than 25% of glomeruli	Tubular atrophy, interstitial infiltrate and sclerosis in less than 25% of the cortical area
	B	Sclerosis up to 50% of glomeruli Adhesions and fibrous crescents up to 50% of glomeruli	Tubular atrophy, interstitial infiltrate and sclerosis up to 50% of the cortical area
	C	Sclerosis more than 50% of glomeruli Adhesions and fibrous crescents in more than 50% of the glomeruli	Tubular atrophy, interstitial infiltrate and sclerosis more than 50% of the cortical area

Grade I: Minimal or minor lesions.

Grade II: Focal-segmental or diffuse proliferative glomerulonephritis (mainly proliferative lesions).

Grade III: Advanced chronic glomerulonephritis or endstage renal disease (mainly sclerotic lesions).

[a] The presence of occasional global sclerotic glomeruli does not remove the biopsy specimen from this category.

[b] The presence of occasional fibrous crescents does not remove the biopsy specimen from this category.

[c] The presence of occasional proliferative lesions does not remove the biopsy specimen from this category.

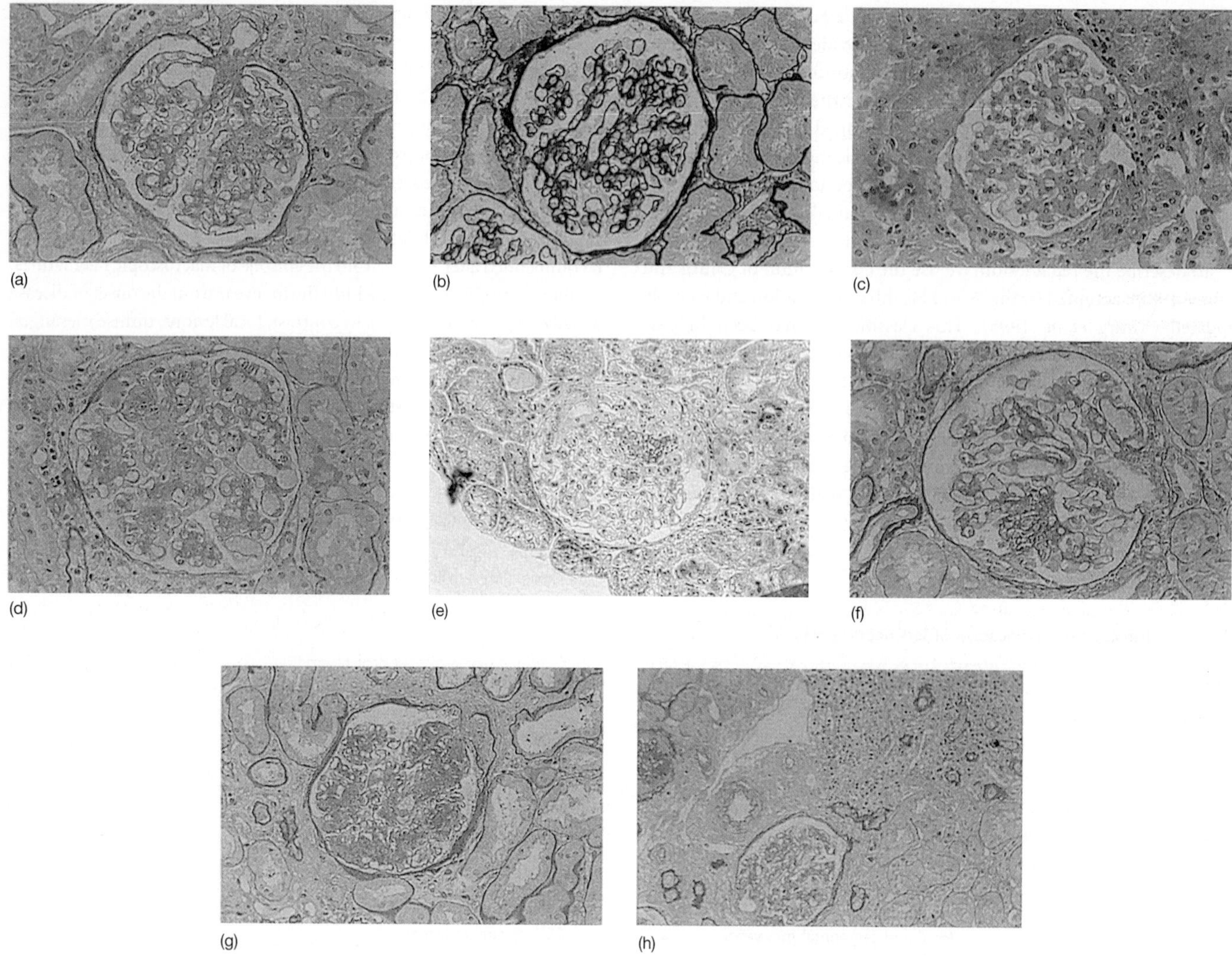

Fig. 3 Elementary renal lesions observed in patients with primary IgA nephropathy are reported according to their gradual and progressive severity. The combination of these lesions defines the five grades of primary IgA nephropathy. (a) Mild expansion of the mesangial matrix and segmental mesangial hypercellularity in the right part of the glomerulus (PAS 500×). (b) Moderate expansion of the mesangial matrix which evidences the mesangial tree in the glomerulus (PASM 500×). (c) Enlargement of the mesangial area caused by mild hypercellularity, increased mesangial matrix, and large fuchsin-positive mesangial deposits (Masson 500×). (d) Severe global expansion of the mesangium caused by increased cell proliferation and matrix deposition (PAS 500×). (e) Segmental necrosis with epithelial proliferation and a small cellular crescent (Masson 500×). (f) Segmental sclerosis with capsular adhesion very close to the fibrotic crescent (PAS 500×). (g) Marked mesangial proliferation with deposits of hyaline substance and capsular adhesion (PAS 400×). (h) Interstitial infiltration with mononuclear cells, tubular atrophy, and glomerular ischaemia (PAS 150×).

longer (>3 years). The multivariate analysis of the difference between urinary abnormality and onset and renal biopsy time showed twice the hazard ratio in patients with more than 3 years of interval. Therefore, the glomerular damage is able to progress for 3 years or longer after the clinical onset of renal disease. Thus, a renal biopsy should be performed within 3 years from the clinical onset of the disease in IgA nephropathy patients demonstrating both haematuria and proteinuria, when such subjects are also suspected of having the disease (Kiyoshi *et al.* 1998). The significant risk of progression in low-grade lesions suggests that the point of no return may occur earlier than perceived and that delayed renal biopsy in these patients may no longer be justified. Combined grade histology and isolated haematuria at the time of renal biopsy enhance the sensitivity to determine early IgA nephropathy and to define a non-early cohort with a higher risk of disease progression appropriate for the recruitment into clinical trials within realistic time frames (Lai *et al.* 2002).

In general, the clinical course of the disease corresponds to the histological course, which makes renal biopsy a good prognostic indicator (Table 3). Patients with asymptomatic microhaematuria and proteinuria detected at a routine medical examination most frequently have minimal or minor changes on the initial renal biopsy. Renal biopsies from patients with episodes of gross haematuria reveal histological changes of grades 1 to 2, whereas patients with the nephrotic syndrome mainly show grade 3 lesions, similar to those found in patients with renal insufficiency. Hypertension is more frequent in patients with grades 2 and 3 histological lesions. Patients admitted with rapidly progressive glomerulonephritis have florid crescents in many glomeruli and diffuse signs of sclerosing glomerulonephritis. Small crescents usually

Table 3 Histologic score of the renal biopsy in IgA nephropathy

Glomeruli	Tubules	Interstitium	Vessels	Total
Mesangial cell proliferation (0–3)	Atrophy (0–3)	Oedema (0–3)	Hyalinosis + intimal fibrosis (0–3)	
Endocapillary proliferation (0–3)	Necrosis (0–3)	Cellular infiltrates (0–3)	Intimal proliferation (0–3)	
Cellular crescents (0–3)		Fibrosis (0–3)	Vascular thrombosis (0–3)	
Mesangial matrix increase (0–3)			Fibrinoid necrosis (0–3)	
Fibrotic crescents (0–3)				
Glomerular sclerosis Segmental (0–3) Global (0–3)				
0–21[a]	0–6[a]	0–9[a]	0–12[a]	0–48[a]

Absent = 0; less than 25% of glomeruli, tubules, interstitium or vessels involved = 1; up to 50% = 2; more than 50% = 3.

[a] Indicates range.

represent an occasional finding in primary IgA nephropathy, but in a small number of patients the histological lesions consist mainly of crescents (crescentic IgA nephropathy). The presence of fibrin and other biologically active substances stimulates the accumulation of monocytes and triggers the local proliferation of visceral and parietal epithelium.

Tubulointerstitial changes are present in a varying percentage of cases. Studies, designed to characterize interstitial cell infiltrates, demonstrated the presence of an increased number of monocytes/macrophages and T-lymphocytes, mainly T-helper/inducer cells, while the amount of T-suppressor/cytotoxic cells was within the normal range (Alexopoulos *et al.* 1989). The severity of tubulointerstitial lesions, as well as glomerulosclerosis, is more common in older patients. In contrast, mesangial proliferation is more frequent in younger patients. Very large macrophages are usually seen in the lumen of renal tubules and in the urine. They frequently have contact with tubular epithelial cells expressing intercellular adhesion molecules and the tubular cells in such lesions often have degenerative changes. The number of these giant macrophages correlates with the degree of haematuria, proteinuria, and serum creatinine value. The existence of very large macrophages in certain active inflammatory sites reflects the activity of the disease and may have a predictive value for the progression of glomerulonephritis (Oda *et al.* 1998).

The renal lesions observed at repeated biopsies are proliferative lesions that change little, and in some cases mesangial cell proliferation is replaced by an increased mesangial matrix. Glomerular sclerosis, interstitial fibrosis, and vessel wall damage increase with time, although there is much variation in the rate of increase among patients.

A strong correlation has been found between the plasma creatinine concentration at the time of biopsy and the degree of global sclerosis, arteriosclerosis, and interstitial fibrosis, and these correlate with age at biopsy and with age at the onset of the disease. In a few cases, an episode of gross haematuria precedes the acute worsening of renal function, which may require temporary dialytic support. The biopsy exhibits benign glomerular morphology, with only some glomeruli showing segmental crescents or sclerosis, but a severe acute tubular necrosis. Most of the tubules are filled with red blood cell casts occluding tubular lumens; erythrophagocytosis, pigment phagocytosis, and/or tubular obstruction are very common (Praga *et al.* 1985).

The most constant abnormality in children with primary IgA nephropathy is a widening of the glomerular mesangium due to a variable combination of mesangial hypercellularity and increased mesangial matrix. Histological examination of Japanese children with primary IgA nephropathy (Yoshikawa *et al.* 1987) revealed that predominant mesangial hypercellularity was almost exclusively seen in the initial biopsy, whereas predominant mesangial matrix expansion was usually seen at the follow-up biopsy. Thus, mesangial hypercellularity is characteristic of an early lesion in children, but progression of the disease leads to a gradual decrease in mesangial cellularity and an increase in matrix with subsequent sclerosis. Focal tubular atrophy, together with interstitial cellular infiltration and fibrosis, are frequently observed. A predominance of mesangial hypercellularity is rare in adult patients. This difference between adults and children may be due to the short interval between the onset of the disease and the renal biopsy in the latter subjects. It is usual to find a very long asymptomatic period preceding the apparent onset of the disease in adults.

Children with primary IgA nephropathy characterized by a predominance of matrix expansion are resistant to treatment: they have persistent proteinuria at follow-up and do not show any modification of matrix accumulation at the second biopsy. This matrix increase is an irreversible glomerular change and eventually leads to glomerular sclerosis.

Immunofluorescence

As immunofluorescent deposits are present in all mesangial regions of both normal and affected glomeruli, the old descriptive histological term of 'focal and segmental glomerulonephritis' is incorrect, since all glomeruli are affected by the immunological process. In the first immunofluorescence studies, Berger and Hinglais (1968) reported mesangial IgA and IgG deposits, but it became evident from subsequent reports that the predominant immunoglobulin is IgA, almost exclusively IgA1 with λ light chain in a polymeric form.

By definition, IgA is the sole or dominant immunoglobulin present in all glomeruli, C3 detectable in up to 70 per cent of renal biopsies has the same distribution as IgA. IgG is present in 50–70 per cent of the renal biopsies (Schena *et al.* 1990), but it often has the same intensity of staining as IgA, a feature that explains why this disease was initially called IgA–IgG nephropathy. IgM deposits are also found, but less commonly (31–66 per cent). The early complement components, such as C1q and C4, are rarely detected, but when present they are invariably associated with IgG and/or IgM.

The spatial distribution of IgA and C3 in mesangial deposits, studied by confocal laser microscopy, is represented by IgA and C3 coated by an outer layer of IgA alone in mild forms of the disease, whereas the IgA layer is absent in severe forms. These findings suggest that a free access of active complement components to cells and/or mesangial matrix receptors could trigger a cytolytic reaction and that IgA seems to act as a protective layer on C3 components (Onetti-Muda *et al.* 1995). A stronger deposition of C3c than C3d has been reported in IgA nephropathy patients with severe haematuria (over 20 urinary red blood cells in high power), high incidence of glomerular endocapillary proliferation, and decreased glomerular filtration rate (GFR). These findings suggest that glomerular deposition of C3c is associated with the inflammatory active phase of disease in IgA nephropathy patients (Nakagawa *et al.* 2000).

Non-specific vascular C3 is associated with renal hyaline arteriolosclerosis as in all renal conditions. The presence of both renal arteriolosclerosis and C3 seems to precede the appearance of hypertension and characterizes progressive cases.

Fibrin/fibrinogen deposits have been observed in 30–40 per cent of cases. Fibrin-related antigen is found in the mesangium and on the endothelium of glomerular capillary loops. Deposition of von Willebrand factor is greater in the endothelium than in the mesangium. Aggregated platelets adhering to the glomerular capillary walls are present. Such a distribution of platelets and von Willebrand factor shows that the endothelium of the non-sclerotic areas of the segmental sclerotic glomeruli is considerably damaged, suggesting that such damage may activate the intraglomerular coagulation, thus contributing to the development of global glomerular sclerosis (Ono *et al.* 2001). The degree of fibrin deposition is strictly correlated with the mesangial proliferation, suggesting that the coagulation/fibrinolysis system plays an important role in the progression of renal damage. Colucci *et al.* (1991) have shown a reduced fibrinolytic activity (plasminogen activator antigen and its activity) in the urine of primary IgA nephropathy patients with plasma creatinine concentrations greater than 1.5 mg/dl.

IgA deposits may be confined to the mesangium (mesangial type), or be present in the glomerular capillary walls as well as in the mesangium (capillary type) (Fig. 4). Changes in the pattern of deposition may occur, so that at repeat biopsy a change from the capillary to the mesangial type or vice versa may be observed. In the latter case, renal function often shows a progressive deterioration. IgA deposits contain the J chain, a subunit of dimeric and polymeric immunoglobulins, the detection of

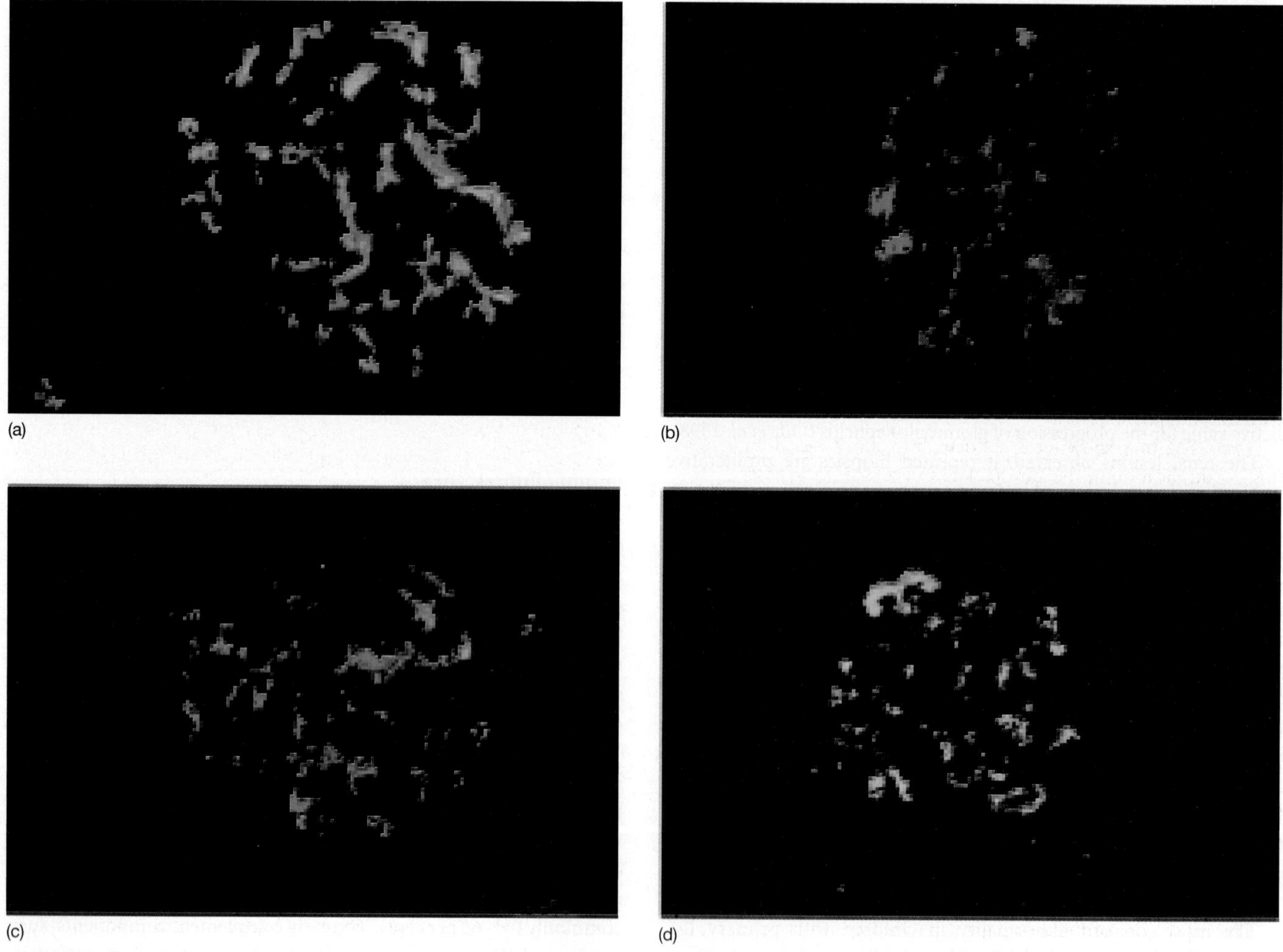

Fig. 4 Immunofluorescent deposits in mesangial proliferative glomerulonephritis. Mesangial depoists of IgA (a), IgG (b), IgM (c), and C3 (d) (×250) (see text).

which, described by Suzuki *et al.* (1990), has been confirmed. A recent *in situ* hybridization study performed in endoscopic duodenal biopsies from primary IgA nephropathy patients has demonstrated a reduction in J chain mRNA expression in duodenal IgA plasma cells. This result argues against the gastrointestinal lamina propria as the source of glomerular IgA (Harper *et al.* 1994a).

The antigen specificity of the IgA in mesangial deposits is unknown. Gregory *et al.* (1988) examined the possible role of infective agents and reported that the deposits contained cytomegalovirus antigen, but conflicting results have been reported by others using polymerase chain reaction (PCR) and *in situ* hybridization techniques. Other groups of viruses (herpes simplex, Epstein–Barr virus, hepatitis B) and bacteria (*Haemophilus parainfluenzae*) have been observed in the kidneys of patients with primary IgA nephropathy and other glomerulonephritides; therefore, these infections may be coincidental rather than causal. Glomerular deposition of food antigens has also been detected by immunofluoresce techniques, but results are inconsistent (Coppo *et al.* 2000).

Electron microscopy

The most characteristic change on electron microscopy is the presence of electron-dense deposits in mesangial and paramesangial areas. The quantity, size, shape, and density of these deposits vary from glomerulus to glomerulus and from one mesangial zone to another. Mesangiolysis is a common phenomenon in primary IgA nephropathy occuring in about 40 per cent of cases. This lesion is related to the chronic damaging mechanism of mesangial overload by IgA immune complexes and is causally associated with glomerulosclerosis. The process of glomerular sclerosis progression initially occurs in the mesangio-subendothelial system (mesangiolysis and subendothelial widening) than proliferating mesangial cells extend into the widened space [between the glomerular basement membrane (GBM) and endothelial cells] and reach the peripheral portion of capillary loop.

A constant finding is an increase of basement membrane-like material in the mesangial matrix. The mesangial matrix is more dense in patients with diffuse mesangial proliferative glomerulonephritis, and in those with minor changes with superimposed focal lesions, than in cases with minimal lesions alone.

The GBM may show local abnormalities, such as thinning, splitting, or duplication of the lamina densa in one-third of cases.

Immunohistochemistry and molecular biology techniques

Mesangial cells may express many surface proteins such as CD34, megsin, and CXCR3. CD34 is a marker of mesangial transdifferentiation, since it is expressed in concomitance with alpha-smooth muscle actin (ASMA) and it increases gradually with severity of renal damage. Megsin-positive cells coincide with mesangial cells and expression is most evident in glomeruli with severe mesangial cell proliferation and slight mesangial matrix expansion (Suzuki *et al.* 1999a). Megsin acts as a functional moderator of mesangial cell function (Inagi *et al.* 2001). CXCR3 is a chemokine receptor expressed by mesangial cells which binds the interferon-γ (IFN-γ) inducible protein of 10 kDa (IP-10) and monokines. These chemoattractants induce infiltration of monocytes and proliferation of mesangial cells (Romagnani *et al.* 1999).

The expression of intrarenal gene transcripts of various cytokines (IL-1β, TNF-α, IL-6, IL-15, IL-2, IFN-γ, IL-10) and chemokines (IL-8, RANTES, MCP-1) are closely interrelated, but not often associated with the pathological grading system of renal lesions. The IFN-γ/IL-10 ratio is greater in patients with renal dysfunction than in those with normal renal function. Gene transcript levels of proinflammatory cytokines are related to the amount of proteinuria. The IFN-γ/IL-10 ratio is greater in patients with severe glomerular sclerosis. IL-10 gene expression is related to the severity of tubulointerstitial damage. IL-10, IFN-γ, and TNF-α gene expression are related to the degree of mesangial matrix expansion and the extent of intrarenal arteriolar changes. Th1/Th2 predominance and the level of proinflammatory cytokines could be responsible for the process of renal lesions (Lim *et al.* 2001).

An upregulation of PDGFβ-receptor mRNA and protein expression at glomerular and interstitial level has been reported by Gesualdo *et al.* (1994). The increased expression of mRNA PDGF BB and its receptor was related to the degree of glomerular proliferation and the extent of fibrosing interstitial lesions.

Transforming growth factor (TGF)-β1 has been shown in the areas of glomerular proliferation in patients with increased proliferative lesions. However, more than a marker of proliferative changes, the glomerular TGF-β1/beta-actin mRNA ratio has been proposed as a marker of glomerulosclerosis (Yang *et al.* 1997). Increased expression of protein and mRNA TGF-β R types I, II, and III has been observed in glomerular and Bowman's capsular cells comprising the tuft adhesions to Bowman capsules. The three TGF-β receptors are also present in glomerular epithelial cells in the vicinity of glomerular sclerotic lesions, in crescent cells, and in some tubules and infiltrative mononuclear cells found in the periglomerular and tubulointerstitial lesions (Yamamoto *et al.* 1998).

Other growth factors have been described: basic fibroblast growth factor (bFGF) has been observed as overexpressed in glomeruli, and in areas of tubulointerstitial damage (Stein-Oakley *et al.* 1997). Positivity for hepatic growth factor (HGF) on epithelial cells of tubules is present in IgAN patients with severe clinical parameters and has been considered as a factor exacerbating the disease (Fidirkin *et al.* 1999). Connective tissue growth factor is upregulated in IgA nephropathy, mainly in those cases with chronic tubulointerstitial damage. Its presence correlates with the degree of renal damage and is co-expressed with ASMA (Ito *et al.* 1998).

ASMA and PDGFβ receptor-positive cells are strikingly increased in patients with moderate and severe renal lesions, particularly in areas of tubulointerstitial fibrosis. PDGF-β R gene and protein expression, at the tubulointerstitial level, parallel that in ASMA. PDGFβ-receptor expression is upregulated in glomeruli and correlates with mesangial cell proliferation, while ASMA is not present (Ranieri *et al.* 2001).

Interstitial myofibroblasts play a significant role in the progression of tubulointerstitial damage. Periglomerular fibroblasts have been seen surrounding non-sclerotic hypertrophic glomeruli in patients with increasing creatinine and, thus, may have a role in the progression of the disease (Oba *et al.* 1998). Tubular epithelial cells can undergo change towards a myofibroblast-like phenotype on the basis of *de novo* ASMA expression, loss of cytokeratin, and *de novo* collagen staining; thus, transdifferentiation of tubular cells has a role in the progression of renal fibrosis (Jinde *et al.* 2001).

ICAM-1 and -3 correlate significantly with interstitial infiltration of LFA1$^+$ cells and CD68$^+$ cells and with interstitial infiltrate of CD3$^+$ cells. The interstitial infiltration of these immune cells correlates with the histological renal lesions such as the index of glomerular damage and the percentage of involved interstitial volume.

ELAM-1 and VCAM-1 with different intensities are present in renal lesions. They are closely related to the major histological changes in IgA nephropathy, including mesangial expansion, formation of crescents and adhesions, and tubulointerstitial injury (Ogawa *et al.* 1997). CD40 and CD40 ligand expression has also been studied in IgA nephropathy. An upregulation of this system in the presence of mononuclear cells has been found (Yellin *et al.* 1997).

A small resident population of macrophage/monocytes ($CD68^+$ cells) is present in glomeruli and interstitium, of which only 1–2 per cent shows evidence of proliferation (positive expression of proliferating cell nuclear antigen—PCNA). This low number of CD68 positive cells is associated with increased deposition of mesangial matrix. It has been postulated that macrophages are responsible for the lack of fast catabolism of the mesangial deposits. This mild macrophage infiltrate is present in IgA nephropathy patients, but it increases with the loss of renal function. Therefore, macrophage proliferation is a marker of progressive renal damage (Yang *et al.* 1998) and local production of MCP-1 by infiltrating monocytes may modulate the monocyte influx and consequently the tubulointerstitial damage (Grandaliano *et al.* 1996).

Mast cells secrete bFGF. Tryptase is localized in the granules of cells. Double labelled immunohistochemistry has revealed that some tryptase-positive mast cells had bFGF in their cytoplasm. Mast cells are associated with fibroblasts and/or T lymphocytes in the interstitium (Ehara and Shigematsu 1998). Mast cells participate in chronic inflammation and tissue fibrosis. In fact, they have been found in the renal cortical tubulointerstitium, periglomerular areas, and medullary interstitium. The number of infiltrating mast cells correlated with serum creatinine at the time of renal biopsy, with intensity of tubulointerstitial injury, and fibrosis. Thus, mast cells contribute to the renal deterioration in IgA nephropathy by inducing chronic tubulointerstitial injury (Hiromura *et al.* 1998). The number of mast cells correlate with the extent of interstitial fibrosis and the degree of renal function. Mast cells may also be present in the non-fibrotic areas and this finding may be one of the predictive factors for the prognosis of IgAN (Kurusu *et al.* 2001).

Diagnosis and differential diagnosis

Primary IgA nephropathy or Berger's disease is characterized by one or more episodes of recurrent macroscopic haematuria in patients with concomitant upper respiratory tract infections or other mucosal infections. The diagnosis cannot be made on clinical grounds, as it needs biopsy-proved evidence of mesangial deposits of IgA with/without IgG, IgM, and C3. Renal biopsy also plays an important role in the prognosis, because different degrees of renal involvement influence the outcome of the disease.

The disease may be asymptomatic initially and may be detected by mass urine screening tests. Persistent microscopic haematuria with mild proteinuria is the main laboratory finding.

The occurrence of a macroscopic haematuria episode may induce the physician to consider other renal diseases such as acute post-infectious glomerulonephritis, Henoch–Schönlein purpura, and thin GBM nephropathy, in which more frequently persistent microscopic haematuria occurs. Acute postinfectious glomerulonephritis (Chapter 3.8) is characterized by macroscopic haematuria and transient hypocomplentaemia (low CH50 and depressed levels of C4 and C3) after a latent period of 1–8 weeks after infection. In these cases, the resolution of glomerulonephritis is common, but in few subjects abnormal microhaematuria may persist. In these cases, renal biopsy performed after the acute phase of the disease shows endocapillary proliferative lesions with mononuclear cell infiltrate in the glomerular flocculus, mainly granulocytes, monocytes, and subepithelial deposits of IgG (sometimes IgM and/or IgA). Renal biopsy performed later may reveal a mesangial proliferative glomerulonephritis without IgA deposits which may explain persistent microscopic haematuria (Yoshizawa *et al.* 1996).

Thin GBM nephropathy (Chapter 16.4.1) shows at presentation persistent microscopic haematuria or proteinuria, and sometimes both. Electron microscope reveals a patchy reduction in the thickness of the glomerular and tubular basement membrane (<150 μm) and the disease may be familial. Urinary erythrocyte counts are higher in IgA nephropathy patients, who also have more proteinuria than subjects with thin glomerular basement membrane nephropathy. The outcome is worse in IgA nephropathy patients (Auwardt *et al.* 1999). However, several cases of association between the two diseases (thinning of GBM together with mesangial IgA deposits) have been reported.

Differential diagnosis with Henoch–Schönlein purpura (Chapter 4.5.2) is more frequent in children than in adults. The peak age ranges from 15–30 years for a diagnosis of IgA nephropathy, whereas Henoch–Schönlein purpura nephritis is mainly seen in childhood. Nephritic and/or nephrotic syndrome are more frequent at presentation in the Henoch–Schönlein purpura nephritis. The most important clinical features for the correct diagnosis are the extrarenal signs such as palpable purpura, often occurring in the lower limbs. In addition, this disease is associated with hypersensitivity to drugs. Endocapillary and extracapillary lesions and fibrin deposits are more frequent in Henoch–Schönlein purpura nephritis (Davin *et al.* 2001). However, in 20–50 per cent of patients with this disease, IgA nephropathy may subsequently occur.

Natural history

Clinical outcome

There is a marked variability in the clinical outcome of primary IgA nephropathy in all geographical areas of the world, with a spectrum ranging from complete disappearance of blood and protein in the urine to the development of chronic renal failure requiring dialysis or transplantation. Microhaematuria disappears spontaneously in 3–25 per cent of patients, although the regression of renal lesions and disappearance of mesangial IgA deposits have never been observed. A small number of patients whose clinical presentation is characterized by macrohaematuria, loin pain, and normal serum creatinine rapidly progress to endstage renal disease over 2–3 years. In these cases, the renal lesions are characterized by persisting crescents and progressive loss of structure in glomeruli. Furthermore, patients with crescentic primary IgA nephropathy have an increased prevalence of hypertension, renal insufficiency, and nephrotic-range proteinuria.

The overall clinical outcome shows that 69–80 per cent of patients continue to have normal renal function after a weighted mean follow-up of 2–5 years (Schena 1990). Renal biopsies from these patients usually reveal either no change or only minimal glomerular lesions. Stable renal function is generally present in subjects with a mild form of mesangial proliferative glomerulonephritis, while deterioration of renal function occurs in patients with advanced histological lesions. After a weighted mean follow-up period of 2–5 years hypertension is more common in

Australian (48 per cent) and European patients (39 per cent) than in Asian (21 per cent) and North American patients (20 per cent).

The prevalence of chronic renal insufficiency appears to be greater in Australian (23 per cent) and European patients (23 per cent) than in patients from Asia and North America (13 and 15 per cent, respectively). The renal impairment is more common in males than in females, but the rate of deterioration varies considerably from subject to subject. Two groups of patients have been identified by their clinical course, one with a slowly progressive disease and another with a more rapid course progressing to renal insufficiency within a few years. Patients in the first group most likely represent the natural history of the nephritis, whereas many patients in the second group have unfavourable prognostic factors, such as severe uncontrolled hypertension.

Patients with normal or stable renal function have mild proteinuria, normal blood pressure, and mild histological lesions. In contrast, patients with progressive renal impairment show heavy proteinuria, hypertension, proliferative lesions, and crescents. Patients with a proteinuria of more than 3.5 g/day and impaired renal function develop chronic renal insufficiency within a short time from the appearance of clinical signs. Furthermore, a few cases have a rapid course to terminal renal failure; they are referred to as having 'malignant IgA nephropathy'.

Endstage kidney disease occurs more frequently in North Americans (15 per cent) and Europeans (11 per cent) than in patients from Asia and Australia (approximately 9 per cent).

The actuarial curves of renal survival from numerous studies show 81–94 per cent of *adult* patients with normal renal function after 10 years in Europe, 87–93 per cent in Australia, 74–87 per cent in Asia, and 57–78 per cent of patients in the United States (D'Amico 2000).

This wide variability is biased by the following factors: (a) the time of observation, which has been considered the apparent onset of the disease in some studies (Wyatt *et al.* 1984; D'Amico *et al.* 1985; Beukhof *et al.* 1986; Woo *et al.* 1986; Kusumoto *et al.* 1987; Noel *et al.* 1987; Velo *et al.* 1987; Alamartine *et al.* 1991; Koyama *et al.* 1997) or the time of the renal biopsy in others (Nicholls *et al.* 1984; D'Amico *et al.* 1986; Katafuchi *et al.* 1988; Rekola *et al.* 1989; Johnston *et al.* 1992; Kang *et al.* 1995; Frimat *et al.* 1997; Haas 1997; Mera *et al.* 2000); (b) wide variability of the renal lesions and degree of renal function at the time of diagnosis; (c) inclusion of patients enrolled at the time of urinary screening as followed in Asian countries, therefore the policy of renal biopsy use is the point of commencement; (d) inclusion of treated and untreated patients.

A meta-analysis, which takes into consideration medical literature published between 1966 and 1989, included 23 articles and demonstrated a different renal survival curve when observations begin at the moment of renal biopsy compared to observations from the first symptoms (Roodnat *et al.* 1991). The mean renal survival at 5, 10, and 15 years from the first symptoms was 92.8, 85, and 75.5 per cent, respectively, while that at 5, 10, 15, and 20 years from the renal biopsy was 88.8, 80.2, 68.1, and 70.6 per cent, respectively. The prognosis of the disease appears to be 'better' when observation begins at the moment of the first symptoms.

The long-term outcome of renal survival in large series of children affected by primary IgA nephropathy has also been described. When considering the natural history of IgA nephropathy in children, long-term analysis including the adult life should be taken into account. After the first report of Levy *et al.* (1985) in which a follow-up of 13.5 years in 91 children demonstrated that only eight children (9 per cent) developed renal failure, other studies from different areas of the world have been performed. In Europe, Linné *et al.* (1991) found the persistence of clinical signs of disease in 47 per cent of their patients, who were followed for a mean period of 10.7 years. Urine abnormalities were present in all patients, proteinuria in 35 per cent, hypertension in 9 per cent, and decreased GFR in 3 per cent. The more common histological lesions in these patients consisted of focal–segmental glomerular changes. In the United States, Hogg *et al.* (1994) observed endstage renal disease in 15 per cent of 80 patients followed for a mean period of 4 years. Seven variables were found predictive of progressive deterioration of the renal function: presence of glomerular sclerotic changes in more than 20 per cent of the glomeruli, Afro-American race, male gender, hypertension at biopsy, proteinuria at biopsy, older age at presentation, and presence of crescents in renal biopsy. Wyatt *et al.* (1995) reported 87 per cent of IgA nephropathy patients with normal renal function after 10 years from the time of apparent onset in a large cohort of 103 paediatric patients who underwent renal biopsy before the age of 18 years. In Japan, Yoshikawa *et al.* (1992) found urinary abnormalities in 38 per cent of patients, persistent heavy proteinuria in 10.5 per cent, and progression to chronic renal failure in 0.5 per cent of 200 children aged less than 15 years who were followed for a mean period of 5 years. The poor outcome was characterized by heavy proteinuria at biopsy; diffuse mesangial proliferation; a high proportion of glomeruli showing sclerosis, crescents, or capsular adhesions in more than 30 per cent of glomeruli; the presence of tubulo-interstitial infiltrates; subepithelial electron-dense deposits; and lysis of the GBM.

In conclusion, paediatric patients have often a more early diagnosis than adults, due to the more frequent onset with gross haematuria, or because of population screening. Hence, the medium-term prognosis is better than that usually found in adult patients since less severe clinical signs (hypertension, proteinuria, impaired renal function) and histological lesions (extent of sclerosis and tubulointerstitial damage) are present at the time of renal biopsy. However, the disease is progressive over decades and the long-term prognosis becomes similar to patients with clinical onset in adult age. Life-long follow-up is needed in these children in order to detect the manifestations of signs of progressive disease and the need to initiate a therapy.

Clinical and histological prognostic markers

A number of *parameters*, evidenced by univariate and multivariate analysis, predict a poor outcome (Table 4).

In the single patient, even the evaluation of the prognostic markers (impairment of renal function, severe proteinuria, blood pressure) sometimes failes to correctly predict outcome, probably because of the heterogeneity of the disease and the discontinuous activity of some injuring mechanisms during its course (D'Amico 2000).

Haematuria

The degree of haematuria, whether gross or microscopic, has no apparent bearing on the severity or likelihood of progression of primary IgA nephropathy. However, there are contrasting results on this finding, since some reports have shown that isolated or recurrent gross haematuria is more common in patients with a benign course. In contrast, others reported that gross haematuria is a poor prognostic sign, since crescents and impaired renal function are often present. Nicholls *et al.* (1984) demonstrated a strong correlation between haematuria

Table 4 Clinical and histological risk factors in patients with primary IgA nephropathy

Risk factor	Univariate analysis[a]	Multivariate analysis[b]
Haematuria	Absence of history of recurrent macrohaematuria	High number of erythrocytes in urine
Proteinuria	>3.5 g/day Nephrotic syndrome	>1 g/day at renal biopsy
Hypertension	At presentation Family history	High values at presentation Family history
Serum creatinine	>1.5 mg/day at presentation	>120 μmol/l at renal biopsy
Renal biopsy	Severe renal damage represented by mesangial hypercellularity, glomerular sclerosis, interstitial infiltration, interstitial fibrosis, tubular atrophy, elevated number of crescents; IgA deposits in the peripheral capillary loops	High total glomerular score, tubulointerstitial lesions
Age	>40 years	Younger age; older age
Gender	Male	
BMI	Excessive value	Excessive value

[a] Nicholls *et al.* (1984); D'Amico *et al.* (1985, 1986); Beukhof *et al.* (1986); Noel *et al.* (1987).

[b] Beukhof *et al.* (1986); D'Amico *et al.* (1986); Bogenschutz *et al.* (1990); Alamartine *et al.* (1991); Johnston *et al.* (1992); Katafuchi *et al.* (1994); Kang *et al.* (1995); Frimat *et al.* (1997); Haas (1997); Koyama *et al.* (1997); Mera *et al.* (2000).

(red blood cells > 10^5/ml) and the presence of crescents. They believe that the major mechanism of progression in the disease is the destruction of glomeruli induced by crescent formation, which occurs both during episodes of gross haematuria and when there is a continuing high count of urinary erythrocytes. The renal survival rate is less in patients with persistent microhaematuria than in those with macroscopic episodes of haematuria.

Proteinuria

The absence of proteinuria at diagnosis is generally a good prognostic sign. However, adverse events in IgA nephropathy patients with haematuria and minimal proteinuria (<0.5 g/day) are represented by proteinuria greater than 1 g/day, hypertension, and impaired renal function. In these cases, age at presentation and histological grade are independent predictors of developing an adverse event in 10 years. Therefore, even mild IgA nephropathy should be considered as a potentially progressive disease, life-long follow-up with regular monitoring of blood pressure and proteinuria is recommended (Schena 2001; Szeto *et al.* 2001; Usui *et al.* 2001).

The presence of moderate (1–3 g/day) or heavy (>3 g/day) proteinuria at the time of biopsy is considered to be an indicator of the eventual progression towards renal insufficiency. This has been certainly proved for proteinuria of more than 2 g/day. In fact, its presence correlates with global sclerosis, interstitial fibrosis, and serum creatinine. Therefore, segmental and global proliferation, glomerular sclerosis, tubulointerstitial damage, and vessel sclerosis increase with increasing proteinuria. Persisting or increasing proteinuria during the course of the disease is associated with an impairment of renal function and sometimes with endstage renal failure.

The nephrotic syndrome is uncommon, but its presence is associated with a variable prognosis, because patients with mild renal lesions respond to steroids, whereas those with advanced changes do not.

The product of duration (years) and urinary protein excretion (g/day) at the time of renal biopsy is significantly correlated with both histological grade (glomerular and tubulointerstitial damage) and plasma creatinine concentration. Therefore, the natural course of the disease is steadily progressive, dependent on the duration and amount of proteinuria. The products of these two factors (proteinuria index) many be a useful predictor for glomerular and interstitial histopathological changes and the fate of renal function in the disease (Eiro *et al.* 2002).

Hypertension

Sodium sensitivity of blood pressure is present before the appearance of hypertension and is related to histological damage. In fact, the sensitivity index evaluated by a diet with an ordinary sodium intake for 1 week and a sodium-restricted diet for another week was greater in patients with glomerular sclerosis, tubulointerstitial damage and normal to high-normal blood pressure than in patients with optimal pressure (Konishi *et al.* 2001).

The development of hypertension is more common in patients with vascular sclerosis, whose appearance may be due to impaired intrarenal haemodynamics with afferent arteriolar vasodilatation. The presence of renal hyaline arteriosclerosis and renal vascular C3 seems to precede the appearance of hypertension. The degree of hypertension increases with duration of symptoms and the age of patients at the time of diagnosis. Patients with macrohaematuria have a lower mean blood pressure than those presenting with proteinuria. Accelerated hypertension develops in about 5 per cent of patients.

IgA nephropathy patients with raised blood pressures (SBP > 140 mmHg; DBP > 90 mmHg) at the time of renal biopsy have a higher percentage of sclerotic glomeruli than patients with optimal blood pressure. In addition, they have lower creatinine clearance. The optimal values proposed by the World Health Organization in 1999 prevents histological evidence of renal damage in these patients, since those with optimal values at the time of renal biopsy have less renal damage (mesangial proliferation and vessel changes) than patients with intermediate or high values of blood pressure (Osawa *et al.* 2001).

The circadian variation of blood pressure is preserved in normotensive IgA nephropathy patients (dippers) whereas no diurnal blood pressure variations are observed in hypertensives who have high night-time blood pressure and high serum creatinine. The lack of circadian rhythm seems to accelerate the progression of the disease (Csiky *et al.* 1999).

Patients with hypertension, both children and adults, have a progressive decrease in renal function. Persistent hypertension develops most frequently in patients who have heavy proteinuria for a long period. Uncontrolled, severe hypertension is a possible cause of rapid deterioration to endstage disease. Hypertension and renal insufficiency at the time of biopsy are unfavourable prognostic signs.

Kusumoto *et al.* (1987) demonstrated that the effect of hypertension in children, who developed signs of the disease at a mean age of 12 years, appeared 21 years or more after the onset of the disease (mean age 30 years). In adults, hypertension influenced kidney survival rate during the first 12 years after the onset of hypertension (mean age 40 years). Therefore, hypertension affects renal function at a mean age of 30–40 years, but the effect of arteriosclerosis and ageing increases after the age of 40 years.

Renal insufficiency

Twenty years after the apparent onset of the disease, chronic renal insufficiency (serum creatinine > 1.5 mg/dl) is present in 50–70 per cent of primary IgA nephropathy patients, while endstage kidney disease occurs in 20–50 per cent of patients. Age and severity of the clinical findings play an important role.

As the disease progresses, renal function decreases further in subjects with initially impaired renal function (serum creatinine 2–4 mg/dl), whereas it remains unchanged in patients who initially have normal renal function. Patients with a decrease in the GFR are, on average, 10 years older than subjects with a preserved GFR, and the known duration of the disease in the former group is longer. Patients with decreased renal function are more frequently hypertensive.

Repeated determinations of GFR with an accurate method [^{51}Cr]EDTA or inulin clearance are valuable tests to predict the final outcome early in the disease. Rekola *et al.* (1991) showed that 32 per cent of their patients with initially normal GFR had a deterioration of renal function within 5 years, and 25 per cent developed endstage renal failure within 20 years. This finding emphasizes that primary IgA nephropathy may be a severe disease in the long-term. However, the rate of progression to renal insufficiency is quite different from case to case, since some patients show a rapid decline of renal function over a few years, while in others there is good preservation of the renal function for over 30 years.

An observational retrospective study identified three groups of IgA nephropathy patients: (a) stable chronic course with constantly normal or only minor elevated serum creatinine lasting years; (b) a progressive course with continuously increasing serum creatinine; (c) a rare early acute course with a short-term increase of serum creatinine followed by a rapid return to the normal range. The existence of a 'point of no return' at 3 mg/dl (265 μmol/l) during the natural course of the disease was indicated. Over 3 mg/dl, the serum creatinine value doubled within 10 months (Scholl *et al.* 1999). Therefore, increased creatinine is a highly significant marker of progressive disease in both adults and children with IgA nephropathy.

Histological lesions

The predictive value of the first renal biopsy must be emphasized, since the histological and immunofluorescence grading are reliable prognostic indicators. The renal survival rate in patients with diffuse proliferative glomerulonephritis and focal crescents is shorter than that of patients with minimal glomerular lesions, focal proliferative glomerulonephritis, and mild to moderate proliferative glomerulonephritis. The patients who develop chronic renal failure have marked capsular adhesions, fibrocellular crescents, glomerular hyalinization, and sclerosis. The extracapillary lesion is especially important since long-term follow-up studies have shown that the renal survival rate decreases as the percentage of crescents increases (Nicholls *et al.* 1984; Abe *et al.* 1986). Renal survival is 40 per cent 5 years after the initial biopsy in patients with more than 50 per cent of crescents and 25 per cent after 10 years, whereas the 5-year survival rate is 91 per cent in patients with less than 50 per cent of crescents and 81 per cent after 10 years. Children have been reported to have a better prognosis, probably because severe mesangial proliferation, sclerotic glomeruli, severe interstitial changes, and renal arteriosclerosis are less frequent. This finding has been confirmed by the meta-analysis study of Roodnat *et al.* (1991).

The best predictive index in primary IgA nephropathy are the glomerular lesions present in the renal biopsy. Therefore, severe mesangial proliferation, frequent sclerotic glomeruli, crescents, a high proportion of glomerular adhesions, vascular sclerosis, and marked interstitial fibrosis are considered histological markers of a poor prognosis. Glomerular sclerosis and progressive renal damage are mediated by vascular sclerosis caused by ischaemia as well as by mesangial production of sclerogenic factors. Sclerosis reflects renal function more closely than proliferative changes, and mesangial sclerosis is the most important histological prognostic factor. Life-table analysis in patients with moderate disease demonstrate that only the degree of proteinuria (>2.0 g/day) and the extent of segmental glomerulosclerosis are of prognostic significance. Mesangial matrix increases with the duration of the disease in adult patients. A predominance of matrix is, therefore, characteristic of the late lesions.

Patients with more extracapillary lesions have more severe proteinuria, decreased renal function, and increased blood pressure. Moreover, a progressive reduction of renal function occurs in patients with recurrent extracapillary lesions. Such lesions are a very important factor because their presence at the time of the initial biopsy is associated with a more than fivefold increase in progression to endstage renal failure.

Patients followed for 2 years after the second biopsy showed that changes in mesangial areas, evaluated by quantitative analysis, were a valuable prognostic indicator. Patients with decreased mesangial sclerosis at the second biopsy had stable renal function and a favourable outcome, whereas those in whom mesangial sclerosis increased had a deterioration in renal function during the follow-up period. In the latter group, there were glomeruli which showed varying degrees of sclerosis, including global sclerosis (Tateno and Kobayashi 1987).

Interstitial sclerosis is highly suggestive of an unfavourable prognosis. Tubulointerstitial infiltrates occur mainly in patients with an evolutive disease and increased serum creatinine. The extent of T-cell infiltration (T-helper and T-suppressor cells) is more marked in patients with impaired renal function at the time of renal biopsy or in those who will present a deterioration of renal function during the follow-up period after biopsy. The liberation of cytokines by T-helper cells may be directly responsible for tubular damage (Alexopoulos *et al.* 1989). Further studies have shown a correlation between the tubulointerstitial damage and the GFR in crescentic primary IgA nephropathy, where the presence of interstitial IL-2R+ monocytes reflects the local production of cytokines by activated cells with damage to adjacent structures (Li *et al.* 1990). The decrease of renal function in primary IgA nephropathy patients over 8–15 years of follow-up correlates with the presence of tubulointerstitial monocytes but not with glomerular monocyte infiltrates; this further suggests the participation of cell-mediated immunity in the evolution of primary IgA nephropathy.

Immunofluorescent deposits

IgA, IgG, and C3 tend to be deposited in the capillary walls in patients with crescents or adhesions of the capillary loop to Bowman's capsule. The capillary IgA deposits, especially IgA–IgG subepithelial deposits, may induce the rupture or an increased permeability of the glomerular capillary walls, in association with thinning and splitting of the lamina densa, and cause the formation of crescents. Thus, capillary IgA deposits can represent a useful marker of insidious progression.

Deposition of IgG and/or IgM appears to coincide with a more severe form of the disease. Extraglomerular vascular IgM deposits, mostly accompanied by C3, are present in 7 per cent of patients; their presence coincides with an increased incidence of vascular lesions, severe glomerulosclerosis, arterial hypertension, and elevated serum creatinine (Zidar *et al.* 1992). A comparison of pathological lesions on repeated renal biopsies in 73 patients revealed that the vascular C3 deposits were responsible for the renal progression in the second renal biopsy (Alamartine *et al.* 1990).

A significant correlation between the decrease of the renal function and the presence of tubulointerstitial deposits of C3 underline the importance of immunologically mediated tubulointerstitial damage induced by complement in the progression of the disease. Studies have shown the local *in vitro* production of C3 by cultured human mesangial cells, which increase after IL-1β and IL-6 (Montinaro *et al.* 1995) and IFN-γ stimulation (Sacks *et al.* 1993a), by human proximal tubular epithelial cells (Brooimans *et al.* 1991), and by glomerular podocytes regulated by IFN-γ (Sacks *et al.* 1993b). These investigations provide evidence for the proinflammatory function of complement in the progression of the renal damage, since the fragments of C3 (C3a and C3b) can stimulate the synthesis of cytokines and other factors by resident cells, thus creating a vicious circle which contributes to tissue injury.

Age

Comparison between IgA nephropathy patients over age 50 and those under the age of 50 showed that older patients had a significantly higher incidence of hypertension. Daily proteinuria, systolic blood pressure, and serum IgA levels were significantly higher, and Ccr was significantly lower in older patients at the time of the renal biopsy (Frimat *et al.* 1996).

The better prognosis in children is attributed to the less frequent occurrence of hypertension and to the lesser degree of glomerular injury found at the initial renal biopsy. Patients with adult-onset of the disease (over 35 years of age) have an unfavourable prognosis since they have greater mean blood pressure, proteinuria, and impaired renal function than patients with juvenile (under 19 years) and young (20–34 years) onset of the disease. Additionally, in patients with adult-onset of the disease mesangial proliferative and sclerotic lesions are more frequent than in younger patients (Yagucki *et al.* 1994).

A recent multicentre nephrology study reviewed clinical and pathological features in 80 children with primary IgA nephropathy who were followed for at least 4 years. Seven markers were found to be predictive of endstage kidney disease in children: the presence of glomerular sclerotic changes, especially when these were associated with proliferation or when sclerosis affected 20 per cent or more of the glomeruli; Afro-American race; hypertension at biopsy; proteinuria at biopsy; age at presentation; crescents; male gender (Hogg *et al.* 1994).

Gender

Men have a worse prognosis than women. No differences between the sexes have been found when haematuria, proteinuria, fibrosis, and arteriosclerosis in the kidney were considered. However, serum creatinine was greater in males. The effect of gender on the progression of chronic glomerulonephritides, including IgA nephropathy, has been examined in a meta-analysis that included 68 studies with a total of 11,345 patients. Results showed that men with chronic renal disease of various aetiologies show a more rapid decline in renal function with time than do women (Neugarten *et al.* 2000).

Race and ethnicity

Primary IgA nephropathy is the most common primary glomerulonephropathy in white-skinned people. It has been observed only in a few cases in Afro-Americans who have a worse prognosis, and it is virtually non-existent among black-skinned Africans. In the United States, primary IgA nephropathy is approximately six times more frequent in the Caucasian than in the Afro-American population (Jennette *et al.* 1985). Immunological abnormalities of Afro-American primary IgA nephropathy patients are similar to, but not identical to, those of Caucasian patients (Crowley-Nowick *et al.* 1994). Of interest, these patients have a predominat IgA2 immune response, and this isotype does not include *O*-linked glycans, whose altered glycosylation seems to be involved in the pathogenesis of the disease. A high proportion of mesangial proliferative glomerulonephritis has been found among Zuni and Navajo Indians who are not uniformly IgA positive (Hoy *et al.* 1993). It is necessary to underline that in this population alcohol abuse is very frequent. Primary IgA nephropathy appears to be very common in those of Oriental origin.

Other risk factors

A case–control study carried out in Japan on risk factors for IgA nephropathy evidenced that a family history of chronic nephritis, susceptibility to the common cold, preference for salty foods, frequent consumption of raw eggs, and a high intake of carbohydrates, including rice, were significantly associated with an increased risk for the disease. Episodes of tonsillitis and exposure to organic solvents are not more frequent in IgA nephropathy patients than in control population. Use of antioxidant vitamin supplements, and a high intake of proteins, fats, monounsaturated fatty acids, and all/*n*-3 polyunsaturated fatty acids were somewhat protective (Wakai *et al.* 1999, 2002). Hypertriglyceridaemia and hyperuricaemia are more frequent at the time of renal biopsy in patients with progressive renal damage than in those with stable disease. In patients with normal renal function at the time of initial diagnosis, hypertriglyceridaemia, hyperuricaemia, hypertension, and proteinuria are independent risk factors for progression of the disease (Syrjanen *et al.* 2000).

Pregnancy

The controversy surrounding pregnancy and primary IgA nephropathy is based on three important aspects: (a) the effect of the disease on fetal outcome; (b) the effect of gestation on maternal health during pregnancy; and (c) the effect of pregnancy on the remote prognosis of patients with underlying primary IgA nephropathy.

Primary IgA nephropathy in women with preserved renal function (GFR > 70 ml/min), mild proteinuria, and minimal or absent hypertension has no adverse effects on the course of gestation and on the fetal outcome. Women with decreased renal function (GFR < 70 ml/min), heavy or moderate proteinuria, and/or hypertension before conception tend to have more obstetric complications. The occurrence and severity of EPH-gestosis is higher in patients with severe renal damage than in those with mild renal lesions. The incidence of IUGR is elevated in patients with advanced renal damage (Koido *et al.* 1998). In patients with hypertension the rate of live birth is very low if hypertension exists before pregnancy and/or is not controlled during gestation. The fetal loss rate ranges between 13 and 20 per cent. The incidence of persistent hypertension, increased proteinuria, and endstage renal failure in these patients is increased significantly (see Chapter 15.3).

Therapy

Primary IgA nephropathy is classified as a slowly progressive renal disease, since 20–50 per cent of patients in long-term follow-up studies develop endstage kidney failure 20 years or more after the apparent onset of the disease. The first reaction of many nephrologists, after the initial histological assessment, is to monitor the clinical signs, such as the frequency of macrohaematuria episodes, the degree of proteinuria, hypertension, and renal function, without starting any drug treatment.

Tonsillectomy and antibiotics have been reported to reduce the number of episodes of macrohaematuria, but its usefulness is questionable. Retrospective studies show contrasting data. Kosaka *et al.* (1998) demonstrated that tonsillectomy was clinically of great value. Since patients after a mean follow-up of approximately 9 years showed clinical remission, stable renal function rate and remission of the minor lesions. In contrast, Rasche *et al.* (1999) revealed that tonsillectomy does not reduce the risk of developing renal failure or prevent progression since the probability of renal survival 10 years after renal biopsy was similar to that of patients without tonsillectomy. Recently, Akagi *et al.* (1999) declared that tonsillectomy is indicated only in patients with mild and moderate renal damage since it reduces proteinuria in more those 50 per cent of patients. This procedure is indicated in patients with frequent tonsillitis and episodes of macroscopic haematuria and clear indication to this surgical treatment. All these conclusions are of limited value since all were obtained from non-controlled randomized studies.

Even though the disease is progressive, various investigators have attempted a pharmacological treatment. Retrospective studies (Lai *et al.* 1985; Mustonen *et al.* 1987; Kobayashi *et al.* 1989) have shown a beneficial effect of corticosteroids in patients with proteinuria of 1–2 g/day, after 10 or more years, renal function was preserved (creatinine clearance more than 70 ml/min) in subjects treated with corticosteroids at the time of renal biopsy for a mean period of 18 months. In contrast, patients with a previous deterioration in renal function had a poor clinical course, irrespective of the use of steroids. A randomized clinical trial (RCT) (Pozzi *et al.* 1999) was carried out in adult patients with moderate lesions, moderate proteinuria (1–3 g/day), and normal renal function. They received methylprednisolone intravenously (1 g/day for 3 consecutive days at the beginning of months 1, 3, and 5) and oral prednisone 0.5 mg/kg on alternate days for 6 months. Steroid treatment protected against deterioration of the renal function and a sustained reduction in urinary protein excretion was observed. However, during the follow-up a certain number of patients showed an increasing proteinuria after the therapy was stopped, thus suggesting a new course of corticosteroids. Considering these data, the authors started a new, ongoing RCT, in which enrolled patients received corticosteroids with further addition of azathioprine to ensure a stable remission (Locatelli *et al.* 1999).

The benefit of early treatment with corticosteroid has been shown in an RCT carried out in patients with diffuse proliferative lesions. A reduction of mesangial cell proliferation, mesangial matrix accumulation, and cellular crescents associated with decreased proteinuria was observed in the renal biopsy repeated after 1 year (Shoji *et al.* 2000). The positive effect of combination therapy (*prednisone* and *cyclophosphamide*) on progression has been reported by other investigators in patients with moderate renal damage (Tsuruya *et al.* 2000; Ballardie *et al.* 2002). In some studies, 6 months of cyclophosphamide was substituted by azathioprine for a further 2 years. Histological improvement was documented by repeated renal biopsy (McIntyre *et al.* 2001). The benefit of a long-term treatment with a low dose of *azathioprine* was demonstrated by a retrospective study of Goumenos *et al.* (1995).

The possibility of benefit from immunosuppressive therapy has been found also in children with IgA nephropathy. A preliminary 7-year-study of long-term alternate-day corticosteroid therapy performed in a group of six children with progressive nephropathy demonstrated the need for a prospective controlled trial, because patients with an intermediate grade of pathology may benefit from such therapy (Waldo *et al.* 1993). The same conclusions were reached by Andreoli and Bergstein (1989), who treated 10 children having severe primary IgA nephropathy with prednisone and azathioprine for 1 year. Combination therapy using prednisolone, azathioprine, heparin-warfarin, and dipyridomole in different combinations was used by Yoshikawa *et al.* (1999) in a controlled trial in children with severe IgA nephropathy. Results showed that combined treatment for 2 years, early in the course of disease, reduced the progression of renal damage. A controlled trial is currently in progress to compare the effects of prednisolone, azathioprine, heparin-warfarin, and dipyridomole with those of prednisolone alone in children with severe IgA nephropathy.

The presence of mild glomerular lesions and normal renal function in many cases with heavy proteinuria indicates a probable good response to drugs. However, the immediate response to corticosteroids and the subsequent tendency to relapse in some cases may suggest that primary IgA nephropathy is superimposed on a pre-existing asymptomatic minimal change disease in some patients. This is supported by the fact that in a few nephrotic children, initial renal biopsies were negative for IgA deposits, but repeat biopsies were positive. In addition, some patients may have a spontaneous remission of their nephrotic syndrome. A long-term controlled trial performed in 34 primary IgA nephropathy patients with nephrotic syndrome suggested that corticosteroid therapy is only beneficial in cases with mild histological lesions; therefore, its indiscriminate use should be discouraged (Lai *et al.* 1986).

Plasma exchange associated with corticosteroids and immunosuppressive drugs have yielded conflicting results in patients with rapidly progressive primary IgA nephropathy. Roccatello *et al.* (1995) demonstrated that this treatment delays the onset of dialysis in patients with florid extracapillary proliferation, but it is inadequate to reverse the inflammatory lesions before the development of chronic changes. In some patients, the extracapillary lesions are associated to segmental areas of necrotizing lesions in glomerular tufts and interstitial accumulation of monocytes and T-lymphocytes, deposition of fibrinogen, and expression of the adhesion molecules. The clinical course is characterized by acute flares and progression to endstage renal failure. In these cases, the aggressive therapy with steroids and cyclophosphamide has probably a beneficial effect (D'Amico *et al.* 2001). Immunosuppressive therapy improves vasculitic lesions and arrests the progress of glomerular scarring (Harper *et al.* 2000).

High-dose immunoglobulin therapy has been used in patients with severe primary IgA nephropathy (heavy proteinuria, hypertension, altered renal function, and severe renal lesions). The 9 months of immunoglobulin therapy improved renal function, but the drawback of this treatment is the obsevation of rebounds shortly after the end of the treatment (Rostoker *et al.* 1998).

Another possible way of slowing the progression of the renal damage in human glomerulonephritis consists in reducing the formation or blocking the action of different mediators involved in the inflammatory process. For this reason, trials in primary IgA nephropathy have been performed by administering anti-inflammatory drugs, anticoagulants, antiplatelet drugs, and fish oil with variable results.

ACE-inhibitors or AT1 receptor blockers have a beneficial effect on patients with impaired renal function and non-selective proteinuria because these drugs administered for a period of more than 1 year reduce proteinuria and improve the selectivity index of the urinary proteins (Woo *et al.* 2000). They probably modify the size of pores of the GBM by reducing the radius of large unselective pores (Remuzzi *et al.* 1999). In addition, they have a protective effect by reducing blood pressure in patients with mild renal insufficiency and hypertension (Kanno *et al.* 2000). A monitoring blood pressure study carried out in patients with chronic glomerulonephritis has shown that hypotensive subjects have an improvement of the renal damage, represented by a slower rate of progression of renal function less than hypertensive patients. The adequate values should be 100–125/55–75 in patients aged 40–60, and 105–140/60–85 mmHg in those over 60 years old (Omata *et al.* 1996).

Even though ACE-inhibitors in various nephropathies of different origins have been proved to significantly reduce proteinuria and progression to ESRF (Maschio *et al.* 1996; Ruggenenti *et al.* 2000), no significant data could be obtained by sub-analysis of IgAN patients. Indeed, in 75 patients enrolled in the REIN study with proteinuria more than 1 g/day, (mean 3 g/day) ACE-inhibitor induced a 35 per cent reduction in GFR decline, but the effect was without statistical significance (Ruggenenti *et al.* 2000). A meta-analysis of ACE-inhibitor results in 240 adult patients with IgAN (Dillon 2001) showed that in seven studies (three short-term, one randomized perspective, and three retrospective in hypertensive patients) ACE-inhibitors decreased proteinuria, but it was significant in four of seven reports only. As for the renoprotective effect, differences in control therapies and deficiencies in study design prevented definitive conclusions regarding an evidence-based benefit of ACE-inhibitors in IgAN, and that a prospective controlled study is warranted, which is ongoing (Coppo *et al.* 2001).

It has been shown that ACE-inhibitors attenuate the expression of TGF-β1 at renal levels in these patients (Shin *et al.* 2000). The antiproteinuric effect of these drugs may be potentiated by the association of indomethacin (Perico *et al.* 1998) or in combining ACE-inhibitors and angiotensin II receptor antagonists (Russo *et al.* 1999). The former association needs a frequent and accurate control of the renal function by the evaluation of creatinine clearance, the latter combination is more remarkable in reducing proteinuria than either drug administered alone. Probably, the combination therapy has an additive dose-dependent antiproteinuric effect that is likely to be induced by the drug-related reduction in intraglomerular haemodynamics (Russo *et al.* 2001).

The randomized-controlled trials on *fish-oil therapy* showed contrasting results on the beneficial effect of this drug (Bennett *et al.* 1989; Donadio *et al.* 1994; Pettersson *et al.* 1994). A meta-analysis indicated that a modest positive effect was observed (Dillon 1997). Thus, studies enrolling larger numbers of IgA nephropathy patients are necessary to detect the benefit, and treatment should be planned for a longer period.

A recent overview on the most important randomized controlled trials analysed their quality according to the Consolidated Standards of Reporting Trials (CONSORT) statement and the duration of the follow-up (Strippoli *et al.* 2003). The analysis showed a wide heterogeneity among the RCTs and the meta-analysis indicated only corticosteroids and immunosuppressive drugs may be potentially beneficial to the outcome of the renal function. Nevertheless, when the results of meta-analysis were adjusted for the duration of the follow-up, it was found that this effect decreased and became null as follow-up increased. In conclusion, further RCTs are necessary, relating specifically to more homogeneous groups of IgA nephropathy patients and therapeutic regimens with a long-term follow-up. In addition, the clinical trials should be designed within a standard quality protocol if we want to be able to pool these data into useful meta-analyses.

Recurrence of primary IgA nephropathy in renal transplants

The first report in which recurrence of the disease was observed in transplanted subjects with biopsy-proven IgA nephropathy in the native kidney was published by Berger *et al.* (1975), a finding confirmed by many subsequent reports.

IgA nephropathy is the second most common recurrent glomerulonephritis after focal segmental glomerular sclerosis. It is likely that initially, in the majority of patients, recurrent mesangial IgA deposits are clinically unimportant. With time (more than approximately 6 years) a significant percentage of patients with primary IgA nephropathy in native kidneys develop mesangial proliferative glomerulonephritis, progressive allograft dysfunction characterized by proteinuria of more than 1 g/day, and mesangial deposits of IgA in the graft. The incidence is greater in living-related donor grafts (20 per cent) than in cadaveric donor grafts (4 per cent) (Andressdottir *et al.* 2001). Younger patients are more prone to the risk of recurrence (Ponticelli *et al.* 2001). Recurrence increases to 44 per cent with longer follow-up, but this does not limit the graft outcome. Recurrence is not influenced by the type of living donor; therefore, both live-related and unrelated kidneys may be offered to IgA nephropathy patients (Kim *et al.* 2001).

Despite the potential for recurrence, IgA nephropathy patients have good long-term graft survival (Bumgardner *et al.* 1998).

Cumulative graft survival difference is not reduced in living versus cadaveric donor recipients. The 10-year graft survival rate is 63 per cent for a graft from a living related donor versus 93 per cent from an unrelated donor. Graft loss occurs with long-term follow-up.

Cyclosporin does not reduce the incidence and severity of the disease recurrence. The analysis of IgA production by PBMC in transplanted IgA nephropathy patients, studied by ELISPOT and intracytoplasmic immunofluorescence, shows a low number of IgA spot forming cells, thus suggesting that immunosuppressive therapy could interfere with the anomalies of IgA metabolism (Kennel *et al.* 1997).

A beneficial effect of ACE-inhibitors has been observed in patients with post-transplant IgA nephropathy because histopathological lesions indicative of acute inflammatory insults were suppressed, and glomerular hypertrophy, which may relate to haemodynamic burden such as hyperfiltration, was prominent. A future long-term follow-up study is required to establish the effectiveness of ACE-i in the treatment of post-transplant IgA nephropathy (Oka *et al.* 2000).

Epidemiology and immunogenetics

Geographical distribution

Primary IgA nephropathy represents the most frequent glomerulonephritis among patients undergoing renal biopsy in Asia (29.2 per cent), Australia (12 per cent), Europe (10.7 per cent), and North America (5 per cent) (Schena 1990). The differences in the prevalence of distribution in different geographic regions of the world are strongly biased by the biopsy policy and use of health-screening urinary tests. The concept that the prevalence of primary IgA nephropathy may be influenced by the policy for renal biopsy is also supported by the epidemiological data reported in the literature in the last 20 years in different regions of the world (Table 5). Thus, it is misleading to compare 'prevalence' of primary IgA nephropathy between various regions of the world, unless the indications for renal biopsy are taken into consideration, or proper population-based studies are carried out.

Urinary screening policy strongly influences the apparent prevalence of primary IgA nephropathy. In fact, in the Asian area, there is a large difference between the apparent prevalence in Japan, Singapore, Korea, and Hong Kong because in 1973 the Japanese School Health Law imposed urinalysis screening in schoolchildren. In Singapore, army recruits undergo a regular medical examination and subjects with recurrent micro- or macrohaematuria receive renal biopsy. Such screenings, in conjunction with frequent renal biopsy examination of subjects who present with recurrent microscopic, as well as macroscopic haematuria, could contribute to the increased prevalence of primary IgA nephropathy observed in these populations. Thus, IgA nephropathy is the most frequent disease diagnosed by renal biopsy in the Orient: the frequency of IgA nephropathy among all biopsied patients with primary glomerulonephritis increases from the Western (United States 16.7 per cent, Italy 35.9 per cent) to the Eastern (Japan 47 per cent, Singapore 45 per cent) regions. Nevertheless, small number of registries of renal biopsies in the rest of the world (Italy, Spain, Australia) show that IgA nephropathy is the most frequent glomerulonephritis in both children and in adults (Schena *et al.* 1997; Coppo *et al.* 2000).

Males have a much greater incidence of primary IgA nephropathy worldwide, except for Hong Kong, and the male–female ratio has been reported to be from 2 : 1 to 6 : 1. However, when the disease occurs in those of African origin, females are much more frequently affected. In some Indian tribes of New Mexico, such as the Zunis, IgA nephropathy occurs with the same frequency in the two sexes.

Table 5 Differences in prevalence of the IgA nephropathy in two consecutive periods in different geographical areas

Country	Prevalence (%)	Prevalence (%)
United States	1.5 (Lee *et al.* 1982)	16.7 (Braden *et al.* 2000)
United Kingdom	4 (Sisson *et al.* 1975)	21.1 (Propper *et al.* 1988)
The Netherlands	5 (Van der Peet 1997)	22 (Tieboch *et al.* 1987)
Japan	40 (Shirai *et al.* 1978)	47.4 (RGPCRD 1999)
Singapore	33.7 (Sinniah *et al.* 1981)	45 (Woo *et al.* 1999)

Family studies

After the first report by Tolkoff-Rubin *et al.* (1978) on the possible presence of relatives with biopsy-proven IgA nephropathy in the family of a patient with primary IgA nephropathy, other much larger studies have been reported (Julian *et al.* 1988; Scolari *et al.* 1999; Hsu *et al.* 2000). Affected members were either parent–offspring or siblings and, in addition, other relatives frequently showed clinical glomerulonephritis. Some may suffer from mild urinary abnormalities, such as persistent microhaematuria and or proteinuria, whereas others show recurrent macrohaematuria or chronic renal failure.

The true incidence of familial primary IgA nephropathy is unknown because few renal units systematically examine the urine of family members and perform renal biopsy in those subjects with persistent microhaematuria. However, a recent epidemiological study (Schena *et al.* 2002), in a large series of families of IgA nephropathy patients showed that familial clustering of the disease occurred in more than 50 per cent of patients. Thus, the disease clusters in families more frequently than we may expect: the relative risk was greater in first-degree (16.4) than in second-degree relatives (2.4). This finding suggests that examination of family members might avoid a late referral of subjects with persistent urinary abnormalities and late diagnosis of the disease. In a case–control study in Japan, Wakai *et al.* (1999) found a deterioration of the renal function in more than 40 per cent of subjects in whom IgA nephropathy was diagnosed by the school screening programme. Therefore, the epidemiologic studies urgently recommend a rapid and early diagnosis of the disease and the differentiation of IgA nephropathy from other benign diseases such as thin-membrane disease or normal renal parenchyma.

Taking into consideration that IgA nephropathy may occur in a sporadic or familial form, three generations of a cohort of 110 patients with biopsy-proven IgA nephropathy were checked for urinalysis and renal survival was estimated in patients from familial and sporadic disease (Schena *et al.* 2002). The 20-year renal survival rate from the apparent onset of the disease was significantly poorer in patients with familial (41 per cent) than in patients with sporadic (94 per cent) IgA nephropathy. Furthermore, 15-year renal survival from the time of renal biopsy was significantly worse in familial disease: endstage renal disease was present in 64 per cent of familial and only in 8 per cent of patients with sporadic IgA nephropathy. Therefore, familial IgA nephropathy should not be considered a benign disease, and an accurate family history and urinalysis in all family members is recommended in clinical practice.

Immunological serum abnormalities in relatives

Abnormalities in the immune regulation of the IgA system have been observed in both primary IgA nephropathy patients and their relatives (Table 6). On the basis of these findings, it is reasonable to hypothesize that a common genetic substrate affects B-lymphocyte function in patients and their relatives. It is noteworthy that peripheral blood mononuclear cells isolated from relatives show an increased mitogen-induced synthesis of IgA and IgA1 compared to normal subjects. On the contrary, they lack the spontaneous hyperproduction of IgA1 that specifically characterizes the patients (Scivittaro *et al.* 1994a). Thus, the reduced suppressor activity which is claimed to explain basal IgA1 and IgM hyperproduction in IgA nephropathy patients may be superimposed upon a general hyperactivity of specific IgA1 in relatives, as revealed by *in vitro* stimulation with mitogens.

These findings support the view that the unbalanced regulation of immunoglobulin synthesis is not limited to an altered switch from IgM to IgA1 production. An altered production of cytokines may play an important role within this framework. Many cytokines, mainly IL-4, IL-5, and TGF-β may regulate isotype production. Peripheral blood mononuclear cells from patients and their relatives with microhaematuria showed increased spontaneous production of IL-2, whereas IL-4, IL-6, and IFN-γ were normal (Scivittaro *et al.* 1994b). PHA stimulation induced an increased production of all the cytokines tested. Interestingly, relatives of primary IgA nephropathy patients who had themselves microhaematuria had the same profile of cytokine production as primary IgA nephropathy patients. Conversely, relatives with normal urinanalysis did not display any significant difference in cytokine synthesis from normal individuals.

It is noteworthy that some of these cytokines play a key role in immunoglobulin class switching and influence the synthesis of IgA and IgE by peripheral blood mononuclear cells from patients with primary IgA nephropathy. Thus, this abnormality could favour an imbalance in the distribution of isotypes in the antibody response of patients and relatives. Such an imbalance expressed as a loss of mucosal balance might underlie defects in the population of antigen-specific IgA+ cells in the mucosal lamina propria, promoting antigen penetration of the mucosal barrier (Emancipator 1992). Immunoglobulin class switch recombination allows B-cells to express sequentially antibodies that have identical specificities but that differ in class and, thus, in effector function.

Table 6 Immunological abnormalities observed in family members of primary IgA nephropathy patients

Occurrence of increased serum levels
IgA, IgA1
Polymeric IgA
IgA rheumatoid factor
IgA1–IgG, IgA1–IgM immune complexes
Increased percentage
IgA-bearing cells
Tα4 cells
In vitro mitogen-stimulated peripheral blood mononuclear cells over-produce
IgA, IgA1
Polymeric IgA
Cytokines (IL-2, IL-4, IFN-γ)

Immunogenetic associations

The occurrence of the disease in two or more family members suggests that an heritable trait for IgA nephropathy could be present in certain families and may contribute to the risk of developing renal disease. Considering this aspect different genetic approaches have been performed, such as association studies and familial studies. Early studies showed an association between some HLA antigens and the disease, but there is a discrepancy among these studies because of a bias in the selection of patients, and of differences in the geographical situation. HLA antigen associations vary from country to country and, in some countries, from area to area (Schena 1998). In addition, it is likely that more than one gene exerts its influence in determining susceptibility to the disease and, conversely, the effects of these genes are modified by different environmental factors in the population. Of particular interest is the report of a strong association of HLA–DR4 with primary IgA nephropathy, the relative risk ranging between 2.1 and 4.7. Since the DR locus appears to influence various aspects of humoral and cellular immune response, particularly the efficiency of interaction among T-cells, B-cells, and macrophages, it is reasonable to hypothesize that the sequence of immunological processes in primary IgA nephropathy may be controlled genetically by the HLA–DR genes. Several findings, such as increased serum IgA, mainly in polymeric (p) form, increased IgA-bearing cells, and an increased *in vitro* spontaneous production of IgA by peripheral blood mononuclear cells, argue in favour of an abnormal IgA immune response. Several investigators studied the influence of DR4 antigen at the onset of the disease, but contrasting data have been published.

The application of HLA polymorphism analysis at the gene level has overcome the limitation of traditional typing methods. Since some alleles do not contain a unique sequence, they need to be identified with a combination of probes able to detect sequences present in two or more alleles. Three class II products, DP, DQ, and DR, are crucial for presentation of processed antigen to specific T-cells. In the past 4 years, several investigators have studied the gene polymorphism of these class II products in primary IgA nephropathy patients and different results were obtained. It is possible that putative gene(s) could reside within or adjacent to the DQ and DR subregions. Therefore, a linkage disequilibrium between the DR and DQ loci, in which DQ alleles can be inherited more frequently together with certain DR alleles, may contribute to the susceptibility of the disease.

Association studies with candidate genes, which may be responsible for the onset of the disease, have been carried out, but data are contradictory. In fact, studies on the population of genes which modulate T-cell receptor of lymphocytes (TCR β, α) have shown different data in European and Asian populations (Table 7a). Other studies on gene polymorphism listed in Table 7b have shown contrasting data on their effect on the progression of the disease. The influence of ACE I/D gene polymorphism on the onset of the disease in Caucasian and Asian patients has not been confirmed in a series of studies enrolling a large number of patients (Suzuki *et al.* 2000; Schena *et al.* 2001) (Table 7c). The bias of many studies is represented by the low number

Table 7 Association studies in IgA nephropathy: (a) part I; (b) part II; (c) part III (the renin–angiotensin system)

Candidate genes	Polymorphisms	Onset	Progression	No. of pts	Population
(a)					
TcR Cβ	RFLP (Bgl II)	n		40	German
			y	34	Japanese
TcR Cα	RFLP (Taq I)	y	n	53	Chinese
		n		213	Japanese
			y	84	Japanese
(b)					
ecNOS	ecNOS4 b/a	n	y	68	Japanese
		n	n	115	Korean
		n	n	70	German
NPYY1	Y/y	n	y	68	Japanese
IL-1ra	VNTR	y	y	111	Chinese
TNF-α	−308 A/G	n	y	111	Chinese
TNF-β	RFLP (NcoI)	y		77	British
Sμ, Sα	RFLP (SacI)	n	y	78	Chinese
PAF	G994T	n	y	89	Japanese
UTR	G38A	n	y	110	German
Megsin	C2093T	n	n	110	German
α1	α1 hs1/2	n	y	104	French
(c)					
AGT	M235T		y	168	Canadian
			n	64	American
		n	n	247	Italian
			n	274	French
AT1R	A1166C		n	64	American
			n	168	Canadian
			n	274	French
ACE	I/D		y	53	Japanese
		n	y	48	Japanese
			y	97	Japanese
		n	y	100	Scottish
		n	n	204	German
			y	64	American
			y	168	Canadian
		n	n	70	German
		n	n	247	Italian
			n	274	French
			n	527	Japanese
		n	n	110	German

y = yes; n = no.

of patients enrolled in the studies, population stratification, and ethnic differences.

The occurrence of the disease in more than two relatives in families suggests extensive genetic studies in a large number of IgA nephropathy families. A multicentre study in which 30 IgA nephropathy families (24 from Italy and 6 from the United States) were analysed by whole-genome scanning revealed by linkage analysis a close association with the trait 6q 22–23 in 60 per cent of familial IgA nephropathy (Gharavi *et al.* 2000). But other suspected traits of the chromosomes were identified. These findings support the hypothesis that familial IgA nephropathy is a multifactorial or 'complex' disease in which one or more genes, probably in combination with environmental factors, may be responsible for the onset of the disease.

Pathogenesis

Although more than 3800 papers have been published in the last 35 years from the first description of a new glomerulonephritis by Berger *et al.* (1967) (Fig. 5), and several excellent reviews (listed in the bibliography) and proceedings of symposia (Table 8) have covered various aspects of primary IgA nephropathy, the pathogenesis of this disease remains to be elucidated.

IgA nephropathy is a worldwide disease which is characterized by (a) increased serum IgA, mainly IgA1 in polymeric form, in more than 50 per cent of patients; (b) increased IgA-bearing B lymphocytes and activated Tα helper cells; (c) overexpression of TGF-β and IL-4 mRNA in $CD4^+$ cells; and (d) IgA deposits in the mesangium. Considering

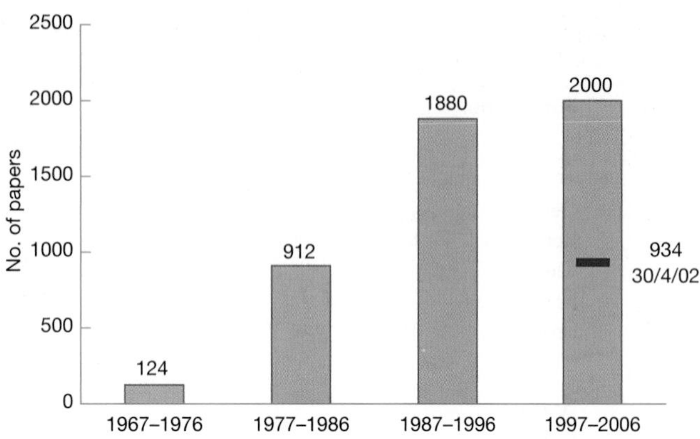

Fig. 5 Number of papers published after the first description of primary IgA nephropathy by Berger *et al.* (1967).

Table 8 Proceedings of the International Symposia on IgA nephropathy

1983	Milan	*Contributions to Nephrology*, Vol. 40, 1984
1986	Bari	*Seminars in Nephrology*, Vol. 7, No. 4, 1987
1988	Washington DC	*American Journal of Kidney Diseases*, Vol. 12, No. 5, 1988
1990	Tokyo	Hartcourt Brace Jovanovich, Japan, 1990
1992	Nancy	*Contributions to Nephrology*, Vol. 104, 1993
1994	Adelaide	*Contributions to Nephrology*, Vol. 111, 1995
1996	Singapore	*Nephrology*, Vol. 3, 1997
1998	Noordwijkerhout	No publication available
2001	Kyongiu	*Nephrology*, Vol. 7, 2002

these abnormalities, probably four systems such as blood, bone marrow, mucosa, and kidney are involved in the pathogenesis of the disease.

Structural alterations of IgA

The predominance of IgA in the mesangial deposits of glomeruli suggests a role for this protein in the pathogenesis of the disease.

IgA is the most abundant class of antibody in humans, and its structure is different from that of other mammals including rodents and logomorphes; therefore, only data from human IgA studies can be considered useful. IgA exists in the blood as two isotypes, IgA1 and IgA2. The IgA1 molecule is the predominant isotype which is present in the glomerular deposits of IgA nephropathy. The presence of the hinge region between CH1 and CH2 domains represents the major structural difference between the two IgA subclasses. This region, lacking in IgA2, consists of 18 amino acids. The amino acid sequence shows three threonine and three serine residues occupied by *O*-glycans (Fig. 6).

The *O*-glycosylation consists of a core *N*-acetyl galactosamine (GalNAc) which occurs alone or extended with β1,3-linked Gal or further with sialic acid in α2, 3 and/or α2, 6 linkage. Thus, each glycan may consist of one of four different forms, A–D (Fig. 7). Glycans A and B have neutral charge while C and D are negative charge for the presence of one or two sialic acid units. The form B is named T antigen by the team Thomsen–Friedenrich while the agalactosyl GalNAc moiety (form B) is referred to as Tn antigen. The IgA1 *O*-glycans are short mucin-type carbohydrate chains, which are unusual in serum proteins.

Normally, serum IgA1 consists of a mixture of molecules with different *O*-glycoforms, whereas an abnormal IgA1 *O*-glycoform pattern has been shown in IgA nephropathy patient serum by using different techniques such as lectin binding assay, matrix-assisted laser desorption spectroscopy, gas–liquid chromatography, and, more recently, fluorophore-assisted carbohydrate electrophoresis which has evidenced a high frequency of *O*-glycans consisting of GalNAc alone (Tomana *et al.* 1997; Hiki *et al.* 1998; Allen *et al.* 1999).

Undergalactosylation of IgA1 hinge region causes (a) increased binding to GalNac-specific lectins such as Vicia Villosa; (b) decreased binding to Jacalin; (c) self-aggregation of IgA1 molecules which constitute macroaggregates; and (d) adhesion to extracellular matrix proteins such as type IV collagen, fibronectin, and laminin. Kokubo *et al.* (1998) demonstrated that the removal of carbohydrates from the normal IgA1 molecule by digestion with neuraminidase caused self-aggregation of the molecules so called as macroaggregates and increased adhesion activity. The desialylation is a prerequisite for the self-aggregation while the undergalactosylation is very important for the adhesion to extracellular matrix proteins. The undergalactosylated IgA1 isolated from the serum of IgAN patients, fractionated according to their electric charge and the degree of the affinity with Jacalin, were injected into the left kidney of Wistar rats. Desialyted or degalactosylated IgA1 accumulated in the glomeruli and induced polymorphonuclear cell infiltration. In contrast, untreated native IgA1 did not accumulate. Therefore, the glomerulophilic IgA1 are undergalactosylated in the hinge region. Not only sialic acid, but other *O*-glycans are also lacking in these IgA1 macromolecules. An abnormal glycosylation of pIgA1 has been found in patients with IgAN and in those with Henoch–Schönlein nephritis, whereas such abnormality was not present in children with Henoch–Schönlein purpura and no evidence of renal involvement (Allen *et al.* 1998).

Since the peptide epitope of the IgA1 hinge region is aberrantly exposed by the undergalactosylation, the humoral immune response in IgA nephropathy is characterized by the presence of anti-IgA1 hinge peptide antibodies, IgG and IgM class, in the serum of IgAN patients (Kokubo *et al.* 2000). The production of these antibodies could cause the formation of IgA1–IgG and IgA1–IgM immune complexes that are present at high levels in the blood of IgAN patients. The reactivity of these antibodies was greatest in the naked, followed by the agalacto, sialo, and native IgA1; thus, the more carbohydrates removed from the hinge region, the greater the reactivity. Therefore, the absence of carbohydrates in the hinge region does not protect this piece of Fc segment of IgA1 and the peptide epitope increase the B-cell to be activated and produce anti-α1 HP antibodies.

Undergalactosylation of IgA-1 decreases the negative charge to this immunoglobulin. In fact, the densitometric analysis of serum IgA1 by two-dimensional gel electrophoresis reveals that alpha-heavy chains have low mean ratio of anionic charges as compared to healthy controls. This means a low content of sialic acid residues in IgA1 which causes easy interactions with other proteins such as other immunoglobulins, complement components, extracellular matrix, and antigens. The catabolism of asialylated and asialylated–agalactosylated IgA1 should involve the

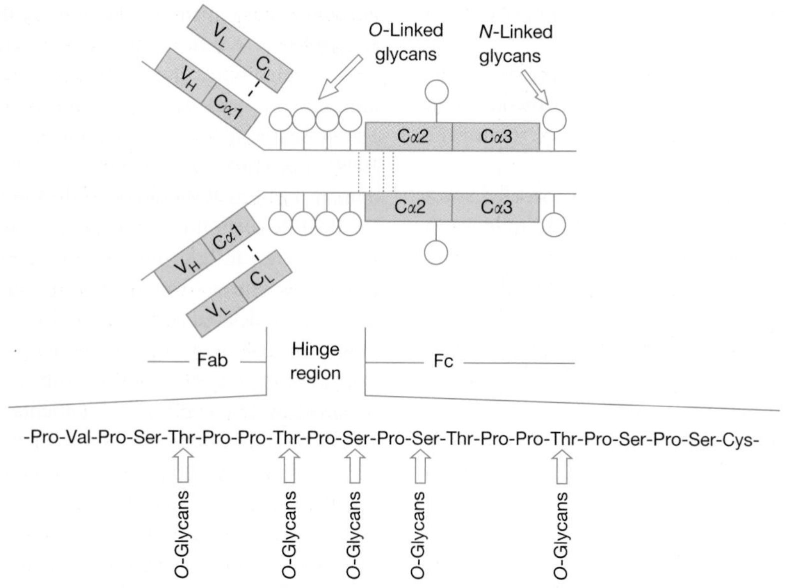

Fig. 6 The IgA1 molecule, with particular magnification of the hinge region.

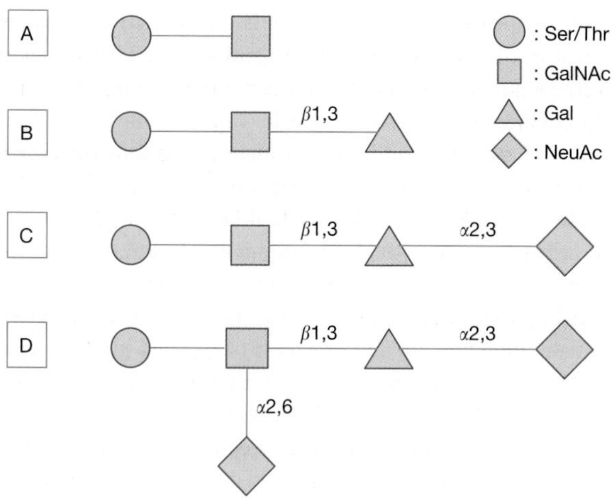

Fig. 7 *O*-Glycoforms.

hepatic asioglycoprotein receptor. However, aberrantly glycosylated IgA1, circulating in macromolecular form—either due to auto-aggregation or complexes, escape this specific clearance system (Roccatello *et al.* 1993) possibly because the size of the aggregates excludes them from the Dissie space, where the asialoglycoprotein receptors (ASGP-Rs) are located (Tomana *et al.* 1997).

The possibility of DNA point mutations or deletions in the nucleotide sequence which codifies the core amino acid sequence of IgA1 in IgAN patients was investigated in DNA of these subjects. Even though IgA nephropathy patients showed in this study an abnormal *O*-glycosylation, there was no difference in the nucleotide sequence of the $\alpha 1$ hinge region in these patients in comparison with race- and sex-matched controls (Greer *et al.* 1998). In addition, no difference was found in the mRNA transcripts derived from genomic DNA sequence of the IgA nephropathy patients. These data suggest that a post-translational defect may occur in these subjects.

The addition of Gal to GalNAc is modulated by glycosyltransferases. For this reason the activity of β1,3 galactosyltransferase (β1,3 GT), an enzyme responsible for galactosylation of *O*-linked sugars, was measured in cell lysates from B-, T-cells, and monocytes (Allen *et al.* 1997). Interestingly, a reduced β1,3 GT activity was found in B-cell lysates. This finding supports the hypothesis that increased degalactosylated IgA1 may be the consequence of reduced β1,3 GT activity. Unfortunately, the assay used for this study cannot indicate whether this defect is represented by low levels of enzyme or compromised activity. The gene of β1,3 GT has been recently cloned and sequenced and there is some evidence that multiple isotypes of this enzyme with some tissue specificity exists in humans. Therefore, gene expression and polymorphism studies are under way. Defect of *O*-glycosylation of a membrane protein is present in a haematological disorder, the so-called Tn polyagglutinability syndrome, in which the Thomsen–Freidenrich antigen (T antigen) is agalactosylated. This abnormality is caused by the loss of β1,3 GT activity in the affected cells due to repression of a functional gene.

It has been shown that stimulation of murine B-cells with IL-4 and IL-5 alters the terminal glycosylation of secreted IgA. The alteration in terminal glycosylation is more profound in IgA secreted from surface IgM^+ than from surface IgA^+ CH12LX cells. Therefore, increased production of IL-4 and IL-5 by PBMC of IgA nephropathy patients may explain the production of abnormally glycosylated IgA1 which deposit in the glomeruli. A relative or absolute increased production of Th2 cytokines in response to mucosal infections may be the pathogenic factor responsible for profound reduction of terminal galactosylation and sialylation (Chintalacharuvu and Emancipator 1997; Chintalacharuvu *et al.* 2001).

Elevated levels of lambda-IgA1 with reduced k/λ ratio are present in the blood of IgA nephropathy patients. The unusual glycosylation and sialylation of the lambda-IgA1 hinders their clearance by the ASGP-R of hepatocytes. Therefore, the negative charge of lambda-IgA1 and high serum levels favour mesangial deposition in the glomeruli for a selective binding (Leung *et al.* 2002).

Normal or low levels of secretory components are present in the blood of IgA nephropathy patients. These data support the idea that circulating IgA do not originate from epithelial compartment of the mucosal immunoglobulins.

Circulating immune complexes consist of undergalactosylated, most polymeric IgA1, and IgG antibodies specific for GalNAc residues in *O*-linked glycans of the hinge region of the IgA1 heavy chains. Antibodies are present in the IgG (predominantly IgG2 subclass) and less frequently in the IgA1 isotype. The deficiency of Gal in the hinge region of IgA1 molecules induces the exposition of GalNAc residues that are recognized by naturally occurring IgG and IgA1 antibodies (Tomana *et al.* 1999). Serum IgG3 subclass bind preferentially to asialo–agalacto IgA1 and this solves the question of why the IgG3 is co-present with deposited IgA1 in IgA nephropathy (Iwase *et al.* 1999).

Blood

The biological functions of IgA depend primarily on their interaction with cell surface receptors. Many receptors have been characterized.

IgAFc receptor (R) (CD89) is present in approximately 20 per cent of circulating mononuclear cells (B lymphocytes, monocytes/macrophages) in healthy subjects. It is a class-specific receptor because it is not inhibited in the binding of IgA by high concentrations of other immunoglobulins. Adachi *et al.* (1983), for the first time, described an abnormal expression of Fcα R on lymphocytes of IgA nephropathy patients which was further confirmed by Kashem *et al.* (1994) in polymorphonuclear leucocytes and monocytes by using monoclonal antibody (My-43) in flow cytometry. Fcα R is expressed as multiple isoforms named a-1, a-2, and a-3, which differ by deletions in the extracellular domains. FcαR protein and mRNA expression on blood monocytes and granulocytes of IgA nephropathy patients were analysed by Toyabe *et al.* (1997). They demonstrated that the whole molecule of Fcα R on monocytes had a higher molecular weight and the protein core also had a higher molecular weight. This was due to the expression pattern of mRNA which showed predominantly the transcript Fcα R a-1. They concluded that the specific expression of Fcα R a-1 on IgA nephropathy monocytes may be related to delayed FcαR-mediated endocytosis in monocytes from the disease. The expression of Fcα Rs on the surface of circulating blood cells is downregulated by polymeric IgA. This contributes to the persistence of circulating IgA1 and IgA1-immune complexes due to the impaired binding and degradation (Grossetete *et al.* 1998). The pathogenic role of this receptor was recently evidenced in generating transgenic mice highly expressing human CD89 on monocyte/macrophages. These mice spontaneously developed massive mesangial IgA deposits, glomerular and intestitial macrophage infiltration, mesangial matrix expansion, haematuria, and mild proteinuria (Launay *et al.* 2000). It was shown that CD89 after interaction with IgA released from cells and circulate in the blood in soluble form complexed with IgA. These complexes were responsible for renal damage, in fact depletion of soluble CD89 form from serum abolished this effect.

Monteiro's group demonstrated a down-regulation of Fcα R on blood cells (monocytes and granulocytes) caused by the presence of elevated serum IgA (Grossetete *et al.* 1998). When autologous plasma was removed from the cells *in vitro* FcαR was upregulated. These data show a negative regulatory role of serum IgA on the surface of Fcα R expression and persistence of circulating IgA1 and IgA1-immune complexes in the blood, thus impairing their binding and degradation. Human Fcα R is encoded by a gene of five exons located on chromosome 19q 13.4. This receptor binds transiently monomer IgA, while is avid for IgA-immune complexes. Histidil 85 and arginyl 82 in the FG loop of domain 1 are essential for the IgA-binding activity of the Fcα R (Wines *et al.* 1999). Therefore, the mutagenesis of these residues in the FG loop of domain 1 of Fcα R should be studied in IgA nephropathy patients.

ASGP-R is another candidate receptor involved in IgA catabolism and clearance of IgA1-immune complexes from the circulation. This receptor is expressed by hepatocytes and binds IgA via its *O*-linked moieties. A delayed and impaired clearance of IgA1-immune complexes in IgA nephropathy patients has been demonstrated by Roccatello *et al.* (1993). In this study, the authors used aggregated IgA obtained by IgA nephropathy patients. In another study, Rifai *et al.* (1989) by administering myeloma aggregated IgA in IgA nephropathy patients demonstrated a normal clearance of these complexes.

These different results may be explained by the presence of a glycosylation defect of serum IgA1 in IgA nephropathy patients. In addition, *in vivo* studies in mice have shown that underglycosylated human IgA1 binds preferentially to the kidneys rather than to the liver (Mestecky *et al.* 1993). Considering these data, it is possible to conclude that aberrantly underglycosylated IgA1 escapes the specific hepatic clearance by the ASGP-R and has a favoured deposition in the kidney.

Blood of IgA nephropathy patients is characterized by increased number of IgA-bearing B-lymphocytes and activated Tα helper cells. The expression of intracellular cytokines in these cells is represented by a predominance of IL-4, IL-10, and IL-13 belonging to Th2 subset (Ebihara *et al.* 2001). In addition, an increased mRNA expression of IL-5 and IL-6 produced by Th2 cells has been observed (Ichinose *et al.* 1996). This increased production of IL-4 by peripheral blood mononuclear cells may explain the hyperproduction of IgA. Stimulation of murine B-cells with IL-4 and IL-5 decreases the terminal glycosylation of secreted IgM and increases that of IgA. Thus, Th2-derived cytokines differentially influence the glycosylation of secreted glycoproteins by B-cells. This might elucidate the basis of aberrant glycosylation in IgA nephropathy (Chintalecharuvu and Emancipator 2000).

Purified gamma delta T-cells of IgA nephropathy patients induced expression of IgA on naive IgD$^+$B-cells more efficiently than alpha beta T-cells. Since the proportion of gamma delta T-cells in peripheral blood mononuclear cells of these patients is high and correlates with the proportion of surface IgA-positive B-cells, there is an enhanced production IgA. In addition, gamma delta T-cells produce a large amount of TGF-β1, which is one of the main cytokines that induces IgA class switching on B-cells (Toyabe *et al.* 2001).

Bone marrow

Most patients with IgA nephropathy have a higher memory repertoire of IgA1 producing B-lymphocytes in the bone marrow together with high plasma IgA1. The connection between the bone marrow compartment and the mucosal immune system is probably based on traffic of either antigen-presenting cells or antigen-specific lymphocytes.

Bone marrow is the most important source of plasma cells producing IgA and IgA1 in IgA nephropathy patients (Van den Wall Bake *et al.* 1988). An increased synthesis of both monomeric and polymeric IgA1 in bone marrow culture has been found (Van den Wall Bake *et al.* 1989). A shift in the IgA subclass distribution towards IgA1 is present, therefore the IgA1 in the circulation and mesangial deposits may mainly originate from the bone marrow (Harper *et al.* 1994b). Cytokines play an important role on the proliferation and differentiation of lymphoid cells. An increased production IL-10 by PBMC after stimulation may be responsible for an increased number of IgAproducing B-lymphocytes in the bone marrow. Therefore, high levels of endogenous IL-10 may downregulate the effector function of monocytes, or possible antigen-presenting cells in general and consequently the IgA response at the mucosal level (de Fijter *et al.* 1998).

High serum levels of IgA, IgA-immune complexes, and hyperresponsiveness of patient lymphocytes to antigens, shown *in vitro* and *in vivo*, are present in IgA nephropathy patients. An abnormal systemic response to immunization has been demonstrated in IgA nephropathy patients when it was induced by the administration of tetanus toxoid (Layward *et al.* 1992). These data suggest that the excess bone marrow production of IgA may be of 'mucosal' type pIgA, which has abnormal access to the circulation and hence the mesangium.

Mucosa

Patients with IgA nephropathy often present macroscopic haematuria in concomitance with upper respiratory tract infections, mainly tonsillitis and pharyngitis.

Palatine tonsils in IgA nephropathy patients have a reduced reticulation which exceed 50 per cent of total crypt epithelia in those with advance stage of renal damage. The low level of reticulation in tonsillar crypts may induce an unusual immunity (Sato *et al.* 1996). In addition, an increased expression of CD31 and CD54 on endothelial venules of tonsils may explain the increased lymphocyte recruitment observed in tonsils of these patients (Kennel-De March *et al.* 1997a,b). Bené *et al.* (1983) were the first to evidence, using quantitative immunohistomorphometry, an increased number of dimeric IgA-producing plasma cells, stained for cytoplasmic IgA and J chain in the tonsils of IgA nephropathy patients. Egido *et al.* (1984) showed an increased number of tonsillar IgA bearing lymphocytes which produced in culture, after pokewed mitogen stimulation, a large amount of polymeric IgA. These investigators concluded that pIgA deposited in the kidneys of IgA nephropathy patients may be of mucosal origin since an immunoregulatory dysfunction in the secretory immune system is present. Bené *et al.* (1991) confirmed these tonsillar anomalies in a multicentre study which analysed 303 tonsils obtained from 70 IgA nephropathy patients and 142 controls. The immunohistomorphometric study evidenced an increased percentage and number of IgA positive cells in patients. A further immunohistochemical and electron microscopy study demonstrated that the germinal centres of the tonsil were constituted by follicular dendritic cells with preferential IgA1 localization (Kusakari *et al.* 1994). B-cells were isolated from germinal centres and the number of B-1- and B-2-cells was determined by flow cytometry. An increased number of B-1-cells, likely producing IgA1 antibody, was found. These cells showed a reduced susceptibility to Fas-mediated apoptosis. Therefore, activated B-1-cells survive in the germinal centres due to this impaired apoptosis and thus produce abnormal amount of antibodies (Kodama *et al.* 2001). In conclusion, immune response of these cells could have an important impact in the pathogenesis of the disease.

An increased concentration of IgA has been found in the *nasal washings* of IgA nephropathy patients. Similar data were also found in *pharyngeal washings*. Furthermore, these authors demonstrated a cytopathic effect of extracts from pharyngeal cells of IgA nephropathy patients on fibroblasts, thus concluding that some antigenic substances may exist in epithelial cells of the upper respiratory tract in these patients (Tomino *et al.* 1986).

Elevated *salivary IgA levels* were also found in a large percentage of patients with IgA deposit. Further, high salivary IgA1 was demonstrated by other investigators (Rostoker *et al.* 1992) both in IgA nephropathy patients and in those with other forms of primary glomerulonephritis. These data were not confirmed by Layward *et al.* (1993).

Quantification of immunoglobulin-producing cells was done in *small intestinal mucosa* of IgA nephropathy patients and a normal distribution of immunocytes producing IgA, IgM, and IgG was found (Westberg *et al.* 1983). Similar data on IgA1 and IgA2-containing plasma cells were found in the *jejunum* of patients by Hené *et al.* (1988). Harper *et al.* (1994a) demonstrated a reduced expression of J chain mRNA in *duodenal* IgA plasma cells of patients with IgA nephropathy. Clinical exacerbation of the disease is frequently associated with mucosal infection.

Kidney

Mesangial cells play an important role in monitoring the structure and function of the glomerulus. A new mesangium predominant gene termed 'megsin', which belongs to the serpin superfamily, has been discovered. Megsin is predominantly expressed in human mesangial cells. It is overexpressed in the expanded mesangium of glomeruli of IgA nephropathy patients and correlates with mesangial cell proliferation (Miyata *et al.* 1998).

The IgA1 fragments of serum IgA nephropathy patients have a decrease of GalNAc, Gal, and sialic acid. The decreased galactosylation and sialylation of the IgA1 hinge region is responsible for its glomerular deposition in IgA nephropathy (Odani *et al.* 2000). IgA1 eluted from IgA mesangial deposits have a more pronounced lectin binding activity than serum IgA1 of some patients (Allen *et al.* 2001). Some studies have demonstrated that *in vitro* produced desialylated and degalactosylated IgA as well as IgA glycoforms isolated from sera of IgA nephropathy patients are active in modulating mesangial cell reactivity even more than macromolecular aggregated IgA (Coppo *et al.* 2000).

Mesangial cell integrin regulates cell growth and survival, extracellular matrix production, and organization. Mesangial cells express mostly $\alpha v\beta 3$ and some $\alpha 3\beta 1$. *In vitro* desialylated and degalactosylated IgA enhanced $\alpha v\beta 3$ expression on cultured mesangial cells as well as IgA from IgA nephropathy patients with high exposure of internal sugars, suggesting that truncation of terminal sugars of IgA glycan chains upregulates the expression of these receptors of matrix components. This integrin hyperexpression may increase matrix synthesis and accumulation and transmission of contractile forces to the capillary wall, thus favouring capillary stretching (Peruzzi *et al.* 2000). Moreover, these IgA1 glycoforms (desialylated and degalactosylated) either prepared *in vitro* or isolated from sera of IgAN patients decrease the mesangial cell proliferation rate, enhance the apoptosis rate of human mesangial cells, downregulate VEGF-A messanger RNA (Amore *et al.* 2000) and increase NOS activity and iNOS RNA (Amore *et al.* 2001).

The presence of Fcα R in cultured human mesangial cells was reported by Gomez-Guerrero *et al.* (1993). The expression of this receptor was enhanced by the overnight incubation with IgA in the culture medium. Parallel experiments showed this receptor in human and rat mesangial cells and peritoneal macrophages (Gomez-Guerrero *et al.* 1993). Dimeric and polymeric IgA bind the Fcα R since they induce the local production of IL-6 by rat mesangial cells (Van den Dobbelsteen *et al.* 1994). This higher affinity of polymeric IgA than monomeric IgA was observed also in human mesangial cells. The binding was specific for the IgA1. Fcα R binds the CH2 domain of the Fc region of IgA1. Aggregated IgA induce stimulation of Fcα R in human mesangial cells and synthesis of the inflammatory mediators such as IL-6, TNF-α, MCP-1, IP-10, and IL-8, via the transcription factor NF-κB (Duque *et al.* 1997).

The binding of serum polymeric IgA to human mesangial cells is charge dependent. In fact, pIgA1 from IgA nephropathy patients with the highest net negative charge binds more to human mesangial cells. Preincubation with polyanion decrease the binding of pIgA1 to human mesangial cells. Therefore, the anionic charge of IgA1 plays an important role in kidney mesangial cell deposition (Leung *et al.* 2001). Mass spectrometry proves an under *O*-glycosylation of IgA1 deposited in the glomeruli, because the number of carbohydrates composing *O*-glycans (GalNAc, Gal, and NANA) in the deposited IgA1 are significantly low. This underglycosylation of the *O*-glycan side chains in the hinge region (decreased sialylation and galactosylation) may explain the crucial role in the glomerular deposition (Hiki *et al.* 2001). The increased expression of Fcα R is associated with severity of proteinuria and haematuria.

Five years after the description of Fcα R in human mesangial cells, other investigators demonstrated that monomeric and polymeric IgA1 also bind mesangial cells independently of Fcα R1 (CD 89), which is different from ASGP-R (Diven *et al.* 1998). Recently, Barratt *et al.* (2000) identified a novel Fcα R expressed by human mesangial cells which was distinct from the CD 89 previously described, although the two proteins may share a common molecular origins.

Gómez-Guerrero *et al.* (1998) also reported the presence of the ASGP-R with high affinity for galactose residues of aggregated IgA1 in rat and human mesangial cells. They suggested that the catabolism of dimeric and polymeric IgA1 is modulated by the binding of Fc region of IgA1 to the Fcα R and by the affinity of the hinge region carbohydrates to the ASGP-R. In this case, if a defective galactosylation process at the hepatic and renal level occurs in IgA nephropathy patients, deglycosylated IgA1 have reduced affinity for the mesangial ASGP-R. They persist as circulating IgA1 immune complexes in the blood and accumulate in the kidney. In addition, the high deposition of IgA-immune complexes induces the local production of cytokines, chemokines, and growth factors.

Transferrin receptor (CD71) is a novel receptor which binds selectively IgA1 antibodies, monomeric better than polymeric forms. This binding is inhibited by transferrin. The transferrin receptor is overexpressed in culture mesangial cells of IgA nephropathy patients (Moura *et al.* 2001).

In vitro studies have shown that aggregated IgA1 induce c-jun expression in human mesangial cells, which express on the surface Fcα R and Fcγ R (Diven *et al.* 1998; Suzuki *et al.* 1999b). However, other investigators have failed to demonstrate Fcα R and they concluded that the binding of IgA to human mesangial cells occur via an IgA receptor distinct from CD89 (Westerhuis *et al.* 1999; Leung *et al.* 2000). Sublytic complement injury to mesangial cells, mediated by terminal membrane attack complex of complement (C5b-9), is a potential initiating mechanism in IgAN. This injury induces the production of inflammatory molecules and growth factors, including many regulated by the transcription of factor NF-κB (Mudge *et al.* 2000).

In conclusion, exposure to antigen(s) induces abnormal production of IgA antibody at the bone marrow level by B-cells, localized firstly in the mucosa axis of the upper respiratory tract and then in the bone marrow after cell migration. The synthesized IgA1 antibodies are undergalactosylated and they produce anti-IgA1 hinge peptide antibodies, IgG and IgM classes, which could cause the formation of IgA1–IgG and IgA1–IgM immune complexes. These complexes deposit in the kidney at the mesangial level. The downregulation of Fcα R on blood cells and in mesangial cells (binding of Fc region IgA1) or the reduced binding of the undergalactosylated IgA1 (hinge region) to the ASGP-R in hepatic and mesangial cells may cause delayed and impaired clearance of IgA1-immune complexes in IgA nephropathy patients. The persistence of IgA1-immune complexes could cause deposition at renal level and local production of cytokines, chemokines, and growth factors, which are responsible for glomerular lesions and progression of renal damage in the disease.

Experimental models of IgA nephropathy

Although the pathogenetic mechanisms of IgAN are unknown, clinical and experimental observations suggest that the renal deposition of circulating IgA-immune complexes may play a central role (Novak *et al.* 2001). In order to clarify the disease factors, several experimental models of IgA nephropathy have been established (listed in Table 9). We refer the reader to a specific review for more details (Montinaro *et al.* 1999).

IgA nephropathy associated with liver disease

This condition is usually clinically silent, characterized by mild microhaematuria, proteinuria, and glomerular lesions associated with mesangial IgA deposits and smaller amounts of other immunoglobulins and complement components. It is found most commonly in patients with alcoholic liver cirrhosis and in non-cirrhotic portal fibrosis after the insertion of a splenorenal shunt for portal hypertension. IgA nephropathy sometimes occurs in other liver diseases not related to alcohol, such as viral and cryptogenic chronic hepatitis, and chronic hepatosplenic schistosomiasis. Postmortem studies and renal biopsies (Newell 1987) demonstrated that glomerular abnormalities occur in 50–100 per cent of patients with liver cirrhosis.

Clinical features

Macrohaematuria may occur, but much less frequently than in patients with Berger's disease. Renal insufficiency is rare and does not correlate with the glomerular lesions. A few cases present heavy proteinuria, which may be associated with the nephrotic syndrome. Since the increase of systemic blood pressure is rare in patients with cirrhosis and portal hypertension, the occurrence of arterial hypertension is suggestive of an underlying liver glomerulonephritis. In patients with non-cirrhotic portal fibrosis, there is an increase in the incidence of proteinuria, microhaematuria, and high serum creatinine after splenorenal shunting operation (Dash *et al.* 1997).

Laboratory findings

Urinalysis reveals microhaematuria and proteinuria, which is in the nephrotic range in a small percentage of cases, particularly in those with membranoproliferative glomerulonephritis. In general, there are mild urine abnormalities in patients with minimal glomerular lesions, whereas heavy proteinuria, cylindruria, and microhaematuria are associated with severe proliferative lesions.

Increased serum IgA, mainly in the polymeric form, is present in 77–91 per cent of the patients, although high values are also found in 54 per cent of subjects with liver cirrhosis and without nephritis. Antibodies against dietary and bacterial antigens have often been found.

Reduced C3 (and rarely C4) may be observed in these patients. It is not known whether hypocomplementaemia is due to reduced hepatic synthesis or to increased catabolism. Increased C3d is present in the blood. However, no correlation between hypocomplementaemia and the degree of liver abnormalities has been observed, and reduced C3 occurs in both mesangial and proliferative forms of glomerulonephritis.

Circulating immune complexes have been detected in the blood of cirrhotic patients (Coppo *et al.* 1985). They are mainly of IgA type, both IgA1 and IgA2 subclasses, and do not directly correlate with renal abnormalities. Mixed cryoglobulins containing IgA have also been found in these patients.

Table 9 Experimental models of IgA nephropathy in animals

Animals	Models
Active models	
Swiss Webster mice	Intraperitoneal injection of dextran (1981)
Mice	Intraperitoneal injection of apoferritin (1982)
BALB/c mice	Oral administration of ovalbumin, bovine gamma-globulins (1983)
Mice	Bile-duct ligation (1983)
C3H/NeJ and C3H/cB mice	Oral administration of ferritin and bovine serum albumin (1986)
DdY mice	Spontaneous IgA nephropathy model (1985)
Rat	IV injection of monoclonal antibody to Thy-1.1 antigen (1987)
DdY mice	Oral administration of lactalbumin with RES blockage (1986)
BALB/c mice	Oral administration of crude gluten (1989)
Rats	Alcohol intoxication (1990)
B6C3F1 mice	Dietary exposure to trichothecene vomitoxin (1991)
C3H/HeN mice	Intraperitoneal injection of Gram-negative bacteria (1993)
129/J mice	Intranasal administration of inactivated Sendai virus (1992)
Mice	Oral administration of nivalenol (mycotoxin) (1997)
Marmots	Dietary exposure to gladine-like cereal proteins (1999)
Passive models	
BALB/c mice	IV injection of anti-DNP–DNP–BSA immune complexes (1979)
Swiss Webster mice	IV injection of dextran–antidextran immune complexes (1983)
C56BL/6 mice	IV injection of IgA anti-DNP/DNP–IgA anti-PC complexes and PC-containing antigens (pneumococcal C polysaccharide and other synthetic antigens) (1991)

DNP–BSA, dinitrophenylated bovine serum albumin; DNP, dinitrophenol; IV, intravenous; RES, reticuloendothelial; PC, phosphorocholine.

Renal biopsy

The characteristic glomerular lesions in the kidney of patients with liver disease are widening of the mesangial matrix, thickening of the capillary wall, a small increase in mesangial cellularity, and electron-dense deposits in the mesangium. Thickening of the GBM with areas of rarefaction is occasionally present. Proliferative lesions similar to those found in mesangiocapillary and rapidly progressive glomerulonephritis may be observed in some patients and would indicate that there are two forms of the disease. However, it is not clear whether non-proliferative lesions evolve into proliferative disease, or if the two forms represent different pathological responses to the same insult.

Immunofluorescence reveals IgA deposits associated with IgG and/or IgM and/or C3. They are present both in proliferative lesions and in non-proliferative glomerulonephritis. IgA is the main immunoglobulin present. It contains the J chain and is able to bind the secretory component. IgA2 is the major component of the mesangial deposits. This finding suggests that the immunoglobulin is derived from the gastrointestinal tract. The co-deposition of C3 in granular pattern indicates an immune complex type of glomerulonephritis. In fact, the demonstration of electron-dense deposits in the mesangium suggests immune complexes and not mere trapping of IgA in the glomeruli.

Pathogenesis

Various mechanisms, listed in Table 10, have been suggested for the pathogenesis of liver glomerulonephritis, but there is no clear evidence for any of them. The interaction between IgA produced by intestinal plasma cells and food antigens that cross the intestinal mucosa damaged by alcohol causes the formation of immune complexes. Smith *et al.* (1990) demonstrated that the infusion of a liquid diet containing alcohol in Wistar rats induced immune dysfunction in the mucosal immune system which is responsible for an IgA nephropathy. In addition, the incidence of renal disease is dependent on the time frame of alcohol ingestion (Smith and Tsukamoto 1992). Moreover, the combination of a lipotrope-deficient diet with an increased intake of alcohol may promote hepatic and renal changes, leading to hepatocellular injury and to a secondary form of IgA nephropathy (Amore *et al.* 1994). The impaired liver catabolism of immune complexes could be responsible for their persistence in the blood of patients with liver cirrhosis. Abnormal levels of IgA immune complexes occur only after alcohol-induced hepatic damage, since chronic alcoholics without biochemical evidence of liver damage have normal values of IgA immune complexes.

Table 10 Factors involved in the pathogenesis of liver

Arteriolar sclerosis
Choline deficiency
Alcohol abuse
Hyperoestrogenaemia
Hyperaldosteronism
Toxic substances
Lecithin cholesterol acyltransferase deficiency
Circulating immune complexes

The increased circulating immune complexes may be secondary to portacaval shunting of bacterial or food antigens, which bypass hepatic Kupffer cells. This hypothesis is supported by the presence of serum antibodies against bacteria and food and by an abnormal antibody production by peripheral blood lymphocytes after stimulation with these antigens. In addition, the splenorenal shunt procedure enhances the direct porto systemic circulation and partly bypasses the hepatic reticuloendothelial system. Therefore, immune complexes coming from the gastrointestinal tract bypass the liver and their excessive delivery causes their glomerular deposition in the systemic circulation. However, the splenorenal shunting procedure *per se* is not the predisposing factor because the presence of a poor reticuloendothelial system is necessary. The major pathway for the clearance of IgA2 is the liver throughout the ASGP-R. The dysfunction of this receptor may account for elevated serum levels of circulating IgA immune complexes in liver disease (Rifai *et al.* 2000).

HIV-associated IgA nephropathy

The human immunodeficiency virus (HIV) infection may be associated with different forms of glomerulonephritis, such as glomerulosclerosis, as well as diffuse mesangial proliferative, endocapillary proliferative, membranous, and membranoproliferative glomerulonephritis. IgA nephropathy may occur in the course of HIV infection (Kimmel *et al.* 1992).

HIV-associated glomerulosclerosis has a striking predilection for Afro-American patients and Caucasian men with normal or low CD4 cell counts. Although the large number of HIV-infected cases overwhelm the Asian countries, no cases of HIV-associated nephropathy are documented in the literature. Recently, Praditpornsilpa *et al.* (1999) described 26 cases of HIV-infected patients with associated nephropathy. The disease can be rare in Black and White children (Cachat *et al.* 1998).

HIV patients with associated nephropathy have micro- or macrohaematuria with minimal or moderate renal insufficiency, proteinuria more or less than 1 g/day, and increased serum IgA and circulating immune complexes. The renal biopsy, in addition to IgA nephropathy, reveals tubuloreticular inclusions which appear to be a general marker of HIV infection. Kimmel *et al.* (1992) isolated circulating immune complexes composed of idiotypic IgA antibody reacting with anti-HIV IgG or IgM. In addition, they eluted the same immune complex from the renal tissue and identified HIV DNA by PCR. These findings are in favour of an IgA nephropathy caused by the deposition of circulating IgA–anti-HIV antibody complexes in the glomeruli (see Chapter 3.13).

IgA nephropathy and associated systemic disorders

Since the first description of Berger *et al.* (1967), primary IgA nephropathy has been found typically in association with liver diseases and Henoch–Schönlein purpura, but in the past few years other associations have been reported, mainly with systemic disorders, such as lupus erythematosus, cryoglobulinaemia, rheumatic diseases, and other illnesses involving the upper respiratory tract, gastrointestinal tract, skin, and other organs.

Table 11 Diseases associated with IgA nephropathy

Mucosal diseases
Angle-closure glaucoma
Anterior uveitis
Bronchial and pulmonary diseases
Bronchiolitis obliterans
Coeliac disease
Crohn's disease
Cystic fibrosis
Dermatitis herpetiformis
Diffuse panbronchiolitis
Enteric fever
Episcleritis
Keratoconjunctivitis sicca
Oral mucosa sensitization in prosthesis implantation
Scleritis
Ulcerative colitis
Whipple's disease
Neoplasia
B-cell lymphoma
Bronchial carcinoma
Cutaneous T-cell lymphoma
Hepatocellular carcinoma
Multiple myeloma
Mycosis fungoides
Renal cell carcinoma
Small cell lung cancer
Immunological and systemic disorders
Acquired reactive perforating collagenosis
Anaphylactoid purpura
Ankylosing spondylitis
Antiphospholipid syndrome
Behçet's disease
Bullous pemphigoid
Churg–Strauss syndrome
Haemolytic anaemia and bullous dermatosis
Haemolytic uraemic syndrome
HIV
Idiopathic thrombocytopenic purpura
Inflammatory demyelinating polyradiculoneuropathy
Juvenile rheumatoid arthritis
Leucocytoclastic cutaneous vasculitis
Mixed cryoglobulinaemia
Myasthenia gravis
Paroxysmal nocturnal haemoglobinaemia
Polyarteritis nodosa
Psoriatic arthritis
Reiter's disease
Rheumatoid arthritis
Sarcoidosis
Henoch–Schönlein purpura
Sjögren's syndrome
Systemic lupus erythematosus
Takayasu's arteritis
Wegener's granulomatosis
Others
Aortitis syndrome
Acute interstitial nephritis
Chronic alcoholic liver disease
Cystic fibrosis
Clostridium difficile colitis

Table 11 (continued)

C9 congenital deficiency
Diabetic glomerulosclerosis
Diabetes mellitus
Eosinophilic fascitis
Epidermolysis bullosa
Fabry's disease
Factor V deficiency
Graves' disease
Hepatitis A virus infection
Hereditary angioedema
Hermansky–Pudlak syndrome
HTLV-1 associated myelopathy
Hypercalciuria
Hypoaldosteronism
Intramembranous dense deposits
Kimura's disease
Late heredodegenerative hearing loss
Lepromatius leprosy
Lymphoedema precox
Membranous nephropathy
Myelodysplastic syndrome
Nail-patella syndrome
Pemphigus foliaceus
Pernicious anaemia
Poems syndrome
Polychondritis
Polycythaemia vera
Porphyria
Psoriasis vulgaris
Pulmonary haemorrhage
Pustolosis palmaris and plantaris
Renal hypouricaemia
Retinal vasculopathy
Rhabdomyolysis associated with *Streptococcus viridans* bacteraemia
Simple renal cyst
Silicosis
Thin basement membrane disease
Tuberculosis
Vitiligo
Whipple's disease
Wilson's disease
α-Antitrypsin deficiency
β-Thalassaemia

Coeliac disease is frequently associated with IgA nephropathy. It has been hypothesized that circulating immune complexes originating in the small intestine could be responsible for the renal disease. The antigen could be derived from the damaged mucosa, a product of gluten, or increased mucosal permeability to antigens. The introduction of a gluten-free diet in patients with IgA nephropathy due to coeliac disease induces the resolution of proteinuria and the improvement of renal function (Woodrow *et al.* 1993). Therefore, there may be a small subgroup of IgA nephropathy patients who have underlying coeliac disease; in these patients treatment with a gluten-free diet may have a beneficial effect on a renal disease that is usually not responsive to any other therapy.

Table 11 lists the diseases associated with IgA nephropathy. Patients may develop these diseases before or during the clinical course of the nephritis.

Some associations have been reported in isolated cases and may be purely coincidental, whereas others appear to be the result of concomitant mucosal infection, as in bronchial and pulmonary disease, disseminated tuberculosis, *Mycoplasma pneumoniae* pneumonia, sarcoidosis, silicosis, enteric fever, or coeliac disease. Finally, the appearance of IgA nephropathy after the placement of nickel-alloy base dental crowns suggests that the prosthesis implantation might stimulate the oral mucosa to produce IgA, with resultant immune complex formation and renal deposition. The description of remission after the removal of the prosthesis supports this hypothesis.

Proliferative and/or sclerosing glomerulonephritis is considered very unusual in patients with neoplastic diseases. IgA nephropathy has been reported in patients with neoplasia and the cases are listed in Table 11. It occurs in older age groups and the presence of increased serum IgA suggests that an abnormal IgA response to chronic mucosal irritation or to a specific tumour antigen might be responsible for the onset of IgA nephropathy.

Several diseases may be accompanied by a dysregulation of IgA system, implying the presence of increased serum polymeric IgA or of circulating IgA immune complexes, and their consequent deposition within the kidney. In this context, IgA nephropathy may only represent one of the complications brought about by IgA deposition, as demonstrated by the common involvement of extrarenal vessel walls. These conditions occur mainly in immunological and systemic disorders, such as ankylosing spondylitis, psoriatic arthritis, juvenile rheumatoid arthritis, and arthritis after Yersinia infection. Furthermore, the association of various rheumatic disorders with scleritis may explain the appearance of IgA nephropathy in patients with scleritis. An immunofluorescence study demonstrated numerous infiltrating plasma cells secreting dimeric IgA in episcleral inflammatory infiltrate (Bené *et al.* 1984). Increased serum IgA may occur in the presence of other immunological and proliferative disorders, such as mixed cryoglobulinaemia, the Sjögren syndrome, and immunothrombocytopenia.

Bibliography

Allen, A. C. and Feehally, J. (1999). IgA1 glycosylation and the pathogenesis of IgA nephropathy. *American Journal of Kidney Diseases* **35**, 551–556.

Coppo, R., Amore, A., Hogg, R., and Emancipator, S. (2000). Idiopathic nephropathy with IgA deposits. *Pediatric Nephrology* **15**, 139–150.

D'Amico, G. (2000). Natural history of idiopathic IgA nephropathy: role of clinical and histological prognostic factors. *American Journal of Kidney Diseases* **36**, 227–237.

Dillon, J. J. (2001). Treating IgA nephropathy. *Journal of the American Society of Nephrology* **12**, 846–847.

Feehally, J. (2001). Predicting prognosis in IgA nephropathy. *American Journal of Kidney Diseases* **38**, 881–883.

Floege, J. and Feehally, J. (2000). IgA nephropathy: recent developments. *Journal of the American Society of Nephrology* **11**, 2395–2403.

Galla, J. H. (2001). Molecular genetics in IgA nephropathy. *Nephron* **88**, 107–112.

Glassock, R. J. (1999). The treatment of IgA nephropathy: status at the end of the millenium. *Journal of Nephrology* **12**, 288–296.

Hogg, R. J. and Waldo, B. (1996). Advances in treatment: immunoglobulin A nephropathy. *Seminars in Nephrology* **16**, 511–516.

Julian, B. A. (1999). Treatment of IgA nephropathy. *Seminars in Nephrology* **20**, 277–285.

Kincaid-Smith, P. (1999). Treatment of mesangial immunoglobulin A glomerulonephritis. *Seminars in Nephrology* **19**, 166–172.

Koyama, A., Igarashi, M., and Kobayashi, M. (1997). Natural history and risk factors for immunoglobulin A nephropathy in Japan. Research Group on Progressive Renal Diseases. *American Journal of Kidney Diseases* **29**, 526–532.

Nolin, L. and Courteau, M. (1999). Management of IgA nephropathy: evidence-based recommendations. *Kidney International* **70** (Suppl.), S56–S62.

Pettersson, E. (1997). IgA nephropathy: 30 years on. *Journal of Internal Medicine* **242**, 349–353.

Radford, M. G., Jr., Donadio, J. V., Jr., Bergstralh, E. J., and Grande J. P. (1997). Predicting renal outcome in IgA nephropathy. *Journal of the American Society of Nephrology* **8**, 199–207.

Rantala, I. *et al.* (2001). Pathogenetic aspects of IgA nephropathy. *Nephron* **88**, 193–198.

Scheinman, J. I. *et al.* (1997). IgA nephropathy: to treat or not to treat? *Nephron* **75**, 251–258.

Schena, F. P. (1995). Immunogenetic aspects of primary IgA nephropathy. *Kidney International* **48**, 1998–2013.

Scolari, F. (1999). Familial IgA nephropathy. *Journal of Nephrology* **12**, 213–219.

Shigematsu, H. (1997). Histological grading and staging of IgA nephropathy. *Pathology International* **47**, 194–202.

Waldo, F. B. *et al.* (1998). Current concepts and controversies in IgA nephropathy. *Pediatric Nephrology* **12**, 498–504.

Yoshikawa, N., Iijima, K., and Ito, H. (1999). IgA nephropathy in children. *Nephron* **83**, 1–12.

Yoshikawa, N., Tanaka, R., and Iijima, K. (2001). Pathophysiology and treatment of IgA nephropathy in children. *Pediatric Nephrology* **16**, 446–457.

References

Abe, T. *et al.* (1986). Participation of extracapillary lesions (ECL) in progression of IgA nephropathy. *Clinical Nephrology* **25**, 37–41.

Adachi, M. *et al.* (1983). Altered expression of lymphocyte Fc alpha receptor in selective IgA deficiency and IgA nephropathy. *Journal of Immunology* **131**, 1246–1251.

Akagi, H. *et al.* (1999). Prognosis of tonsillectomy in patients with IgA nephropathy. *Acta Oto Laryngologica Supplement* **540**, 64–66.

Alamartine, E., Sabatier, J. C., and Berthoux, F. C. (1990). Comparison of pathological lesions on repeated biopsies in 73 patients with primary IgA glomerulonephritis: value of quantitative scoring and approach to prognosis. *Clinical Nephrology* **34**, 45–51.

Alamartine, E. *et al.* (1991). Prognostic factors in mesangial IgA glomerulonephritis: an extensive study with univariate and multivariate analyses. *American Journal of Kidney Diseases* **18**, 12–19.

Alexopoulos, E. *et al.* (1989). The role of interstitial infiltrates in IgA nephropathy: a study with monoclonal antibodies. *Nephrology, Dialysis, Transplantation* **4**, 187–195.

Allen, A. C., Topham, P. S., Harper, S. J., and Feehally, J. (1997). Leucocyte beta 1,3 galactosyltransferase activity in IgA nephropathy. *Nephrology, Dialysis, Transplantation* **12**, 701–706.

Allen, A. C., Willis, F. R., Beattie, T. J., and Feehally, J. (1998). Abnormal IgA glycosylation in Henoch–Schönlein purpura restricted to patients with clinical nephritis. *Nephrology, Dialysis, Transplantation* **13**, 930–934.

Allen, A. C. *et al.* (1999). Analysis of IgA1 *O*-glycans in IgA nephropathy by fluorophore-assisted carbohydrate electrophoresis. *Journal of the American Society of Nephrology* **10**, 1763–1771.

Allen, A. C. *et al.* (2001). Mesangial IgA1 in IgA nephropathy exhibits aberrant *O*-glycosylation: observations in three patients. *Kidney International* **60**, 969–973.

Allmaras, E. *et al.* (1997). Rapidly progressive IgA nephropathy with anti-myeloperoxidase antibodies benefits from immunosuppression. *Clinical Nephrology* **48**, 269–273.

Amore, A. *et al.* (1994). Experimental IgA nephropathy secondary to hepato cellular injury induced by dietary deficiencies and heavy alcohol intake. *Laboratory Investigation* **70**, 68–77.

Amore, A. *et al.* (2000). Aberrantly glycosylated IgA molecules downregulate the synthesis and secretion of vascular endothelial growth factor in human mesangial cells. *American Journal of Kidney Diseases* **36**, 1242–1252.

Amore, A. *et al.* (2001). Glycosylation of circulating IgA in patients with IgA nephropathy modulates proliferation and apoptosis of mesangial cells. *Journal of the American Society of Nephrology* **12**, 1862–1871.

Andreoli, S. P. and Bergstein, J. M. (1989). Treatment of severe IgA nephropathy in children. *Pediatric Nephrology* **3**, 248–253.

Andresdottir, M. B., Hoitsma, A. J., Assmann, K. J., and Wetzels, J. F. (2001). Favorable outcome of renal transplantation in patients with IgA nephropathy. *Clinical Nephrology* **56**, 279–288.

Auwardt, R., Savige, J., and Wilson, D. (1999) A comparison of the clinical and laboratory features of thin basement membrane disease (TBMD) and IgA glomerulonephritis (IgA GN). *Clinical Nephrology* **52**, 1–4.

Ballardie, F. W. and Roberts, I. S. (2002). Controlled prospective trial of prednisolone and cytotoxics in progressive IgA nephropathy. *Journal of the American Society of Nephrology* **13**, 142–148.

Barratt, J. *et al.* (2000). Identification of a novel Fcalpha receptor expressed by human mesangial cells. *Kidney International* **57**, 1936–1948.

Bené, M. C. *et al.* (1983). Quantitative immunohistomorphometry of the tonsillar plasma cells evidences an inversion of the immunoglobulin A versus immunoglobulin G secreting cell balance. *Journal of Clinical Investigation* **71**, 1342–1347.

Bené, M. C. *et al.* (1984). IgA nephropthy: dimeric IgA secreting cells are present in episcleral infiltrate. *American Journal of Clinical Pathology* **82**, 608–611.

Bené, M. C., Hurault De Ligny, B., Kessler, M., and Faure, G. C. (1991). Confirmation of tonsillar anomalies in IgA nephropathy: a multicenter study. *Nephron* **58**, 425–428.

Bennett, W. M., Walker, R. G., and Kincaid-Smith, P. (1989). Treatment of IgA nephropathy with eicosapentanoic acid (EPA): a two-year prospective trial. *Clinical Nephrology* **31**, 128–131.

Berger, J. and Hinglais, N. (1968). Les depots intercapillaires d'IgAIgG. *Journal d' Urologie et Nephrologie* **74**, 694–695.

Berger, J., De Montera, H., and Hinglais, N. (1967). Classification des glomerulo-nephrites en pratique biopsique. *Proceedings of the Third International Congress on Nephrology, Washington 1966*, Vol. 2, pp. 198–221.

Berger, J., Yaneva, H., Nabarra, B., and Barbanel, C. (1975). Recurrence of mesangial deposition of IgA after renal transplantation. *Kidney International* **7**, 232–241.

Beukhof, J. R. *et al.* (1986). Toward individual prognosis of IgA nephropathy. *Kidney International* **29**, 549–556.

Brooimans, R. A. *et al.* (1991). Interleukin-2 mediates stimulation of complement C3 biosynthesis in human proximal tubular epithelial cells. *Journal of Clinical Investigation* **88**, 379–384.

Bumgardner, G. L., Amend, W. C., Ascher, N. L., and Vincenti, F. G. (1998). Single-center long-term results of renal transplantation for IgA nephropathy. *Transplantation* **65**, 1053–1060.

Cachat, F., Cheseaux, J. J., and Guignard, J. P. (1998). HIV-associated nephropathy in children. *Archives de Pediatrie* **5**, 1353–1358.

Chintalacharuvu, S. R. and Emancipator, S. N. (1997). The glycosylation of IgA produced by murine B cells is altered by Th2 cytokines. *Journal of Immunology* **159**, 2327–2333.

Chintalacharuvu, S. R. and Emancipator, S. N. (2000). Differential glycosylation of two glycoproteins synthesized by murine b cells in response to IL-4 plus IL-5. *Cytokine* **12**, 1182–1188.

Chintalacharuvu, S. R. *et al.* (2001). T cell cytokines determine the severity of experimental IgA nephropathy by regulating IgA glycosylation. *Clinical and Experimental Immunology* **126**, 326–333.

Churg, J. and Sobin, L. H. *Renal Disease. Classification and Atlas of Glomerular Disease.* Tokyo, New York: Igaku-Shoin, 1982.

Churg, J., Bernstein, J., and Glassock, R. *Glomerular Disease* 2nd edn. Tokyo, New York: Igaku-Shoin, Medical Publisher, Inc, 1995.

Colucci, M. *et al.* (1991). Urinary procoagulant and fibrinolytic activity in human glomerulonephritis. Relationship with renal function. *Kidney International* **39**, 1213–1217.

Coppo, R. *et al.* (1982). Circulating immune complexes containing IgA, IgG and IgM in patients with primary IgA nephropathy and with Henoch–Schöenlein nephritis. Correlation with clinical and histologic signs of activity. *Clinical Nephrology* **18**, 230–239.

Coppo, R. *et al.* (1985). Presence and origin of IgA1 and IgA2 containing circulating immune complexes in chronic alcoholic liver diseases with and without glomerulonephritis. *Clinical Immunology and Immunopathology* **35**, 1–8.

Coppo, R. *et al.* (1995). Macromolecular IgA and abnormal IgA reactivity in sera from children with IgA nephropathy. Italian Collaborative Paediatric IgA Nephropathy Study. *Clinical Nephrology* **43**, 1–13.

Coppo, R., Amore, A., Hogg, R., and Emancipator, S. (2000). Idiopathic nephropathy with IgA deposits. *Pediatric Nephrology* **15**, 139–150.

Coppo, R., Chiesa, M., Peruzzi, L., and Amore, A. (2001). Treatment of IgAN with converting enzyme inhibitors: design of a prospective randomized multicenter trial. *Journal of Nephrology* **14**, 447–452.

Crowley-Nowick, P. A. *et al.* (1994). Immunological studies of IgA nephropathy in blacks reveal elevations of serum IgA2 as well as IgA1. *Nephrology, Dialysis, Transplantation* **9**, 1324–1329.

Csiky, B. *et al.* (1999). Ambulatory blood pressure monitoring and progression in patients with IgA nephropathy. *Nephrology, Dialysis, Transplantation* **14**, 86–90.

D'Amico, G. *et al.* (1985). Idiopathic IgA mesangial nephropathy. Clinical and histological study of 374 patients. *Medicine* **64**, 49–60.

D'Amico, G. *et al.* (1986). Prognostic indicators in idiopathic IgA mesangial nephropathy. *Quarterly Journal of Medicine* **59**, 363–378.

D'Amico, G. *et al.* (2001). Idiopathic IgA nephropathy with segmental necrotizing lesions of the capillary wall. *Kidney International* **59**, 682–692.

Dash, S. C. *et al.* (1997). Increased incidence of glomerulonephritis following spleno-renal shunt surgery in non-cirrhotic portal fibrosis. *Kidney International* **52**, 482–485.

Davin, J. C., Ten Berge, I. J., and Weening, J. J. (2001). What is the difference between IgA nephropathy and Henoch–Schönlein purpura nephritis? *Kidney International* **59**, 823–834.

de Fijter, J. W., Daha, M. R., Schroeijers, W. E., van Es, L. A., and Van Kooten, C. (1998). Increased IL-10 production by stimulated whole blood cultures in primary IgA nephropathy. *Clinical and Experimental Immunology* **111**, 429–434.

Dillon, J. J. (1997). Fish oil therapy for IgA nephropathy: efficacy and interstudy variability. *Journal of the American Society Nephrology* **8**, 1739–1744.

Dillon, J. J. (2001). Treating IgA nephropathy. *Journal of the American Society of Nephrology* **12**, 846–847.

Diven, S. C. *et al.* (1998). IgA induced activation of human mesangial cells: independent of FcalphaR1 (CD 89). *Kidney International* **54**, 837–847.

Donadio, J. V., Jr. *et al.* (1994). A controlled trial of fish oil in IgA nephropathy. Mayo Nephrology Collaborative Group. *New England Journal of Medicine* **331**, 1194–1199.

Duque, N., Gomez-Guerrero, C., and Egido, J. (1997). Interaction of IgA with Fc alpha receptors of human mesangial cells activates transcription factor nuclear factor-kappa B and induces expression and synthesis of monocyte chemoattractant protein-1, IL-8, and IFN-inducible protein 10. *Journal of Immunology* **159**, 3474–3482.

Ebihara, I. *et al.* (2001). Th2 predominance at the single-cell level in patients with IgA nephropathy. *Nephrology, Dialysis, Transplantation* **16**, 1783–1789.

Egido, J. *et al.* (1984). Immunological abnormalities in the tonsils of patients with IgA nephropathy: inversion in the ratio of IgA : IgG bearing lymphocytes and increased polymeric IgA synthesis. *Clinical and Experimental Immunology* **57**, 101–106.

Ehara, T. and Shigematsu, H. (1998). Contribution of mast cells to the tubulointerstitial lesions in IgA nephritis. *Kidney International* **54**, 1675–1683.

Eiro, M. *et al.* (2002). The product of duration and amount of proteinuria (proteinuria index) is a possible marker for glomerular and tubulointerstitial damage in IgA nephropathy. *Nephron* **90**, 432–441.

Emancipator, S. N. (1992). Aspects of the pathogenesis of IgA nephropathy. *Clinical Immunological News* **12**, 149–156.

Fidirkin, A. *et al.* (1999). Tubulointerstitial lesions in IgA nephropathy and localization of hepatocyte growth factor. *International Urology and Nephrology* **31**, 557–562.

Frimat, L. *et al.* (1996). IgA nephropathy in patients over 50 years of age: a multicentre, prospective study. *Nephrology, Dialysis, Transplantation* **11**, 1043–1047.

Frimat, L. *et al.* (1997). IgA nephropathy: prognostic classification of end stage renal failure. *Nephrology, Dialysis, Transplantation* **12**, 2569–2575.

Gesualdo, L. *et al.* (1994). Expression of platelet-derived growth factor in normal and diseased human kidney. An immunohistochemistry and *in situ* hybridization study. *Journal of Clinical Investigation* **94**, 50–58.

Gharavi, A. G. *et al.* (2000). IgA nephropathy, the most common cause of glomerulonephritis, is linked to 6q22–23. *Nature Genetics* **26**, 354–357.

Gomez-Guerrero, C., Gonzalez, E., and Egido, J. (1993). Evidence for a specific IgA receptor in rat and human mesangial cells. *Journal of Immunology* **151**, 7172–7181.

Gomez-Guerrero, C., Duque, N., and Egido, J. (1998). Mesangial cells possess an asialoglycoprotein receptor with affinity for human immunoglobulin A. *Journal of the American Society of Nephrology* **9**, 568–576.

Goumenos, D., Ahuja, M., Shortland, J. R., and Brown, C. B. (1995). Can immunosuppressive drugs slow the progression of IgA nephropathy? *Nephrology, Dialysis, Transplantation* **10**, 1173–1181.

Grandaliano, G. *et al.* (1996). Monocyte chemotactic peptide-1 expression in acute and chronic human nephritides: a pathogenetic role in interstitial monocytes recruitment. *Journal of the American Society of Nephrology* **7**, 906–913.

Greer, M. R. *et al.* (1998). The nucleotide sequence of the IgA1 hinge region in IgA nephropathy. *Nephrology, Dialysis, Transplantation* **13**, 1980–1983.

Gregory, M. C., Hammond, M. E., and Brewer, E. D. (1988). Renal deposition of cytomegalovirus antigen in immunoglobulin-A nephropathy. *Lancet* **i**, 11–14.

Grossetete, B. *et al.* (1998). Down-regulation of Fc alpha receptors on blood cells of IgA nephropathy patients: evidence for a negative regulatory role of serum IgA. *Kidney International* **53**, 1321–1335.

Haas, M. (1997). Histologic subclassification of IgA nephropathy: a clinicopathologic study of 244 cases. *American Journal of Kidney Diseases* **29**, 829–842.

Haas, M. *et al.* (2000). ANCA-associated crescentic glomerulonephritis with mesangial IgA deposits. *American Journal of Kidney Diseases* **36**, 709–718.

Hara, M. *et al.* (1998). Urinary excretion of podocytes reflects disease activity in children with glomerulonephritis. *American Journal of Nephrology* **18**, 35–41.

Harper, S. J. *et al.* (1994a). Expression of J chain mRNA in duodenal IgA plasma cells in IgA nephropathy. *Kidney International* **45**, 836–844.

Harper, S. J. *et al.* (1994b). Increased immunoglobulin A and immunoglobulin A1 cells in bone marrow trephine biopsy specimens in immunoglobulin A nephropathy. *American Journal of Kidney Diseases* **24**, 888–892.

Harper, L. *et al.* (2000). Treatment of vasculitic IgA nephropathy. *Journal of Nephrology* **13**, 360–366.

Hené, R. J., Schurman, H. J., and Kater, L. (1988). Immunoglobulin A subclass-containing plasma cells in the jejunum in primary IgA nephropathy and in Henoch–Schönlein purpura. *Nephron* **48**, 4–7.

Hiki, Y. *et al.* (1998). Analyses of IgA1 hinge glycopeptides in IgA nephropathy by matrix-assisted laser desorption/ionization time-of-flight mass spectrometry. *Journal of the American Society of Nephrology* **9**, 577–582.

Hiki, Y. *et al.* (2001). Mass spectrometry proves under-*O*-glycosylation of glomerular IgA1 in IgA nephropathy. *Kidney International* **59**, 1077–1085.

Hiromura, K., Kurosawa, M., Yano, S., and Naruse, T. (1998). Tubulointerstitial mast cell infiltration in glomerulonephritis. *American Journal of Kidney Diseases* **32**, 593–599.

Hogg, R. J. *et al.* (1994). Prognostic indicators in children with IgA nephropathy—Report of the Southwest Pediatric Nephrology Study Group. *Pediatric Nephrology* **8**, 15–20.

Hotta, O. *et al.* (1999). Detection of urinary macrophages expressing the CD16 (Fc gamma RIII) molecule: a novel marker of acute inflammatory glomerular injury. *Kidney International* **55**, 1927–1934

Hoy, W. E., Hughson, M. D., Smith, S. M., and Megill, D. M. (1993). Mesangial proliferative glomerulonephritis in Southwestern American Indians. *American Journal of Kidney Diseases* **21**, 486–496.

Hsu, S. I. *et al.* (2000). Evidence for genetic factors in the development and progression of IgA nephropathy. *Kidney International* **57**, 1818–1835.

Ichinose, H. *et al.* (1996). Detection of cytokine mRNA-expressing cells in peripheral blood of patients with IgA nephropathy using non-radioactive *in situ* hybridization. *Clinical and Experimental Immunology* **103**, 125–132.

Inagi, R. *et al.* (2001). Specific tissue distribution of megsin, a novel serpin, in the glomerulus and its up-regulation in IgA nephropathy. *Biochemical and Biophysical Research Communications* **286**, 1098–1106.

Ito, Y. *et al.* (1998). Expression of connective tissue growth factor in human renal fibrosis. *Kidney International* **53**, 853–861.

Iwase, H. *et al.* (1999). Human serum immunoglobulin G3 subclass bound preferentially to asialo-, agalactoimmunoglobulin A1/Sepharose. *Biochemical and Biophysical Research Communications* **264**, 424–429.

Jennette, J. C., Wall, S. D., and Wilkman, A. S. (1985). Low incidence of IgA nephropathy in blacks. *Kidney International* **28**, 944–950.

Jinde, K. *et al.* (2001). Tubular phenotypic change in progressive tubulointerstitial fibrosis in human glomerulonephritis. *American Journal of Kidney Diseases* **38**, 761–769.

Johnston, P. A., Brown, J. S., Barumholtz, D. A., and Davison, A. M. (1992). Clinico-pathological correlations and long-term follow-up of 253 United Kingdom patients with IgA nephropathy. A report from the MRC glomerulonephritis registry. *Quarterly Journal of Medicine* **84**, 619–627.

Julian, B. A. *et al.* (1988). Familial clustering and immunogenetic aspects of IgA nephropathy. *American Journal of Kidney Diseases* **12**, 366–370.

Kang, S. W. *et al.* (1995). Prognostic factors and renal survival in IgA nephropathy. *Yonsey Medical Journal* **36**, 45–52.

Kanno, Y., Okada, H., Saruta, T., and Suzuki, H. (2000). Blood pressure reduction associated with preservation of renal function in hypertensive patients with IgA nephropathy: a 3-year follow-up. *Clinical Nephrology* **54**, 360–365.

Kashem, A. *et al.* (1994). Fc alpha R expression on polymorphonuclear leukocyte and superoxide generation in IgA nephropathy. *Kidney International* **45**, 868–875.

Katafuchi, R., Takebayshi, S., and Taguchi, T. (1988). Hypertension-related aggravation of IgA nephropathy: a statistical approach. *Clinical Nephrology* **30**, 261–269.

Kennel-De March, A. *et al.* (1997a). Low levels of spontaneously activated peripheral IgA-secreting cells in nontransplanted IgA nephropathy patients. *America Journal of Kidney Diseases* **30**, 64–70.

Kennel-De March, A. *et al.* (1997b). Enhanced expression of CD31 and CD54 on tonsillar high endothelial venules in IgA nephropathy. *Clinical Immunology and Immunopathology* **84**, 158–165.

Kim, Y. S. *et al.* (2001). Live donor renal allograft in end-stage renal failure patients from immunoglobulin A nephropathy. *Transplantation* **71**, 233–238.

Kimmel, P. L. *et al.* (1992). Brief report: idiotypic IgA nephropathy in patients with human immunodeficiency virus infection. *New England Journal of Medicine* **327**, 702–706.

Kiyoshi, Y., Hisano, S., and Takebayashi, S. (1998). Importance of the duration from the onset of a urinary abnormality until a biopsy is performed: a multivariate analysis on the application of renal biopsy for patients with IgA nephropathy. *Nippon Jinzo Gakkai Shi* **40**, 547–554.

Kobayashi, Y. *et al.* (1983). IgA nephropathy: prognostic significance of proteinuria and hitological alterations. *Nephron* **34**, 146–153.

Kobayashi, Y. *et al.* (1989). Moderately proteinuric IgA nephropathy: prognostic prediction of individual clinical courses and steroid therapy in progressive cases. *Nephron* **53**, 250–256.

Kodama, S., Suzuki, M., Arita, M., and Mogi, G. (2001). Increase in tonsillar germinal centre B-1 cell numbers in IgA nephropathy (IgAN) patients and reduced susceptibility to Fas-mediated apoptosis. *Clinical Expert Immunology* **123**, 301–308.

Koido, S., Makino, H., Iwazaki, K., and Makino, T. (1998). IgA nephropathy and pregnancy. *Tokai Journal Experimental Clinical Medicine* **23**, 31–37.

Kokubo, T., Hiki, Y., Iwase, H., Tanaka, A., Toma, K., Hotta, K., and Kobayashi, Y. (1998). Protective role of IgA1 glycans against IgA1 self-aggregation and adhesion to extracellular matrix proteins. *Journal of the American Society of Nephrology* **9**, 2048–2054.

Kokubo, T. *et al.* (2000). Humoral immunity against the proline-rich peptide epitope of the IgA1 hinge region in IgA nephropathy. *Nephrology, Dialysis, Transplantation* **15**, 28–33.

Konishi, Y. *et al.* (2001). Sodium sensitivity of blood pressure appearing before hypertension and related to histological damage in immunoglobulin a nephropathy. *Hypertension* **38**, 81–85.

Kosaka, M. (1998). Long-term prognosis for tonsillectomy patients with IgA nephropathy. *Nippon Jibiinkoka Gakkai Kaiho* **101**, 916–923.

Koyama, A., Igarashi, M., Kobayashi, M., and Members and Coworkers of the Research Group on Progressive Renal Disease (1997). Natural history and risk factors for immunoglobulin A nephropathy in Japan. *American Journal of Kidney Diseases* **29**, 526–532.

Kurusu, A. *et al.* (2001). Relationship between mast cells in the tubulointerstitium and prognosis of patients with IgA nephropathy. *Nephron* **89**, 391–397.

Kusakari, C. *et al.* (1994). Immunopathological features of palatine tonsil characteristic of IgA nephropathy: IgA1 localization in follicular dendritic cells. *Clinical and Experimental Immunology* **95**, 42–48.

Kusumoto, Y. *et al.* (1987). Long-term prognosis and prognostic indices of IgA nephropathy in juvenile and in adult Japanese. *Clinical Nephrology* **28**, 118–124.

Lai, K. N. *et al.* (1985). Nephrotic range proteinuria—a good predictive index of disease in IgA nephropathy? *Quarterly Journal of Medicine* **57**, 677–688.

Lai, K. N., Lai, F. M., Ho, C. P., and Chan, K. W. (1986). Corticosteroid therapy in IgA nephropathy with nephrotic syndrome: a long-term controlled trial. *Clinical Nephrology* **26**, 174–180.

Lai, F. M. *et al.* (2002). Primary IgA nephropathy with low histologic grade and disease progression: is there a 'point of no return'? *American Journal of Kidney Diseases* **39**, 401–406.

Launay, P. *et al.* (2000). Fcalpha receptor (CD89) mediates the development of immunoglobulin A (IgA) nephropathy (Berger's disease). Evidence for pathogenic soluble receptor-Iga complexes in patients and CD89 transgenic mice. *Journal of Experimental Medicine* **191**, 1999–2009.

Layward, L. *et al.* (1992). Increased and prolonged production of specific polymeric IgA after systemic immunization with tetanus toxoid in IgA nephropathy. *Clinical Experimental Immunology* **88**, 394–398.

Layward, L., Finnemore, A. M., Allen, A. C., Harper, S. J., and Feehally, J. (1993). Systemic and mucosal IgA responses to systemic antigen challenge in IgA nephropathy. *Clinical Immunology and Immunopathology* **69**, 306–313.

Lee, S.-M. K. *et al.* (1982). IgA nephropathy: morphologic predictors of progressive renal disease. *Human Pathology* **13**, 314–322.

Leung, J. C., Tsang, A. W., Chan, D. T., and Lai, K. N. (2000). Absence of CD89, polymeric immunoglobulin receptor, and asialoglycoprotein receptor on human mesangial cells. *Journal of the American Society of Nephrology* **11**, 241–249.

Leung, J. C. *et al.* (2001). Charge-dependent binding of polymeric IgA1 to human mesangial cells in IgA nephropathy. *Kidney International* **59**, 277–285.

Leung, J. C. *et al.* (2002). Increased sialylation of polymeric lambda-IgA1 in patients with IgA nephropathy. *Journal of Clinical Laboratory Analysis* **16**, 11–19.

Levy, M. *et al.* (1985). Beyer's disease in children. Natural history and outcome. *Medicine* **64**, 157–180.

Li, H. L. *et al.* (1990). Mononuclear cell activation and decreased renal function in IgA nephropathy with crescents. *Kidney International* **37**, 1552–1556.

Lim, C. S. *et al.* (2001). Thl/Th2 predominance and proinflammatory cytokines determine the clinicopathological severity of IgA nephropathy. *Nephrology, Dialysis, Transplantation* **16**, 269–275.

Linné, T., Berg, U., Bohman, S.-O., and Sigstrom, L. (1991). Course and long-term outcome of idiopathic IgA nephropathy in children. *Pediatric Nephrology* **5**, 383–386.

Locatelli, F. *et al.* (1999). Combined treatment with steroids and azathioprine in IgA nephropathy: design of a prospective randomised multicentre trial. *Journal of Nephrology* **12**, 308–311.

Maschio, G. *et al.* (1996). Effect of the angiotensin-converting-enzyme inhibitor benazepril on the progression of chronic renal insufficiency. The angiotensin-converting-enzyme inhibition in progressive renal insufficiency study group. *New England Journal of Medicine* **11**, 334, 939–945.

McIntyre, C. W., Fluck, R. J., and Lambie, S. H. (2001). Steroid and cyclophosphamide therapy for IgA nephropathy associated with crescenteric change: an effective treatment. *Clinical Nephrology* **56**, 193–198.

Meadow, S. R. *et al.* (1972). Schönlein–Henoch nephritis. *Quarterly Journal of Medicine* **41**, 241–258.

Mera, J., Uchida, S., and Nagase, M. (2000). Clinicopathologic study on prognostic markers in IgA nephropathy. *Nephron* **84**, 148–157.

Mestecky, J. *et al.* (1993). Defective galactosylation and clearance of IgA1 molecules as a possible etiopathogenic factor in IgA nephropathy. *Contributions to Nephrology* **104**, 172–182.

Mina, S. N. and Murphy, W. M. (1985). IgA nephropahy. A comparative study of the clinicopathologic features in children and adults. *American Journal of Clinical Patology* **83** (6), 669–675.

Miyata, T. *et al.* (1998). A mesangium-predominant gene, megsin, is a new serpin upregulated in IgA nephropathy. *Journal of Clinical Investigation* **102**, 828–836.

Montinaro, V. *et al.* (1995). Biosynthesis of C3 by human mesangial cells. Modulation by proinflammatory cytokines. *Kidney International* **47**, 829–836.

Montinaro, V., Gesualdo, L., and Schena, F. P. (1999). The relevance of experimental models in the pathogenetic investigation of primary IgA nephropathy. *Annales de Medecine Interne (Paris)* **150**, 99–107.

Moura, I. C. *et al.* (2001). Identification of the transferrin receptor as a novel immunoglobulin (Ig)A1 receptor and its enhanced expression on mesangial cells in IgA nephropathy. *Journal of Experimental Medicine* **194**, 417–425.

Mudge, S. J. *et al.* (2000). Sublytic complement injury does not activate NF-kappa B, or induce mitogenesis in rat mesangial cells. *Experimental Nephrology* **8**, 291–298.

Mustonen, J., Pasternack, A., and Helin, H. (1987). The course of disease in patients with nephrotic syndrome and IgA nephropathy. *Seminars in Nephrology* **7**, 374–376.

Nakagawa, H. *et al.* (2000). Significance of glomerular deposition of C3c and C3d in IgA nephropathy. *American Journal of Nephrology* **20**, 122–128.

Neugarten, J., Acharya, A., and Silbiger, S. R. (2000). Effect of gender on the progression of nondiabetic renal disease: a meta-analysis. *Journal of the American Society of Nephrology* **11**, 319–329.

Newell, G. C. (1987). Cirrhotic glomerulonephritis: incidence, morphology, clinical features and pathogenesis. *American Journal of Kidney Diseases* **9**, 183–190.

Nicholls, K. M., Fairley, K. F., Dowling, J. P., and Kincaid-Smith, P. (1984). The clinical course of mesangial IgA associated nephropathy in adults. *Quarterly Journal of Medicine* **53**, 22–50.

Noel, L. H., Droz, D., Gascon, M., and Berger, J. (1987). Primary IgA nephropathy: from the first-described cases to the present. *Seminars in Nephrology* **7**, 351–354.

Novak, J., Julian, B. A., Tomana, M., and Mesteck, J. (2001). Progress in molecular and genetic studies of IgA nephropathy. *Journal of Clinical Immunology* **21**, 310–327.

Oba, S. *et al.* (1998). Relevance of periglomerular myofibroblasts in progression of human glomerulonephritis. *American Journal of Kidney Diseases* **32**, 419–425.

Oda, T. *et al.* (1998). Clinicopathological significance of intratubular giant macrophages in progressive glomerulonephritis. *Kidney International* **53**, 1190–1200.

Odani, H. *et al.* (2000). Direct evidence for decreased sialylation and galactosylation of human serum IgA1 Fc *O*-glycosylated hinge peptides in IgA nephropathy by mass spectrometry. *Biochemical and Biophysical Research Communications* **271**, 268–274.

Ogawa, T. *et al.* (1997). Precise ultrastructural localization of endothelial leukocyte adhesion molecule-1, vascular cell adhesion molecule-1, and intercellular adhesion molecule-1 in patients with IgA nephropathy. *Nephron* **75**, 54–64.

Oka, K. *et al.* (2000). A clinicopathological study of IgA nephropathy in renal transplant recipients: beneficial effect of angiotensin-converting enzyme inhibitor. *Nephrology, Dialysis, Transplantation* **15**, 689–695.

Omata, K. *et al.* (1996). Therapeutic advantages of angiotensin converting enzyme inhibitors in chronic renal disease. *Kidney International* **55** (Suppl.), S57–S62.

Onetti-Muda, A. O., Feriozzi, S., Rahimi, S., and Faraggiana, T. (1995). Spatial arrangement of IgA and C3 as a prognostic indicator of IgA nephropathy. *Journal of Pathology* **177** (2), 201–208.

Ono, T. *et al.* (1991). Relationship of intraglomerular coagulation and platelet aggregation to glomerular sclerosis. *Nephron* **58**, 429–436.

Osawa, Y. *et al.* (2001). Determination of optimal blood pressure for patients with IgA nephropathy based on renal histology. *Hypertension Research* **24**, 89–92.

Perico, N. *et al.* (1998). The antiproteinuric effect of angiotensin antagonism in human IgA nephropathy is potentiated by indomethacin. *Journal of the American Society of Nephrology* **9**, 2308–2317.

Peruzzi, L. *et al.* (2000). Integrin expression and IgA nephropathy: *in vitro* modulation by IgA with altered glycosylation and macromolecular IgA. *Kidney International* **58**, 2331–2340.

Pettersson, E. E. *et al.* (1994). Treatment of IgA nephropathy with omega-3-polyunsaturated fatty acids: a prospective, double-blind, randomized study. *Clinical Nephrology* **41**, 183–190.

Pirani, C. L. and Salinas-Marrigal, L. (1968). Evaluations of percutaneous renal biopsy. *Pathology Annual* **3**, 249.

Ponticelli, C. *et al.* (2001). Kidney transplantation in patients with IgA mesangial glomerulonephritis. *Kidney International* **60**, 1948–1954.

Pozzi, C. *et al.* (1999). Corticosteroids in IgA nephropathy: a randomised controlled trial. *Lancet* **353**, 883–887.

Praditpornsilpa, K. *et al.* (1999). Renal pathology and HIV infection in Thailand. *American Journal of Kidney Diseases* **33**, 282–286.

Praga, M. *et al.* (1985). Acute worsening of renal function during episodes of macroscopic hematuria in IgA nephropathy. *Kidney International* **28**, 69–74.

Ranieri, E., Gesualdo, L., Petrarulo, F., and Schena, F. P. (1996). Urinary IL-6/EGF ratio: a useful prognostic marker for the progression of renal damage in IgA nephropathy. *Kidney International* **50**, 1990–2001.

Ranieri, E. *et al.* (2001). The role of alpha-smooth muscle actin and platelet-derived growth factor-beta receptor in the progression of renal damage in human IgA nephropathy. *Journal Nephrology* **14**, 253–262.

Rasche, F. M., Schwarz, A., and Keller, F. (1999). Tonsillectomy does not prevent a progressive course in IgA nephropathy. *Clinical Nephrology* **51**, 147–152.

Rekola, S., Bergstrand, A., and Bucht, H. (1989). IgA Nephropathy. A retrospective evaluation of prognostic indices in 176 patients. *Scandinavian Journal of Urology and Nephrology* **23**, 27–50.

Rekola, S., Bergstrand, A., and Bucht, H. (1991). Deterioration of GFR in IgA nephropathy as measured by ^{51}Cr-EDTA clearance. *Kidney International* **40**, 1050–1054.

Remuzzi, A. *et al.* (1999). ACE inhibition and ANG II receptor blockade improve glomerular size-selectivity in IgA nephropathy. *American Journal of Physiology* **276**, 457–466.

Rifai, A. *et al.* (1989). Clearance kinetics and fate of macromolecular IgA in patients with IgA nephropathy. *Laboratory Investigation* **61**, 381–388.

Rifai, A., Fadden, K., Morrison, S. L., and Chintalacharuvu, K. R. (2000). The *N*-glycans determine the differential blood clearance and hepatic uptake of human immunoglobulin (Ig)A1 and IgA2 isotypes. *Journal of Experimental Medicine* **191**, 2171–2182.

Roccatello, D. *et al.* (1993). Removal systems of immunoglobulin A and immunoglobulin A containing complexes in IgA nephropathy and cirrhosis patients. The role of asialoglycoprotein receptors. *Laboratory Investigation* **69**, 714–723.

Roccatello, D. *et al.* (1995). Report on intensive treatment of extracapillary glomerulonephritis with focus on crescentic IgA nephropathy. *Nephrology, Dialysis, Transplantation* **10**, 2054–2059.

Romagnani, P. *et al.* (1999). Role for interactions between IP-10/Mig and CXCR3 in proliferative glomerulonephritis. *Journal of the American Society of Nephrology* **10**, 2518–2526.

Roodnat, J. I. *et al.* (1991). What do we really know about the long-term prognosis of IgA-nephropathy? *Journal of Nephrology* **3**, 145–151.

Rostoker, G. *et al.* (1992). Secretory IgA are elevated in both saliva and serum of patients with various types of primary glomerulonephritis. *Clinical and Experimental Immunology* **90**, 305–311.

Rostoker, G. *et al.* (1998). Imbalances in serum proinflammatory cytokines and their soluble receptors: a putative role in the progression of idiopathic IgA nephropathy (IgAN) and Henoch–Schönlein purpura nephritis, and a potential target of immunoglobulin therapy? *Clinical and Experimental Immunology* **114**, 468–476.

Ruggenenti, P. *et al.* (2000). Chronic proteinuric nephropathies. II. Outcomes and response to treatment in a prospective cohort of 352 patients: differences between women and men in relation to the ACE gene polymorphism. Gruppo Italiano di Studi Epidemiologici in Nefrologia (Gisen). *Journal of the American Society of Nephrology* **11** (1), 88–96.

Russo, D. *et al.* (1999). Additive antiproteinuric effect of converting enzyme inhibitor and losartan in normotensive patients with IgA nephropathy. *American Journal of Kidney Diseases* **33**, 851–856.

Russo, D. *et al.* (2001). Coadministration of losartan and enalapril exerts additive antiproteinuric effect in IgA nephropathy. *American Journal of Kidney Diseases* **38**, 18–25.

Sacks, S. H., Zhou, W., Campbell, R. D., and Martin, J. (1993a). C3 and C4 gene expression and interferon-gamma-mediated regulation in human glomerular mesangial cells. *Clinical and Experimental Immunology* **93**, 411–417.

Sacks, S. H. *et al.* (1993b). Complement C3 gene expression and regulation in human glomerular epithelial cells. *Immunology* **79**, 348–354.

Sato, Y. *et al.* (1996). IgA nephropathy with poorly developed lymphoepithelial symbiosis of the palatine tonsils. *Nephron* **74**, 301–308.

Schena, F. P. (1990). A retrospective analysis of the natural history of primary IgA nephropathy worldwide. *American Journal of Medicine* **89**, 209–215.

Schena, F. P. (1998). Immunogenetic aspects of primary IgA nephropathy—Nephrology Forum. *Kidney International* **48**, 1998–2013.

Schena, F. P. (2001). Immunoglobulin a nephropathy with mild renal lesions: a call in the forest for physicians and nephrologists. *American Journal of Medicine* **110**, 499–500.

Schena, F. P. and Gesualdo, L. (2001). Markers of progression in IgA nephropathy. *Journal of Nephrology* **14**, 554–574.

Schena, F. P. *et al.* (1989). Increased serum levels of IgA1–IgG immune complexes and anti-F(ab′) 2 antibodies in patients with primary IgA nephropathy. *Clinical and Experimental Immunology* **77**, 15–20.

Schena, F. P., Montenegro, M., and Scivittaro, V. (1990). Meta-analysis of randomised controlled trials in patients with primary IgA nephropathy (Berger's disease). *Nephrology, Dialysis, Transplantation* **51**, 47–52.

Schena, F. P. *et al.* (1997). Survey of the Italian registry of renal biopsies. Frequency of the renal diseases for 7 consecutive years. *Nephrology, Dialysis, Transplantation* **12**, 418–426.

Schena, F. P. *et al.* (2001). ACE gene polymorphism and IgA nephropathy. An ethically homogeneous study and a meta-analysis review. *Kidney International* **60**, 732–740.

Schena, F. P. *et al.* (2002). Increased risk of end-stage renal disease in familial IgA nephropathy. *Journal of the American Society of Nephrology* **13**, 453–460.

Scholl, U. *et al.* (1999). The 'point of no return' and the rate of progression in the natural history of IgA nephritis. *Clinical Nephrology* **52**, 285–292.

Scivittaro, V. *et al.* (1994a). *In vitro* immunoglobulin production in relatives of patients with IgA nephropathy. *Clinical Nephrology* **42**, 1–8.

Scivittaro, V. *et al.* (1994b). Profiles of immunoregulatory cytokine production *in vitro* in patients with IgA nephropathy and their kindred. *Clinical and Experimental Immunology* **96**, 311–316.

Scolari, F. *et al.* (1999). Familial clustering of IgA nephropathy: further evidence in an Italian population. *American Journal of Kidney Diseases* **33**, 857–865.

Shin, G. T. *et al.* (2000). ACE inhibitors attenuate expression of renal transforming growth factor-beta1 in humans. *American Journal of Kidney Disease* **36**, 894–902.

Shoji, T. *et al.* (2000). Early treatment with corticosteroids ameliorates proteinuria, proliferative lesions, and mesangial phenotypic modulation in adult diffuse proliferative IgA nephropathy. *American Journal of Kidney Diseases* **35**, 194–201.

Sinniah, R. (1985). IgA mesangial nephropathy: Berger's disease. *American Journal of Nephrology* **5**, 73–83.

Smith, S. M. and Tsukamoto, H. (1992). Time dependency of IgA nephropathy induction in alcohol ingestion. *Alcocholism—Clinical and Experimental Research* **16**, 471–473.

Smith, S. M., Yu, G. S. M., and Tsukamoto, H. (1990). IgA nephropathy in alcohol abuse. An animal model. *Laboratory Investigation* **62**, 179–184.

Southwest Pediatric Nephrology Study Group (1985). Association of IgA nephropathy with steroid-responsive nephrotic syndrome. *American Journal of Kidney Diseases* **3**, 157–164.

Stein-Oakley, A. N., Maguire, J. A., Dowling, J., Perry, G., and Thomsom, N. M. (1997). Altered expression of fibrogenic growth factors in IgA nephropathy and focal and segmental glomerulosclerosis. *Kidney International* **51**, 195–204.

Strippoli, G. F., Manno, C., and Schena, F. P. (2003). An 'evidence-based' survey of therapeutic options for IgA nephropathy: assessment and criticism. *American Journal of Kidney Diseases* **41**, 1129–1139.

Suzuki, S., Kobayashi, H., Sato, H., and Arakawa, M. (1990). Immunohistochemical characterization of glomerular IgA deposits in IgA nephropathy. *Clinical Nephrology* **34**, 93–94.

Suzuki, D. *et al.* (1999a). Expression of megsin mRNA, a novel mesangium-predominant gene, in the renal tissues of various glomerular diseases. *Journal of the American Society of Nephrology* **10**, 2606–2613.

Suzuki, Y. *et al.* (1999b). Expression and physical association of Fc alpha receptor and Fc receptor gamma chain in human mesangial cells. *Nephrology, Dialysis, Transplantation* **14**, 1117–1123.

Suzuki, S. *et al.* (2000). Insertion/deletion polymorphism in ACE gene is not associated with renal progression in Japanese patients with IgA nephropathy. *American Journal of Kidney Diseases* **35** (5), 896–903.

Syrjanen, J., Mustonen, J., and Pasternack, A. (2000). Hypertriglyceridaemia and hyperuricaemia are risk factors for progression of IgA nephropathy. *Nephrology, Dialysis, Transplantation* **15**, 34–42.

Szeto, C. C. *et al.* (2001). The natural history of immunoglobulin a nephropathy among patients with hematuria and minimal proteinuria. *American Journal of Medicine* **110** (6), 434–437.

Tateno, S. and Kobayashi, Y. (1987). Quantitative analysis of mesangial areas in serial biopsied patients with IgA nephropathy. *Nephron* **46**, 28–33.

Tolkoff-Rubin, N. E. *et al.* (1978). IgA nephropathy in HLA-identical siblings. *Transplantation* **26**, 430–433.

Tomana, M. *et al.* (1997). Galactose-deficient IgA1 in sera of IgA nephropathy patients is present in complexes with IgG. *Kidney International* **52**, 509–516.

Tomana, M. *et al.* (1999). Circulating immune complexes in IgA nephropathy consist of IgA1 with galactose-deficient hinge region and antiglycan antibodies. *Journal of Clinical Investigation* **104**, 73–81.

Tomino, Y. *et al.* (1986). Cytopathic effects of antigens in patients with IgA nephropathy. *Nephron* **42**, 161–166.

Toyabe, S. *et al.* (1997). IgA nephropathy-specific expression of the IgA Fc receptors (CD89) on blood phagocytic cells. *Clinical and Experimental Immunology* **110**, 226–232.

Toyabe, S., Harada, W., and Uchiyama, M. (2001). Oligoclonally expanding gammadelta T lymphocytes induce IgA switching in IgA nephropathy. *Clinical and Experimental Immunology* **124**, 110–117.

Tsuruya, K. *et al.* (2000). Combination therapy using prednisolone and cyclophosphamide slows the progression of moderately advanced IgA nephropathy. *Clinical Nephrology* **53**, 1–9.

Usui, J. *et al.* (2001). Heterogeneity of prognosis in adult IgA nephropathy, especially with mild proteinuria or mild histological features. *Internal Medicine* **40**, 697–702.

van den Dobbelsteen, M. E. *et al.* (1994). Binding of dimeric and polymeric IgA to rat renal mesangial cells enhances the release of interleukin 6. *Kidney International* **46** (2), 512–519.

van der Wall Bake, A. W. L. *et al.* (1988). The bone marrow as production site of the IgA deposited in the kidneys of patients with IgA nephropathy. *Clinical and Experimental Immunology* **72**, 321–325.

van der Wall Bake, A. W. *et al.* (1989). Elevated production of polymeric and monomeric IgA1 by the bone marrow in IgA nephropathy. *Kidney International* **35**, 1400–1404.

Velo, M. *et al.* (1987). Natural history og IgAN nephropathy in patients followed up for more than ten years in Spain. *Seminars in Nephrology* **7**, 346–350.

Wakai, K. *et al.* (1999). Risk factors for IgA nephropathy: a case–control study in Japan. *American Journal of Kidney Diseases* **33**, 738–745.

Wakai, K. *et al.* (2002). Risk factors for IgA nephropathy: a case–control study with incident cases in Japan. *Nephron* **90**, 16–23.

Waldo, F. B. *et al.* (1993). Treatment of IgA nephropathy in children: efficacy of alternate-day oral prednisone. *Pediatric Nephrology* **7**, 529–532.

Westberg, N. G. *et al.* (1983). Quantitation of immunoglobulin-producing cells in small intestinal mucosa of patients with IgA nephropathy. *Clinical Immunology and Immunopathology* **26**, 442–445.

Westerhuis, R. *et al.* (1999). Human mesangial cells in culture and in kidney sections fail to express Fc alpha receptor (CD89). *Journal of the American Society of Nephrology* **10**, 770–778.

Wines, B. D. *et al.* (1999). Identification of residues in the first domain of human Fc alpha receptor essential for interaction with IgA. *Journal of Immunology* **162** (4), 2146–2153.

Woo, K. T. *et al.* (1986). The natural history of IgA nephritis in Singapore. *Clinical Nephrology* **25**, 15–21.

Woo, K. T. *et al.* (1989). Protein selectivity: a prognostic index in IgA nephritis. *Nephron* **52**, 300–306.

Woo, K. T. *et al.* (1991). Pattern of proteinuria in IgA nephritis by SDS-PAGE: clinical significance. *Clinical Nephrology* **36**, 6–11.

Woo, K. T., Lau, Y. K., Wong, K. S., and Chiang, G. S. (2000). ACEI/ATRA therapy decreases proteinuria by improving glomerular permselectivity in IgA nephritis. *Kidney International* **58**, 2485–2491.

Woodrow, G., Innes, A., Boyd, S. M., and Burden, R. P. (1993). A case of IgA nephropathy with coeliac disease responding to a gluten-free diet. *Nephrology, Dialysis, Transplantation* **8** (12), 1382–1383.

Wyatt, R. J. *et al.* (1982). Partial H (β1H) deficiency and glomerulonephritis in two families. *Journal of Clinical Immunology* **2**, 110–117.

Wyatt, R. J. *et al.* (1984). IgA nephropathy: presentation, clinical course, and prognosis in children and adults. *American Journal of Kidney Diseases* **4**, 192–200.

Wyatt, R. J. *et al.* (1987). Complement activation in IgA nephropathy. *Kidney International* **31**, 1019–1023.

Wyatt, R. J. *et al.* (1995). IgA nephropathy: long-term prognosis for pediatric patients. *Journal of Pediatrics* **127**, 913–919.

Wyatt, R. J. *et al.* (1997). IgA nephropathy databank: development of a system for management of renal biopsy acquired data. *American Journal of Kidney Diseases* **29**, 817–828.

Yagucki, Y. *et al.* (1994). Comparative studies of clinicalpathologic changes in patients with adult and juvenile-onset of IgA nephropathy. *Journal of Nephrology* **7**, 182–185.

Yamamoto, T. *et al.* (1998). Expression of types I, II, and III TGF-beta receptors in human glomerulonephritis. *Journal of the American Society of Nephrology* **9**, 2253–2261.

Yang, C. W. *et al.* (1997). Glomerular transforming growth factor-beta1 mRNA as a marker of glomerulosclerosis-application in renal biopsies. *Nephron* **77**, 290–297.

Yang, N. *et al.* (1998). Local macrophage proliferation in human glomerulonephritis. *Kidney International* **54**, 143–151.

Yellin, M. J. *et al.* (1997). Immunohistologic analysis of renal CD40 and CD40L expression in lupus nephritis and other glomerulonephritides. *Arthritis and Rheumatism* **40**, 124–134.

Yokoyama, H. *et al.* (1998). Urinary levels of chemokines (MCAF/MCP-1, IL-8) reflect distinct disease activities and phases of human IgA nephropathy. *Journal of Leukocyte Biology* **63**, 493–499.

Yoshikawa, N. *et al.* (1987). Mesangial changes in IgA nephropathy in children. *Kidney International* **32**, 585–589.

Yoshikawa, N., Ito, H., and Nakamura, H. (1992). Prognostic indicators in childhood IgA nephropathy. *Nephron* **60**, 60–67.

Yoshikawa, N. *et al.* (1999). A controlled trial of combined therapy for newly diagnosed severe childhood IgA nephropathy. The Japanese Pediatric IgA Nephropathy Treatment Study Group. *Journal of the American Society of Nephrology* **10**, 101–109.

Yoshioka, T. *et al.* (1992). IgA nephropathy in patients with congenital C9 deficiency. *Kidney International* **42** (5), 1253–1258.

Yoshizawa, N. *et al.* (1996). Asymptomatic acute poststreptococcal glomerulonephritis following upper respiratory tract infections caused by Group A streptococci. *Clinical Nephrology* **46**, 296–301.

Zidar, N. *et al.* (1992). Renal extraglomerular vascular immune deposits in IgA glomerulonephritis. *Kidney International* **42**, 144–149.

Zwirner, J. *et al.* (1997). Activated complement C3: a potentially novel predictor of progressive IgA nephropathy. *Kidney International* **51**, 1257–1264.

3.7 Membranous nephropathy

Heather Reich and Daniel Cattran

Introduction

Membranous glomerulonephritis (MGN) is the most common cause of adult-onset nephrotic syndrome, and remains among the leading causes of endstage renal disease (ESRD) due to glomerulonephritis. Despite its relatively high prevalence in nephrologists' practice, there remains debate regarding many aspects of its management. Determining, for instance, which patients will progress and how long to wait in order to determine a patient's prognosis, continue to be areas of intense speculation. Furthermore, the role of immunomodulatory therapy and the success rate of various medication regimens remain the subject of many reviews. This chapter will address the epidemiology as well as the clinical and pathological features of MGN, and discuss some of the ongoing areas of debate in this important cause of renal disease.

Epidemiology

MGN has historically been the most common cause of nephrotic syndrome observed in adult populations, accounting for approximately 25 per cent of biopsies done for the investigation of this clinical syndrome (Haas *et al.* 1995, 1997; Schena 1997). In large biopsy series, its overall frequency is 10 per cent of all histological diagnoses (Davison *et al.* 1984; Zucchelli *et al.* 1996). Due to its relatively high incidence as a cause of glomerular disease, it is the second or third most common primary GN to lead to ESRD in the industrialized nations (USRDS 1999; Maisonneuve *et al.* 2000). The majority of cases of MGN are idiopathic in nature (idiopathic or primary MGN), however, up to one-third of cases are related to systemic diseases (secondary MGN) (Gluck *et al.* 1973; Row *et al.* 1975; Ehrenreich *et al.* 1976; Abe *et al.* 1986; Adu and Cameron 1989; Cahen *et al.* 1989; Glassock 1992). The major causes of secondary MGN are listed in Table 1.

Table 1 Conditions and medications associated with secondary MGN

Immunologic
SLE and mixed connective tissue disease
Rheumatoid arthritis
Antiphospholipid antibody syndrome
Sjögren's syndrome
Sarcoidosis
Autoimmune hepatitis
Autoimmune thyroiditis (Hashimoto)
Graft-versus-host disease following bone marrow transplantation
Neoplasm
Solid tumours—lung, breast, gastrointestinal, renal
Haematological—lymphoma, usually non-Hodgkin's
Infection
Viral—Hepatitis, usually hepatitis B, also C; HIV
Bacterial—syphilis
Mycobacterial—leprosy
Parasitic—malaria, schistosomiasis, filariasis
Medication
D-Penicillamine
Gold
Captopril
Probenecid
NSAID
Bucillamine
Other
Renal allografts—*de novo* disease
Mercury
Sickle-cell disease
Diabetes

Differences in incidence of MGN have recently been observed over time and across different ethnic and geographic populations. Although for the past 50 years, MGN has been the most common cause of nephrotic syndrome in industrialized countries, focal–segmental glomerulosclerosis (FSGS) has been emerging in some studies as the new number one. Some of this trend is related to the inclusion of larger numbers of subjects of African origin, in whom FSGS has a higher incidence than MGN (D'Agati 1994; Korbet 1996), but an increasing proportion of FSGS has also been observed in non-African ethnic groups (Haas 1997). One large recent biopsy series in an American metropolitan setting has documented a halving of the prevalence of MGN in biopsies done between 1990 and 1994 (14.5 per cent) compared with the period 1975–1979 (38.3 per cent), with a proportionate increase in the relative frequency of FSGS (Braden *et al.* 2000). In elderly populations, however, MGN remains the most common type of primary glomerulonephritis (Abrass 1985; Donadio 1990; Passerini *et al.* 1993).

Secondary MGN in association with solid tumours approaches 22 per cent in patients over 60 years of age (Keur *et al.* 1989; Burstein *et al.* 1993). In a recent series of 155 patients 10 per cent of patients over 60 years of age had MGN associated with a malignancy, versus only 1 per cent of patients under 60 (O'Callaghan *et al.* 2002). The aetiology also differs depending upon the geographic location of the affected MGN population, for instance in areas where the local prevalence of associated infectious diseases including hepatitis and malaria are high.

MGN consistently occurs more frequently in males. They account for up to 70 per cent of patients with MGN in several large series (Mallick *et al.* 1983; Davison *et al.* 1984; Honkanen 1986; Kida *et al.* 1986; MacTier *et al.* 1986). The peak age of onset of MGN is the fourth or fifth decade of life (Rosen 1971; Gluck *et al.* 1973; Ehrenreich *et al.* 1976; Noel *et al.* 1979; Davison *et al.* 1984; Honkanen 1986; Honkanen *et al.* 1992).

MGN may be associated with familial clustering, and it has been documented to occur in cases of identical twins (Guella *et al.* 1997). In addition, various geographic populations have a higher frequency of specific HLA haplotypes associated with the disease. Japanese patients have the HLA-DR2 allele (Hiki *et al.* 1984), whereas patients with idiopathic MGN from England and Greece more frequently have DR3 (Vaughan *et al.* 1995). Furthermore, the HLA haplotype has been correlated with disease progression. DR3+ B8− has been associated with remissions in an Italian population (Papiha *et al.* 1987), and DR3 and DR5 have been more frequently associated with ESRD in an Afro-American and Caucasian-American population (Freedman *et al.* 1994). Clustering of certain HLA antigens by geographic region may explain some of the international differences in disease prevalence and clinical course.

Clinical features

The clinical features present at diagnosis or at the time of biopsy of patients with primary MGN will be discussed first, secondary forms will be discussed later. It is important to note that the characteristics of patients at the time of biopsy will vary from study to study, given differing thresholds and criteria for biopsy at various centres. Therefore, although the development of MGN may be quite insidious, it is often the presence of 'full-blown' nephrotic syndrome that prompts referral and biopsy. Table 2 illustrates the range in clinical features present in patients at the time of diagnosis or biopsy in several of the larger studies of patients with MGN containing predominantly subjects with idiopathic MGN.

The definition of nephrotic syndrome has varied in the many studies that have described the clinical characteristics of MGN, but for the most part, a combination of peripheral oedema and proteinuria of greater than 3 g/24 h have been required. The majority of patients with MGN, ranging from half to over 90 per cent, have the 'nephrotic syndrome' at the time of biopsy. The remaining patients often had significant proteinuria, but within the non-nephrotic range (likely what prompted medical attention).

The absence or presence of haematuria is of little help in the diagnosis of MGN, as it is present in approximately half the patients surveyed. The haematuria is almost exclusively microscopic in nature, although macroscopic haematuria has also been reported on rare occasions (Ramzy *et al.* 1981; MacTier *et al.* 1986).

The presence of hypertension at presentation has also varied widely. A significant proportion of patients in these studies, 30–50 per cent had elevated blood pressure at presentation, often in the absence of renal insufficiency. The finding of systolic hypertension at presentation is noted particularly frequently in older patients although its relationship to the disease as opposed to age *per se* is not clear (O'Callaghan *et al.* 2002).

The percentage of patients with impairment of renal function at diagnosis varies widely in the studies reviewed, as illustrated in Table 2. In general, a minority of patients, likely in the range of 20 per cent,

Table 2 Clinical features present at diagnosis or time of biopsy, expressed as per cent (%) of patients

Study	Number	Nephrotic syndrome (%)	Non-nephrotic proteinuria (%)	Haematuria (%)	Hypertension (%)	Renal insufficiency (%)
Gluck et al. (1973)	38	92	N/A	42	N/A	18
Noel et al. (1979)	116	76	24	55	6[a]	6
Ramzy et al. (1981)	35	74	26	54	~50	46
Davison et al. (1984)	64	81	19	19	N/A	33
Honkanen (1986)	67	76	N/A	28	27	8
Kida et al. (1986)	104	54	30	N/A	N/A	29
MacTier et al. (1986)	37	93	7	71	45	N/A
Murphy et al. (1988)	139	54	N/A	33	40	18
Donadio et al. (1988)	140	83	N/A	N/A	30	N/A[b]
Hay et al. (1992)	51	92	8	N/A	33[c]	16
Schieppati (1993)	100	~63	37	N/A	55	N/A[b]

[a] Seven of 116 subjects had hypertension in absence of renal insufficiency. A further seven had moderate renal insufficiency.

[b] Mean creatinine 1.2 ± 0.5 mg/dl in Donadio study, clearance 95.5 ± 36 ml/min/1.73 m^2 in Schieppati study.

[c] An additional 22% had 'controlled' blood pressure on medications.

N/A—not available.

will have depressed renal function. This impairment, however, is usually mild in severity, and in some cases may be due to hypoalbuminaemia and changes in intra- and extracellular volume rather than parenchymal disease. The finding of acute renal failure is very rare in MGN, and should direct investigation towards other diagnoses or related conditions, such as bilateral renal vein thrombosis, excessive diuresis, or the use of nephrotoxic medications.

There are several features that should prompt the clinician to suspect a secondary cause of MGN. Extremes of age at presentation (i.e. over 60 or under 20 years), presence of weight loss, gastrointestinal disturbances, rash, arthritis, or risk factors for hepatitis, raise the likelihood that the MGN is secondary in nature. Due to the wide range of causes of secondary MGN, the clinical features present at diagnosis are more variable than in the primary form. Laboratory testing may reveal positive autoimmune serology (i.e. antinuclear and anti-DNA antibodies, and/or low complement), positive hepatitis serology, or cryoglobulin tests, in contrast with primary MGN, in which these investigations are negative or normal.

The characteristics of patients presenting with systemic lupus erythematosus (SLE)-associated MGN are well summarized in a recent review article (Kolasinski *et al.* 2002). Overall, a pure membranous lesion on biopsy is rare in SLE, present in only 14 per cent of biopsies (GISNEL Study 1992). Furthermore, up to 50 per cent of patients with renal involvement will change histological classification on later biopsies (Ponticelli and Moroni 1998). Similar to idiopathic MGN, the majority of patients with MGN due to SLE have nephrotic-range proteinuria (64 per cent) and normal renal function at diagnosis (90 per cent). Haematuria is variable; a large number of red cell casts should lead the clinician to suspect proliferative activity, and the possible presence of a mixed lesion on biopsy.

Hepatitis B virus (HBV)-associated MGN is usually associated with nephrotic-range proteinuria, and normal renal function (Lin 1990; Lai *et al.* 1991; Pena *et al.* 2001).

Clinical evidence of liver disease is not required for the development of MGN, and although the worldwide prevalence of HBV is quite high, the development of MGN as a result of this infection is relatively infrequent. The features of this condition are described more extensively in paediatric populations, who may have a different natural history compared with adults (see section on 'Natural history' below). The development of antibodies to HBV surface antigen has been related to clinical remission (Hsu *et al.* 1989).

The majority, although not all patients with HBV who develop MGN, are also seropositive for hepatitis Be antigen (HBeAg) (Lin 1990; Lai *et al.* 1991). The correlation of the presence of HBeAg and clinical outcome is debatable, although remission of MGN with the development of antibodies to this antigen has been reported.

Patients with MGN associated with malignancy tend to be older—in one study of nine patients the mean age was 63 years with all patients over 52 (Burstein *et al.* 1993). In this series of Burstein, all patients had nephrotic-range proteinuria, and six out of nine had evidence of renal insufficiency at presentation (one was related to obstruction). Other studies have reported the prevalence of malignancy in subjects with the nephrotic syndrome between 6 and 11 per cent (Lee *et al.* 1966; Row *et al.* 1975; Yamauchi *et al.* 1985; Cahen *et al.* 1989). Most patients manifested proteinuria prior to or at the time of diagnosis of the malignancy. Reappearance of proteinuria may herald relapse of the malignancy.

Pathology

The hallmark finding in MGN is the presence of subepithelial immune deposits, best seen on electron microscopy (EM). These are found in cases of both primary and secondary forms of the disease. The principal findings evident in MGN by conventional diagnostic techniques will be described in this section. Although many of the features are common to both primary and secondary forms of MGN, there are some characteristics described that are highly suggestive of a secondary cause.

Light microscopy

Early in the disease, glomeruli may appear normal, and changes may only be evident on EM or immunofluorescence (IF). One of the earliest changes seen by LM is a 'moth eaten' appearance of the basement membrane when observed 'en face' using silver stains (Kern *et al.* 1999). Silver staining is also useful to observe the linear 'spike' projections protruding from the outer (epithelial) surface of the glomerular basement membrane (GBM). With disease progression, and larger numbers of immune deposits, capillary walls and the GBM may appear globally thickened. The mesangium usually exhibits normal cellularity in idiopathic MGN. Segmental and global glomerulosclerosis may be observed with advanced disease.

The tubulointerstitial compartment and vessels are usually unremarkable in early disease. With disease chronicity, however, tubulointerstitial atrophy and fibrosis are frequently observed. Vascular injury with arterial and arteriolar sclerosis may be evident with associated hypertension.

Immunofluorescence

The characteristic finding on IF microscopy in MGN is granular capillary wall staining for immunoglobulin and complement. IgG is the most common immunoglobulin, and is found in more than 70 per cent of cases. C3 is also very commonly present. The finding of intense C1q staining, and the presence of other immunoglobulins such as IgM and IgA are suggestive of lupus-associated membranous nephropathy (Jennette *et al.* 1983).

Electron microscopy

EM is the best modality for diagnosing MGN, and is especially useful in detecting changes that may suggest SLE as a cause. Several 'staging' systems have been used to describe the pathological changes observed (Ehrenreich and Churg 1968; Bariety *et al.* 1970; Gartner *et al.* 1977). A modified version of the Ehrenreich and Churg scale, which includes the addition of a Stage V lesion, is the most widely used system to describe the histopathological variations seen on biopsy.

Stage I—subepithelial deposits

At this stage of disease, light microscopy (LM) findings are frequently normal. The GBM is usually normal in thickness, with minimal evidence of spike formation. A few small, flat, electron-dense deposits are seen on the epithelial surface of the GBM.

Stage II—'spike' formation

'Spikes' protruding from epithelial surface of GBM become clearly visible. The spikes extend between the electron-dense deposits, and are present in virtually every capillary loop. With progression, the spike tips may have a widened or clubbed appearance. The number and size of deposits are increased compared with Stage I.

Stage III—incorporation of deposits

Electron-dense deposits become surrounded by and incorporated into the GBM. This results in an irregular thickening of the GBM, and capillary wall. The capillary wall may appear to have a split appearance due to interruption of the GBM by this immune-complex material.

Stage IV—disappearing deposits

The deposits incorporated within the GBM lose their electron density. As a result, the GBM has a very irregular, thickened appearance. Areas of the GBM occupied by deposit material that has lost electron density will have a vacuolated or lucent appearance.

Stage V—reparation stage

During this 'healing' phase, the deposits have become completely rarified, and the GBM appearance is returning to normal. The GBM appears partially thickened, and may still contain areas of lucency. Some consider Stage V to include an 'endstage' appearance, with glomerular obsolescence and sclerosis (Donadio *et al.* 1988).

In addition to the pathological changes described by the staging system, diffuse effacement of visceral epithelial cell foot processes is frequently observed on EM in MGN. This finding may be associated with particularly heavy proteinuria.

A review of 350 biopsies of patients with primary MGN at the University of Carolina reveals that 70 per cent of patients present with Stage I or II biopsy findings (Falk *et al.* 2000). Some disagreement exists regarding whether a biopsy should be staged according to the predominant lesion observed in the majority of glomerulae, versus the most advance lesion evident in the specimen. Tornroth *et al.* (1987) demonstrated that in biopsies of patients with a protracted clinical course, lesions representing all stages of disease are often present in one specimen. They suggested that based upon serial biopsies of patients with MGN, the presence of subepithelial deposits correlate with an 'active' clinical stage, whereas replacement by lucent intramembranous lesions occurred during clinical remission. Cessation of formation of immune complexes may result in the presence of intramembranous healing changes, such as in a patient who has one 'flare' of proteinuria, then achieves a complete remission. However, ongoing formation of immune complexes, as may occur in the patient with a more protracted and progressive course, may result in the continued formation of new subepithelial deposits that will be seen in addition to more 'chronic' intramembranous lesions. In addition, he suggested that deposits which are large and extend from the subepithelial space deep into the membrane may indicate continuous deposition of immune complex material.

Pathological findings in secondary MGN

There are several features which are highly suggestive of a secondary aetiology. A large series of 170 biopsies from patients with a (histological) diagnosis of MGN were examined in one series (Jennette *et al.* 1983). Twenty-eight of the subjects eventually received a diagnosis of SLE based upon serological or clinical criteria. The location of immune deposits differed in these patients. The findings of mesangial, subendothelial, and tubular basement membrane-dense deposits in addition to the subepithelial deposits were highly suggestive of SLE-related MGN. Evidence from animal studies (see section on 'Pathophysiology') suggests that in idiopathic MGN, immune-complex formation occurs *in situ*, along the basal surface of the podocyte. Secondary forms of MGN, however, are associated with immune-complex formation in the circulation, and therefore, deposits are more likely to be found throughout the glomerulus, as opposed to only in the subepithelial zone. As previously mentioned, mesangial hypercellularity is uncommon in idiopathic MGN, and its presence suggests an underlying systemic disease. Other findings that are highly suggestive of a secondary cause of MGN include tubuloreticular inclusions (which may be found in association with viral or SLE-associated MGN), and intense C1q staining (which correlates with SLE-associated disease). Although not routinely checked, various hepatitis antigens may be found in the glomerulus of MGN due to hepatitis B; in one study, 100 per cent of biopsies were positive for hepatitis core antigen, and 88 per cent for the e-antigen, with only a minority of biopsies demonstrating the presence of surface antigen deposition (Lin 1990).

Pathophysiology

The morphological changes seen on biopsy in MGN suggest that the podocyte injury and subepithelial immune deposits are central in the pathogenesis of the disease. The Heymann model of experimental membranous nephropathy in rats bears many similarities to both the clinical and pathological findings observed in human MGN. First described over 40 years ago, the immunization of susceptible strains of rats with Freund's adjuvant and 'rat kidney suspension' consisting of material extracted from the brush border of proximal convoluted tubule cells known as Fx1A, produces proteinuria and subepithelial deposits identical to that seen in human MGN (Heymann *et al.* 1959). Much of the focus of research in the Heymann nephritis model has been related to the identification of the responsible antigen(s) and the subsequent immune response (Shankland 2000). The deposition of immune complexes results in the activation of many mediators of injury, including leucocytes, complement, products of arachidonic acid metabolism, a variety of cytokines, adhesion molecules, and growth factors.

The initial subject of intense investigation involving the Heymann nephritis model was the antigenic target(s) of the immune response stimulated by injection of the nephritogenic kidney membrane extract. The target has been identified as a large membrane glycoprotein, gp330, which is also known as megalin due to its large size of 515 kDa (Kerjaschki and Farquhar 1982; Saito *et al.* 1994). The protein is a polyspecific receptor, and is a member of the low-density lipoprotein receptor family (Herz *et al.* 1988; Raychowdhury *et al.* 1989; Kerjaschki and Neale 1996). It complexes with a specific epitope of the 44 kDa protein known as receptor associated protein (RAP), and can be found expressed in the clathrin-coated pits on the bases of podocyte foot processes (Kerjaschki and Farquhar 1982; Pietromonaco *et al.* 1990; Kerjaschki *et al.* 1992; Orlando *et al.* 1992; Farquhar 1996). The anatomic location of megalin supports its role in receptor-mediated endocytosis. RAP likely functions as a chaperone assisting in the folding of megalin in the endoplasmic reticulum of the cell, and facilitating its transport to the cell surface.

Circulating antibodies directed against megalin likely penetrate the GBM and bind to megalin/RAP forming immune complexes *in situ*.

Megalin was confirmed to be the putative antigen based on the following criteria: (a) active immunization of rats with megalin produces subepithelial immune deposits (active Heymann nephritis), (b) injection of autologous antimegalin antibodies produces similar deposits (passive Heymann nephritis), and (c) antibodies eluted from affected rat glomeruli recognize only megalin (Kerjaschki and Farquhar 1982; Farquhar *et al.* 1995). Furthermore, a binding site for immunoglobulin G has been localized to the LDL-receptor-like domain of megalin, and Heymann nephritis has been reproduced using recombinant segments of this domain (Raychowdhury *et al.* 1996; Saito *et al.* 1996). Despite the extensive advances describing the antigens involved in the Heymann nephritis model, the identification of a parallel system in humans with MGN remains elusive.

Complement is required for the development of tissue injury and proteinuria, as illustrated by the fact that antiFx1A antibodies and immune complex deposition in the presence of C6 or C8 deficient rats do not result in proteinuria (Salant *et al.* 1980; Cybulsky *et al.* 1986; Baker *et al.* 1989). After the deposition of immune complexes, the complement system is activated, leading to insertion of the C5b–9 membrane attack complex (MAC) into the podocyte plasma membrane (Couser *et al.* 1992). The MAC is formed after proteolytic cleavage of C5 and combination with components C6–C9. Its insertion into the cell membranes of nucleated cells results in sublytic activity (Koski *et al.* 1983), and in combination with other stimuli, is capable of causing cell death. The MAC has been localized to the subepithelial deposits and along the surface of podocytes, particularly in the clathrin-coated pits of glomerular epithelial cells in passive Heymann Nephritis. It is probably endocytosed and transported intracellularly in multivescicular bodies, and then exocytosed into the urinary space (Kerjaschki *et al.* 1987). Podocyte injury and resulting proteinuria has been shown to be dependent upon the presence of the MAC, as depletion of complement with cobra venom factor is associated with lack of proteinuria, despite the formation of immune deposits. The MAC has been documented in the urine of Heymann nephritis animals, and may be a marker of disease activity (Pruchno *et al.* 1989; Schulze *et al.* 1989).

In human MGN studies, the presence of C5b–9 has been documented within immune complex deposits (Hinglais *et al.* 1986). In one biopsy study, MAC was found in 50 per cent of biopsies of idiopathic MGN, 75 per cent of MGN secondary to lupus, and a minority of MGN due to hepatitis B (Lai *et al.* 1989). The presence of MAC on biopsy in one recent study was not, however, found to be correlated with the severity of proteinuria or the presence of the nephrotic syndrome; it was suggested that rather than MAC deposition, glomerular expression of various adhesion molecules may be more reflective of advanced disease (Honkanen *et al.* 1998; Papagianni *et al.* 2002). As in the Heymann nephritis model, the MAC has also been identified in the urine of human subjects with MGN. The clinical course of the disease has been shown to have some association with the presence of urinary C5b–9 in human studies; two studies have found that the presence of MAC is correlated with an 'active' clinical course with ongoing proteinuria, and declining function (Coupes *et al.* 1992, 1993; Kon *et al.* 1995). One study, however, correlated its presence with a shorter duration of disease, lower creatinine, but more proteinuria (Schulze *et al.* 1991). The differences may relate to small sample sizes, cross-sectional design, and differing statistical methods used to prove the association.

Although it appears that epithelial cell injury is dependent upon the presence of the MAC, the mechanism by which the MAC causes injury, and the podocyte's maladaptive response to this injury remain areas of ongoing active investigation. Several mechanisms have been proposed to account for the cellular consequences of MAC insertion in the podocyte which ultimately lead to the destruction of the glomerular filtration barrier. The role of the production of reactive oxygen species (ROS) and products of the arachidonic acid pathway in the presence of the MAC has been the focus of much investigation. Injury to both the epithelial cell and the basement membrane is hypothesized to be mediated in part by ROS whose production is stimulated by the presence of the MAC. The presence of ROS in tissue has been correlated with the development of proteinuria, and the administration of ROS scavengers (antioxidants) has been documented to cause a decrease in this proteinuria (Shah 1988, 1989). The ROS may in fact be produced locally, as is suggested by *in vitro* experiments in which the application of C5b–9 to cultured epithelial cells results in the production of ROS (Adler *et al.* 1986). Subsequent injury to the filtration barrier may then be induced by peroxidation of membrane proteins and collagen (Kerjaschki 1996). The MAC has also been documented to activate epithelial cell cytosolic phospholipase A2 *in vivo* and *in vitro*, resulting in the production of free arachidonic acid by post-translational regulation of the enzyme (Cybulskly *et al.* 1995, 2000). Arachidonic acids are known to be precursors of eicosanoids (e.g. prostaglandins, leukotrienes, and thromboxanes), that have potential haemodynamic effects within the glomerulus, and are present in increased levels in the Heymann model. The MAC has been also been implicated in activating a variety of stress-associated pathways, including protein kinase C and the extracellular signal-related kinase ERK2 (Cybulsky *et al.* 1998).

The podocyte reaction to injury induced by the MAC is one of hypertrophy, rather than proliferation. In addition, an increase in extracellular matrix is observed, and can be appreciated at a microscopic level as thickening of the basement membrane. It is postulated that interruption of cell cycle regulation may cause the lack of proliferation of podocytes (Shankland *et al.* 1997, 1999). The accumulation of extracellular matrix may be mediated to a large extent by transforming growth factor-β (TGF-β). Recent experiments further indicated that only certain TGF-β/receptor isoforms lead to matrix expansion in the Heymann model (Shankland 1996). In addition, urinary levels of this cytokine have been found to be elevated in patients with MGN (Honkanen *et al.* 1997).

A final interesting observation from the Heymann model relates to structural changes in the podocyte and interconnecting slit diaphragms that occur with the immune-complex formation. This change seems to permit the passage of protein through the filtration barrier. Microscopically, foot process effacement is easily appreciable. This may be related to disruption of the actin cytoskeleton that has been documented to be mediated by MAC exposure (Topham *et al.* 1999). Recently, it has been demonstrated that indeed nephrin dissociates from the actin cytoskeleton in experimental membranous nephropathy, resulting in prominent changes in the morphology of the slit diaphragm (Yuan *et al.* 2002).

Slit diaphragms have also been observed to undergo morphological changes, confirmed by documentation in human samples of decreased mRNA levels of nephrin, the primary component of the diaphragm (Furness *et al.* 1999).

Although much of the focus thus far has been on complement-mediated injury, cellular and humoral-mediated pathways are also thought to be important factors, at least in the experiment model. The complement activation and glomerular immunoglobulin deposition are CD4+ T-cell-dependant humoral responses. The CD4+ help for antibody response is a function of the Th2 cell, which produces interleukin (IL)-4, -5, -6, -10, and -13. Early in the course of the disease, both glomerular and interstitial T-cells as well as macrophage infiltrates are found. A role for cell-mediated injury is supported by the observations that depletion of the cytotoxic CD8+ T-cell reduces the injury and that monoclonal anti-CD4 and anti-CD8 treatment modifies the disease (Penny *et al.* 1998).

There are early data suggesting that both susceptibility to and progression of MGN may have a genetic basis, however the mechanism remains unclear (Vaughan *et al.* 1995). Advances in laboratory technology that allow a broader look at changes in gene expression may help to elucidate the alterations responsible for the injury that produces MGN. In addition, further investigation into the factors responsible for an individual's susceptibility to either progression or spontaneous remission in this type of immunological injury is required.

Natural history

The natural history of idiopathic MGN remains difficult to characterize due to a limited number of studies of untreated subjects. Furthermore, a methodological review of the quality of studies classically used to describe the natural history of this condition reveals multiple inconsistencies in the literature that contribute to the difficulty establishing the natural history (Marx and Marx 1997). This review emphasizes the lack of uniformity with respect to diagnostic criteria, selection of end-points, baseline severity, statistical techniques, and assessment of treatment effects used in assessing the course of MGN.

Table 3 includes a group of studies examining the natural history of MGN. These studies were selected from a large number of available articles, based upon relatively large patient sample size, and a significant percentage of patients who received only supportive therapy. In addition, these studies provided data regarding the clinical status at diagnosis, and clear statistics regarding patient outcomes. The disease course of MGN is considered to be indolent when left untreated, as is evident in most of the studies quoted in this table. Figure 1 illustrates the overall survival rates extracted from some of the studies in Table 3. The 10-year survival rates are favourable, averaging 82 per cent. The study by Murphy *et al.* (1988) also provides information regarding survival if the patients had nephrotic syndrome at presentation; the 5- and 8-year survival were slightly lower at 85 and 82 per cent, respectively. This relatively good prognosis may be an underestimate of today's outcome, given the introduction within the last decade of more potent antihypertensive medications, angiotensin-converting enzyme (ACE) inhibitors, and lowered ideal levels for target blood pressure. However,

Table 3 Selected studies examining the natural history of idiopathic MGN

Study (year, country)	Number of subjects	Mean follow-up (months)	Outcomes
Noel *et al.* (1979, France)	116	54	CR 23.5%, PR 14.5%, NR 43%, deterioration 19% (9.5% ESRD)
Davison *et al.* (1984, Great Britain)	64	N/A—range 2–15 years	47% no change, 42% doubling creatinine, or reaching >400 μmol/l, 8% slow deterioration, 3% excluded
Kida *et al.* (1986, Japan)	104 (59—no treatment)	138	CR 40%, PR 30%, 10–15% persistent disease
MacTier *et al.* (1986, Scotland)	37	64	30% CR, 16% persistent proteinuria, 19% proteinuria and CRF, 22% ESRD, 13% non-renal mortality
Donadio *et al.* (1988, USA)	140 (89—no treatment)	127.4	64% stable, 20% ESRD, 16% CRF
Murphy *et al.* (1988, Australia)	139 (79—no treatment)	52	Overall, 50% alive, normal function, 13% CRF, 6% ESRD, 11% non-renal death, 20% lost to follow-up Patients with NS had 9% CR, 20% PR, 20% still nephrotic, without NS had 19% CR, 21% PR, 6% still nephrotic
Cattran *et al.* (1989, Canada)	158 (77—no treatment)	48	31% CR, 38% PR, 29% NR, 7% ESRD or death
Schieppati *et al.* (1993, Italy)	100	52	68% normal function, 18% CRF, 14% ESRD (including 6% mortality)

See text regarding the criteria used for selection of the studies included in this table.

CR, complete remission; PR, partial remission; NR, no response; CRF, chronic renal failure; ESRD, endstage renal disease; NS, nephrotic syndrome.

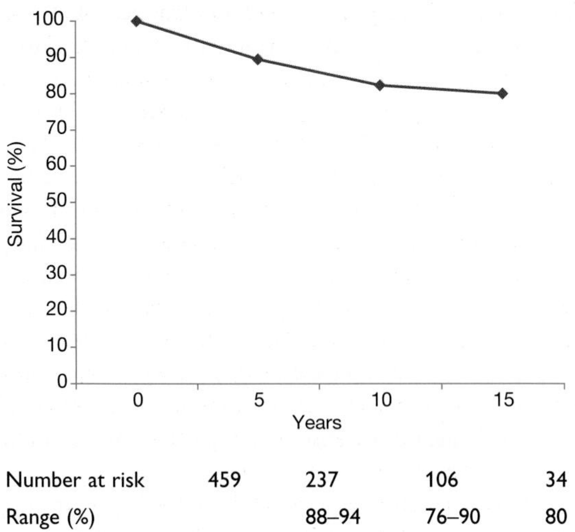

Fig. 1 Average overall survival, based upon studies by Noel *et al.* (1979); Kida *et al.* (1986); Murphy *et al.* (1988); and Schieppati *et al.* (1993). Number at risk, and range in survival rates provided below graph.

this assumption is speculative, as there are still no data indicating that these advances have yielded an improvement in the natural history of this disease.

Despite purposeful selection of studies in Table 3 based upon some degree of uniformity in data and sample size, the variability in outcome evident in the table illustrate some of the shortcomings of the available literature. For example, the year of diagnosis and entry into study has important implications; the accuracy of the diagnosis may even be questioned, given the lack of electron microscopy prior to the early 1970s. In addition, some discrepancies in outcome may reflect differences in the quality of 'conservative therapy' that have evolved over time. The study by Noel *et al.* (1979), for instance, included patients diagnosed between 1958 and 1975, and is potentially subject to inconsistencies in diagnosis, that may explain their differences in outcome compared with the other studies. Another element to be considered when interpreting the data is the presence or absence of nephrotic syndrome at diagnosis. In the Donadio study, 83 per cent had nephrotic syndrome at diagnosis, compared to only 60 per cent in the study by Kida *et al.* (1986). This may explain part of the differences in survival observed, given that the presence of the nephrotic syndrome impacts negatively on prognosis. One large study by Zucchelli *et al.* (1987) including 82 subjects with at least 10 years of follow-up reported a far more ominous prognosis, with 20 per cent reaching ESRD, 17 per cent chronic renal insufficiency, and 20 per cent of patients suffering from non-renal mortality. These results may be due to the methodological differences described. For instance, all patients were diagnosed prior to 1976, and 100 per cent had the nephrotic syndrome. A final element to be considered is the control group used for comparison (if available). The study by Donadio *et al.* (1988) compares survival to actuarial life tables in normal individuals, as opposed to the focus of the Zuchelli paper, in which the comparison is patients that did versus those that did not receive treatment.

Another approach to understanding the natural history is to examine reviews combining studies of pooled treated and untreated patients. A review of 11 such reports of idiopathic MGN revealed an overall renal survival of 65–90 per cent by 10 years (Cattran *et al.* 1992). Similarly, a large pooled analysis of 32 studies examined the course of 1189 patients, estimated renal survival at 86 per cent at 5 years, 65 per cent at 10 years, and 60 per cent at 15 years (Hogan *et al.* 1995).

Non-renal related morbidity and mortality in patients with idiopathic MGN is difficult to determine from the literature. There are, however, quite alarming mortality rates in several of the earlier studies of the natural history of the disease. Recent reviews of these earlier papers have indicated that a high proportion of deaths in this population—up to 60 per cent—are non-renal-related (Donadio *et al.* 1988; Laluck and Cattran 1999). One early study of 32 subjects, for instance, indicated 41 per cent mortality in the follow-up period (Franklin *et al.* 1973). A high mortality rate was confirmed in larger more recent series as well, where 6–20 per cent of patients died by the end of the follow-up period (Kida *et al.* 1986; Zucchelli *et al.* 1987; Murphy *et al.* 1988; Wehrmann *et al.* 1989). These deaths tend to occur at a young age (mean 51), and are most often due to cardiovascular disease or malignancy (Honkanen 1986). The reasons for this high rate of premature non-renal deaths may be due to comorbid conditions, the effects of the disease itself or of the treatment. The precise cause of death in many of the aforementioned studies is unclear. An as yet unidentified element of glomerulonephritis may increase the risk of mortality. A compelling review of 2380 subjects who underwent biopsy for evaluation of their glomerulonephritis revealed that by 10 years following diagnosis, 32 per cent of the subjects had died (Heaf *et al.* 1999). Further analysis indicated that MGN is a 'low risk' group, as the relative mortality was only three times that of the general population. This is an area in the natural history of MGN about which little information exists, and where further investigation is certainly warranted.

Natural history—secondary MGN

The data regarding the natural history of MGN secondary to systemic diseases is equally complex; the major determinant of the course is, as expected, the primary condition involved. The most common aetiologies, SLE, malignancy, HBV, and medication-related MGN will be discussed.

The natural history of SLE-related MGN is summarized in a recent review of the available data. This study pooled together 157 patients with SLE and a predominant membranous lesion on biopsy (WHO Class V), with follow-up ranging from 25 to 279 months (Kolasinski *et al.* 2002). Only 23 per cent of patients with 'pure' MGN had complete resolution of proteinuria at follow-up. Most patients (84.5 per cent) continue to have normal renal function, but the numbers with abnormal renal function (14.6 per cent) and with ESRD (5.1 per cent) are not negligible. When data were available, subjects were also examined according to WHO classification subgroups where the MGN lesion was accompanied by diffuse proliferative changes (previously WHO Classes Vc and Vd) or focal proliferative changes (previously WHO Va and Vb). Those with WHO Vc and Vd had a higher rate of ESRD (35.7 versus 24.6 per cent), but WHO subclass generally does not appear to be an independent predictor of renal failure when adjusted for renal function at presentation, proteinuria, anaemia, and age (Donadio *et al.* 1995). Much of the prognosis of SLE–MGN seems related to the subsequent development of proliferative changes on biopsy (Pasquali *et al.* 1993; Sloan *et al.* 1996). It is interesting to note that although there are limited data on the subject, there was a rather striking rate of non-renal-related deaths of 8.2 per cent due to a variety of causes, emphasizing the serious prognostic implications of renal involvement in SLE. Although overall survival in SLE patients has improved over time, the 5-year survival of patients with SLE of all histological types is worse if there is renal involvement (not specifically MGN) (Cameron 1999).

HBV-associated MGN has a variable natural history, depending upon the population studied. The majority of information is available from paediatric populations. In children, the disease generally has a benign course. The cumulative probability of remission at 4 years is 64 per cent (Gilbert and Wiggelinkhuizen 1994), and is usually associated with younger age, and smaller burden of subepithelial immune deposits (Hsu *et al.* 1989). The membranous lesion has been documented to actually resolve with the gradual spontaneous remission of the nephrotic syndrome (Gonzalo *et al.* 1999). The natural history in adults may not be as benign. One study of adults infected in an endemic area (therefore vertical transmission possible) indicated that spontaneous remission was uncommon in this population with progressive renal failure seen in 29 per cent, with 10 per cent reaching ESRD by the end of the average 60-month follow-up period (Lai *et al.* 1991).

There are fewer data regarding the natural history of MGN associated with malignancy. There are several reported cases of resolution of the MGN with treatment of the primary malignancy by resection or medical therapy (Robinson *et al.* 1984; Coltharp *et al.* 1991; Burstein *et al.* 1993).

With regard to medications associated with MGN, it is generally held that discontinuation of the causative agent results in a resolution of the nephrotic syndrome. This has been documented in a relatively large series of patients with MGN related to gold therapy for rheumatoid arthritis (Hall *et al.* 1987). All patients had a remission of their proteinuria, although a period of up to 18 months was required for complete resolution. Renal function remained stable during the course of the illness.

Prognostic factors

Given the overall favourable natural history of MGN, it is useful to isolate factors that identify individual patients at risk of progressive renal insufficiency. These patients would be the ones who would derive the greatest benefit from potentially hazardous immunosuppressive therapy. Several risk factors for progression have been identified, and used to create a semiquantitative algorithm that is useful in identifying those at greatest risk. This equation is described further in the next section. In univariate analysis, gender, advanced age, hypertension, renal insufficiency at presentation, and severity of urinary protein excretion all appear to be predictive.

Gender has a significant influence on progression of MGN—with males having a worse prognosis. The first observation that gender may affect prognosis was reported as a trend towards more rapid deterioration of renal function in a study of prednisone for treatment of MGN (Collaborative Study 1979). This was later confirmed in a case series (Hopper *et al.* 1981). Two studies in 1984 confirmed by univariate analysis that male gender is associated with an unfavourable prognosis (Davison *et al.* 1984; Tu *et al.* 1984). The gender ratio at presentation versus at the endstage of the disease also illustrates this effect. In several populations, it has been observed that the gender ratio is almost equal at presentation of MGN (Abe *et al.* 1986; Harrison *et al.* 1986; Simon *et al.* 1994), whereas at ESRD it is consistently 2–3 : 1, male : female (USRDS 1999 Annual Data Report; The National Institutes of Health, National Institute of Diabetes and Digestive and Kidney Disease, Bethesda, 1999; Maisonneuve *et al.* 2000). This would fit with our own long-term observational data that indicate by multivariate analysis that the only two factors associated with spontaneous remission are persistent subnephrotic proteinuria, and female gender (Laluck and Cattran 1999). The role of gender in the progression of MGN has been closely studied in a large meta-analysis, which included 21 studies containing 1894 patients followed for an average of 84 months (Neugarten *et al.* 2000). The pooled analysis confirmed that male gender is highly significantly associated with a more rapid rate of progression in MGN (standardized effect size estimate 0.30, 95 per cent CI 0.16–0.36, $p < 0.00001$).

Older age is generally associated with a higher risk of development of chronic renal insufficiency. We recently performed a retrospective study of 74 patients over 60 years of age at time of diagnosis of idiopathic MGN and compared them to 249 younger subjects in the same registry (Zent *et al.* 1997). Older subjects had significantly greater median serum creatinine (1.3 versus 1.0 mg/dl, $p < 0.001$), and lower calculated creatinine clearance values (55 versus 95 ml/min, $p < 0.0001$) than those in the younger-onset group. The incidence of chronic renal insufficiency defined as a clearance of less than 50 ml/min was significantly more in the elderly after a mean observation time of nearly 4 years (59 versus 25 per cent, $p < 0.0001$), but the rate of deterioration in renal function was not different. The observed difference in rates of chronic renal failure may therefore be due in large part to loss of reserve of functional nephron mass with age, such that there is less remaining to compensate for the additive detrimental effects of a glomerular disease. A more recent retrospective study including 44 patients presenting over 60 years of age confirmed that older patients more often have worse renal impairment at presentation than a younger cohort, and also a worse prognosis for renal survival (O'Callaghan *et al.* 2002). Smaller individual studies have found a somewhat more variable association with age and renal prognosis (Row *et al.* 1975; Davison *et al.* 1984; Tu *et al.* 1984; Zuchelli *et al.* 1987; Schieppati *et al.* 1993; Honkanen *et al.* 1994).

The nephrotic syndrome and nephrotic-range proteinuria were shown early on to be associated with a worse prognosis, when analysed in univariate analysis (Row *et al.* 1975; Noel *et al.* 1979; Mallick *et al.* 1983; Davison *et al.* 1984; Tu *et al.* 1984; Gerstoft *et al.* 1986; Donadio *et al.* 1988; Murphy *et al.* 1988; Wehrmann *et al.* 1989). Multivariate analysis, however, does not consistently reveal that the degree of proteinuria at the time of diagnosis predicts outcome (Tu *et al.* 1984; Schieppati 1993; Marx and Marx 1999). On the other hand, a complete or partial remission in proteinuria is associated with a favourable outcome (Ponticelli *et al.* 1992a; Laluck and Cattran 1999). Inconsistencies in these findings may be related to the fact subjects received biopsies at different stages of diagnosis, and therefore using time of biopsy or time of diagnosis as 'baseline' may yield inconsistent results. In addition, given the variable course of the disease, a dynamic view of proteinuria over time is likely more indicative of prognosis (see below). Hypertension and renal insufficiency at the time of biopsy have shown similar results to proteinuria with respect to prediction of outcome. There is general agreement that impaired function at the time of biopsy and hypertension do not portend a favourable prognosis, however, studies have again shown variable results when incorporating these factors in multivariate analysis (same reference as above).

Biopsy findings may correlate with prognosis, particularly when examining the degree of tubulointerstitial damage. More 'advanced' stages of pathology have been found to correlate with an adverse prognosis in some studies. For instance, subjects with stage III and IV lesions have been found to correlate with an adverse prognosis, compared with stages I and II in most (Franklin *et al.* 1973; Gluck *et al.* 1973; Noel *et al.* 1979; Zucchelli *et al.* 1986, 1987; Tornroth 1987; Hay 1992), but not all studies (Abe *et al.* 1986). The finding of tubulointerstitial damage is more consistently associated with a poor prognosis (Noel *et al.* 1979; Ramzy *et al.* 1981) even in multivariate analysis (Wehrmann *et al.* 1989). Most recently, an analysis of histological features and clinical correlation in 19 patients with MGN revealed that tubulointerstitial changes including the number of interstitial cells, particularly the number of CD45RO-positive cells, and increases of interstitial collage IV and VI were the most important pathological features predictive of prognosis (Wu *et al.* 2001).

Several other factors have been correlated with outcome, but are not yet part of the usual diagnostic assessment. Urinary excretion of IgG and α1-microglobulin has been correlated with outcome more closely than total proteinuria (Bazzi 2001). In addition, there has been significant investigation into the role of genetic factors that are associated with the course of MGN. HLA genotype has been shown to influence disease course, depending upon the population, as discussed in the section on epidemiology (Abe *et al.* 1986; Kida *et al.* 1986; Papiha *et al.* 1987; Freedman *et al.* 1994). These associations, however, have not been consistent and were not found in the most recent sizeable British MRC trial (Cameron *et al.* 1990). Finally, the finding of mesangial immune deposits may suggest a favourable prognosis in idiopathic MGN (Davenport *et al.* 1994).

Predicting prognosis

Given the potential toxicities of the medications involved in treating MGN, as well as the significant potential for a patient to undergo a spontaneous remission, it is valuable to be able to predict the clinical course of an individual patient before making therapeutic decisions. Ideally, the data required to provide prognostic information should be obtainable as soon as possible after diagnosis. The difficulty associating the above factors with long-term outcome is their poor specificity, and the fact that they reflect only cross-sectional data at diagnosis. In addition, these factors are in general, qualitative in nature. Another approach is to use dynamic changes in clinical parameters over time to produce a semi-quantitative risk of progression (Pei *et al.* 1992; Cattran 2001). The equation used for this calculation is presented in Fig. 2(a), with sample calculations in Fig. 2(b). This approach incorporates the clinical parameters of proteinuria and creatinine clearance estimates over fixed periods of time. The approach demonstrates an impressive overall accuracy of predicting progression to chronic renal failure. When the sensitivity, specificity, positive and negative predictive values are considered, the accuracy of this formula, meaning its ability to predict whether or not a patient will progress, can be determined. This accuracy changes according to the severity of proteinuria values over a 6-month observation period; when values were persistently greater than 4 g/day, for instance, the algorithm can accurately predict whether a patient will or will not progress with a rate of 71 per cent. At more than or equal to 6 g/day, the accuracy rises to 84 per cent, and at more than or equal to 8 g/day, reaches 84 per cent (Cattran *et al.* 1997). If the patient's renal function was impaired or deteriorated over the 6 months, sensitivity and specificity were even higher in regards to progression. In addition, the regression formula has been validated in two populations—101 patients from Italy, and 78 patients from Finland (Cattran *et al.* 1997).

There are several advantages to this algorithm. First, all of the factors are easily obtainable standard laboratory measurements. In addition, the dynamic nature of the algorithm allows it to be recalculated and reapplied over the course of a patient's disease. It is important to note that the individual risk factors of age, gender, biopsy findings, and presence of hypertension were not found to be independent of the factors in the model, and although relevant to each individual case, they do not add to the predictive value of the algorithm.

(a) Logistic regression model:

$$X = 1.26 + (0.3 \times \text{PP}) - (0.3 \times \text{slope Ccr}) - 0.05 \times \text{Ccr}_i$$

PP: The level of persistent proteinuria in g/24 h. The number used is the lowest level observed over a period of 6 months

Slope Ccr: The slope of the creatinine clearance over the period used to observe persistent proteinuria (e.g. 6 months). Measured in ml/min/month^{-1}

Ccr_i: The initial creatinine clearance documented at the beginning of the observation period, in ml/min

Use the calculated X to obtain a probability of progression (R) by substituting as follows:

$$R = \frac{e^X}{(1 + e^X)}$$

(b)

Patient A:

Month	Proteinuria (g/24 h)	Creatinine clearance (ml/min)
0	10	90
3	6	90
6	4	90

Would like to know patient A's risk of progression. One requires 6 months of follow-up for the calculation

$$\text{PP} = 4 \text{ g/24 h}$$

$$\text{Slope Ccr} = \frac{\text{Ccr final} - \text{Ccr initial}}{\text{Time}} = \frac{90 \text{ ml/min} - 90 \text{ ml/min}}{6 \text{ months}} = 0$$

Initial Ccr = 90 ml/min

$$X = 1.26 + (0.3 \times \text{PP}) - (0.3 \times \text{slope Ccr}) - (0.05 \times \text{Ccr}_i)$$
$$= 1.26 + (0.3 \times 4) - (0.3 \times 0) - (0.05 \times 90)$$
$$X = -2.04$$
$$e^X = 0.13$$
$$R = (0.13/1.13) \times 100 = 11\% \text{ risk of progression}$$

On the other hand, if his proteinuria remained at 10 g/day and his initial Ccr was only 80 ml/min, but his creatinine clearance did not change over 6 months, his estimated risk of progression would rise to:

$$X = 1.26 + (0.3 \times 10) - (0.3 \times 0) - (0.05 \times 80) = 0.26$$
$$e^X = 1.30$$
$$R = 1.3/(1 + 1.3)$$
$$R = 56\% \text{ risk of progression}$$

Fig. 2 (a) Prediction model for risk of progression in idiopathic MGN. (b) Sample calculation of risk of progression.

Treatment

The focus of treatment will relate to idiopathic MGN; the treatment of secondary MGN will be briefly discussed in the next section. In consideration of the therapy for idiopathic MGN, it is useful to divide treatment into four categories:

1. non-immunological therapy;
2. specific immunotherapy;
3. treatment of secondary effects/complications of the nephrotic syndrome;
4. strategies to reduce complications of the immunosuppressive therapy.

Non-immunological therapy

These treatments tend to carry a low risk of adverse effects, and are applicable to most patients presenting with primary or secondary MGN. Dietary protein restriction remains an area of some debate in the treatment of proteinuric glomerular disease (see Chapter 3.4), as these patients are at a significant risk of malnutrition, especially if they develop progressive renal insufficiency. Dietary manipulation alone has not been shown to induce a complete remission of the nephrotic syndrome in idiopathic MGN. However, there are data to suggest that protein restriction results in a reduction in both proteinuria and progression of disease, demonstrated specifically in patients with MGN, and as well in patients with other causes of the nephrotic syndrome (Cupisti *et al.* 1990; D'Amico *et al.* 1991; D'Amico and Gentile 1992; Pedrini *et al.* 1996; Kopple *et al.* 1997). Dietary modification has been shown to be additive to the anti-proteinuric effects of antihypertensives (Gansevoort *et al.* 1995a), and to have a favourable effect on the lipid profile (D'Amico and Gentile 1992). A target protein intake of 0.8 g/kg/day plus replacement of urinary protein losses (based upon MDRD data, Kopple *et al.* 1997) is probably reasonable, as long as close attention is paid to ensure patients maintain adequate overall nutrition.

Antihypertensive treatment improves proteinuria, and slows the progression of renal disease. Multiple studies have shown the additional benefit of ACE inhibitors, above the effect of blood pressure lowering alone (Peterson *et al.* 1995; Gansevoort *et al.* 1995a,b; Ruggenenti *et al.* 1998, 1999). This benefit is likely related to both the lowering of intraglomerular pressure, and the anti-inflammatory/antiproliferative effects of these agents. The additional benefit of ACE inhibition has been demonstrated specifically in idiopathic MGN (Thomas *et al.* 1991; Rostoker *et al.* 1995). An equivalent benefit of angiotensin-receptor blocking agents to ACE inhibitors specifically in MGN has not yet been confirmed.

Specific immunotherapy

The majority of trials in idiopathic MGN do not meet rigorous standards; they are often non-controlled, have small patient numbers, and short observation periods (Geddes and Cattran 2000).

The regimens examined in controlled trials include corticosteroids alone or in combination with chlorambucil, cyclophosphamide, or cyclosporin, and the latter three drugs used as single agents. These medications all have significant adverse effects, and therefore the decision to subject a patient to these risks, must be weighed against the potential benefits. Given the variable clinical outcomes of patients, it is useful to first establish categories of progression, as determined by the factors in the previously discussed algorithm. This requires an initial observation period of 6 months, during which time non-immunological interventions should be maximized. In order to determine the categories of progression, specific therapeutic trials were retrospectively divided according to their subjects' initial laboratory characteristics. This allows the separation of the effectiveness of any one therapy to be judged by the category of risk of progression of the patients in that trial. Once these risk categories are established, one can assign any individual patient into their risk category and a treatment strategy can be developed based on best evidence with a clearer picture of the risk–benefit ratio for both the patient and the physician. Figure 3 outlines the approach to therapy that will be discussed.

Risk of progression categories

Low risk of progression

Symptomless with a normal creatinine clearance at presentation, peak proteinuria less than 4 g/day, and stable creatinine clearance over 6 months of observation.

The prognosis of these patients is generally excellent. Our study of three cohorts of patients from Canada ($n = 184$), Finland ($n = 78$), and Italy ($n = 101$) showed that 17–28 per cent of patients present in this category. Of these, only 6, 0, and 24 per cent respectively, developed sustained renal insufficiency (clearance < 60 ml/min/1.73 m^2) after a mean follow-up of 70, 104, and 59 months. The average overall risk of progression was only 5 per cent. Blood pressure management, and antiproteinuric strategies with agents such as ACE inhibitors are very important in this group. However, given the generally favourable

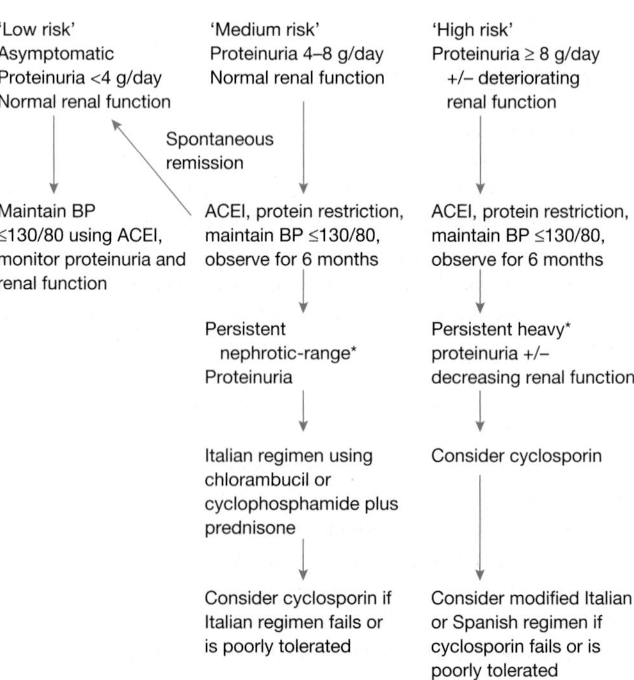

Fig. 3 Algorithm for the treatment of idiopathic MGN. Patients may change from one category to another during the course of follow-up. Abbreviations: BP, blood pressure; ACEI, angiotensin-converting-enzyme inhibiting drug. * Introduce appropriate risk reduction strategies.

outcome, immunosuppressive therapy is not recommended. A small percentage of individuals will progress, so ongoing monitoring of renal function, proteinuria, and blood pressure is necessary. Their risk of progression may change, and therefore should be periodically reassessed.

Medium risk of progression

Normal creatinine clearance at presentation and during the 6 months of observation, but proteinuria consistently 4–8 g/day, over that period.

Corticosteroids alone have been shown to be ineffective in inducing remission, and while some have indicated transient improvement in proteinuria, they have not been found to prevent progression in all but one controlled studies to date (Collaborative Study of the Adult Idiopathic Nephrotic Syndrome 1979; Kobayashi *et al.* 1982; Cattran *et al.* 1989). Entry criteria in these trials would have placed the participants into the 'medium risk' category. Although the total follow-up periods were less than 4 years, and the protocol for administration differed, it is generally held that corticosteroids alone do not have a role in treatment of idiopathic MGN (Lewis 1993; Muirhead 1999).

There is evidence of benefit, however, when corticosteroids in combination with a cytotoxic agent are used in this risk group. A significant increase in both remission of proteinuria and renal survival was demonstrated, with follow-up out to 10 years in a trial comparing a regimen of prednisone and chlorambucil to symptomatic treatment (Ponticelli *et al.* 1984, 1992b, 1995). The regimen is given over a 6-month period. It consists of 1 g of IV methylprednisolone daily for the first 3 days of months 1, 3, and 5 followed by 27 days of oral methylprednisolone 0.5 mg/kg/day for the remainder of the month. In alternating months (months 2, 4, 6), chlorambucil 0.2 mg/kg/day is used instead of the corticosteroid. At 10 years, the probability of survival without dialysis was 92 per cent in the treatment group, and 60 per cent in the group receiving symptomatic therapy ($p = 0.004$). During the follow-up, the probability of achieving a complete or partial remission was 83 per cent in the treated group, and only 38 per cent in the controls ($p = 0.000$) and at last follow-up, 62 per cent of treated patients were in either a complete or partial remission, compared with 33 per cent of controls ($p < 0.05$). Chlorambucil is difficult to obtain and not often used in some countries, and cyclophosphamide is commonly substituted. A further trial from the same group (Ponticelli *et al.* 1998) compared the original regimen employing chlorambucil, with a similar regimen substituting cyclophosphamide 2.5 mg/kg/day. Short-term benefits similar to those found in the first trial were demonstrated. There was, however, a substantial rate of relapse of nephrotic syndrome. At 2 years, up to 30 per cent of patients in both groups had relapsed to nephrotic range proteinuria. Overall, the regimens were surprisingly well-tolerated, with only 10 per cent of patients discontinuing treatment due to adverse effects.

A recent trial examined the effectiveness of cyclosporin in combination with low dose prednisone in this risk category (Cattran *et al.* 2001). Fifty-one subjects were enrolled in this multicentre, placebo-controlled trial. All had failed to achieve remission after at least 8 weeks of therapy with prednisone 1 mg/kg/day. Study subjects receiving active treatment ($n = 28$) were given cyclosporin in a liquid formulation starting at 3.5 mg/kg/day divided in two doses, and adjusted to achieve whole blood 12 h trough levels of 125–225 μg/l (monoclonal assay). Control subjects ($n = 23$) received a placebo liquid, and all subjects were given prednisone at a dose of 0.15 mg/kg/day to a maximum of 15 mg/day. Subjects received 26 weeks of therapy, after which the cyclosporin/placebo was stopped, and steroid dose was tapered. By 26 weeks, 75 per cent of treated subjects had reached a partial or complete remission, compared with only 22 per cent of controls ($p = 0.001$). By week 52, 43 per cent of treatment subjects, and 40 per cent of control subjects had relapsed—this difference was not statistically significant. The fraction of patients remaining in remission, however, remained significantly different at the 1-year mark—39 per cent of cyclosporin-treated subjects remained in remission, versus 13 per cent in the placebo group ($p = 0.007$). This improvement in remission rate was not at the expense of a change in renal function, since there was no significant change noted in creatinine clearance in either group. Further studies are necessary to determine if a longer course of treatment, higher dose, or retreatment of relapses may increase the rate and perhaps the duration of response.

High risk of progression

Persistent proteinuria not less than 8 g/day over the 6 months of observation with or without deteriorating renal function This subgroup of patients is small, and very few trials have exclusively studied subjects in this risk category. Corticosteroid treatment alone was examined in the subgroup of 55 patients with renal insufficiency from the relatively large randomized trial of Canadian subjects (Cattran *et al.* 1989). All in this subgroup had an initial creatinine clearance of less than 72 ml/min. Those treated with prednisone (dose of 45 mg/m^2 on alternate days for 6 months) did not demonstrate an improvement in rate of deterioration of renal function. In the one randomized study of corticosteroids alone in high risk subjects (mean proteinuria was 10.6 g/day) (Cameron *et al.* 1990), prednisolone at 100–150 mg on alternate days given for 8 weeks and then tapered did not confer benefit with respect to rate of deterioration of function or proteinuria. Somewhat in contrast, an earlier small retrospective uncontrolled study of 15 patients with declining function suggested that 5 days of 1 g methylprednisolone IV followed by a tapering course of prednisolone was associated with an initial stabilization in function in nine of the subjects (Short *et al.* 1987). At last follow-up, however, two patients had died, and five had reached ESRD, suggesting that any positive effects of the treatment were transient.

Four studies have examined the utility of chlorambucil, utilizing modified versions of the Italian regimen in patients with a high risk of progression. A substantial improvement in renal function in more than half of patients, and a decline in proteinuria was noted in one study of eight patients (Mathieson *et al.* 1988). Similarly, half of the 21 subjects in a subsequent study were noted to have a stabilization or improvement in renal function (Warwick *et al.* 1994), but subjects with an initial creatinine between 180 and 480 μmol/l continued to show deterioration in function. When the outcome of these subjects was compared to historical controls, however, there did appear to be a trend to improved renal survival (Stirling *et al.* 1998). The success noted by these small studies must, however, be balanced by the high incidence of serious complications; in the aforementioned study by Stirling, for instance, half of the patients had significant side-effects related to therapy (infectious and myelosuppressive), necessitating discontinuation of medications in six of 19 patients. This study population, particularly those with significantly impaired renal function, may be the group most vulnerable to drug toxicity. Most recently, one retrospective study of 39 subjects compared conservative therapy in patients treated between 1975 and 1989, to a group treated with a regimen of oral chlorambucil (0.15 mg/kg/day for 14 weeks) plus oral prednisone for 6 months between 1990 and 2000 (Torres *et al.* 2002). At 4 years of follow-up, those receiving the chlorambucil/prednisone routine had a 90 per cent probability of renal survival at 4 years of follow-up, compared with only a 55 per cent probability in subjects receiving only conservative therapy ($p < 0.001$).

Monthly pulse cyclophosphamide for 6 months plus prednisone compared to prednisone alone produced no additional benefit in a randomized trial that included 36 who qualified as 'high risk' by virtue of renal insufficiency (Falk *et al.* 1992). Two non-randomized case–control studies in similar populations involving long-term oral cyclophosphamide with or without prednisone did indicate a benefit to the therapy (Bruns *et al.* 1991; Jindal *et al.* 1992). However, apart from the limitations of the non-randomized design, long-term cyclophosphamide exposure carries the significant risks of infertility, infection, and malignancy, limiting the applicability of these trials. Direct comparison of cyclophosphamide and chlorambucil was undertaken in two trials that included patients with progressive deterioration in renal function. The first compared a traditional Italian regimen with chlorambucil to a modified routine with IV cyclophosphamide pulses at months 2, 4, 6, and thrice daily 1 g IV methylprednisolone pulses at months 1, 3, and 5 (Reichert *et al.* 1994). The authors concluded that cyclophosphamide administered in this manner was not beneficial after 6–36 months of follow-up. The same group then examined a group of patients receiving one of two treatment strategies. The first ($n = 15$) received a regimen of 3 days of IV methylprednisolone followed by 0.5 mg/kg/day of oral prednisone given in months 1, 3, and 5 alternating with oral chlorambucil 0.15 mg/kg/day in months 2, 4, and 6. The comparison group ($n = 17$) received cyclophosphamide 1.5–2.0 mg/kg/day for 1 year, and steroids in comparable doses to the first group (Branten *et al.* 1998). Those treated with cyclophosphamide showed a greater benefit with a greater reduction in serum creatinine (121 versus 61 μmol/l fall, $p < 0.01$), lower incidence of ESRD (4 versus 1 patients, $p < 0.05$), and more frequent remission of proteinuria, and fewer short-term side-effects.

Cyclosporin has been examined in detail in this population by more than one investigator. In our randomized controlled trial of patients with documented progressive renal insufficiency (mean creatinine was 195 μmol/l), 1 year of cyclosporin was administered at a dose of 3.8 mg/kg, and compared with placebo (Cattran *et al.* 1995). Cyclosporin-treated patients demonstrated significantly reduced proteinuria, and a slower rate of progression of renal failure ($p = 0.02$ and $p < 0.02$, respectively). These positive results were sustained in more than half of the patients as late as 2 years after treatment. The number of patients in the study, however, was small, and there was a trend towards transient increases in creatinine noted in the cyclosporin treatment group. A similar benefit was noted in an uncontrolled study of 15 individuals with steroid-resistant progressive disease, however, their relapse rate was higher (Rostoker *et al.* 1993). A recent retrospective review from a large collaborative group treated 41 patients considered high risk due to the severity of proteinuria (>10 g/day), and resistance to other immunosuppressive drugs (Fritsche *et al.* 1999). Thirty-four per cent achieved a complete remission after a mean treatment time of 225 days, at a mean dose of 3.3 mg/kg. This helps to confirm the drug's efficacy, but also the need for prolonged therapy before assuming resistance to the medication.

Mycophenolate Mofetil (MMF), an immunosuppressive agent that preferentially inhibits purine synthesis in activated lymphocytes, has been used successfully in the realm of transplantation, and is emerging as a potential new agent for use in glomerulonephritis. Two uncontrolled studies have employed MMF in the treatment of idiopathic MGN. The first trial included 16 patients with nephrotic syndrome due to MGN who would be categorized as either medium or high risk by virtue of their renal parameters alone (Miller *et al.* 2000). Nearly all had steroid-resistant disease, and half had failed cytotoxic and cyclosporin therapy. Moderate success was noted after a mean of 8 months of treatment, with six patients achieving a halving in their proteinuria. No difference was noted with respect to deterioration in their renal function. A second study included 17 patients with MGN amongst a group of 46 subjects with primary glomerulonephritis, treated for a minimum of 3 months with MMF (Choi *et al.* 2002). Patients were more heterogeneous with regard to risk profile, and received variable doses of prednisone in addition to the MMF. There was, however, a significant decrease in proteinuria, and trend towards improved renal function. Side-effects in both of these studies were infrequent, and further controlled trials with this agent are warranted.

Another promising new agent described is rituximab, a monoclonal antibody directed against the surface antigen CD20 of B-cells. The drug is believed to interfere with B cell function, thereby inhibiting production of antibodies to the putative unknown human autoantigen involved in the pathogenesis of MGN. An uncontrolled trial of this intravenous medication in seven patients was recently reported (Remuzzi *et al.* 2002). All were on full doses of ACE inhibitors, and had not reached remission after an observation of 1 year following biopsy. The mean creatinine clearance was 68.7 ml/min/1.73 m^2, and mean proteinuria was 8.6 g/day (all had over 3.5 g/day). By 20 weeks (the last follow-up), urine protein had decreased to a mean of 3.7 g/day. Two patients achieved a full remission, and three, a partial remission. Adverse effects were mild, and infusion-related.

Treatment of secondary MGN

There are few data to guide the treatment of MGN related to SLE and hepatitis, due to their variable natural history, and a paucity of randomized controlled trials. The general conservative measures described for the treatment of primary MGN (ACE inhibition, blood pressure control, lipid-lowering therapy, etc.) are, in our opinion, also recommended for the treatment of secondary forms of MGN, despite a lack of clear evidence from controlled trials.

In the case of MGN secondary to SLE, as discussed earlier, the prognosis seems very dependent upon the coexistence of proliferative lesions on biopsy. The therapy is therefore usually guided by the degree of proliferation seen, or by the presence of systemic features. An isolated pure membranous nephropathy in the absence of any systemic features or proliferation on biopsy is relatively rare. Although patients with pure membranous lesion are generally regarded as having a lower risk of ESRD, morbidity associated with the persistence of nephrotic syndrome has prompted interest in the role of immunosuppression for this scenario (Donadio 1992). There is evidence of favourable response rates with modified versions of the Italian regimen of combination steroids and cytotoxic agents (Paasquali *et al.* 1993; Moroni *et al.* 1998; Chan *et al.* 1999). More recently, evidence regarding the utility of cyclosporin has emerged (Radhakrishnan *et al.* 1994; Austin *et al.* 1997). Although these studies included small numbers of patients, and one included patients with proliferative lesions, there appeared to be high response rates, with minimal nephrotoxicity. Given the overall lack of data on this subject, no clear recommendations can be made regarding the optimal therapy for a pure membranous lesion in SLE (see also Chapter 4.7.2).

Data regarding therapy for HBV-related MGN are largely from paediatric populations. As discussed in the section on natural history, spontaneous remissions are relatively common in children, but perhaps less frequent in adults. The use of immunosuppressants in this condition carries the risk of allowing uncontrolled viral replication, and possible future exacerbation of hepatitis (Lai *et al.* 1990). A small study initially suggested the efficacy of interferon-alpha in membranous GN due to HBV in inducing serologic, biochemical and renal remission (Listen-Melman *et al.* 1989). In children, the utility of α-interferon (IFN) following trials of prednisone was been studied in a relatively large group of 40 patients (Lin 1995). Twenty received IFN therapy for 12 months, and 20 received supportive treatment only. Both groups had failed steroid therapy. At the end of the study period, all patients in the IFN group were completely free of proteinuria, compared to none in the control group. Disappearance of HBeAg occurred more frequently in the treatment group. In adults, one study of the natural history of HBV-related MGN documented a poor response to IFN in the five patients who received the therapy (Lai *et al.* 1991). A study assessing the long-term outcome of 15 patients, indicated that half of those treated with interferon had a sustained remission in their liver disease with loss of HBV DNA and HBeAg, as well as favourable aminotransferase levels (Conjeevaram *et al.* 1995). The 'responders', all of whom had MGN as the associated renal lesion, also demonstrated marked improvement in proteinuria. From the limited data available, there appears to be a role for interferon, particularly in the presence of serological markers of active liver disease. Further data are needed regarding the concomitant use of antiviral agents in HBV-related MGN.

Treatment of secondary effects/ complications of the nephrotic syndrome

The burden of cardiovascular disease is clearly evident in both the dialysis and transplant populations, necessitating attention to any modifiable risk factors in the predialysis stage (USRDS 1995 Annual Data Report. The National Institutes of Health National Institute of Diabetes and Digestive and Kidney Diseases, Bethesda, 1995). The increased cardiovascular mortality observed in patients with persistent nephrotic-range proteinuria may in part be related to the associated lipid disorders (Ordonez *et al.* 1993; Wheeler and Bernard 1994). In addition to an established role in cardiovascular disease, lipids may play a role in the progression of renal disease (Wheeler 1995) (see Chapter 3.4 for further discussion). Various patterns of lipid abnormalities have been associated with the nephrotic syndrome, the most consistent being an increased total cholesterol due to elevations in VLDL, IDL, and LDL fractions. HDL tends to remain normal or low (Joven *et al.* 1990). As previously mentioned, dietary manipulation (using soy-protein diet) has been shown to lower total cholesterol, and may merit a role in treatment (D'Amico *et al.* 1992). The HMG–CoA reductase inhibitor class of lipid-lowering drugs has clearly been shown to be effective in the management of dyslipidaemia due to nephrotic syndrome when studied in a randomized, prospective, blinded, placebo-controlled manner (Spitalewitz *et al.* 1993). To date, there have been no trials examining the effect of lipid management on cardiovascular mortality in the nephrotic syndrome, due to the large sample size and duration of follow-up that would be required (see also Chapter 3.4).

Thrombotic complications pose a significant risk in patients with nephrotic syndrome, particularly when the syndrome is due to MGN (see Chapter 3.4). The frequency of these complications has varied widely in reports due to differences in methods of screening and detection, however the incidence in MGN appears to be particularly high (Trew *et al.* 1978; Wagoner *et al.* 1983; Llach 1985; Bellomo and Atkins 1993; Rabelink *et al.* 1994). The prevalence has been documented to be in the range of 20–50 per cent when all thromboembolic events are included. An increase in mortality has also been associated. Renal vein thrombosis has been found most recently in up to 35 per cent of patients with idiopathic MGN (Bellomo and Atkins 1993). Multiple factors appear to contribute to this hypercoagulable state including platelet abnormalities, decreased coagulation inhibitors, and hyperfibrinogenaemia (Vaziri 1983; Rabelink *et al.* 1994). Patients with serum albumin less than 2.5 g/l may be at greatest risk. It remains difficult, however, to predict which patients will develop thromboembolic complications, even when screening for additional heritable thrombophilic tendency is included in the work-up (Robert *et al.* 1987; Fabri *et al.* 1998). Given the risks of bleeding, the potential benefit of prophylactic anticoagulation has been considered formally by decision analyses. One examination of the topic (Bellomo *et al.* 1993) compared the risks of prophylactic anticoagulation with the current approach of secondary prevention. They calculated an overall reduction in morbid events of 32 per cent in favour of prophylactic anticoagulation. However, their analysis was limited by difficulties ascertaining estimates necessary to calculate event rates, due to limitations of the available literature. A subsequent study used Markov-based analysis model, estimated that the number of fatal embolic events prevented by anticoagulation would exceed fatal bleeding events (Sarasin and Schifferli 1994). Nevertheless, given the difficulties establishing bleeding risks in this population, prophylactic anticoagulation even in the high-risk group has not been adopted by all clinicians.

The oedema associated with nephrotic syndrome is one of the most troubling symptoms for patients (see Chapter 3.4). A tendency to sodium retention in part related to an abnormal responsiveness to atrial natriuretic peptide and an increased distal nephron reabsorption has been documented both clinically and in experimental studies (Peterson *et al.* 1988; Perico *et al.* 1989; Plum *et al.* 1996; Van de Walle *et al.* 1996). Loop diuretics are the mainstay of oedema management. The addition of a distally acting diuretic may be of particular benefit given the pathophysiological mechanisms involved in the sodium avidity associated with nephrotic syndrome. Attention must be paid to avoid depletion of effective circulating volume or 'overdiuresis'.

Strategies to reduce the side-effects of immunosuppressive therapy

Bone disease and infections are two potentially avoidable complications of the immunosuppressive agents most often used to treat idiopathic MGN. Bone loss due to corticosteroid treatment, is related to both dose and duration of therapy, and is greatest in the first 3–6 months of treatment. Prolonged low-dose exposure, however, has also been associated with significant loss of bone density (Canalis 2001). The effects of steroids on the intestinal absorption of calcium, and promotion of calciuria suggest that calcium and vitamin D should be incorporated into the treatment regimen. There are, as well, significant data indicating the protective effects of antiresorptive medications on bone loss and fractures induced by glucocorticoids. Several agents, including etidronate and alendronate, have been shown in multicentred well-designed trials, to improve these outcomes, and should be used when prolonged glucocorticoid treatment is anticipated (Adachi *et al.* 1997; Saag *et al.* 1998). Ongoing monitoring in patients at risk for renal stones and/or renal insufficiency is mandatory when biphosphonates are given in this population. Avascular necrosis of the femoral head is another potentially serious skeletal complication of prednisone. Patients must be informed of this potential side-effect, as it is not preventable, and is not necessarily dose-related.

Individuals receiving prolonged immunosuppressive therapy are at substantial risk of infectious complications, particularly *Pneumocystis carinii* pneumonia (PCP). The use of trimethoprim–sulfamethoxazole (TMP–SMX) significantly reduces the incidence of PCP in this population (Ognibene *et al.* 1995). Ongoing monitoring for excessive myelosuppression should also be employed in order to reduce the potential for infections.

Gonadal toxicity due to cyclophosphamide is of significant concern to patients. Daily oral cyclophosphamide causes permanent ovarian failure in over 70 per cent of women after 1 year, and in up to 45 per cent of women who receive the intravenous form, depending upon dose and timing of administration (Janssen and Genta 2000). Impairment of gonadal function may be more frequent in men, but may be more readily reversible. Cumulative doses of greater than 7.5 g/m^2 have been associated with permanent gonadal dysfunction and when assessed by weight, as little as 100 mg/kg has been reported to be harmful in mature males (Rivkees and Crawford 1988; Meistric *et al.* 1992). In women, therapy with gonadotropin-releasing agonists to inhibit ovulation appears to offer some protection regarding maintenance of fertility, and should be considered in ovulatory women receiving alkylating agents (Blumenfield and Haim 1997). Similarly, one study of men receiving cyclophosphamide for nephrotic syndrome suggested that intramuscular injections of testosterone given biweekly preserves fertility (Masala *et al.* 1997). Cryopreservation of sperm or oocytes should also be considered prior to initiation of therapy.

Acrolein the toxic metabolite produced from cyclophosphamide, induces urothelial damage. Pretreatment with hydration and MESNA should be used particularly, if administering the intravenous formulation of cyclophosphamide. Given the cumulative toxicity of the drug, and the long-latency period between exposure and development of side-effects, it has been recommended that urinalysis to screen for new haematuria be performed every 3–6 months for up to 11 years after initiation of the drug (Vlaovic and Jewett 1999). A long-term risk of other malignancies, including skin cancers, and haematological malignancy has been documented in patients treated with cyclophosphamide for non-oncological indications, and should be discussed with patients before therapy is initiated (Radis *et al.* 1995).

Conclusion

Idiopathic MGN remains an important cause of nephrotic syndrome in adults. Due to the relatively high prevalence of the condition, it remains the second or third most common type of primary glomerular disease to cause endstage renal failure and need for dialysis or transplantation. The non-renal morbidity and mortality associated with MGN are also significant. Although advances have been made in understanding the pathogenesis of this condition, its treatment remains similar to that of other glomerulonephritides–conservative management focusing on risk-reduction, with or without the use of broad-spectrum immunosuppression.

The variable clinical course of the condition makes decisions regarding therapy a particular challenge. Establishing which patients are at high risk of disease progression is an important part of this decision-making process. We have proposed the utilization of a validated predictive model involving 6 months of surveillance of the patient's clinical status that can be used to better quantify a patient's risk of progression, and aid in balancing the renal disease risks versus the risks of therapy. The clinician may also use the risk stratification method to then ascertain the therapy with the most favourable track record in patients with a similar clinical presentation. The trials assessing immunotherapy often do not meet rigorous standards; small sample sizes and case–control design are often employed due to the relatively low prevalence of the disease. It has been estimated that approximately 600 patients with a follow-up period of 5 years or more would be required for studies to be sufficiently powered to detect a 50 per cent difference between 'active' and 'supportive' therapy in MGN, if one assumes a median survival of 200 months (Remuzzi *et al.* 1994). The future of clinical trials of therapy for MGN are likely therefore to require international collaboration.

The therapy for MGN is not benign, and close attention must be paid to complications associated with both the nephrotic syndrome, and the therapy used to treat it. Until we have more specific therapy, or a more benign treatment, the decision to treat a patient with immunosuppression must be made with caution. The tremendous growth of genomic data and instruments with which to detect changes in gene expression in the course of disease, is likely to extend our understanding of the pathogenesis of this complex condition in the near future. The emergence of these technologies may also provide new methods of diagnosing this condition, detecting which patients are at risk, and help guide treatment.

References

Abe, S. *et al.* (1986). Idiopathic membranous glomerulonephritis: aspects of geographical differences. *Journal of Clinical Pathology* **39**, 1193–1198.

Abrass, C. K. (1985). Glomerulonephritis in the elderly. *American Journal of Nephrology* **5**, 409–418.

Adachi, J. D. *et al.* (1997). Intermittent etidronate therapy to prevent corticosteroid-induced osteoporosis. *New England Journal of Medicine* **337**, 382–387.

Adler, S. *et al.* (1986). Complement membrane attack complex stimulates production of reactive oxygen metabolites by cultured rat mesangial cells. *Journal of Clinical Investigation* **77**, 762–767.

Adu, D. and Cameron, J. S. (1989). Aetiology of membranous nephropathy. *Nephrology, Dialysis, Transplantation* **4**, 757–758.

Austin, H. A. *et al.* (2000). Lupus membranous nephropathy: controlled trial of prednisone, pulse cyclophosphamide, and cyclosporine A. *Journal of the American Society of Nephrology* **11**, A439 (abstract).

Baker, P. J. *et al.* (1989). Depletion of C6 prevents development of proteinuria in experimental membranous nephropathy in rats. *American Journal of Pathology* **135**, 185–194.

Bariety, J. *et al.* (1970). 'Extra-membranous' glomerulopathies (E.M.G.). Morphological study with optic microscopy, electron microscopy and immunofluoresence. *Pathologie et Biologie (Paris)* **18**, 5–32.

Bazzi, C. (2001). Urinary excretion of IgG and alpha(1)-microglobulin predicts clinical course better than extent of proteinuria in membranous nephropathy. *American Journal of Kidney Diseases* **38**, 240–248.

Bellomo, R. and Atkins, R. C. (1993). Membranous nephropathy and thromboembolism: is prophylactic anticoagulation warranted? *Nephron* **63**, 249–254.

Bellomo, R. *et al.* (1993). Idiopathic membranous nephropathy in an Australian population: the incidence of thromboembolism and its impact on the natural history. *Nephron* **63**, 240–241.

Blumenfeld, Z. and Haim, N. (1997). Prevention of gonadal damage during cytotoxic therapy. *Annals of Medicine* **29**, 199–206.

Braden, G. L. *et al.* (2000). Changing incidence of glomerular diseases in adults. *American Journal of Kidney Diseases* **35**, 878–883.

Branten, A. J. *et al.* (1998). Oral cyclophosphamide versus chlorambucil in the treatment of patients with membranous nephropathy and renal insufficiency. *Quarterly Journal of Medicine* **91**, 359–366.

Bruns, F. J. *et al.* (1991). Sustained remission of membranous glomerulonephritis after cyclophosphamide and prednisone. *Annals of Internal Medicine* **114**, 725–730.

Burstein, D. M., Korbet, S. M., and Schwartz, M. M. (1993). Membranous glomerulonephritis and malignancy. *American Journal of Kidney Diseases* **22**, 5–10.

Cahen, R. *et al.* (1989). Aetiology of membranous glomerulonephritis: a prospective study of 82 adult patients. *Nephrology, Dialysis, Transplantation* **4**, 172–180.

Cameron, J. S. (1999). Lupus nephritis. *Journal of the American Society of Nephrology* **10**, 413–424.

Cameron, J. S., Healy, M. J., and Adu, D. (1990). The Medical Research Council trial of short-term high-dose alternate day prednisolone in idiopathic membranous nephropathy with nephrotic syndrome in adults. The MRC Glomerulonephritis Working Party. *Quarterly Journal of Medicine* **74**, 133–156.

Canalis, E. and Giustina, A. (2001). Glucocorticoid-induced osteoporosis: summary of a workshop. *Journal of Clinical Endocrinology and Metabolism* **86**, 5681–5685.

Cattran, D. C. (2001). Idiopathic membranous glomerulonephritis. *Kidney International* **59**, 1983–1994.

Cattran, D. C. *et al.* (1989). A randomized controlled trial of prednisone in patients with idiopathic membranous nephropathy. *New England Journal of Medicine* **320**, 210–215.

Cattran, D. C., Pei, Y., and Greenwood, C. (1992). Predicting progression in membranous glomerulonephritis. *Nephrology, Dialysis, Transplantation* **7** (Suppl. 1), 48–52.

Cattran, D. C. *et al.* (1995). A controlled trial of cyclosporine in patients with progressive membranous nephropathy. Canadian Glomerulonephritis Study Group. *Kidney International* **47**, 1130–1135.

Cattran, D. C. *et al.* (1997). Validation of a predictive model of idiopathic membranous nephropathy: its clinical and research implications. *Kidney International* **51**, 901–907.

Cattran, D. C. *et al.* (2001). Cyclosporine in patients with steroid-resistant membranous nephropathy: a randomized trial. *Kidney International* **59**, 1484–1490.

Chan, T. *et al.* (1999). Treatment of membranous lupus nephritis with nephrotic syndrome by sequential immunosuppression. *Lupus* **8**, 545–551.

Choi, M. J. *et al.* (2002). Mycophenolate mofetil treatment for primary glomerular diseases. *Kidney International* **61**, 1098–1114.

Collaborative Study of the Adult Idiopathic Nephrotic Syndrome (1979). A controlled study of short-term prednisone treatment in adults with membranous nephropathy. *New England Journal of Medicine* **301**, 1301–1306.

Coltharp, W. H. *et al.* (1991). Nephrotic syndrome complicating adenocarcinoma of the lung with resolution after resection. *Annals of Thoracic Surgery* **51**, 308–309.

Conjeevaram, H. S. *et al.* (1995). Long-term outcome of hepatitis B virus-related glomerulonephritis after therapy with interferon alfa. *Gastroenterology* **109**, 540–546.

Coupes, B. *et al.* (1992). Clinical aspects of C3dg and C5b-9 in human membranous nephropathy. *Nephrology, Dialysis, Transplantation* **7** (Suppl. 1), 32–34.

Coupes, B. M. *et al.* (1993). The temporal relationship between urinary C5b-9 and C3dg and clinical parameters in human membranous nephropathy. *Nephrology, Dialysis, Transplantation* **8**, 397–401.

Couser, W. G., Schulze, M., and Pruchno, C. J. (1992). Role of C5b-9 in experimental membranous nephropathy. *Nephrology, Dialysis, Transplantation* **7** (Suppl. 1), 25–31.

Cupisti, A. *et al.* (1990). Dietary proteins affect proteinuria in primary membranous glomerulonephritis with nephrotic syndrome and normal renal function. *Contributions to Nephrology* **83**, 166–169.

Cybulsky, A. V. *et al.* (1986). Complement-induced glomerular epithelial cell injury. Role of the membrane attack complex in rat membranous nephropathy. *Journal of Clinical Investigation* **77**, 1096–1107.

Cybulsky, A. V. *et al.* (1995). Complement C5b-9 activates cytosolic phospholipase A2 in glomerular epithelial cells. *American Journal of Physiology* **269**, F739–F749.

Cybulsky, A. V., Papillon, J., and McTavish, A. J. (1998). Complement activates phospholipases and protein kinases in glomerular epithelial cells. *Kidney International* **54**, 360–372.

Cybulsky, A. V. *et al.* (2000). Complement-induced phospholipase A2 activation in experimental membranous nephropathy. *Kidney International* **57**, 1052–1062.

D'Agati, V. (1994). The many masks of focal segmental glomerulosclerosis. *Kidney International* **46**, 1223–1241.

D'Amico, G. and Gentile, M. G. (1992). Effect of dietary manipulation on the lipid abnormalities and urinary protein loss in nephrotic patients. *Mineral and Electrolyte Metabolism* **18**, 203–206.

D'Amico, G. *et al.* (1991). Effect of dietary proteins and lipids in patients with membranous nephropathy and nephrotic syndrome. *Clinical Nephrology* **35**, 237–242.

D'Amico, G. *et al.* (1992). Effect of vegetarian soy diet on hyperlipidaemia in nephrotic syndrome. *Lancet* **339**, 1131–1134.

Davenport, A. *et al.* (1994). Do mesangial immune complex deposits affect the renal prognosis in membranous glomerulonephritis? *Clinical Nephrology* **41**, 271–276.

Davison, A. M. *et al.* (1984). The natural history of renal function in untreated idiopathic membranous glomerulonephritis in adults. *Clinical Nephrology* **22**, 61–67.

Donadio, J. V., Jr. (1990). Treatment of glomerulonephritis in the elderly. *American Journal of Kidney Diseases* **16**, 307–311.

Donadio, J. V., Jr. (1992). Treatment of membranous nephropathy in systemic lupus erythematosus. *Nephrology, Dialysis, Transplantation* **7** (Suppl. 1), 97–104.

Donadio, J. V., Jr. *et al.* (1988). Idiopathic membranous nephropathy: the natural history of untreated patients. *Kidney International* **33**, 708–715.

Donadio, J. V., Jr. *et al.* (1995). Prognostic determinants in lupus nephritis: a long-term clinicopathologic study. *Lupus* **4**, 109–115.

Ehrenreich, T. and Churg, J. Pathology of membranous nephropathy. In *Pathology Annual* (ed. S. C. Scommers), pp. 145–186. New York: Appleton-Century-Crofts, 1968.

Ehrenreich, T. *et al.* (1976). Treatment of idiopathic membranous nephropathy. *New England Journal of Medicine* **295**, 741–746.

Fabri, D. *et al.* (1998). Inherited risk factors for thrombophilia in children with nephrotic syndrome. *European Journal of Pediatrics* **157**, 939–942.

Falk, R. J. *et al.* (1992). Treatment of progressive membranous glomerulopathy. A randomized trial comparing cyclophosphamide and corticosteroids with corticosteroids alone. The Glomerular Disease Collaborative Network. *Annals of Internal Medicine* **116**, 438–445.

Falk, R., Jennette, J. C., and Nachman, P. H. Primary glomerular disease. In *The Kidney* (ed. B. M. Brenner and F. C. Rector), pp. 1263–1292. Philadelphia, PA: W. B. Saunders, 2000.

Farquhar, M. G. (1996). Molecular analysis of the pathological autoimmune antigens of Heymann nephritis. *American Journal of Pathology* **148**, 1331–1337.

Farquhar, M. G. *et al.* (1995). The Heymann nephritis antigenic complex: megalin (gp330) and RAP. *Journal of the American Society of Nephrology* **6**, 35–47.

Franklin, W. A., Jennings, R. B., and Earle, D. P. (1973). Membranous glomerulonephritis: long-term serial observations on clinical course and morphology. *Kidney International* **4**, 36–56.

Freedman, B. I. *et al.* (1994). HLA associations in end-stage renal disease due to membranous glomerulonephritis: HLA-DR3 associations with progressive renal injury. Southeastern Organ Procurement Foundation. *American Journal of Kidney Diseases* **23**, 797–802.

Fritsche, L. *et al.* (1999). Treatment of membranous glomerulopathy with cyclosporin A: how much patience is required? *Nephrology, Dialysis, Transplantation* **14**, 1036–1038.

Furness, P. N. *et al.* (1999). Glomerular expression of nephrin is decreased in acquired human nephrotic syndrome. *Nephrology, Dialysis, Transplantation* **14**, 1234–1237.

Gansevoort, R. T., de Zeeuw, D., and de Jong, P. E. (1995a). Additive antiproteinuric effect of ACE inhibition and a low-protein diet in human renal disease. *Nephrology, Dialysis, Transplantation* **10**, 497–504.

Gansevoort, R. T. *et al.* (1995b). Antiproteinuric effect of blood-pressure-lowering agents: a meta-analysis of comparative trials. *Nephrology, Dialysis, Transplantation* **10**, 1963–1974.

Gartner, H. V. *et al.* (1977). Correlations between morphologic and clinical features in idiopathic perimembranous glomerulonephritis. A study on 403 renal biopsies of 367 patients. *Current Topics in Pathology* **65**, 1–29.

Geddes, C. C. and Cattran, D. C. (2000). The treatment of idiopathic membranous nephropathy. *Seminars in Nephrology* **20**, 299–308.

Gerstoft, J. *et al.* (1986). Prognosis in glomerulonephritis. II. Regression analyses of prognostic factors affecting the course of renal function and the mortality in 395 patients. Calculation of a prognostic model. Report from a Copenhagen study group of renal diseases. *Acta Medica Scandinavica* **219**, 179–187.

Gilbert, R. D. and Wiggelinkhuizen, J. (1994). The clinical course of hepatitis B virus-associated nephropathy. *Pediatric Nephrology* **8**, 11–14.

Glassock, R. J. (1992). Secondary membranous glomerulonephritis. *Nephrology, Dialysis, Transplantation* **7** (Suppl. 1), 64–71.

Gluck, M. C. *et al.* (1973). Membranous glomerulonephritis. Evolution of clinical and pathologic features. *Annals of Internal Medicine* **78**, 1–12.

Gonzalo, A. *et al.* (1999). Membranous nephropathy associated with hepatitis B virus infection: long-term clinical and histological outcome. *Nephrology, Dialysis, Transplantation* **14**, 416–418.

Gruppo Italiano per lo Studio della Nefrite Lupica (GISNEL) (1992). Lupus nephritis: prognostic factors and probability of maintaining life-supporting renal function 10 years after the diagnosis. *American Journal of Kidney Diseases* **19**, 473–479.

Guella, A., Akhtar, M., and Ronco, P. (1997). Idiopathic membranous nephropathy in identical twins. *American Journal of Kidney Diseases* **29**, 115–118.

Haas, M., Spargo, B. H., and Coventry, S. (1995). Increasing incidence of focal–segmental glomerulosclerosis among adult nephropathies: a 20-year renal biopsy study. *American Journal of Kidney Diseases* **26**, 740–750.

Haas, M. *et al.* (1997). Changing etiologies of unexplained adult nephrotic syndrome: a comparison of renal biopsy findings from 1976–1979 and 1995–1997. *American Journal of Kidney Diseases* **30**, 621–631.

Hall, C. L. *et al.* (1987). The natural course of gold nephropathy: long term study of 21 patients. *British Medical Journal (Clinical Research Edition)* **295**, 745–748.

Harrison, D. J., Thomson, D., and MacDonald, M. K. (1986). Membranous glomerulonephritis. *Journal of Clinical Pathology* **39**, 167.

Hay, N. M. *et al.* (1992). Membranous nephropathy: a 19 year prospective study in 51 patients. *New Zealand Medical Journal* **105**, 489–491.

Heaf, J., Lokkegaard, H., and Larsen, S. (1999). The epidemiology and prognosis of glomerulonephritis in Denmark 1985–1997. *Nephrology, Dialysis, Transplantation* **14**, 1889–1897.

Herz, J. *et al.* (1988). Surface location and high affinity for calcium of a 500-kD liver membrane protein closely related to the LDL-receptor suggest a physiological role as lipoprotein receptor. *EMBO Journal* **7**, 4119–4127.

Heymann, W. *et al.* (1959). Production of the nephrotic syndrome in rats by Freund's adjuvants and a rat kidney suspension. *Proceedings of the Society of Experimental Biology and Medicine* **100**, 660–664.

Hiki, Y. *et al.* (1984). Strong association of HLA-DR2 and MT1 with idiopathic membranous nephropathy in Japan. *Kidney International* **25**, 953–957.

Hinglais, N. *et al.* (1986). Immunohistochemical study of the C5b-9 complex of complement in human kidneys. *Kidney International* **30**, 399–410.

Hogan, S. L. *et al.* (1995). A review of therapeutic studies of idiopathic membranous glomerulopathy. *American Journal of Kidney Diseases* **25**, 862–875.

Honkanen, E. (1986). Survival in idiopathic membranous glomerulonephritis. *Clinical Nephrology* **25**, 122–128.

Honkanen, E., Tornroth, T., and Gronhagen-Riska, C. (1992). Natural history, clinical course and morphological evolution of membranous nephropathy. *Nephrology, Dialysis, Transplantation* **7** (Suppl. 1), 35–41.

Honkanen, E. *et al.* (1994). Long-term survival in idiopathic membranous glomerulonephritis: can the course be clinically predicted? *Clinical Nephrology* **41**, 127–134.

Honkanen, E. *et al.* (1997). Urinary transforming growth factor-beta 1 in membranous glomerulonephritis. *Nephrology, Dialysis, Transplantation* **12**, 2562–2568.

Honkanen, E. *et al.* (1998). Adhesion molecules and urinary tumor necrosis factor-alpha in idiopathic membranous glomerulonephritis. *Kidney International* **53**, 909–917.

Hopper, J., Jr., Trew, P. A., and Biava, C. G. (1981). Membranous nephropathy: its relative benignity in women. *Nephron* **29**, 18–24.

Hsu, H. C. *et al.* (1989). Membranous nephropathy in 52 hepatitis B surface antigen (HBsAg) carrier children in Taiwan. *Kidney International* **36**, 1103–1107.

Janssen, N. M. and Genta, M. S. (2000). The effects of immunosuppressive and anti-inflammatory medications on fertility, pregnancy, and lactation. *Archives of Internal Medicine* **160**, 610–619.

Jennette, J. C., Iskandar, S. S., and Dalldorf, F. G. (1983). Pathologic differentiation between lupus and nonlupus membranous glomerulopathy. *Kidney International* **24**, 377–385.

Jindal, K. *et al.* (1992). Long-term benefits of therapy with cyclophosphamide and prednisone in patients with membranous glomerulonephritis and impaired renal function. *American Journal of Kidney Diseases* **19**, 61–67.

Joven, J. *et al.* (1990). Abnormalities of lipoprotein metabolism in patients with the nephrotic syndrome. *New England Journal of Medicine* **323**, 579–584.

Kerjaschki, D. and Farquhar, M. G. (1982). The pathogenic antigen of Heymann nephritis is a membrane glycoprotein of the renal proximal tubule brush border. *Proceedings of the National Academy of Sciences USA* **79**, 5557–5581.

Kerjaschki, D. and Neale, T. J. (1996). Molecular mechanisms of glomerular injury in rat experimental membranous nephropathy (Heymann nephritis). *Journal of the American Society of Nephrology* **7**, 2518–2526.

Kerjaschki, D., Miettinen, A., and Farquhar, M. G. (1987). Initial events in the formation of immune deposits in passive Heymann nephritis. gp330–anti-gp330 immune complexes form in epithelial coated pits and rapidly become attached to the glomerular basement membrane. *Journal of Experimental Medicine* **166**, 109–128.

Kerjaschki, D. *et al.* (1992). Identification of a pathogenic epitope involved in initiation of Heymann nephritis. *Proceedings of the National Academy of Sciences USA* **89**, 11179–11183.

Kern, W. F. *et al. Atlas of Renal Pathology*, Philadelphia, PA: W.B. Saunders, 1999.

Keur, I., Krediet, R. T., and Arisz, L. (1989). Glomerulopathy as a paraneoplastic phenomenon. *Netherlands Journal of Medicine* **34**, 270–284.

Kida, H. *et al.* (1986). Long-term prognosis of membranous nephropathy. *Clinical Nephrology* **25**, 64–69.

Kobayashi, Y. *et al.* (1982). Prednisone treatment of non-nephrotic patients with idiopathic membranous nephropathy. A prospective study. *Nephron* **30**, 210–219.

Kolasinski, S. L., Chung, J. B., and Albert, D. A. (2002). What do we know about lupus membranous nephropathy? An analytic review. *Arthritis and Rheumatism* **47**, 450–455.

Kon, S. P. *et al.* (1995). Urinary C5b-9 excretion and clinical course in idiopathic human membranous nephropathy. *Kidney International* **48**, 1953–1958.

Kopple, J. D. *et al.* (1997). Effect of dietary protein restriction on nutritional status in the Modification of Diet in Renal Disease Study. *Kidney International* **52**, 778–791.

Korbet, S. M. *et al.* (1996). The racial prevalence of glomerular lesions in nephrotic adults. *American Journal of Kidney Diseases* **27**, 647–651.

Koski, C. L. *et al.* (1983). Cytolysis of nucleated cells by complement: cell death displays multi-hit characteristics. *Proceedings of the National Academy of Sciences USA* **80**, 3816–3820.

Lai, K. N., Lo, S. T., and Lai, F. M. (1989). Immunohistochemical study of the membrane attack complex of complement and S-protein in idiopathic and secondary membranous nephropathy. *American Journal of Pathology* **135**, 469–476.

Lai, K. N. *et al.* (1990). The therapeutic dilemma of the usage of corticosteroid in patients with membranous nephropathy and persistent hepatitis B virus surface antigenaemia. *Nephron* **54**, 12–17.

Lai, K. N. *et al.* (1991). Membranous nephropathy related to hepatitis B virus in adults. *New England Journal of Medicine* **324**, 1457–1463.

Laluck, B. J., Jr. and Cattran, D. C. (1999). Prognosis after a complete remission in adult patients with idiopathic membranous nephropathy. *American Journal of Kidney Diseases* **33**, 1026–1032.

Lee, J. C., Yamauchi, H., and Hopper, J., Jr. (1966). The association of cancer and the nephrotic syndrome. *Annals of Internal Medicine* **64**, 41–51.

Lewis, E. J. (1993). Idiopathic membranous nephropathy—to treat or not to treat? *New England Journal of Medicine* **329**, 127–129.

Lin, C. Y. (1990). Hepatitis B virus-associated membraneous nephropathy: clinical features, immunological profiles and outcome. *Nephron* **55**, 37–44.

Lin, C. Y. (1995). Treatment of hepatitis B virus-associated membranous nephropathy with recombinant alpha-interferon. *Kidney International* **47**, 225–230.

Lisker-Melman, M. *et al.* (1989). Glomerulonephritis caused by chronic hepatitis B virus infection: treatment with recombinant human alpha-interferon. *Annals of Internal Medicine* **111**, 479–483.

Llach, F. (1985). Hypercoagulability, renal vein thrombosis, and other thrombotic complications of nephrotic syndrome. *Kidney International* **28**, 429–439.

MacTier, R. *et al.* (1986). The natural history of membranous nephropathy in the West of Scotland. *Quarterly Journal of Medicine* **60**, 793–802.

Maisonneuve, P. *et al.* (2000). Distribution of primary renal diseases leading to end-stage renal failure in the United States, Europe, and Australia/New Zealand: results from an international comparative study. *American Journal of Kidney Diseases* **35**, 157–165.

Mallick, N. P., Short, C. D., and Manos, J. (1983). Clinical membranous nephropathy. *Nephron* **34**, 209–219.

Marx, B. E. and Marx, M. (1997). Prognosis of idiopathic membranous nephropathy: a methodologic meta-analysis. *Kidney International* **51**, 873–879.

Marx, B. E. and Marx, M. (1999). Prediction in idiopathic membranous nephropathy. *Kidney International* **56**, 666–673.

Masala, A. *et al.* (1997). Use of testosterone to prevent cyclophosphamide-induced azoospermia. *Annals of Internal Medicine* **126**, 292–295.

Mathieson, P. W. *et al.* (1988). Prednisolone and chlorambucil treatment in idiopathic membranous nephropathy with deteriorating renal function. *Lancet* **2**, 869–872.

Meistric, M. L. *et al.* (1992). Impact of cyclophosphamide on long-term reduction in sperm count in men treated with combination chemotherapy for Ewing and soft tissue sarcomas. *Cancer* **70**, 2703–2712.

Miller, G. *et al.* (2000). Use of mycophenolate mofetil in resistant membranous nephropathy. *American Journal of Kidney Diseases* **36**, 250–256.

Moroni, G. *et al.* (1998). Treatment of membranous lupus nephritis. *American Journal of Kidney Diseases* **31**, 681–686.

Muirhead, N. (1999). Management of idiopathic membranous nephropathy: evidence-based recommendations. *Kidney International Supplement* **70**, S47–S55.

Murphy, B. F., Fairley, K. F., and Kincaid-Smith, P. S. (1988). Idiopathic membranous glomerulonephritis: long-term follow-up in 139 cases. *Clinical Nephrology* **30**, 175–181.

Neugarten, J., Acharya, A., and Silbiger, S. R. (2000). Effect of gender on the progression of nondiabetic renal disease: a meta-analysis. *Journal of the American Society of Nephrology* **11**, 319–329.

Noel, L. H. *et al.* (1979). Long-term prognosis of idiopathic membranous glomerulonephritis. Study of 116 untreated patients. *American Journal of Medicine* **66**, 82–90.

O'Callaghan, C. A. *et al.* (2002). Characteristics and outcome of membranous nephropathy in older patients. *International Urology and Nephrology* **33**, 157–165.

Ognibene, F. P. *et al.* (1995). *Pneumocystis carinii* pneumonia: a major complication of immunosuppressive therapy in patients with Wegener's granulomatosis. *American Journal of Respiratory and Critical Care Medicine* **151**, 795–799.

Ordonez, J. D. *et al.* (1993). The increased risk of coronary heart disease associated with nephrotic syndrome. *Kidney International* **44**, 638–642.

Orlando, R. A. *et al.* (1992). gp330 associates with a 44-kDa protein in the rat kidney to form the Heymann nephritis antigenic complex. *Proceedings of the National Academy of Sciences USA* **89**, 6698–6702.

Papagianni, A. A. *et al.* (2002). C5b-9 and adhesion molecules in human idiopathic membranous nephropathy. *Nephrology, Dialysis, Transplantation* **17**, 57–63.

Papiha, S. S. *et al.* (1987). HLA-A, B, DR and Bf allotypes in patients with idiopathic membranous nephropathy (IMN). *Kidney International* **31**, 130–134.

Pasquali, S. *et al.* (1993). Lupus membranous nephropathy: long-term outcome. *Clinical Nephrology* **39**, 175–182.

Passerini, P. *et al.* (1993). Idiopathic membranous nephropathy in the elderly. *Nephrology, Dialysis, Transplantation* **8**, 1321–1325.

Pedrini, M. T. *et al.* (1996). The effect of dietary protein restriction on the progression of diabetic and nondiabetic renal diseases: a meta-analysis. *Annals of Internal Medicine* **124**, 627–632.

Pei, Y., Cattran, D., and Greenwood, C. (1992). Predicting chronic renal insufficiency in idiopathic membranous glomerulonephritis. *Kidney International* **42**, 960–966.

Pena, A. *et al.* (2001). Membranous nephropathy associated with hepatitis B in Spanish children. *Clinical Nephrology* **55**, 25–30.

Penny, M. J., Boyd, R. A., and Hall, B. M. (1998). Mycophenolate mofetil prevents the induction of active Heymann nephritis: association with Th2 cytokine inhibition. *Journal of the American Society of Nephrology* **9**, 2272–2282.

Perico, N. *et al.* (1989). Blunted excretory response to atrial natriuretic peptide in experimental nephrosis. *Kidney International* **36**, 57–64.

Peterson, C. *et al.* (1988). Atrial natriuretic peptide and the renal response to hypervolemia in nephrotic humans. *Kidney International* **34**, 825–831.

Peterson, J. C. *et al.* (1995). Blood pressure control, proteinuria, and the progression of renal disease. The modification of diet in renal disease study. *Annals of Internal Medicine* **123**, 754–762.

Pietromonaco, S. *et al.* (1990). Molecular cloning of a cDNA encoding a major pathogenic domain of the Heymann nephritis antigen gp330. *Proceedings of the National Academy of Sciences USA* **87**, 1811–1815.

Plum, J., Mirzaian, Y., and Grabensee, B. (1996). Atrial natriuretic peptide, sodium retention, and proteinuria in nephrotic syndrome. *Nephrology, Dialysis, Transplantation* **11**, 1034–1042.

Ponticelli, C. and Moroni, G. (1998). Renal biopsy in lupus nephritis—what for, when and how often? *Nephrology, Dialysis, Transplantation* **13**, 2452–2454.

Ponticelli, C. *et al.* (1984). Controlled trial of methylprednisolone and chlorambucil in idiopathic membranous nephropathy. *New England Journal of Medicine* **310**, 946–950.

Ponticelli, C. *et al.* (1992a). Remissions and relapses in idiopathic membranous nephropathy. *Nephrology, Dialysis, Transplantation* **7** (Suppl. 1), 85–90.

Ponticelli, C. *et al.* (1992b). Methylprednisolone plus chlorambucil as compared with methylprednisolone alone for the treatment of idiopathic membranous nephropathy. The Italian Idiopathic Membranous Nephropathy Treatment Study Group. *New England Journal of Medicine* **327**, 599–603.

Ponticelli, C. *et al.* (1995). A 10-year follow-up of a randomized study with methylprednisolone and chlorambucil in membranous nephropathy. *Kidney International* **48**, 1600–1604.

Ponticelli, C. *et al.* (1998). A randomized study comparing methylprednisolone plus chlorambucil versus methylprednisolone plus cyclophosphamide in idiopathic membranous nephropathy. *Journal of the American Society of Nephrology* **9**, 444–450.

Pruchno, C. J. *et al.* (1989). Urinary excretion of C5b-9 reflects disease activity in passive Heymann nephritis. *Kidney International* **36**, 65–71.

Rabelink, T. J. *et al.* (1994). Thrombosis and hemostasis in renal disease. *Kidney International* **46**, 287–296.

Radhakrishnan, J. *et al.* (1994). Cyclosporine treatment of lupus membranous nephropathy. *Clinical Nephrology* **42**, 147–154.

Radis, C. D. *et al.* (1995). Effects of cyclophosphamide on the development of malignancy and on long-term survival of patients with rheumatoid arthritis. A 20-year followup study. *Arthritis and Rheumatism* **38**, 1120–1127.

Ramzy, M. H. *et al.* (1981). The long-term outcome of idiopathic membranous nephropathy. *Clinical Nephrology* **16**, 13–19.

Raychowdhury, R. *et al.* (1989). Autoimmune target in Heymann nephritis is a glycoprotein with homology to the LDL receptor. *Science* **244**, 1163–1165.

Raychowdhury, R. *et al.* (1996). Induction of Heymann nephritis with a gp330/megalin fusion protein. *American Journal of Pathology* **148**, 1613–1623.

Reichert, L. J. *et al.* (1994). Preserving renal function in patients with membranous nephropathy: daily oral chlorambucil compared with intermittent monthly pulses of cyclophosphamide. *Annals of Internal Medicine* **121**, 328–333.

Remuzzi, G., Schieppati, A., and Garattini, S. (1994). Treatment of idiopathic membranous glomerulopathy. *Current Opinion in Nephrology and Hypertension* **3**, 155–163.

Remuzzi, G. *et al.* (2002). Rituximab for idiopathic membranous nephropathy. *Lancet* **360**, 923–924 (letter).

Rivkees, S. A. and Crawford, J. D. (1998). The relationship of gonadal activity and chemotherapy-induced gonadal damage. *Journal of the American Medical Association* **259**, 2123–2125.

Robert, A. *et al.* (1987). Clinical correlation between hypercoagulability and thrombo-embolic phenomena. *Kidney International* **31**, 830–835.

Robinson, W. L. *et al.* (1984). Remission and exacerbation of tumor-related nephrotic syndrome with treatment of the neoplasm. *Cancer* **54**, 1082–1084.

Rosen, S. (1971). Membranous glomerulonephritis: current status. *Human Pathology* **2**, 209–231.

Rostoker, G. *et al.* (1993). Long-term cyclosporin A therapy for severe idiopathic membranous nephropathy. *Nephron* **63**, 335–341.

Rostoker, G. *et al.* (1995). Low-dose angiotensin-converting-enzyme inhibitor captopril to reduce proteinuria in adult idiopathic membranous nephropathy: a prospective study of long-term treatment. *Nephrology, Dialysis, Transplantation* **10**, 25–29.

Row, P. G. *et al.* (1975). Membranous nephropathy. Long-term follow-up and association with neoplasia. *Quarterly Journal of Medicine* **44**, 207–239.

Ruggenenti, P. *et al.* (1998). Renal function and requirement for dialysis in chronic nephropathy patients on long-term ramipril: REIN follow-up trial. Gruppo Italiano di Studi Epidemiologici in Nefrologia (GISEN). Ramipril efficacy in nephropathy. *Lancet* **352**, 1252–1256.

Ruggenenti, P. *et al.* (1999). Renoprotective properties of ACE-inhibition in non-diabetic nephropathies with non-nephrotic proteinuria. *Lancet* **354**, 359–364.

Saag, K. G. *et al.* (1998). Alendronate for the prevention and treatment of glucocorticoid-induced osteoporosis. Glucocorticoid-Induced Osteoporosis Intervention Study Group. *New England Journal of Medicine* **339**, 292–299.

Saito, A. *et al.* (1994). Complete cloning and sequencing of rat gp330/'megalin', a distinctive member of the low density lipoprotein receptor gene family. *Proceedings of the National Academy of Sciences USA* **91**, 9725–9729.

Saito, A. *et al.* (1996). Mapping rat megalin: the second cluster of ligand binding repeats contains a 46-amino acid pathogenic epitope involved in the formation of immune deposits in Heymann nephritis. *Proceedings of the National Academy of Sciences USA* **93**, 8601–8605.

Salant, D. J. *et al.* (1980). A new role for complement in experimental membranous nephropathy in rats. *Journal of Clinical Investigation* **66**, 1339–1350.

Sarasin, F. P. and Schifferli, J. A. (1994). Prophylactic oral anticoagulation in nephrotic patients with idiopathic membranous nephropathy. *Kidney International* **45**, 578–585.

Schena, F. P. (1997). Survey of the Italian Registry of Renal Biopsies. Frequency of the renal diseases for 7 consecutive years. The Italian Group of Renal Immunopathology. *Nephrology, Dialysis, Transplantation* **12**, 418–426.

Schieppati, A. *et al.* (1993). Prognosis of untreated patients with idiopathic membranous nephropathy. *New England Journal of Medicine* **329**, 85–89.

Schulze, M. *et al.* (1989). Increased urinary excretion of C5b-9 distinguishes passive Heymann nephritis in the rat. *Kidney International* **35**, 60–68.

Schulze, M. *et al.* (1991). Elevated urinary excretion of the C5b-9 complex in membranous nephropathy. *Kidney International* **40**, 533–538.

Shah, S. V. (1988). Evidence suggesting a role for hydroxyl radical in passive Heymann nephritis in rats. *American Journal of Physiology* **254**, F337–F344.

Shah, S. V. (1989). Role of reactive oxygen metabolites in experimental glomerular disease. *Kidney International* **35**, 1093–1106.

Shankland, S. J. (2000). New insights into the pathogenesis of membranous nephropathy. *Kidney International* **57**, 1204–1205.

Shankland, S. J. *et al.* (1996). Differential expression of transforming growth factor-beta isoforms and receptors in experimental membranous nephropathy. *Kidney International* **50**, 116–124.

Shankland, S. J. *et al.* (1997). Cyclin kinase inhibitors are increased during experimental membranous nephropathy: potential role in limiting glomerular epithelial cell proliferation *in vivo*. *Kidney International* **52**, 404–413.

Shankland, S. J., Pippin, J. W., and Couser, W. G. (1999). Complement (C5b-9) induces glomerular epithelial cell DNA synthesis but not proliferation in vitro. *Kidney International* **56**, 538–548.

Short, C. D. *et al.* (1987). Methylprednisolone in patients with membranous nephropathy and declining renal function. *Quarterly Journal of Medicine* **65**, 929–940.

Simon, P. *et al.* (1994). Epidemiology of primary glomerular diseases in a French region. Variations according to period and age. *Kidney International* **46**, 1192–1198.

Sloan, R. P. *et al.* (1996). Long-term outcome in systemic lupus erythematosus membranous glomerulonephritis. Lupus Nephritis Collaborative Study Group. *Journal of the American Society of Nephrology* **7**, 299–305.

Spitalewitz, S. *et al.* (1993). Treatment of hyperlipidemia in the nephrotic syndrome: the effects of pravastatin therapy. *American Journal of Kidney Diseases* **22**, 143–150.

Stirling, C. M., Simpson, K., and Boulton-Jones, J. M. (1998). Immunosuppression and outcome in idiopathic membranous nephropathy. *Quarterly Journal of Medicine* **91**, 159–164.

Thomas, D. M. *et al.* (1991). Enalapril can treat the proteinuria of membranous glomerulonephritis without detriment to systemic or renal hemodynamics. *American Journal of Kidney Diseases* **18**, 38–43.

Topham, P. S. *et al.* (1999). Complement-mediated injury reversibly disrupts glomerular epithelial cell actin microfilaments and focal adhesions. *Kidney International* **55**, 1763–1775.

Tornroth, T., Honkanen, E., and Pettersson, E. (1987). The evolution of membranous glomerulonephritis reconsidered: new insights from a study on relapsing disease. *Clinical Nephrology* **28**, 107–117.

Torres, A. *et al.* (2002). Conservative versus immunosuppressive treatment of patients with idiopathic membranous nephropathy. *Kidney International* **61**, 219–227.

Trew, P. A. *et al.* (1978). Renal vein thrombosis in membranous glomerulonephropathy: incidence and association. *Medicine (Baltimore)* **57**, 69–82.

Tu, W. H. *et al.* (1984). Membranous nephropathy: predictors of terminal renal failure. *Nephron* **36**, 118–124.

Van de Walle, J. G. *et al.* (1996). Renal sodium handling in children with nephrotic relapse: relation to hypovolaemic symptoms. *Nephrology, Dialysis, Transplantation* **11**, 2202–2208.

Vaughan, R. W. *et al.* (1995). An analysis of HLA class II gene polymorphism in British and Greek idiopathic membranous nephropathy patients. *European Journal of Immunogenetics* **22**, 179–186.

Vaziri, N. D. (1983). Nephrotic syndrome and coagulation and fibrinolytic abnormalities. *American Journal of Nephrology* **3**, 1–6.

Vlaovic, P. and Jewett, M. A. (1999). Cyclophosphamide-induced bladder cancer. *Canadian Journal of Urology* **6**, 745–748.

Wagoner, R. D. *et al.* (1983). Renal vein thrombosis in idiopathic membranous glomerulopathy and nephrotic syndrome: incidence and significance. *Kidney International* **23**, 368–374.

Warwick, G. L., Geddes, C. G., and Boulton-Jones, J. M. (1994). Prednisolone and chlorambucil therapy for idiopathic membranous nephropathy with progressive renal failure. *Quarterly Journal of Medicine* **87**, 223–229.

Wehrmann, M. *et al.* (1989). Long-term prognosis of chronic idiopathic membranous glomerulonephritis. An analysis of 334 cases with particular regard to tubulo-interstitial changes. *Clinical Nephrology* **31**, 67–76.

Wheeler, D. C. (1995). Lipids—what is the evidence for their role in progressive renal disease? *Nephrology, Dialysis, Transplantation* **10**, 14–16.

Wheeler, D. C. and Bernard, D. B. (1994). Lipid abnormalities in the nephrotic syndrome: causes, consequences, and treatment. *American Journal of Kidney Diseases* **23**, 331–346.

Wu, Q. *et al.* (2001). Analysis of prognostic predictors in idiopathic membranous nephropathy. *American Journal of Kidney Diseases* **37**, 380–387.

Yamauchi, H. *et al.* (1985). Cure of membranous nephropathy after resection of carcinoma. *Archives of Internal Medicine* **145**, 2061–2063.

Yuan, H. *et al.* (2002). Nephrin dissociates from actin, and its expression is reduced in early experimental membranous nephropathy. *Journal of the American Society of Nephrology* **13**, 946–956.

Zent, R., Nagai, R., and Cattran, D. C. (1997). Idiopathic membranous nephropathy in the elderly: a comparative study. *American Journal of Kidney Diseases* **29**, 200–206.

Zucchelli, P. *et al.* (1986). Clinical and morphologic evolution of idiopathic membranous nephropathy. *Clinical Nephrology* **25**, 282–288.

Zucchelli, P. *et al.* (1987). Long-term outcome of idiopathic membranous nephropathy with nephrotic syndrome. *Nephrology, Dialysis, Transplantation* **2**, 73–78.

Zucchelli, P. and Pasquali, S. Membranous nephropathy. In *Oxford Textbook of Clinical Nephrology* (ed. A. M. Davison). Oxford: Oxford University Press, 1996.

3.8 Mesangiocapillary glomerulonephritis

Vijay Kher and Sanjeev Gulati

Introduction

Mesangiocapillary glomerulonephritis (MCGN) is a morphological entity characterized by diffuse mesangial cellular proliferation and thickening of capillary walls due to subendothelial extension of mesangium. It has varied clinical manifestations, ranging from persistent microscopic haematuria or recurrent gross haematuria at one end to acute nephritic syndrome, nephrotic syndrome, and chronic renal failure at the other. Most cases are idiopathic, although a few are due to infections. A characteristic association of this entity is prolonged hypocomplementaemia, with evidence of activation of alternate complement pathway by nephritic factors.

This is certainly not a recent entity as is evident from the reappraisal of three postmortem kidney specimens originally described by Richard Bright—two of which have been established as the earliest known examples of MCGN (Weller and Nester 1972). However, even nearly two centuries later it continues to be an enigma for nephrologists the world over. Though the incidence of MCGN has declined in Europe, North America, and Japan (Simon *et al.* 1987; Itaka *et al.* 2000), it continues to be a common form of nephritis in the developing countries (Asinob *et al.* 1999; Gulati *et al.* 1999). Even in the developed countries, there has been a renewed interest in this entity with the emergence of viral infections like hepatitis C. We are still unsure as to the precise role of complement in the condition and sadly its management still remains a therapeutic dilemma.

Terminology

MCGN has been known by several other names. The most commonly used have been *membranoproliferative glomerulonephritis* (MPGN), *lobular glomerulonephritis*, and *chronic persistent hypocomplementaemic glomerulonephritis*. The term MCGN is a more precise and accurate anatomical description of the histological appearance, and will be used in this chapter.

MCGN has been subdivided on the basis of histopathological appearance into types I, II, and III. *Type I MCGN* ('classical' MPGN), the commonest of these, is morphologically an immune complex mediated glomerulonephritis in which the classic complement pathway is activated. Histologically, it is characterized by the presence of subendothelial deposits.

Type II MCGN, also known as *dense deposit disease*, resembles the earlier variety in its clinical features, association with hypocomplementaemia, and appearance on light microscopy. It differs from type I, however, in the involvement of the alternate complement pathway and presence of intramembranous dense deposits.

The term *Type III* has been used to describe other morphological variants of type I characterized by the presence of additional subepithelial deposits and complex glomerular basement membrane (GBM) alterations. Clinically, the affected patients are older, less often hypocomplementaemic, and have a more favourable prognosis.

Thus, histopathology forms the basis of differentiating these subtypes from each other although the clinical features are more or less similar. Thus, we will first describe the histopathological features.

Histopathology

Type I (classic) MCGN with subendothelial deposits (Fig. 1)

Glomeruli

The glomeruli show uniform changes and are all enlarged, with a diffuse increase in glomerular cellularity. The hypercellularity is usually global. The increase in cellularity within each glomerular lobule creates an accentuation of the lobular pattern or lobulation (Fig. 1a). The mesangial hypercellularity and the increase in the amount of mesangial matrix create a much larger mesangial or centrilobular area, with the lobules sometimes assuming a club shape. In some patients, however, the glomerular hypercellularity is associated with very little accentuation of the lobular pattern. It has been postulated that the severity of the mesangial lesion relates to the duration of renal disease. As the lobular lesion progresses, the cellularity tends to diminish and is replaced by an increase in mesangial matrix and sclerosis (Bohle *et al.* 1974).

There is diffuse thickening of the glomerular capillary walls; the thickening can be more prominent in some glomeruli and in some capillary loops than in others. Periodic acid-Schiff (PAS) and silver methenamine stains show that the thickened glomerular capillary walls often have two basement membranes with a clear or non-argyrophilic region between them (Figs 1c and 2). This double contour is sometimes termed as *tram tracking, splitting, or duplication of the GBM*. In some capillaries, the replication of basement membranes is very complex, resulting in multiple laminations. The double contour is brought about by the outward migration of mesangial cells along the inside of the capillary walls. Because mesangial cells produce basement membrane-like material, the cytoplasm of these cells is covered on the outside by the original basement membrane and on the inside by the newly formed membrane. Both the membranes stain positively with silver and give rise to the double contour.

Crescents may be noted also in some 10 per cent of patients. These crescents may be small and focal, or larger, affecting most of the

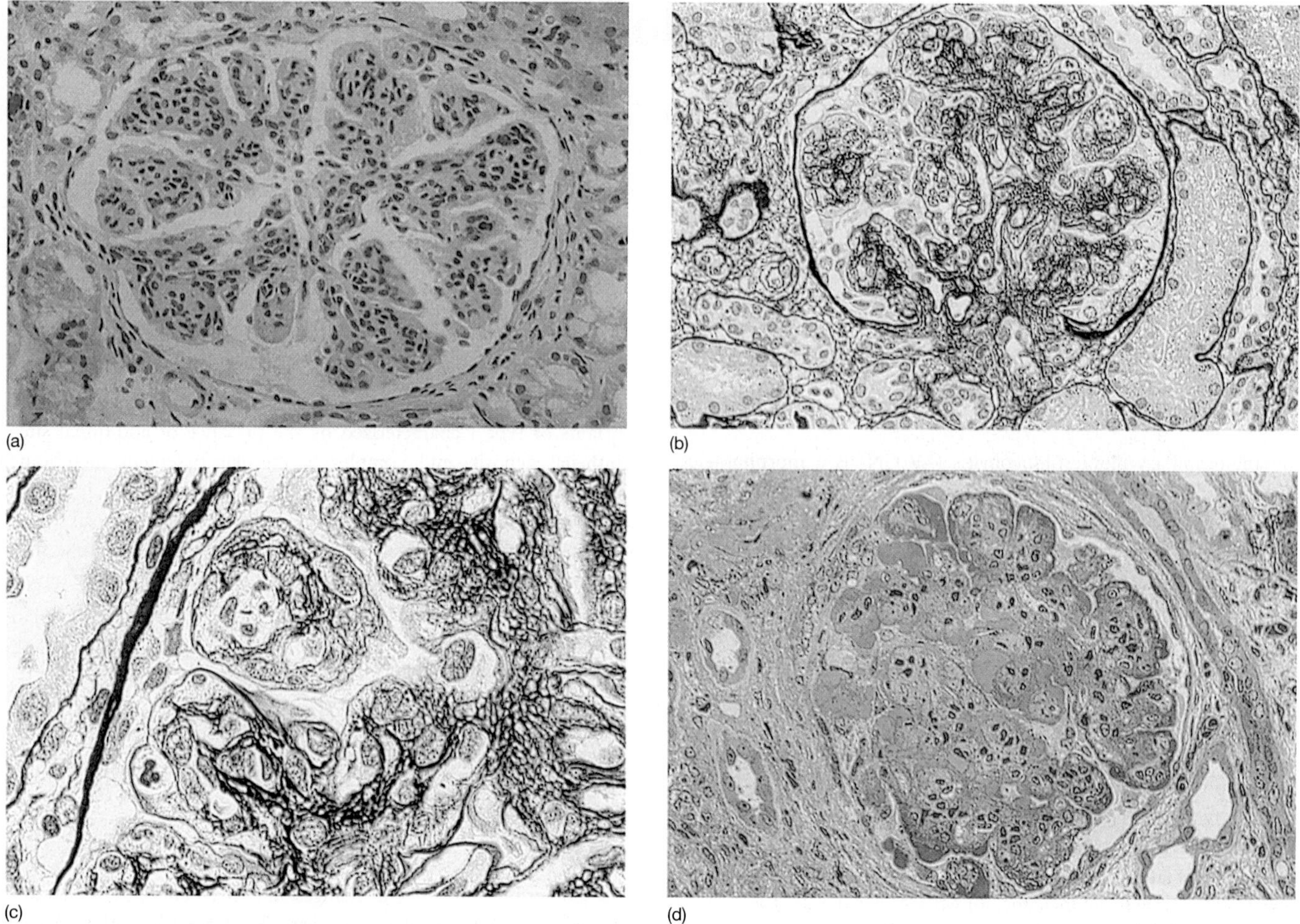

Fig. 1 (a) Glomerulus stained with haematoxylin and eosin. The extreme lobularity and increased mesangial cellurlarity of the glomerulus is shown—hence the now obsolete term 'lobular' glomerulonephritis. The extra cellularity is the result of both an increase in the number of mesangial cells and an infiltration with leucocytes, including polymorphonuclear neutrophils, which can be prominent in some cases (original magnification ×280). (b) Glomerulus stained with silver methenamine to show the diffuse increase in silver-positive mesangial matrix and the double contour' appearance of the glomerular capillary walls on silver staining (original magnification ×280). (By courtesy of Dr Barrie Hartley.) (c) A higher power view of a silver-stained preparation to show the complex thickening of the glomerular capillary walls. Nuclei of mesangial cells infiltrating between the true basement membrane (outer contour), and secreting mesangial matrix (inner contour), can be seen (original magnification ×980). (By courtesy of Dr Barrie Hartley.) (d) A 1-μm plastic-embedded section stained with toluidine blue, which shows the darker blue staining immune aggregates beneath the capillary basement membrane (original magnification ×100).

glomeruli. They often indicate a poorer prognosis (Jha *et al.* 1994; Kumar *et al.* 1996). In several studies of crescentric glomerulonephritis in children, type I MCGN accounts for up to approximately one-fourth of all cases (Jardim *et al.* 1992).

Blood vessels

Involvement of arteries and arterioles is common in patients who have renal failure and hypertension. There is marked arterial intimal thickening in patients with long-standing renal disease and in those in whom dialysis has been instituted. The presence of a vasculitis is strongly associated with underlying cryoglobulinaemia or hepatitis B or C related MCGN.

Electron microscopic findings

Electron microscopy has helped to distinguish type I MCGN from other glomerular lesions with features like MCGN, and to clarify the findings of light microscopy (Donadio *et al.* 1979). Ultrastructural studies have shown native GBM accompanied by subendothelial dense deposits and other glomerular deposits (Fig. 3). There is mesangial hypercellularity and increased mesangial matrix, both of which are often present between the normal-appearing GBM and glomerular endothelium (mesangial interposition). The new mesangial matrix-like material produced by the migrating mesangial cells creates an inner basement membrane. The thickened capillary wall is therefore composed of two or more layers of basement membrane-like material, interposed mesangial cells, and electron-dense, discrete immune-type deposits. In some cases, the double contour of the peripheral glomerular capillary wall is related to the interposition not of mesangial cells but of monocytes. This finding is characteristic of cryoglobulinaemic MCGN (Monga *et al.* 1987) (see Chapter 4.6). The electron-dense deposits are generally described as 'subendothelial' but are in fact nearly within the inner aspect of the original basement membrane.

Some patients have scattered, small glomerular subepithelial deposits quite similar to the humps noted in classic acute postinfectious (poststreptococcal) glomerulonephritis. They are found in as many as 30–50 per cent of cases studied (Lévy *et al.* 1979). Small subepithelial deposits may have accompanying protruding spikes of GBM-like material similar to that noted in membranous glomerulonephritis. The presence of large number of glomerular subepithelial deposits form part of the pattern of type III MCGN. Occasionally, intramembranous deposits are noted in type I MCGN and fragmentation of the GBM can occur. The application of silver impregnation on renal electron microscopy may help resolve the various patterns of MCGN. It may also be important to perform the ultrastructural studies at high magnification (e.g. 30,000×) to determine if the deposits have a microtubular substructure such as those seen with cryoglobulinaemia.

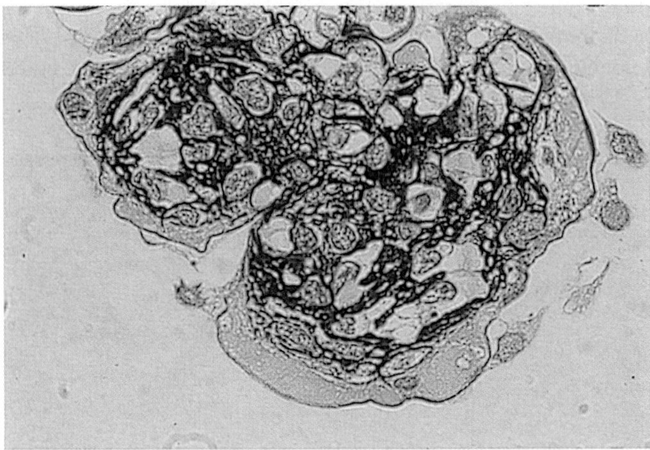

Fig. 2 Mesangiocapillary glomerulonephritis type I. A high-power view of the appearances in the capillary wall, showing the thin, silver-positive, true basement membrane on the outer surface of the capillary lobule, with a more irregular inner deposit of silver-staining, basement membrane-like material, secreted by interposed mesangial cells, within the lobule, which creates and nuclei, and silver-negative immune aggregates. Silver methanamine counterstained with haematoxylin and eosin; original magnification ×500. (By courtesy of Dr Barrie Hartley.)

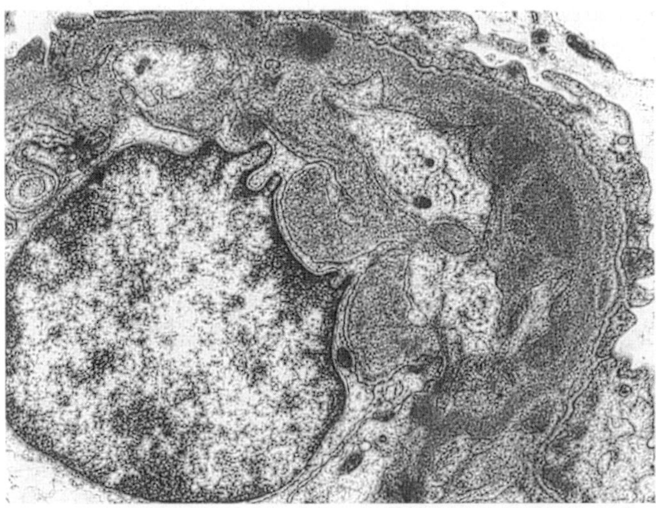

Fig. 3 Mesangiocapillary glomerulonephritis type I. This electron micrograph of the capillary wall shows the complex thickening to consist of the normal-looking basement membrane on the outside, with subendothelial electron-dense material representing immune aggregates in a subendothelial position. Within this are electron-lucent areas of interposed mesangial cell cytoplasm, and new basement membrane-like material abutting the capillary lumen filled by a large mononuclear cell. Original magnification ×9747. (By courtesy of Dr Barrie Hartley.)

Immunofluorescence findings

Immunofluorescence staining is generally quite typical (Belgiojoso *et al.* 1976). The most consistent finding is a strongly positive staining for C3 in a fine to coarse granular pattern along the glomerular capillaries (Fig. 4). A characteristic picture is produced, with the glomerular capillaries around the periphery of the expanded lobules predominantly, and often solely, affected, so that the lobules stand out quite clearly as a negative zone, cloaked by strongly positive glomerular capillaries that may impart a broken, wide, band-like pattern (Davis *et al.* 1978). C3 may also sometimes be noted, however, in the glomerular mesangium as well. When there is a great increase in the amount of mesangial matrix, mesangial deposits are often obscured or absent (Davis and Cavallo 1976). Mesangial C3 is less common than in dense deposit disease (type II MCGN). Early components of the classic pathway of complement activation (especially C1q) are sometimes visible and are present in about half to two-thirds of patients. There is no correlation between the immunofluorescent pattern and the serum complement profile (Silva 1998).

Immunoglobulins are noted in most patients; although the immunofluorescent staining is usually present in regions similar to those where C3 is evident, it is generally fainter than with C3. IgG is the immunoglobulin most commonly found, in some two-thirds of biopsies. The staining for IgG is thought to decrease as the disease progresses and the deposits become replaced or obscured by increase in mesangial matrix and sclerosis. IgM is less commonly evident than IgG, and is seen in 60–80 per cent of the patients (Donadio *et al.* 1979). A predominance of IgM is typically observed in type I MCGN from chronic

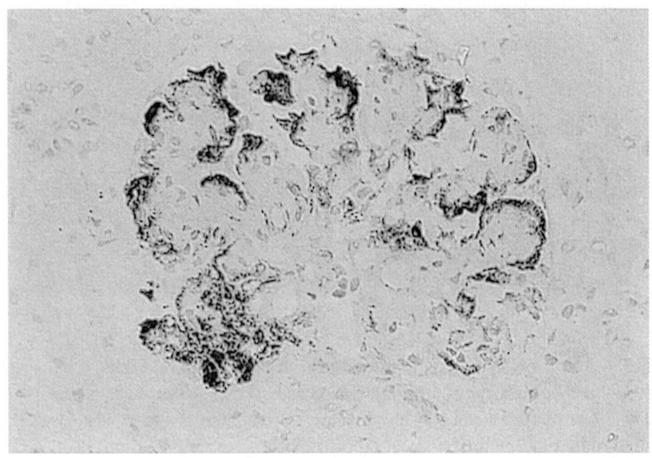

Fig. 4 Mesangiocapillary glomerulonephritis type I. Frozen section stained with immunoperoxidase conjugated, anti-IgM serum to demonstrate the lumpy aggregates of immune material present around the capillary walls. Original magnification ×200. (By courtesy of Dr Barrie Hartley.)

bacterial infection, such as osteomyelitis or infected ventriculoatrial shunt (see Chapter 3.12). IgA is found even less often. It is important to ascertain whether IgA is the predominant or co-dominant immunoreactant, in order to diagnose a mesangiocapillary form of IgA nephropathy, which is rare. IgD has been recorded, but it is usually accompanied by other immunoglobulins (Donadio *et al.* 1979).

Dense deposit disease (type II MCGN)

This has been reported to account for 15–33 per cent of all patients with (Figs 5–7) MCGN (Habib *et al.* 1975; Donadio *et al.* 1979) although its indicence seems to be declining.

Glomeruli

The designation 'dense deposit disease' is probably more precise than type II MCGN, as proliferative changes are not always present. The characteristic feature is the presence of semicontinuous 'deposits' within the glomerular capillary wall (specifically the GBM). Some degree of mesangial hypercellularity or sclerosis may be seen, although it is often less than that noted in type I MCGN. The thickening of the glomerular capillary walls is caused by these elongated, irregular intramembranous deposits (Habib *et al.* 1975; Donadio *et al.* 1979). The deposits are often ribbon-like, and stain strongly with eosin and appear somewhat refractile. They are intensely PAS-positive, and the trichrome stain shows them to be fuchsinophilic. These glomerular intramembranous deposits appear dark blue with toluidine blue in 0.5 or 1.0 mm plastic embedded sections (Campbell-Boswell *et al.* 1979). A double contour appearance of the glomerular capillary wall is noted

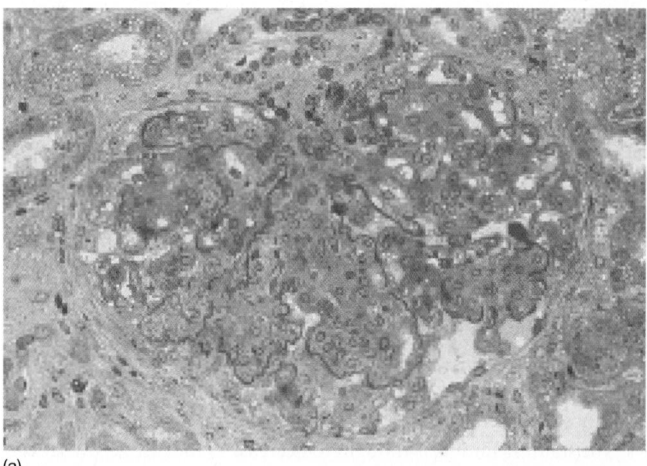
(a)

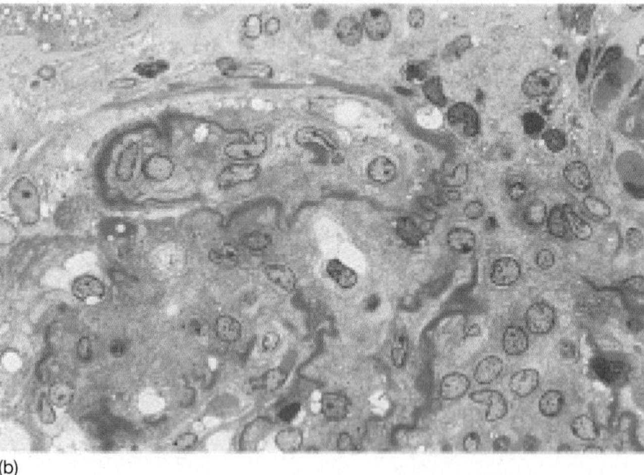
(b)

Fig. 5 Mesangiocapillary type II (dense-deposit disease). (a) Plastic-embedded section cut at 1-μm thickness and stained with toluidine blue. The linear material following the basement membrane of the capillary wall is also evident in Bowman's capsule (bottom). Original magnification ×400. (b) A higher magnification of a portion of the field in (a). The reflection of the dense material into Bowman's capsule is seen on the left (arrow). 'Breaks' in the continuity of the material within the basement membrane of the capillary wall can also be seen. Original magnification ×500. (By courtesy of Dr Barrie Hartley.)

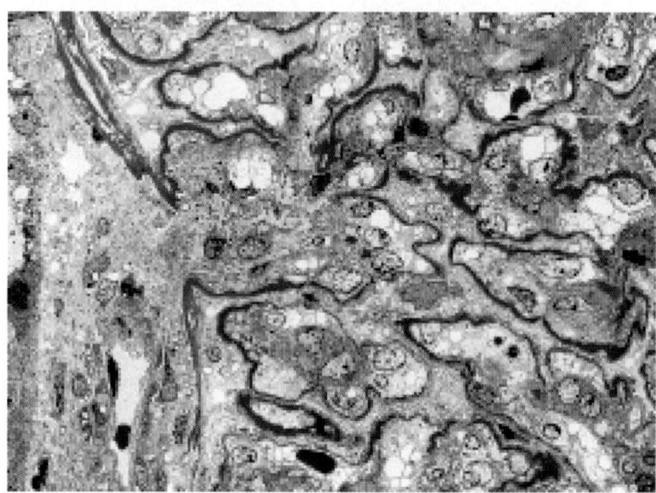

Fig. 6 Mesangiocapillary type II (dense-deposit disease). The glomerular hilus is at the centre left of the figure. The capillary basement membranes and Bowman's capsule (left) are replaced with a rather irregular, electron-dense, osmiophilic material, which occupies the lamina densa continuously with only a few breaks. Electron microphotograph; original magnification ×1200. (By courtesy of Dr Barrie Hartley.)

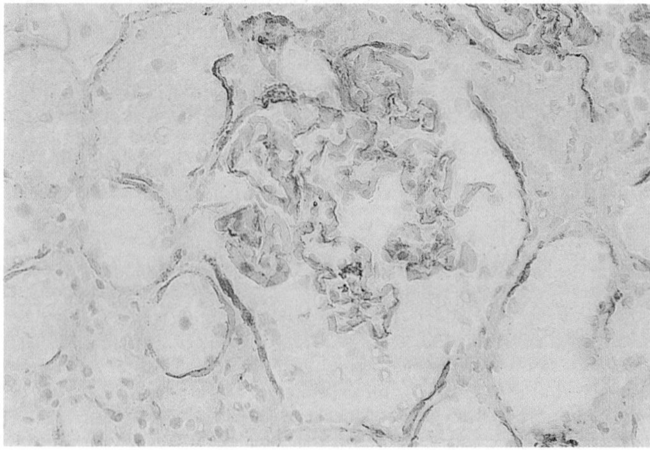

Fig. 7 Mesangiocapillary type II. Frozen section stained with immunoperoxidase conjugated, anti-Clq antibody to show the staining of the inner and outer basement membrane (lamina rara interna and externa) with complement components. Original magnification ×200. (By courtesy of Dr Barrie Hartley.)

in approximately half of the patients. The glomerular intramembranous deposits may also stain with the fluorochrome dye thioflavin T (Churg *et al.* 1979; Date *et al.* 1982). They vary greatly in size and number, and it is this feature that determines the extent of the glomerular capillary wall thickening. Although some authors believe that dense deposit disease can be diagnosed by light microscopy, in many cases electron microscopy will be needed to establish the presence of deposits with certainty. Glomerular subepithelial electron-dense discrete deposits similar to the subepithelial 'humps' noted in the classic acute postinfectious (poststreptococcal) glomerulonephritis may be seen in dense deposit disease (Joh *et al.* 1993). Bowman's capsule is often infiltrated with the material also.

Tubules

The same type of deposits noted in the GBM may be identified along the proximal and distal tubular basement membranes. With progression of glomerular sclerosis, there is tubular atrophy and interstitial fibrosis.

Blood vessels

Intimal thickening of the arteries becomes evident as the disease progresses, probably resulting from accompanying hypertension. Electron-dense deposits may be identified in a few interstitial capillaries and arterioles (Habib *et al.* 1975; Joh *et al.* 1993).

Interstitium

There may be interstitial inflammation, mostly caused by chronic inflammatory cells (i.e. lymphocytes). Foam cells are sometimes present, indicative of a persisting nephrotic syndrome. Interstitial fibrosis appears as renal failure develops. Tubulointerstitial nephritis may be seen.

Electron microscopy (Fig. 6)

Electron microscopy reveals unique alterations in the GBM. The disease takes the name 'dense deposit disease' from the characteristic ultrastructural appearance of the glomerular intramembranous deposits. The hallmark is the presence of dense osmiophilic material in the GBM (Joh *et al.* 1993), basal lamina of Bowman's capsule, tubular basement membrane—mostly proximal but also involving distal tubules and mesangial regions. Involvement of the glomerular capillary walls is variable and may show a variety of patterns. The deposits may replace the entire width of the lamina dense. In the latter instance, the remnant or native GBM can be identified on one or both sides of the dense deposits. The nature of the electron-dense deposit is still not known. The use of the word 'deposit' (as hitherto in this chapter) to describe the abnormality gives the impression that some extraneous material, usually by implication an antibody or antigen–antibody complexes, has been laid down in the GBM. There is, however, no evidence that this is so, from the details of abnormal membrane or immunohistological findings or serological studies. It is therefore likely that the GBM may have undergone a chemical change *in situ*. There is some suggestion that alteration in galactosyl residues has occurred.

Immunofluorescence findings

Immunofluorescence microscopy reveals intense staining for C3, noted along the glomerular capillary walls and often in the glomerular mesangial regions. The immunofluorescence pattern has been variously described as linear, pseudolinear, smooth, ribbon-like granular, or nodular (Habib *et al.* 1973, 1975; Davis *et al.* 1978; Kim *et al.* 1979; Joh *et al.* 1993). The C3 deposition is usually diffuse, global, and, as noted previously, intense. The staining may be continuous or discontinuous. The mesangial deposits may stain either as scattered granules or as heavy, coarse granules. The early components of complement, CIq and C4, are usually absent, although occasionally CIq is found (Fig. 7).

Differentiation of type I from type II MCGN generally poses little problem when light, immunofluorescence, and electron microscopy are all performed. The type I variety is characterized by interposed mesangial cytoplasm and subendothelial deposits while type II has intramembranous deposits and mesangial deposits (The Southwest Pediatric Nephrology Study Group 1985). However, when intramembranous deposits are focal and segmental, there may be some difficulty. Use of thioflavine T stains, immunofluorescence, and electron microscopic localization will facilitate the differentiation. Light-chain disease may also show similar findings, but the deposits are generally coarser and immunofluorescence microscopy of light chains is generally diagnostic (see Chapter 4.3) , and on occasion amyloidosis (see Chapter 4.2.1) and diabetes (see Chapter 4.1) may cause confusion on light microscopy using non-specific stains (see below).

Type III MCGN (mixed membranous and proliferative glomerulonephritis) (Fig. 8)

Burkholder *et al.* (1970) first described a subtype of MCGN with features of both membranous and proliferative glomerulonephritis. This pattern has some features of typical MCGN type I, such as thickening of the glomerular capillary walls, double contours, mesangial

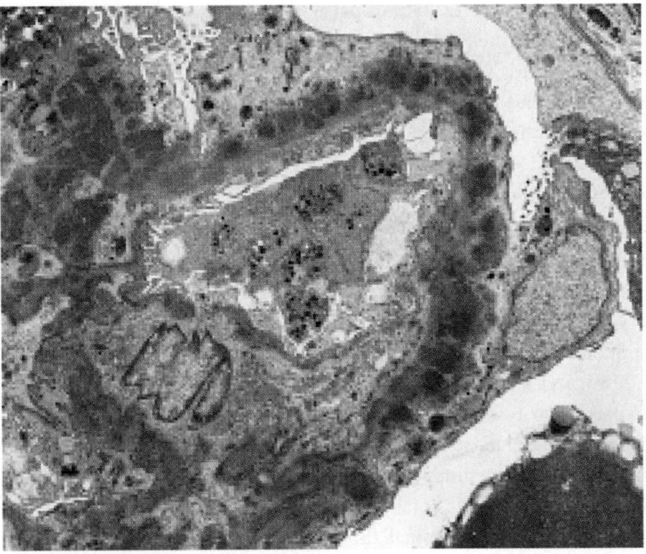

Fig. 8 Mesangiocapillary glomerulonephritis type III. This electron micrograph shows the irregular appearance of electron-dense, presumed immune aggregates within, outside, and under the glomerular capillary basement membrane. Many observers regard this as a late variant of type I mesangiocapillary glomerulonephritis, but others as a distinct histopathological entity. This appearance may be easily confused with a late membranous nephropathy. Original magnification ×3822. (By courtesy of Dr Barrie Hartley.)

interposition, and subendothelial deposits. In addition, however, there were silver-positive spikes along the GBM and trichrome positive subepithelial humps such as are seen in stage III membranous glomerulonephritis. Ultrastructural studies reveal the presence of glomerular electron-dense deposits, and immunofluorescent staining showed a heavy granular pattern along the glomerular capillary walls and mesangium for C3 and sometimes for IgG and IgM. There are glomerular subendothelial and subepithelial deposits, which are often contiguous or connect through the lamina densa of the GBM (Burkholder *et al.* 1970; Anders and Thoenes 1975). These deposits sometimes have a 'washed-out' appearance together with a layering of the lamina-densa-like material. This pattern was initially described on the basis of ultrathin silver-impregnated plastic embedded sections studied with optical and electron microscopy. There is complex disruption of the GBM (lamina densa), often with thickening and expansion of the basement membrane and layering by a silver-negative basement membrane-like material.

Differential diagnosis

Apart from morphological lesions identical to MCGN being described in numerous forms with recognizable aetiologic agents, or occurring in association with other diseases (Table 1 and see below) as mentioned above, several other histological appearances may easily be confused with idiopathic MCGN, especially on light microscopy using non-specific stains such as haematoxylin and eosin. These can, however, be differentiated on the basis of clinical features, laboratory findings, and characteristic histological, immunohistological, and ultrastructural features. In addition, several other conditions may mimic the appearances of MCGN closely.

Diabetes mellitus (Chapter 4.1)

Patients with diabetic nephropathy have small nodular lesions and lobular enlargement, which may give an appearance similar to the lobular form of MCGN. However, the diffuse distribution of these lesions in MCGN and the immunohistology helps in distinguishing it from diabetic nephropathy.

Mixed cryoglobulinaemia (Chapter 4.6)

This entity is characterized by reversible precipitation of immunoglobulins at cold temperatures. In type II mixed cryoglobulinaemia (MC) a particularly well-defined pattern of glomerular involvement called cryoglobulinaemic glomerulonephritis has been described, in which the monoclonal rheumatoid factor usually is an IgM-k (Monga *et al.* 1985; D'Amico *et al.* 1989). This is characterized by massive endocapillary hypercellularity due to an infiltration of monocytes (Mazzucco *et al.* 1986; Monga *et al.* 1986). Another typical morphological feature is the frequent and sometimes massive presence of amorphous, eosinophilic, PAS-positive deposits totally filling the capillary lumina, giving the appearance of 'intraluminal thrombi' (Tarantino *et al.* 1981; Monga *et al.* 1986; Castiglione *et al.* 1988). Thickening of the GBM, with a double contoured appearance is due to a characteristic *peripheral interposition of monocytes* (Mazzucco *et al.* 1986; D'Amico *et al.* 1989). In at least one-third of the patients with MC, vasculitis of small and medium-sized arteries is found. Immunohistological features follow a predictable pattern and the pattern of deposition. The identity of the prevailing immunoreactants is particularly important in the differential diagnosis (Ben Bassat *et al.* 1983). The pattern is characterized by large deposits in capillary lumina as intraluminal thrombi and diffuse granular staining of peripheral capillary walls (subendothelial deposits). IgM and lgG are the prevailing immunoreactants, suggesting that the deposits are locally trapped or precipitated cryoglobulins.

Table 1 Clinical associations of mesangiocapillary glomerulonephritis

Disease	MCGN type	Cross references
Infections		
Streptococcal (serological)	I and II	Chapter 3.12
Infective endocarditis (mainly streptococcal)	I	Chapter 3.12
Shunt nephritis (staphylococcal)	I	Chapter 3.12
Abscesses	I	Chapter 3.12
Buckley's syndrome (raised serum IgE, dermatitis)	I	
Sinusitis	I	
Cystic fibrosis	I	
Tuberculosis	I	Chapter 3.14
Leprosy	I	Chapter 3.14
Mycoplasma	I	
Hepatitis B	I	Chapter 3.12/3.14
Hepatitis C	I	Chapter 4.6
Hepatitis G?	I	
Filariasis	I	Chapter 3.12/3.14
Malaria	I	Chapter 3.12/3.14
Schistosomiasis	I	Chapter 3.12/3.14
Candidiasis	II	
Autommunity		
Systemic lupus erythematosus	I (II)	Chapter 4.7.1/4.7.2
Systemic sclerosis	I	Chapter 4.8
Mixed cryoglobulinaemia	I	Chapter 4.10
Castleman's disease	I	
Sjögren's syndrome	I	
Hypocomplementaemic urticarial vasculitis	I	
Neoplasia/dysproteinaemia		
Carcinoma	I	Chapter 3.13
Leukaemias	I	Chapter 3.13
Lymphoma (Hodgkin's and non-Hodgkin's)	I	Chapter 3.13
Ovarian dysgerminoma	I	
Myeloma	I	Chapter 4.3
Light-chain nephropathy	I	Chapter 4.3
Waldenstrom's macroglobulinaemia		Chapter 4.3
Metabolic		
Alpha 1-antitrypsin deficiency	I	
Complement deficiency	I and II	
Hypogammaglobulinaemia		
Miscellaneous		
Sickle-cell disease	I	Chapter 4.11
Cyanotic heart disease	I	
Sarcoidosis	I	Chapter 4.4
Partial lipodystrophy (with complement deficiency)	II (and occasionally I)	
Hydatidiform mole	I	
Ulcerative colitis		
Downs' syndrome		

Amyloidosis (Chapter 4.2.1)

On haematoxylin and eosin staining, the nodular deposits of amyloid may resemble MCGN. However, specific amyloid stains (Congo red), the failure of the material in MCGN to take silver stains, immunohistochemistry, and electron microscopy help in distinguishing the two.

Systemic lupus erythematosus (Chapter 4.7.1)

Renal morphological features similar to those of idiopathic MCGN, with marked and homogeneous mesangial proliferation and a diffuse double-contoured appearance of thickened capillary walls, are present but uncommon in systemic lupus erythematosus (SLE). In fact, in type IV diffuse SLE nephritis, the proliferation is usually much more irregular and patchy than the diffuse changes found in idiopathic MCGN (Austin *et al.* 1984; Balow and Austin 1988). Intraglomerular leucocyte infiltration is present with segmental distribution on the tuft, often in areas with necrotic changes (Alexoupoulos *et al.* 1990). Intracapillary necrosis is common and confined mainly to a single lobule, whereas in idiopathic MCGN this has never been described. Often, pyknotic nuclear debris is seen in and around the necrotic segment. It is in these areas that the so-called haematoxylin bodies are most frequently recognized. Typically, the capillary walls are quite irregularly involved; the capillary loops may be markedly thickened and have a rigid, refractile appearance on routine haematoxylin and eosin staining, the classic 'wire loop' (Austin *et al.* 1984). The diffuse double contour of thickened basement membranes is rare in SLE. The intense positivity for Clq in SLE nephritis is an important feature in the differential diagnosis with regard to other forms of MCGN. Simultaneous presence of deposits in *subepithelial, mesangial, subendothelial, and intramembranous sites* on electron microscopy is suggestive of lupus nephritis. Finally, serology helps in the distinction of both the complement profile (see below) and the presence or absence of anti-DNA antibodies.

Light-chain nephropathy (Chapter 4.3)

The appearance of glomerular lesions occurring in light-chain disease may be variable, but the most common feature is massive mesangial nodules, similar to those seen in the nodular form of type I MCGN (Gallo *et al.* 1980). The staining characteristics of the glomerular nodules, however, are different in the two diseases; those found in light-chain disease are *more PAS-positive, and negative on silver staining*. Moreover, the constant presence in light-chain disease of tubular basement membrane, vascular, and interstitial deposits is frequently sufficient to trigger the suspicion that the underlying cause of the nephropathy is systemic deposition of immunoglobulin fragments. Immunofluorescence allows a further differentiation, with a *strong staining for k light chains* in glomeruli, tubular basement membrane, vessels, and interstitium (Gallo *et al.* 1980; Silver *et al.* 1986). Finally, electron microscopy shows *typical fine granular deposits of extremely electron-dense material* distributed through the mesangial area and along the GBM (Seymour *et al.* 1980).

Liver disease

A pattern of MPGN has been described in a number of forms of liver disease (Montoliu *et al.* 1986). The morphological picture is often indistinguishable from the glomerular lesions of classic type I MCGN. The prevalence and intense *positivity for IgA in the mesangium and capillary walls* is the most important characteristic finding in all these examples.

Henoch–Schönlein purpura (Chapter 4.5.2)

Some of these patients may have a variant of MCGN (pseudo-MCGN). However, this differs from the idiopathic variety by its characteristic mesangial deposition of IgA.

Postinfectious nephritis (Chapters 3.9 and 3.12)

Sometimes patients with postinfectious nephritis may have histological lesions similar in appearance to MCGN. However, the intramembranous deposits are seen in short stretches, and never diffuse as in MCGN.

Evolution of histological changes

Most patients of types I and II MCGN who have more than 50 per cent of glomeruli affected remain in this category if repeat biopsies are examined, although a decrease in affected glomeruli can occur (Taguchi and Bohle 1989). Most patients with less than 50 per cent of glomeruli involved show an increase but again reversal may occur. In type I MCGN, focal changes may become diffuse or may remit. The majority of cases have diffuse changes on presentation and these remain. Proliferation and lobularity tend to diminish with time. The number and distribution of deposits in type I vary with time but type II deposits tend to persist. Spontaneous improvement resulting in return of glomeruli to normal have been noted, particularly in those associated with infections that regress but also in apparently idiopathic cases of type I. Clinical observation shows that most patients with type II MCGN have continuing and progressive disease; recorded histological regression of the dense deposits is rare (Habib *et al.* 1973).

'Secondary' forms of MCGN (Rennke 1995)

In addition to the idiopathic forms of MCGN discussed above, this form of glomerulonephritis may be found in many other conditions, shown in Table 1. The important points to note from Table 1 are the prominent part played by infections, with the corollary that secondary forms are more common than the idiopathic form in developing countries. The majority of secondary forms—and almost exclusively those caused by infections—are MCGN of type I. These cases also account for the majority of patients reported to have spontaneous regression.

A special relationship has long been known to exist between MCGN, almost always of type II, hypocomplementaemia from nephritic factor, and *partial (upper body) lipodystrophy*, both of which may precede the onset of the renal disease or appear at about the same time (Fig. 9). Only recently has the relationship of the loss of subcutaneous fat become clearer (Mathieson and Peters 1997), in that adipocytes play a major role in complement metabolism through production of complement factor D, which as a serine protease cleaves factor B of the alternative pathway. Nephritic factor can induce complement-mediated lysis of adipocytes *in vitro* and possibly *in vivo* if infection triggers cytokine release—a common prelude to the onset of lipodystrophy.

Aetiology and pathogenesis of MCGN

The aetiology and pathogenesis of this glomerular transformation is largely unknown. The following information needs to be considered before trying to explain the pathogenesis.

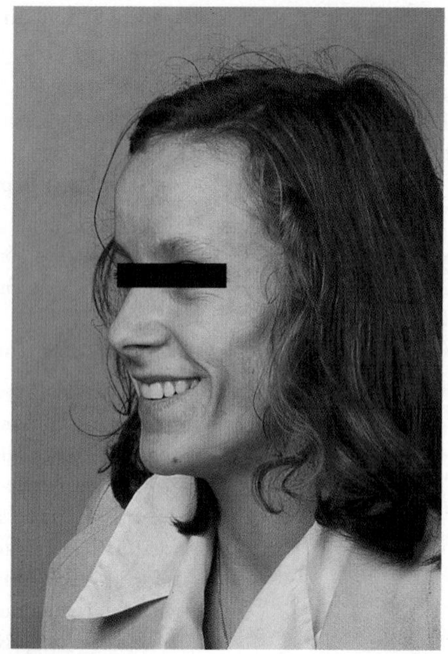

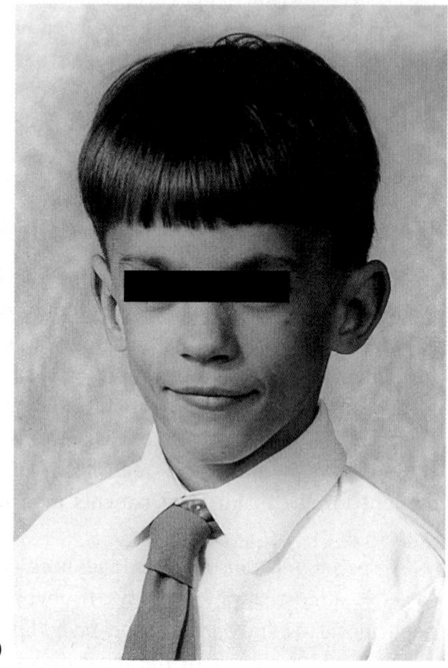

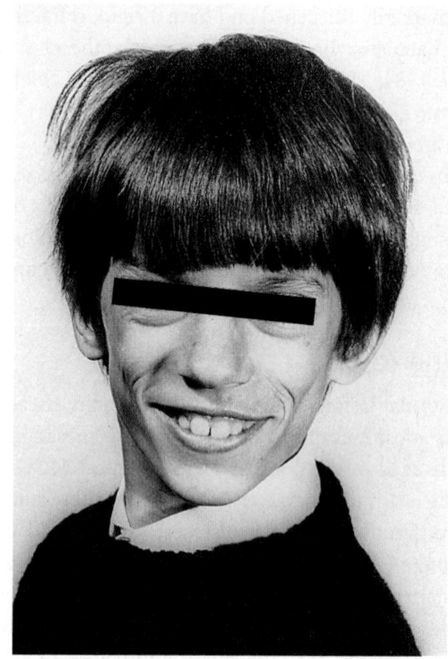

Fig. 9 (a) A young woman with facioscapular partial lipodystrophy. The 'paper-thin' smile is seen. (b) Family photographs of a normal young boy (left) who developed partial lipodystrophy (right) following an attack of measles. He went on to have mesangiocapillary glomerulonephritis and renal failure.

Natural and experimental animal models of MCGN

Naturally occurring animal models of MCGN include forms found in cats, beagle dogs, and Finnish-Landrace lambs, all of which have been reported to develop a spontaneous type I MCGN. In Yorkshire piglets also, homozygous deficiency of factor H is always associated with a fatal chronic glomerulonephritis, which resembles in some respects type II MCGN (Jansen *et al.* 1993, 1998). Their 50 per cent survival of 37 days could be extended to 82 days by weekly transfusions of normal porcine plasma. Glomerular complement deposition starts *in utero*. Postnatally, the GBM becomes greatly thickened by material that contains C3 as well as terminal complement components. Jansen *et al.* (1998) speculate that complement activation occurs *in situ* within the GBM, which if true has important implications for the pathogenesis of human type II MCGN.

Genetic studies in human MCGN

MCGN has been reported in siblings from several families (Bogdanovic *et al.* 2000) and in successive generations of a family with either X-linked recessive (Stutchfield *et al.* 1986) or autosomal dominant modes of inheritance (Sherwood *et al.* 1987). There have been reports also of an association between type I MCGN and the genotype HLA-B8, -DR3 SC01,-G402 (Welch *et al.* 1986). There may be an impairment of closely linked B-cell alloantigens (also called Ia antigens) that are concerned with the genetic control of specific immunological responses. This impairment could affect antigen recognition or the ability to respond to that antigen. A specific B-lymphocyte determinant (or surface antigen) has been suggested to be associated with MCGN by Friend *et al.* (1977). In another study, an increase in the number of IgM immunoglobulin-bearing lymphocytes was observed in patients with type I MCGN and dense deposit disease, as well as in certain family members of patients who had no renal disease (Sakai *et al.* 1979).

Infection and chronic antigenaemia

Information on the aetiologic agents in all types of MCGN (types I, II, and III) is scarce, and the exact pathogenesis remains unclear. It is believed that type I MCGN results from chronic antigenaemia and generation of nephritogenic immune complexes (a chronic serum sickness-like response). The precise nature of the putative antigen(s) in most patients with type I MCGN is unknown, however, and these are classified as 'idiopathic'. However, there are many examples of secondary type I MCGN that appear to be caused by immune complexes generated by infections or autoimmune or neoplastic diseases (Table 1). The incidence of type I MCGN has declined in the West in accordance with a decline in the incidence of infections and of postinfectious nephritis in general, including poststreptococcal disease, which may be associated also with type I MCGN. The origin and nature of type II MCGN, dense deposit disease is completely unknown.

The role of platelets

In experimental models of MCGN, platelets have been found to participate in glomerular damage along with other mediators (Kasai *et al.* 1981; Cameron 1984). Platelets contain potent mitogenic proteins like platelet specific protein factor 4 and platelet derived growth factor (PDGF), which have chemotactic activity for neutrophils and monocytes. Activated platelets also release transforming growth factor β, which plays a predominant role in the evolution of glomerular sclerosis by stimulating matrix protein deposition and inhibiting its resorption. Patients with MCGN have enhanced platelet activation, as established by lower intraplatelet concentration of serotonin, higher levels of free plasma serotonin, and non-thrombin platelet-aggregating material (Parbatni *et al.* 1980; Kasai *et al.* 1981) and although there is some correlation with disease activity, there is considerable overlap between normal and abnormal values. Donadio *et al.* (1984) provided evidence of diminished platelet survival in more than two-thirds of their patients; the glomerular filtration rate (GFR) stabilized or improved after treatment with antiplatelet drugs (dipyridamole and aspirin) (see below). Platelet antigens have been demonstrated in glomeruli (Miller *et al.* 1980). However, the actual role and importance of *in vivo* platelet activation remains unclear as it does in glomerulonephritis in general.

Role of circulating immune complexes and humoral immunity

There is considerable evidence to suggest that MCGN, especially type I, is an immune complex-mediated glomerulonephritis. This includes the finding of immunoreactants in the glomeruli, the presence of serum and glomerular cryoglobulins, and the presence of circulating immune complexes (CICs) in the serum in about half of the patients. To add to this is the occurrence of secondary type I MCGN in patients with known immune complex diseases, such as SLE, shunt nephritis, chronic bacteraemia, and chronic hepatitis B or C infections (see Chapter 3.12). The proportion of B-lymphocyte subsets with surface IgG or other determinants is increased in a number of primary glomerular diseases, including MCGN, which suggests enhanced antibody production that could contribute to immune complex formation.

The role of cellular immunity

There is some evidence that cellular immunity may play a role in the pathogenesis of MCGN. Patients with MCGN have been documented to have high titres of lymphocytotoxic antibodies (Nabakayashi *et al.* 1985). Other studies have documented depression of Natural Killer cell-mediated immunity, and antibody-dependent cell mediated cytotoxicity (Dobrin *et al.* 1975; Hruby *et al.* 1985). Alternatively, these defects may be only epiphenomena.

The role of complement deficiency

MCGN has been associated with a number of complement deficient states, such as partial lipodystrophy with acquired persistently low plasma C3 concentrations (see below), as well as genetic deficiencies of Clq, C2, C3, C6, C7, C8, factor B, and the complement degradation inhibitor factors H and l (Pickering *et al.* 1971; Coleman *et al.* 1983) (Fig. 9). Some studies have suggested that complement depletion represents an immune deficiency state that predisposes the individual to chronic bacterial and viral infections and subsequent immune complex formation (Coleman *et al.* 1983). It is also possible that complement deficiency impairs the solubilization, disaggregation, and clearance of deposited immune complexes.

Takahashi *et al.* (1978) and Coleman *et al.* (1983) noted a significantly higher incidence of all complement deficiencies (23 per cent) in patients with MCGN types I and III than among normal subjects (7 per cent) or patients with other types of glomerulonephritis (5 per cent). These complement deficiencies in patients with MCGN were either partial (heterozygous) or complete (homozygous) and were present for long periods of time as well as in healthy family members. Inhibition of immune complex solubilization in the sera of patients with MCGN has been found. The inhibition was more dramatic in those with active disease, but it did not correlate with the form of therapy, proteinuria, level of CICs, or serum level of complement.

Hypocomplementaemia

Hypocomplementaemia, usually persistent, is frequently present in all types of MCGN. Cross-sectional studies show that 50–60 per cent of all patients have a low concentration of C3, and consequently also a low serum level of haemolytic complement (CH50) (Habib *et al.* 1973, 1975; Cameron *et al.* 1983; Schwertz *et al.* 2001). The concentration of C4 tends to be normal, which helps in diagnosis from other hypocomplementaemic states. Thus, the hypocomplementaemia is produced through activation of the *alternative pathway* C3 convertase, C3b.Bb, whose persistence in the circulation is stabilized by autoantibodies known as 'nephritic factors'. Although a nephritic factor was first described nearly 30 years ago, there is little clinical evidence that this autoantibody is by itself nephritogenic. There are no studies to date that have demonstrated correlations between hypocomplementaemia (assumed to indicate the presence of nephritic factor) and onset or progression of type II MCGN. As a result, nephritic factors have usually been considered as epiphenomena. The hypocomplementaemia could operate by allowing persistent infection due to inefficient opsonization and continuous immune-complex formation, and/or by a relative failure of the complement-mediated solubilization of immune complexes.

Various studies (Pangburn and Muller-Eberhard 1984a,b; West and McAdams. 1995) show that active C3 convertase circulating in excess is associated with glomerular deposits. These glomerular deposits are basic to nephritogenesis, and thus convertase in excess is associated with nephritis. Production of the alternative pathway convertase C3b.Bb, proceeds continually in the circulation, by combination of C3 nephritic factor to C3b.Bb in the presence of magnesium (Pangburn and Muller-Eberhard 1984a,b; West 1994). The binding of C3 nephritic factors to C3b.Bb does not allow enzymatic inactivation of this complex, thus resulting in continuous C3 breakdown. The instability of native C3b.Bb makes its direct measurement in serum difficult, and its presence in excess must be inferred from the presence of factor H dysfunction. In a study of 27 individuals with factor H deficiency (who have continuous activation of the alternative pathway, with convertase present in excess in the circulation), 14 (52 per cent) had signs of nephritis, a frequency significantly above the norm. In 10 of these patients, the nephritis was mild and in some transient, but four had severe disease resulting in renal failure (Strife *et al.* 1977; Meri *et al.* 1992; Deschenes *et al.* 1996). The nephritis was not of immune complex origin, however, and IgG and C4 were not found in the glomerular deposits.

Nephritic factors have been shown to be responsible for the hypocomplementaemia in types II and III MCGN. The factor found in type II MCGN was originally known as 'C3 nephritic factor' or C3NeF, but to distinguish it from nephritic factors described later, it has been subsequently designated as the nephritic factor of the amplification loop, or Nf_a. It is an IgG autoantibody which reacts with an epitope on the activated factor B of native convertase to form a complex of C3b.Bb.Nf_a (Scott *et al.* 1978). Complexing with this autoantibody both increases the stability of the convertase and makes it resistant to dissociation by factor H. In the absence of factor H, the stabilized convertase has a half-life 16-fold greater than that of native C3b.Bb (Weiler *et al.* 1976). Most of the patients with circulating Nf_a have type II MCGN, a few have partial lipodystrophy with or without type II MCGN, and some apparently healthy individuals have been reported who had neither of the above. Because C3b.Bb.Nf_a activates only C3, it can produce marked depression of the serum C3 level with little or no depression of other complement components (Mollnes *et al.* 1986; Ng and Peters 1986; West and McAdams 1999).

The nephritic factor of the terminal pathway (NF_t) produces the hypocomplementaemia in type III MCGN (West and McAdams 1999). It differs from Nf_a in that it activates terminal components. Because activation of C5 requires at least two C3b molecules in close proximity, NF_t-stabilized convertase is thought to have the composition: C3bn.Bb.P.NF_t. Compatible with the *in vitro* observations, patients with NF_t have depressed plasma concentrations of both C3 and C5, and many have reduced concentrations of one or more of the other terminal components (West and McAdams 1999). Concentrations of properdin are also depressed. For reasons not clear, about 20 per cent of the patients with type I MCGN (33 per cent of the hypocomplementaemic patients) have evidence for circulating NF_t, although their disease otherwise has the characteristics of being circulating immune complexed in origin (Daha *et al.* 1977; Pangburn and Muller-Eberhard 1984a,b).

In types II and III MCGN, paramesangial deposits correlate with a depressed level of C3, or a depressed level in the recent past, and in type III MCGN, subendothelial deposits strongly correlate with hypocomplementaemia (West and McAdams 1998).

Type I can be distinguished from type III by differences in the frequency of subendothelial and paramesangial deposits in specimens obtained during normo- and hypocomplementaemia. Thus, absence of subendothelial deposits in biopsies obtained when the C3 level is low is evidence for type III MCGN while their presence when the C3 level is normal is evidence for type I. The reverse, however, does not apply. Also, the presence of paramesangial deposits, regardless of the C3 level at biopsy, would be strong evidence for type III.

On follow-up, C3 levels were persistently normal in 62 per cent of patients with type I and in 43 per cent of patients with type III but in only 18 per cent of patients with type II. There was no significant difference in renal survival probability in patients with or without C3NeF activity (Schwertz *et al.* 2001). The distribution of different types of C3 nephritic factors is given in Table 2.

Hepatitis B antigenaemia

MCGN has been well documented to occur in patients with chronic hepatitis B virus (HBV) infection (Johnson and Couser 1990) although overall, membranous glomerulonephritis is the commonest histopathological lesion seen in hepatitis B antigenaemia (see Chapter 3.7). Conversely, patients with classical MCGN type I have a significantly higher carrier rate of hepatitis B surface antigen (HBsAg) than the normal population. In a study of 46 adult patients with MCGN from Hong Kong (Chan *et al.* 1989), 20 per cent of the tested showed positive results for HBsAg (twice the incidence in the general population). However, there was no difference in the cumulative renal survival between those MCGN patients with HBsAg and those without. Hepatitis B positive patients with renal disease most commonly have nephrotic range proteinuria and microscopic haematuria. Hypertension (50 per cent) and renal insufficiency (20 per cent) are the other clinical features. Serum complement levels (C3 and C4) are often depressed, and circulating complexes may be present. HBsAg and antibodies to hepatitis B core antigen (HBcAg) are usually present in the serum. Patients often have no history of clinical hepatitis in spite of having elevated transaminase levels. Liver biopsy often shows either chronic active or chronic persistent hepatitis (Kneiser *et al.* 1974), although cirrhosis can be present. On rare occasions acute fulminant hepatitis may be present. Light microscopic examination of the renal biopsy shows type I MCGN (or occasionally type III MCGN). HBsAg has been demonstrated in the capillary walls.

Table 2 Characteristics of C3 nephritic factor

	$C3NeF_a$	$C3NeF_t$
Main disease association	Type II	Type III
Activation of complement	C3	C3; C5–9
Speed of action	Rapid	Slow

The pathogenesis most likely involves glomerular mesangial and subendothelial trapping of CICs that are at least in part composed of HBV antigens (Johnson and Couser 1990). These HBV-containing immune complexes presumably localize in the glomerulus either as a result of passive trapping of immune complexes or due to local *in situ* immune complex formation at this site. There is some *in vitro* and *in vivo* evidence in humans that HBV can directly infect the mesangial cell and possibly other resident glomerular cells (Johnson and Couser 1990). It is also possible that the HBV antigens are not pathogenetically related, and that the immune deposits develop by another virally induced mechanism such as autoimmunity. There still remains, however, the possibility that HBV infection and the glomerular process are pathogenetically unrelated. Treatment with beta interferon can lead to a decrease in the severity of proteinuria (Johnson and Couser 1990).

Hepatitis C antigenaemia (see also Chapter 4.6)

Hepatitis C infection has been well documented to be associated with essential MC (Misiani *et al.* 1992) and MCGN (Burstein and Rodby 1993; Parsquarielo *et al.* 1993; Johnson *et al.* 1993, 1994). A high titre of antihepatitis C virus antibodies has been reported in the serum and cryoprecipitate along with serum HCV RNA, which suggests a close aetiologic relationship between essential MC (Misiani *et al.* 1992; Ohsawa *et al.* 1999). Liver biopsies often show advanced chronic active hepatitis or cirrhosis (Johnson *et al.* 1993). However, the overall prevalence of MCGN in patients with HCV infection is low. In a retrospective review of 114 autopsies of patients with HCV, only three were found to have MCGN on renal histology (Gopalani and Ahuja 2001).

These patients usually have signs of moderate to severe proteinuria and impaired renal function. Renal biopsy usually discloses type I MCGN, although other patterns, such as membranous glomerulonephritis, have been noted (Roth 1995). This form of MCGN is quite similar to that noted in cryoglobulinaemic glomerulonephritis, and the pattern is possibly caused, at least, in part, by the cryoglobulins. There may be massive infiltration of the glomeruli by monocytes (Monga *et al.* 1981; D'Amico and Fornasieri 1995), and the diffuse thickening of the glomerular capillary wall with its double-contoured appearance is mainly due to the peripheral interposition of monocytes, with less obvious mesangial expansion/interposition (Monga *et al.* 1981; D'Amico and Fornasieri 1995). In some cases, large eosinophilic refractile 'hyaline thrombi' are noted by light microscopy within the glomerular capillary lumina. These may be intensely PAS-positive hyaline masses and may even involve small arteries or arterioles. The light microscopic appearance may also be one of acute exudative and proliferative glomerulonephritis or MCGN type.

The standard therapy for chronic HCV infection remains interferon alpha-2b (Johnson *et al.* 1994). Treatment may suppress viraemia, reduce proteinuria, and stabilize renal function. Cyclophosphamide treatment has also been reported to be of benefit (Quigg *et al.* 1995). The demonstration of a response to interferon treatment, with a decrease in proteinuria and clearance of HCV RNA, also suggests the aetiologic role of HCV in the pathogenesis of this renal disease (Roth 1995). A concomitant improvement in renal histological parameters too has been reported. Some studies suggest that more than half (and possibly <90 per cent) of mixed 'essential' cryoglobulinaemias are associated with chronic liver disease due to HCV infection (Peschre Bertschi and Schifferli 1993).

The precise role of HCV in the pathogenesis of MCGN remains unknown. It has been postulated that chronic infection with HCV may stimulate the production of anti-HCV antibodies and monoclonal rheumatoid factor in type II cryoglobulins, which then deposit in the glomeruli. None of the studies have been able to document viral antigen(s) in the glomeruli, although there have been a few reports claiming to show virus-like particles in the mesangial regions by electron microscopy (Johnson *et al.* 1993).

Shunt nephritis and endocarditis (see also Chapter 3.12)

Staphylococcus epidermidis is the most common organism responsible for glomerulonephritis associated with infected ventriculoatrial shunts. The histological picture resembles that of type I MCGN. However, in contrast to idiopathic type I MCGN, IgM is usually the predominant immunoglobulin in glomerular immune deposits (Dobrin *et al.* 1975). Another major difference from the classic idiopathic form of type I MCGN is that there is disappearance of the clinical abnormalities when the infected shunts are replaced, in contrast to the inexorable progression seen in most patients with the idiopathic form of type I MCGN.

Comment

Having gleaned all these various possible clues from the presumed aetiological association, and adding the knowledge from histological and immunological studies, it is apparent that no single pathogenetic mechanism emerges. Three main possibilities are:

- The association with infections and the site of deposits in type I, with the associated immune reactants, suggest an antigen–antibody type of disease, either with circulating complexes or with *in situ* immune complex formation. However, circulating antigen–antibody complexes are detected in only a minority of cases and a significant proportion do not have detectable deposition of immunoglobulin (type I).
- Hypocomplementaemia is the cause of MCGN. This may occur through the activation of complement cascade and its attendant inflammatory sequelae in the kidney. Against this hypothesis is the general inability to induce nephritis in experimental animals by complement activation with the exception of a mild glomerulitis with C3 deposition in one report using levan in rabbits, and the occurrence of MCGN, particularly in transplanted kidneys without evidence of complement activation. Alternatively, hypocomplementaemia may predispose to infection, the failure of efficient elimination of exogenous antigen and the persistence of antigen–antibody complexes, manifest as nephritis. The latter explanation obviously relates to the first.
- The abnormalities in the glomerular tubular and capillary basement membranes in type II may be structural arising from a biochemical defect due either to some primary defect in the membrane or possibly induced by a foreign antigen deposited in the kidney. The altered basement membrane, in common with other surface activators, may be able to activate complement predominantly via the alternate pathway. In type II particularly, it is conceivable that the mesangial proliferation of cells and matrix and their extension into the glomerular loops, is secondary to complement activation and its inflammatory sequelae.

None of these suggested mechanisms is mutually exclusive, nor is any one particularly favoured by the genetic and hereditary data. These could be associated with a predisposition for any of the mechanisms, either directly or by linkage to other, as yet undefined genes.

Clinical features and diagnosis

Incidence

Type I MCGN has been reported in patients of all ages except in infancy, the youngest reported case being a boy aged 15 months, although it is described most commonly in children (Habib *et al.* 1973; Davis *et al.* 1978; Levy *et al.* 1979; Magil *et al.* 1979). MCGN is one of the important histopathological patterns found in children with an idiopathic nephrotic syndrome, accounting for approximately 7.5 per cent cases of idiopathic nephrotic syndrome in the report of International Study of Kidney Disease in Children (1978). In adults it accounts for 10 per cent of all patients of nephrotic syndrome. In earlier studies MCGN had been reported to account for 10–20 per cent of primary glomerulonephritis. However, recent studies from the developed world document a much lower incidence, of the order of 2–6 per cent (Belgiojoso *et al.* 1985; Simon *et al.* 1987; Itaka *et al.* 2000). Most of this decrease has been due to a decline in the incidence of type I MCGN. This decrease in incidence is believed to parallel a decline in the incidence of infections—mainly streptococcal and hepatitis. In contrast, in developing countries MCGN continues to be a significant entity (Mota-Hernandez *et al.* 1985), accounting for 40 per cent of all cases in this study from Mexico. In our experience too, it was an important cause of INS, accounting for 16 per cent of all children in a recent series (Gulati *et al.* 1999).

The incidence of type I MCGN is much greater than type II, probably because of its association with infection. In a study by Date *et al.* (1983) from India, type I accounted for 94 per cent of all subtypes of MCGN.

Clinical features

Mesangiocapillary proliferative glomerulonephritis type I (with subendothelial deposits, classic type, MCGN)

The clinical characteristics are varied but centre on a nephritic urinary sediment together with proteinuria. Patients may have clinical symptoms of acute nephritic or nephrotic syndrome, or both. Others have a clinical picture resembling acute glomerulonephritis with microscopic haematuria and red blood cell casts (Lévy *et al.* 1979). Proteinuria is almost uniformly present, the nephrotic syndrome is a typical mode of presentation and has been noted in over half of the patients in most series (Habib *et al.* 1973; Donadio *et al.* 1979; Magil *et al.* 1979). Persistent microscopic haematuria (which is usually accompanied with proteinuria) is a frequent presentation (20–30 per cent). An acute nephritic syndrome is seen in another 10–20 per cent of patients (Lévy *et al.* 1979) and is characterized by oliguria, oedema, haematuria, hypertension, and renal insufficiency. Attacks of gross haematuria occur in a minority of patients, and are more usual in children than in adults (Cameron *et al.* 1983). Hypertension is commonly present at the clinical onset (noted in about one-third of the patients) but usually of mild degree. It is usually only transient and decreases to normal levels within several weeks in most patients (Lévy *et al.* 1979). Hypertension is typically observed as the renal disease progresses, and is more common in adults than in children (Cameron *et al.* 1983). Occasionally, MCGN may be asymptomatic and only detected, for example, in school urinary screening of children (Itaka *et al.* 1994). Anaemia out of proportion to the degree of renal failure may occur in MCGN, and such patients usually present with tiredness, breathlessness, and pallor. This anaemia is perhaps due to the presence of activated complement binding to the CR1 receptor present on the surface of human red cells.

Blood urea nitrogen (BUN) and serum creatinine levels are elevated at clinical onset in about a fourth of the patients. These values may stay elevated and progress to chronic renal failure (CRF) or return to normal over a few weeks in about half the patients. Depression of GFR is more often noted in adults than in children (Cameron *et al.* 1983). The clinical onset is not uncommonly preceded by a history of a respiratory infection, which is noted in about half the patients. Although group A streptococcal infections are not thought to play a role in the genesis of this pattern of renal disease, two studies have shown elevated antistreptolycin O (ASO) titres in 38 per cent (Cameron *et al.* 1970) and 25 per cent (Lévy *et al.* 1979) of patients, respectively.

Depressed levels of serum C3 have been found at the time of diagnosis in approximately one-third to half of the patients (Habib *et al.* 1973). In most patients serial determinations usually reveal hypocomplementaemia some time during the course of renal disease. In some patients a normal level may persist throughout the course of illness; alternatively the level may drop at a later time (Cameron *et al.* 1970). In the series of Habib *et al.* (1973), in as many as 40 per cent of patients, MCGN did not have depressed serum complement. Serum concentrations of the early components of classic pathway of complement activation (i.e. Clq, C4, and C2) and components of the alternative pathway (i.e. factor B, properdin) are also frequently low, but less commonly or severely than in systemic lupus or cryoglobulinaemia.

Type II MCGN (dense deposit disease)

The clinical features of type II MCGN are more or less similar to type I and it is difficult to differentiate them purely on this basis. However, there are certain differences which give some clues (Table 3). Acute nephritic syndrome is common in type II than in type I and has been reported in 20–40 per cent of patients (Antoine and Faye 1972; Vargas *et al.* 1976). Gross haematuria is also a common feature at the time of presentation and has been reported in 11–57 per cent of patients (Vargas *et al.* 1976; Davis *et al.* 1978). Proteinuria too is almost always observed. About half of these patients have nephrotic syndrome at presentation and more than 80 per cent develop it during the course of the disease (Habib *et al.* 1975; Vargas *et al.* 1976). Deranged renal function at onset is more common and a majority progress to endstage renal disease (ESRD). Clinical remissions are uncommon. Hypertension is almost always found at onset or during the course of the disease (Cameron *et al.* 1970; Habib *et al.* 1975). Persistently low serum levels of C3 are found in most patients (80 per cent). In contrast to type I, serum levels of the early components of the complement pathway are almost always normal. Serum concentrations of factor B and properdin of the alternative pathway are low.

Ocular changes in type II MCGN

Abnormalities of the optic fundi have been described in the form of diffuse bilateral symmetrical yellow lesions, similar to the drusen at the posterior pole (Fig. 10) which may be useful in diagnosis also. As the duration of disease increases (>10 years), these become more prominent.

Table 3 Comparison between type I MCGN and dense deposit disease

Features	Type I MCGN	Dense deposit disease
Age (at clinical onset)	Older	Younger
Asymptomatic urinary findings (at clinical onset)	Asymptomatic proteinuria and haematuria	Less common
Nephrotic syndrome	Less common	More common
Acute nephritic syndrome	Less common	More common
Gross haematuria	Less common	More common
Low serum complement	Less common (less severe, less persistent)	Common (severe, persistent)
C3NeF	Less common	More common
Partial lipodystrophy (with hypocomplementaemia and C3NeF)	Rare	Mainly associated with this type
Recurrence in renal transplants	Less common (ca. 25%)	Frequent (80+%)
Renal prognosis	Better	Worse

Drusen are deposits of extracellular material, lying between the basement membrane of the retinal pigment epithelium and the inner collagenous zone of Bruch's membrane. Clinically, drusen are seen as yellowish deposits lying deep inside the retina (Sarks and Sarks 1994). Patients with prominent drusen are predisposed to the more severe manifestations of macular degeneration (Sarks and Sarks 1994). Drusen are identified in more than 86–96 per cent of patients of type II MCGN with history of renal disease lasting more than 16 months or more (Leys *et al.* 1991). The type of fundus lesions correlated statistically with the duration of renal disease, but not with age, gender, or renal insufficiency. Histological examination reveals electron-dense deposits in the basement membranes of capillaries and Bruch's membrane (Duvall-Young *et al.* 1989a,b). Foci of new vessels and disciform scarring were seen in patients with history of renal disease of 15 years or more. Choroidal neovascularization may occur with haemorrhage and loss of vision.

The identification of drusen in a young patient with chronic glomerulonephritis contributes to the diagnosis of dense deposit disease. Patients with type II MCGN should have their ocular fundus examined on a regular basis (Leys *et al.* 1996).

Type III MCGN

The clinical and laboratory features are similar to patients with type I and dense deposit disease. Patients with type III are more frequently detected by chance discovery of haematuria and proteinuria in apparently healthy patients. Thus, the onset may be insiduous. Nephrotic syndrome is the other common mode of presentation (Jackson *et al.* 1987; Meyers *et al.* 1998). Serum C3, C5, and properdin levels are low in about half of the patients, but the early classic pathway complement components are normal suggesting alternative pathway activation. As compared to type I, patients with type III have longer lasting hypocomplementaemia, haematuria, and proteinuria (Braun *et al.* 1999).

Clinical diagnosis

The diagnosis of MCGN is histological, as the clinical features do not distinguish it from other types of glomerular disorder. Thus, clinical diagnosis is not practicable; however, certain features are suggestive of its presence. For example, suspicion of MCGN should be aroused in a child or adult with episodes of microscopic haematuria and proteinuria with anaemia out of proportion to the degree of renal failure. If the patient has associated persistent (>8 weeks) hypocomplementaemia in absence of features of systemic lupus, the likelihood of MCGN is very great. Careful ophthalmoscopic examination may reveal the characteristic retinopathy of type II MCGN (Fig. 10).

Recurrence of MCGN in renal allografts (see Chapter 13.3.4)

Recurrence of MCGN has been well documented in renal allografts. In type I the recurrence rate is of the order of 20–30 per cent. In contrast, type II MCGN recurs in about 80–90 per cent of patients (Cameron and Turner 1977). Serum complement levels or presence of C3 nephritic factor have not been found to be useful in predicting recurrence in these patients. However, the disease may have a more benign clinical course when it recurs. HCV-associated MCGN can also occur *de novo* or recur in renal transplant recipients, and has been observed in HCV infected patients after liver transplantation (Nakopoulou 2001).

Natural and treatment history of MCGN

Natural history

Knowledge of the natural history of the untreated condition is essential before the effects of therapy can be assessed for any condition, especially in the absence of large controlled trials. Many studies available indicate that the renal survival in MCGN at 10 years (from diagnosis) is about 50 per cent, at least in adults. Chronic renal disease is generally progressive, and overall renal prognosis is poor. The clinical course of patients can be quite variable in both adults (Donadio *et al.* 1979) and children (Habib *et al.* 1973; Lévy *et al.* 1979). The nephrotic syndrome persists in some, while others have nephrotic or nephritic episode with abnormal findings on urinalysis between the episodes. As compared to type I, patients with type III have longer lasting hypocomplementaemia,

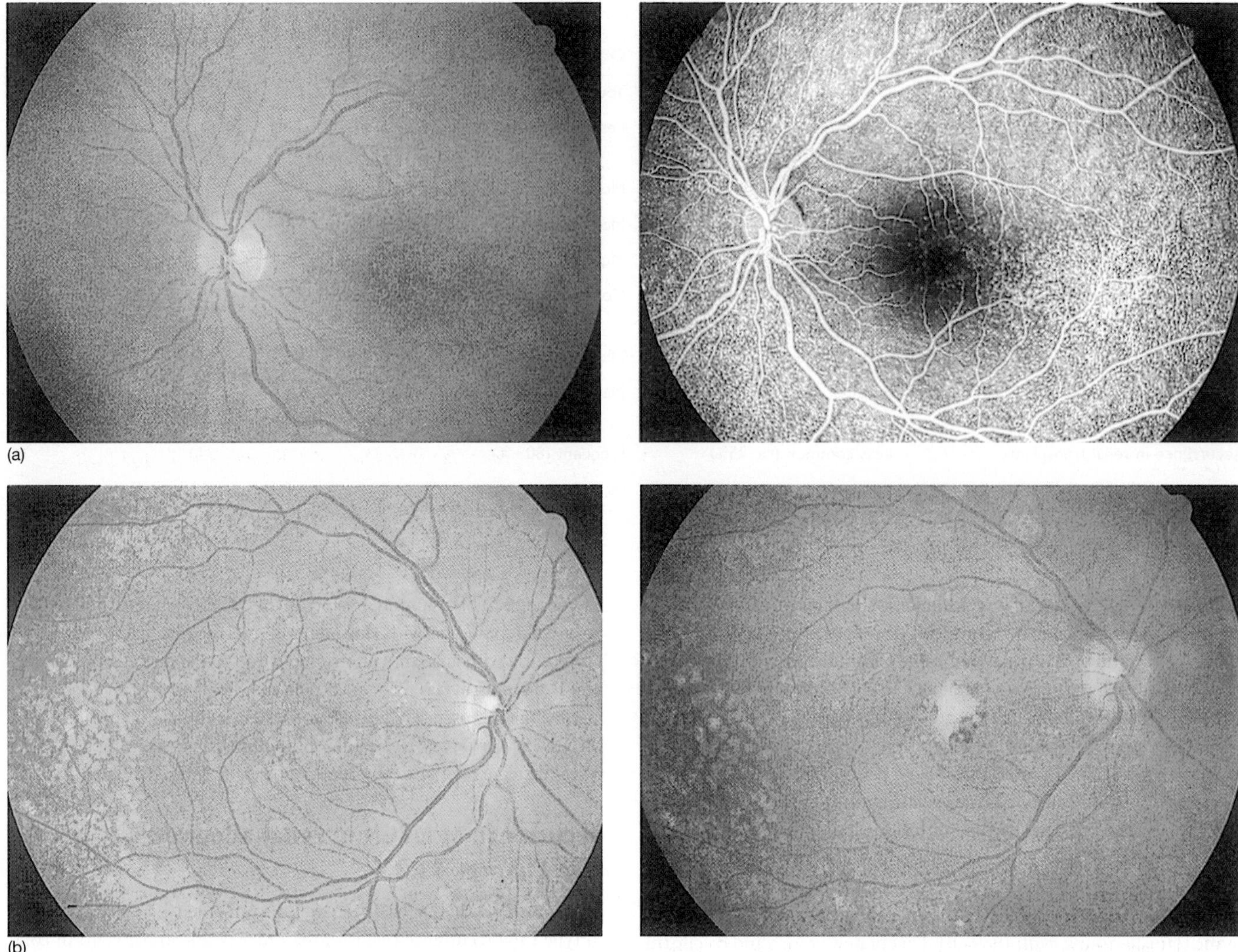

Fig. 10 (a) Early changes of the ocular fundus in a child with membranoproliferative glomerulonephritis type II. The colour photography of the left eye shows numerous small yellow deposits (small hard drüsen) and mottled pigmentation. These changes are more easily detected with fluorescein angiography (right). (b) Metamorphosia and blurred vision of the right eye and evolution to a central scotoma in a 50-year-old patient with chronic glomerulonephritis and biopsy-proven dense-deposit disease. Note serous detachment of the retina and haemorrhages caused by subfoveal choroidal neovascularization, and evolution to a fibrovascular scar. Note also larger drüsen occupying most of the fundus. [By courtesy of Anita Leys and Willem Proesmans, U.Z. Leuven, Belgium and reproduced from Leys *et al.* (1991, 1996), with permission.]

haematuria, and proteinuria, more disease relapses, and significantly greater loss of renal function during therapy (Braun *et al.* 1999). In type I clinical remission has been noted in 5–20 per cent of patients (Lévy *et al.* 1979; Cameron *et al.* 1983). The series of Lévy *et al.* (1979) showed complete remission in only four of 84 children. In this study, 17 children went into remission, but 13 relapsed; in only four patients was the remission maintained for periods of upto 4 years. In type II, although temporary remissions may occur, it is unusual for them to be permanent. In a series of 44 patients, only one patient achieved remission.

As regards the long-term outcome of MCGN (both types I and II), ESRD develops in majority of the patients (Davis *et al.* 1978; Donadio *et al.* 1979; Lévy *et al.* 1979; Magil *et al.* 1979; Cameron *et al.* 1983; Schmitt *et al.* 1990). In the study by Cameron *et al.* (1983) the actuarial survival was 50 per cent at 11 years, which was similar to survival rate found by Habib *et al.* (1973). In a large series of children from Paris (Lévy *et al.* 1979), 84 were followed for periods of upto 18 years: about 25 per cent died from renal insufficiency or are on long-term haemodialysis, 11 per cent continued to have chronic renal failure, 21 per cent had persistent nephrotic syndrome, 38 per cent had isolated proteinuria, and only 5 per cent appeared to experience spontaneous remission. Donadio *et al.* (1979) studied mainly adults and observed that ESRD developed in 40 per cent during the course of follow-up: the mean time of onset of renal failure was just over 5 years. In the large series of 220 mainly adult patients with type I MCGN from Germany with an average follow-up of 5 years, 23 per cent of patients died during follow-up, 26 per cent experienced ESRD, 24 per cent suffered chronic renal failure, and only 27 per cent remained normal in terms of renal function (Schmitt *et al.* 1990). A number of patients have persistent proteinuria with no renal insufficiency.

Prognosis in treated patients

There appears to be no major difference in clinical outcome between children and adults, although the data are often difficult to interpret because of possible difference in biopsy policies between children and adults. Children tend to have a more acute presentation and a slower decline in renal function, although on prolonged follow-up, the overall renal survival is similar to that in adults. Children were found to have 50 per cent of survival time of 76 months, whereas in adults it was 44 months (Magil *et al.* 1979). Men tended to experience renal failure in a relatively shorter time than women and children.

The prognosis differs between the three subtypes of MCGN, with type II carrying the greatest risk of the development of endstage renal failure (ESRF): in one recent study the median time to ESRF in types I, II, and III were, respectively, 15.3, 8.7, and 15.9 years (Scwertz *et al.* 1996).

The presence of a nephritic syndrome at clinical onset has been reported to be indicative of a poor prognosis in most studies (Lévy *et al.* 1979; Magil *et al.* 1979; Cameron *et al.* 1983). Since presentation with the nephrotic syndrome carries a substantially increased risk of ESRF compared with other milder clinical syndromes (Somers *et al.* 1995), the adverse prognosis of type II MCGN may simply reflect the greater likelihood of nephrotic presentation with this histological type. The other features suggestive of a poor prognosis include the absence of clinical remission during the course of the disease, renal dysfunction at onset (Bohle *et al.* 1992), persistent hypertension (Ito *et al.* 1986; Schmitt *et al.* 1990; Bohle *et al.* 1992; Kumar *et al.* 1996), and the presence of gross haematuria (Donadio *et al.* 1979; Lévy *et al.* 1979). Patients with hypocomplementaemia do not fare worse than those with normal level of complement (Cameron *et al.* 1973). The histological indicators of a poor prognosis include presence of mesangial deposits, glomerular sclerosis, tubulointerstitial fibrosis, and crescents (Vargas *et al.* 1976; Lévy *et al.* 1979; Cameron *et al.* 1983; Kumar *et al.* 1996) (Table 4).

Table 4 Factors heralding a poor prognosis in MCGN

Clinical
Acute nephritic presentation
Hypertension
Nephrotic range proteinuria
Renal dysfunction at onset
Absence of clinical remission
Histological
Dense-deposit disease (type II)
Crescents
Tubulointerstitial fibrosis
Mesangial deposits
Glomerular sclerosis

Treatment of MCGN

The problems relating to the evaluation of treatment of patients with MCGN are similar to the difficulties that beset studies of treatment of other types of chronic nephritis. The condition is not common, lasts many years, may remit spontaneously, and even when progressive it may fluctuate markedly and quickly. There are no serological markers for disease activity. Moreover, various studies include a varying mix of types I, II, and III, which may influence the outcome of therapeutic trials. Most studies contain only small numbers of patients, and are uncontrolled. Despite these limitations several studies have been reported and are summarized in Tables 5 and 6.

Table 5 Uncontrolled trials of various drugs in patients with MCGN

Reference	Drugs	Patients *n*; types I/II	Renal function			Follow-up (years)
			Increased	Stable	Decreased	
Habib *et al.* (1973)	Prednisone, chlorambucil	28; NK 66; NK	3 20	13 33	12 13	
Vanrenterghem (1975)	Non-steroidal anti-inflammatory drug + cyclophosphamide,	9; NK	4	3	2	1.7
McEnery *et al.* (1980)	Prednisolone	27; 15/5 + 7-III	7	16	4	6
Abreo and Moorthy (1982)	Prednisone, dipyridamole, warfarin, cyclophosphamide	9; NK	3	4	2	7.8
Cameron *et al.* (1983)	Prednisone, azathioprine, cyclophosphamide	38	7	19	12	—
Strife *et al.* (1984)	Prednisone	16; all III	1	9	6	5
Warade *et al.* (1985)	Prednisone	6; 6/0	4	2	0	5
Blainey *et al.* (1986)	Prednisone, cyclophosphamide	69; NK	7	20	42	6.8

NK, not known.

Table 6 Controlled trials of various drugs in patients with MCGN

Reference	Drugs	Patients *n*; types I/II	Renal function			Follow-up (years)	Controls *n*; types	Renal function		
			Increased	Stable	Decreased			Increased	Stable	Decreased
Kincaid-Smith (1972)	Cyclophosphamide + dipyridamole + warfarin	16; NK	10	3	3	3	13; NK	0	0	13
Lagrue *et al.* (1975)	Chloambucil, azathioprine	25; NK	1	4	20	2	9; NK	1	2	6
Donadio *et al.* (1984)	Dipyridamole + acetylsalicylic acid	21; 21/2	0	18	3	7	19; 19/0	0	10	9
Zimmerman *et al.* (1983)	Dipyridamole + warfarin	13; NK	0	13	0	1	13; NK	0	9	4
Cattran *et al.* (1985)	Cyclophosphamide + dipyridamole + coumadin	22; 17/5	4	12	6	1.5	25; 18/5	6	13	6
Mota-Hernandez *et al.* (1985)	Prednisolone	10; 10/0	1	9	0	6.5	8; 7/1	1	3	4
Tarshish *et al.* (1992)	Prednisolone on alternate days	80; 42/14	0	53	27	3.5	33; 26/5+	0	20	13
Zauner (1994)	Acetylsalicylic acid + dipyridamole	18; 15/3	0	18	0	3	8; 8/0	0	8	0+

NK, not known.

Corticosteroid treatment

The Cincinnati group was the first to advocate the long-term use of alternate-day high-dose prednisone (McEnery 1990; West 1992). Unfortunately, this suggestion was not based on controlled trials, relying instead on retrospective comparisons with 'control' series published from other centres in the past. Nevertheless, the results do suggest that prednisone treatment may alter the natural history. In a study involving 71 prednisone-treated childhood patients followed for a mean of over 10 years, the renal survival was 82 per cent at 10 years from onset, and 75 per cent from start of treatment; figures substantially better than that would be predicted from the known natural history (West 1992). The recommended schedule involves oral administration of 2–2.5 mg/kg (~60 mg/m^2, maximum dose 80 mg) of prednisone on alternate days, reducing slowly thereafter with average doses of 1.75, 1.5, 1.0, and 0.6 mg/kg in the 2nd, 3rd, 4th, and 5th years, respectively. The beneficial effect was more evident after 3 years of treatment and if prednisone was started within 12 months of clinical onset. Clearly the long-term use of corticosteroids in young individuals has the potential to have major adverse effects on growth, metabolism, and skeletal integrity. Alternate-day schedules probably reduce the adverse effects, but the price that may be paid for this 'successful' therapy remains so high that many nephrologists remain reluctant to adopt the Cincinnati approach.

The International Study of Kidney Disease in children ISKDC attempted to address the efficacy of this regime of alternate-day prednisone in a double-blind randomized prospective controlled trial (Tarshish *et al.* 1992). The dose used was 40 mg/m^2, maximum dose 60 mg, smaller than that recommended by the Cincinnati group in an attempt to minimize side-effects. Eighty patients were randomized (42 type I, 14 type II, 17 type III, and seven not classified); 47 received prednisone and 33 received placebo (lactose). The mean duration of treatment was 41 months with a mean follow-up of 63 months. There was a modest overall difference in treatment failures (development of renal failure or withdrawal due to adverse effects): 40 per cent in the prednisone group and 55 per cent with placebo. The effect of treatment was more impressive when subjected to life-table analysis: at 130 months, renal survival was 61 per cent in the prednisone group and 12 per cent in the placebo group. An important caveat in the interpretation of this trial was the considerable and significant difference in the duration of disease before entry between the controls (18 years) and the treated group (9 years) since outcome of disease is related to this period. Other less well-designed studies have corroborated the findings that corticosteroids may be beneficial in the treatment of children with MCGN (Habib *et al.* 1973; McEnery and McAdams 1988; Ford *et al.* 1992).

Alkylating agents

The data regarding the efficacy of these agents are scarce and uncontrolled. The Guy's group reported good results in 6 out of 10 patients (children and adults) with aggressive MCGN treated with cyclophosphamide as part of a combined treatment regimen (Chapman *et al.* 1980). Faedda *et al.* (1994) treated 19 patients with methylprednisone followed by oral prednisone and cyclophosphamide. Of the 19 patients, 15 achieved complete remission and three achieved a partial remission and the results were similar to those achieved with prednisone alone in other series. The survival rate after a mean follow-up of 4 years was 79 per cent (Faedda *et al.* 1994). However, there are no studies to suggest whether addition of cyclophosphamide to prednisolone provides any added advantage.

Combination therapy

Initial enthusiasm for combination therapy was based on the report by Kincaid-Smith (1979) on the effects of cyclophosphamide, warfarin, and dipyridamole in 16 patients with MCGN whose renal function was impaired: renal survival was substantially better than that in a retrospectively analysed group of 13 untreated patients. However, the apparent benefits of therapy were magnified by the unexpectedly poor outcome in the (retrospective) control group, in which all 13 patients progressed to ESRF. If the outcome in the treated patients is compared to that predicted from other studies of the natural history of MCGN, the effects are less impressive. Two subsequent controlled trials of 'triple therapy' did not show any significant benefit, and highlighted some major adverse effects (Tiller *et al.* 1981; Cattran *et al.* 1985).

The combination of aspirin plus dipyridamole was reported to have useful effects in a randomized, double-blind, placebo-controlled trial in 40 patients by Donadio *et al.* (1984) from the Mayo clinic, and this resulted in this form of therapy for MCGN being popular for some years, perhaps because of its relative safety. However, in the control group, the rate of deterioration was more rapid than expected and has led to concerns about the representativeness of the control group. Moreover, a later report by the same authors (Donadio and Offord 1989) showed no significant difference in the survival curves between the two groups. More recently, Zauner (1994) reported beneficial effects of aspirin plus dipyridamole on proteinuria in patients with nephrotic syndrome due to MCGN, but little effect on renal function. Zimmerman *et al.* (1983) used warfarin and dipyridamole together in a crossover trial in 18 patients. There was a reduction in proteinuria but very little change in the GFR; furthermore, there was a high rate of haemorrhagic complications.

Thus, in 215 patients involved in robust randomized controlled trials, little benefit has been found in adults with any immunosuppressive therapy, but the data do suggest a possible benefit of antiplatelet therapy (Levin 1999). Reduction of proteinuria has been used as a surrogate marker and may be an important clinical outcome in these patients. Well-designed controlled trials comparing high-dose steroids (the effective regimen in children) with aspirin and dipyridamole in high-risk adults have not been done.

Other approaches

Long-term treatment with non-steroidal anti-inflammatory drugs (NSAIDs) has been advocated by Lagrue *et al.* (1998) who reported observations in 53 patients, again without a control group. The effect of these agents on proteinuria, as seen in other conditions such as membranous nephropathy (Velosa *et al.* 1985), may be explained by an effect on intrarenal haemodynamics. Angiotensin-converting enzyme inhibitors (ACEI) have recently been shown to have useful renoprotective effects in patients with renal diseases, irrespective of the nature of the primary condition (The GISEN Group 1997). Hypertension in patients with MCGN should be treated aggressively, and ACEI may be the agents of first choice; they may have additional non-specific renoprotective effects by reducing the proteinuria. There is little information on the effects of cyclosporin in MCGN; anecdotal reports suggest beneficial effects (Cattran 1991). One recent study from Turkey included six patients with MCGN, and suggested that the majority of patients showed some improvement, at least in the short-term (Noyan *et al.* 1995). Given the evidence for the presence of circulating factors causing complement activation in MCGN (considered further below), measures aimed at removal of these from the circulation would seem to offer a logical approach.

Plasmapheresis has not been studied in a controlled manner, but one early report of its use in patients with MCGN whose renal function was deteriorating rapidly reported stabilization in some patients (McGinley *et al.* 1985).

Treatment of MCGN associated with hepatitis B or C

The recognition of HBV and HCV as probable causes for type I MCGN provides the opportunity of treating the disease by eliminating the antigens. The interferons alpha and beta are agents that suppress viraemia.

Alpha-interferon

Alpha-interferon (IFN-α) is a multifunctional cytokine with antiviral, anti-inflammatory, and immunomodulatory activities. Early studies of HCV patients uncomplicated by renal disease treated with 6-month courses of IFN-α (3 million units × 3/week) revealed response rates with roughly 40 per cent achieving viral clearance (HCV RNA < 100 copies/ml). However, after discontinuation of treatment, a sustained response was achieved in only 10–15 per cent (Davis *et al.* 1989; Camma *et al.* 1999). A modest improvement in sustained response could be achieved with prolonged courses of IFN-α (Poynard *et al.* 1996). Factors predicting a poor response to treatment include a high viral load (>2 million copies/ml) and viral genotype 1, liver cirrhosis, hepatic iron deposition in the liver, and longstanding infection (Davis and Lau 1997).

The treatment of HCV-associated MCGN with IFN-α also suffers from a poor sustained response once treatment is stopped. Renal disease improves initially in the 50–60 per cent who achieve clearance of viraemia. However, the HCV viraemia rebounds after cessation of treatment and is followed by a clinical flare 1–3 months later. Johnson *et al.* (1994) reported 14 patients treated with IFN-α for 6–12 months. In those who achieved viral clearance, proteinuria decreased by 60 per cent without change in renal function, however, once the IFN-α was discontinued, the viraemia and proteinuria recurred. The most common side-effects of IFN-α include flu-like symptoms, weight loss, hypoalbuminaemia, and anaemia. IFN-α also has an immunostimulatory effect which may induce autoimmune disorders such as thyroid (Watanabe *et al.* 1994) or liver disease or even worsen the underlying glomerular disease in patients who do not achieve viral clearance (Cattran *et al.* 1999; Ohta *et al.* 1999). IFN may also cause an acute interstitial nephritis (Nassar *et al.* 1998) or rarely nephritic syndrome and acute renal failure (Dimitrov *et al.* 1997).

Ribavirin

This is an antiviral nucleoside analogue with broad activity against both RNA and DNA viruses; however, its exact mechanism of action remains unclear. The drug is taken orally and is generally well tolerated, although the dose is often limited by the development of a reversible haemolytic anaemia. (Bodenheimer *et al.* 1997). When given alone in HCV infection, ribavirin therapy may improve liver function tests (transaminases), but does not improve viraemia and the response is not maintained (Bodenheimer *et al.* 1997). Recently, promising results have been reported with a combination of IFN-α and ribavirin. In HCV infection without renal disease significant improvements in response compared with IFN-α alone have been described with a sustained response rate of 31–38 per cent (McHutchison *et al.* 1998; Poynard *et al.* 1998; Reichard *et al.* 1998). The greatest improvement in response over IFN-α alone has been in patients with high viral loads. The standard dose of ribavirin used was 1000–1200 mg orally per day with IFN-α 3 million units three times per week for 6 months. There also appears to be benefit in those who have relapsed following initial INF-α therapy (Davis *et al.* 1998) and even in those who are resistant to IFN-α alone (Brillanti *et al.* 1994). This combination therapy has not been investigated in patients with renal disease, although one case report describes successful treatment (Misiani *et al.* 1999).

Analysis of treatment results by subtypes of MCGN

Most of the reported trials of treatment predominantly consists of patients with type I and type III MCGN, these being the more common forms, so that any conclusions regarding therapy can most safely be applied to those types. Type II MCGN is considered to carry the worst prognosis, and the available information is conflicting on whether this type is as responsive (or as unresponsive!) to treatment as the others. One analysis from the Cincinnati group reported clinical and histological improvement in a group of six childhood patients with type II MCGN treated with alternate-day prednisone (Oberkircher *et al.* 1988). There was a suggestion in the ISKDC study (Bergstein and Andreoli 1995), that children with type II fared less well, there being little difference between prednisone and placebo in these individuals. However, the numbers were very small, only 14 of the 80 patients had type II. If the type II patients were excluded, and the 66 others analysed together, the effect of prednisone was greater than for the study group as a whole. In the uncontrolled study of plasmapheresis of Cattran *et al.* (1991), apparent benefit occurred only in patients with type I MCGN. Only two patients with hypocomplementaemic type II MCGN were included, but it is of interest that neither of these showed any response to plasmapheresis, especially since the evidence for a causative role of a circulating factor is strongest for this type of MCGN. There is one case report describing a patient with recurrent type II MCGN in a renal transplant who apparently improved after plasmapheresis (Faedda *et al.* 1994).

Summary of treatment options

The present-day treatment of patients with renal disease is inadequate and sometimes dangerous, a statement still true for glomerulonephritis half a century after it was made by Thomas Addis. However, there now seems to be a move towards finding that MCGN is not untreatable. The current recommendations of treatment have been summarized by Levin (1999) as follows:

1. Children with idiopathic MCGN who have nephrotic range proteinuria or impaired renal functions may respond to high dose steroid therapy which should be maintained for at least 6–12 months (grade A evidence).
2. Adults with idiopathic MCGN, proteinuria (>3 g/day), or impaired renal functions should undergo a trial of therapy with dipyridamole or aspirin (grade B evidence).
3. Patients (both children and adults) with rapidly progressive renal failure or a recent deterioration in renal function especially those

with crescents on histopathology should be treated with pulse methylprednisolone therapy followed by oral prednisone and cyclophosphamide (grade B evidence).

4. Patients (both children and adults) with microscopic haematuria, proteinuria ($<$3 g), and normal renal function should be followed up every 3 months. They can be treated with ACE inhibitors.

5. Patients (both children and adults) with chronic renal failure should be managed conservatively.

6. Patients with HCV-associated MCGN should be treated with IFN-α and immunosuppressive agents should be avoided.

Mesangiocapillary glomerulonephritis—how many diseases?

Having reviewed the pathological, immunological, clinical, and treatment features of MCGN, we should now address the question of whether we are studying a single disease or not. As with any disease in which the pathogenesis is unknown, it is not possible to answer the question satisfactorily. Since 'mesangiocapillary glomerulonephritis' is a histological diagnosis and types I and II are designated by major histological differences it would seem self-evident that it represents more than one disease, especially in view of the profound and totally definitive electron-microscopic differences between the two types. Enhancing this difference are the contrasts in immunohistology, the greater incidence of—and more marked—hypocomplementaemia with the increased frequency of C3 nephritic factors in types II and III, the segregation of the different types of C3 nephritic factor with types I and II, the association of type II with partial lipodystrophy, and the mounting evidence from hepatitis B and C infections that type I can represent immune-complex disease. Thus, despite the similarities in the light microscopic appearances and the clinical features that originally led us to regard the two types as the same disease, the time has now come to approach types I and II as different conditions with some similarities. Clinicians, pathologists, immunologists, and geneticists should now clearly state, when studying this disease, whether the patients are type I or type II and abandon the unqualified term 'mesangiocapillary glomerulonephritis'.

References

Alexopoulos, E. *et al.* (1990). Lupus nephritis: correlation of interstitial cells with glomerular function. *Kidney International* **37**, 100–109.

Anders, D. and Thoenes, W. (1975). Basement membrane changes in membranoproliferative glomerulonephritis: a light and electron microscopic study. *Virchows Archives (A) Pathology Anatomy Histology* **369**, 87–109.

Antoine, B. and Faye, C. (1972). The clinical course associated with dense deposits in the kidney basement membranes. *Kidney International* **1**, 420–427.

Asinob, A. O. *et al.* (1999). Predominance of membranoproliferative glomerulonephritis in childhood nephrotic syndrome in Nigeria. *African Journal of Medicine* **18**, 203–206.

Austin, H. *et al.* (1984). Diffuse proliferative lupus nephritis: identification of specific pathologic features affecting renal outcome. *Kidney International* **25**, 689–695.

Balow, J. E. and Austin, H. A. (1988). Renal disease in systemic lupus erythematosus. *Rheumatic Disease Clinics of North America* **14**, 117–137.

Belgiojoso, G. B. *et al.* (1976). Immunofluorescence patterns in chronic membranoproliferative glomerulonephritis. *Clinical Nephrology* **6**, 303–310.

Belgiojoso, G. B. *et al.* (1985). Is membranoproliferative glomerulonephritis really decreasing? *Nephron* **40**, 380–381.

Ben Bassat, M. *et al.* (1983). The clinicopathologic features of cryoglobulinemic nephropathy. *American Journal Clinical Pathology* **79**, 147–156.

Bergstein, J. M. and Andreoli, S. P. (1995). Responses of type I membranoproliferative glomerulonephritis to pulse methylprednisolone and alternate-day prednisone therapy. *Pediatric Nephrology* **9**, 268–271.

Blainey, J. D., Brewer, D. B., and Hardwick, J. (1986). Proteinuric glomerular disease in adults: cumulative life tables over twenty years. *Quarterly Journal of Medicine* **59**, 555–567.

Bodenheimer, H. C. *et al.* (1997). Tolerance and efficacy of oral ribavirin treatment of chronic hepatitis C: a multicenter trial. *Hepatology* **26**, 473–477.

Bogdanovic, R. M. *et al.* (2000). Membranoproliferative glomerulonephritis in two siblings: report and literature review. *Pediatric Nephrology* **14**, 400–405.

Bohle, A. *et al.* (1974). The morphological and clinical features of membranoproliferative glomerulonephritis in adults. *Virchows Archives: An International Journal of Pathology* **363**, 213–224.

Bohle, A. *et al.* (1992). The long term prognosis of primary glomerulonephritis: a morphological and clinical analysis of 1747 cases. *Pathology, Research and Practice* **188**, 908–924.

Braun, M. C., West, C. D., and Strife, C. F. (1999). Differences between membranoproliferative glomerulonephritis types I and III in long term response to alternate day prednisone regimen. *American Journal of Kidney Diseases* **34**, 1022–1032.

Brillanti, S. *et al.* (1994). A pilot study of combination therapy with ribavirin plus interferon alpha for interferon alpha-resistant chronic hepatitis C. *Gastroenterology* **107**, 812–817.

Burkholder, P. M., Marchand, A., and Kryeger, R. P. (1970). Mixed membranous and proliferative glomerulonephritis: a correlative light, immunofluorescence and electron microscopic study. *Laboratory Investigation* **23**, 459–479.

Burstein, D. M. and Rodby, R. A. (1993). Membranoproliferative glomerulonephritis associated with hepatitis C virus. *Journal of the American Society of Nephrology* **4**, 1288–1293.

Cameron, J. S. (1984). Platelets in glomerular disease. *Annual Reviews of Medicine* **35**, 175–180.

Cameron, J. S. and Turner, D. R. (1977). Recurrent glomerulonephritis in transplanted kidneys. *Clinical Nephrology* **7**, 47–54.

Cameron, J. S. *et al.* (1970). Membranoproliferative glomerulonephritis and persistent hypocomplementemia. *British Medical Journal* **4**, 7–14.

Cameron, J. S., Ogg, C. S., White, R. H. R., and Glasgow, E. F. (1973). The clinical features and prognosis of normocomplementemic glomerulonephritis. *Clinical Nephrology* **1**, 8–13.

Cameron, J. S. *et al.* (1983). Idiopathic mesangiocapillary glomerulonephritis: comparison of types I and II in children and adults and long term prognosis. *American Journal of Medicine* **74**, 175–192.

Camma, C. *et al.* (1999). Chronic hepatitis C and interferon alpha: conventional and cumulative meta-analyses of randomized controlled trials. *American Journal of Gastroenterology* **94**, 581–595.

Campbell-Boswell, M. V., Linder, D., Naylor, B. R., and Brooks, R. E. (1979). Kidney tubule basement membrane alterations in type II membranoproliferative glomerulonephritis. *Virchows Archives (A) Pathology Anatomy Histology* **382**, 49–61.

Castiglione, A. *et al.* (1988). The relationship of infiltrating renal leukocytes to disease activity in lupus and cryoglobulinemic glomerulonephritis. *Nephron* **50**, 14–23.

Cattran, D. C. (1991). Current status of cyclosporine A in the treatment of membranous, IgA and membranoproliferative glomerulonephritis. *Clinical Nephrology* **35** (Suppl. 1), S43–S47.

Cattran, D. C. (1999). Interferon therapy: a double-edged sword? *American Journal of Kidney Diseases* **33**, 1174–1176.

Cattran, D. C. *et al.* (1985). Results of controlled drug trial in membranoproliferative glomerulonephritis. *Kidney International* **27**, 436–441.

Chan, M. K. *et al.* (1989). Adult onset mesangiocapillary glomerulonephritis: a disease with a poor prognosis. *Quarterly Journal of Medicine* **72**, 599–608.

Chapman, S. J. *et al.* (1980). The treatment of mesangiocapillary glomerulonephritis in children with combined immunosuppression and anticoagulation. *Archives of Disease in Childhood* **55**, 446–451.

Churg, J., Duffy, J. L., and Bernstein, T. (1979). Identification of dense deposit disease: a report for the International Study of Kidney Diseases in Children. *Archives of Pathology and Laboratory Medicine* **103**, 67–72.

Coleman, T. H., Forristal, J. K., Kosaka, T., and West, C. D. (1983). Inherited complement deficiencies in membranoproliferative glomerulonephritis. *Kidney International* **24**, 681–690.

D'Amico, G. and Fornasieri, A. (1995). Cryoglobulinemic glomerulonephritis: a membranoproliferative glomerulonephritis induced by hepatitis C virus. *American Journal of Kidney Diseases* **25** (3), 361–369.

D'Amico, G. *et al.* (1989). Renal involvement in essential mixed cryoglobulinemia. *Kidney International* **35**, 1004–1014.

Daha, M. R., Austen, K. F., and Fearon, D. T. (1977). The incorporation of C3 nephritic factor (C3NeF), into a stabilized C3 convertase C3b, Bb (C3NeF), and its release after decay of convertase function. *Journal of Immunology* **119**, 812–817.

Date, A., Neela, P., and Shastry, J. C. (1982). Thioflavin T fluorescence in membranoproliferative glomerulonephritis. *Nephron* **32**, 90–92.

Date, P. A., Neela, P., and Shastry, J. C. M. (1983). Membranoproliferative glomerulonephritis in a tropical environment. *Annals of Tropical Medicine and Parasitology* **3**, 1004–1014.

Davis, B. K. and Cavallo, T. (1976). Membranoproliferative glomerulonephritis: localisation of early components of complement in glomerular deposits. *American Journal of Pathology* **84**, 283–298.

Davis, G. L. and Lau, J. Y. (1997). Factors predictive of a beneficial response to therapy of hepatitis C. *Hepatology* **26**, S122–S127.

Davis, A. E. *et al.* (1978). Membranoproliferative glomerulonephritis (MCGN type I) and dense deposit disease in children. *Clinical Nephrology* **9**, 184–193.

Davis, G. L. *et al.* (1989). Treatment of chronic hepatitis C with recombinant interferon alfa. A multicenter randomized, controlled trial. Hepatitis Interventional Therapy Group. *New England Journal of Medicine* **321**, 1501–1506.

Davis, G. L. *et al.* (1998). Interferon alpha-2b alone or in combination with ribavirin for the treatment or relapse of chronic hepatitis C. International Hepatitis Interventional Therapy Group. *New England Journal of Medicine* **339**, 1493–1499.

Deschenes, G. *et al.* (1996). Glomerulonephritis with collagen deposits, hemolytic anemia and inherited factor H deficiency. *Journal of American Society of Nephrology* **7**, 1331 (abstract).

Dimitrov, Y. *et al.* (1997). Acute renal failure and nephrotic syndrome with alpha interferon therapy. *Nephrology, Dialysis, Transplantation* **12**, 200–203.

Dobrin, R. S. *et al.* (1975). The role of complement, immunoglobulin and bacterial antigen in coagulase negative staphylococcal shunt nephritis. *American Journal of Medicine* **59**, 660–673.

Donadio, J. V. and Offord, K. P. (1989). Reassessment of treatment results in membranoproliferative glomerulonephritis, with emphasis on life-table analysis. *American Journal of Kidney Diseases* **14**, 445–451.

Donadio, J. V., Jr. *et al.* (1979). Idiopathic membranoproliferative (mesangiocapillary) glomerulonephritis, a clinicopathologic study. *Mayo Clinic Proceedings* **54**, 141–150.

Donadio, J. V. *et al.* (1984). Membranoproliferative glomerulonephritis: a prospective trial of platelet inhibitor therapy. *New England Journal of Medicine* **310**, 1421–1426.

Duvall-Young, J., MacDonald, M. K., and McKechine, N. M. (1989a). Fundus changes in (type II) mesangiocapillary glomerulonephritis simulating drusen: a histopathology report. *British Journal of Ophthalmology* **73**, 297–302.

Duvall-Young, J. *et al.* (1989b). Fundus changes in mesangiocapillary glomerulonephritis type II: clinical and fluorescein angiography findings. *British Journal of Ophthalmology* **73**, 900–906.

Faedda, R. *et al.* (1994). Immunosuppressive treatment of membranoproliferative glomerulonephritis. *Nephron* **67**, 59–65.

Ford, D. M. *et al.* (1992). Childhood membranoproliferative glomerulonephritis type I limited steroid therapy. *Kidney International* **41**, 1606–1612.

Friend, P. S., Yunis, E. J., Noreen, H. J., and Michael, A. F. (1977). B cell alloantigen associated with chronic mesangiocapillary glomerulonephritis. *Lancet* **1**, 562–564.

Gallo, G. R. *et al.* (1980). Nodular glomerulopathy associated with nonamyloidotic kappa light chain deposits and excess immunoglobulin light chain synthesis. *American Journal of Pathology* **99**, 621–644.

Gopalani, A. and Ahuja, T. S. (2001). Prevalence of glomerulopathies in autopsies of patients infected with hepatitis C virus. *American Journal of Medical Sciences* **322** (2), 57–60.

Gulati, S. *et al.* (1999). Changing trends of histopathology in childhood nephrotic syndrome. *American Journal of Kidney Diseases* **34** (4), 1–6.

Habib, R., Kleinknecht, C., Gubler, M. C., and Levy, M. (1973). Idiopathic membranoproliferative glomerulonephritis in children: a report of 105 cases. *Clinical Nephrology* **1**, 194–214.

Habib, R. *et al.* (1975). Dense deposit disease: a variant of membranoproliferative glomerulonephritis. *Kidney International* **7**, 204–215.

Hruby, Z., Kopec, W., and Szewezyk, Z. (1985). Activity of circulating monocytes in patients with chronic glomerulonephritis. *International Nephrology and Urology* **17**, 379–387.

International Study of Kidney Disease in Children (1978). Nephrotic syndrome in children: prediction of histopathology from clinical and laboratory characteristics at time of diagnosis. *Kidney International* **13**, 159–165.

Itaka, K., Igarashi, S., and Sakai, T. (1994). Hypocomplementemia and membranoproliferative glomerulonephritis in school urinary screening in Japan. *Pediatric Nephrology* **8**, 420–422.

Itaka, K., Sakai, T., Yagisawa, K., and Aoki, Y. (2000). Decreasing hypocomplementemia and membranoproliferative glomerulonephritis in Japan. *Pediatric Nephrology* **14**, 794–796.

Ito, Y. *et al.* (1986). Hypertension and renal insufficiency in children with chronic glomerulonephritis. *International Journal of Pediatric Nephrology* **7**, 187–190.

Jackson, E. C. *et al.* (1987). Differences between types I and III in clinical presentation, glomerular morphology and complement perturbation. *American Journal of Kidney Diseases* **9**, 115–120.

Jansen, J. H., Hogasen, K., and Mollness, T. E. (1993). Extensive complement activation in hereditary porcine membranoproliferative glomerulonephritis type II (porcine dense deposit disease). *American Journal of Pathology* **143**, 1356–1365.

Jansen, J. H., Hogasen, K., Harboe, M., and Hovig, T. (1998). *In situ* complement activation in porcine membranoproliferative glomerulonephritis. *Kidney International* **53**, 331–349.

Jardim, H. M. *et al.* (1992). Crescentric glomerulonephritis in children. *Pediatric Nephrology* **6**, 231–235.

Jha, R. *et al.* (1994). Prognosis of adult MPGN—significance of clinical parameters and therapy. *Indian Journal of Nephrology* **4** (Suppl. 3), 53–57.

Joh, K. *et al.* (1993). Morphologic variations of dense deposit disease, light and electron microscopic, immunohistochemical and clinical findings in 10 patients. *Acta Pathologica Japonica* **43**, 552–565.

Johnson, R. J. and Couser, W. G. (1990). Hepatitis B and infection and renal disease: clinical, immunopathogenetic and therapeutic considerations. *Kidney International* **37**, 663–676.

Johnson, R. J. *et al.* (1993). Membranoproliferative glomerulonephritis associated with hepatitis C virus infection. *New England Journal of Medicine* **328**, 465–470.

Johnson, R. J. *et al.* (1994). Hepatitis C virus-associated glomerulonephritis. Effect of alpha-interferon therapy. *Kidney International* **46**, 1700–1704.

Kasai, N. *et al.* (1981). Platelet aggregating immune complexes and intraplatelet serotonin in idiopathic glomerulonephritis and systemic lupus. *Clinical and Experimental Immunology* **43**, 64–72.

Kim, Y., Vernier, R. L., Fish, A. J., and Michael, A. F. (1979). Immunofluorescence studies of dense deposit disease: the presence of rail road tracks and mesangial rings. *Laboratory Investigation* **40**, 474–480.

Kincaid-Smith, P. (1972). The treatment of chronic mesangiocapillary (membranoproliferative) glomerulonephritis with impaired renal function. *Medical Journal of Australia* **2**, 589–592.

Kincaid-Smith, P. (1979). The treatment of chronic mesangiocapillary (membranoproliferative) glomerulonephritis with impaired renal function. *Medical Journal of Australia* **2**, 587–592.

Kneiser, M. R. *et al.* (1974). Pathogenesis of renal disease associated with viral hepatitis. *Archives of Pathology* **97**, 193–200.

Kumar, P. *et al.* (1996). Clinicopathological determinants of outcome in childhood MCGN. *Indian Journal of Nephrology* **6**, 14–18.

Lagrue, G., Bernard, D., Bariety, J., Druet, P., and Guevel, J. (1975). Traitement par le chlorambucil et Pazathioprine dans les glomerulonephritis primitives. Resultats d'une etude controlee. *Journal d' Urologic et Nephrologic* **9**, 655–672.

Lagrue, G., Laurent, J., and Belghiti, D. (1998). Renal survival in membranoproliferative glomerulonephritis (MCGN): role of long-term treatment with non-steroid anti-inflammatory drugs (NSAID). *International Nephrology and Urology* **20**, 669–677.

Levin, A. (1999). Management of membranoproliferative glomerulonephritis: evidence-based recommendations. *Kidney International* **70** (Suppl.), S41–S46.

Lévy, M., Gubler, M. C., and Habib, R. New concepts in a membranoproliferative glomerulonephritis. In *Progress in Glomerulonephritis* (ed. P. Kincaid-Smith, A. J. F. d' Apice, and R. C. Atkins), p. 177. New York: Wiley, 1979.

Leys, A., Proesmans, W., Van Damme-Lombaerts, R., and Van Damme, B. (1991). Specific eye fundus lesions in type II membranoproliferative glomerulonephritis. *Pediatric Nephrology* **5**, 189–192.

Leys, A., Van Damme, B., and Verberckmoes, R. (1996). Ocular complications of type 2 membranoproliferative glomerulonephritis. *Nephrology, Dialysis, Transplantation* **11**, 211–214.

Magil, A. B. *et al.* (1979). Membranoproliferative glomerulonephritis type I: comparison of natural history in children and adults. *Clinical Nephrology* **11**, 234–244.

Mathieson, P. W. and Peters, D. K. (1997). Lipodystrophy in MCGN type II: the clue to links between the adipocyte and the complement system. *Nephrology, Dialysis, Transplantation* **12**, 1804–1805.

Mazzucco, G. *et al.* (1986). Cell interposition in glomerular capillary walls in cryoglobulinemic glomerulonephritis: ultrastructural investigation of 23 cases. *Ultrastructural Pathology* **10**, 355–361.

McEnery, P. T. (1990). Membranoproliferative glomerulonephritis the Cincinnati experience—cumulative renal survival from 1957 to 1989. *Journal of Pediatrics* **116**, S109–S114.

McEnery, P. T. and McAdams, A. J. (1988). Regression of membranoproliferative glomerulonephritis type II (dense deposit disease): observations in six children. *American Journal of Kidney Diseases* **12**, 138–146.

McEnery, P. T., McAdams, A. I., and West, C. D. (1980). Membranoproliferative glomerulonephritis: improved survival with alternate day prednisone therapy. *Clinical Nephrology* **13**, 117–124.

McGinley, E., Watkins, R., McLay, A., and Boulton-Jones, J. M. (1985). Plasma exchange in the treatment of mesangiocapillary glomerulonephritis. *Nephron* **40**, 385–390.

McHutchison, J. G. *et al.* (1998). Interferon alfa-2b alone or in combination with ribavirin as initial treatment for chronic hepatitis C. Hepatitis Interventional Therapy Group. *New England Journal of Medicine* **339**, 1485–1492.

Meri, S., Koistinen, V., Miettinen, A., Tornroth, T., and Seppala, I. J. (1992). Activation of the alternative pathway of complement by monoclonal λ light chains in membranoproliferative glomerulonephritis. *Journal of Experimental Medicine* **175** (4), 939–950.

Meyers, K. E., Finn, L., and Kaplan, B. S. (1998). Membranoproliferative glomerulonephritis type III. *Pediatric Nephrology* **12** (6), 512–522.

Miller, K., Dressner, I. G., and Michael, A. F. (1980). Localization of platelet antigens in human kidney disease. *Kidney International* **18**, 472–477.

Misiani, R. *et al.* (1992). Hepatitis C virus infection in patients with essential mixed cryoglobulinemia. *Annals of Internal Medicine* **117**, 573–577.

Misiani, R. *et al.* (1999). Successful treatment of HCV-associated cryoglobulinemic glomerulonephritis with a combination of interferon-alpha and ribavirin. *Nephrology, Dialysis, Transplantation* **14**, 155–160.

Mollnes, T. E. *et al.* (1986). Effect of nephritic factor on C3 and the terminal pathway of complement in vivo and in vitro. *Clinical and Experimental Immunology* **65**, 73–79.

Monga, G., Mazzucco, G., di Belgiojoso, G. B., and Busnach (1981). Monocyte infiltration and glomerular hypercellularity in human acute and persistent glomerulonephritis. Light and electron microscopic, immunofluorescence, and histochemical investigation on twenty-eight cases. *Laboratory Investigation* **44** (4), 381–387.

Monga, G., Mazzucco, G., and Castello, R. (1985). Glomerular monocyte infiltration in human nephropathies: prevalence and correlation with clinical and morphological variables. *Virchows Archives (A) Pathology Anatomy Histology* **405** (4), 483–496.

Monga, G. *et al.* (1986). Monocyte infiltration and glomerular hypercellularity in human acute and persistent glomerulonephritis: light and electron microscopic, immunofluorescence and histochemical investigation on 28 cases. *Laboratory Investigation* **44**, 381–387.

Monga, G. *et al.* (1987). Ultrastructural findings in cryoglobulinemic glomerulonephritis. *Applied Pathology* **5**, 108–115.

Montoliu, J. *et al.* (1986). Glomerular disease in the cirrhosis of liver: low frequency of IgA deposits. *American Journal of Nephrology* **6**, 199–205.

Mota-Hernandez, F. *et al.* (1985). Prednisone versus placebo in membranoproliferative glomerulonephritis: long term clinico-pathological correlations. *International Journal of Pediatric Nephrology* **6**, 25–28.

Nabakayashi, K., Arimura, Y., Yoshida, M., and Nagasawa, T. (1985). Anti T cell antibodies in primary glomerulonephritis. *Clinical Nephrology* **23**, 74–80.

Nakopoulou, L. (2001). Membranoproliferative glomerulonephritis. *Nephrology, Dialysis, Transplantation* **16** (Suppl. 6), 71–73.

Nassar, G. M. *et al.* (1998). Reversible renal failure in a patient with the hypereosinophilia syndrome during therapy with alpha interferon. *American Journal of Kidney Diseases* **31**, 121–126.

Ng, Y. C. and Peters, D. K. (1986). C3 nephritic factor (C3NeF): dissociation of cell-bound and fluid phase stabilization of alternative pathway C3 convertase. *Clinical and Experimental Immunology* **65**, 45–47.

Noyan, A. *et al.* (1995). Efficacy and side effects of cyclosporine A in nephrotic syndrome of childhood. *Nephron* **70**, 410–415.

Oberkircher, O. R. *et al.* (1988). Regression of recurrent membranoproliferative glomerulonephritis type II in a transplanted kidney after plasmapheresis therapy. *Transplantation Proceedings* **20** (Suppl.1), 418–423.

Ohsawa, I. *et al.* (1999). High prevalence of Hepatitis C virus antibodies in older patients with membranoproliferative glomerulonephritis. *Nephron* **82** (4), 366–367.

Ohta, S. *et al.* (1999). Exacerbation of glomerulonephritis in subjects with chronic hepatitis C virus infection after interferon therapy. *American Journal of Kidney Diseases* **33**, 1040–1048.

Pangburn, M. K. and Muller-Eberhard, H. J. (1984a). The alternative pathway of complement. *Springer Seminars Immunopathology* **7**, 163–192.

Pangburn, M. K. and Muller-Eberhard, H. J. (1984b). The C3 convertase of the alternative pathway of human complement. *Biochemical Journal* **235**, 723–730.

Parbatni, A. *et al.* (1980). Platelet and plasma serotonin concentrations in glomerulonephritis. *Clinical Nephrology* **14**, 112–117.

Parsquariello, A. *et al.* (1993). Cryoglobulinemic membranoproliferative glomerulonephritis associated with hepatitis C virus. *American Journal of Nephrology* **13**, 300–304.

Peschre Bertschi, A. and Schifferli, J. A. (1993). Cryoglobulinémie essentielle. *Schweizerische Rundschau Medidiziniche Praxis* **82** (6), 163–167.

Pickering, R. J. *et al.* (1971). The complement system in chronic glomerulonephritis: three newly associated observations. *Journal of Pediatrics* **78**, 30–43.

Poynard, T. *et al.* (1996). Treatment of chronic hepatitis C by interferon for longer duration than six months. *Digestive Disease Sciences* **41** (Suppl. 12), S99–S102.

Poynard, T. *et al.* (1998). Randomized trial of interferon alpha2b plus ribavirin for 48 weeks or for 24 weeks versus interferon alpha2b plus placebo for 48 weeks for treatment of chronic infection with hepatitis C virus. International Hepatitis Interventional Therapy Group (IHIT). *Lancet* **352**, 1426–1432.

Quigg, R. J. *et al.* (1995). Successful treatment of cryoglobulinemic membranoproliferative glomerulonephritis associated with hepatitis C virus infection. *American Journal of Kidney Diseases* **25**, 798–800.

Reichard, O. *et al.* (1998). Randomised, double blind, placebo-controlled trial of interferon alpha-2b with and without ribavirin for chronic hepatitis C. The Swedish Study Group. *Lancet* **351**, 83–87.

Rennke, H. G. (1995). Nephrology forum: secondary membranoproliferative glomerulonephritis. *Kidney International* **47**, 643–656.

Roth, D. (1995). Hepatitis C virus: the nephrologists's view. *American Journal of Kidney Diseases* **25**, 3–16.

Sakai, H. *et al.* (1979). Increase of IgM bearing peripheral blood lymphocytes in patients with idiopathic membranoproliferative glomerulonephritis and their family members. *Clinical Nephrology* **12**, 210–215.

Sarks, S. H. and Sarks, J. P. Age-related macular degeneration atrophic form. In *Retina* (ed. J. Ryan), pp. 1071–1102. St Louis: C.V. Mosby, 1994.

Schmitt, H. *et al.* (1990). Long term prognoses of type I membranoproliferative glomerulonephritis significance of clinical and morphological parameters. An investigation of 220 cases. *Nephron* **55**, 242–250.

Schwertz, R. *et al.* (1996). Outcome of idiopathic membranoproliferative glomerulonephritis in children. *Acta Paediatrica Scandinavica* **85**, 308–312.

Schwertz, R. *et al.* (2001). Complement analysis in children with idiopathic membranoproliferative glomerulonephritis: long term follow up. *Pediatric Allergy Immunology* **12** (3), 166–172.

Scott, D. M. *et al.* (1978). The immunoglobulin natures of nephritic factor (NeF). *Clinical and Experimental Immunology* **32**, 12–17.

Seymour, A. E. *et al.* (1980). Kappa light chain glomerulosclerosis in multiple myeloma. *American Journal of Pathology* **101**, 557–580.

Sherwood, M. C., Pincott, J. R., Goodwin, F. J., and Dillon, M. J. (1987). Dominantly inherited glomerulonephritis and an unusual skin disease. *Archives of Disease in Childhood* **62** (12), 1278–1280.

Silva, F. G. Membranoproliferative glomerulonephritis. In *Pathology of the Kidney* (ed. R. H. Heptinstall), pp. 309–368. Philadelphia, PA: Lippincott-Raven Company, 1998.

Silver, M. M. *et al.* (1986). Renal and systemic kappa light chain deposits and their plasma cell origin identified by immunoelectron microscopy. *American Journal of Pathology* **122**, 17–27.

Simon, P. *et al.* (1987). Variations of primary glomerulonephritis incidence in a rural area of 40,000 inhabitants in the last decade. *Nephron* **45**, 171–174.

Somers, M. *et al.* (1995). Non-nephrotic children with membranoproliferative glomerulonephritis: are steroids indicated? *Pediatric Nephrology* **9**, 140–144.

Strife, C. F. *et al.* (1977). Membranoproliferative glomerulonephritis with disruption of the glomerular basement membrane. *Clinical Nephrology* **7**, 65–72.

Strife, C. F., Jackson, R. J., and McAdams, A. J. (1984). Type III membranoproliferative glomerulonephritis: long term clinical and morphological evaluation. *Clinical Nephrology* **21**, 323–334.

Stutchfield, P. R. *et al.* (1986). X linked mesangiocapillary glomerulonephritis. *Clinical Nephrology* **26**, 150–156.

Taguchi, T. and Bohle, A. (1989). Evaluation of change with time of glomerular morphology in membranoproliferative glomerulonephritis: a serial biopsy study of 33 cases. *Clinical Nephrology* **31**, 297–306.

Takahashi, M., Bernstein, J., Tobin, J. N., and Edelman, C. M. Jr. (1978). Requirements for the solubilization of immune aggregates by complement: the role of the classical pathway. *Journal of Clinical Investigation* **62**, 349–358.

Tarantino, A. *et al.* (1981). Renal disease in essential mixed cryoglobulinemia long term follow up of 44 patients. *Quarterly Journal of Medicine* **50**, 1–30.

Tarshish, P., Bernstein, J., Tobin, J. N., and Edelmann, C. M., Jr. (1992). Treatment of mesangiocapillary glomerulonephritis with alternate-day prednisone—a report of the International Study of Kidney Disease in children. *Pediatric Nephrology* **6** (2), 123–130.

The GISEN Group (1997). Randomised placebo-controlled trial of effect of ramipril on decline in glomerular filtration rate and risk of terminal renal failure in proteinuric, non-diabetic nephropathy. *Lancet* **349**, 1857–1863.

The Southwest Pediatric Nephrology Study Group (1985). Dense deposit disease in children: prognostic value of clinical and pathologic indicators. *American Journal of Kidney Diseases* **6**, 161–169.

Tiller, D. J. *et al.* A prospective randomized trial in the use of cyclophosphamide, dipyridamole and warfarin in membranous and mesangiocapillary glomerulonephritis. In *Advances in Basic and Clinical Nephrology* (ed. W. Zurukzoglu, *et al.*), pp. 345–351. Eighth International Congress of Nephrology, Basel: Karger, 1981.

Vanrenterghem, Y., Roels, L., Verbeckmoes, R., and Michielsen, P. (1975). Treatment of chronic glomerulonephritis with a combination of indomethacin and cyclophosphamide. *Clinical Nephrology* **4**, 218–222.

Vargas, A. R. *et al.* (1976). Mesangiocapillary glomerulonephritis with dense deposits in the basement membranes of the kidney. *Clinical Nephrology* **5**, 73–82.

Velosa, J. A. *et al.* (1985). Treatment of severe nephrotic syndrome with meclofenamate: an uncontrolled pilot study. *Mayo Clinic Proceedings* **60**, 586–592.

Warady, B. A., Guggenheim, S., Sedman, A., and Lum, G. M. (1985). Prednisone therapy of membranoproliferative glomerulonephritis in children. *Journal of Pediatrics* **107**, 702–707.

Watanabe, U. *et al.* (1994). The risk factor for development of thyroid disease during interferon-alpha therapy for chronic hepatitis C. *American Journal of Gastroenterology* **89**, 399–403.

Weiler, J. M., Daha, M. R., Austen, K. F., and Fearon, D. T. (1976). Control of the amplification convertase of complement by the plasma protein factor H. *Proceedings National Academy of Sciences USA* **73**, 3268–3272.

Welch, T. *et al.* (1986). Major histocompatibility-complex extended haplotypes in membranoproliferative glomerulonephritis. *New England Journal of Medicine* **314**, 1476–1481.

Weller, R. O. and Nester, B. (1972). Histological reassessment of three kidneys originally described by Richard Bright in 1827–1836. *British Medical Journal* **2**, 761–763.

West, C. D. (1992). Idiopathic membranoproliferative glomerulonephritis in childhood. *Pediatric Nephrology* **6**, 96–103.

West, C. D. (1994). Nephritic factors predispose to chronic glomerulonephritis. *American Journal of Kidney Diseases* **24**, 956–963.

West, C. D. and McAdams, A. J. (1995). Paramesangial glomerular deposits in membranoproliferative glomerulonephritis type II correlate with hypocomplementemia. *American Journal of Kidney Diseases* **25**, 853–861.

West, C. D. and McAdams, A. J. (1998). Glomerular paramesangial deposits: association with hypocomplementemia in membranoproliferative glomerulonephritis type I and type III. *American Journal of Kidney Diseases* **31**, 427–434.

West, C. D. and McAdams, A. J. K. (1999). The alternative pathway C3 convertase and glomerular deposits. *Pediatric Nephrology* **13**, 1448–1453.

Zauner, I. (1994). Effect of aspirin and dipyridamole on proteinuria in idiopathic membranoproliferative glomerulonephritis: a multicentre prospective clinical trial. *Nephrology, Dialysis, Transplantation* **9**, 619–622.

Zimmerman, S. *et al.* (1983). Prospective randomized trial of warfarin and dipyridamole in patients with membranoproliferative glomerulonephritis. *American Journal of Medicine* **75**, 920–927.

3.9 Acute endocapillary glomerulonephritis

Bernardo Rodríguez-Iturbe

Definition and general considerations

Acute endocapillary glomerulonephritis is characterized by an increased number of cells within the glomerular tuft. Endocapillary proliferation may occur without apparent cause (idiopathic), but is often a feature of primary renal diseases, such as IgA nephropathy (see Chapter 3.6), and of glomerulonephritis observed in systemic diseases, such as lupus erythematosus and cryoglobulinaemia. In addition, endocapillary glomerulonephritis is associated with a large number of bacterial, viral, and fungal infections, as well as with parasitic infestations (Table 1). Poststreptococcal glomerulonephritis (PSGN) is the prototype disease entity of endocapillary glomerulonephritides.

In the same disease entity, different periods of the natural history may be associated with different pathological characteristics. For example, hepatitis B may present initially with a self-limited acute mesangial proliferative glomerulonephritis and a serum sickness-like syndrome, while the chronic carrier state results in membranoproliferative glomerulonephritis in adults and membranous glomerulonephritis in children. Furthermore, diseases that in their typical presentation have exclusively endocapillary proliferation, such as PSGN, may at times present a mixed pathological appearance, including mesangial sclerosis or extensive crescent formation. This lack of uniformity in the pathology results from the variability of antigen load, size, and charge, the characteristics of antibody response, and the efficiency of immune-complex removal. As demonstrated in serum sickness experimental models, circulating immune-complexes are usually deposited in subendothelial and mesangial regions and, if the condition is self-limited, induce a transient glomerulonephritis. *In situ* immune complex formation is characterized by penetration of the antigen, followed by antibody, through the basement membrane to subendothelial locations. This pathogenetic modality is favoured in circumstances of antigen excess, when immune-complexes are easily dissociated, and when antigens are cationic, since they are attracted by the negatively charged glomerular basement membrane (see Chapter 3.1).

Several investigations have suggested that the severity of proliferative changes may be inferred from urinary investigations. Urinary monocyte chemoattractant protein-1 (MCP-1) (Rovin *et al.* 1996) and urinary proinflammatory macrophages expressing CD16 (Fcγ receptor III) correlate with proliferative activity (Hotta *et al.* 1999). In IgA nephropathy (Chapter 3.6), acute proliferative changes are associated with high levels of urinary interleukin 8 (IL-8) (Yokohama *et al.* 1998). Reduced glycosaminoglycan/creatinine urinary concentration ratio is characteristic of acute endocapillary glomerulonephritis (Tencer *et al.* 1997). Yet, it should be recognized that isolated glomerular disease is not associated with increased serum creatinine and the degree of interstitial involvement is the critical variable correlated with uraemia (Bohle *et al.* 1998).

Table 1 Infectious agents associated with endocapillary glomerulonephritis

Associated with infectious syndromes
Skin and throat (*Streptococcus group A*)
Bacterial endocarditis (*Staphylococcus aureus, Streptococcus viridans*)
Pneumonia (*Diplococcus pneumoniae, Mycoplasma*)
Meningitis (*Meningococcus pneumoniae, Mycoplasma*)
Visceral abscesses and osteomyelitis (*S. aureus, Escherichia coli, Pseudomonas aeruginosa, Proteus mirabilis, Klebsiella, Clostridium perfringens*)
'Shunt' nephritis (*S. aureus, Staphylococcus albus, S. viridans*)
Infected vascular prosthesis (*S. aureus*)
Guillain–Barré syndrome (*G–B infectious agent?*)
Associated with specific bacterial diseases
Typhoid fever (*Salmonella typhi*)
Leprosy
Yerisiniosis
Brucellosis
Leptospirosis
Associated with viral infections
Hepatitis A, B, and C
Epstein–Barr virus
Parvovirus B19
Cytomegalovirus
Measles
Mumps
Varicella
Coxsackie virus
Associated with parasitic infestation
Malaria (*Plasmodium falciparum, P. malariae*)
Schistosomiasis (*Schistosoma haematobium, S. mansoni*)
Toxoplasmosis
Trichinosis (*Trichinella spiralis*)
Filiarasis (*Onchocerca volvulus, Loa Loa*)
Associated with other infectious organisms
Rickettsiae (Coxiella)
Fungi (*Candida albicans, Coccidioides immitis, Histoplasma capsulatum*)

Epidemiology

Endocapillary glomerulonephritis remains a common form of presentation of renal disease but the epidemiology has changed. In a study of nephrology admissions in a suburban borough of Paris, 44 of 76 adult patients had endocapillary glomerulonephritis, but staphylococcus and Gram-negative infections, rather than streptococci, were usually the infectious cause and 45 per cent of the patients were alcoholics, diabetics, or intravenous drug users (Montseny *et al.* 1995). The association between postinfectious glomerulonephritis with alcoholism has also been emphasized by Keller *et al.* (1994). Endocapillary glomerulonephritis in children is a common histological presentation of primary renal disease in Africa, India, Pakistan, Uganda, Malaysia, and Papua New Guinea. It accounts for 20 per cent of the cases with nephritic syndrome in Namibia (van Buuren *et al.* 1999) and of the cases with proteinuria in Zimbabwe (Borok *et al.* 1997). Aetiological associations with streptococcal infections and malaria are suspected in some countries but not in others.

The incidence of PSGN is decreasing in the United States, the United Kingdom, and Central Europe, where it has virtually disappeared in certain regions (Simon *et al.* 1994). Nevertheless, PSGN continues to have a worldwide distribution. Poststreptococcal nephritis is common among aboriginal communities in Australia (Currie and Brewster 2001) and still represents more than 70 per cent of children admitted with glomerulonephritis in Singapore (Yap *et al.* 1990) and in Venezuela (Orta and Moriyón 2001).

PSGN results usually from upper respiratory and skin infections. Pharyngitis and tonsillitis are the usual sites of antecedent infection in winter and spring in temperate climates and impetigo is more frequent in the tropics in the summer months. In African-American children, PSGN usually follows pyoderma (Roy and Stapleton 1990).

The disease is most common between the ages of 2 and 12 years, but can occur at any age; in a large series, 5 per cent of the patients are usually younger than 2 years and 5–10 per cent are older than 40 years. The clinically overt cases of PSGN are twice more common in males than in females, but subclinical disease occurs with equal frequency in both genders.

Sporadic cases occur in clusters in poor urban and rural areas. Epidemic outbreaks occur in closed communities or in densely populated areas. These epidemics tend to be cyclic in certain areas with low socioeconomic status and poor hygienic conditions, such as in the Red Lake Indian Reservation in Minnesota (Anthony *et al.* 1969), Port of Spain, Trinidad (Poon-King *et al.* 1967), and Maracaibo, Venezuela (Rodríguez-Iturbe 1984). The attack rate of nephritis after streptococcal infection is variable, ranging from 5 to 25 per cent in reported epidemics. Isolated outbreaks also have been reported in New South Wales, Australia (Muscatello *et al.* 2001), in rugby team members with infected skin abrasions (Ludlam and Cookson 1986), and, more recently, by the ingestion of unpasteurized cheese infected with *Streptococcus zooepidemicus* from bovine mastitis in a farm in Quilombo do Gaia, Brazil (Balter *et al.* 2000).

Clinical aspects

The infection preceding nephritis

As emphasized in Table 1, certain infections appear to be more commonly associated with glomerulonephritis. The clinical characteristics of infection with nephritogenic group A streptococci are well known. The usual site of infection is the skin or throat, but other locations are possible. Unusual sites of infection include spider bites (Lung and Mallory 2000) and infected circumcision wound (Tasic and Polenakovic 2000).

Streptococcal pharyngitis may cause only sore throat or it may be accompanied by tonsillar exudate, fever, and cervical lymphadenopathy. The likelihood of a streptococcal aetiology is less than 3 per cent when none of these is present and about 50 per cent when all three are present (Komaroff *et al.* 1986). Scarlatinal rash is due to an erythrogenic toxin that is produced by the bacteria. Vomiting may be a prominent symptom in scarlet fever.

Streptococcal impetigo is characterized by groups of small vesicles that appear in exposed skin areas. They break rapidly and leave lesions covered with a thick crust; this distinguishes them from staphylococcal impetigo that usually starts with larger vesicles that leave a thin friable crust when they break. Regional lymphadenopathy is usually present in patients with active infection. Streptococcal impetigo does not affect deeper tissues and heals without scarring, unless it originates as a superinfection of lesions produced by the scratching associated with scabies. A history of intense itching, particularly if it is also present in other family members, is a diagnostic clue and careful inspection of the skin in the interdigital spaces and flexor surface of the wrists may reveal scabies.

Nephritis follows throat infections after a latent period of 1 or 2 weeks; the latent period after skin infections is typically 3–6 weeks. When impetigo and pharyngitis are present at the same time, the infection in the throat is usually due to contamination from the skin (Anthony *et al.* 1969). One-third of the patients have microscopic haematuria during the latent period.

Clinical features of acute nephritis

Subclinical disease is manifested by microscopic haematuria and a reduction in serum complement. Blood pressure may or may not be elevated. Biopsy studies demonstrated that these patients invariably have endocapillary proliferation and their prognosis is excellent. Anthony *et al.* (1969) have reported that patients with subclinical nephritis outnumber the patients with clinical disease in epidemics by a factor of 1.5. Two prospective studies in families of index cases revealed a remarkably similar ratio of subclinical/clinical disease of 5.3 (Dodge *et al.* 1967) and 4.0 (Rodríguez-Iturbe *et al.* 1981b). The acute nephritic syndrome is the classic clinical presentation of PSGN. It was first described as a feared complication of the convalescent period of scarlet fever in the epidemics of the eighteenth century when, at times, the urine became 'dark and scanty' (von Plenciz 1792). The typical patient is a boy, 2–14 years of age, who suddenly develops puffiness of the eyelids and facial oedema; his urine output is reduced and the urine acquires a tea colour. When examined, his blood pressure is found to be elevated. Forty per cent of children have the full clinical picture of the acute nephritic syndrome: oedema, haematuria, hypertension, and oliguria. At least two of these symptoms are present in more than 96 per cent of the children with acute PSGN (Rodríguez-Iturbe 1984).

In a typical case of poststreptococcal nephritis, improvement is observed after 2–7 days when the urine volume increases, followed rapidly by resolution of oedema and return of the blood pressure to normal.

Haematuria is a universal finding. Only exceptionally the diagnosis of acute glomerulonephritis may be made if the urine sediment is normal. Gross haematuria is present in one-third of the patients and microscopic haematuria is found in the rest. Gross haematuria, if present, usually disappears when urine output increases. Microscopic haematuria usually persists for many months after the acute attack and disappears usually within 1 year and always within 4 years (Kasahara *et al.* 2001). Red blood cell casts and dysmorphism of more than 80 per cent of the erythrocytes in the urine are characteristic of glomerular haematuria. Phase-contrast microscopy is valuable in evaluating the shape of erythrocytes, which becomes distorted as a consequence of their transit through the nephron (Fairley and Birch 1982) (see Chapters 1.2 and 3.3). However, the diagnostic usefulness of this finding has been limited by the definitions of dysmorphism and different observers may disagree in the interpretation of red cell morphology in 38 per cent of occasions (Raman *et al.* 1986). The morphology that is more specific and sensitive for the diagnosis of glomerular haematuria is the doughnut-like red cell shapes with one or more blebs (Tomita *et al.* 1992). Microscopic examination of the urine should be performed as soon as possible after voiding, since red blood cells are destroyed rapidly, particularly in alkaline urine.

Oedema is the chief complaint in most patients. This is well recognized since the earliest accounts of the disease that described the 'dropsy which succeeds scarlet fever' (Wells 1812). Oedema is usually confined to the face and legs in adolescents, while generalized oedema is more common in younger children. Ascites is unusual in patients with the acute nephritic syndrome. Fluid retention in acute glomerulonephritis has long been associated with a decreased glomerular filtration rate resulting from the inflammatory reaction in the glomeruli. Renal blood flow is normal and, consequently, the filtration fraction is depressed. Traditionally, the reduced glomerular filtration rate is thought to be responsible for sodium retention as it diminishes the filtered sodium. This is clearly an oversimplification because a reduced glomerular filtration rate is seen in a variety of other conditions where fluid retention does not occur. Furthermore, profound sodium retention can occur in patients with a mildly reduced glomerular filtration rate and spontaneous diuresis can occur before the glomerular filtration rate has improved. Therefore, the pathogenesis of sodium retention necessarily implies loss of the compensatory glomerulotubular 'balance' and an impaired pressure-natriuresis response. Micropuncture studies demonstrate that proximal tubular reabsorption is decreased in proportion to the fall in glomerular filtration rate and, therefore, it is assumed that the defect is localized in distal segments of the nephron inaccessible to micropunture. Endothelial and/or mesangial vasoactive factors released by glomerular injury may induce sodium retention at the collecting duct (Juncos 2002). It appears likely that the infiltrating inflammatory cells that release vasoactive mediators which promote sodium retention (Johnson *et al.* 2002) play a role in the pathogenesis of primary renal sodium retention, but this possibility has not been explored. At any rate, the fractional sodium excretion is usually less than 1 per cent and the urine–plasma creatinine concentration ratio more than 40.

Hypertension is present in more than 80 per cent of patients, but only 50 per cent require drug treatment. Haemodynamic measurements indicate that increased plasma volume, increased cardiac output, and elevated peripheral vascular resistance contribute to the hypertension in the acute nephritic syndrome. These findings are consistent with the volume-dependent nature of arterial hypertension in the acute nephritic syndrome. Rarely, hypertensive encephalopathy may complicate the clinical course and constitutes a medical emergency. A recent report describes a reversible leucoencephalopathy associated with severe hypertension (Soylu *et al.* 2001). Because these are rare events, if a patient presents evidence of central nervous system involvement, such as somnolence or convulsions, the possibility of systemic lupus erythematosus or haemolytic uraemic syndrome should be considered.

Oliguria is referred as a symptom on admission by less than half of the children or their parents/guardians. Non-specific symptoms, such as dull lumbar pain, malaise, weakness, and nausea, frequently accompany the cardinal manifestations of the acute nephritis syndrome.

Congestive heart failure may develop during the acute nephritic syndrome and the severity of the fluid retention and hypertension are determining factors in the development of this complication. Nevertheless, there is a long-standing observation that some patients can develop heart failure with moderate hypertension and a minor degree of oedema (Murphy and Murphy 1954) and, more recently, echocardiographic studies have demonstrated myocardial dysfunction in some patients (Balat *et al.* 1993). Therefore, close monitoring of seemingly mild disease is advisable, particularly in elderly patients.

Proteinuria of 3 g/day/1.73 m^2 or more, with or without other features of the nephrotic syndrome, is seen in only 4 per cent of the clinically overt cases of acute PSGN in children, which contrasts with the prevalence of massive proteinuria in adult patients with this disease and with the incidence of severe proteinuria in the acute nephritic syndrome that may be caused by systemic lupus erythematosus, 'shunt' nephritis, and nephritis associated with visceral abscess.

The course of acute glomerulonephritis in elderly patients is different from that in children (Table 2). Dyspnoea and pulmonary congestion, oliguria, massive proteinuria, azotaemia, and early mortality are substantially more common in the adult population. Prognosis is poorer and may be related to the coexistence of diabetes mellitus, cardiovascular or liver disease rather than to the severity of the renal disease itself since the serological and histological characteristics of acute glomerulonephritis do not differ in the various age groups (Washio *et al.* 1994).

Table 2 Clinical manifestations of acute poststreptococcal glomerulonephritis in children and elderly adults

	Children (%)	Elderly patients (%)
Haematuria	100	100
Proteinuria	80	92
Oedema	90	75
Hypertension[a]	60–80	80–86
Oliguria	10–50	58
Dyspnoea/heart failure	<5	43
Nephrotic proteinuria	<4	20
Azotaemia	25–40	70–83
Early mortality	<0.1	25

Data in elderly patients taken from the review of Melby *et al.* (1987) and Washio *et al.* (1994). Data in children taken from several studies reviewed in the text.

[a] At discharge, hypertension persists in 43% of the elderly patients and exceptionally, if ever, in children.

Hormonal systems—the pathogenesis of oedema and hypertension

Hormonal systems involved in the regulation of extracellular volume are appropriately modified in response to the extracellular expansion that occurs in PSGN. Plasma renin activity and plasma aldosterone levels are depressed in the acute oedematous phase; concomitantly, the atrial natriuretic factor increases three- to fivefold. Both the suppression of plasma renin activity and the stimulation of atrial natriuretic peptide are correlated with the weight gained in the acute oedematous phase (Rodríguez-Iturbe 1984; Rodríguez-Iturbe *et al.* 1990). Endothelin is also increased and may contribute to a postulated tubular unresponsiveness to atrial natriuretic peptide (Ozdemir *et al.* 1992). The hormonal profile suggests a compensatory response to primary fluid retention. Nevertheless, despite the low plasma renin, treatment with converting enzyme inhibitors induce a transient increase in the glomerular filtration rate, suggesting that some degree of preglomerular vasoconstriction exists in acute glomerulonephritis, possibly resulting from increased intrarenal angiotensin II activity.

Urinary prostaglandins E2 and F2α and kallikrein excretion are reduced in the acute nephritic syndrome, presumably because of decreased renal synthesis. It is unlikely that reduction of prostaglandins and kallikrein play a determinant role in circulatory congestion and hypertension of these patients since improvement occurs in most patients despite persistence of low levels of these hormones.

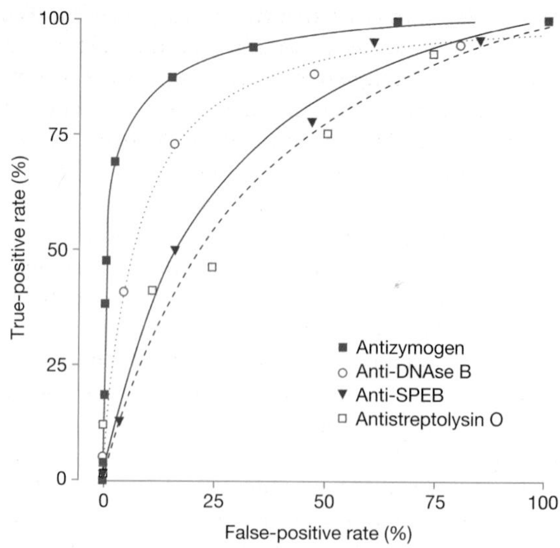

Fig. 1 Receiving operating characteristics curves of a multicentric study comparing serum titres of antistreptolysin O, anti-DNAse B, antistreptococcal pyrogenic exotoxin B (SPEB), and antizymogen (used with permission of *Kidney International* 1998: **54**, 509–517).

Diagnosis

Endocapillary glomerulonephritis is a pathological description that requires, whenever possible, an aetiological diagnosis. A poststreptococcal origin is suggested by the history but needs confirmation of a streptococcal infection. The frequency with which positive cultures may be obtained in patients with PSGN is variable. In epidemics, it may be as high as 70 per cent and in sporadic cases it is about 25 per cent. The evidence of recent infection is frequently obtained from the demonstration of increasing titres of one or more antistreptococcal serum antibodies. Historically, antistreptolysin O (ASO) titres were found elevated in nearly 80 per cent of the patients with streptococcal throat infection but the frequency is much less in pyodermitis. A recent study found elevated ASO titres in only one-third of the patients, while anti-DNAse titres were high in 73 per cent of postimpetigo cases (Parra *et al.* 1998). The streptozyme test, which includes four antigens (DNAse B, Streptolysin O, hyaluronidase, and streptokinase), is elevated in nearly 80 per cent of the cases. Antibodies against a nephritis-associated plasmin receptor (NAPLr) (Yamakami *et al.* 2000) and antibodies against the zymogen precursor of streptococcal pyrogenic exotoxin B (Parra *et al.* 1998), both of which are assumed to be nephritogenic antigens (see later), are more sensitive and specific than the rest but they are not clinically available. Receiving operating characteristics (ROC) curves of antizymogen serum titres are consistently superior to ASO and anti-DNAse B titres as markers for streptococcal infection in acute PSGN (Parra *et al.* 1998; Fig. 1).

Additional serological findings in the first week of nephritis in children include depressed C3 in 90 per cent of the patients. Circulating immune-complexes and increased IgG are present in almost two-thirds of the patients with acute PSGN (Rodríguez-Iturbe 1984). Interestingly, elevated serum IgG are found more frequently in patients without glomerular immunoglobulin deposits (West and McAdams 1998).

The diagnosis of subclinical glomerulonephritis (transient drop in complement, microscopic haematuria, and, at times, arterial hypertension) is only possible if patients at risk are placed under prospective surveillance. This may be done in household members and siblings of index cases or in closed communities in epidemic conditions since in the general population the possibility of developing the disease after streptococcal infection is remote. However, recent evidence indicates that the assumption may not be correct. In Japan, the prospective follow-up of 49 patients with Group A streptococcal infection in the upper respiratory tract uncovered 12 patients who developed subclinical glomerulonephritis (Yoshizawa *et al.* 1997b). Renal biopsy is not indicated in subclinical cases since all patients who develop haematuria and a fall in serum complement have endocapillary proliferation and because subclinical nephritis has an excellent immediate and long term prognosis.

The bedside differential diagnosis between nephrotic syndrome and acute nephritic syndrome in an oedematous child can be helped by the examination of the ear cartilage that has a soft, paper-like consistency in young children with nephrotic syndrome as a result of long-standing hypoalbuminaemia (Heymann *et al.* 1963). Another clue may be the existence of ascites, which is frequent in the nephrotic syndrome and rare in acute nephritic syndrome, as noted almost two centuries ago (Wells 1812).

The differential diagnosis of a patient presenting with acute nephritic syndrome may be approached considering whether the clinical picture is due to a primary renal disease or is the initial manifestation of an otherwise silent systemic disease. Systemic lupus erythematosus, Goodpasture's syndrome, essential cryoglobulinaemia, subacute and acute bacterial endocarditis, 'shunt' nephritis, visceral abscess, 'microscopic' polyarteritis glomerulonephritis, and Wegener's granulomatosis may occasionally present as an isolated nephritis.

Measurement of serum complement activity (CH_{50}) has been suggested as a first-line test in evaluation of acute glomerulonephritis because low serum complement is a feature of 90 per cent or more of the cases of acute PSGN, type II mesangiocapillary glomerulonephritis, diffuse proliferative lupus nephritis, subacute bacterial endocarditis, 'shunt' nephritis, and essential cryoglobulinaemia. The finding of a normal serum complement would make any of these diagnoses unlikely. A low serum complement, on the other hand, excludes IgA nephropathy, polyarteritis nodosa, and antiglomerular basement disease (Table 3). Additional diagnostic insight may be gained if determination of C3 and C4 are done concomitantly: very low C3 and normal or mildly depressed values of C4 is typical of diseases in which there is preferential activation of the alternative pathway, such as mesangiocapillary glomerulonephritis type II and poststreptococcal nephritis. In fact, mesangiocapillary glomerulonephritis presenting with the acute nephritic syndrome may be difficult to differentiate from PSGN, especially since some cases of PSGN may present mesangial interposition in the capillaries and occasional intramembranous electron-dense deposits. The lack of widespread intramembranous deposits in PSGN and the rapid recovery of complement levels would help in the differential diagnosis in most instances. In mesangiocapillary glomerulonephritis, the persisting activation of complement is due to an IgG autoantibody (C3 nephritic factor, C3 NeF) with specificity for the alternative pathway C3 convertase C3bBb, which renders this enzyme resistant to its natural inhibitors. In PSGN, Fremeaux-Bacchi *et al.* (1994) have found C3 NeF autoantibody activity of the IgG class, suggesting that the activation of the alternate complement pathway is mediated by transient expression of C3 NeF autoantibody. In contrast, with these diseases, a low C4 in association with relatively preserved levels of C3 is characteristic of cryoglobulinaemia type II. Finally, a proportional decrease in C3 and C4 is found in lupus erythematosus and bacterial endocarditis. In Third-World countries where caloric and protein malnutrition is endemic, it is worthwhile to keep in mind that severe malnutrition, *per se*, is a cause of depressed C3 concentrations. Serial determinations of serum complement are of clinical value in glomerulonephritis associated with bacterial infections. Serum complement returns to normal in 12 weeks in all patients with uncomplicated PSGN (Kasahara *et al.* 2001) and persistence of low levels should raise the possibility of membranoproliferative glomerulonephritis or lupus nephritis.

Table 3 Serum complement and proteinuria in diseases that may present with features of acute nephritic syndrome

Proteinuria	Serum complement (CH_{50})	
>3.5 g/day/1.73 m^2	Normal (>90%)	Low (>90%)
Likely (70–90%)	Visceral abcesses	Mesangiocapillary GN I and II Lupus nephritis Shunt nephritis
Unlikely (<10%)	IgA nephritis Henoch–Schönlein purpura Microscopic polyarteritis nodosa	Acute PSGN Essential mixed cryoglobulinaemia
No help (40–60%)	Anti-GBM disease	

Numbers refer to the percentage of cases with the corresponding finding. PSGN, poststreptococcal glomerulonephritis; GN, glomerulonephritis; GBM, glomerular basement membrane.

The existence of proteinuria in the nephritic range (≤3.5 g/day/1.73 m^2) may also be helpful in the differential diagnosis. Massive proteinuria is frequent in lupus nephritis, mesangiocapillary glomerulonephritis types I and II, shunt nephritis, and nephritis associated with visceral abscess, but is unusual in other renal diseases, particulary in acute PSGN.

Indications for renal biopsy

Renal biopsy may contribute in specific circumstances to the management of PSGN. The acute disease has a self-limited course with an excellent prognosis and the risks of a biopsy, however small, are better avoided if the case is typical. However, biopsy is justified on clinical grounds if unusual features cast substantial doubt on the presumptive diagnosis. For example, renal biopsy may be advised when massive proteinuria is present in the acute stage, or if the serum complement is normal, or if the complement is persistently reduced after 3–4 months. These characteristics are sufficiently unusual in acute PSGN that other diagnostic possibilities should be entertained. A biopsy should also be considered when the serum creatinine increases progressively, because a biopsy showing crescentic glomerulonephritis might lead to aggressive modalities of treatment, such as steroid bolus and immunosuppressive drugs.

Aetiopathogenesis of poststreptococcal glomerulonephritis

The vast majority of acute endocapillary glomerulonephritis is thought to be immunologically mediated. The nature of the antigens involved, the characteristics of the antibody response, the site of the immune reaction, and the role of cellular immune mechanisms are of obvious relevance and are considered elsewhere. Only those aspects directly relevant to PSGN will be discussed here.

It is usual to start the historical perspective with the landmark observations of Schick (1907), who noted the latent period between scarlet fever and nephritis and suggested pathogenetic similarities between postscarlatinal nephritis and experimental serum sickness. When the streptococcal aetiology of scarlet fever was established (Dochez and Sherman 1924), the nephritis that followed was ascribed to an 'allergic' reaction to the bacterium. Acute rheumatic fever and glomerulonephritis are both non-infectious complications of streptococcal infection, but have epidemiological and biological differences and only rarely occur in the same patient. Therefore, Seegal and Earle (1941) postulated the existence of rheumatogenic and nephritogenic strains of the bacterium. Since recurrence of poststreptococcal nephritis is a very rare event (Watanabe and Yoshizawa 2001), it is likely that the putative antigen is shared between nephritogenic strains and that it confers long-lasting immunity.

Streptococcal antigens

Over the years, many investigations have attempted to define the nephritogenic antigen(s) in PSGN. Group A streptococci are the usual infective agents and nephritogenic strains include M types 1, 2, 4, and 12 in throat infections and M types 25, 45, 47, 55, 57, and 60 in skin infections. Group C streptococci have been also the cause of recent epidemics of glomerulonephritis (Francis *et al.* 1993; Balter *et al.* 2000; Nicholson *et al.* 2000).

M protein, M protein–fibrinogen complexes, streptokinase, and streptococcal cell membrane antigens of M types 6 and 12 have all been suspected to have a nephritogenic role on the basis of the antibody profiles of patients and the ability of a given antigen to bind to the glomeruli. Yet, none of these antigens have been reproducibly localized in biopsies of patients with acute PSGN and numerous attempts to induce nephritis with streptococcal products in experimental animals have yielded inconsistent results.

Two antigenic fractions are at present actively studied (reviewed by Yoshizawa 2000): the NAPLr, originally named 'endostreptosin' by Lange *et al.* (1983), which was identified as glyceraldehyde-3-phosphate dehydrogenase (GAPDH), and a cationic (p*K* 8.0) streptococcal antigen (Vogt *et al.* 1983, 1990), identified as the zymogen precursor of the streptococcal pyrogenic exotoxin B (SPEB) (Poon-King *et al.* 1993). NAPLr (Yamakami *et al.* 2000) as well as SPEB (Cu *et al.* 1998) have been identified in the early biopsies (less than a month from the onset of symptoms) of patients with acute PSGN and, as discussed earlier, antibody titres to these antigens are present in the serum of the vast majority of patients with the disease. Both these antigens injected intravenously have affinity for the glomeruli. Streptococcal extracts, likely containing NAPLr, induced histological features of acute nephritis and activation of the alternative complement pathway (Yoshizawa *et al.* 1997a). Yoshizawa (2000) has proposed that NAPLr could bind to the glomeruli and capture circulating plasmin activated by streptokinase. Plasmin bound to the glomeruli, inaccessible to physiological inhibitors, could cause direct tissue destruction and inflammation. The participation of streptokinase in the pathogenesis of PSGN is suggested by studies showing that allele substitution of the streptokinase gene reduces the nephritogenic potential of group A streptococci (Nordstrand *et al.* 2000).

With respect to the potential pathogenetic role of zymogen, Vogt (1990) has emphasized that cationic antigens, such as SPEB and its zymogen precursor, are attracted by the negatively charged glomerular basement membrane, and penetrate towards a subepithelial location where they react *in situ* with antibody. The resulting subepithelial location of the immune complexes found in experimental nephritis induced by cationic antigens resemble the 'humps' that are characteristic lesions of PSGN. Recent studies indicate that SPEB/zymogen are proapoptotic to leucocytes (Viera *et al.* 2001) and induce leucocyte infiltration in the kidney, possibly as a result of the induction of chemotactic and migration inhibition factor (MIF) activities (Romero *et al.* 1999).

Another cationic components that could have pathogenetic relevance are the streptococcal histones that may readily accumulate in the glomeruli (Choi *et al.* 1995). After streptococcal lysis, histones can enter the blood and bind to the anionic proteoglycans to trigger an *in situ* immune complex formation or directly induce the production of proinflammatory cytokines (Zhang *et al.* 1999).

Superantigens

Increasing evidence suggests the possible participation of superantigens in the pathogenesis of some glomerulonephritis. Bacterial superantigens can activate autoreactive T cells and lead to the induction or aggravation of autoimmune reactivity. Superantigens may stimulate large numbers of lymphocytes expressing the same V domain and inflammatory mediators released by these activated T cells may exert intense local damage. Methicillin-resistant *Staphylococcus aureus* are the classical microorganisms that trigger a superantigen response. Such a response is characterized by polyclonal gammopathy and can explain the development of immune-complex glomerulonephritis with normal complement (Yoh *et al.* 2000). Acute PSGN typically present low complement; nevertheless, it has been postulated that streptococcal protein M could act as a superantigen in the induction of PSGN, as well as rheumatic fever and scarlet fever (reviewed by Schafer and Sheil 1995).

Autoimmune reactivity

Autologous antigen–antibody complexes may play a role in PSGN. Autoimmune nephrogenicity may be related to similarities between streptococcal cell membrane antigens and the glomerular basement membrane (Zelman and Lange 1995) or result from systemic autoimmune reactivity. Anti-immunoglobulin reactivity has been studied since McIntosh *et al.* (1972) showed that streptococcal neuraminidase (sialidase) could react with IgG, and that autologous sialic acid-depleted IgG could induce the formation of antiglobulins and subsequent nephritis in rabbits. Nephritogenic streptococci produce neuraminidase and neuraminidase activity and free sialic acid have been detected in the plasma of patients with acute PSGN (Rodríguez-Iturbe *et al.* 1981a; Asami *et al.* 1985).

These experimental findings were followed by observations that serum rheumatoid factor activity, particularly IgG-rheumatoid factor, was present in 32–43 per cent of patients with poststreptococcal nephritis (Rodríguez-Iturbe 1984; Sesso *et al.* 1986). The possibility of an autoimmune response to altered immunoglobulin received additional support from the finding of anti-IgG reactivity in the antibody eluted from the kidney of a fatal case of PSGN and in the immune deposits detected by immunofluorescence in renal biopsies from such patients (reviewed by Rodriguez-Iturbe 1984).

Neuraminidase reduction of surface sialic acid in circulating leucocytes may facilitate their accumulation in the kidney. Studies of Marín *et al.* (1995) have demonstrated that neuraminidase treatment of circulating leucocytes induces the binding of neutrophils, monocytes, and T lymphocytes to the glomerulus and interstitium of normal kidneys, a phenomenon that could be relevant to the nephritogenicity associated with infections with some neuraminidase-producing bacteria. Further, evidence of a role for neuraminidase comes from the finding that desialized leucocytes are, in fact, infiltrating the kidney in early biopsies of acute PSGN (Marín *et al.* 1997). Recently, Duvic *et al.* (2000) reported the simultaneous presentation of acute PSGN and thrombotic microangiopathy and suggested a role for neuraminidase in the combined clinical picture.

Another possible mechanism for the production of antiglobulins is the binding of the Fc fragment of IgG to receptors in the surface of group A streptococcus. This binding induces intense anti-IgG reactivity and glomerulonephritis with anti-IgG deposits. Burova *et al.* (1998) have postulated that PSGN might be triggered by this mechanism.

Additional clinical evidence of autoimmune reactivity in PSGN includes the demonstration of DNA–anti-DNA complexes (Vilches and Williams 1984), anticardiolipin antibodies that do not seem to correlate with the glomerular disease (Ardiles *et al.* 1999), and antineutrophil cytoplasmic autoantibodies that are more frequently observed in patients with crescentic glomerulonephritis and uraemia (Ardiles *et al.* 1997).

Characteristics of the immune reactivity and complement activation

Traditionally, the pathogenesis of acute glomerulonephritis has been centred on the renal deposition of circulating immune complexes. This assumption is based on similarities between PSGN and acute serum sickness. In fact, human acute PSGN and experimental acute serum sickness share the characteristics of a brisk antibody response, circulating immune complexes, transient reduction of serum complement, immune deposits in the kidney, and clinical nephritis. Both conditions have a complete resolution in a short period of time. Nevertheless, the nephritogenicity of preformed immune complexes is difficult to prove experimentally. Complement-dependent, proliferative glomerulonephritis mediated by leucocytes occurs when preformed immune-complexes are administered, but large amounts of complexes are needed and their glomerular location is largely subendothelial since they cannot traverse the glomerular basement membrane.

Since the original studies by Vogt and his associates (reviewed by Vogt 1984), numerous investigators have shown that the charge of the antigen, antibody, or immune complex has an important influence on its penetration through the glomerular basement membrane. Neutral or negatively charged molecules are excluded if their size exceeds that of serum albumin (effective radius of 35.5 Å), whereas cationic molecules penetrate the glomerular basement membrane freely, attracted by its negative electrostatic charge. Subepithelial deposits readily result from the administration of small quantities of cationic antigens, and are associated with injury mediated by the membrane attack complex of complement. These findings have particular relevance in acute PSGN in view of the typical subepithelial location of immune deposits in this disease.

Clearly, nephritogenicity is not restricted to cationic molecules. Inflammatory reactions in the glomerular basement membrane may reduce its anionic sites and favour the penetration of antigens and immune complexes of neutral or anionic charge. Furthermore, the subendothelial and mesangial locations of the immune complexes, favoured by non-cationic complexes, are associated with increased capability of recruiting circulating leucocytes, than are subepithelial deposits.

Complement activation has long been accepted as playing a role in immune-complex-induced nephritis, since glomerular immune deposits are capable of activating the complement system and components of the complement system are localized in the renal tissue. In PSGN, serum C3 is more frequently and more intensively depressed than C4; therefore, a preferential activation of the alternate complement pathway is assumed. Recently, new mechanisms of complement activation of potential relevance in PSGN have been disclosed. Berge *et al.* (1997) have demonstrated that protein H, a surface protein of *Streptococcus pyogenes*, by itself, reduced complement deposition on bacterial surfaces but in association with IgG is capable of activating the classic complement pathway. Oshawa *et al.* (1999) have demonstrated that the newly recognized lectin complement pathway is activated in PSGN, likely as a result of the recognition of the starter molecule mannose-binding lectin by the *N*-acetyl glucosamine residues of the bacterial wall or, less likely, by galactosamine radicals in the glomerular wall, if they had been exposed by neuraminidase.

The complement system recruits inflammatory cells but, in addition, individual components have direct nephritogenicity. C3a and C5a cause histamine release and increased permeability, and the terminal C5b–C9 complex (membrane attack complex) has a direct effect on the glomerular capillary membrane. Matsell *et al.* (1994) has shown that plasma terminal C5b–C complement complexes are consistently elevated at the onset of acute PSGN. Non-lytic effects of the membrane attack complex may result from their potential to stimulate platelets to secrete serotonin and thromboxane B, the macrophages to secrete phospholipids and arachidonic acid, and the mesangial cells to secrete proteases, and phospholipases, and generate oxygen reactive radicals. Damage inflicted directly by the C5b–C9 complex has potential importance in a variety of proliferative glomerulonephritides in which it is prominently deposited in the glomeruli, such as PSGN, IgA nephropathy, lupus nephritis, Henoch–Schönlein purpura, and membranoproliferative glomerulonephritis.

The role of platelet activation and consumption in the pathogenesis of PSGN has been studied by Mezzano *et al.* (1990, 1993, 1995), who showed a reduction in platelet counts and survival time and in plasma serotonin in these patients. These findings are related to a platelet-activating factor present in almost all patients with acute PSGN (Mezzano *et al.* 1993).

Infiltrating cells and production of cytokines

Significant numbers of infiltrating cells are present in postinfectious glomerulonephritis. Macrophages and lymphocytes are present in glomeruli and in tubulointerstitial regions and their participation in the acute inflammatory reaction as well as in the non-immune mechanisms of scarring that characterize the progressive renal damage have been recently reviewed (Rodríguez-Iturbe *et al.* 2001).

Several lines of evidence suggest the importance of cellular immune mechanisms in poststreptococcal nephritis. Nearly two decades ago, Parra *et al.* (1984) demonstrated CD4 (helper) lymphocytes and macrophages in early renal biopsies of PSGN. The importance of cell-mediated mechanisms is underlined by the report that PSGN can occur in patients with congenital C9 deficiency (Maruyama *et al.* 1995). Infiltration of mononuclear cells is accomplished by the production of chemotactic mediators in combination with the expression of intracellular adhesion molecules that facilitate the migration of cells from the circulation. Several complement components are well-known chemotactic factors and, in addition, macrophages can bind to the Fc portion of the immunoglobulins deposited in the glomerulus. However, the number of infiltrating macrophages is not correlated with the deposits of complement or immunoglobulin and other mechanisms are likely playing a more relevant role in promoting intrarenal cellular accumulation. The influence of T cells in facilitating macrophage infiltration is indicated by the studies of Parra *et al.* (1990), who showed that supernatants of glomerular cultures had MIF activity that correlated with the severity of proteinuria and with the intensity of intraglomerular lymphocyte and macrophage accumulation.

The role of intracellular adhesion molecules is evidenced by the overexpression of ICAM-1 and LFA-1 in the glomeruli as well as in the cells infiltrating tubulointerstitial areas of the kidney (Parra *et al.* 1994). Augmented local production of cytokines, such as IL-1 and tumour necrosis factor-α (TNF-α), are capable of inducing increased endothelial expression of intercellular adhesion molecules and in proliferative glomerulonephritis. Yokohama *et al.* (1997) have reported a direct correlation between serum TNF-α levels and glomerular ICAM-1 expression.

The production of cytokines is a central event in the pathophysiology of cell-mediated damage. IL-6, IL-1, and TNF-α, can be produced by resident mesangial cells and by infiltrating cells. A pathogenic role has been proposed for IL-6 in mesangial proliferative nephritis, specifically in lupus nephritis and IgA nephropathy (Horii *et al.* 1993; Yoshioka *et al.* 1993). Increased plasma levels of TNF-α and increased plasma and urinary levels of IL-6 are present in the first week of PSGN (Otha *et al.* 1992; Soto *et al.* 1997a,b). Glomerular IL-8 immunoreactivity correlates with neutrophil infiltration and the expression of transforming growth factor-β correlates with mesangial expansion (Mezzano *et al.* 1997).

Genetic aspects

The increased familial incidence of acute PSGN has been noted since Wells (1812) noted that postscarlatinal nephritis occurred more frequently among siblings of index cases as a result of 'similarity of constitution derived from common parents'. Dodge *et al.* (1967) also noted an increased familial incidence of PSGN. In prospective family studies, we found that PSGN developed in almost 38 per cent of the siblings of index cases with sporadic disease (Rodriguez-Iturbe *et al.* 1981b). This incidence is greater than the attack rate of children at risk in epidemics, estimated to range between 28 per cent for throat infections and 5 per cent for skin infections (Anthony *et al.* 1969). Nevertheless, definite associations between acute PSGN and HLA antigens have been elusive, and only DR4 and DR1 have been found to be more common in unrelated patients with the disease in Venezuela (Layrisse *et al.* 1983) and Japan (Naito *et al.* 1987), respectively.

Pathology

Acute endocapillary glomerulonephritis is typical of PSGN. The glomerular tuft shows an increased number of cells and appears to fill up Bowman's space (Fig. 2a). The basement membrane is normal. Oda *et al.* (1997) have shown intense proliferative activity in resident glomerular cells by double immunohistochemical staining studies. Initially, 80 per cent of the proliferating cells were endothelial cells and as the disease continued, mesangial cells represented half of the glomerular cells in active proliferation (Fig. 2b and c). The glomerular hypercellularity is increased by infiltration of cells from the circulation. Polymorphonuclear leucocyte infiltration may be intense ('exudative' glomerulonephritis) in early biopsies. Macrophages and lymphocytes also infiltrate glomeruli and tubulointerstitial areas in variable numbers. Within the glomerular tuft, macrophages predominate and helper T cells are in higher proportion in early biopsies (Parra *et al.* 1984). Overexpression of ICAM-1 is observed in glomeruli, peritubular capillaries, and tubular cells and LFA-1 positive cells are increased threefold in glomeruli and 10-fold in interstitium, where the infiltrates observed in early biopsies have a focal pattern of distribution (Parra *et al.* 1994).

Ultrastructural studies demonstrate subepithelial, subendothelial, and intramembranous immune aggregates as well as proliferating and infiltrating cells. Electron-dense subepithelial deposits (humps) are the hallmark lesion of acute PSGN (Fig. 2d), but also occur in glomerulonephritis of other aetiologies, such as systemic lupus erythematosus, bacterial endocarditis, and cryoglobulinaemia.

Immune deposits of the granular type are found in the capillary loops and in the mesangium. Granular deposits of IgG, IgM, anti-IgG, and C3 are usually prominent. Deposits of other complement components, including the terminal membrane attack complex, C5b–C9, usually accompany C3 deposits. Anti-IgG deposits are also found in the glomeruli. Findings of immune deposits and characteristics of the infiltrating cells in acute PSGN are shown in Table 4.

Clinicopathological correlations have emerged from the careful studies of Sorger (1986), who noted three distinct immunofluorescence patterns in postinfectious glomerulonephritis. The finely granular '*starry sky*' pattern of immune deposition (Fig. 2e) in the capillary walls, and to a lesser degree in the mesangium, may be seen in the first week of the disease. The '*mesangial pattern*' (Fig. 2f), is characterized by lumpy deposits of C3; immunoglobulins are sometimes absent, and this pattern is frequently found in biopsies taken 4–6 weeks later. The '*garland pattern*' is formed by heavy confluent deposits of IgG and C3, which tend to outline the glomerular capillaries (Fig. 2g). The garland pattern correlates with a large number of subepithelial humps in electron microscopy and is associated with massive proteinuria. Heavy proteinuria is associated with worse long-term prognosis.

Resolution of endocapillary glomerulonephritis depends on the disappearance of the immune disease, which, in postinfectious nephritis, depends on the eradication of the infecting microorganism. Soto *et al.* (1997a,b) have shown that apoptosis is the usual form of resolution in postinfectious glomerulonephritis. When the number of apoptotic cells is related to the number of proliferating cells, biopsies of acute PSGN had shown a striking direct relationship. This, in contrast with the findings in proliferative lupus nephritis, shows a relative reduction in apoptosis. Lu *et al.* (2000) reported recently essentially similar findings. Transformation of histological characteristics may occur, and is

Table 4 Immune deposits and infiltrating cells in acute poststreptococcal glomerulonephritis

Glomerular immune deposits	Positive/total biopsies	
Complement C3	53/53	
Complement C5b–C9[a]	6/7	
IgG	32/52	
IgM	38/50	
IgA	1/40	
IgE	0/34	
Antihuman IgG	16/55	
Infiltrating cells[a]	**Cells per 100 glomerular cells (normal)**	**Cells per mm^2 of interstitium (normal)**
Polymorphonuclear neutrophils	4.94 (0.1)	
Monocytes	3.35 (0)	58 ± 21 (36 ± 5)
T lymphocytes	0.48 (0.12)	136 ± 12 (26 ± 11)
CD_4 + lymphocytes	0.25 (0)	
CD_8 + lymphocytes	0.07 (0.06)	
CD_4/CD_8 ratio	3.57 (–)	

Data obtained from biopsies taken less than 1 month after the beginning of symptoms.

[a] Data from Parra *et al.* (1984, 1994).

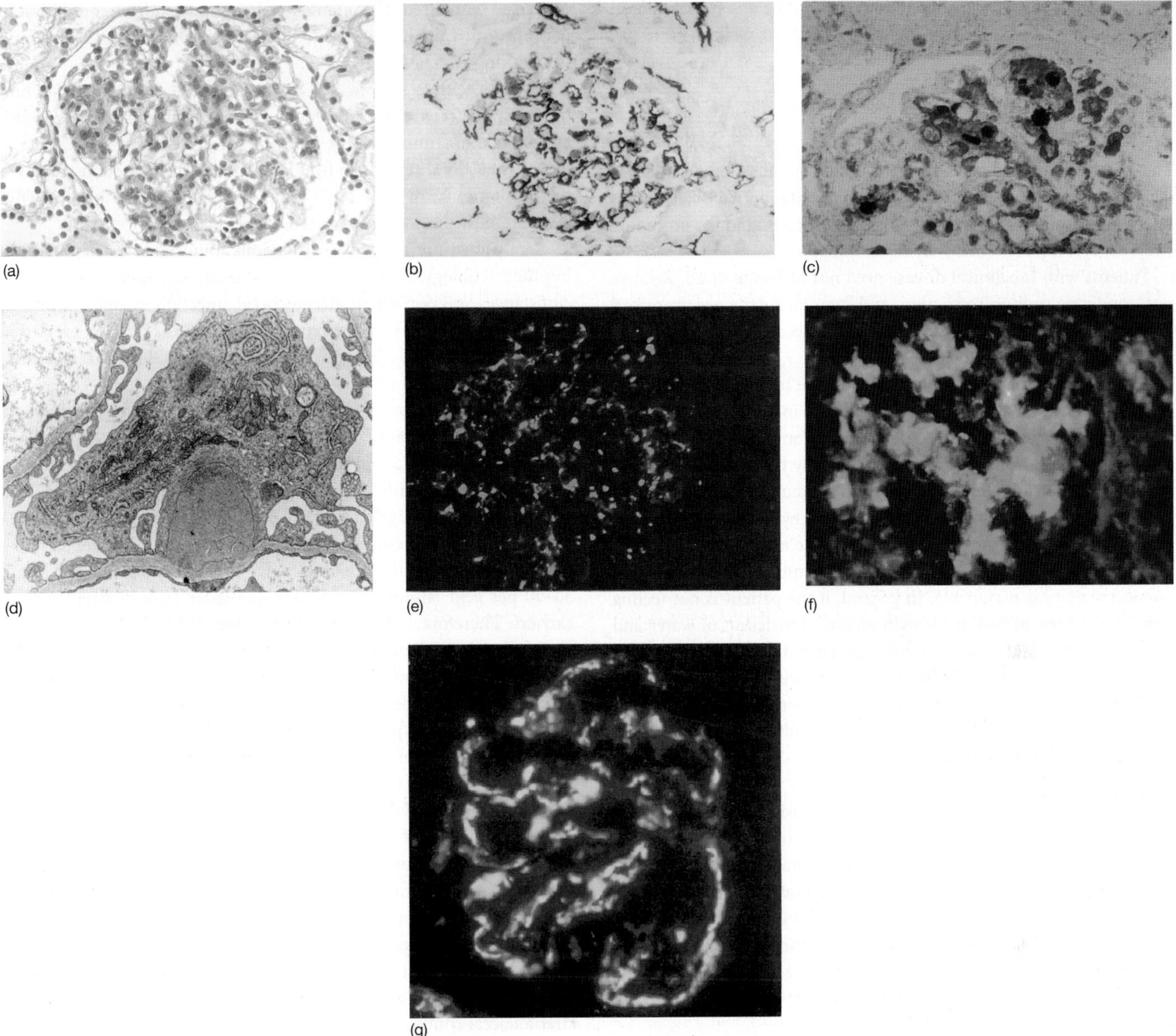

Fig. 2 Acute endocapillary glomerulonephritis of poststreptococcal aetiology. (a) Increased number of mesangial cells and infiltration with neutrophils. Basement membrane is normal. (b) Proliferation of endothelial cells shown in double staining for proliferating cell nuclear antigen (PCNA) in brown (immunoperoxidase-DAB) and staining for endothelial cells in blue (anti-CD31 polyclonal antibody, immunoalkaline phosphatase). Biopsy taken 6 days after onset. [Reproduced with permission from Yoshizawa *et al.* (1997). *Journal of Pathology* **183**, 359–368.] (c) Proliferation of mesangial cells shown with double staining for PCNA in black (immunoperoxidase-DAB $NiCl_2$) and staining for phenotypically changed mesangial cells in red (α-smooth muscle actin Mab, immunoperoxidase-EAC). Biopsy taken 9 days after onset. [Reproduced with permission from Yoshizawa *et al.* (1997). *Journal of Pathology* **183**, 359–368.] (d) Large electron-dense subepithelial deposit ('hump') shown by electron microscopy (4000×) (courtesy of N. Yoshizawa). (e) '*Starry sky*' pattern of C3 deposition (FITC-labelled anti-C3 staining). (f) '*Mesangial*' pattern of immunoglobulin deposits (FITC-labelled anti-IgG staining). (g) '*Garland*' pattern of immune deposits (FITC-labelled anti-IgG staining) (courtesy of Dr N. Yoshisawa).

the rule in cases that do not resolve completely. In acute PSGN, endocapillary proliferation in an early biopsy may change to focal segmental sclerosis or mesangiocapillary glomerulonephritis after some months or, more rarely, progress to a crescentic form of nephritis (reviewed in Fairley *et al.* 1987). Similar observations were made more than two decades ago by Beaufils *et al.* (1981) in glomerulonephritis associated with severe infections. These authors noted that the proliferative morphology is typical of cases occurring within 2 months of infection, while cases showing mesangioproliferative changes and crescent formation appear after a longer delay. Prolonged oligoanuria, lasting longer than 1 week in acute PSGN, has been associated with mesangiolysis (Drut and Drut 1992).

Follow-up studies, performed several years after the initial episode of acute PSGN, have revealed immune deposits and a variable degree of mesangial sclerosis and obliteration, even in the absence of clinical manifestations of renal disease (Baldwin *et al.* 1980; Gallo *et al.* 1980).

Treatment

The treatment of endocapillary proliferative glomerulonephritis will depend on the aetiology and the clinical presentation. We shall discuss only the treatment of the acute nephritic syndrome and the preceding streptococcal infection that may result in nephritis.

Patients with subclinical disease need not be hospitalized. Relative rest, moderate sodium restriction, and keeping a daily weight record are recommended. No specific treatment is needed and the family is advised to report any sudden weight gain.

Patients with the acute nephritic syndrome usually need hospitalization. This is always the case in adults and also in most children. Home management may be considered if a nurse or family physician is available to do a daily home call and the child only has mild oedema and normal serum creatinine. Nevertheless, the parents of the child should be warned that oliguria may develop and severe hypertension may occasionally complicate a course that appeared quite mild at the outset.

Strict bed rest is of doubtful value but a moderate restriction of physical activity is reasonable. In general, if the patient is not feeling well he will keep to bed of his own accord. Restriction of water and sodium intake should be prescribed to all patients with the acute nephritic syndrome. Our usual practice is to withhold oral intake in the first 12–24 h to define with accuracy the urinary volume before deciding on fluid allowance. This practice results, in addition, in an early and desirable weight loss.

Loop diuretics may benefit approximately 80 per cent of the patients with acute nephritis syndrome. Establishment of an effective diuresis is important because it reduces the cardiovascular congestion and helps in the control of hypertension. Several studies have shown that furosemide increases urine output several fold in PSGN and reduces the hospital stay from 7–10 to 4–5 days. Furosemide, 40 mg intravenously or orally, may be given initially and repeated every 12 h. It is unusual that diuretic therapy is needed longer than 48 h. Thazide diuretics have been used by some but we find them to be of limited use in these patients.

Antihypertensive medication may be used when the blood pressure is significantly elevated and it is judged unwise to wait for the effect of the diuretic therapy. This is the case in approximately half the children with PSGN and nearly 80 per cent of adults. Nifedipine (10 mg orally in adults and 5 mg in children, every 4–6 h) is usually effective. Some patients require parenteral hydralazine, but the development of important tachycardia, especially if the baseline heart rate is more than 100 per minute, is a potential complication. Diazoxide (1–3 mg/kg, maximum 150 mg) may be used in some resistant patients but it causes sodium retention and should be used in conjunction with furosemide that is best maintained for at least a day after stopping the diazoxide. Nitroprusside may be used when there is hypertensive encephalopathy. A rare patient with convulsions will require sedation and intubation.

Pulmonary oedema may complicate the clinical course and should be treated with oxygen, loop diuretics, and rotating tourniquets. Digitalis is ineffective and carries an increased risk of intoxication. Dialysis should be used early if there is raising azotaemia or hyperkalaemia. Peritoneal dialysis should be avoided in dyspnoeic patients or started with a reduced quantity of liquid and shorter equilibration periods until a significant negative balance is achieved and the patient is breathing effortlessly.

Patients with crescentic PSGN usually need dialysis. It has not been demonstrated that intravenous steroids, immunosuppression, or anticoagulation improves the outcome of crescentic PSGN. Nevertheless, anecdotal reports indicate that bolus of intravenous methylprednisolone, 0.5 g daily for 3 days, may improve the patient with severe rapidly progressive glomerulonephritis.

Removal of the antigen is of obvious importance in nephritis of immune aetiology. In the case of PSGN, treatment and, in certain circumstances, prevention of streptococcal infection is often possible. Oral phenoxymethyl or phenoxyethyl penicillin G (125 mg, every 6 h for 7–10 days) should eradicate the bacterium from the throat and skin. Oral benzylpenicillin (200,000 units four times daily for 7–10 days) is equally effective. Better compliance and similar results may be obtained with a single injection of 1.2 million units of benzathine benzylpenicillin in adults and half this dose in small children. In persons allergic to penicillin, erythromycin in doses of 250 mg every 6 h in adults, and 40 mg/kg in children, given for 7–10 days, is an appropriate alternative.

Only 10–15 per cent of throat infections in the adult are streptococcal in origin, and throat cultures give 10 per cent false-negative and 30–50 per cent false-positive results; the latter arise in streptococcal carriers. Therefore, certain clinical clues may help decide when to use antibiotics. Streptococcal aetiology of a sore throat can be practically ruled out if there is no fever, or tonsillar exudate, or cervical adenitis. In contrast, 40–50 per cent of the patients with all three symptoms have a streptococcal pharyngitis. Because of the rate of false-positive and false-negative throat cultures, the patients who present the mentioned clinical triad should be treated, and those who have none of these findings should not be treated, and cultures need not be obtained. However, in the vast majority of patients with sore throat who have one or two of these signs, culture should be done and treatment given to those patients with a positive result (Komaroff *et al.* 1986). Rapid high-sensitivity streptococcal tests are useful if positive, but the culture confirmation of negative results is generally advised. However, a recent report indicates that the decision of not to treat, based only on a negative test, was not associated with increased incidence of post-streptococcal complications (Webb *et al.* 2000).

Preventive antibiotic treatment is justified in populations at risk during epidemics, and in siblings of index cases. The latter show evidence of streptococcal infection within 2–3 weeks after the presentation of the index case in a vast majority of cases, and over one-third will develop nephritis (Rodriguez-Iturbe *et al.* 1981b). A recent study has reported success in treating a community to prevent new cases of PSGN and suggest that household members of index cases should receive benzathine penicillin G (Johnston *et al.* 1999).

Prognosis

The early mortality of acute endocapillary glomerulonephritis is very low in children but significant in adults (Table 2). Cardiovascular complications are the main cause of death in acute PSGN. Irreversible renal failure may follow acute glomerulonephritis if widespread extracapillary (crescentic) proliferation develops, but crescentic PSGN has a more favourable prognosis than other types of rapidly progressive glomerulonephritis.

The natural history of PSGN has been extensively studied. Initial reports in 1930 and 1940 indicated an excellent prognosis but follow-up periods were relatively short. Subsequent studies have given controversial results. The incidence of abnormal laboratory findings during the follow-up varies from 3.5 (Potter *et al.* 1982) to 60 per cent (Baldwin *et al.* 1980). Discrepancies may result, in part, from the different prognosis of PSGN in adults and in children, which is not always taken into account in the reported series. Also, a worse prognosis is associated with the clinical presentation of nephrotic syndrome and with alcoholism (Keller *et al.* 1994). In fact, a subgroup of adult patients who were nephrotic at presentation may have an incidence of chronic renal failure as high as 77 per cent (Vogl *et al.* 1986). A recent study with a specific outbreak of PSGN in adults, resulting from consumption of cheese contaminated with *S. zooepidemicus*, reports an alarming incidence of chronicity: impaired renal function was found in 30 per cent of the patients after 2 years of follow-up (10 per cent of them in chronic dialysis therapy) (Pinto *et al.* 2001). The worse prognosis in adults may result, in part, from age-related impairment of the Fc-receptor function of the mononuclear phagocyte system (Mezzano *et al.* 1991). The association of several risk factors superimposed on an initial attack of acute PSGN may have a definite influence in the long-term prognosis. Hoy *et al.* (1998) have reported, in Australian aborigines, an incidence of endstage renal disease of 2700 patients per million and that the incidence of albuminuria was directly correlated with a history of PSGN, hypertension, and heavy drinking and inversely correlated with birth weight.

Studies after 1970 reporting the findings in children, 10–20 years after the acute episode, found that approximately 20 per cent of the patients have an abnormal urine analysis or creatinine clearance, but less than 1 per cent have azotaemia. Proteinuria and hypertension occur in 8–13 per cent of the patients in most studies (range 1.4–46 per cent).

The incidence of glomerular sclerosis and fibrosis is nearly 50 per cent (Gallo *et al.* 1980), but their clinical relevance is uncertain. Our own data, which include 110 children with epidemic and sporadic PSGN followed prospectively 15–18 years after the acute episode, indicate an incidence of 7.2 per cent of proteinuria, 5.4 per cent of microhaematuria, 3.0 per cent of arterial hypertension, and 0.9 per cent of azotaemia. These values are essentially similar to those found in the general population. We have also followed 10 cases of subclinical PSGN for 10–11 years and the prognosis is excellent.

References

Anthony, B. F. *et al.* (1969). Attack rates of acute nephritis after type 49 streptococcal infections of the skin and of the respiratory tract. *Journal of Clinical Investigation* **48**, 1697–1704.

Ardiles, L. *et al.* (1997). Incidence and studies on antigenic specificities of anti-neutrophil cytoplasmatic autoantibodies (ANCA) in poststreptococcal glomerulonephritis. *Clinical Nephrology* **48**, 389–390.

Ardiles, L. *et al.* (1999). Anticardiolipin antibodies in acute poststreptococcal glomerulonephrhitis and streptococcal impetigo. *Nephron* **83**, 47–53.

Asami, T. *et al.* (1985). Elevated serum and urine sialic acid levels in renal diseases of childhood. *Clinical Nephrology* **23**, 112–119.

Balat, A., Baysal, K., and Kocak, H. (1993). Myocardial functions of children with acute poststreptococcal glomerulonephritis. *Clinical Nephrology* **39**, 151–155.

Baldwin, D. S. *et al.* Natural history of poststreptococcal glomerulonephritis. In *Streptococcal Diseases and the Immune Response* (ed. J. B. Zabriskie and S. E. Read), pp. 563–579. New York: Academic Press, 1980.

Balter, S. *et al.* (2000). Epidemic nephritis in Nova Serrana, Brazil. *Lancet* **355**, 1776–1780.

Beaufils, M. (1981). Glomerular disease complicating abdominal sepsis (Nephrology Forum). *Kidney International* **19**, 609–618.

Berge, A. *et al.* (1997). Streptococcal protein H forms soluble complement-activating complexes with IgG, but inhibits complement activation by IgG-coated targets. *Journal of Biological Chemistry* **272**, 20774–20781.

Bohle, A. *et al.* (1998). Human glomerular structure under normal conditions and isolated glomerular diseases. *Kidney International* **54** (Suppl. 67), S186–S188.

Borok, M. Z. *et al.* (1997). Clinicopathological features of Zimbabwean patients with sustained proteinuria. *Central African Journal of Medicine* **43**, 152–158.

Burova, L. A. *et al.* (1998). Triggering of renal tissue damage in the rabbit by IgG Fc receptor-positive group A streptococci. *Acta Pathologica Microbiologica et Immunologica Scandinavica* **106**, 277–287.

Choi, S. H., Zhang, X., and Stinton, M. W. (1995). Dynamics of streptococcal histone retention by mouse kidneys. *Clinical Immunology and Immunopathology* **6**, 68–74.

Cu, G.A. *et al.* (1998). Immunohistochemical and serological evidnce for the role of streptococcal proteinase in acute post-sreptococcal glomerulonephritis. *Kidney International* **54**, 819–825.

Currie, B. J. and Brewster, D. R. (2001). Chilodhood infections in the tropical north of Australia. *Journal of Paediatrics and Childhood Health* **37**, 326–330.

Dochez, A. R. and Sherman, L. (1924). The significance of *Streptococcus hemolyticus* in scarlet fever and the preparation of a specific antiscarlatinal serum by immunization of the horse to *Streptococcus hemolyticus scarlatinae*. *Journal of the American Medical Association* **2**, 542–544.

Dodge, W. F., Spargo, B. F., and Travis, L. B. (1967). Occurrence of acute glomerulonephritis in sibling contacts of children with sporadic acute glomerulonephritis. *Pediatrics* **40**, 1028–1030.

Drut, R. and Drut, R. M. (1992). Mesangiolytic poststreptococcal glomerulonephritis. *Pediatric Pathology* **12**, 113–117.

Duvic, C. *et al.* (2000). Acute poststreptococcal glomerulonephritis associated with thrombotic microangiopathy in an adult. *Clinical Nephrology* **54**, 169–173.

Fairley, K. and Birch, D. F. (1982). Hematuria: a simple method for identifying glomerular bleeding. *Kidney International* **21**, 105–108.

Farley, C., Mathews, D. C., and Becker, G. J. (1987). Rapid development of diffuse crescents in post-streptococcal glomerulonephritis. *Clinical Nephrology* **28**, 256–260.

Francis, A. J. *et al.* (1993). Investigation of milk-borne *Streptococcus zooepidemicus* infection associated with glomerulonephritis in Australia. *Journal of Infection* **27**, 317–323.

Frémeaux-Bacchi, V. *et al.* (1994). Hypocomplementaemia of poststreptococcal acute glomerulonephritis is associated with a C3 nephritic factor (C3NeF) IgG autoantibody activity. *Nephrology, Dialysis, Transplantation* **9**, 1747–1750.

Gallo, G. R. *et al.* (1980). Role of intrarenal vascular sclerosis in progression of poststreptococcal glomerulonephritis. *Clinical Nephrology* **13**, 449–457.

Heymann, W. *et al.* (1963). Decreased elasticity of auricular cartilage in the nephrotic syndrome of children. *Journal of Pediatrics* **62**, 74–76.

Horii, Y. *et al.* (1993). Role of interleukin-6 in the progression of mesangial proliferative glomerulonephritis. *Kidney International* **39** (Suppl.), S71–S75.

Hotta, O. *et al.* (1999). Detection of urinary macrophages expressing CD16 (Fcγ) molecule: a novel marker of acute glomerular injury. *Kidney International* **55**, 1927–1934.

Hoy, W. E. *et al.* (1998). The multidimensional nature of renal disease: rates and association of albuminuria in an Australian aboriginal community. *Kidney International* **54**, 1269–1304.

Johnson, R. J. *et al.* (2002). Subtle acquired renal injury as a mechanism for salt-sensitive hypertension. *New England Journal of Medicine* **346**, 913–923.

Johnston, F. *et al.* (1999). Evaluating the use of penicillin to control outbreaks of acute poststreptococcal glomerulonephritis. *Pediatric Infectious Disease Journal* **18**, 327–332.

Juncos, L. I. (2002). Intrarenal mechanisms of salt and water retention in the nephritic syndrome. *Kidney International* **61**, 1182–1195.

Kasahara, T. *et al.* (2001). Prognosis of acute poststreptococcal glomerulonephritis (APSGN) is excellent in children, when adequately diagnosed. *Pediatrics International* **43**, 364–367.

Keller, C. K. *et al.* (1994). Postinfectious glomerulonephritis—is there a link to alcoholism? *Quarterly Journal of Medicine* **87**, 97–102.

Komaroff, A. L., Pass, T. M., and Aronson, M. D. (1986). The prediction of streptococcal pharyngitis in adults. *Journal of General Internal Medicine* **1**, 1–7.

Lange, K., Seligson, G., and Cronin, W. (1983). Evidence for the *in situ* origin of poststreptococcal glomerulonephritis: glomerular localization of endostreptosin and clinical significance of the subsequent antibody response. *Clinical Nephrology* **19**, 3–10.

Layrisse, Z. *et al.* (1983). Family studies of the HLA system in acute poststreptococcal glomerulonephritis. *Human Immunology* **7**, 177–185.

Lu, F. *et al.* (2000). Dysregulation of apoptosis: a possible mechanism leading to chronic progressive renal histologic changes in lupus nephritis. *Chinese Medical Journal* **113**, 1082–1086.

Ludlam, H. and Cookson, B. (1986). Scrum kidney: epidemic pyoderma caused by a nephritogenic streptococcus pyogenes in a rugby team. *Lancet* **ii**, 331–333.

Lung, J. M. and Mallory, S. B. (2000). A child with spider bite and glomerulonephritis: a diagnostic challenge. *International Journal of Dermatology* **39**, 287–289.

Marín, C., Mosquera, J., and Rodríguez-Iturbe, B. (1995). Neuraminidase promotes neutrophil, lymphocyte and macrophage infiltration in the normal rat kidney. *Kidney International* **47**, 88–95.

Marín, C., Mosquera, J., and Rodríguez-Iturbe, B. (1997). Histological evidence of neuraminidase activity in acute nephritis: desialized lymphocytes infiltrate the kidney in acute poststreptococcal glomerulonephritis. *Clinical Nephrology* **47**, 217–221.

Maruyama, K. *et al.* (1995). C9 deficiency in a patient with poststreptococcal glomerulonephritis. *Pediatric Nephrology* **9**, 746–748.

Matsell, D. G., Wyatt, R. J., and Glaber, L. W. (1994). Terminal complement complexes in acute poststreptococcal glomerulonephritis. *Pediatric Nephrology* **8**, 671–676.

McIntosh, R. M. *et al.* (1972). Glomerular lesions produced in rabbits by autologous serum and autologous IgG modified by treatment with a culture of hemolytic streptococcus. *Journal of Medical Microbiology* **5**, 1–5.

Melby, P. C. *et al.* (1987). Poststreptococcal glomerulonephritis in the elderly. Report of a case and review of the literature. *American Journal of Nephrology* **7**, 235–240.

Mezzano, S. *et al.* (1990). Decrease in mean platelet survival time in acute poststreptococcal glomerulonephritis (APSGN). *Clinical Nephrology* **34**, 147–151.

Mezzano, S. *et al.* (1991). Age influence on mononuclear phagocyte system Fc-receptor function in poststreptococcal nephritis. *Nephron* **57**, 16–22.

Mezzano, S. *et al.* (1993). Detection of platelet-activating factor activity in plasma of patients with streptococcal nephritis. *Journal of the American Society of Nephrology* **4**, 235–242.

Mezzano, S. *et al.* (1995). Decreased platelet counts and decreased platelet serotonin in poststreptococcal nephritis. *Nephron* **69**, 135–139.

Mezzano, S. *et al.* (1997). Immunohistochemical localization of IL-8 and TGF-beta in streptococcal glomerulonephritis. *Journal of the American Society of Nephrology* **8**, 234–241.

Montseny, J. J. *et al.* (1995). The current spectrum of infectious glomerulonephritis. Experience with 76 patients and review of the literature. *Medicine (Baltimore)* **74**, 63–73.

Murphy, T. R. and Murphy, F. D. (1954). The heart in acute glomerulonephritis. *Annals of Internal Medicine* **41**, 510–532.

Muscatello, D. J. *et al.* (2001). Acute poststreptococcal glomerulonephritis: public health implications of recent clusters in New South Wales and epidemiology of hospital admissions. *Epidemiology and Infectology* **126**, 365–372.

Naito, S., Hohara, M., and Arakawa, K. (1987). Associations of class II antigens of HLA with primary glomerulopathies. *Nephron* **45**, 111–114.

Nicholson, M. L. *et al.* (2000). Analysis of immunoreactivity to a *Streptococcus equi* subsp. *zooepidemicus* M-like protein to confirm an outbreak of poststreptococcal glomerulonephritis, and sequences of M-liked proteins from isolates obtained from different host species. *Journal of Clinical Microbiology* **38**, 4126–4130.

Nordstrand, A. *et al.* (2000). Allele substitution of the streptokinase gene reduces the nephritogenic capacity of group A streptococcal strain NZ131. *Infection and Immunity* **68**, 1019–1025.

Oda, T. *et al.* (1997). Glomerular proliferatinig cell kinetics in acute poststreptococcal glomerulonephritis. *Journal of Pathology* **183**, 359–368.

Orta, N. and Moriyón, J. C. (2001). Epidemiología de las enfermedades renales en niños en Venezuela. *Archivos Venezolanos de Puericultura y Pediatría* **64**, 76–83.

Oshawa, I. *et al.* (1999). Evidence of lectin complement pathway activation in postsreptococcal glomerulonephritis. *Kidney International* **56**, 1158–1159.

Otha, K. *et al.* (1992). Detection and clinical usefulness of urinary interleukin-6 in the diseases of the kidney and the urinary tract. *Clinical Nephrology* **38**, 185–189.

Ozdemir, S. *et al.* (1992). Plasma atrial natriuretic peptide and endothelin levels in acute poststreptococcal glomerulonephritis. *Pediatric Nephrology* **6**, 519–522.

Parra, G., Mosquera, J., and Rodríguez-Iturbe, B. (1990). Migration inhibition factor in acute serum sickness nephritis. *Kidney International* **38**, 1118–1124.

Parra, G. *et al.* (1984). Cell populations and membrane attack complex in glomeruli and patients with poststreptococcal glomerulonephritis: indentification using monoclonal antibodies by indirect immunofluorescence. *Clinical Immunology and Immunopathology* **33**, 324–332.

Parra, G. *et al.* (1994). Expression of adhesion molecules in poststreptococcal glomerulonephritis. *Nephrology, Dialysis, Transplantation* **9**, 1412–1417.

Parra G. *et al.* (1998). Antibody to streptococcal zymogen in the serum of patients with acute glomerulonephritis: a multicentric study. *Kidney International* **54**, 509–517.

Pinto, S. L. W. *et al.* (2001). Follow-up of patients with epidemic poststreptococcal glomerulonephritis. *American Journal of Kidney Diseases* **38**, 249–255.

Poon-King, T. *et al.* (1967). Recurrent epidemic nephritis in South Trinidad. *New England Journal of Medicine* **277**, 728–733.

Poon-King, T. *et al.* (1993). Identification of an extracellular plasmin binding protein from nephritogenic streptococci. *Journal of Experimental Medicine* **178**, 759–763.

Potter, E. V. *et al.* (1982). Twelve to seventeen-year follow-up of patients with poststreptococcal acute glomerulonephritis in Trinidad. *New England Journal of Medicine* **307**, 725–729.

Raman, G. V. *et al.* (1986). A blind controlled trial of phase contrast microscopy by two observers for evaluating the source of hematuria. *Nephron* **44**, 304–308.

Rodriguez-Iturbe, B. (1984). Epidemic poststreptococcal glomerulonephritis (Nephrology Forum). *Kidney International* **25**, 129–136.

Rodriguez-Iturbe, B., Katiyar, V. N., and Coello, J. (1981a). Neuraminidase activity and free sialic acid levels in the serum of patients with acute poststreptococcal glomerulonephritis. *New England Journal of Medicine* **304**, 1506–1510.

Rodriguez-Iturbe, B., Rubio, L., and Garcia, R. (1981b). Attack rate of poststreptococcal glomerulonephritis in families. A prospective study. *Lancet* **i**, 401–403.

Rodríguez-Iturbe, B. *et al.* (1990). Atrial natriuretic factor in the acute nephritic and nephrotic syndromes. *Kidney International* **38**, 512–517.

Rodríguez-Iturbe, B. *et al.* (2001). The role of immunocompetent cells in nonimmune renal diseases. *Kidney International* **59**, 1626–1640.

Romero, M. *et al.* (1999). Erythrogenic toxin type B and its precursor isolated from streptococci induce leukocyte infiltration in normal rat kidneys. *Nephrology, Dialysis, Transplantation* **14**, 1867–1874.

Rovin, B. H., Doe, N., and Tan, L. C. (1996). Monocyte chemoattractant protein-1 levels in patients with glomerular disease. *American Journal of Kidney Diseases* **27**, 640–646.

Roy, S. and Stapleton, F. B. (1990). Changing perspectives in children hospitalized with poststreptococcal glomerulonephritis. *Pediatric Nephrology* **4**, 585–588.

Schick, B. (1907). Die Nachkrankheiten des Scharlach. *Jahrbuch der Kinderheilkunde* **65** (Suppl.), 132–173.

Seegal, D. and Earle, D. P. (1941). A consideration of certain biological differences between glomerulonephritis and rheumatic fever. *American Journal of Medical Sciences* **201**, 528–539.

Sesso, R. C. C., Ramos, O. L., and Periera, A. B. (1986). Detection of IgG-rheumatoid factor in sera of patients with acute poststreptococcal glomerulonephritis and its relation with circulating immunocomplexes. *Clinical Nephrology* **26**, 55–60.

Schafer, R. and Sheil, J. M. (1995). Superantigens and their role in infectious diseases. *Advances in Pediatric Infectious Diseases* **10**, 369–390.

Simon, P. *et al.* (1994). Epidemiology of primary glomerular diseases in a French region. Variations according to period and age. *Kidney International* **46**, 1192–1198.

Sorger, K. (1986). Postinfectious glomerulonephritis. Subtypes, clinico-pathological correlations and follow-up studies. *Veröffentlichungen aus der Pathologie* **125**, 1–105.

Soto, H. *et al.* (1997a). Apoptosis in proliferative glomerulonephritis: descreased apoptosis expression in lupus nephritis. *Nephrology, Dialysis, Transplantation* **12**, 273–280.

Soto, H. M., Parra, G., and Rodríguez-Iturbe, B. (1997b). Circulating levels of cytokines in poststreptococcal glomerulonephritis. *Clinical Nephrology* **47**, 6–12.

Soylu, A. *et al.* (2001). Posterior leukoencephalopathy syndrome in poststreptococcal acute glomerulonephritis. *Pediatric Nephrology* **16**, 601–603.

Tasic, V. and Polenakovic, M. (2000). Acute poststreptococcal glomerulonephritis following circumcision. *Pediatric Nephrology* **15**, 274–275.

Tencer, J. *et al.* (1997). Decreased excretion of glycosaminoglycans in patients with primary glomerular diseases. *Clinical Nephrology* **48**, 212–219.

Tomita, M. *et al.* (1962). A new morphological classification of urinary erythrocytes for the differential diagnosis of glomerular hematuria. *Clinical Nephrology* **37**, 84–97.

vanBuuren, A. J., Bates, W. D., and Muller, N. (1999). Nephrotic syndrome in Namibian children. *South African Medical Journal* **89**, 1088–1091.

Viera, N. T. *et al.* (2001). Streptococcal erythrogenic toxin B induces apoptosis and proliferation in human leukocytes. *Kidney International* **59**, 950–958.

Vilches, A. R. and Williams, D. G. (1984). Persistent anti-DNA antibodies and DNA-anti complexes in poststreptococcal glomerulonephritis. *Clinical Nephrology* **22**, 97–101.

Vogl, W. *et al.* (1986). Long-term prognosis for endocapillary glomerulonephritis of poststreptococcal type in children and adults. *Nephron* **44**, 58–65.

Vogt, A. *et al.* (1983). Cationic antigens in poststreptococcal glomerulonephritis. *Clinical Nephrology* **20**, 271–279.

Vogt, A. *et al.* (1990). The role of cationic proteins in the pathogenesis of immune complex glomerulonephritis. *Nephrology, Dialysis, Transplantation* **5** (Suppl. 1), 6–9.

Von Plenciz, M. A. (1792). Tractatus III de Scarlatina. Vienna: J.A. Trattner. Cited by Becker, C.G. and Murphy, G.E. (1968). The experimental induction of glomerulonephritis like that in man by infection with group A streptococcus. *Journal of Experimental Medicine* **127**, 1–23.

Washio, M. *et al.* (1994). Clinicopathological study of poststreptococcal glomerulonephritis in the elderly. *Clinical Nephrology* **41**, 265–270.

Watanabe, T. and Yoshizawa, N. (2001). Recurrence of acute poststreptococcal glomerulonephritis. *Pediatric Nephrology* **16**, 598–600.

Webb, K. H., Needham, C. A., and Kurtz, S. R. (2000). Use of a high-sensitivity rapid strep test without culture confirmation of negative results: 2 years' experience. *Journal of Family Practice* **49**, 34–38.

Wells, W. C. (1812). Observation on the dropsy which succeeds scarlet fever. *Transactions of the Society for the Improvement in Medical and Chirurgical Knowledge* **3**, 167–186.

West, C. D. and McAdams, A. J. (1998). Serum and glomerular IgG in post-streptococcal glomerulonephritis are correlated. *Pediatric Nephrology* **12**, 392–396.

Yamakami, K. *et al.* (2000). The potential role for nephritis-associated plasmin receptor in acute poststreptococcal glomerulonephritis. *Methods* **21**, 185–197.

Yap, H.-K. *et al.* (1990). Acute glomerulonephritis—changing patterns in Singapore children. *Pediatric Nephrology* **4**, 482–484.

Yoh, K. *et al.* (2000). Cytokines and T-cell responses in superantigen-related glomerulonephritis following methicillin-resistant *Staphylococcus aureus* infection. *Nephrology, Dialysis, Transplantation* **15**, 1170–1174.

Yokohama, H. *et al.* (1997). Glomerular ICAM-1 expression related to circulating TNF-alpha in human glomerulonephritis. *Nephron* **76**, 425–433.

Yokohama, H. *et al.* (1998). Urinary levels of chemokines (MCAF/MCP-1) reflect distinct disease activities and phases of human IgA nephropathy. *Journal of Leukocyte Biology* **63**, 493–499.

Yoshizawa, N. (2000). Acute glomerulonephritis. *Internal Medicine* **39**, 687–694.

Yoshizawa, N. *et al.* (1997a). Experimental acute glomerulonephritis induced in the rabbit with a specific streptococcal antigen. *Clinical and Experimental Immunology* **107**, 61–67.

Yoshizawa, N. *et al.* (1997b). Asymptomatic acute poststreptococcal glomerulonephritis following upper respiratory tract infections causes by group A streptococci. *Clinical Nephrology* **46**, 296–301.

Zelman, M. F. and Lange, C. F. (1995). Immunochemical studies of streptococcal cell membrane antigens immunologically related to glomerular basement membrane. *Hybridoma* **14**, 529–536.

Zhang, L. *et al.* (1999). Streptococcal histone induces murine macrophages to produce interleukin-1 and tumor necrosis factor alpha. *Infection and Immunity* **67**, 6473–6477.

3.10 Crescentic glomerulonephritis

Jeremy Levy and Charles D. Pusey

Introduction and definition

The term 'crescentic glomerulonephritis' originated in the era of descriptive pathology, and despite its lack of precision regarding underlying aetiopathogenesis of glomerular inflammation, remains to this day a useful descriptive term. It is the pathological correlate of the clinical syndrome of rapidly progressive glomerulonephritis (RPGN). However, both labels provide no clue as to the pathophysiological processes contributing to the often catastrophic renal damage, and the same crude histological appearances and clinical presentation can be found in a wide range of conditions. The formation of crescents seems to represent a final common pathway of severe glomerular inflammation. Hence the term 'crescentic nephritis' should now always be accompanied by a more precise aetiopathological label which describes the underlying cause.

In 1914, Volhard and Fahr provided beautiful descriptions of severe glomerular destruction, and commented on the extracapillary proliferation of cells in Bowman's capsule (Fig. 1). These cells appear as a crescent within the glomerulus in cross-section. It was not until 1942 that the term rapidly progressive glomerulonephritis was introduced for patients who developed renal failure over weeks or months, most of whom were found to have crescentic nephritis (Ellis 1942). At the time it was thought the major cause was poststreptococcal disease.

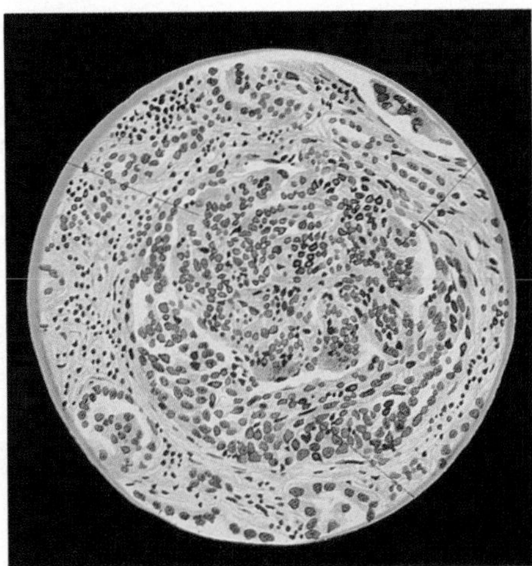

Fig. 1 Crescentic nephritis as illustrated by Volhard and Fahr (1914). The glomerular tuft shows proliferation, and a cellular crescent occupies the lower segment of Bowman's capsule.

Within the next few years, a number of reports had identified crescentic nephritis in patients with vasculitis, and suggested that this might be the major underlying cause (Davson *et al.* 1948).

Over the next 30 years, the development of renal biopsy and then immunohistology allowed many workers to appreciate that crescents were a feature of different forms of nephritis, and that, in general, they were a very poor prognostic sign. Most patients were dead within months or a few years, and recovery of renal function was rare (Couser 1982; Glassock 1985). During the 1970s, immunohistology, in particular, allowed patients with crescentic nephritis to be categorized into three groups according to glomerular findings on immunofluorescent staining for IgG and complement within the glomerular tuft, which continue to form the basis of contemporary classifications (Whitworth *et al.* 1976; Beirne *et al.* 1977; Morrin *et al.* 1978; Neild *et al.* 1983):

(1) patients with linear staining caused by anti-GBM antibodies (anti-GBM disease, GBM = glomerular basement membrane) (Chapter 3.11);

(2) those in whom glomerular immunoglobulin deposition was scarce or absent [now known to be almost universally associated with antineutrophil cytoplasmic antibodies (ANCA)] (Chapters 4.5.1 and 4.5.3);

(3) those with prominent granular deposits (and an underlying primary glomerulonephritis) (see especially Chapters 3.6, 3.8, 3.9, 3.12, 3.14, 4.6, 4.7.2).

In all three groups, the severity of renal failure at presentation was recognized as a poor prognostic sign, as was the proportion of glomeruli containing crescents (Whitworth *et al.* 1976; Beirne *et al.* 1977; Morrin *et al.* 1978). Much of the literature from the period debated the precise definition of 'crescentic nephritis', although it should be obvious that the precise appearance of a crescent (circumferential, partial, focal) will be dictated by the plane through which the glomerulus has been cut (Fig. 2). More recently, it has become clear that in almost all the crescentic nephritides, prognosis is more dependent on the extent of tubulointerstitial scarring and fibrosis, and the number of normal glomeruli, rather than any measure of crescentic glomeruli. Both human and animal studies have shown that glomerular inflammation can evolve rapidly—further obscuring the usefulness of crescent scores *per se*. Prognosis is crucially dependent on the precise diagnosis rather than the crescentic nature of the glomerular injury. This was not fully appreciated in many of the early clinical reports of the treatment of crescentic nephritis, which often included heterogeneous groups of patients with crescentic histology (Glockner *et al.* 1988; Keller *et al.* 1989).

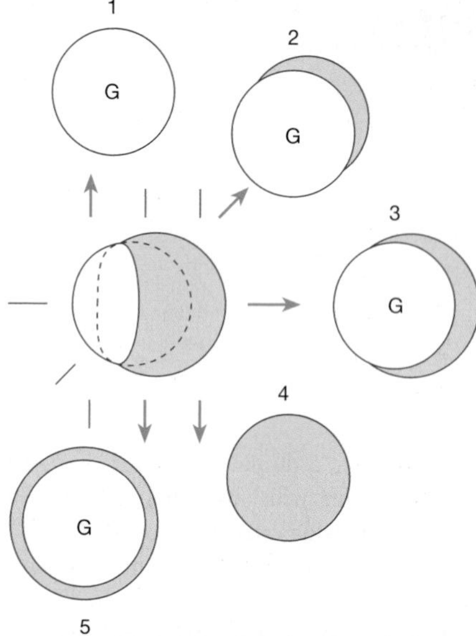

Fig. 2 The effect of the direction of the section on the appearance of a single 'crescent'. The centre figure represents a glomerulus partially surrounded by a crescent. The arrows indicate various sections, and point to the appearance seen in each section: G, glomerular tuft; the shaded area represents the crescent. The crescent can appear to be absent, segmental, or circumferential depending on which plane the section takes.

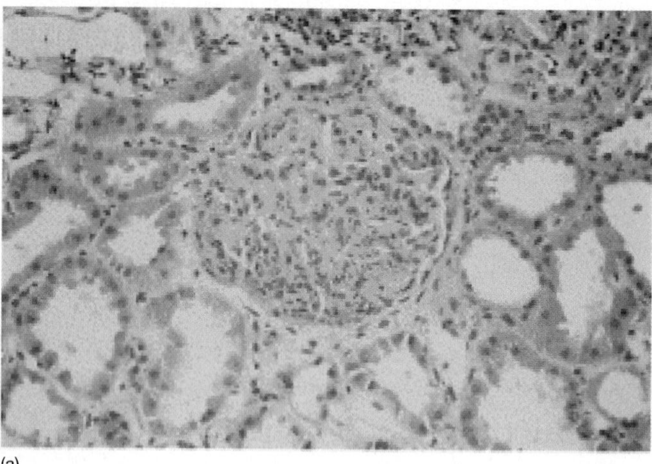

(a)

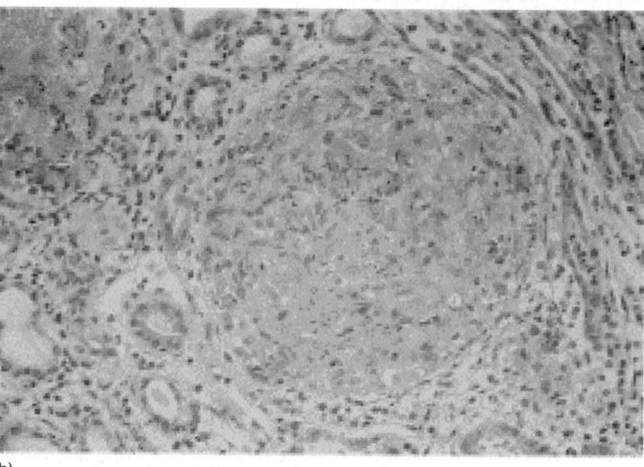

(b)

Fig. 3 Renal biopsies taken 5 days apart from a patient with Alport's syndrome who developed *de novo* anti-GBM disease in a renal allograft. (a) Occasional glomeruli in the first biopsy showed mild segmental proliferation but there was no necrosis or extracapillary proliferation. (b) Five days later there was extensive necrosis and all glomeruli in the second biopsy had circumferential crescents (from Professor Cameron).

Diagnosis, therefore, depends on the integration of clinical data, renal biopsy findings (Fig. 3), and serological tests such as anti-GBM antibodies, ANCA, systemic lupus erythematosus (SLE) antibodies, and cryoglobulins. In this way, anti-GBM disease or ANCA-associated vasculitis can be clearly distinguished from other causes of crescentic nephritis, with significant implications for therapy. Thus, for example, most patients with crescentic RPGN will not recover renal function from dialysis dependency if they have anti-GBM disease, but may do so if they have ANCA-associated disease (Levy *et al.* 2001; Zauner *et al.* 2002). The term 'idiopathic' crescentic glomerulonephritis has been widely used in the literature with a variety of meanings, but now generally recognized as synonymous with pauci-immune glomerulonephritis or renal limited vasculitis. Since the discovery of ANCA, there has been much debate as to the reality of truly idiopathic crescentic glomerulonephritis (Falk and Jennette 1988) (see Chapter 4.5.2). Anganco *et al.* (1994) retrospectively reanalysed all their patients with crescentic nephritis ($n = 89$) and found only one patient without systemic features or circulating ANCA who might have been truly 'idiopathic', but even this patient had a positive ANCA assay on one occasion. Similarly, Ferrario *et al.* (1994) re-examined their patients with histologically defined crescentic glomerulonephritis and made the useful distinction between those with and without segmental necrosis. Biopsies without necrosis had immunoglobulin and complement deposition detectable by immunohistology, and should therefore be regarded as primary glomerulonephritides with superimposed crescentic change. Patients with segmental necrosis had circulating ANCA and pauci-immune immunohistology, and could all be regarded as having renal limited or systemic ANCA-associated vasculitis. Occasional population-based studies of RPGN or crescentic nephritis have reported small numbers of patients in whom ANCA are never detected (Cohen and Clark 2000; Hedger *et al.* 2000). However, it should be remembered that some patients only have a fleetingly detectable ANCA, and ANCA may disappear rapidly with treatment. Overall, we would favour the view that patients with crescentic pauci-immune glomerulonephritis *all* have a small vessel vasculitis, which will almost always be found to be associated with ANCA, and there is little to separate these patients clinically or by histological findings (Falk *et al.* 1990; Andrassy *et al.* 1991; Bindi *et al.* 1993; Ferrario *et al.* 1994).

Varieties of crescentic nephritis

Crescents occur when breaks in glomerular capillaries allow leakage of cells and plasma proteins into Bowman's space. Crescents can therefore occur in almost any disease leading to glomerular inflammation, and sometimes in renal diseases that do not primarily affect the glomerulus. Widespread crescent formation, however, requires active and specific attack on glomerular capillaries, and is found in a more restricted set of diseases (Table 1).

Table 1 Underlying diagnoses in all patients with crescentic glomerulonephritis seen at Hammersmith Hospital between 1990 and 2000

Diagnosis	Number (%)
ANCA-associated vasculitis	53 (37)
SLE	33 (23)
IgA disease	17 (12)
MCGN	9 (6)
Focal–segmental glomerulonephritis	9 (6)
Anti-GBM disease	8 (6)
Postinfectious glomerulonephritis	5 (3)
Membranous glomerulonephritis	3 (2)
Focal–segmental glomerulosclerosis	3 (2)
Henoch–Schönlein purpura	2 (1)
Others	4 (3)

Three broad groups of crescentic nephritis can be distinguished:

(1) Anti-GBM disease, characterized by circulating anti-GBM antibodies and linear deposition of antibody along the membrane; this constitutes about 10 per cent of cases (see Chapter 3.11).

(2) Renal microscopic vasculitis characterized by scanty glomerular deposits of immunoglobulin and circulating ANCA; comprises about 60 per cent of cases (see Chapters 4.5.1 and 4.5.3).

(3) A heterogeneous group usually associated with obvious granular deposits of immunoglobulin, in which crescent formation complicates an identifiable form of nephritis, usually proliferative in type; causes around 30 per cent of cases (see Sections 3 and 4, *passim*).

Pauci-immune glomerulonephritis is the most common cause of crescentic pathology with RPGN, followed in most series by SLE and anti-GBM disease (Neild *et al.* 1983; Jennette 1999). IgA disease is the most common primary glomerulonephritis in which to find crescents (Chapter 3.6), but rarely presents clinically with RPGN. Table 2 shows the diseases presenting with a clinical diagnosis of RPGN, regardless of the presence of crescents on renal biopsy.

Anti-GBM disease

In principle, this is easy to diagnose on the basis of linear deposition of antibody along the GBM on immunohistology of the renal biopsy, and detection of circulating anti-GBM antibodies (see Chapter 3.11). However, occasionally linear immunoglobulin can be found in other

Table 2 Underlying causes of RPGN from recent published series (numbers given as percentages)

	Heilmann *et al.* (1987); (*n* = 64)	Keller *et al.* (1989); (*n* = 46)	Ritz *et al.* (1991); (*n* = 38)	Levy *et al.* (1994); (*n* = 48)	Angangco *et al.* (1994); (*n* = 82)
Pauci-immune crescentic nephritis (including microscopic polyangiitis, Wegener's granulomatosis, renal limited and systemic vasculitis)	68	65	52	56	44
Polyarteritis nodosa		4		4	
Churg–Strauss syndrome				2	
Anti-GBM disease	20	20	8	15	12
Systemic lupus erythematosus	0	7	8	6	2
Henoch–Schönlein purpura	3	2	13	8	17
Postinfectious GN			13	2	4
Cryoglobulinaemia	2			2	1
Mixed connective tissue disease				4	1
Rheumatoid arthritis					5
Primary GN (IgA, membranous, MCGN)	6	2	5		12

ANCA, antineutrophil cytoplasmic antibody; GN, glomerulonephritis; MCGN, mesangiocapillary glomerulonephritis.

conditions, and rarely circulating antibodies are undetectable using conventional assays (Salama *et al.* 2002). It is an important diagnosis to make rapidly since recovery is rare once patients become dialysis dependent (Levy *et al.* 2001).

Renal microscopic vasculitis (Chapters 4.5.1 and 4.5.2)

This is the most common cause of crescentic glomerulonephritis and may present with isolated renal disease or with evidence of more widespread systemic vasculitis (see Chapters 4.5.1 and 4.5.2). It is now clear that most patients have detectable circulating ANCA, whether or not they have systemic disease. The vasculitides can be classified on the basis of the size of the blood vessels involved or by clinical features, but almost all forms have been reported to cause crescentic glomerulonephritis. Microscopic polyangiitis, Wegener's granulomatosis, and isolated renal vasculitis are the most common diagnoses; Churg–Strauss syndrome (Clutterbuck *et al.* 1987), relapsing polychondritis (Neild *et al.* 1978; Chang-Miller *et al.* 1987), Takayasu's disease (Hellmann *et al.* 1987; Logan *et al.* 1994), giant-cell arteritis (Droz *et al.* 1979), rheumatoid vasculitis (Breedveld *et al.* 1985; Naschitz *et al.* 1989; Kiyama *et al.* 1991), and vasculitis associated with narcotic abuse (Citron *et al.* 1970) are all well recognized. There have been isolated case reports of crescentic glomerulonephritis in juvenile polymyositis (Kamata *et al.* 1982), acute rheumatic fever (Mustonen *et al.* 1983), and Behçet's disease (Donnelly *et al.* 1989; Tietjen and Moore 1990).

Crescentic nephritis with granular immune deposits

These patients form a heterogeneous group in which a variety of stimuli lead to a proliferative nephritis with crescents. Immunohistology shows granular deposits of immunoglobulin and complement along capillary walls and in the mesangium. Causes include infection, systemic immune complex diseases (especially SLE), and most commonly underlying pre-existing primary glomerulonephritides. This group is the most common cause of crescentic glomerulonephritis in children.

Systemic infections (see also Chapter 3.12)

Poststreptococcal nephritis can rarely present with crescentic histology (Löhlein 1907; Lewy *et al.* 1977; Southwest Pediatric Nephrology Study Group 1985; Edelstein and Bates 1992; Srivastava *et al.* 1992; Tapaneya-Olarn *et al.* 1992) or sometimes progress to a crescentic phase (Morel-Maroger *et al.* 1974; Gill *et al.* 1977; Old *et al.* 1984; Modai *et al.* 1985; Fairley *et al.* 1987). Some of these patients have been reported to recover spontaneously even with quite extensive crescent formation (Nakamoto *et al.* 1965; Leonard *et al.* 1970; Whitworth *et al.* 1976; Southwest Pediatric Nephrology Study Group 1985), especially when electron microscopy shows subepithelial humps rather than subendothelial or intramembranous deposits (Sonsino *et al.* 1972; Hinglais *et al.* 1974; Neild *et al.* 1983). However, extensive crescents (>60 per cent) are associated with a poor outcome (Srivastava *et al.* 1992; Montseny *et al.* 1995).

Infective endocarditis rarely causes crescentic pathology (Beaufils *et al.* 1976), although there are occasional exceptions (Neugarten *et al.* 1984; Rovzar *et al.* 1986; Kannan and Mattoo 2001; Kodo *et al.* 2001), in contrast to children with infected atrioventricular shunts, in whom crescentic membranoproliferative nephritis is not uncommon (Niaudet and Levy 1983; Southwest Pediatric Nephrology Study Group 1985; Wakabayshi *et al.* 1985). Eradication of infection is important in both situations. Removal of the infected shunt leads to recovery of renal function in almost all cases (Wakabayashi *et al.* 1985). Endocarditis can also present with systemic vasculitis and crescentic glomerulonephritis (Kodo *et al.* 2001).

There are case reports of patients with visceral abscesses developing crescentic nephritis (Beaufils *et al.* 1976; Whitworth *et al.* 1976; Connelly and Gallacher 1987), but in many instances, the infection may simply have exacerbated an underlying pre-existing renal disease. This has been well documented in anti-GBM disease and its animal models, in which local or systemic infection can exacerbate nephritis probably via the release of proinflammatory cytokines (Rees *et al.* 1977). Similarly, patients with methicillin resistant *Staphylococcus aureus* (MRSA) sepsis have also been identified with crescentic nephritis, but clearly the same caveats apply. Individual patients with human immunodeficiency virus (HIV), hepatitis B virus, Ross river virus, leprosy, legionella, mycoplasma, and syphilis infections have also occasionally been reported to have crescentic glomerulonephritis on renal biopsy. In all these cases, patients have also been exposed to a variety of drugs, and may have had pre-existing renal disease.

Systemic immune complex disease

Systemic lupus erythematosus (see also Chapters 4.7.1. and 4.7.2)

Crescents are a common feature of lupus nephritis in patients with class IV proliferation, less common in type III, and rare in patients with isolated membranous histology (Yeung *et al.* 1984; Williams *et al.* 1985; Leaker *et al.* 1987). A single study of the outcome of patients with crescentic nephritis demonstrated a four- to sixfold increased risk of renal failure in 45 patients (95% confidence interval 1.29–14.7; Magil *et al.* 1988). Uncontrolled studies have also suggested a poorer prognosis in patients with class IV disease and crescents (Leaker *et al.* 1987; Sumethkul *et al.* 2000). The natural history of such crescents is unclear.

Henoch–Schönlein purpura (see also Chapter 4.5.2)

Moderate crescentic change is a common feature of Henoch–Schönlein purpura (HSP) in both adults and children (Niaudet *et al.* 1984; Southwest Pediatric Nephrology Study Group 1985; Jardim *et al.* 1992; Flynn *et al.* 2001), but most series will be biased towards patients with more severe disease in whom renal biopsies have been performed. Extensive crescent formation may be associated with a poorer prognosis, and patients are more likely to receive immunosuppression.

Others

Individual patients with Reiter's syndrome, myeloma, cryoglobulinaemia, light chain deposit disease, familial Mediterranean fever, hypocomplementaemic urticarial vasculitis, and amyloid have also been reported with crescentic glomerulonephritis on renal biopsy, although these are rare presentations of renal disease in each case.

Primary glomerulonephritis

Mesangial IgA disease (see also Chapter 3.6)

Small focal crescents are a common feature of IgA disease, being found in up to 35 per cent of biopsies (Nicholls *et al.* 1984; D'Amico *et al.* 1985; Boyce *et al.* 1986; Lai *et al.* 1987). More extensive cellular crescents are rare (Abuelo *et al.* 1984; Welch *et al.* 1988; D'Amico 2000). In our own series of 145 patients with crescentic glomerulonephritis, IgA disease was the third most common underlying cause after ANCA-associated vasculitis and SLE (see Table 1), but only 24 per cent of the biopsies with IgA disease had more than 50 per cent crescents. D'Amico *et al.* (1985) found only 2.4 per cent of biopsies with extensive crescents in their study of 374 patients with IgA disease, although 30 per cent of patients had at least one crescent. Crescents are known to be found commonly after episodes of macroscopic haematuria, and subsequently resolve, and these patients have a better long-term prognosis (Bennett and Kincaid-Smith 1983). Hotta *et al.* (2002) reported that 32 of 35 patients with IgA disease had cellular crescents on first biopsy, which had completely resolved in all by the time of a second biopsy (a mean of 77 months later). Patients had received a variety of treatments. The clinical syndrome of RPGN with crescentic histology is rare.

The effect of crescents themselves on the prognosis of patients with IgA disease is unclear. Abe *et al.* (1986) documented a poor prognosis in patients with extensive crescents, with a high incidence of endstage renal failure. Seventeen of twenty six patients with more than 50 per cent crescents reached dialysis over 7.9 years follow-up compared with none of those without crescents. Haas (1997) suggested that crescents were a significant negative predictive indicator for renal survival in patients only with focal proliferative IgA disease, while Daniel *et al.* (2000) found crescents were associated with a poor outcome overall. Frequently, however, patients with extensive crescents also have marked tubulointerstitial scarring, and the poor prognosis might, therefore, be independent of the crescentic change itself (Daniel *et al.* 2000). Our own data support this view since most patients with extensive crescent formation also had severe tubular scarring and fibrosis. Patients with fresh cellular crescents and little tubular damage have been reported to respond to immunosuppression with improved renal function.

Mesangiocapillary and membranous glomerulonephritis (see also Chapters 3.7 and 3.8)

Crescents are found in about 15 per cent of patients with mesangiocapillary nephritis and rarely in membranous nephropathy. The few patients with crescentic mesangiocapillary glomerulonephritis (MCGN) tend to have extensive crescents (McCoy *et al.* 1975; Davis *et al.* 1978; Chapman *et al.* 1980; Neild *et al.* 1983; Southwest Pediatric Nephrology Study Group 1985; Korzets and Bernheim 1987). In membranous nephropathy, crescents either occur late in the disease (Klassen *et al.* 1974; Nicholson *et al.* 1975; Tateno *et al.* 1981; Kurki *et al.* 1984; Koethe *et al.* 1986; Nguyen *et al.* 1988) or in patients with coexistent anti-GBM antibodies (Hill *et al.* 1978). Crescents themselves are not a prognostic predictor of outcome in idiopathic membranous nephropathy (Wu *et al.* 2001).

Drugs (see also Chapter 19.2)

Penicillamine is the most common drug that has been shown unequivocally to cause crescentic nephritis, when used to treat rheumatoid arthritis (Gibson *et al.* 1976; Gavaghan *et al.* 1981; Swainson *et al.* 1982; Sadjadi *et al.* 1985; Macarron *et al.* 1992; Nanke *et al.* 2001), Wilson's disease (Sternlieb *et al.* 1975), primary biliary cirrhosis (Matloff and Kaplan 1980), or systemic sclerosis (Ntoso *et al.* 1986). Many of the patients have had a full-blown pulmonary-renal syndrome with RPGN and pulmonary haemorrhage, sometimes with the development of ANCA (Gaskin *et al.* 1995). Interestingly, none of the large number of patients taking the drug for cystinuria has been reported to develop this complication. Penicillamine is a potent polyclonal B cell activator and can induce synthesis of pathogenic autoantibodies, which may be the mechanism for crescentic nephritis. The related drug bucillamine has also been reported to cause crescentic nephritis (Yoshida *et al.* 1992).

Propylthiouracil has been linked repeatedly with crescentic nephritis with the development of antimyeloperoxidase ANCA in both adults and children, systemic features of vasculitis, and a generally good prognosis with immunosuppressive treatment (Fujieda *et al.* 2002). Hydralazine similarly has been found to induce P-ANCA and crescentic glomerulonephritis (Mason and Lockwood 1986; Almroth *et al.* 1992) as well as the much more common lupus syndrome (see Chapters 4.7.1 and 4.7.2). Case reports have also implicated phenylbutazone, rifampicin, streptokinase, enalapril, and interleukin-2 as causing crescentic nephritis.

Miscellaneous causes

Small numbers of patients with crescentic nephritis have been found to have malignancies, either at presentation or developing later, including carcinomas and lymphomas (Whitworth *et al.* 1976; Beirne *et al.* 1977; Neild *et al.* 1983; Biava *et al.* 1984; Weinstein *et al.* 1990; Dussol *et al.* 1992; Westman *et al.* 1998) (see Chapter 3.13). Whether there is any causal link remains unclear. Individual case reports have apparently implicated hydrocarbons, snake envenoming, α1-antitrypsin deficiency, pancreatitis, and silicosis in the genesis of crescentic nephritis (Tervaert *et al.* 1998). α1-Antitrypsin is a natural inhibitor of serine proteinases such as proteinase 3, and partial deficiency has also been associated with Wegener's granulomatosis (see Chapter 4.5.2). Exposure to organic solvents has also been implicated in the development of anti-GBM antibody disease. One study has reported that 13 per cent of patients with renal amyloidosis had crescents on biopsy, predominantly in patients with AA amyloid (Nagata *et al.* 2001).

Crescentic nephritis in children

Crescentic glomerulonephritis is rare in children but can be caused by all the diseases already discussed in adults (Anand *et al.* 1975; Cunningham *et al.* 1980; Miller *et al.* 1984; Southwest Pediatric Nephrology Study Group 1985; Heilman *et al.* 1987; Walters *et al.* 1988; Jardim *et al.* 1992; Srivastava *et al.* 1992; Tapenaya-Olarn *et al.* 1992; Hattori *et al.* 2001). Poststreptococcal glomerulonephritis, HSP, and mesangiocapillary glomerulonephritis are the most common causes with marked variation in incidence between different series (Cunningham *et al.* 1980; Walters *et al.* 1988). All are rare in children under 4 years. ANCA-associated disease and anti-GBM disease are extremely uncommon. Children with ANCA-associated crescentic glomerulonephritis, however, behave similarly to adults in both presentation, response to treatment, and outcome (Hattori *et al.* 2001). Hypertension is more common than in adults. Diagnosis needs to be made rapidly to allow appropriate treatment.

Epidemiology

The overall incidence of crescentic glomerulonephritis is between 2 and 5 per cent of unselected renal biopsies, regardless of the country of origin, be it France, England, America, India, or China (Whitworth *et al.* 1976; Neild *et al.* 1983; Woo *et al.* 1986; Date *et al.* 1987; Heilman *et al.* 1987; Parag *et al.* 1988; Tang *et al.* 2001; Vendemia *et al.* 2001). Men are affected twice as commonly as women, and Afro-Caribbeans are relatively rarely affected, except by crescentic SLE. In one study from South Africa, idiopathic crescentic glomerulonephritis and anti-GBM disease were more common in White than Black patients (Parag *et al.* 1988). There is an increased incidence in the elderly—data from the Italian registry of renal biopsies suggests a threefold increase (Vendemia *et al.* 2001).

Clinical aspects

Clearly, the precise clinical features of patients with RPGN vary with the underlying disease, and it is not particularly useful to provide an amalgamated clinical overview. Full details of the individual diseases can be found in the following chapters. Some features are relatively common to all causes of crescentic nephritis; hypertension is rare, loin pain not uncommon, constitutional symptoms found in approximately 50 per cent, urine almost always contains blood, red cell casts, granular casts, and protein, but nephrotic range proteinuria is rare. Leucocytes are also a common finding in the urine, often with more than 30,000/ml (Segasothy *et al.* 1989). Rate of progression to renal failure is variable from hours (e.g. in anti-GBM disease) to months (some cases of MCGN).

Non-specific markers of inflammation are usually raised, including C-reactive protein (CRP), peripheral blood leucocytes, alkaline phosphatase, immunoglobulins and platelets, and serum albumin is usually depressed. There may be a normochromic normocytic anaemia. Specific investigations include ANCA [detected both by immunofluorescence and enzyme-linked immunosorbent assay (ELISA)] and anti-GBM antibodies, and markers for SLE [ANA, anti-double-stranded DNA (dsDNA) antibodies, serum complement]. These are the crucial investigations in all patients with RPGN.

Imaging is usually non-specifically abnormal. Ultrasound will show swollen, echogenic kidneys with loss of the corticomedullary junction. Intravenous urography is rarely performed now and simply shows poor renal uptake of contrast because of renal failure. Angiography is usually normal as the large vessels are rarely effected, aside from polyarteritis nodosa. Nuclear imaging simply shows poor renal perfusion and filtration, although DMSA scans may occasionally show peripheral infarcts in larger vessel vasculitides (especially in polyarteritis nodosa).

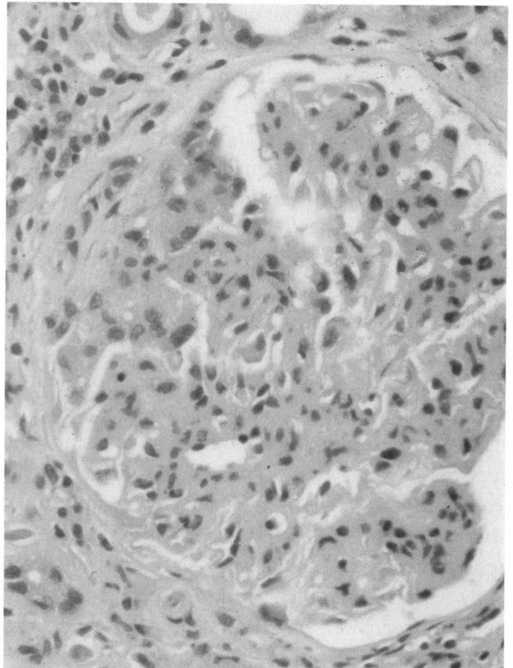

Fig. 4 A small segmental crescent in a patient with IgA nephropathy (haematoxylin and eosin).

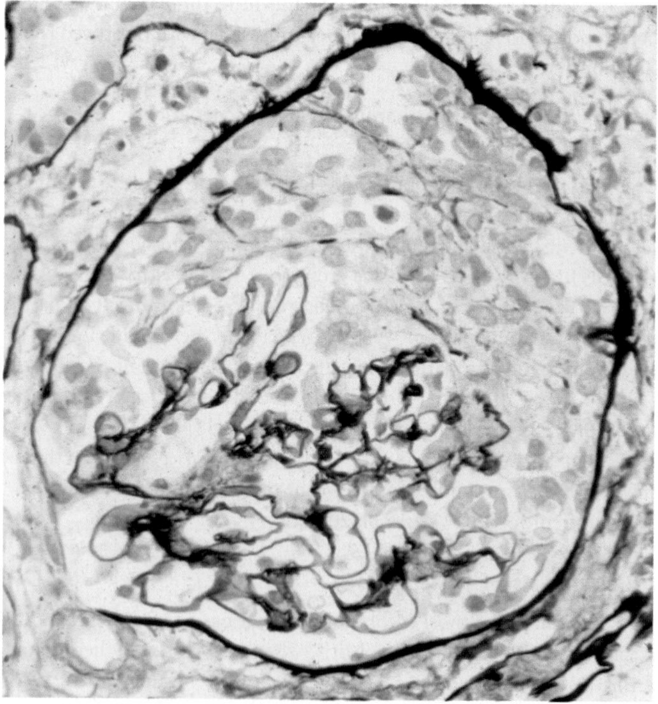

Fig. 5 A large cellular crescent compressing the glomerular tuft from a patient with ANCA-associated vasculitis (methenamine silver–haematoxylin and eosin).

Pathology of crescentic nephritis

Histopathology

Some of the pathological changes seen in crescentic glomerulonephritis are found regardless of the precise underlying diagnosis, whilst other changes are much more specifically associated with individual disease entities. This distinction is crucial since the cellular crescents in IgA disease (Fig. 4) or ANCA-associated vasculitis (Fig. 5), for example, may have very different implications but look histologically identical. In general, the kidney in acute crescentic glomerulonephritis is swollen, and petechial haemorrhages are commonly seen along the core of a renal biopsy. The crescent itself is an accumulation of cells in Bowman's capsule which can vary from circumferential to segmental, and floridly cellular to completely fibrosed. Although the precise geometry of an individual crescent is a reflection of the tissue section (see above), crescents are more likely to be extensive and circumferential in some diseases such as anti-GBM disease or ANCA-associated vasculitis, and more often segmental and sparse in IgA disease or membranous nephropathy. Although the formal definition of a crescent is of two or more layers of cells that are partially or completely filling Bowman's capsule, it can be difficult sometimes to distinguish an adhesion between the glomerular capillary loop and Bowman's capsule from genuine but localized extracapillary cellular proliferation.

The precise nature of the cells making up the cellular crescent has generated much debate over the last few decades, but has become more clearly defined using cell line specific markers, immunohistochemistry, and molecular techniques (Monga *et al.* 1981; Jennette and Hipp 1985; Bolton *et al.* 1987; Hooke *et al.* 1987; Nolasco *et al.* 1987). One of the problems in this field has been the very heterogeneity of the crescentic glomeruli themselves, with regard to underlying stimulus, age, and surrounding inflammatory pathology. The majority of cells within the crescent are proliferating parietal epithelial cells and infiltrating macrophages (see below). The degree of proliferation can vary hugely. Extensive crescents subsequently compress the glomerular tuft and in some diseases [e.g. anti-GBM disease (Fig.6)] can cause complete obliteration of the glomerular capillary loops. Cellular crescents have two possible fates, either complete resolution or scarring (total or segmental) with fibrosis, and little is known about the processes determining these outcomes in an individual crescent. Crescents, which undergo fibrosis, initially accumulate reticulin and fibrin before subsequently transforming into acellular fibrous tissue rich in type I collagen. This process can occur in as little as a few days, but more commonly takes weeks (Downer *et al.* 1988). Type I collagen gene expression, however, is upregulated in cells within crescents 48 h after the initial stimulus in some animal models of crescentic glomerulonephritis (He *et al.* 2001). Fibrosed crescents can then be seen within biopsies for years after the acute nephritis, for example, in ANCA-associated disease. Alternatively crescents can resolve completely, leaving no fibrous ghost nor cellular elements. This is best documented in IgA disease in which serial biopsies can show large numbers of cellular crescents at time of macroscopic haematuria (or an episode of acute renal impairment), but no evidence of crescents on repeat biopsy. Patients having serial biopsies in crescentic IgA disease who have received immunosuppressive treatment can also be shown to have complete resolution of crescents (Hotta *et al.* 2002). It has been suggested that resolution is more likely in glomeruli with intact capillary loops, and in which there has not been rupture of the glomerular basement membrane or Bowman's capsule. Cellular crescents can vary within an individual patient. In some diseases, for example, anti-GBM disease, the characteristic histological appearance is of similar crescents in all glomeruli, usually large and cellular, suggesting an acute single insult causing the renal damage. In contrast, the glomeruli of patients with ANCA-associated diseases usually show crescents at all stages within a single biopsy, from circumferential and cellular to fibrosed. The supposition in these cases is that an ongoing process is inducing crescent formation over several months either continuously or episodically. The histology in ANCA-negative renal limited vasculitis is identical.

Crescents in membranous glomerulonephritis and MCGN are rarely extensive, and do not usually obscure the underlying characteristic microscopic changes characteristic of the individual disease. Focal and segmental necrosis is common in renal microscopic vasculitis, anti-GBM disease and SLE, and is also seen in HSP. It is uncommon in postinfectious glomerulonephritis. Interstitial changes (Fig. 7) are also very common in patients with acute crescentic glomerulonephritis ranging from an acute interstitial infiltrate with prominent macrophages, lymphocytes, and occasional eosinophils, to more chronic interstitial scarring and tubular atrophy. Given the nature of the blood supply to the tubules, it is not surprising that when glomerular capillary loops becomes compressed by a cellular crescent, the tubules dependent on capillary blood from that efferent glomerular arteriole will become ischaemic. In fact, in most glomerular diseases tubular damage is a better prognostic marker for long-term renal function than

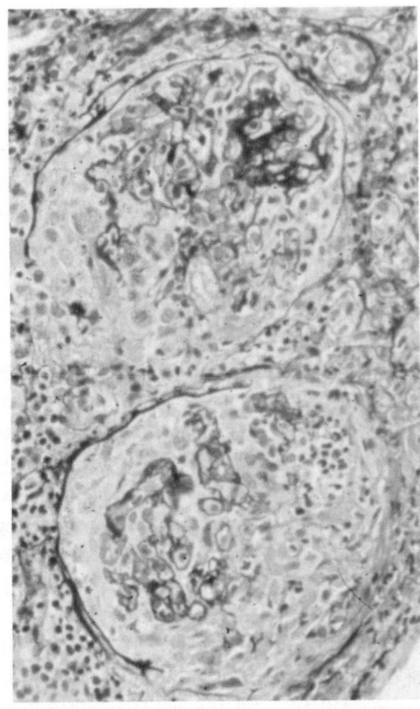

Fig. 6 Two adjacent glomeruli from a patient with anti-GBM disease showing almost identical crescents in each glomerulus.

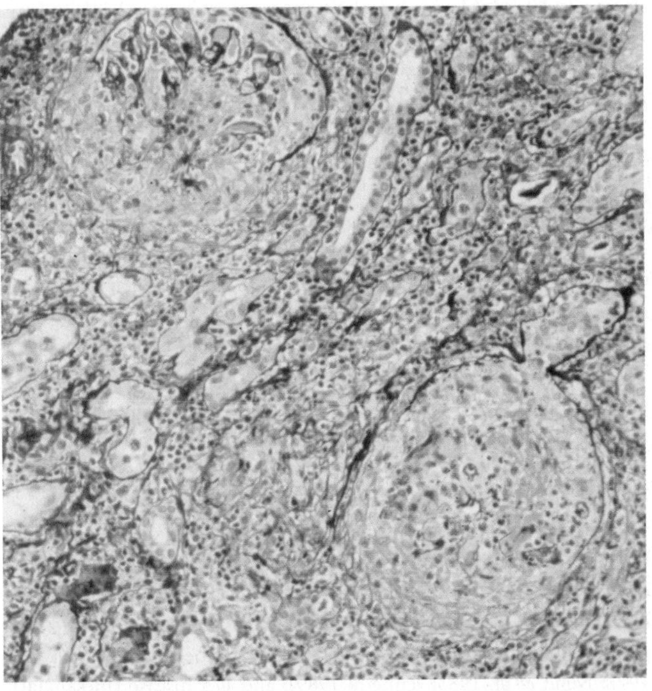

Fig. 7 A marked acute interstitial infiltrate in severe crescentic nephritis from a patient with anti-GBM disease, comprised predominantly of lymphocytes and monocytes.

the extent of glomerular damage, and is almost universally better than a crescent score. A cluster analysis of multiple features in 109 patients with crescentic glomerulonephritis showed that no single factor regulated prognosis, which was instead determined by a complex combination of factors including crescent scores, glomerulosclerosis, tubulointerstitial disease, hypertension, and proteinuria (Sasatomi *et al.* 1999). Large numbers of eosinophils in the interstitium with a crescentic glomerulonephritis might suggest a diagnosis of Churg–Strauss syndrome (Clutterbuck *et al.* 1987). Finally, some patients also show true vasculitis in blood vessels within the renal biopsy, with fibrinoid necrosis in arteriole walls, rupture of the internal elastic lamina and perivascular inflammation. Clearly the segmental necrosis within glomeruli may represent a similar process in a smaller blood vessel within the glomerulus.

Immunohistology

Immunohistology is the key pathological investigation in patients with crescentic glomerulonephritis and RPGN, together with appropriate serological tests. Findings will clearly distinguish ANCA-associated renal vasculitis, anti-GBM disease, and many primary glomerulonephritides in crescentic phase. Historically, the development of immunochemistry was paramount in the understanding of the aetiology of many of these disease. Linear staining of the GBM with immunoglobulin and complement C3 is characteristic of anti-GBM disease (Fig. 8). Antibody is also deposited along Bowman's capsule and distal tubular membranes. Less intense linear staining can be seen in diabetes, myeloma, and in renal allografts, none of which show crescentic glomerulonephritis on light microscopy. Glomeruli, which have sustained severe damage, may have such extensive disruption to the GBM that it is difficult to see intact capillary walls, and hence the staining pattern may not be easy to recognize. IgG is most commonly found, but occasional patients have been described with concomitant or even isolated IgM or IgA deposition (see also Chapter 3.11). In contrast, the glomeruli of patients with ANCA-associated renal vasculitis do not have any substantial deposits of antibody or complement, hence the term 'pauci-immune'. In reality, there are often scanty deposits of IgG and C3, but of low intensity. ANCA-negative renal limited vasculitis shows identical immunohistology. Patients with primary glomerular disease show the characteristic findings of the underlying disease, such as mesangial IgA deposits in IgA disease, granular capillary wall deposits of IgG and C3 in postinfectious glomerulonephritis and widespread granular IgG, IgM, C3, C4, and C1q in capillary walls and the mesangium in SLE. Complement C3 may be found in isolation in type II MCGN, and together with IgM in necrotic regions of glomeruli. The crescent itself usually stains strongly for fibrin, and macrophages are detectable immunohistochemically.

Electron microscopy

The findings on electron microscopy (Fig. 9) reflect those on immunohistology. Immune deposits are not found in ANCA-associated diseases, in renal limited vasculitis or in anti-GBM disease, but are common in SLE (where they are widely distributed), postinfectious glomerulonephritis (subepithelial or subendothelial) (Beirne *et al.* 1977; Neild *et al.* 1983; Jennette 1989), and IgA disease (mesangial). Electron microscopic changes reflecting the extensive damage occurring in crescentic nephritis include clear views of the ruptures of Bowman's capsule and GBMs, wrinkling of the GBM and areas of mesangiolysis (Bonsib 1988). Scanning electron microscopy clearly shows holes in Bowman's capsule and capillary walls. Fibrin is easily visualized in the crescent itself.

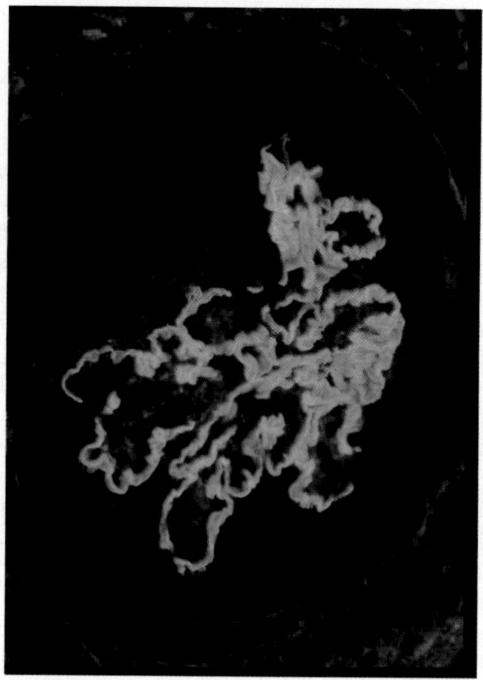

Fig. 8 Glomerulus from a patient with anti-GBM disease stained with fluorescein-conjugated anti-IgG antibody. Linear deposition of IgG is seen along the capillary walls, with minor deposition along Bowman's capsule. The glomerular tuft is compressed by a circumferential crescent (not visualized).

Pathogenesis

It is likely that a final common pathway drives crescent formation in the different diseases, despite the disparate range of underlying causes for these conditions. Hence, the initial insult in a kidney may be somewhat irrelevant, but at some point the process initiates cellular proliferation and infiltration into Bowman's space and the appearance of a cellular crescent (Fig. 10). This critical nidus at which different diseases converge is probably the development of breaches in the GBM, and subsequent leakage of intravascular contents (including cells) into Bowman's space. Bonsib (1985) has shown beautifully these holes by direct electron microscopy. The precise cause of the initial disruption of the basement membrane is probably irrelevant; hence the rare patients with amyloid and crescent formation can be shown to have amyloid fibrils disrupting the GBM (Nagata *et al.* 2001), while in anti-GBM disease, it is antibody, complement, and infiltrating leucocytes (Fig. 11). Crescents themselves vary from freshly cellular to completely fibrosed, and there is an extensive literature describing the phenomenology of the crescent, from human biopsy specimens and various animal models (Fig. 12). This has actually added to the confusion, since a wide range of different experimental protocols can induce crescentic glomerulonephritis. Although all the models may indeed have crescents in the glomeruli, the underlying cause will have varied, and hence

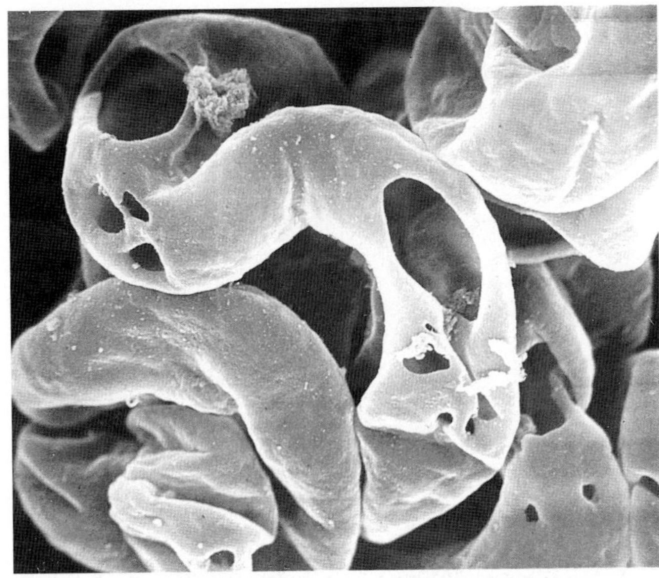

(a)

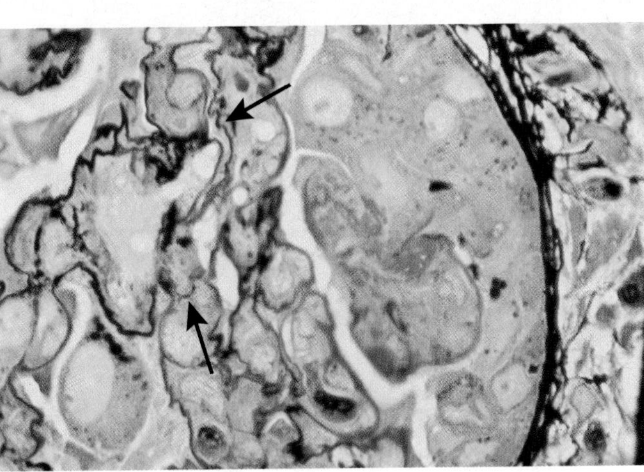

(b)

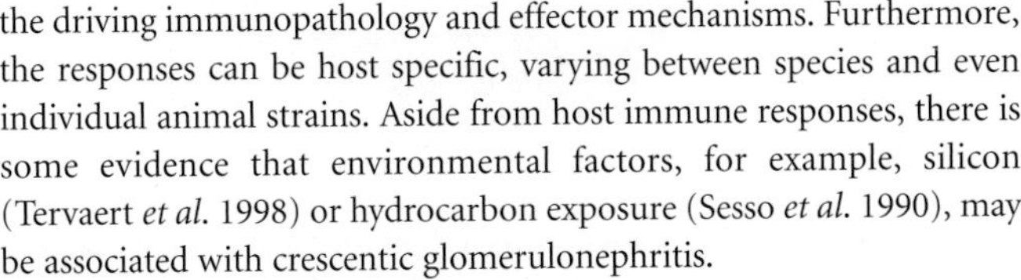

Fig. 9 (a) Holes in the basement membrane in crescentic glomerulonephritis. The scanning electron microscopy preparation is a glomerulus from a renal biopsy which has been treated to remove all cells. (Reproduced with permission from Bonsib 1985.) (b) Shows in conventional sectioning the efflux of fibrin (F) through a gap in the sliver-stained basement membrane (arrows), with cells around the exuded fibrin. (Silver methenamine–haematoxylin and eosin; magnification 167×.)

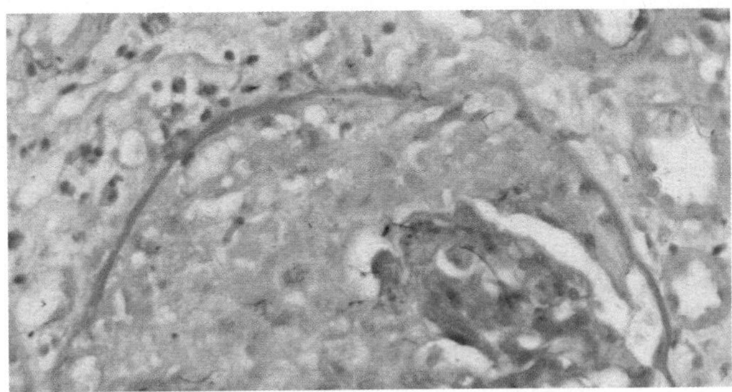

Fig. 10 A detailed view of a cellular crescent causing disruption of Bowman's capsule and beginning to stimulate a periglomerular inflammatory reaction, from a patient with Wegener's granulomatosis.

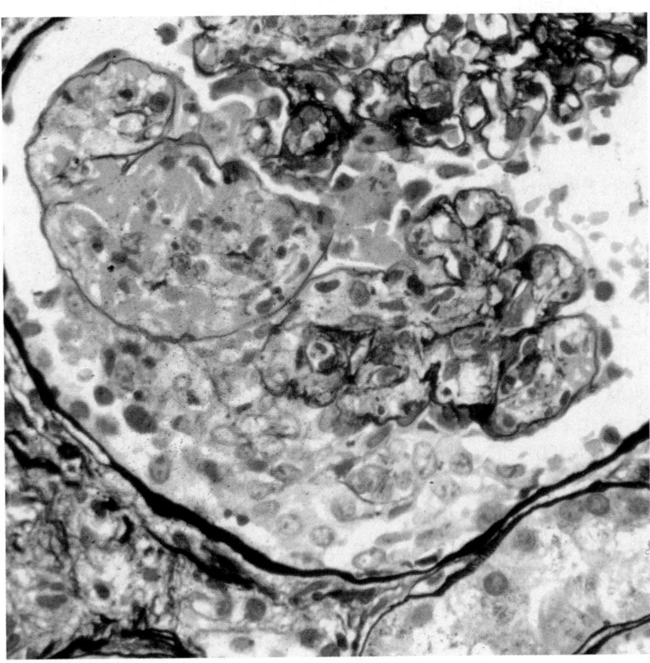

Fig. 11 A cellular segmental crescent abutting but not disrupting Bowman's capsule in a patient with HSP.

the driving immunopathology and effector mechanisms. Furthermore, the responses can be host specific, varying between species and even individual animal strains. Aside from host immune responses, there is some evidence that environmental factors, for example, silicon (Tervaert *et al.* 1998) or hydrocarbon exposure (Sesso *et al.* 1990), may be associated with crescentic glomerulonephritis.

Langerhans first suggested in 1885 that crescents in human disease were predominantly proliferating glomerular epithelial cells. Subsequent analysis using electron microscopy, immunohistology, and molecular identification of cell specific mRNA species has confirmed that parietal epithelial cells are important constituents of all crescents. However, it has also emerged that many crescents also contain abundant monocytes/macrophages and less frequently lymphocytes (Ferrario *et al.* 1985). Schiffer and Michael (1978) showed the presence of male cells (lacking Barr bodies), probably macrophages, within crescents in the glomeruli of two male patients with renal transplants from female donors. In the late 1970s, Atkins *et al.* were able to culture macrophages from glomeruli of patients with crescentic glomerulonephritis (Atkins *et al.* 1976, 1980). Thus crescents are formed both from locally resident cells lining Bowman's space and from intravascularly derived infiltrating cells. Macrophages within crescents can also be shown to be actively proliferating (Yang *et al.* 1998). The precise balance of macrophages and intrinsic glomerular epithelial cells within an individual crescent will vary depending on the underlying initiating disease, the immune response of the host and the time period since the original insult (Bolton *et al.* 1987). A very recent electron microscopic analysis in experimental

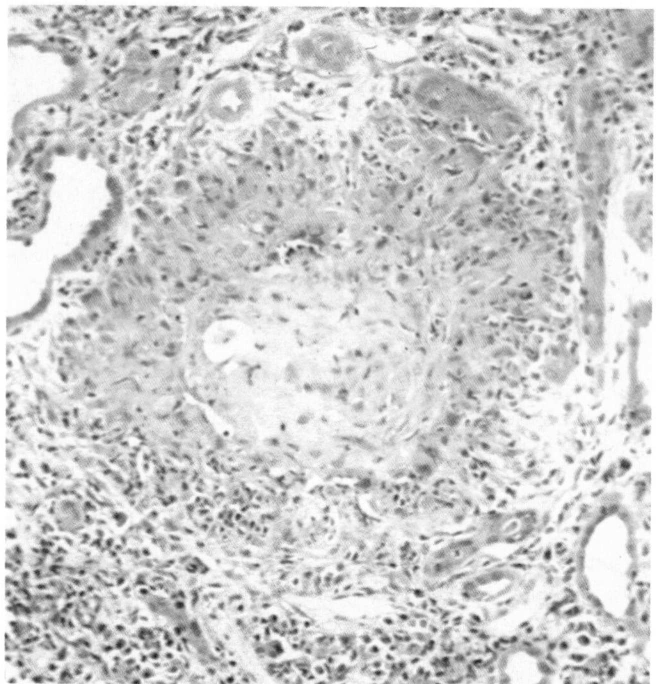

Fig. 12 An extensive crescent completely obliterating Bowman's capsule in a patient with microscopic polyangiitis (haematoxylin and eosin).

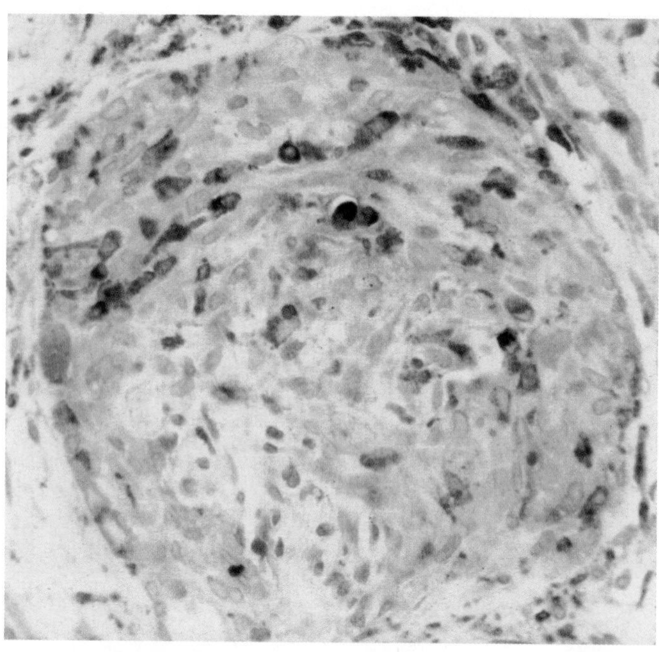

Fig. 13 A single glomerulus from a patient with ANCA-associated disease stained with anti-CD68 monoclonal antibody, which recognizes activated macrophages (immunoperoxidase). The crescent itself contains large numbers of macrophages, and only a few within the glomerular capillary loops.

crescentic glomerulonephritis in mice has shown that in the first 3 days after the initiation of disease, the major abnormalities are endothelial, with subsequent podocyte changes preceding the formation of crescents (Figs 13 and 14). Intriguingly, podocyte bridges were clearly seen between parietal epithelial cells and as a component of crescents (Le Hir *et al.* 2001). The spreading of podocytes onto the parietal basement membrane may well, therefore, also be a drive to crescent formation. Other cell types which have been found in crescents include antigen specific T cells in rat models of anti-GBM disease (Wu *et al.* 2002). Another factor determining the cellular response is whether Bowman's capsule and the GBM have been disrupted (Boucher *et al.* 1987). Where breaches in the basement membranes are more extensive, the macrophage and leucocyte influx is greater, and conversely, when breaches are rare (as in many immune complex crescentic glomerulonephritides) epithelial cells predominate.

A whole pantheon of experimental data has emerged in the last decade to suggest that even in diseases thought to be antibody mediated (especially anti-GBM disease), the cellular immune response is crucial in the formation of crescents. Furthermore, it seems to be the Th1-type of immune response which is absolutely required for the development of crescentic glomerulonephritis (Holdsworth *et al.* 1999; Kitching *et al.* 2000). This data has been derived from both animal models, and from studies on the cytokines and cells detectable in human biopsy samples. In almost all model systems, crescentic glomerulonephritis requires the classical Th1 cytokines, interleukin-12 (IL-12) and γ-interferon, whilst administration of IL-4 or IL-10 (Th2 cytokines) improves or prevents disease (Kitching *et al.* 1997a,b, 1999; Cook *et al.* 1999). IL-12-deficient mice are protected from the development of crescents and a cellular influx into the kidney, although they can often mount antibody responses, and sometimes deposit antibody in the kidney (Kitching *et al.* 1999; Timoshanko *et al.* 2001). The Th1 costimulatory protein B7.1 has also been identified as a crucial

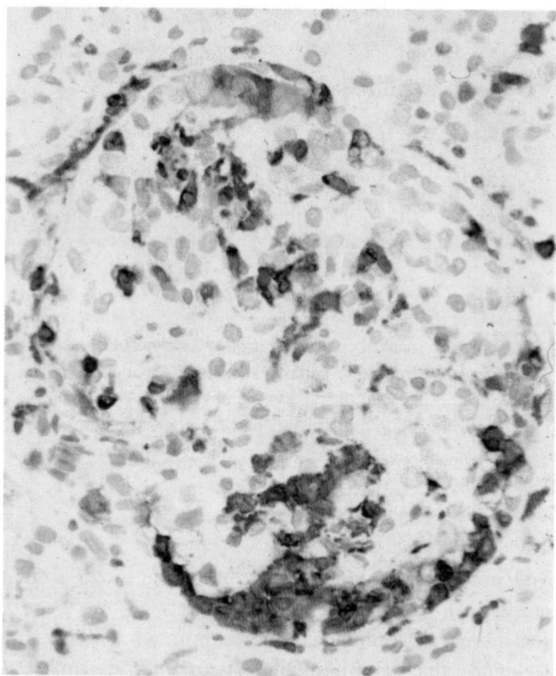

Fig. 14 A single glomerulus from a patient with ANCA-associated disease stained with anti-calprotectin monoclonal antibody, which also recognizes activated macrophages (immunoperoxidase). The small crescent (in the lower portion of the glomerulus) contains large numbers of macrophages.

factor for the development of crescentic glomerulonephritis, and blockade diminishes renal injury (Li *et al.* 2000; Reynolds *et al.* 2000). Tumour necrosis factor (TNF)-α and IL-1 may also play pivotal roles, and are both increased in glomeruli of patients and animals with crescentic glomerulonephritis. Blockade of either TNF-α or IL-1 experimentally can prevent crescent formation, and also decrease its extent, and TNF-deficient mice do not get crescentic glomerulonephritis (Ryffel *et al.* 1998; Karkar *et al.* 2001). Trials have begun in patients using various blocking strategies against both TNF and IL-1. Cytokines increasing macrophage accumulation in glomeruli also augment crescentic nephritis. Macrophage migration inhibitory factor (MIF) is increased in the biopsies of patients and animals with crescentic disease (Brown *et al.* 2002), and experimentally blocking antibodies prevent crescent formation and decrease leucocyte influx into kidneys despite normal antibody responses (Yang *et al.* 1998). Similarly, macrophage chemoattractant protein (MCP1) and macrophage inflammatory protein (MIP1) are found in cellular crescents and the interstitium, and may be synthesized both by infiltrating leucocytes and the parietal epithelium (Wada *et al.* 1999; Segerer *et al.* 2000). Further requirements for crescent formation include CD4 positive T cells in several animal models; deficient mice are protected from crescentic glomerulonephritis, and therapeutic blockade can abrogate disease (Tipping *et al.* 1998). The important role for CD4 T cells and cell-mediated immunity is also supported by the observation of upregulation of MHC class II molecules in glomeruli, and by the absolute requirement for local expression of MHC class II molecules within the kidney—mice without major histocompatibility complex (MHC) class II molecules in tissues (including the kidney) in whom circulating leucocytes have normal class II expression (because of bone marrow reconstitution) are protected from crescentic glomerulonephritis (Li *et al.* 1998).

Non-cytokine proteins important in the aetiology of crescentic glomerulonephritis include extracellular matrix proteoglycans such as versican, decorin, biglycan, laminin, and heparin (Stokes *et al.* 2001). Fibrin and type I collagen are also major constituents of crescents, the former synthesized and deposited early in crescent formation, and the latter as a later phenomenon, although collagen expression is initially upregulated early in crescentic glomerulonephritis (He *et al.* 2001). Fibrinogen-deficient animals have markedly reduced disease (Drew *et al.* 2001).

Treatment

General considerations

Objective assessment of the response to treatment of crescentic glomerulonephritis has been confounded by the heterogeneity of diseases included in most studies. It has become very clear over the last decade that the underlying immunopathological drive to crescent formation makes a substantial contribution to the outcome, but more importantly other biopsy features predict outcome much more than crescents themselves (Evans *et al.* 1986; Sasatomi *et al.* 1999). As with other primary glomerulonephritides, the extent of tubulointerstitial scarring is a better marker of poor prognosis than a crescent score in almost all diseases causing crescentic glomerulonephritis. In anti-GBM disease, high crescent scores are associated with a worse outcome, but interstitial scarring better predicts lack of reversibility. In ANCA-associated vasculitis, the number of normal glomeruli and not the number of crescents is associated with renal recovery, and in IgA disease most studies have not demonstrated a worse outcome in patients with crescents in glomeruli. Renal function at presentation independent of histology is also a powerful predictor of outcome, and in clinical trials patients should be stratified by renal function as well as by precise diagnosis (McLaughlin *et al.* 1998). Furthermore, there are few controlled studies of treatment in crescentic glomerulonephritis, and almost all older series include a huge range of diseases (Jindal 1999). It is only in the last 5 years or so that a number of well controlled randomized controlled trials in specific diseases have been conducted.

In general, treatment is often divided into two phases in crescentic glomerulonephritis. First, induction of remission during the acute phase, followed by maintenance therapy to control the underlying immunopathology in the longer term. The induction phase of treatment should both suppress the acute inflammatory features of crescentic glomerulonephritis and control the underlying aberrant immune response, while the maintenance phase should prevent scarring and prevent recrudescence of acute inflammation. Thus, in anti-GBM disease, plasma exchange removes circulating pathogenic autoantibodies, while prednisolone and cyclophosphamide (and possibly other effects of plasma exchange) suppress the acute inflammatory response, cell infiltration, and further antibody synthesis. Prior to the use of any immunosuppressive therapies, the mortality from crescentic glomerulonephritis was 100 per cent (Cameron 1971). Steroids improved the survival but only 25 per cent of patients escaped the need for dialysis. Patients with crescentic glomerulonephritis due to poststreptococcal glomerulonephritis had a better outcome. Various other treatments were tried during the 1970s and 1980s including anticoagulation and antiplatelet therapies (given the importance of fibrin in the crescent), but no controlled trials were performed, and combination therapy with immunosuppressive drugs was usual (Cameron 1973; Hind *et al.* 1983). More recently, the prognosis for renal recovery has improved with the earlier diagnosis of crescentic glomerulonephritis, more precise disease characterization, and more carefully targeted treatments (Zauner *et al.* 2002), although some studies fail to demonstrate any improvement in renal or patient survival over the last two decades (McLaughlin *et al.* 1998). The mainstay of therapy has remained relatively non-specific immunosuppression with combination therapies including steroids, cyclophosphamide and azathioprine, with or without methylprednisolone and plasma exchange. The era of specific immunoregulation is only just about to begin.

Plasma exchange in crescentic nephritis

Plasma exchange has been used to treat almost all causes of crescentic glomerulonephritis, but with little controlled data in most instances. In anti-GBM disease, the rationale is clearly to remove pathogenic autoantibodies, but the process also has effects on inflammatory mediators and possibly cell-mediated immune function. Prior to the introduction of plasma exchange, almost all patients died and renal recovery was rare (Lockwood *et al.* 1976). There has only been one small controlled trial in Goodpasture's disease which showed a small beneficial effect on renal recovery (Johnson *et al.* 1985). The largest experience of plasma exchange was reported by Levy *et al.* (2001) in 71 patients treated intensively with plasma exchange, prednisolone and cyclophosphamide, with excellent renal and patient survival in patients presenting with mild or moderate renal failure. Patients presenting with dialysis-dependent renal failure rarely, but occasionally, recovered renal function. Other groups have used less intensive regimens, which may well affect the potential benefit of therapy.

The benefits of plasma exchange in anti-GBM disease subsequently led to the more widespread use of the treatment in other crescentic glomerulonephritides, especially in pauci-immune vasculitis

(Rifle *et al.* 1981; Muller *et al.* 1986). The identification of the pathogenic role of ANCA antibodies has strengthened the rationale for plasma exchange in this setting. There have been a number of controlled trials reported since 1988, but unfortunately most have included patients with a wide range of underlying renal diseases in crescentic phase (Glockner *et al.* 1988; Cole *et al.* 1992). The most cohesive study was reported by Pusey *et al.* (1991) in which only patients with non-anti-GBM pauci-immune crescentic nephritis were enrolled into a prospective, randomized trial. Plasma exchange was of significant benefit to patients presenting with severe renal failure requiring dialysis, but not to those with lesser degrees of renal impairment. The overall consensus from all these studies was that plasma exchange may offer benefit to patients with severe renal failure, but not to those with creatinine less than 500 μmol/l (Jindal 1999; Zauner *et al.* 2002). This data prompted the multi-centre prospective randomized controlled MEPEX trial, in which 151 patients with ANCA-associated crescentic glomerulonephritis and creatinine greater than 500 μmol/l were randomized to plasma exchange or intravenous methylprednisolone as induction treatment in addition to conventional oral immunosuppression. The results clearly showed the benefit of plasma exchange in this group of patients with severe renal failure, with around 70 per cent coming off dialysis when treated with plasma exchange, but only 50 per cent recovering renal function when treated with methylprednisolone. A single study comparing plasma exchange with immunoadsorption in 44 patients with crescentic glomerulonephritis showed no difference between the two modalities, with 70 per cent of patients with ANCA-associated disease coming off dialysis (Stegmayr *et al.* 1999).

Evidence for the benefit of plasma exchange in all other crescentic nephritides is poor (Jindal 1999). A controlled trial of plasma exchange (performed relatively infrequently) in SLE with moderate renal dysfunction has shown no benefit, but case reports in patients with severe renal failure have shown occasional benefit (see Chapter 4.7.2). One small series of patients with crescentic IgA disease has been reported in whom plasma exchange may have improved outcome (Roccatello *et al.* 1995). Individual cases reporting the success of plasma exchange have been published in almost all forms of crescentic glomerulonephritis (Lockwood *et al.* 1977).

Methylprednisolone in crescentic nephritis

Intravenous methylprednisolone has been used extensively in all forms of crescentic nephritis (O'Neill *et al.* 1979; Oredugba *et al.* 1980; Rondeau *et al.* 1993; Jindal 1999). The only controlled comparison is the MEPEX study comparing plasma exchange with methylprednisolone in ANCA-associated crescentic glomerulonephritis with severe renal failure (see above) in which methylprednisolone was significantly worse at improving renal function. There have been no controlled comparisons of oral versus intravenous steroids, and there is a suggestion that intravenous steroids may be associated with an increased risk of osteoporosis, avascular necrosis and infection. However, Bolton and Sturgill (1989) and Andrassy *et al.* (1991) have both reported good recovery of renal function with methylprednisolone at 30 mg/kg/day and 250 mg/day, respectively, in patients with pauci-immune crescentic glomerulonephritis and severe renal failure, and a number of smaller uncontrolled studies have reported good outcomes in crescentic glomerulonephritis treated with intravenous steroids. In an animal model of crescentic glomerulonephritis, 30 mg/kg methylprednisolone was most effective in reducing crescent formation, cellular influx, and intraglomerular chemokine expression (Ou *et al.* 2001). Roccatello *et al.* (2000) have reported 12 patients with crescentic IgA disease treated with intravenous methylprednisolone followed by oral immunosuppression, in whom the 5-year renal survival was significantly improved compared to an untreated group (91.6 per cent versus 37.5 per cent). This was not, however, a randomized prospective controlled study. A retrospective study separating patients with insidious crescentic glomerulonephritis from those with acute disease suggested that pulse therapy may be more beneficial in insidious disease (Takeda *et al.* 1998).

Other induction treatments

All treatment regimens for crescentic glomerulonephritis now include cyclophosphamide, since the demonstration of greater efficacy than azathioprine in patients with Wegener's granulomatosis (Fauci *et al.* 1983) and microscopic polyangiitis (Fauci *et al.* 1979), but there is continued debate as to the benefit of oral versus intravenous treatment. A number of trials have been performed with ambiguous results, and a randomized controlled multi-centre trial is currently underway across Europe. In general, it seems that toxicity and side-effects are less with an intravenous regimen, but that efficacy in controlling renal inflammation is also reduced (Adu *et al.* 1997; Haubitz *et al.* 1998; de Groot *et al.* 2001). De Groot's meta-analysis of the rather sparse data (143 patients enrolled into a number of studies) showed that pulse cyclophosphamide was significantly less likely to fail to induce remission (OR 0.29; 95% CI 0.12–0.73) and had a significantly lower risk of infection and leucopenia, but relapses occurred slightly (but not statistically significantly) more often. Intravenous immunoglobulin (at 2 g/kg over 3–5 days) has been used in a number of studies and appears to be beneficial in the short term, but with a risk of an acute deterioration in renal function (Jayne *et al.* 2000). Treatment with chlorambucil, cyclosporin, mycophenolate, and anti-lymphocyte globulin have also been reported anecdotally in a few patents with crescentic glomerulonephritis. Anti-TNF therapy with either blocking antibodies (infliximab) or soluble receptors (eternacept) may be of benefit in ANCA-associated diseases.

Maintenance therapy

The need for maintenance therapy in crescentic glomerulonephritis depends on the underlying disease. Long-term maintenance therapy is needed in almost all patients with ANCA-associated disease, since 50 per cent will relapse either with local or systemic disease, and long-term treatment can reduce relapses significantly (Gordon *et al.* 1993). The recent CYCAZAREM trial clarified the optimum therapeutic regimen by demonstrating that oral azathioprine after induction of remission was as effective as oral cyclophosphamide with a trend to less short-term toxicity, and undoubted longer-term benefits (Jayne *et al.* 2003). Few, if any, patients with ANCA-associated crescentic glomerulonephritis should now remain on cyclophosphamide beyond 3 months. Patients relapsing on azathioprine may require further cyclophosphamide. Alternative agents include mycophenolate, anti-TNF therapy, cyclosporin, leflunomide, deoxyspergualin, and methotrexate (if renal function preserved). In contrast, anti-GBM disease is not a relapsing disease, and patients do not require long-term maintenance therapy. Patients can stop cyclophosphamide at 3 months and be 'weaned' off steroids by approximately 6 months. There are no good data on the length of immunosuppression needed in patients with primary glomerulonephritis in crescentic phase, but where treatment has been initiated, we would continue low-dose maintenance immunosuppression (prednisolone and azathioprine) for 1–2 years. In addition to ongoing immune-mediated damage, patients are also at risk of progressive renal decline from haemodynamic factors and progressive scarring, independent of the initial insult. This seems more likely in all crescentic glomerulonephritides if patients make only a partial recovery after induction treatment, and if their serum creatinine does not reduce to less than 250 μmol/l (Savage *et al.* 1985; Keller *et al.* 1989). Distinguishing relapse from progressive scarring can be very difficult, but is clearly an important distinction. Rebiopsy will help, and monitoring circulating ANCA may also be useful, although there are few studies to support the use of serial ANCA alone in guiding decisions about immunosuppression (Jayne *et al.* 1995; Oliveira *et al.* 1995).

Both long- and short-term immunosuppression carry risks of infection especially, and all patients need to be carefully advised, monitored, and treated with prophylactic antimicrobials especially against *Pneumocystis carinii*, oral fungi, and probably cytomegalovirus (CMV) (Cohen *et al.* 1982; Adu *et al.* 1987). Patients are also at risk of cataracts, gastric ulcers, bone marrow suppression, avascular necrosis, osteoporosis, dyslipidaemia, hypertension, cancers, and diabetes (Boitard and Bach 1989). Hence, patients require very careful monitoring and long-term follow-up (Westman *et al.* 1998; Aaserod *et al.* 2000).

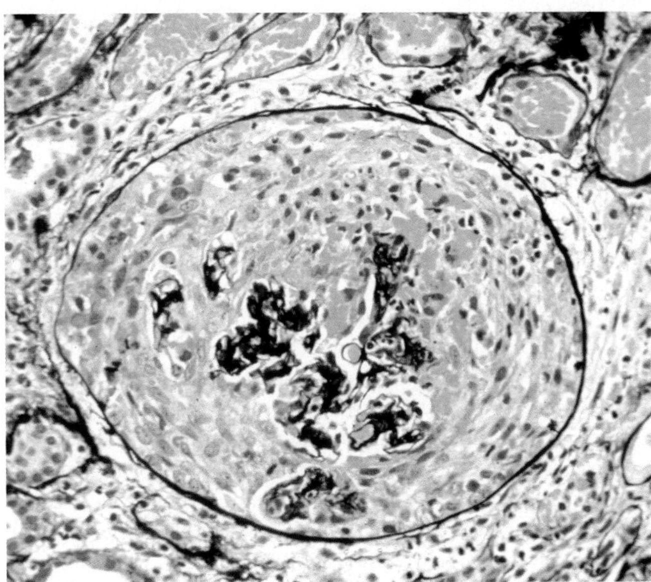

Fig. 15 A highly cellular circumferential crescent in a patient with anti-GBM disease (silver methenamine).

Specific diseases

Anti-GBM disease

Plasma exchange removes circulating antibodies rapidly, and immunosuppressive regimens based on plasma exchange have led to excellent renal and patient survival if patients are treated before they require dialysis (Fig. 15). More controversial is the treatment of patients with severe renal failure, as many studies have reported no recovery of renal function in this setting. Levy *et al.* (2001), however, demonstrated that over 50 per cent of patients with creatinine greater than 500 μmol/l but not requiring dialysis were able to significantly improve renal function in the long term with full treatment. Dialysis requiring patients rarely recovered. A decision about treatment in severe renal failure should be based on the biopsy appearances, length of history, and presence of confounding factors such as tubular necrosis. Pulmonary haemorrhage in itself is an indication for plasma exchange (see Chapter 3.11).

Renal microscopic vasculitis

The outcome for patients with microscopic polyangiitis, Wegener's granulomatosis, and isolated renal vasculitis has improved enormously in the last decades, such that now over 70 per cent of patients with severe renal failure should recover renal function, maintained in the long term, even if dialysis dependent at presentation (Bruns *et al.* 1989; Westman *et al.* 1998; Aasarod *et al.* 2000). Patients with less severe renal failure respond well to cyclophosphamide and steroids, but patients with creatinine greater than 500 μmol/l should be treated additionally with plasma exchange (based on the large MEPEX trial, and cumulative data from the previous smaller trials). All of these patients probably require long-term maintenance immunosuppression to minimize relapses. Age and crescent score do not predict outcome, however, older patients tend to have higher mortality and morbidity, predominantly from infective complications (Aaserod *et al.* 2000) (see also Chapter 4.5.2).

Crescentic nephritis complicating primary glomerulonephritis

Crescentic nephritis associated with membranous nephropathy is rare, and has been associated in some cases with the development of anti-GBM antibodies. Treatment has generally been as for anti-GBM disease but with poor outcomes. Case reports of isolated crescentic membranous nephritis have not responded well to immunosuppression. Crescentic IgA disease is much more common. A distinction must be made between small crescents found incidentally in patients with IgA nephropathy, which is common and has a good prognosis; crescents found after episodes of macroscopic haematuria, which can resolve fully; and a true crescentic glomerulonephritis causing RPGN. The latter is uncommon, and the outcome is more associated with tubulointerstitial scarring than the crescentic changes *per se*. Some patients have responded to immunosuppression, with or without plasma exchange, but rarely make a full recovery. McIntyre *et al.* (2001) reported beneficial effects of oral steroids and cyclophosphamide in nine patients with crescentic IgA nephritis, but most did not have severe renal failure (mean creatinine 149 μmol/l). Harper *et al.* (2000) demonstrated healing of vasculitic lesions in crescentic IgA disease when treated with steroids and cyclophosphamide or azathioprine, but 25 per cent of their patients still ended up on dialysis after 2–7 years. Intravenous methylprednisolone (three pulses of 1 g) followed by oral immunosuppression may have improved the renal outcome in a small series of patients with crescentic IgA disease treated by Roccatello *et al.* (2000). Finally a number of reports from Japan demonstrate improved proteinuria and histological features in patients with proliferative IgA disease (including crescents) when treated with steroids (Shoji *et al.* 2000). Crescentic mesangiocapillary glomerulonephritis has been reported in a number of small series and case reports, with generally a very poor response to immunosuppression with or without plasma exchange.

Poststreptococcal nephritis

True poststreptococcal glomerulonephritis is a rare entity now, but can present with extensive crescents. Early series reported complete resolution in up to 50 per cent of patients given supportive treatment only (Anand *et al.* 1975; Whitworth *et al.* 1976), but also high mortality. More recently, patients have often also received immunosuppression when a biopsy reveals extensive crescents, with possibly improved recovery rates; Southwest Pediatric Nephrology Study Group (1985). However, the benefit of immunosuppression in this setting remains unclear since many patients recover spontaneously (Roy *et al.* 1981). Follow-up biopsies have shown a mixture of fibrosed crescents, complete glomerulosclerosis and normal glomeruli, suggesting that crescents can resolve fully (Roy *et al.* 1981). Patients who have later deterioration in renal function have interstitial scarring. There are even fewer data available in adults, but most recent case reports have used steroids alone or in combination with other immunosuppressives in patients with extensive crescents (see Chapter 3.9).

Infective endocarditis and postinfectious crescentic glomerulonephritis

There are no trial data, nor even any large series of patients with infectious causes of crescentic glomerulonephritis (Fig. 16), hence recommending treatments is impossible. Infection must be rigorously controlled before contemplating immunosuppression, and patients requiring cardiac valve replacement should have this performed early. Individual cases have been reported in whom renal recovery was coincident with the institution of immunosuppression after treatment of infection. Plasma exchange has also been used, especially in patients with persistent hypocomplementaemia and progressive decline in renal function (Daimon *et al.* 1998; Kannan and Mattoo 2001).

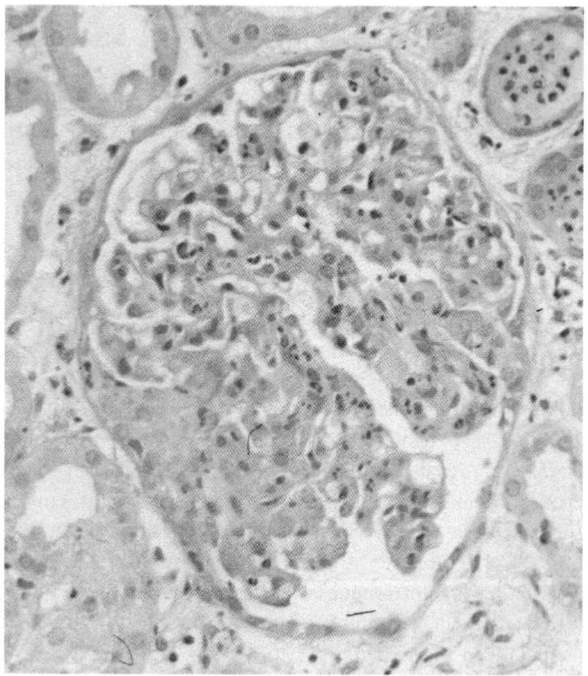

Fig. 16 A segmental cellular crescent from a patient with endocarditis-associated crescentic glomerulonephritis (haematoxylin and eosin).

Conclusions

Many forms of crescentic glomerulonephritis can now be successfully treated. Hence, it is no longer sufficient to describe a patient as simply having a crescentic nephritis, since both acute and long-term treatments will vary depending on the precise underlying immunopathological diagnosis. Patients should be given a precise diagnosis on the basis of serological investigations and immunohistology. The recognition of ANCA as a major cause of most crescentic glomerulonephritides has led to the possibility of more targeted treatments and a better understanding of immunopathology. The last decade has seen the completion of a number of excellent randomized controlled trials which have answered some fundamental questions for patients with crescentic glomerulonephritis—plasma exchange is of definite benefit in patients with ANCA-associated RPGN who present with creatinine greater than 500 μmol/l; azathioprine is the drug of choice for long-term maintenance immunosuppression after induction of remission in ANCA-associated disease. It is also clear that markers of chronic damage are better indicators of outcome than crescent scores, and that prevention of scarring by early intensive treatment will produce better long-term survival.

References

Aasarod, K. *et al.* (2000). Wegener's granulomatosis: clinical course in 108 patients with renal involvement. *Nephrology, Dialysis, Transplantation* **15**, 611–618.

Abe, T. *et al.* (1986). Participation of extracapillary lesions (ECL) in progression of IgA nephropathy. *Clinical Nephrology* **25**, 7–41.

Abuelo, J. G. *et al.* (1984). Crescentic IgA nephropathy. *Medicine* **63**, 396–406.

Adu, D. *et al.* (1987). Polyarteritis and the kidney. *Quarterly Journal of Medicine* **239**, 221–237.

Adu, D. *et al.* (1997). Controlled trial of pulse versus continuous prednisolone and cyclophosphamide in the treatment of systemic vasculitis. *Quarterly Journal of Medicine* **90**, 401–409.

Almroth, G. *et al.* (1992). Autoantibodies and leucocyte antigens in hydralazine-associated nephritis. *Journal of Internal Medicine* **231**, 37–42.

Anand, S. K., Trygstrad, C. W., Sharma, H. M., and Northway, J. D. (1975). Extracapillary proliferative glomerulonephritis in children. *Pediatrics* **56**, 434–442.

Andrassy, K., Kuster, S., Waldherr, R., and Ritz, E. (1991). Rapidly progressive glomerulonephritis: analysis of prevalence and clinical course. *Nephron* **59** (2), 206–212.

Anganco, R. *et al.* (1994). Does truly 'idiopathic' crescentic glomerulonephritis exist? *Nephrology, Dialysis, Transplantation* **9**, 630–636.

Atkins, R. C., Holdsworth, S. R., Glasgow, E. F., and Mathews, F. E. (1976). The macrophage in human rapidly progressive glomerulonephritis. *Lancet* **i**, 830–832.

Atkins, R. C. *et al.* (1980). Tissue culture of isolated glomeruli from patients with glomerulonephritis. *Kidney International* **17**, 515–527.

Beaufils, M. *et al.* (1976). Acute renal failure of glomerular origin during visceral abcesses. *New England Journal of Medicine* **295**, 185–189.

Beirne, G. J. *et al.* (1977). Idiopathic crescentic glomerulonephritis. *Medicine* **56**, 349–381.

Bennett, W. M. and Kincaid-Smith, P. (1983). Macroscopic haematuria in mesangial IgA nephropathy: clinical pathologic correlations. *Kidney International* **23**, 393–400.

Biava, C. G., Gonwa, T. A., Naughton, J. L., and Hopper, J., Jr. (1984). Crescentic glomerulonephritis associated with nonrenal malignancies. *American Journal of Nephrology* **4**, 208–214.

Bindi, P. *et al.* (1993). Necrotizing crescentic glomerulonephritis without significant immune deposits: a clinical and serological study. *Quarterly Journal of Medicine* **86** (1), 55–68.

Boitard, C. and Bach, J.-F. (1989). Long term complications of conventional immunosuppressive treatment. *Advances in Nephrology* **18**, 335–354.

Bolton, W. K. and Sturgill, B. C. (1989). Methylprednisolone therapy for acute crescentic rapidly progressive glomerulonephritis. *American Journal of Nephrology* **9**, 368–375.

Bolton, W. K., Innes, D. J., Jr., Sturgill, B. C., and Kaiser, D. L. (1987). T-cells and macrophages in rapidly progressive glomerulonephritis: clinicopathologic correlations. *Kidney International* **32**, 869–876.

Bonsib, S. M. (1985). GBM discontinuities. Scanning electron microscopic study of a cellular glomeruli. *American Journal of Pathology* **119**, 357–360.

Bonsib, S. M. (1988). GBM necrosis and crescent organization. *Kidney International* **33**, 966–974.

Boucher, A., Droz, D., Adafer, E., and Noel, L. H. (1987). Relationship between the integrity of Bowman's capsule and the composition of cellular crescents in human crescentic glomerulonephritis. *Laboratory Investigation* **56**, 526–533.

Boyce, N. W., Holdsworth, S. R., Thomson, N. M., and Atkins, R. C. (1986). Clinicopathological associations in mesangial IgA nephropathy. *American Journal of Nephrology* **6**, 246–252.

Breedveld, F. C., Valentin, R. M., Westdt, M. L., and Weening, J. J. (1985). Rapidly progressive glomerulonephritis with glomerular crescent formation in rheumatoid arthritis. Rapidly progressive renal failure in a child (clinical conference). *Scottish Medical Journal* **30**, 184–189.

Brown, F. G. *et al.* (2002). Urine macrophage migration inhibitory factor reflects the severity of renal disease in human glomerulonephritis. *Journal of the American Society of Nephrology* **13** (Suppl. 1), S7–S13.

Bruns, F. J., Adler, S., Fraley, D. S., and Segel, D. P. (1989). Long-term follow-up of aggressively treated idiopathic rapidly progressive glomerulonephritis. *American Journal of Medicine* **86**, 400–406.

Cameron, J. S. (1971). Immunosuppressant agents in the treatment of glomerulonephritis. 2. Cytotoxic drugs. *Journal of the Royal College of Physicians* **5**, 301–322.

Cameron, J. S. (1973). Are anticoagulants beneficial in the treatment of rapidly progressive glomerulonephritis. *Proceedings of the European Dialysis and Transplant Association* **10**, 57–90.

Chang-Miller, A. *et al.* (1987). Renal involvement in relapsing polychondritis. *Medicine* **66**, 202–217.

Chapman, S. J., Cameron, J. S., Chantler, C., and Turner, D. (1980). Treatment of mesangiocapillary glomerulonephritis in children with combined immunosuppression and anticoagulation. *Archives of Disease of Childhood* **55**, 446–451.

Citron, B. P. *et al.* (1970). Necrotising angiitis associated with drug abuse. *New England Journal of Medicine* **283**, 1003–1011.

Clutterbuck, E. J., Evans, D. J., and Pusey, C. D. (1987). Renal involvement in Churg–Strauss syndrome. *Nephrology, Dialysis, Transplantation* **71**, 158–163.

Cohen, B. A. and Clark, W. F. (2000). Pauci-immune renal vasculitis: natural history, prognostic factors, and impact of therapy. *American Journal of Kidney Diseases* **36**, 914–924.

Cohen, J., Pinching, A. J., Rees, A. J., and Peters, D. K. (1982). Infection and immunosuppression: a study of the infective complications in 75 patients with immunologically medicated disease. *Quarterly Journal of Medicine* **201**, 1–15.

Cole, E. *et al.* (1992). A prospective randomized trial of plasma exchange as additive therapy in idiopathic crescentic glomerulonephritis. The Canadian Apheresis Study Group. *American Journal of Kidney Diseases* **20**, 261–269.

Connelly, C. E. and Gallacher, B. (1987). Acute crescentic glomerulonephritis as a complication of a *Staphylococcus aureus* abscess of hip joint prosthesis. *Journal of Clinical Pathology* **40**, 1486 (letter).

Cook, H. T. *et al.* (1999). Interleukin 4 ameliorates crescentic glomerulonephritis in Wistar Kyoto rats. *Kidney International* **55**, 1319–1326.

Couser, W. G. (1982). Idiopathic rapidly progressive glomerulonephritis. *American Journal of Nephrology* **2**, 57–69.

Cunningham, R. J. *et al.* (1980). Rapidly progressive glomerulonephritis in children: a report of thirteen cases and a review of the literature. *Pediatric Research* **14**, 128–132.

Daimon, S. *et al.* (1998). Infective endocarditis induced crescentic glomerulonephritis dramatically improved by plasmapheresis. *American Journal of Kidney Diseases* **32**, 309–313.

D'Amico, G. (2000). Natural history of idiopathic IgA nephropathy: role of clinical and histological prognostic factors. *American Journal of Kidney Diseases* **36**, 227–237.

D'Amico, G. *et al.* (1985). Idiopathic IgA mesangial nephropathy. Clinical and histological study of 374 patients. *Medicine (Baltimore)*, **64**, 49–60.

Daniel, L. *et al.* (2000). Tubular lesions determine prognosis in IgA nephropathy. *American Journal of Kidney Disease* **35**, 13–20.

Date, A. *et al.* (1987). Renal disease in adult Indians: a clinicopathological study of 2827 patients. *Quarterly Journal of Medicine* **64**, 729–737.

Davis, C. A. *et al.* (1978). Observations on the evolution of idiopathic rapidly progressive glomerulonephritis. *Clinical Nephrology* **9**, 91–101.

Davson, J., Ball, J., and Platt, R. (1948). The kidney in periarteritis nodosa. *Quarterly Journal of Medicine* **67**, 175–202.

De Groot, K., Adu, D., and Savage, C. O. S. (2001). The value of pulse cyclophosphamide in ANCA associated vasculitis: meta-analysis and critical review. *Nephrology, Dialysis, Transplantation* **16**, 2018–2027.

Donnelly, S., Jothy, S., and Barre, P. (1989). Crescentic glomerulonephritis in Behçet's syndrome—results of therapy and review of the literature. *Clinical Nephrology* **31**, 213–218.

Downer, G., Phan, S. H., and Wiggins, R. C. (1988). Analysis of renal fibrosis on a rabbit model of crescentic nephritis. *Journal of Clinical Investigation* **82**, 998–1006.

Drew, A. F. *et al.* (2001). Crescentic glomerulonephritis is diminished in fibrinogen deficient mice. *American Journal of Physiology: Renal Physiology* **281**, F1157–F1163.

Droz, D., Noel, L. H., Leibowitch, M., and Barbanel, C. (1979). Glomerulonephritis and necrotizing angiitis. *Advances in Nephrology* **8**, 343–363.

Dussol, B., Berland, Y., and Casanova, P. (1992). Crescentic glomerulonephritis associated with gastric adenocarcinoma. *Nephrologie* **13**, 163–165.

Edelstein, C. L. and Bates, W. D. (1992). Subtypes of acute postinfectious glomerulonephritis: a clinico-pathological correlation. *Clinical Nephrology* **38** (6), 311–317.

Ellis, A. (1942). Natural history of Bright's disease. Clinical, histological and experimental observations. *Lancet* **i**, 34–36.

Evans, D. J. *et al.* (1986). Renal biopsy in prognosis of treated 'glomerulonephritis with crescents'. *Abstracts of the 10th International Congress of Nephrology*, p. 60.

Fairley, C., Mathewson, D. C., and Becker, G. J. (1987). Rapid development of diffuse crescents in post-streptococcal glomerulonephritis. *Clinical Nephrology* **28**, 256–260.

Falk, R. J. and Jennette, J. C. (1988). Anti-neutrophil cytoplasmic autoantibodies with specificity for myeloperoxidase in patients with systemic vasculitis and idiopathic necrotizing and crescentic glomerulonephritis. *New England Journal of Medicine* **318**, 1651–1657.

Falk, R. J., Hogan, S., Carey, T. S., and Jennette, C. (1990). Clinical course of anti-neutrophil cytoplasmic autoantibody-associated glomerulonephritis and vasculitis. *Annals of Internal Medicine* **113**, 656–663.

Fauci, A. S., Katz, P., Haynes, B. F., and Wolff, S. M. (1979). Cyclophosphamide therapy of severe systemic necrotizing vasculitis. *New England Journal of Medicine* **301**, 235–238.

Fauci, A. S., Haynes, B. F., Katz, P., and Wolff, S. M. (1983). Wegener's granulomatosis: prospective clinical and therapeutic experience with 85 patients for 21 years. *Annals of Internal Medicine* **98**, 76–85.

Ferrario, F. *et al.* (1985). The detection of monocytes in human glomerulonephritis. *Kidney International* **28**, 513–519.

Ferrario, F. *et al.* (1994). Critical re-evaluation of 41 cases of 'idiopathic' crescentic glomerulonephritis. *Clinical Nephrology* **41**, 1–9.

Flynn, J. T. *et al.* (2001). Treatment of Henoch Schönlein purpura glomerulonephritis in children with high dose corticosteroids plus oral cyclophosphamide. *American Journal of Nephrology* **21**, 128–133.

Fujieda, M., Hattori, M., Kurayama, H., and Koitabashi, Y. (2002). Clinical features and outcomes in children with anti-neutrophil cytoplasmic antibody positive glomerulonephritis associated with propylthiouracil. *Journal of the American Society of Nephrology* **13**, 437–445.

Gaskin, G., Thomspon, E. M., and Pusey, C. D. (1995). Goodpasture-like syndrome associated with anti-myeloperoxidase antibodies following penicillamine treatment. *Nephrology, Dialysis, Transplantation* **10**, 1925–1928.

Gavaghan, T. E. *et al.* (1981). Penicillamine-induced 'Goodpasture syndrome'; successful treatment of a fulminant case. *Australian and New Zealand Journal of Medicine* **11**, 261–265.

Gibson, T., Burry, H. C., and Ogg, C. S. (1976). Goodpasture's syndrome. *Annals of Internal Medicine* **84**, 100–101.

Gill, D. G. *et al.* (1977). Progression of acute proliferative post-streptococcal glomerulonephritis to severe epithelial crescent formation. *Clinical Nephrology* **8**, 449–452.

Glassock, R. J. (1985). Natural history and treatment of primary proliferative glomerulonephritis: a review. *Kidney International* **17** (Suppl.), 136–142.

Glockner, W. M. *et al.* (1988). Plasma exchange and immunosuppression in rapidly progressive glomerulonephritis: a controlled, multi-center study. *Clinical Nephrology* **29**, 1–8.

Gordon, M. *et al.* (1993). Relapses in patients with a systemic vasculitis. *Quarterly Journal of Medicine* **86**, 779–789.

Haas, M. (1997). Histological subclassification of IgA nephropathy: a clinicopathological study of 244 cases. *American Journal of Kidney Diseases* **29**, 829–842.

Harper, L. *et al.* (2000). Treatment of vasculitic IgA nephropathy. *Journal of Nephrology* **13**, 360–366.

Hattori, M., Kurayama, H., and Koitabashi, Y. (2001). Antineutrophil cytoplasmic antibody-associated glomerulonephritis in children. *Journal of the American Society of Nephrology* **12**, 1493–1500.

Haubitz, M. *et al.* (1998). Intravenous pulse administration of cyclophosphamide versus daily oral treatment in patients with antineutrophil cytoplasmic antibody associated vasculitis and renal involvement: a prospective randomised study. *Arthritis and Rheumatism* **41**, 1835–1844.

He, J. S. *et al.* (2001). Identification of cellular origin of type I collagen in glomeruli of rats with crescentic glomerulonephritis induced by anti-glomerular basement membrane antibody. *Nephrology, Dialysis, Transplantation* **16**, 704–711.

Hedger, N. *et al.* (2000). Incidence and outcome of pauci-immune rapidly progressive glomerulonephritis in Wessex, UK: a 10 year retrospective study. *Nephrology, Dialysis, Transplantation* **15**, 1593–1599.

Heilman, R. L., Offord, K. P., Holley, K. E., and Velosa, J. A. (1987). Analysis of risk factors for patient and renal survival in crescentic glomerulonephritis. *American Journal of Kidney Diseases* **9**, 98–107.

Hellmann, D. B., Hardy, K., Lindenfeld, S., and Ring, E. (1987). Takayasu's arteritis associated with crescentic glomerulonephritis. *Arthritis and Rheumatism* **30**, 451–454.

Hill, G. S. *et al.* (1978). An unusual variant of membranous nephropathy with abundant crescent formation and recurrence in the transplanted kidney. *Clinical Nephrology* **10**, 114–120.

Hind, C. R. *et al.* (1983). Prognosis after immunosuppression of patients with crescentic nephritis requiring dialysis. *Lancet* **i**, 263–265.

Hinglais, N., Garcia-Torres, R., and Kleinknecht, D. (1974). Long term prognosis of acute glomerulonephritis. The predictive value of early clinical and pathological features observed in 65 patients. *American Journal of Medicine* **56**, 52–60.

Holdsworth, S. R., Kitching, A. R., and Tipping, P. G. (1999). Th1 and Th2 helper cell subsets affect patterns of injury and outcomes in glomerulonephritis. *Kidney International* **55**, 1198–1216.

Hooke, D. H., Gee, D. C., and Atkins, R. C. (1987). Leukocyte analysis using monoclonal antibodies in human glomerulonephritis. *Kidney International* **31**, 964–972.

Hotta, O. *et al.* (2002). Regression of IgA nephropathy: a repeat biopsy study. *American Journal of Kidney Disease* **39**, 493–502.

Jardim, H. M. *et al.* (1992). Crescentic glomerulonephritis in children. *Pediatric Nephrology* **6**, 231–235.

Jayne, D. *et al.* (2003). A randomized trial of maintenance therapy for vasculitis associated with antineutrophil cytoplasmic antibodies. *New England Journal of Medicine* **349**, 36–44.

Jayne, D. R. W. and Rasmussen, N. (2000). European collaborative trials in vasculitis: EUVAS update and latest results. *Clinical and Experimental Immunology* **120** (Suppl.), 13–15.

Jayne, D. R. W., Gaskin, G., Pusey, C. D., and Lockwood, C. M. (1995). ANCA and prediction of relapse in systemic vasculitis. *Quarterly Journal of Medicine* **88**, 127–133.

Jayne, D. R. W. *et al.* (2000). Intravenous immunoglobulin for ANCA associated systemic vasculitis with persistent disease activity. *Quarterly Journal of Medicine* **93**, 433–439.

Jennette, J. C. Crescentic glomerulonephritis. In *Heptinstall's Pathology of the Kidney* (ed. J. C. Jennette, J. L. Olson, and M. M. Schwartz). Philadelphia: Lippincott-Raven, 1999.

Jennette, J. C. and Hipp, C. G. (1985). The epithelial cell antigen phenotype of glomerular crescent cells. *American Journal of Clinical Pathology* **86**, 274–280.

Jennette, J. C., Wilkman, A. S., and Falk, R. J. (1989). Anti-neutrophil cytoplasmic autoantibody—associated glomerulonephritis and vasculitis. *American Journal of Pathology* **135**, 921–930.

Jindal, K. K. (1999). Management of idiopathic crescentic and diffuse proliferative glomerulonephritis: evidence based recommendations. *Kidney International Supplement* **70**, S33–S40.

Johnson, J. P., Whitman, W., Briggs, W. A., and Wilson, C. B. (1985). Plasmapheresis and immunosuppressive agents in antibasement membrane antibody-induced Goodpasture's syndrome. *American Journal of Medicine* **64**, 354–359.

Kamata, K., Kobayashi, Y., Shigematsu, H., and Saito, T. (1982). Childhood type polymyositis and rapidly progressive glomerulonephritis. *Acta Pathologica Japonica* **32**, 801–806.

Kannan, S. and Mattoo, T. K. (2001). Diffuse crescentic glomerulonephritis in bacterial endocarditis. *Pediatric Nephrology* **16**, 423–428.

Karkar, A. M., Smith, J., and Pusey, C. D. (2001). Prevention and treatment of experimental crescentic glomerulonephritis by blocking tumour necrosis factor alpha. *Nephrology, Dialysis, Transplantation* **16**, 518–524.

Keller, F. *et al.* (1989). Long-term treatment and prognosis of rapidly progressive glomerulonephritis. *Clinical Nephrology* **31**, 190–197.

Kitching, A. R. *et al.* (1997a). Interleukin 4 and interleukin 10 attenuate established crescentic glomerulonephritis in mice. *Kidney International* **52**, 52–59.

Kitching, A. R., Tipping, P. G., and Holdsworth, S. R. (1997b). IL12 directs severe renal injury, crescent formation and Th1 responses in murine glomerulonephritis. *European Journal of Immunology* **29**, 1–10.

Kitching, A. R., Holdsworth, S. R., and Tipping, P. G. (1999). IFN-gamma mediates crescent formation and cell-mediated immune injury in murine glomerulonephritis. *Journal of the American Society of Nephrology* **10**, 752–759.

Kitching, A. R., Holdsworth, S. R., and Tipping, P. G. (2000). Crescentic glomerulonephritis—a manifestation of a nephritogenic Th1 response? *Histology and Histopathology* **15**, 993–1003.

Kiyama, S. *et al.* (1991). Crescentic glomerulonephritis associated with renal amyloidosis. *Japanese Journal of Medicine* **30** (3), 238–242.

Klassen, J. *et al.* (1974). Evolution of membranous nephropathy into anti-glomerular-basement-membrane glomerulonephritis. *New England Journal of Medicine* **290**, 319–325.

Kodo, K. *et al.* (2001). Vasculitis associated with septicaemia: case report and review of the literature. *Pediatric Nephrology* **16**, 1089–1092.

Koethe, J. D., Gerig, J. S., Glickman, J. L., Sturgill, B. C., and Bolton, W. K. (1986). Progression of membranous nephropathy to acute crescentic rapidly progressive glomerulonephritis and response to pulse methylprednisolone. *American Journal of Nephrology* **6**, 224–228.

Korzets, Z. and Bernheim, J. (1987). Rapidly progressive glomerulonephritis (crescentic glomerulonephritis) in the course of type I idiopathic membranoproliferative glomerulonephritis. *American Journal of Kidney Diseases* **10**, 56–61.

Kurki, P. *et al.* (1984). Transformation of membranous glomerulonephritis into crescentic glomerulonephritis with GBM antibodies: serial determinations of anti-GBM before the transformation. *Nephron* **38**, 134–137.

Lai, K. N. *et al.* (1987). Plasma exchange in patients with rapidly progressive idiopathic IgA nephropathy: a report of two cases and review of literature. *American Journal of Kidney Diseases* **10**, 66–70.

Langerhans, T. (1885). Über die entzundlichen Veranderungen der Glomeruli und die acute Nephritis. *Virchows Archiv (Pathology and Anatomy)* **99**, 193–204.

Leaker, B., Fairley, K. F., Dowling, J., and Kincaid-Smith, P. (1987). Lupus nephritis: clinical and pathological correlation. *Quarterly Journal of Medicine* **62**, 163–179.

Le Hir, M. *et al.* (2001). Podocyte bridges between the tuft and Bowman's capsule: an early event in experimental crescentic glomerulonephritis. *Journal of American Society of Nephrology* **12**, 2060–2071.

Leonard, C. D. *et al.* (1970). Acute glomerulonephritis with prolonged oliguria: an analysis of 29 cases. *Annals of Internal Medicine* **73**, 703–711.

Levy, J. B. and Winearls, C. G. (1994). Rapidly progressive glomerulonephritis: what should be first line therapy? *Nephron* **67**, 402–407.

Levy, J. B., Turner, A. N., Rees, A. J., and Pusey, C. D. (2001). Long term outcome of anti-glomerular basement membrane antibody disease treated with plasma exchange and immunosuppression. *Annals of Internal Medicine* **134**, 1033–1042.

Lewy, J. E. *et al.* (1977). Clinico-pathologic correlations in acute post-streptococcal nephritis. *Medicine* **50**, 453–501.

Li, S., Kurts C., Kontgen, F., Holdsworth, S. R., and Tipping, P. G. (1998). Major histocompatibility complex class II expression by intrinsic renal cells is required for crescentic glomerulonephritis. *Journal of Experimental Medicine* **188**, 597–602.

Li, S., Holdsworth, S. R., and Tipping, P. G. (2000). B7.1 and B7.2 co-stimulatory molecules regulate crescentic glomerulonephritis. *European Journal of Immunology* **30**, 1394–1401.

Lockwood, C. M. *et al.* (1976). Immunosuppression and plasma exchange in the treatment of Goodpasture's syndrome. *Lancet* **i**, 711–715.

Lockwood, C. M. *et al.* (1977). Plasma-exchange and immunosuppression in the treatment of fulminating immune-complex crescentic nephritis. *Lancet* **i**, 63–67.

Logan, D. *et al.* (1994). Arteritis of both carotid arteries in a patient with focal, crescentic glomerulonephritis and anti-neutrophil cytoplasmic autoantibodies. *British Journal of Rheumatology* **33** (2), 167–169.

Löhlein, M. *Ueber die entzundlichen Veranderungen der Glomeruli der menschlichen Nieren und ihre Gedeuting fur die Nephritis.* Arbeiten aus dem pathologischen institut zu Leipzig 1, Leipzig: Hirzel, 1907.

Macarron, P., Garcia Diaz, J. E., Azofra, J. A., and Martin de Francisco, J. (1992). D-Penicillamine associated with rapidly progressive glomerulonephritis. *Nephrology, Dialysis, Transplantation* **7**, 161–164.

McCoy, R., Clapp, J., and Seigler, H. F. (1975). Membranoproliferative glomerulonephritis. Progression from the pure form to the crescentic form with recurrence after transplantation. *American Journal of Medicine* **59**, 288–292.

Magil, A. *et al.* (1988). Prognostic factors in diffuse proliferative lupus nephritis. *Kidney International* **34**, 511–517.

Mason, P. D. and Lockwood, C. M. (1986). Rapidly progressive nephritis in patients taking hydralazine. *Journal of Clinical Laboratory Immunology* **20**, 151–153.

Matloff, D. S. and Kaplan, M. M. (1980). D-Penicillamine-induced bilary cirrhosis: successful treatment with plasmapheresis and immunosuppressives. *Gastroenterology* **78**, 1046–1049.

McIntyre, C. W., Fluck, R. J., and Lambie, S. H. (2001). Steroid and cyclophosphamide therapy for IgA nephropathy associated with crescentic change: an effective treatment. *Clinical Nephrology* **56**, 193–198.

McLaughlin, K. *et al.* (1998). Has the prognosis for patients with pauci-immune necrotising glomerulonephritis improved? *Nephrology, Dialysis, Transplantation* **13**, 1696–1701.

Miller, M. N., Baumal, R., Poucell, S., and Steele, B. T. (1984). Incidence and prognostic importance of glomerular crescents in renal diseases of childhood. *American Journal of Nephrology* **4**, 244–247.

Modai, D. *et al.* (1985). Biopsy proven evolution of post streptococcal glomerulonephritis to rapidly progressive glomerulonephritis of a post infectious type. *Clinical Nephrology* **23**, 198–202.

Monga, G., Mazzucco, G., Belgiojoso, B., and Bushach, G. (1981). Monocyte infiltration and glomerular hypercellularity in human acute and persistent glomerulonephritis: light and electron microscopic, immunofluorescent and histochemical investigation on twenty eight patients. *Laboratory Investigation* **44**, 381–387.

Montseny, J. J., Meyrier, A., Kleinknecht, D., and Callard, P. (1995). The current spectrum of infectious glomerulonephritis. Experience with 76 patients and review of the literature. *Medicine (Baltimore)* **74**, 63–73.

Morel-Maroger, L., Kourilsky, O., Midnon, F., and Richet, G. (1974). Antitubular basement membrane antibodies in rapidly progressive post-streptococcal glomerulonephritis: report of a case. *Clinical Immunology and Immunopathology* **2**, 185–194.

Morrin, P. A., Hinglais, N., Nabarra, B., and Kreis, H. (1978). Rapidly progressive glomerulonephritis. A clinical and pathologic study. *American Journal of Medicine* **65**, 446–460.

Muller, G. A., Seipel, L., and Risler, T. (1986). Treatment of non anti-GBM-antibody mediated, rapidly progressive glomerulonephritis by plasmapheresis and immunosuppression. *Klinische Wochenschrift* **64**, 231–238.

Mustonen, J., Helin, H., Pasternack, A., and Vanttinen, T. (1983). Acute rheumatic fever with extracapillary glomerulonephritis and the nephrotic syndrome. *Annals of Clinical Research* **15**, 92–94.

Nagata, M. *et al.* (2001). Glomerular crescents in renal amyloidosis: an epiphenomenona or distinct pathology? *Pathology International* **51**, 179–186.

Nakamoto, S., Dunea, G., Kolff, W., and McCormack, L. (1965). Treatment of oliguric glomerulonephritis with dialysis and steroids. *Annals of Internal Medicine* **63**, 359–368.

Nanke, Y., Akama, H., Terai, C., and Kamatani, N. (2000). Rapidly progressive glomerulonephritis with D-penicillamine. *American Journal of Medical Science* **320**, 398–402.

Naschitz, J. E. *et al.* (1989). Recurrent massive alveolar hemorrhage, crescentic glomerulonephritis, and necrotizing vasculitis in a patient with rheumatoid arthritis. *Archives of Internal Medicine* **149**, 406–408.

Nassberger, L., Johansson, A.-C., Bjorck, S., and Sjoholm, A. G. (1991). Antibodies to neutrophil granulocyte myeloperoxidase and elastase: autoimmune responses in glomerulonephritis due to hydralazine treatment. *Journal of Internal Medicine* **229**, 261–265.

Neild, G. H. *et al.* (1978). Relapsing polychondritis with crescentic glomerulonephritis. *British Medical Journal* **i**, 743–745.

Neild, G. H. *et al.* (1983). Rapidly progressive glomerulonephritis with extensive glomerular crescent formation. *Quarterly Journal of Medicine* **52**, 395–416.

Neugarten, J., Gallo, G. R., and Baldwin, D. S. (1984). Glomerulonephritis in bacterial endocarditis. *American Journal of Kidney Disease* **3**, 371–379.

Nguyen, B. P., Reisen, E., and Rodriguez, F. H. J. R. (1988). Idiopathic membranous glomerulopathy complicated by crescentic glomerulonephritis and renal vein thrombosis. *American Journal of Kidney Disease* **12**, 326–368.

Niaudet, P., Levy, M., Broyer, M., and Habib, R. (1984). Clinicopathologic correlations in severe forms of Henoch–Schönlein purpura nephritis. *Contributions to Nephrology* **40**, 250–254.

Nicholls, K. M., Fairley, K. F., Dowling, J. P., and Kincaid-Smith, P. (1984). The clinical course of mesangial IgA nephropathy. *Quarterly Journal of Medicine* **53**, 227–250.

Nicholson, G. D., Amin, U. F., and Alleyne, G. A. (1975). Membranous glomerulonephropathy with crescents. *Clinical Nephrology* **4**, 198–201.

Nolasco, F. E. B. *et al.* (1987). Intraglomerular T cells and monocytes in nephritis: study with monoclonal antibodies. *Kidney International* **31**, 1160–1166.

Ntoso, K. A., Tomaszewski, J. E., Jimenez, S. A., and Neilson, E. G. (1986). Penicillamine-induced rapidly progressive glomerulonephritis in patients with progressive systemic sclerosis: successful treatment of two patients and a review of the literature. *American Journal of Kidney Diseases* **8**, 159–163.

Old, C. W., Herrera, G. A., Reimann, B. E., and Latham, R. D. (1984). Acute post-streptococcal glomerulonephritis progressing to rapidly progressive glomerulonephritis. *Southern Medical Journal* **77**, 1470–1472.

Oliviera, D. J. *et al.* (1995). Relationship between disease activity and ANCA concentration by ELISA in long term management of systemic vasculitis. *American Journal of Kidney Diseases* **25**, 380–389.

O'Neill, W. M., Jr., Etheridge, W. B., and Bloomer, H. A. (1979). High-dose corticosteroids: their use in treating idiopathic rapidly progressive glomerulonephritis. *Archives of Internal Medicine* **139**, 514–518.

Oredugba, O., Mazumdar, D. C., Meyer, J. S., and Lubowitz, H. (1980). Pulse methylprednisolone therapy in idiopathic, rapidly progressive glomerulonephritis. *Annals of Internal Medicine* **92**, 504–506.

Ou, Z. L. *et al.* (2001). Effective methylprednisolone dose in experimental crescentic glomerulonephritis. *American Journal of Kidney Diseases* **37**, 411–417.

Parag, K. B. *et al.* (1988). Profile of crescentic glomerulonephritis in Natal-a clinicopathological assessment. *Quarterly Journal of Medicine* **68**, 629–636.

Pusey, C. D. *et al.* (1991). A randomised controlled trial of plasma exchange in rapidly progressive glomerulonephritis without anti-GBM antibodies. *Kidney International* **40**, 757–763.

Rees, A. J., Lockwood, C. M., and Peters, D. K. (1977). Enhanced allergic tissue damage in Goodpasture's syndrome by intercurrent bacterial infection. *British Medical Journal* **ii**, 723–726.

Reynolds, J. *et al.* (2000). CD28-B7 blockade prevents the development of experimental autoimmune glomerulonephritis. *Journal of Clinical Investigation* **105**, 643–651.

Rifle, G. *et al.* (1981). Treatment of idiopathic acute crescentic glomerulonephritis by immunodepression and plasma-exchange: a prospective randomised study. *Proceedings of the European Dialysis and Transplantation Association* **18**, 493–502.

Roccatello, D. *et al.* (1995). Report on intensive treatment of extracapillary glomerulonephritis with focus on crescentic IgA nephropathy. *Nephrology, Dialysis, Transplantation* **10**, 2054–2059.

Roccatello, D. *et al.* (2000). Steroid and cyclophosphamide in IgA nephropathy. *Nephrology, Dialysis, Transplantation* **15**, 833–835.

Rondeau, E. *et al.* (1993). Methylprednisolone and cyclophosphamide pulse therapy in crescentic glomerulonephritis: safety and effectiveness. *Renal Failure* **15** (4), 495–501.

Rovzar, M. A., Logan, J. L., Ogden, D. A., and Graham, A. R. (1986). Immunosuppressive therapy and plasmapheresis in rapidly progressive glomerulonephritis associated with bacterial endocarditis. *American Journal of Kidney Diseases* **7**, 428–433.

Roy, S., Murphy, W. M., and Arant, B. S. (1981). Post-streptococcal glomerulonephritis in children: comparison of quintuple therapy versus supportive care. *Pediatrics* **98**, 403–410.

Ryffel, B., Eugster, H., Haas, C., and Le Hir, M. (1998). Failure to induce anti-glomerular basement membrane glomerulonephritis in TNF alpha/beta deficient mice. *International Journal of Experimental Pathology* **79**, 453–460.

Sadjadi, S. A., Seelig, M. S., Berger, A. R., and Milstoc, M. (1985). Rapidly progressive glomerulonephritis in a patient with rheumatoid arthritis during treatment with high-dosage D-penicillamine. *American Journal of Nephrology* **5**, 212–216.

Salama, A. *et al.* (2002). Goodpasture's disease in the absence of circulating anti-glomerular basement membrane antibodies using standard techniques. *American Journal of Kidney Diseases* **39**, 1162–1167.

Sasatomi, Y., Kiyoshi, Y., and Takabeyashi, S. (1999). A clinical and pathological study on the characteristics and factors influencing the prognosis of crescentic glomerulonephritis using a cluster analysis. *Pathology International* **49**, 781–785.

Savage, C. O. S. *et al.* (1985). Microscopic polyarteritis: presentation, pathology and prognosis. *Quarterly Journal of Medicine* **56**, 467–483.

Schiffer, M. C. and Michael, A. (1978). Renal cell turnover studied by the Y chromosome (Y body) staining of the transplanted human kidney. *Journal of Laboratory and Clinical Medicine* **92**, 841–848.

Segasothy, M., Fairley, K. F., Birch, D. F., and Kincaid Smith, P. (1989). Immunoperoxidase identification of nucleated cells in urine in glomerular and acute tubular disorders. *Clinical Nephrology* **31**, 281–291.

Segerer, S. *et al.* (2000). Expression of the chemokine monocyte chemoattractant protein 1 and its receptor chemokine receptor 2 in human crescentic glomerulonephritis. *Journal of the American Society of Nephrology* **11**, 2231–2242.

Sesso, R. *et al.* (1990). Exposure to hydrocarbons and rapidly progressive glomerulonephritis. *Brazilian Journal of Medical and Biological Research* **23** (3–4), 225–233.

Shoji, T. *et al.* (2000). Early treatment with corticosteroids ameliorates proteinuria, proliferative lesions, and mesangial phenotypic modulation in adult diffuse proliferative IgA nephropathy. *American Journal of Kidney Diseases* **35**, 194–201.

Sonsino, E. *et al.* (1972). Extracapillary proliferative glomerulonephritis so-called malignant glomerulonephritis. *Advances in Nephrology* **2**, 121–163.

Southwest Pediatric Nephrology Study Group (1985). A clinicopatholgical study of crescentic glomerulonephritis in 50 children. *Kidney International* **27**, 450–498.

Srivastava, R. N. *et al.* (1992). Crescentic glomerulonephritis in children: a review of 43 cases. *American Journal of Nephrology* **12** (3), 155–161.

Stegmayr, B. G. *et al.* (1999). Plasma exchange or immunoadsorption in patient with rapidly progressive crescentic glomerulonephritis. A Swedish multi-center study. *International Journal of Artificial Organs* **22**, 81–87.

Sternlieb, I., Bennett, B., and Scheinberg, I. H. (1975). D-Penicillamine induced Goodpasture's syndrome in Wilson's disease. *Annals of Internal Medicine* **82**, 673–676.

Stokes, M. B. *et al.* (2001). Up-regulation of extracellular matrix proteoglycans and collagen type I in human crescentic glomerulonephritis. *Kidney International* **59**, 532–542.

Sumethkul, V., Chalermsanyakorn, P., Changsirikulchai, S., and Radinahamed, P. (2000). Lupus nephritis: a challenging cause of rapidly progressive crescentic glomerulonephritis. *Lupus* **9**, 424–428.

Swainson, C. P. *et al.* (1982). Plasma exchange in the successful treatment of drug induced renal disease. *Nephron* **30**, 244–249.

Tervaert, J. W., Stegeman, C. A., and Kallenberg, C. G. (1998). Silicon exposure and vasculitis. *Current Opinion in Rheumatology* **10**, 12–17.

Takeda, S. *et al.* (1998). Methylprednisolone pulse therapy in two clinical types of crescentic glomerulonephritis. *Internal Medicine* **37**, 585–591.

Tang, Z. *et al.* (2001). The clinical and pathological characteristics of Chinese patients with pauci-immune crescent glomerulonephritis. *Chinese Medical Journal* **114**, 374–378.

Tapaneya-Olarn, W., Tapaneya-Olarn, C., Boonpucknavig, V., and Boonpucknavig, S. (1992). Rapidly progressive glomerulonephritis in Thai children. *Journal of the Medical Association of Thailand* **75** (Suppl. 1), 32–37.

Tateno, S., Sakai, T., Kobayashi, Y., and Shigematsu, H. (1981). Idiopathic membranous glomerulonephritis with crescents. *Acta Pathologica Japonica* **31**, 211–219.

Tietjen, D. P. and Moore, W. J. (1990). Treatment of rapidly progressive glomerulonephritis due to Behçet's syndrome with intravenous cyclophosphamide. *Nephron* **55**, 69–73.

Timoshanko, J. R., Kitching A. R., Holdsworth, S. R., and Tipping, P. G. (2001). Interleukin 12 from intrinsic cells is an effector of renal injury in crescentic glomerulonephritis. *Journal of the American Society of Nephrology* **12**, 464–471.

Tipping, P. G. *et al.* (1998). Crescentic glomerulonephritis in CD4- and CD8-deficient mice. Requirement for CD4 but not CD8 cells. *American Journal of Pathology* **152**, 1541–1548.

Vendemia, F., Gesualdo, L., Schena, F. P., and D'Amico, G. (2001). Epidemiology of primary glomerulonephritis in the elderly. Report from the Italian Registry of Renal Biopsy. *Journal of Nephrology* **14**, 340–352.

Volhard, F. and Fahr, T. *Die Brightsche Nierenkrankheit.* Berlin: Springer, 1914.

Wada, T. *et al.* (1999). MIP-1 alpha and MCP-1 contribute to crescents and interstitial lesions in human crescentic glomerulonephritis. *Kidney International* **56**, 995–1003.

Wakabayashi, Y., Kobayashi, Y., and Shigematsu, H. (1985). Shunt nephritis: histological dynamics following removal of the shunt. *Nephron* **40**, 111–117.

Walters, M. D. *et al.* (1988). Antineutrophil cytoplasm antibody in crescentic nephritis. *Archives of Disease in Childhood* **63**, 814–817.

Weinstein, T. *et al.* (1990). Unusual case of crescentic glomerulonephritis associated with malignant lymphoma. A case report and review of the literature. *American Journal of Nephrology* **10** (4), 329–332.

Welch, T. R., McAdams, A. J., and Berry, A. (1988). Rapidly progressive IgA nephropathy. *American Journal of Diseases of Childhood* **142**, 789–793.

Westman, K. W. A. *et al.* (1998). Relapse rate, renal survival and cancer morbidity in patients with Wegener's granulomatosis or microscopic polyangiitis with renal involvement. *Journal of the American Society of Nephrology* **9**, 842–852.

Whitworth, J. A., Morel-Maroger, L., Mignon, F., and Richet, G. (1976). The significance of extracapillary proliferation. Clinicopathological review of 60 patients. *Nephron* **16**, 1–19.

Williams, W. W., Shah, D. J., Morgan, A. G., and Alleyne, G. A. O. (1985). Membranous glomerulopathy with crescents in systemic lupus erythematosus. *American Journal of Nephrology* **5**, 158–162.

Woo, K. T. *et al.* (1986). Glomerulonephritis in Singapore: an overview. *Annals of the Academy of Medicine, Singapore* **15**, 20–31.

Wu, J. *et al.* (2002). CD4(+) T cells specific to a glomerular basement membrane antigen mediate glomerulonephritis. *Journal of Clinical Investigation* **109**, 517–524.

Wu, Q. *et al.* (2001). Analysis of prognostic predictors in idiopathic membranous nephropathy. *American Journal of Kidney Disease* **37**, 380–387.

Yang, N. *et al.* (1998a). Reversal of established rat crescentic glomerulonephritis by blockade of macrophage migration inhibitory factor (MIF): potential role of MIF in regulating glucocorticoid production. *Molecular Medicine* **4**, 413–424.

Yang, N. *et al.* (1998b). Local macrophage proliferation in human glomerulonephritis. *Kidney International* **54**, 143–151.

Yeung, C. K. *et al.* (1984). Crescentic lupus glomerulonephritis. *Clinical Nephrology* **21**, 251–258.

Yoshida, A., Morozumi, K., Takeda, A., and Koyama, K. (1992). A case of rapidly progressive glomerulonephritis associated with bucillamine-treated rheumatoid arthritis. *American Journal of Kidney Diseases* **20**, 411–413.

Zauner, I. *et al.* (2002). Predictive value of initial histology and effect of plasmapheresis on long term prognosis of rapidly progressive glomerulonephritis. *American Journal of Kidney Diseases* **39**, 28–35.

3.11 Antiglomerular basement disease

A. Neil Turner and Andrew J. Rees

Definition

Human antiglomerular basement membrane (anti-GBM) disease is an autoimmune disorder characterized by the presence of autoantibodies directed against a target restricted to the glomerular and a few other specialized basement membranes. Its classical manifestations are rapidly progressive nephritis and lung haemorrhage, a syndrome known as Goodpasture's syndrome. The Goodpasture eponym is best reserved for spontaneous human anti-GBM disease, 'Goodpasture's disease', as the clinical syndrome of rapidly progressive glomerulonephritis and pulmonary haemorrhage is more commonly caused by systemic vasculitis, usually associated with antineutrophil cytoplasmic antibodies (ANCA; Chapters 4.5.1 and 4.5.2). The differential diagnosis of pulmonary–renal syndromes is considered further in the section on pulmonary manifestations, below (and see Tables 1 and 2).

Ernest Goodpasture described an 18-year-old man with lung haemorrhage and crescentic nephritis at autopsy during an epidemic of influenza (Goodpasture 1919). Nearly 40 years later, Stanton and Tange (1958) described a group of nine patients with similar findings, and applied Goodpastures name to it before the immunological heterogeneity of the syndrome was appreciated. The disorder may also cause renal or pulmonary disease in isolation.

The classical linear staining of the GBM on direct immunofluorescence was first recognized in human biopsies by Scheer and Grossman (1964), following on from the observations made in experimental anti-GBM disease by Ortega and Mellors (1956). The pathogenicity of these antibodies was shown by Lerner *et al.* in 1967 (Lerner *et al.* 1999). Goodpasture's disease is now known to be caused by autoimmunity to a specific basement membrane antigen, identified as the carboxy-terminal globular (NC1) domain of a tissue-specific type IV collagen chain, the $\alpha3$ chain, hence the Goodpasture antigen may be abbreviated to $\alpha3$(IV)NC1.

Table 1 Causes of rapidly progressive glomerulonephritis with alveolar haemorrhage (Goodpasture's syndrome). Systemic vasculitis (all types) accounts for about two-thirds of cases

Goodpasture's (anti-GBM) disease
ANCA-associated small vessel vasculitis Microscopic polyangiitis Wegener's disease Drug-associated: hydralazine, penicillamine
Uncommonly in other vasculitis Systemic lupus erythematosus Henoch–Schönlein purpura Behçet's disease Mixed essential cryoglobulinaemia Rheumatoid vasculitis

Sources: Leatherman *et al.* (1984); Holdsworth *et al.* (1985); Clutterbuck and Pusey (1987); Leatherman (1987); Vats (1999).

Epidemiology

Incidence

Goodpasture's disease is rare, with an estimated incidence of up to 1 case per million per annum in the United Kingdom, based on the identification of anti-GBM antibodies by immunoassay and renal biopsy. It has been estimated to cause up to 5 per cent of glomerulonephritis (Wilson and Dixon 1973; New Zealand Glomerulonephritis Study Group 1989) though recent figures are variable—1 per cent in Denmark (Heaf *et al.* 1999); 1.5 per cent of biopsies in Italy (Schena 1997); but 2.4 per cent of biopsies in Ireland (Daly *et al.* 1996). It causes 10–20 per cent of crescentic nephritis (Couser 1988; Andrassy *et al.* 1991; Heaf *et al.* 1999).

The disease is more common in White races, and seems to be particularly rare in Asian Indian and Black races, although cases in Black Americans have been described (e.g. Kelly and Haponik 1994). Although there are no large studies of incidence, cases have been reported from Japan (Wakui *et al.* 1992) and China. A New Zealand study (Teague *et al.* 1978) reported a relatively high proportion of

Table 2 Diseases recurrently associated with Goodpasture's disease. Alport's syndrome following transplantation is bracketed as it is not 'true' Goodpasture's disease (see section at end of this chapter)

Disease	Number of reports (approx.)
ANCA–associated vasculitis (mostly with antimyeloperoxidase ANCA)	Hundreds
Membranous nephropathy	<20
Diabetes mellitus	10
Malignancy—lymphoma, bronchial carcinoma	10
Lithotripsy to intrarenal stones	3
(Alport's syndrome following renal transplantation)	(tens)

Maoris (five of 29 cases or 17 per cent, although they only made up 7 per cent of the population).

The disease may occur from childhood to old age. The youngest reported case was 11 months old; several patients in their 80s have been described. Early series showed a marked preponderance of young men. The wider use of immunoassays and immunohistology, and greater awareness of the disease, have led to later series showing greater proportions of women and older patients, although it is still more common in men. Our data show a second peak in incidence in the sixth and seventh decades; this pattern has also been seen in series from Sweden, France, and Germany (Segelmark *et al.* 1991; Herody *et al.* 1993; Merkel *et al.* 1994; Daly *et al.* 1996) (Fig. 1; see also Table 6 below). This age and gender distribution is notably dissimilar to those of other organ-specific autoimmune disorders.

Lung haemorrhage is more common in younger patients and in men (Fig. 1). Glomerulonephritis alone is more common in older patients and in women. The male–female ratio in 71 cases from the United Kingdom in 1980–1984 (Savage *et al.* 1986) was 1.4, but for those with pulmonary haemorrhage as well as glomerulonephritis it was 3.0, and for those with nephritis alone it was 0.9. These differences were probably related to smoking habit.

Clustering of cases has been described in three reports: 15 cases in 3 years from Auckland, New Zealand (Simpson *et al.* 1982), four cases within a 25 mile radius during one winter in Connecticut, USA (Perez *et al.* 1974), and 13 cases within 8 months in Northwest England (Williams *et al.* 1988). Two of our own cases presenting a few months apart recently were unrelated individuals who lived next door to each other. Such reports lend support to the hypothesis that exposure to an infective or other exogenous agent is involved in the pathogenesis. Influenza virus has been specifically mentioned in a number of reports, including Goodpasture's original description, but infection with the virus is common. Wilson and coworkers studied patients with influenza but did not find evidence of anti-GBM antibodies, and many have looked for influenza antibodies in patients with Goodpasture's disease, rarely with any success (Wilson and Smith 1972; Wilson and Dixon 1973). A wider survey looking for antibodies to 13 viruses in 22 patients found no evidence of a disease association with any particular infection (Wilson *et al.* 1973). An almost insuperable problem in analysing anecdotal reports is that an infection may non-specifically exacerbate tissue injury caused by the disease, leading to its clinical presentation in association with an infection that is not causally related to it.

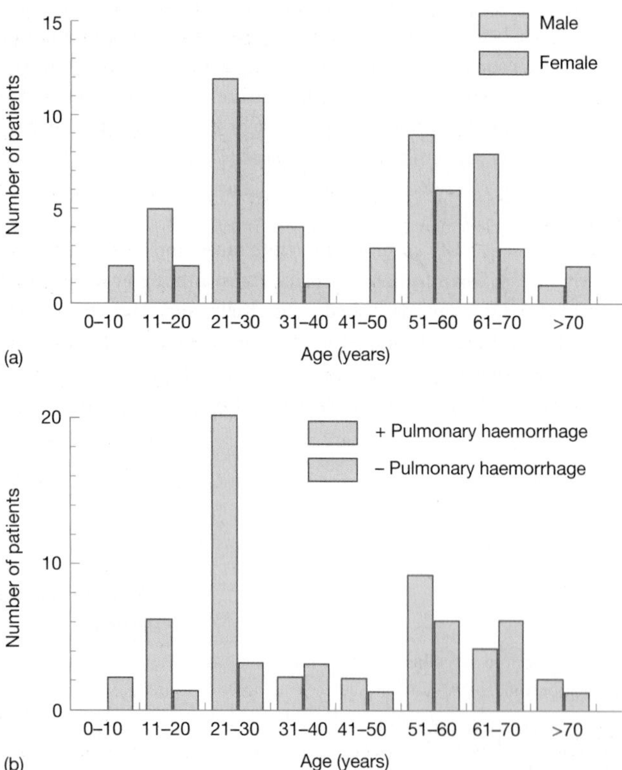

Fig. 1 (a) Age and gender of 68 patients with Goodpasture's disease treated at Hammersmith Hospital, London. (b) Pulmonary haemorrhage in 68 patients with Goodpasture's disease treated at Hammersmith Hospital, London.

Disease associations

There are not only many isolated case reports of Goodpasture's disease occurring in association with other diseases, but also a number of recurrent associations that may reflect important pathogenetic mechanisms (Table 2).

Reports of anti-GBM disease occurring in association with small vessel vasculitis antedate the availability of ANCA assays, and include examples of apparently typical microscopic polyarteritis (Relman *et al.* 1971), an eosinophilic systemic vasculitis (Komadina *et al.* 1988), and Wegener's granulomatosis (Wahls *et al.* 1987). Numerous later reports have documented this association. In the great majority the ANCA have had specificity for myeloperoxidase, and many patients have had clinical features of vasculitis. Some patients with isolated rapidly progressive glomerulonephritis also have positive results in assays for both antibodies and linear binding of antibodies to the GBM. How much contribution to glomerular damage is made by the anti-GBM antibodies is not known, but the titre in some patients can be very high. On average though the anti-GBM antibody titres in double-positive patients may be relatively lower (Jayne *et al.* 1990; Bosch *et al.* 1991; Saxena *et al.* 1991) and relatively easily suppressed by treatment. Some reports suggest (others do not) that double-positive patients are more likely to have recoverable renal function despite oliguria or severe renal impairment at presentation, features usually associated with a poor outcome in anti-GBM disease. These observations suggest that the anti-GBM response could occur in genetically predisposed patients following damage to the glomerular or alveolar basement membrane by small vessel vasculitis. However, there are occasional instances where the clinical history suggests that anti-GBM disease antedated the development of vasculitis (O'Donoghue *et al.* 1989; Peces *et al.* 2000). It is nevertheless possible that these instances were 'double-positive' from the outset (as in Paueksakon *et al.* 1999; Verburgh *et al.* 1999), but that this was not apparent clinically and not identified by the assays.

The true incidence of double positivity for both autoantibodies has varied in different studies, at least in part because of different techniques used to define ANCA. Hellmark (1997) found anti-GBM positivity in less than 12 per cent (8–12 per cent) of samples positive for ANCA; but in samples positive for anti-GBM antibodies, 38 per cent were positive for ANCA. The ANCA specificity of two-thirds of dually positive samples was for myeloperoxidase (MPO). They and others found no difference between the characteristics of the anti-GBM antibodies in the two patient groups. Short *et al.* (1995) identified ANCA in the serum of 21 per cent of patients with anti-GBM antibodies, and that the ANCA specificity was for MPO in 73 per cent. However, only 2.5 per cent of patients with ANCA had anti-GBM antibodies. Their lower rate of double positivity was arrived at after tests of specificity (Western blotting or inhibition assays) that eliminated half of the putative double positives.

An association with idiopathic membranous nephropathy was first described in 1974 (Klassen *et al.* 1974), but many descriptions have followed. Occasionally, this disease undergoes a transformation to a crescentic pattern with rapidly deteriorating renal function. In some of the reported cases, a sudden deterioration of previously diagnosed membranous nephropathy has been associated with anti-GBM antibodies, whereas in others the crescentic change has not been associated with either anti-GBM antibodies or ANCA. In other examples, both membranous nephropathy and anti-GBM disease were present on initial assessment (Fig. 2). Only one of the reported cases has been associated with lung haemorrhage (Takeuchi 1997). Almost all have progressed to ESRF, but the diagnosis has usually been made at a late stage. The amount of Goodpasture antigen is increased in the thickened basement membranes of membranous nephropathy (Kim *et al.* 1991; Haramoto *et al.* 1994), and it is possible that the GBM may sometimes become damaged in membranous nephropathy, triggering immunity to the Goodpasture antigen.

Diabetes mellitus is commonly associated with weak to moderate linear fluorescence for immunoglobulin along the GBM, in the absence of evidence of glomerular inflammation. No specific anti-GBM antibodies can usually be demonstrated in the serum in these circumstances. It is interesting though that a number of recent case reports have described the development of overt anti-GBM disease and the presence of circulating anti-GBM antibodies in 10 patients with diabetes (e.g. Ahuja *et al.* 1998; Curioni *et al.* 2002). Only in one case were ANCA also identified. Most have been type I diabetics and all have had a long history of diabetes with changes of diabetic nephropathy on renal biopsy. As in membranous nephropathy, the thickened GBM of diabetic nephropathy increases the amount of Goodpasture antigen present.

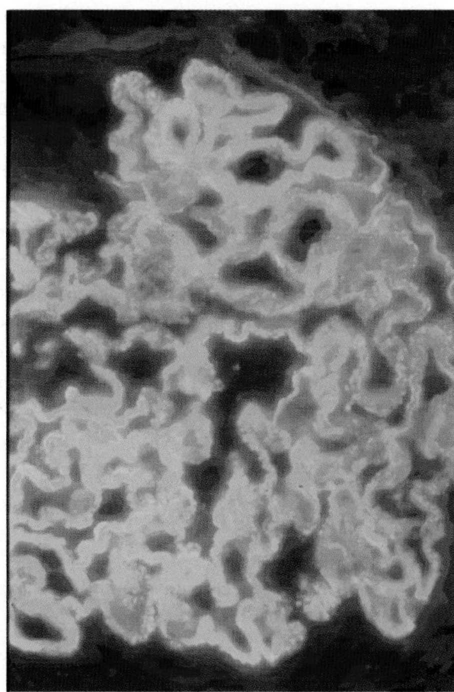

Fig. 2 Direct immunofluorescence for IgG on the glomerulus of a 65-year-old man with nephrotic syndrome that deteriorated rapidly to severe renal failure. Linear binding to the endothelial surface of the GBM is accompanied by granular deposits of IgG subepithelially, typical of membranous nephropathy. This was confirmed by electron microscopy. Typical anti-GBM antibodies were detected in serum.

There are now three published examples of anti-GBM disease following some weeks to months after lithotripsy [Guerin *et al.* 1990; Umekawa *et al.* 1993 (this case appears in at least two other publications); Xenocostas *et al.* 1999]. The patients in all these examples carried HLA-DR15 or DR2, and in that way were already predisposed to developing the disease.

Goodpasture's disease has been associated with lymphoma in six patients, but all in old reports. The two for whom details are available developed Goodpasture's disease at a time when their lymphoma was in remission or cured (Ma *et al.* 1978; Kleinknecht *et al.* 1980; Wilson and Dixon 1981). One had received both chemotherapy and full-mantle radiotherapy, whereas the other had received upper-mantle radiotherapy alone. Some other examples in association with malignancy in both the published literature and in the authors' experience have been associated with predominantly IgA autoantibodies (Maes *et al.* 1999; Carreras *et al.* 2002) (and see Chapter 3.13). In all these cases the tumours have been bronchial carcinomas.

Anti-GBM disease may occur after renal transplantation, when it is usually either recurrent Goodpasture's disease, or develops in patients with Alport's syndrome, which may not have been suspected previously. There are many reports of both, and these are considered in more detail at the end of this chapter.

There are numerous but mostly isolated reports of anti-GBM disease occurring in association with other autoimmune or other possibly relevant diseases, including myasthenia gravis (Drube *et al.* 1997 and our series), coeliac disease (Savage *et al.* 1986), partial lipodystrophy (Blake *et al.* 1980), thyroiditis (Kalderon *et al.* 1973), B12 deficiency anaemia (Wüthrich 1994), dermatomyositis (Kelly and Haponik 1994), after pneumococcal vaccination (Tan and Cumming 1993), in patients on penicillamine therapy (Bindi *et al.* 1997; R. Lechler, unpublished observation), in primary biliary cirrhosis (Komatsu *et al.* 1998), multiple sclerosis (Henderson *et al.* 1998), and in the nail-patella syndrome (Curtis *et al.* 1976). The latter is interesting in view of recent confirmation that the expression of Goodpasture antigen is reduced (but not absent) in nail-patella syndrome (Morello *et al.* 2001).

Clinical features

General manifestations

The clinical features of Goodpasture's disease have been well established from the relatively large series of immunologically defined cases published over the last 30 years (listed in Table 6). Affected individuals often give a history of malaise, and sometimes of arthralgia and weight loss, but these are generally mild. This is in contrast to most cases of systemic vasculitis in which other aspects of the clinical presentation may be identical. Anaemia is common and frequently symptomatic, even in patients who have had little or no haemoptysis. The anaemia is usually microcytic and hypochromic, but sometimes shows evidence of microangiopathy as can be the case with other types of rapidly progressive glomerulonephritis. The iron deficiency probably reflects subclinical pulmonary haemorrhage, but can on occasion be confused with gastrointestinal disease, especially if uraemia is causing nausea and vomiting. Anaemia is also common in systemic vasculitis, but is characteristically normochromic and normocytic. In either disease anaemia can be wrongly attributed to chronic renal failure, which leads to inappropriate treatment.

Pulmonary manifestations

Pulmonary haemorrhage used to be reported in two-thirds of patients, but more recent series suggest the prevelance has fallen to around 50 per cent. Typically, pulmonary haemorrhage presents as haemoptysis that may be episodic. However, pulmonary haemorrhage can occur without haemoptysis. Haemoptysis varies from the trivial to torrential and is a poor reflection of the actual quantity of pulmonary bleeding. Occasional patients give a history of repeated episodes of haemoptysis over many years—even for more than a decade. Pulmonary haemorrhage shows a marked tendency to remit and relapse spontaneously (e.g. Schindler *et al.* 1998; Schmidt *et al.* 1999), a fact which has complicated the interpretation of various therapeutic interventions.

In contrast with renal injury, lung disease shows a very poor correlation with antibody titre (Wilson and Dixon 1981; Simpson *et al.* 1982) even though the Goodpasture antigen is present in alveolar as well as glomerular basement membrane (McPhaul and Dixon 1970; Cashman *et al.* 1988; Kleppel *et al.* 1989; Gunwar *et al.* 1991). This may reflect the lack of direct contact between circulating antibodies and the alveolar basement membrane, either because α3(IV)NC1 is less accessible due to the intrinsic properties of the alveolar basement membrane, or because the unfenestrated (or thinly fenestrated) endothelium that lines the alveolar capillaries constitutes a greater barrier than the fenestrated endothelium in glomeruli (Lerner *et al.* 1967; McPhaul and Dixon 1970; Steblay and Rudofsky 1983), and requires injury by a second insult before it permits the passage of circulating antibodies (Jennings *et al.* 1981; Downie *et al.* 1982; Yamamoto and Wilson 1987).

The latter possibility is consistent with the clear association between cigarette smoking and pulmonary haemorrhage in Goodpasture's disease identified by Donaghy and Rees (1983), and subsequently confirmed by most but not all others. A prompt recurrence of pulmonary haemorrhage has been noted immediately following resumption of smoking in patients in whom the disease was apparently under control (Heale *et al.* 1969; Donaghy and Rees 1983; Daly *et al.* 1996; and Fig. 3 describes a further case). Patients with pulmonary haemorrhage may also give a history of exposure to other inhaled toxins, notably gasoline or other hydrocarbons (D'Apice *et al.* 1978), which may act in a similar manner (Yamamoto and Wilson 1987) (see Chapter 3.12.2). Interestingly, there is no association between smoking and pulmonary haemorrhage in patients with small vessel vasculitis (Wegener's disease or microscopic polyangiitis) (Haworth *et al.* 1985), presumably reflecting different mechanisms of tissue injury. Fluid overload and pulmonary infections have also been shown to provoke lung haemorrhage in Goodpasture disease (Briggs *et al.* 1979; Rees *et al.* 1979; Bailey *et al.* 1981; Simpson *et al.* 1982), and remote or systemic infections can have similar effects (Rees *et al.* 1977; Johnson *et al.* 1978) (see also Fig. 8).

Physical examination can be normal in patients with mild to moderate pulmonary haemorrhage, but the more severely affected are usually tachypnoeic and may be cyanosed. They may expectorate fresh blood and have rather dry-sounding inspiratory crackles on auscultation that are most prominent over the lower lung fields and may be accompanied by areas of bronchial breathing.

Remitting and relapsing lung disease alone may be confused with idiopathic pulmonary haemosiderosis, and isolated pulmonary haemorrhage may be confused with other causes of pulmonary haemorrhage (Morgan and Turner-Warwick 1981; Leatherman *et al.* 1984). The transition to rapidly progressive disease may occur even in patients with a long history, and it can develop over hours rather than days (Briggs *et al.* 1979; Rees *et al.* 1979; Bergrem *et al.* 1980). The factors responsible are only partially understood. It is the rapidity of this deterioration, and the rapidly changing prognosis for renal recovery, that makes prompt diagnosis and therapy of Goodpasture's disease imperative.

The lung lesions resolve almost completely and clinically apparent pulmonary failure does not occur in patients who have survived life-threatening pulmonary haemorrhage. Radiological evidence of fibrosis is exceptional, but patients may have a reduced *K*CO, the diffusion coefficient for carbon monoxide (CO) (Conlon *et al.* 1994).

It is important to distinguish the syndrome of lung haemorrhage and rapidly progressive glomerulonephritis (RPGN) from other causes of renal and pulmonary failure (Table 3).

Radiological changes

Most episodes of pulmonary haemorrhage are associated with changes in the chest radiograph (Bowley *et al.* 1979a,b). Usually the shadows involve the central lung fields, with peripheral and upper-lobe sparing (Fig. 3). The abnormalities are generally symmetrical, but can be markedly asymmetrical. Changes range from ill-defined nodules of size 1–4 mm to confluent consolidation with an air bronchogram, although usually some nodular shadows are still visible at the edge of confluent areas. Shadowing is rarely limited or entirely confined by a fissure, and radiographs that show this or those that demonstrate shadowing at the apex strongly suggest infection, either alone or

Table 3 Other important causes of acute renal and respiratory failure: differential diagnosis of the pulmonary–renal syndrome. The first two causes are common

Pulmonary oedema secondary to hypervolaemia in acute renal failure of any aetiology
Severe cardiac failure with pulmonary oedema
Severe pneumonia (including Legionella pneumonia) with acute tubular necrosis
Infections with pulmonary syndrome and acute interstitial nephritis: hantavirus, leptospirosis, (Legionella)
Paraquat poisoning
Thrombosis of renal vein/inferior vena cava with pulmonary emboli
Antiphospholipid syndrome with pulmonary emboli
Thrombotic microangiopathy (HUS) with acute lung syndrome
Fibrillary glomerulonephritis

Additional sources: Masson (1992); Calls Ginesta (1995); Espinosa (2002).

superimposed on pulmonary haemorrhage. Shadows caused by bleeding are usually start to clear within 48 h, but may last longer when confluent. Residual minor changes are usually gone within 2 weeks. Interpretation may be considerably complicated by the coexistence of infection or fluid overload, especially as both can precipitate haemorrhage.

(a)

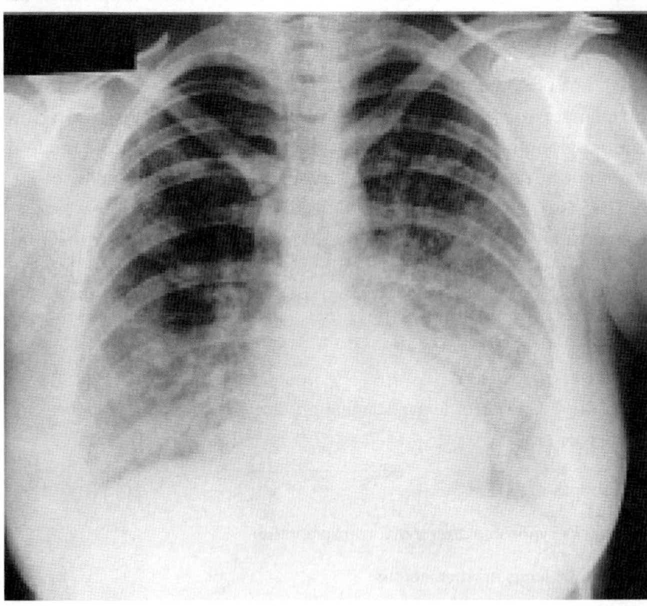

(b)

Fig. 3 Chest radiographs of a 23-year-old woman who presented with pulmonary haemorrhage (a) 1 week before admission and (b) on admission with a 2-week history of breathlessness and three minor episodes of haemoptysis over 3 months, the last 4 days previously. She had a haemoglobin of 5.4 g/dl with indications of iron deficiency. Her renal biopsy is shown in Fig. 6; she had microscopic haematuria, but her serum creatinine was normal at 69 μmol/l. Circulating anti-GBM antibodies were detected by radioimmunoassay, and direct immunofluorescence of the renal biopsy showed linear fixation of IgG and C3 to the GBM. The radiological changes resolved following treatment with cyclophosphamide, prednisolone, and plasma exchange; but 2 weeks later she had a relapse with pulmonary haemorrhage 1 day after resuming smoking.

Diagnosis of pulmonary haemorrhage

The diagnosis of pulmonary haemorrhage presents few problems in the majority of patients, and difficulties only arise in the minority, some with severe disease, in whom haemoptysis is absent. Other indicators include a sudden otherwise unexplained drop in haemoglobin, new shadows on the chest radiograph. Bleeding into the lung also causes an acute increase in the transfer factor corrected for lung volumes and patient's haemoglobin (*K*CO). This is the most specific test for fresh pulmonary haemorrhage (Ewan *et al.* 1976; Bowley *et al.* 1979b). The cause is the additional free haemoglobin within the alveoli that is able to bind inspired CO and so increase values for *K*CO. These results contrast with the usual situation in renal failure in which the *K*CO is about 30 per cent lower than predicted (Lee and Stretton 1975), and for most patients with pulmonary oedema who also show reduced values.

Renal manifestations

One-third to one-half of patients with Goodpasture's disease have no evidence of pulmonary haemorrhage at presentation. Some of these develop clinical or subclinical pulmonary haemorrhage later, but most never do. The renal disease appears to have much less tendency to remit and relapse, although this difference may be largely illusory and associated with the stage of the disease. The renal lesion can improve spontaneously when mild, but rarely does so once significant renal damage has occurred, and deterioration can be extremely rapid (Fig. 4). Patients dying of pulmonary haemorrhage usually have evidence of advanced renal disease, although this may have developed from a mild renal lesion in days or hours. It may simply be that minor tissue injury is more evident in the lungs than in the kidney—for example, bleeding may occlude unaffected alveoli, and haemoptysis is a dramatic symptom, whereas microscopic haematuria is not—or it may be that with the right cofactors the lung can suffer significant immunologically mediated

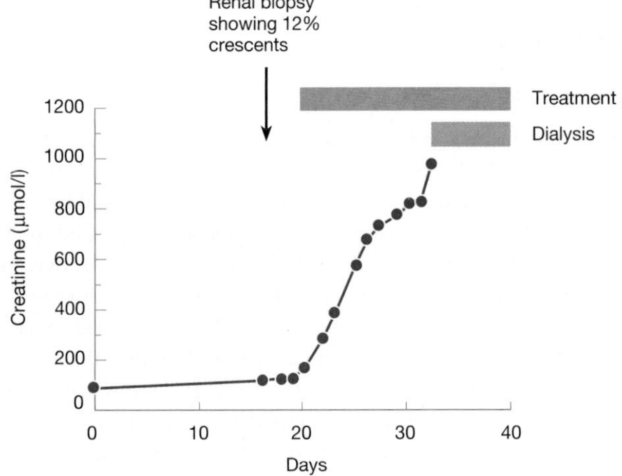

Fig. 4 Very rapid progression of renal injury in one patient in association with infection, despite treatment with cyclophosphamide, prednisolone, and plasma exchange.

damage at an earlier stage in the disease than the kidneys. Occasional patients have a history and findings suggestive of subacutely or chronically progressive renal disease (McPhaul and Mullins 1976).

Abnormalities of the urine sediment, usually microscopic haematuria, are the earliest sign of renal damage. At this stage, before the serum urea or creatinine are abnormal, the changes may remit and relapse without specific treatment. Later, the urine contains numerous dysmorphic red blood cells and red cell casts. Proteinuria is generally modest (<3 g/24 h), but it may occasionally be heavy, particularly in subacute disease.

The clinical manifestations of established renal disease commonly include macroscopic haematuria. There may be loin pain when inflammation is very severe. Hypertension is uncommon at presentation in the absence of hypervolaemia. Oliguria is a late feature and a bad prognostic sign. However, the chance of superimposed acute tubular necrosis in hypoxic and severely ill patients is always high.

Kidney size is usually normal or enlarged due to inflammation. There are no specific morphological or other abnormalities on any type of renal imaging.

Other manifestations possibly related to immunopathology

Anti-GBM antibodies fixed to other basement membranes have been shown in individual cases of Goodpasture's disease, but rarely appear to cause much injury (McPhaul and Dixon 1970; McIntosh *et al.* 1975; Cashman *et al.* 1988). An exception is in the eye. Retinal detachments have been described in at least four cases (Jampol *et al.* 1975; Boucher *et al.* 1997; Sharma 1998) together with antibody fixation to Bruch's membrane and the basement membranes of choroidal vessels (Jampol *et al.* 1975). Other ocular abnormalities have occasionally been reported (Rowe *et al.* 1994). Fixation of antibody to the choroid plexus may also be quite common (S. J. Cashman; see Phelps and Turner 2003), and could be related to the convulsions that occur in some patients. However, convulsions may occur in acute renal failure of any aetiology for a variety of possible reasons, and it is not clear that there is an aetiological relationship.

Diagnosis

Immunological features

The specific diagnosis of Goodpasture's disease rests on the demonstration of anti-GBM antibodies in the circulation or fixed to the kidney. Indirect immunofluorescence using sections of normal kidney is insensitive and difficult and has been replaced by solid phase immunoassays. These can be both highly specific and sensitive, but some assays in current use may give false-positive or -negative results with significant frequency (Litwin 1996; Jaskowski 2002; Salama 2002). This largely depends on the antigen preparation that is used and the samples used to calibrate the assay. If there is any doubt, results should be confirmed by Western blotting (see Fig. 11), or other means, at a centre with special expertise. There have been no reports of high titres of circulating antibodies in the absence of disease attributable to them, and false-negative results are rare. The antibodies have not been found in relatives of patients, in those with other autoimmune disorders, or in normal individuals, although it should be noted that large surveys on this subject have not been published. Direct immunofluorescence on the renal biopsy is the most sensitive technique of all, if adequate renal tissue is obtained and glomerular destruction is not severe; this is the main method of diagnosis in many centres. There may be occasional false-positive results, as linear fluorescence not attributable to Goodpasture's disease has been noted in a number of circumstances (Table 4). Direct immunofluorescence is not useful for following disease activity as linear antibody fixation may be demonstrable for a year or more after diagnosis, after circulating antibodies have become undetectable, and in the absence of clinical disease (Teague *et al.* 1978).

Circulating anti-GBM antibodies are predominantly IgG1 and IgG4 (Segelmark *et al.* 1991), although there are reported and unreported cases in which only IgA antibodies could be detected or were predominant despite quite florid disease (Border *et al.* 1979; Espinoza Melendez 1980; Savage *et al.* 1986; Maes *et al.* 1999; Carreras *et al.* 2002). Fivush (1986) and de Caestecker (1990) also reported minimal or mild disease in the presence of linear IgA depositis. Fervenza (1999) reported moderately severe pulmonary and renal disease in association with a monoclonal IgA-kappa antibody that caused linear fixation to the GBM but did not have affinity for the Goodpasture antigen. This is an exceptional example. The association of IgA anti-GBM disease with bronchial carcinoma in several reports was noted above (see Associated diseases). It seems reasonable to rely on techniques that detect only circulating IgG antibodies for most cases, but to look routinely for IgG, IgA, and IgM, as well as C3, on renal biopsies of all patients with rapidly progressive glomerulonephritis.

Anti-GBM specificity has been estimated to account for less than 1 per cent of circulating IgG (Johansson 1994). There are no consistent changes in the concentration of complement factors or serum immunoglobulins, but plasma exchange will deplete both. Rheumatoid factor, antinuclear antibodies, and cryoglobulins are not usually found.

The association of anti-GBM antibodies with ANCA was discussed under Disease Associations, above. ANCA as well as anti-GBM antibodies should always be sought in patients with either clinical picture. The specificity of the anti-GBM antibodies is usually for the

Table 4 Causes of linear staining on direct immunofluorescence of renal tissue[a]

Goodpasture's disease
Alport's syndrome after renal transplantation
Systemic lupus erythematosus
Diabetes mellitus
Normal autopsy kidneys
Cadaver kidneys after perfusion
Transplant biopsies
Fibrillary nephritis

[a] In most cases, the appearances are of weaker binding than in Goodpasture's disease, but confirmation of specificity can only be achieved by elution studies or by testing serum for antibodies to the Goodpasture antigen (Wilson and Dixon 1974; Querin *et al.* 1986; Alpers *et al.* 1987; Peten *et al.* 1991). Interestingly, although the pathology is quite different, fibrillary nephritis has also been associated with lung haemorrhage (Masson *et al.* 1992; Calls Ginesta 1995).

Goodpasture antigen, although some patients with ANCA, like some with systemic lupus erythematosus, may give non-specifically false-positive results (Short *et al.* 1995).

Now that assays for both anti-GBM antibodies and ANCA are widely available, the diagnosis of idiopathic rapidly progressive glomerulonephritis is much less frequently required. How rarely is a matter of some debate, with the differences probably relating mostly to differences in what is defined as rapidly progressive glomerulonephritis and to differences in assays for ANCA.

Renal features

An adequate renal biopsy is as an essential part of the assessment of patients with this disease, and has prognostic as well as diagnostic importance. The glomeruli are often abnormal even in patients with no clinical evidence of renal involvement (Heptinstall 1983). The earliest and mildest changes consist of segmental mesangial matrix expansion and hypercellularity, progressing to a more generalized, but still focal and segmental, proliferative glomerulonephritis with increased numbers of neutrophils in the glomeruli. Later, glomeruli show a diffuse nephritis with segmental or total necrosis and extensive crescent formation (Fig. 5). Glomerular capillary thrombi may be seen; these, and minor degrees of schistocytosis, may be seen in rapidly progressive glomerulonephritis of any aetiology, and they probably do not justify a separate categorization or imply a close relationship to haemolytic uraemic syndrome or thrombotic thrombocytopaenic purpura (Chapter 10.6.3). Glomerular giant cells have been reported in occasional patients (Sabnis *et al.* 1988). Interstitial inflammation is usually present and may be severe; it has been correlated with the extent of antibody fixation to the basement membrane of the distal convoluted tubules (Andres *et al.* 1978).

Vasculitis of small intrarenal vessels has been described in occasional patients with otherwise typical Goodpasture's disease (Wu *et al.* 1980). ANCA assays were not available at the time of these reports, but this appearance should certainly raise the possibility of systemic vasculitis.

Linear binding of antibody to GBM is found in all patients, however mild the renal disease (e.g. Mathew *et al.* 1975; Saraf *et al.* 1978). Antibody can also usually be seen on the basement membrane of the distal convoluted tubule, but not the proximal tubule, the collecting duct, or other sites in renal tissue (Fig. 6). IgG is almost universally detected, and is accompanied by other immunoglobulins (IgA or IgM) in about a third of cases. Linear C3 is seen in 60–70 per cent, and is bright in about 30 per cent. Occasional reports mention IgM alone, IgA alone, or C3 alone [C3 alone has been associated with typical circulating antibodies (Savage *et al.* 1986)]. There are rare reports of patients with linear IgA alone and circulating antibodies of IgA alone, but typical disease with lung haemorrhage and RPGN; see above.

Additional granular deposits, associated with subepithelial or sometimes intramembranous or subendothelial deposits ultrastructurally, have been noted in some patients (e.g. Rajaraman *et al.* 1984). In one case the granular deposits appeared during resolution (Agodoa *et al.* 1976). Usually, the clinical picture is entirely typical, and there is little reason to suspect pre-existing membranous nephropathy. However, as described earlier, there are clear-cut examples of patients with membranous glomerulonephritis developing Goodpasture's disease. It is not clear whether these two groups are related.

Ultrastructurally, the GBM usually shows a widespread irregular broadening, often with mottled thickening of the lamina rara interna.

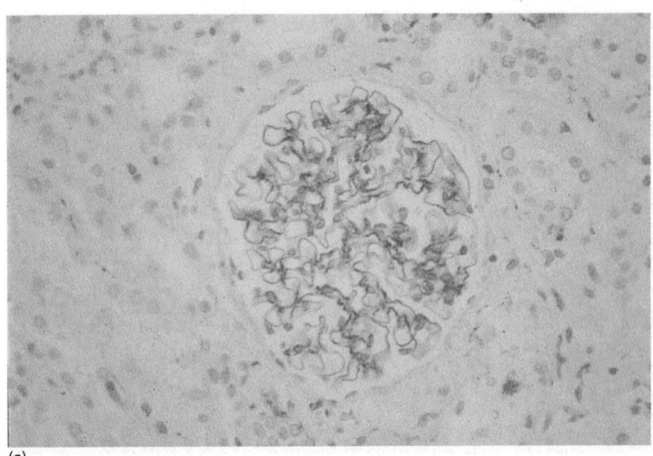
(a)

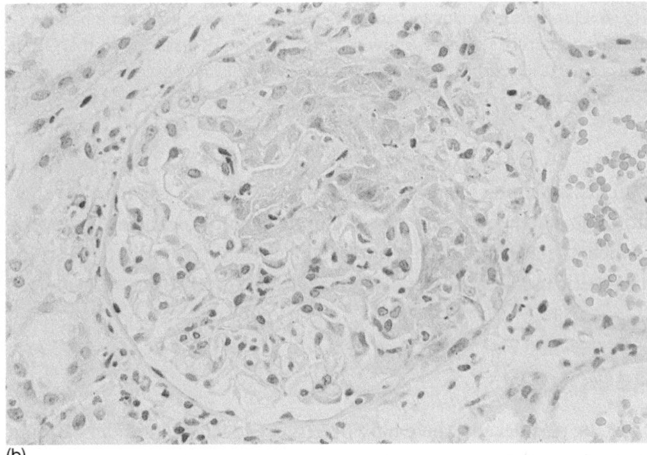
(b)

Fig. 5 (a) A typical glomerulus from the renal biopsy of a patient with very mild renal disease (microscopic haematuria but normal serum creatinine). (b) A glomerulus from a patient with severe renal disease (requiring dialysis at presentation). There is segmental necrosis with extracapillary proliferation. Seventy per cent of the glomeruli showed crescent formation. However, there are still patent capillary loops in this and many other glomeruli, and the crescents are generally cellular. With intensive treatment, renal function improved to a creatinine of 255 at 8 weeks and 168 at 1 year. (By courtesy of Dr Mary Thompson.)

Breaks in the GBM are common. Endothelial and epithelial cells are swollen, and epithelial foot processes may be effaced.

Pulmonary features

At autopsy of patients with pulmonary haemorrhage the lungs are characteristically heavy, showing patchy congestion or haemorrhage. Histologically, intra-alveolar haemorrhage is accompanied by haemosiderin-containing macrophages, deposits of fibrin, and alveolar cell hyperplasia. Electron microscopy shows thickening of the alveolar basement membrane, often with defects (Donald *et al.* 1975). Thickened alveolar walls may show oedema, fibrosis, and modest inflammatory cell infiltration, mainly with polymorphs and lymphocytes.

Immunofluorescence investigations are more difficult in the lung, but linear fixation of immunoglobulin can be detected at autopsy in

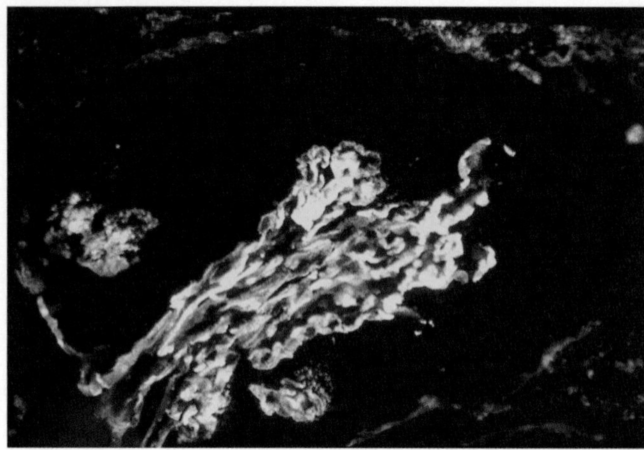

Fig. 6 Direct immunofluorescence for IgG in a glomerulus from a patient with Goodpasture's disease, showing linear fixation of antibody to the GBM. The glomerular tuft has been compressed by a cellular crescent occupying Bowman's space.

patients with lung haemorrhage. However, binding is patchy, so that, although a high success rate in obtaining diagnostic material by transbronchial biopsy has been reported, the technique is too unreliable for diagnostic use (Johnson *et al.* 1985; Nakajima 1999).

Aetiology

Over the past decade, there have been great advances in understanding of how autoimmune disorders arise. Studies in inbred mouse strains have been critical but it is fair to assume that similar mechanisms operate in man, at least in principle. The critical insight has been that loss of tolerance with the consequent development of autoimmune disease requires both an underlying genetic susceptibility and exposure to an environmental trigger. The range of potential triggers is large and their importance relative to inherited susceptibility varies from disease to disease, at least in rodent models. Typically, inheritance predominates in models of generalized autoimmune disease such as systemic lupus, whereas specific triggers are essential in organ specific models such as experimental autoimmune glomerulonephritis (EAG—an analogue of anti-GBM disease), even though not all strains are susceptible (Sado *et al.* 1986). Experimental work has concentrated on two types of trigger: infection with microorganisms that express molecules that induce cross-reactivity immune responses to host proteins—molecular mimicry (reviewed in Wucherpfennig 2001); and presentation of host proteins in the context of stimuli (such as infection or tissue necrosis) that induce strong co-stimulatory responses—the danger hypothesis (Gallucci and Matzinger 2001). EAG for example is induced by immunizing rodents with GBM or its constituents together with adjuvants (Wu *et al.* 2002).

Elucidating the aetiology of autoimmune disease in man is a much more formidable task, but Goodpasture's disease at least provides a model in which pathogenesis has been defined precisely. There is clear evidence of inherited susceptibility from reports of the disease occurring in four sibling pairs (Stanton and Tange 1958; Gossain *et al.* 1972) and two sets of identical twins (D'Apice *et al.* 1978; Simonsen *et al.* 1982). The importance of environmental factors is emphasized by identical twins who are discordant for the disease—two pairs in our series, and others in the literature (Almkuist *et al.* 1981).

Inherited susceptibility

Presently, two genetic regions are known to influence susceptibility to Goodpasture's disease: the HLA complex (reviewed by Phelps *et al.* 2000) and the immunoglobulin heavy chain constant region (Rees *et al.* 1984). In common with other human autoimmune disorders, Goodpasture's disease has been associated with inheritance of specific class II HLA alleles. A strong association with HLA-DR2 specificity (Rees *et al.* 1978) has been confirmed and defined at a molecular level. HLA class II molecules consist of two chains α and β with far greater allelic variability in the β chain. DR specificities are determined exclusively by differences in the β chain, which is encoded by the DRB1 locus. DR2 requires DRB1*15 or DRB1*16 alleles at the B1 locus. DRB1*1501 accounts for over 90 per cent of DR2 specificity in North European caucasoids. Most patients with Goodpasture's disease inherit the B1*1501 allele, and meta-analysis of published series confirms that the primary association is with the DRB1 locus (as opposed to the linked DQ and DP loci) (Phelps *et al.* 2000). It also demonstrates a hierarchy of associations with the DRB1 alleles. These range from a strong positive association with DRB1*1501, through weaker positive associations with DRB1*04 and DRB1*03, to neutral effects and then increasingly strong negative associations with DRB1*01 and DRB1*07. Gene dosage does not affect susceptibility (as reported for DRB1*0401/04 in rheumatoid arthritis); susceptibility is similarly increased in individuals homozygous or heterozygous for the DRB1*1501 allele. By contrast, the susceptibility is abrogated when DR1 or DR7 are inherited together with DR15. Thus, DR1 and 7 alleles confer dominant protection against Goodpasture's disease.

The immunoglobulin heavy chain *Gm* locus which encodes the IgG heavy chain constant region is the second genetic influence on Goodpasture's disease to have been identified (Rees *et al.* 1984a). Association with *Gm* allotypes has been described in various other autoimmune diseases but the reasons for this are undetermined.

Environmental triggers

Clustering of cases in mini-outbreaks; discordance in identical twins; and anecdotal reports of associations with inhaled toxins and infections provide strong evidence for the importance of environmental triggers in Goodpasture's disease. Despite this, no specific triggers have been firmly identified. In part this is because of the difficulty of distinguishing agents that exacerbate previously covert disease from those that initiate it. For example, inhaled cigarette smoke has a non-specific irritant or toxic effect on the lungs and precipitates pulmonary haemorrhage in the presence of circulating anti-GBM antibodies clinically (Donaghy and Rees 1983). In experimental models cigarette smoke and other non-specific irritants (gasoline, oxygen toxicity) act in a similar way (Jennings 1981; Downie *et al.* 1982; Yamamoto and Wilson 1987; Rees unpublished observations). Similarly, intercurrent infection amplifies the intensity of inflammatory responses and can aggravate disease and so make it clinically apparent (Rees *et al.* 1978; Daly *et al.* 1996). Accordingly, it may be impossible to distinguish aggravating effects from true aetiological agents that initiate disease.

Exposure to organic solvents and hydrocarbons has been linked persistently with glomerulonephritis in case reports and case–control studies (Daniell *et al.* 1988; Yaqoob *et al.* 1992). Some of the reports refer specifically to Goodpasture's disease, and one of the pairs of identical twins with Goodpasture's disease makes a particularly compelling case. The twins had not been in direct contact for over 18 months before they each presented shortly after exposure to hydrocarbon fumes (petrol and turpentine fumes, respectively) (D'Apice *et al.* 1978). Other case reports describe anti-GBM nephritis without pulmonary haemorrhage, suggesting that the mechanism might be more than just 'revealing' the disease by precipitating pulmonary haemorrhage (Beirne and Brennan 1972; Kleinknecht *et al.* 1980; Daniell *et al.* 1988). The rarity of Goodpasture's disease makes a prospective study of exposed populations unlikely to succeed, but there is still scope for better case–control studies.

The range of diseases associated with the development of anti-GBM disease were detailed above. Damage to glomerular capillaries is an integral part of the disease process in small vessel vasculitis. Lithotripsy is known to cause intrinsic renal trauma (e.g. Evan *et al.* 1991; Jaeger *et al.* 1995). The sound wave is more tightly focused with modern instruments, but the kidney moves with respiration and it is impossible to avoid causing some tissue damage when fragmenting intrarenal stones. In this case, the timing of the insult is clearly recorded; disease has become apparent after 60–90 days. In diabetes mellitus and membranous nephropathy, the thickened and presumably abnormal GBM contains an increased amount of Goodpasture antigen. Perhaps this alone increases turnover of the antigen and its exposure to the immune system. Explanations for putative associations with other diseases are more speculative.

Pathogenesis

The clearly defined clinical, pathological, and immunological features of Goodpasture's disease have provided the opportunity for a great deal of investigation in attempts to reveal more about the mechanisms underlying human nephritis. Early studies by Scheer and Grossman (1964) identified deposited anti-GBM antibodies in patients with Goodpasture's disease and the ability of these antibodies to transfer disease demonstrated of their pathogenicity (Lerner *et al.* 1967, 1999). Advances since then have shown that the pathogenic antibodies from all patients react with the same component of the GBM and have culminated in the precise delineation of the epitopes they recognize; the identification of HLA alleles that confer susceptibility and resistance to the disease and a basic understanding of why this should be (Phelps *et al.* 1998, 2000); and the characterization of T-cell responses to the Goodpasture antigen. This makes Goodpasture's disease one of the best characterized of all autoimmune diseases.

Glomerular basement membrane and the Goodpasture antigen

Basement membranes are specialized extracellular structures that are usually found at the boundary between cells and connective tissue stroma. The bulk of the components of their matrix is composed of molecules that are common to all basement membranes, while others have a more restricted distribution, presumably related to specific functional roles (Miner 1999). The bulk of the GBM substance is probably synthesized by glomerular epithelial cells. In some other pathologies in which the podocyte is injured by antibodies/immune deposits or metabolic stress (diabetic nephropathy, membranous nephropathy), podocytes may secrete increased amount of normal GBM components, or it is turned over more slowly, to produce a thickened GBM of apparently normal constitution. It is interesting that in these circumstances there may be an increased risk of developing anti-GBM disease (see above).

The target of anti-GBM antibodies in Goodpasture's disease was identified in the late 1980s as a tissue-specific type IV collagen chain, and its precise identity confirmed by cDNA cloning in the early 1990s (Saus *et al.* 1988; Turner *et al.* 1992). It is the 230 amino acid, non-collagenous, carboxy-terminal NC1 domain of the $\alpha3$ chain [$\alpha3$(IV)NC1] (Fig. 7). Type IV collagen molecules are trimeric, and associate into multimolecular networks. The $\alpha3/\alpha4/\alpha5$ network is one of three types of type IV collagen network. It is found only in certain specialized basement membranes, particularly those formed by fusion of epithelial and endothelial cell basement membranes, and/or those involved in gas or fluid exchange or transfer (Table 5). It is remarkable that only this domain is the target of spontaneous autoimmunity, although multiple other tissue-specific molecules can be found in GBM, including the homologous $\alpha4$ chain, which is coexpressed with $\alpha3$(IV).

Two groups have studied *in vitro* cellular behaviour-modifying properties of $\alpha3$(IV)NC1, using either purified protein or peptides synthesized according to its sequence (Fawzi 2000; Maeshima 2002). It has even been labelled 'tumstatin' as a consequence of some of these. It remains to be seen whether these effects have any bearing on the structural and physiological roles of the molecule in its usual location, although it is clear that signalling between matrix and overlying cells is functionally important in most and probably in all tissues.

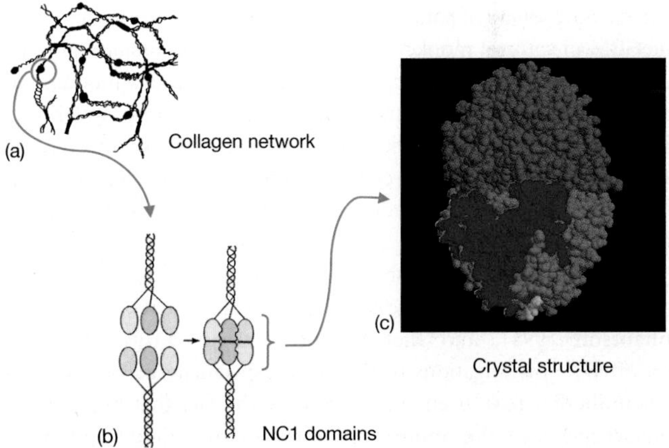

Fig. 7 (a) Cartoon of the network of the type IV collagen network within GBM. (b) An NC1 hexamer, as produced by digestion of GBM with collagenase. (c) The crystal structure of a type IV collagen NC1 domain hexamer. A model of the $\alpha1/\alpha2$ hexamer crystal structure. The NC1 domain of a single type IV collagen chain is shown in blue, with its *N*-terminus (where it joins the collagenous part of the molecule) in light blue. The equivalent location of the major B cell epitope on $\alpha3$(IV)NC1 is shown in red. Modified from Than *et al.* (2002) by Dr R. Phelps. Figure 11 shows the Western blotting pattern of these domains.

Table 5 Distribution of the Goodpasture antigen in human organs by indirect immunofluorescence using serum or antibodies eluted from kidneys of affected patients, Steblay nephritis eluate, monoclonal antibodies or antipeptide antisera (Cashman *et al.* 1988; Kleppel *et al.* 1989; Miner and Sanes 1994; Salama 2001; Wong 2001)

Kidney	GBM, distal TBM, Bowman's capsule
Lung	Alveolar basement membrane
Eye	Bruch's and Descemet's membranes, basement membranes of retinal capillaries, lens capsule, cornea
Ear	Cochlear basement membrane
Brain	Basement membrane of choroidal epithelium
Muscle	Basement membrane at the neuromuscular junction
Thymus	Capillaries and (?) Hassal's corpuscles
Other	Basement membranes of adrenal, breast, pituitary, thyroid

A serine residue at the *N*-terminal region of the $\alpha3$(IV)NC1 domain at the junction with the helical part of the molecule has been shown to be phosphorylated *in vivo* by a specific protein kinase (Revert *et al.* 1995; Raya *et al.* 2000). Intriguingly, this residue is adjacent to an integrin binding 'RGD' (arginine–glycine–aspartate) sequence.

Pathogenicity and epitope of antibodies

Pathogenicity of circulating anti-GBM antibodies in Goodpasture's disease was suggested by their very close association with the disease, and also by the correlation between antibody titre and the severity of renal damage (Simpson *et al.* 1982; Savage *et al.* 1986; Herody *et al.* 1993). Lerner *et al.* (1967, 1999) established the pathogenicity of kidney-fixed antibodies in Goodpasture's disease. They showed that antibody eluted from kidneys of patients with Goodpasture's disease could fix to the GBM of squirrel monkeys *in vivo* and cause pathological glomerular changes. This was expected, as human anti-GBM antibodies are known to be mainly IgG1 and complement fixing, and similar antibodies in animal models exert pathological effects. However, the changes produced in these circumstances by antibodies alone were not of crescentic nephritis, nor would that be expected from observations described below.

Cross-inhibition studies show that the anti-$\alpha3$ antibodies recognize the same epitope or range of epitopes in all patients (Pusey 1987; Johansson 1994), and that the predominant target is always $\alpha3$(IV)NC1. Investigations of the precise specificity of Goodpasture autoantibodies have been complicated by the fact that high-affinity interactions with the antigen are with conformational epitopes—epitopes that depend on the three-dimensional structure rather than the linear sequence of the molecule, possibly involving multiple loops of the protein. The use of peptides and malfolded recombinant antigen made in bacteria has led to a number of contradictory and confusing accounts in the literature. Studies using purified antigens or recombinant antigens made in eukaryotic expression systems have narrowed down the primary epitope to the amino-terminal end of the NC1 domain. Site-directed mutagenesis has identified eight individual residues that seem critical to the epitope at positions 17–31 (Gunnarson *et al.* 2000; Borza *et al.* 2002). In some patients, additional antibodies can be found that bind to other parts of $\alpha3$(IV)NC1, and/or to the NC1 domains of $\alpha4$ or $\alpha5$(IV). These are usually of low titre and subsidiary to major binding to the dominant $\alpha3$(IV) epitope.

Autoantibodies are predominantly directed at a single short region of $\alpha3$(IV)NC1, so it is perhaps not surprising that there is evidence of limited antibody heterogeneity in the immune response, in that some antibody idiotypes are prominently represented (Meyers *et al.* 1998). This may reflect restricted antibody gene usage, but this has not been formally demonstrated. The recent crystallization of $\alpha1$-$\alpha2$ NC1 domain hexamers (Sundaramoorthy *et al.* 2002; Than *et al.* 2002) is likely to provide further impetus to the exploration of these and of other phenomena.

The mechanism by which anti-GBM antibodies cause glomerular injury is discussed further in Chapter 3.2. However it is clear that even in the relatively clear-cut example of nephrotoxic nephritis, outcome is strongly influenced by cell-mediated tissue damage and immunity as well as by direct damage.

T cell responses to the Goodpasture antigen

B cells require T cell help if they are to synthesize antibodies, and tolerance to self-proteins is maintained by regulatory T cells. The $\alpha3$ and $\alpha4$ chains of type IV collagen are both expressed in the thymus, but unlike the $\alpha1$ and $\alpha5$ chains have a highly restricted distribution (Salama 2001; Wong 2001). It is not known what proportion of T cells that recognize the respective α chains are deleted in the thymus, but some are exported to the periphery. Peripheral blood T cells from healthy individuals and from patients with Goodpasture's disease proliferate in response to $\alpha3$(IV)NC1 when incubated with it *in vitro* (Derry *et al.* 1995; Salama *et al.* 2001). Responding T cells from patients and controls have similarly restricted T-cell receptor Vβ gene usage, and common sequences in the TCR regions that interact directly with the peptide bound to MHC class II (complementarity determining region 3—CDR3) (Fisher *et al.* 1994). However, T cells that proliferate in response to $\alpha3$(IV)NC1 are much less abundant in healthy individuals than patients with Goodpasture's disease, and more so in those with active disease than after recovery (Salama 2001). Recent evidence from our laboratory has shown that patients' T cells recognize a different set of epitopes on $\alpha3$(IV)NC1 than T cells from healthy controls (Cairns *et al.* 2003): the nature of the cytokines they secrete and the proportions of anergic and regulatory T cells have yet to be fully determined.

Goodpasture antigen-derived peptides presented to T cells

T cells recognize antigen only when presented in the form of peptides bound to MHC class II molecules on the surface of antigen presenting cells (APCs). Thus, T-cell epitopes are critically dependant on the peptides generated by digestion within the antigen presenting cell ('antigen processing') and the ability of these peptides to bind MHC class II molecules ('antigen presentation'). Knowledge of the precise target of autoimmune attack and the HLA class II molecules involved has provided an exceptional opportunity to examine these processes at a molecular level in man (reviewed in Phelps *et al.* 2000), and in this regard Goodpasture's disease serves as a model human autoimmune disease.

$\alpha3$(IV)NC1-derived peptides have now been characterized that are naturally processed and presented by cells bearing HLA-DR15, the major predisposing MHC molecule. They consist of nested sets centred on core MHC-binding motifs. One set overlaps the major autoantibody epitope (Fig. 7).

Most α3(IV)NC1 derived peptides bound to DR15, DR1, and DR7 molecules with intermediate or high affinity but did so with much higher affinity to DR1 and DR7. Thus, the alleles that confer resistance to Goodpasture's disease bind α3(IV)NC1 derived peptides much more efficiently (Phelps *et al.* 2000).

Helper T cells also have effector functions

Helper T cells also have effector functions by secreting pro- or anti-inflammatory cytokines that influence activation state of macrophages and other inflammatory cells and thus manipulate the relationship between antibody deposition and injury. Studies in experimental autoimmune glomerulonephritis provide direct evidence for such a role, and indeed suggest that crescentic nephritis requires cell-mediated immunity (e.g. Li 1997, 1998; Timoshanko 2002). Despite this, glomerular T cells are rare in Goodpasture's disease, although some are found in the renal cortex (Nolasco *et al.* 1987). Further support for the importance of cell-mediated mechanisms comes from cases in which the fetus has apparently been unaffected by Goodpasture's disease in the mother (Wilson and Dixon 1981; Yankowitz *et al.* 1992; Deubner *et al.* 1995). The predominantly IgG1 anti-GBM antibodies should have been efficiently transported across the placenta, although the accessibility of the antigen in the fetus to circulating antibodies is not known. However, it is well recognized that there can be GBM-fixed antibody, and even significant levels of circulating antibody, with minimal evidence of tissue damage (e.g. Dahlberg *et al.* 1978; Bailey *et al.* 1981), although there could be explanations other those invoking cell-mediated mechanisms. However, at presentation there is a correlation between antibody titre and the severity of renal damage (Simpson *et al.* 1982; Savage *et al.* 1986).

Various downstream events following the initiation of autoimmunity are potential therapeutic targets, and many studies investigating this have been in animal models of anti-GBM disease (see Chapter 3.2).

Resolution of the immune response

An unusual feature of the antibody response in Goodpasture's disease, and one which originally led to hopes for the possible success of a short but intensive course of treatment, is its transient nature. As discussed below, treatment reduces the time to disappearance of the antibody, but even without treatment most patients no longer have detectable circulating antibody after 18–24 months (Wilson and Dixon 1981). The reasons why this autoimmune response is transient, whereas many others are not, is the subject of active investigation. There is emerging evidence that α3(IV)NC1 reactive T cells alter their properties from T helper cells to T regulatory cells during the evolution of the disease (Cairns *et al.* 2003; Salama *et al.* 2003). These could be responsible for terminating the anti-GBM response.

Why is α3(IV)NC1 the target in Goodpasture's disease?

One of the most intriguing questions is why the autoimmune attack on the GBM is always focused on the α3 chain of type IV collagen rather than the other collagen chains with which it forms a macromolecular complex. The unique susceptibility cannot be explained by differential access for circulating anti-GBM antibodies. In animal models of renal disease, injection of antibodies to different GBM components can produce linear staining on direct immunofluorescence and induce pathological effects (Yaar *et al.* 1982; Feintzeig *et al.* 1986; Wick *et al.* 1986). Similarly, antibodies to various GBM components have been described in some human nephritides (Fillit *et al.* 1985; Kefalides *et al.* 1986, 1993; Bygren *et al.* 1989). In the anti-GBM disease that occurs in patients with Alport syndrome after renal transplantation, the target can be the NC1 domain of the α5 chain (see below). However, there is only good evidence that injury mediated by such antibodies is of pathogenic importance in one spontaneous human disease—Goodpasture's disease.

Hypotheses to explain why α3(IV)NC1 is targeted fall into four distinct categories: (a) differences in the distribution of the various type IV collagen chains results in less effective tolerance to α3(IV)NC1 than the other NC1 domains; (b) α3(IV)NC1 possesses additional functional properties that could influence the immune response to it; (c) unique molecular mimicry between α3(IV)NC1 and a microorganism initiates the autoimmune response; and (d) processing of α3(IV)NC1 by antigen presenting cells results in generation of peptides that favour the development of active autoimmunity, rather than tolerance/regulation of the immune response. There is no direct evidence to support any one of these four tolerance-breaking mechanisms, though suggestive or circumstantial evidence supports several of them.

The different distribution of the various type IV collagen chains has already been described. It is notable that the α3 chain has an identical peripheral distribution to the α4 chain, which is not implicated in autoimmunity. The α5 and α6 chains are expressed in the skin, whereas the α3 and α4 chains are not. The skin is an important site for antigen presentation and richly endowed with dendritic cells and individuals develop strong tolerance to antigens expressed there. Importantly, the three type IV collagen chains that predominate in GBM are also to be found in the thymus (Salama 2001; Wong 2001), indicating that the immune system is exposed to all them and not 'immunologically ignorant' of any of these slowly turned over matrix components.

Other influences on tissue injury

A number of investigators have noted the phenomenon first described by Rees *et al.* in 1977, a worsening of clinical condition in association with infection, at a time when the disease seems to be controlled or coming under control (Fig. 8) (Fig. 4 also shows a rapid deterioration in renal function in association with infection). Guillen *et al.* (1995) reported eight exacerbations in association with infection in 11 patients. Comparable phenomena occur in experimental anti-GBM disease, in which activation of inflammatory cells by cytokines is responsible (reviewed in Erwig *et al.* 2001).

Similar effects may occur in other immunologically mediated diseases in which it is impossible to correlate immunopathology with injury. The ability to monitor renal function constantly and to detect lung damage equally readily, and to correlate these with circulating antibody titres, makes Goodpasture's disease exceptionally useful for the study of this phenomenon in humans.

Treatment and outcome

Without treatment, older series show a very poor prognosis for Goodpasture's disease once renal impairment has developed (early series in Table 6); most patients died shortly after diagnosis of

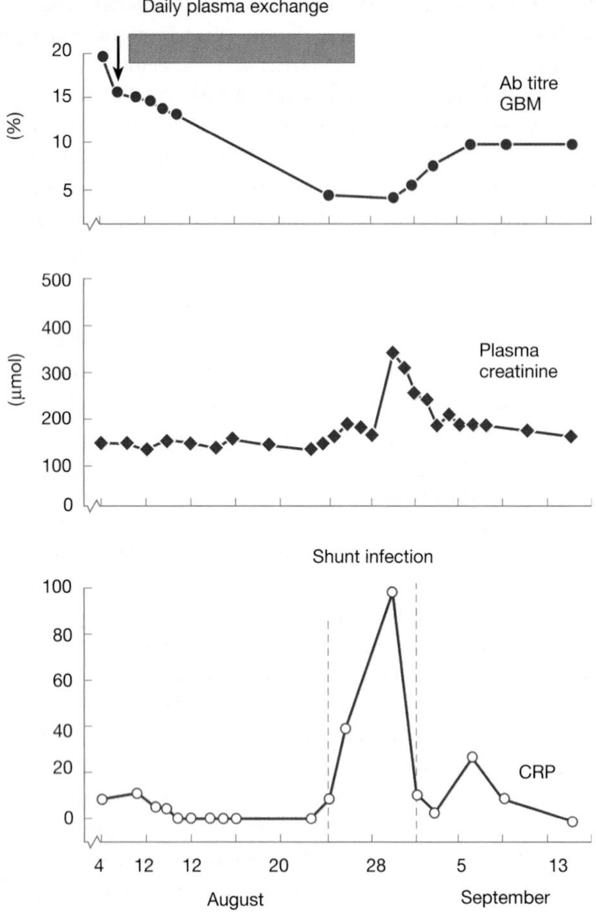

Fig. 8 The effect of intercurrent infection on tissue injury in Goodpasture's disease. Anti-GBM antibody titres (upper panel), creatinine (middle panel), and C-reactive protein (lower panel) in a patient with disease controlled by immunosuppressive agents and plasma exchange, who then developed an infection at the site of an arteriovenous shunt. (Reproduced with permission from Rees *et al.* 1977.)

pulmonary haemorrhage or renal failure. Historically, some authors have ascribed improvement of pulmonary haemorrhage to bilateral nephrectomy or corticosteroid therapy, while others have reported failures of the same treatment. As pulmonary haemorrhage has a tendency to spontaneous remission and relapse, such reports are hard to interpret. Renal function was not improved (Benoit *et al.* 1964). In a later series, retrospective analysis of survivors with preserved renal function suggested that they were more likely to have received corticosteroids than those who had developed endstage renal failure (Wilson and Dixon 1973). Anecdotal reports also suggested that the addition of immunosuppressive agents might confer additional benefit, although numerous failures were also noted (Wilson and Dixon 1973, 1981).

As more effective treatments became available, it became increasingly clear that the severity of disease at presentation was a very powerful influence on outcome, particularly on whether there would be any recovery of renal function. At one extreme, patients with normal serum creatinine values quite frequently show spontaneous resolution of microscopic haematuria (e.g. Schindler *et al.* 1998; Schmidt *et al.* 1999). At the other, those who were oliguric or dialysis-dependent at presentation never regained renal function, and indeed neither did most patients with renal impairment of any severity.

Current treatment regimens

The evidence for the pathogenicity of circulating antibodies in Goodpasture's disease provided the rationale for removal of circulating antibodies as rapidly as possible, whilst simultaneously inhibiting their synthesis. This was behind the introduction of the combination of plasma exchange with more powerful immunosuppressive therapy in the mid-1970s (Lockwood *et al.* 1976) (Table 7). Anecdotally this regimen produced much better results, an experience that was confirmed by others (Johnson *et al.* 1978) (see also the series listed in Table 8).

Most centres now use similar protocols combining cyclophosphamide, moderately high does of prednisolone, and antibody removal by plasma exchange. Pulmonary haemorrhage is usually arrested in 24–48 h, and moderately impaired renal function can be recovered in most patients. The regimen introduced by Lockwood *et al.* (1976) included azathioprine as well as cyclophosphamide, but cyclophosphamide is now generally used alone with equal effect and greater safety. Plasma exchange regimens have differed more substantially, but if removal of antibody is indeed the mode of action, one would expect the more intensive regimens to be most effective. Our current regimen is shown in Table 7; similar regimens have been widely adopted. The improvement in mortality in successive series is illustrated in Table 6; improvements in and greater availability of dialysis, artificial ventilation, and other means of support have undoubtedly also made significant contributions to this. A more detailed comparison of recent series using modern treatment is made in Table 8.

Unfortunately, advanced renal impairment is still not generally salvaged by any current treatment (Fig. 9). It is interesting to contrast these results with those in rapidly progressive glomerulonephritis caused by systemic vasculitis (microscopic polyarteritis or Wegener's disease, for practical purposes), in which oliguric renal failure with a high proportion of crescents is salvageable by similar treatment to that used in Goodpasture's disease (Hind *et al.* 1983; Bolton and Sturgill 1989). It is not clear whether this reflects some subtle and undetermined difference in the damage inflicted by the disease, or whether the results in Goodpasture's disease could be brought up to this level by a future advance in treatment.

Patients with unusual presentations, for example, subacutely with nephrotic syndrome have usually been diagnosed late so it is not surprising that their outcomes have been poor (Andrews *et al.* 1995).

Role of individual elements of treatment

Cytotoxic and immunosuppressive agents

Cyclophosphamide was first used successfully by Couser in 1974, and is probably a key element of therapy. One report describes nonresponse without it (Uezu *et al.* 1999). Early accounts suggested that azathioprine alone did not provide adequate immunosuppression to modify the disease. Alternative immunosuppressive agents have been tried in only a few cases. Cyclosporin use has been described (Querin *et al.* 1992), and seems effective at preventing recurrence after transplantation, but our own experience with this drug has been disappointing (Pepys *et al.* 1982). Mycophenolate mofetil is a better

Table 6 Results of treatment for Goodpasture's disease in larger series since 1964. The first two series included patients with Goodpasture's syndrome of other aetiologies, as the distinction was not then possible

Series	Number of patients	Male/female ratio	Pulmonary haemorrhage (%)	At one year (%)		Remarks
				Mortality (%)	Preserved renal function	
Benoit *et al.* (1964)	52	9.4	100	96	4	43 cases from previous series Mortality figures for 3 years
Proskey *et al.* (1970)	56	3.6	100	77	≤23[a]	51 cases from series 1964–1969
Wilson and Dixon (1973)	53	3.6	60	25	23	Only 11.5% (6 patients) were still off dialysis by the time of analysis
Beirne *et al.* (1977)	26	2.2	54	54	15	3 anti-GBM antibody-negative patients excluded from their data
Teague *et al.* (1978)	29	2.2	100	38	31	This series excluded patients without lung haemorrhage
Briggs *et al.* (1979)	18	8.0	61	17	11	
Peters *et al.* (1982)	41	1.2	56	24	39	
Johnson *et al.* (1985)	17	7.5	94	6	45	
Walker *et al.* (1985)	22	2.1	62	41	45	
Savage *et al.* (1986)	108	1.4	52	21	22	Data from a number of British centres over 10 years
Herody *et al.* (1993)	29	1.6	50	7	45	
Merkel *et al.* (1994)	35	1.7	57	11	40	Results from analysis at 6 months
Daly *et al.* (1996)	40	1.2	67	2.5[b]	20	
Levy *et al.* (2001)	71	1.3	62	21	46	Includes some patients from Savage *et al.* (1986)

[a] Maximum; figures not given.

[b] Minimum; figures not clear.

Table 7 Protocol for treatment of acute Goodpasture's disease (adapted from Lockwood *et al.* 1976)

Prednisolone 1 mg/kg/24 h orally
Cyclophosphamide 3 mg/kg/24 h orally, rounded down to the nearest 50 mg
Daily exchange of 4 l of plasma for 5% human albumin for 14 days or until the circulating antibody is suppressed. In the presence of pulmonary haemorrhage, or within 48 h of an invasive procedure, 300–400 mls of fresh frozen plasma are given at the end of each treatment, or other fractions/factors given according to tests of coagulation.

agent to use in theory. There is a report of its successful use in a patient unable to tolerate cyclophosphamide (Garcia-Canton *et al.* 2000).

Corticosteroids

Prednisolone is probably also a key element of treatment, so the use of bolus doses of methylprednisolone (10 mg/kg intravenously once daily for 1–3 days) has been advocated when there is severe pulmonary haemorrhage or very rapidly declining renal function (Johnson *et al.* 1985). Although this is simpler and cheaper than plasma exchange, it is poorly supported by the available evidence and has not been adequately compared with the rational and proven approach of antibody removal by plasma exchange. Failure of pulmonary haemorrhage to respond to such therapy has been described in several patients (e.g. Williams *et al.* 1988; Uezu *et al.* 1999) and other instances are known. Pulse corticosteroids increase the risk of later infection, a major concern because as well as threatening survival directly, it may exacerbate renal and pulmonary injury, as discussed above. For these reasons, we do not recommend the use of high-dose intravenous corticosteroid pulses.

Antibody removal

Plasma exchange hastens the disappearance of circulating antibody when used in combination with immunosuppressive agents (Johnson *et al.* 1985; Savage *et al.* 1986). There is a strong clinical impression of its efficacy, but proving that it is an essential component in the treatment of severe Goodpasture's disease has been more difficult.

Table 8 Results of treatment in recent series using immunosuppression and plasma exchange. Untreated patients have been excluded. Treated patients are divided into two groups according to their creatinine at the time treatment commenced, or at presentation if this is not available (number in each group in parentheses). The percentage of patients who were alive and not requiring dialysis at 1 year is shown

Series	Percentage with independent renal function at 1 year according to initial creatinine level		Notes on treatment given
	≤600	**>600**	
Briggs *et al.* (1979) (*n* = 15)	36 (11)	0 (4)	Only 4/15 received plasma exchange
Simpson *et al.* (1982) (*n* = 12)	70 (10)	0 (2)	8/12 received plasma exchange
Johnson *et al.* (1985) (*n* = 17)	69 (13)	0 (4)	Less cyclophosphamide than Table 7 Half received plasma exchange, but only every third day, and using frozen plasma
Walker *et al.* (1985) (*n* = 22)	82 (11)	18 (11)	Slightly less cyclophosphamide and plasma exchange than Table 7
Bouget (1990) (*n* = 12)	80 (5)	14 (7)	
Herody *et al.* (1993) (*n* = 22)	93 (14)	0 (15)	Variable amounts of plasma exchange and different immunosuppressive regimens were used
Andrews (1995) (*n* = 15)		7 (15)	Series restricted to those with creatinine > 500
Levy (2001) (*n* = 71)	95 (19)	15 (52)	As Table 7, except some also received azathioprine 1 mg/kg/day

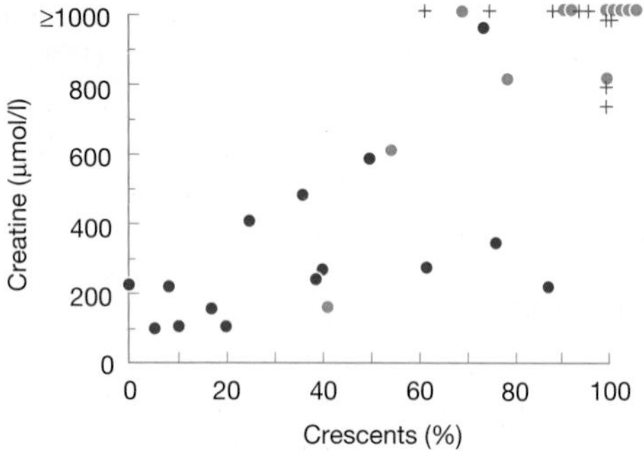

Fig. 9 Plasma creatinine concentration at presentation, and the proportion of glomeruli with crescents, in 38 patients treated at Hammersmith Hospital, London. Those who did not receive the combination of plasma exchange, cyclophosphamide, and prednisolone, or who had less than 10 glomeruli in their renal biopsies, have been excluded. The following are illustrated: (1) the correlation between the creatinine at presentation and histological evidence of glomerular damage, except in one patient with acute tubular necrosis; (2) the close relationship between the severity of renal damage at presentation and outcome; (3) death from pulmonary haemorrhage occurs predominantly in those with severe renal disease.

When used without other agents in Goodpasture's disease it has only a transient effect on antibody titres (Proskey *et al.* 1970; Guillen 1995), and there is no case for using plasma exchange alone.

The role of plasma exchange was examined in the only controlled trial of treatments in Goodpasture's disease (Johnson *et al.* 1985). The group receiving plasma exchange achieved a better outcome than those receiving immunosuppressive agents and prednisolone alone, although the plasma exchange regimen was less intensive and cyclophosphamide doses were lower than in many other centres. However, the authors were justifiably cautious about accepting that plasma exchange had been responsible for the improved outcome, as the group receiving it appeared to have a lesser degree of renal damage when crescent scores were compared. The results did show that patients with mild renal disease (<30 per cent crescents and creatinine < 300 μmol/l) did well on cyclophosphamide and prednisolone whether or not they received plasma exchange, and confirmed that those with severe renal disease (>70 per cent crescents and creatinine > 600 μmol/l) generally fared badly (Fig. 9).

Using immunoadsorption against staphylococcal protein A to adsorb circulating IgG antibodies (Bygren *et al.* 1985; Laczika *et al.* 2000) lowers antibody titres more rapidly than plasma exchange and has a number of theoretical advantages (complement and clotting factors are not depleted; expensive and potentially dangerous replacement colloid solutions are not required). However, it is a more time-consuming and complicated technique, and is not widely available.

The best approach is to use intensive plasma exchange (or immunoadsorption with protein A) in all patients with significant renal impairment that is thought to be retrievable, and in all patients with continuing or recurrent pulmonary haemorrhage. It should be continued until the antibody titre has reached background values, and reintroduced if there is a later increase in creatinine, or recurrence of pulmonary haemorrhage, in association with an elevated antibody titre.

Deciding not to treat

The renal prognosis of patients with severe nephritis on biopsy, severely impaired renal function, or oliguria at presentation is extremely poor. It has been suggested that, in the absence of pulmonary haemorrhage, they should not be given potentially dangerous treatment (Flores *et al.* 1986). However, there are occasional reports of patients who have recovered despite acute renal failure requiring dialysis (Cohen *et al.* 1976; Johnson *et al.* 1978; Walker *et al.* 1985; Maxwell *et al.* 1988; Schindler *et al.* 1998; Laczika *et al.* 2000), and we have treated similar cases, including one who remained on dialysis for 3 months before recovery to a creatinine of under 200 μmol/l. Their hallmark is that they have particularly short histories, rapid renal deterioration, and either surprisingly mild or very recent changes on renal biopsy, with cellular crescents without evidence of fibrosis and patent capillary loops. Some have relatively mild glomerular changes with superimposed acute tubular necrosis. Although uncommon, these patients emphasize the value of an urgent renal biopsy even where the diagnosis has been established serologically.

Some studies report that patients with ANCA in addition to anti-GBM antibodes may have recoverable renal function in severe acute disease, despite oliguria and dialysis dependence.

General and supportive therapy

Evidence from experimental models suggests that oxygen toxicity increases the probability of pulmonary haemorrhage. This makes it prudent to use the minimal acceptable inspired oxygen concentration perhaps particularly for severe lung haemorrhage. Avoidance of fluid overload is important in Goodpasture's disease for the same reason.

Infection is the most important avoidable cause of death. Risks can be minimized by careful monitoring of white blood cell count, avoiding unnecessary intravenous lines and taking care with essential ones, and by avoiding pulse corticosteroid therapy.

Duration and monitoring of treatment

Fortunately, there are relatively simple ways of monitoring the consequences of the disease on both of its major target organs. Serum creatinine is the most useful guide to renal function, as urea will increase considerably with high-dose steroid therapy. Serum creatinine may continue to increase in the first few days of treatment, but usually stabilizes or begins to decline within a week if useful renal function is to be recovered. Haemoptysis, chest radiograph changes, changes in *K*CO, and acute decreases in haemoglobin are guides to the occurrence of pulmonary haemorrhage. Of these, *K*CO is the most sensitive and earliest. A reduction in the titre of anti-GBM antibodies is taken to be an indication of effective therapy, but it does not preclude continuing or worsening disease.

Repeated measurement of the blood count is important both for the detection of haemorrhage (gastrointestinal as well as lung) and to ensure that the cytotoxic agents used are not causing leucopenia. Dose adjustments may be required to allow recovery. The most common time for leucopenia to occur is after 2–3 weeks with daily oral cyclophosphamide, and it is rarely seen before 10 days.

If the disease is coming under control according to these criteria, we generally reduce prednisolone weekly, aiming to stop all treatment at about 3 months in the absence of relapses or resurgences in antibody production.

Relapse and recurrence

Relapses are not uncommon and should be distinguished from recurrent disease, which is rare. Relapse means a worsening of signs or symptoms of the disease before the disease and antibody titre has been totally suppressed. Severity of renal and pulmonary injury may increase early in the course of the disease, either because of inadequate therapy with a rising antibody titre, or because other factors such as infection or fluid overload increase the pathogenicity of low circulating levels of autoantibodies or cell-mediated mechanisms of tissue injury. It is important to identify the reason for the relapse and treat that, while continuing treatment to abrogate the immune response wherever possible. However, it is better to prevent such episodes. Intravascular catheters are now the most common source of significant infection, and attention to them must be rigorous.

Recurrences of pulmonary haemorrhage over many years are well described in the literature; the episodes are usually accompanied by minimal renal disease and resolve spontaneously (e.g. Dahlberg *et al.* 1978; Mehler *et al.* 1987; Klasa *et al.* 1988), but severe renal disease may occur eventually (Levy *et al.* 1996). Recurrent renal disease is exceptional. Recurrence of autoantibody production may occur without signs of tissue damage (Hind *et al.* 1984). Renal transplantation is the best characterized precipitant of recurrence, but many individual case histories are suggestive of infection or exposure to toxic agents at the onset of the illness or of an episode in it. Recurrence needs to be distinguished from the non-immunological decline in renal function that may occur over months and years following an acute glomerular injury (see Chapter 11.1).

Treatment of recurrences is identical to that of initial disease, but probably has a better chance of success as the patients and their physicians make the correct diagnosis more quickly.

Goodpasture's disease in children

A literature review of reports of children with pulmonary–renal syndrome found 13 of 52 cases to have been caused by Goodpasture's disease (von Vigier *et al.* 2000). The major causes of the syndrome in children were Wegener's disease, Goodpasture's disease, SLE, Henoch–Schönlein purpura, and haemolytic–uraemic syndrome.

Anti-GBM disease accounted for two of 30 patients with crescentic nephritis seen over 13 years in a study in London (Jardim *et al.* 1992), and for one of 43 cases seen over 22 years in New Delhi, India (Srivastava *et al.* 1992). While several series of patients with Goodpasture's disease include children, these are not usually described separately; they amount to at least six patients aged less than 15 years. Isolated reports of the disease in children more than double this total. In children the disease seems similar in most respects to that in adults, though some seem to have had other autoimmune phenomena as well. Lung haemorrhage is understandably rare. Diagnosis is often too late to salvage renal function, but there is an impression from the small numbers that children may be more likely to recover from oligoanuria than adults.

Goodpasture's disease after renal transplantation (see also Chapter 13.3.4)

Patients with previous Goodpasture's disease

Patients with previous Goodpasture's disease have been shown to be suitable for transplantation, although cases of recurrence of the disease with graft loss have been noted, particularly where circulating antibodies are present at the time of transplantation (Lerner *et al.* 1967; Beleil *et al.* 1973; Wilson and Dixon 1973; Briggs *et al.* 1979; Simpson *et al.* 1982). Immunosuppressive therapy (and transplant success rates) were substantially less effective in the era of most of these reports, and the incidence of recurrent disease has recently been estimated at about 1 in 40 (2.5 per cent) (Netzer *et al.* 1998). Pulmonary haemorrhage seems to be rare in these circumstances. Recommendations for avoiding recurrence of disease have ranged from simply monitoring the disappearance of circulating antibodies to bilateral nephrectomy. Neither of these precautions is adequate protection, but there is certainly now no immunological reason for performing a nephrectomy. A patient is described (Almkuist *et al.* 1981) who had no detectable circulating antibody for 18 months and a bilateral nephrectomy before receiving the kidney of her identical twin 2 years after her original illness. No immunosuppression was given after the transplant. She developed microscopic haematuria at 2 weeks, and at 6 months circulating antibodies were detectable again and she had crescentic nephritis. Renal function was not seriously impaired, however, and the abnormalities resolved after treatment with azathioprine and corticosteroids. Rarely, Goodpasture's disease has recurred more than a year after transplantation. Trpkov (1998) reported an example in a patient treated with cyclosporin and prednisolone. Another patient (Fonck *et al.* 1998), who was transplanted two years after acute Goodpasture's disease, suffered a recurrence which destroyed the graft after a further 5 years when immunosuppression was discontinued. It is possible that acute allograft rejection may have been the precipitant.

Renal transplantation should be postponed until at least 6 months after the disappearance of circulating antibodies by immunoassay. In patients with persisting antibodies in whom early transplantation is desirable, similar treatment to that used at presentation (Table 7) can be given in preparation for transplantation. With modern immunosuppression and after taking these precautions clinical recurrence should be rare, although linear fixation of IgG to the GBM can occur without overt disease (Couser *et al.* 1973; Wilson and Dixon 1973). In any case, renal function and urine sediment should be closely monitored in all such patients, and anti-GBM titres should be obtained at intervals.

Patients with hereditary nephritis (see Chapters 13.3.4, 16.4.1, and 16.4.3)

When studied by indirect immunofluorescence, the Goodpasture antigen is absent or greatly diminished in most patients with strictly defined hereditary nephritis of the Alport type (Chapter 16.4.1). Transplant of a normal kidney may allow the development of anti-GBM antibodies to foreign antigen(s) (alloantigens) in the donor kidney. Linear IgG fixation to the GBM probably occurs quite commonly, circulating anti-GBM antibodies may develop, and a small proportion of patients have developed crescentic nephritis. Lung haemorrhage does not usually occur. The histological appearances in the kidney and clinical progression are indistinguishable from those of spontaneous Goodpasture's disease (Fig. 10). Many examples of the phenomenon have now been described, and the graft has been lost in the majority (summarized in Brainwood *et al.* 1998).

The molecular defect in Alport's syndrome is now known to be a mutation in a gene encoding one of the tissue-specific type IV collagen chains. The disease is usually X-linked, associated with mutations in the COL4A5 gene encoding the $\alpha5$ chain. Autosomal recessive cases have been shown to be due to mutations on the $\alpha3$ or $\alpha4$ chain genes

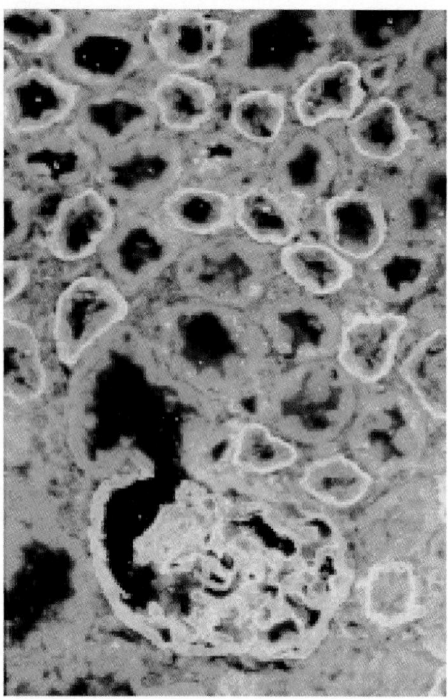

(a)

(b)

Fig. 10 Indirect immunofluorescence of frozen sections of normal kidney (a) and normal skin (b) overlaid with IgG from a patient with Alport's syndrome and post-transplant anti-GBM disease. In the kidney the pattern is almost identical to that obtained with Goodpasture autoantibodies, with binding to GBM and to basement membranes of distal tubules and Bowman's capsule. In the skin, the epidermal basement membrane, which contains $\alpha5$ chains of type IV collagen, is strongly highlighted. Antibodies from patients with Goodpasture's disease do not bind to epidermal basement membrane. This pattern in skin can only clearly be seen around skin appendages or after denaturation of tissue sections with acid and urea. The sections have been counterstained with Evans blue. (By courtesy of Dr Richard Herriot.)

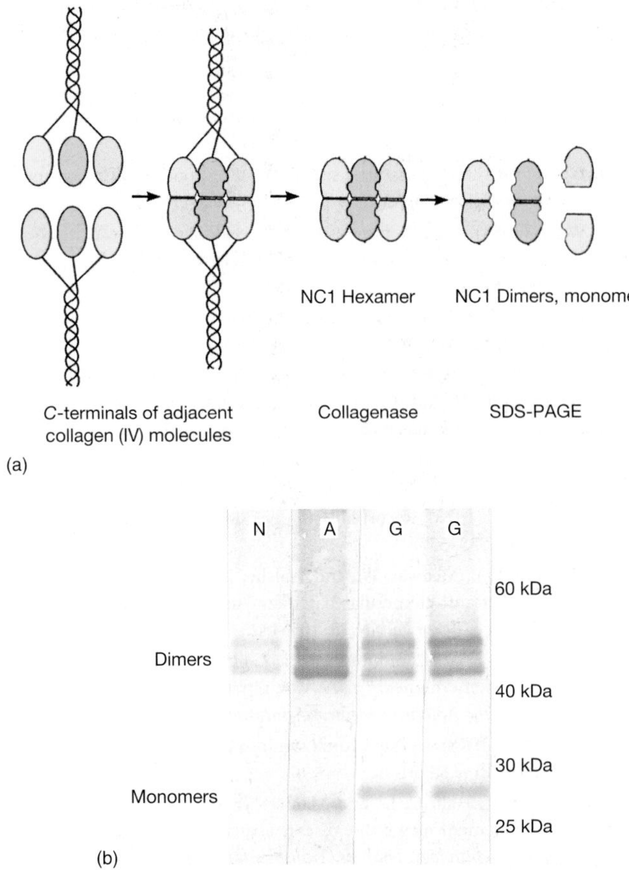

Fig. 11 (a) Western blotting of tissue-specific type IV collagen NC1 domains. Collagenase-solubilised basement membrane from bovine testis has been separated by SDS–PAGE (compare Fig. 7) in non-reducing conditions and transferred to nitrocellulose. (b) Goodpasture sera (lanes marked 'G') recognize monomers of α3(IV)NC1 domains of approximately 28 kDa and a cluster of dimers. Some Alport post-transplant anti-GBM sera (e.g. the lane marked 'A') contain antibodies to α5(IV)NC1, which can be seen as a monomer of approximately 26 kDa. Normal sera ('N') show no monomer recognition but weak staining of dimer regions after prolonged incubation.

on chromosome 2. Presumably mutations in one chain may destabilize a supramolecular network involving all three, producing the degenerative disorder of certain specialized basement membranes that we recognize as Alport's syndrome.

It is now clear that when the α3 chain is absent, so are the α4 and α5 chains (see Chapter 16.4.1). Therefore, in theory any of these chains might be the target of anti-GBM disease after renal transplantation. However, anti-GBM disease develops only rarely; most patients with Alport's syndrome have an entirely routine post-transplant course, although linear antibody fixation may be seen in the absence of nephritis (Querin *et al.* 1986; Peten *et al.* 1991; Byrne *et al.* 2002). Patients with a substantial gene deletion are more likely to develop this complication, perhaps because the antigen in the allograft is then truly foreign to the recipient's immune system (Ding *et al.* 1994). Other genetic factors may also be important, as may the immunosuppression given to prevent rejection of the allograft. Detailed studies show that the target of anti-GBM antibodies in these circumstances is most likely to be the NC1 domain of the α5 chain if the genetic abnormality is in the gene (COL4A5) encoding it (Brainwood *et al.* 1998), that is, different from the classic Goodpasture antigen. In patients with autosomal disease the target may be α3(IV)NC1, the Goodpasture antigen. These differences can be important, as immunoassays developed to identify the anti-α3 chain antibodies that typify Goodpasture's disease may not identify anti-α5 chain antibodies. Therefore it is important to maintain a high index of suspicion, and if there is evidence of glomerular disease to look for linear binding of IgG to the GBM. Reliable techniques for distinguishing anti-α3 from α5 antibodies are not routine, though anti-α5 antibodies are more likely to bind strongly to Bowman's capsule. Sera from patients where the diagnosis is possible are best screened by Western blotting with collagenase-solubilized GBM and/or recombinant proteins (Fig. 11). Once the target has been identified, it should be possible to determine whether a routine anti-GBM antibody assay is adequate for monitoring treatment, and whether antibodies are still present after loss of the graft. If they are, this should preclude a further attempt at transplantation. Treatment is as for spontaneous Goodpasture's disease, and although it has not been successful in most reported cases, success or partial success has been achieved in some. Diagnosis and treatment have often been late, and it is possible that only the most severe examples have been recognized.

Some cases of *de novo* anti-GBM nephritis after transplantation may occur in patients who have this type of hereditary nephritis but who lack a clear family history of renal disease, deafness, or eye changes. If earlier biopsies of native kidneys are available, it is worth re-examining them by immunohistochemical techniques for evidence of the Goodpasture antigen, or examining the patient's skin for evidence of α5(IV) collagen expression (Chapter 16.4.1).

References

Agodoa, L. C. *et al.* (1976). The appearance of nonlinear deposits of immunoglobulins in Goodpasture's syndrome. *American Journal of Medicine* **61**, 407–413.

Ahuja, T. S. *et al.* (1998). Diabetic nephropathy with anti-GBM nephritis. *American Journal of Kidney Diseases* **31**, 127–130.

Almkuist, R. D. *et al.* (1981). Recurrence of anti-glomerular basement membrane antibody mediated glomerulonephritis in an isograft. *Clinical Immunology and Immunopathology* **18**, 54–60.

Alpers, C. E., Rennke, H. G., Hopper, J., and Biava, C. G. (1987). Fibrillary glomerulonephritis: an entity with unusual immunofluorescence features. *Kidney Internationa*l **31**, 781–789.

Andrassy, K., Kuster, S., Waldherr, R., and Ritz, E. (1991). Rapidly progressive nephritis: analysis of prevalence and clinical course. *Nephron* **59**, 206–212.

Andres, G. *et al.* (1978). Histology of human tubulo-interstitial nephritis associated with antibodies to renal basement membranes. *Kidney International* **13**, 480–491.

Andrews, P. A. *et al.* (1995). Unusual presentations of anti-glomerular basement membrane antibody mediated disease are associated with delayed diagnosis and poor outcome. *Clinical Nephrology* **44**, 262–265.

Bailey, R. R. *et al.* (1981). Goodpasture's syndrome with normal renal function. *Clinical Nephrology* **15**, 211–215.

Beirne, G. J. and Brennan, J. T. (1972). Glomerulonephritis associated with hydrocarbon solvents: mediated by antiglomerular basement membrane antibody. *Archives of Environmental Health* **25**, 365–369.

Beleil, O. M., Coburn, J. W., Shinaberger, J. H., and Glassock, R. J. (1973). Recurrent glomerulonephritis due to anti-glomerular basement membrane-antibodies in two successive allografts. *Clinical Nephrology* **1**, 377–380.

Benoit, F. L. *et al.* (1964). Goodpasture's syndrome. A clinicopathological entity. *American Journal of Medicine* **37**, 424–444.

Bergrem, H. *et al.* (1980). Goodpasture's syndrome. A report of seven patients including long-term follow-up of three who received a kidney transplant. *American Journal of Medicine* **68**, 54–58.

Bindi, P. *et al.* (1997). Antiglomerular basement membrane glomerulonephritis following D-penicillamine-associated nephrotic syndrome. *Nephrology, Dialysis, Transplantation* **12**, 325–357.

Blake, D. R., Rashid, H., McHugh, M., and Morley, A. R. (1980). A possible association of partial lipodystrophy with anti-GBM nephritis (Goodpasture's syndrome). *Postgraduate Medical Journal* **56**, 137–139.

Bolton, W. K. and Sturgill, B. C. (1989). Methylprednisolone therapy for acute crescentic rapidly progressive glomerulonephritis. *American Journal of Nephrology* **9**, 368–375.

Border, W. A., Baehler, R. W., Bhathena, D., and Glassock, R. J. (1979). IgA antibasement membrane nephritis with pulmonary hemorrhage. *Annals of Internal Medicine* **91**, 21–25.

Borza, D. B. *et al.* (2002). Quaternary organization of the goodpasture autoantigen, the α3(IV) collagen chain. Sequestration of two cryptic autoepitopes by intrapromoter interactions with the α4 and α5 NC1 domains. *Journal of Biological Chemistry* **277**, 40075–40083.

Bosch, X. *et al.* (1991). Prognostic implication of anti-neutrophil cytoplasmic autoantibodies with myeloperoxidase specificity in anti-glomerular basement membrane disease. *Clinical Nephrology* **36**, 107–113.

Boucher, A., Droz, D., Adafer, E., and Noel, L. H. (1987). Relationship between the integrity of Bowman's capsule and the composition of cellular crescents in human crescentic glomerulonephritis. *Laboratory Investigation* **56**, 526–533.

Bowley, N. B., Hughes, J. M., and Steiner, R. E. (1979a). The chest X-ray in pulmonary capillary haemorrhage: correlation with carbon monoxide uptake. *Clinical Radiology* **30**, 413–417.

Bowley, N. B., Steiner, R. E., and Chin, W. S. (1979b). The chest X-ray in antiglomerular basement membrane antibody disease (Goodpasture's syndrome). *Clinical Radiology* **30**, 419–429.

Brainwood, D., Kashtan, C., Gubler, M. C., and Turner, A. N. (1998). Targets of alloantibodies in Alport anti-glomerular basement membrane disease after renal transplantation. *Kidney International* **53**, 762–766.

Briggs, W. A. *et al.* (1979). Antiglomerular basement membrane antibody-mediated glomerulonephritis and Goodpasture's syndrome. *Medicine (Baltimore)* **58**, 348–361.

Bygren, P., Cederholm, B., Heinegard, D., and Wieslander, J. (1989). Non-Goodpasture anti-GBM antibodies in patients with glomerulonephritis. *Nephrology, Dialysis, Transplantation* **4**, 254–261.

Bygren, P. *et al.* (1985). Goodpasture's syndrome treated with staphylococcal protein A immunoadsorption. *Lancet* **ii**, 1295–1296.

Byrne, M. C. *et al.* (2002). Renal transplant in patients with Alport's syndrome. *American Journal of Kidney Diseases* **39**, 769–775.

Cairns, L. S. *et al.* (2003). The fine specificity and cytokine profile of T-helper cells responsive to the alpha3 chain of type IV collagen in Goodpasture's disease. *Journal of the American Society of Nephrology* **14**, 2801–2812.

Calls Ginesta, J. *et al.* (1995). Fibrillary glomerulonephritis and pulmonary hemorrhage in a patient with renal transplantation. *Clinical Nephrology* **43**, 180–183.

Carreras, L. *et al.* (2002). Goodpasture syndrome during the course of a Schönlein–Henoch purpura. *American Journal of Kidney Diseases* **39**, 1–4.

Cashman, S. J., Pusey, C. D., and Evans, D. J. (1988). Extraglomerular distribution of immunoreactive Goodpasture antigen. *Journal of Pathology* **155**, 61–70.

Clutterbuck, E. J. and Pusey, C. D. (1987). Severe alveolar haemorrhage in Churg–Strauss syndrome. *European Journal of Respiratory Disease* **71**, 158–163.

Cohen, L. H., Wilson, C. B., and Freeman, R. M. (1976). Goodpasture syndrome: recovery after severe renal insufficiency. *Archives of Internal Medicine* **136**, 835–837.

Conlon, P. J. *et al.* (1994). Antiglomerular basement membrane disease: the long-term pulmonary outcome. *American Journal of Kidney Diseases* **23**, 794–796.

Couser, W. G. (1974). Goodpasture's syndrome: a response to nitrogen mustard. *American Journal of Medical Science* **268**, 175–179.

Couser, W. G. (1988). Rapidly progressive glomerulonephritis: classification, pathogenetic mechanisms, and therapy. *American Journal of Kidney Diseases* **11**, 449–464.

Couser, W. G., Wallace, A., Monaco, A. P., and Lewis, E. J. (1973). Successful renal transplantation in patients with circulating antibody to glomerular basement membrane: report of two cases. *Clinical Nephrology* **1**, 381–383.

Curioni, S. *et al.* (2002). Anti-GBM nephritis complicating diabetic nephropathy. *Journal of Nephrology* **15**, 83–87.

Curtis, J. J. *et al.* (1976). Goodpasture's syndrome in a patient with the nail-patella syndrome. *American Journal of Medicine* **61**, 401–416.

Dahlberg, P. J. *et al.* (1978). Recurrent Goodpasture's syndrome. *Mayo Clinic Proceedings* **53**, 533–537.

Daly, C., Conlon, P. J., Medwar, W., and Walshe, J. J. (1996). Characteristics and outcome of anti-glomerular basement membrane disease: a single-center experience. *Renal Failure* **18**, 105–112.

Daniell, W. E., Couser, W. G., and Rosenstock, L. (1988). Occupational solvent exposure and glomerulonephritis. A case report and review of the literature. *Journal of the American Medical Association* **259**, 2280–2283.

D'Apice, A. J. *et al.* (1978). Goodpasture's syndrome in identical twins. *Annals of Internal Medicine* **88**, 61–62.

de Caestecker, M. P., Hall, C. L., and MacIver, A. G. (1990). Atypical anti-glomerular basement membrane disease associated with thin membrane nephropathy. *Nephrology, Dialysis, Transplantation* **5**, 909–913.

Derry, C. J. *et al.* (1995). Analysis of T cell responses to the autoantigen in Goodpasture's disease. *Clinical and Experimental Immunology* **100**, 262–268.

Deubner, H., Wagnild, J. P., Wener, M. H., and Alpers, C. E. (1995). Glomerulonephritis with antiglomerular basement membrane antibody during pregnancy potential role of the placenta in amelioration of disease. *American Journal of Kidney Diseases* **25**, 330–335.

Ding, J., Zhou, J., Tryggvason, K., and Kashtan, C. E. (1994). *COL4A5* deletions in three patients with Alport syndrome and posttransplant antiglomerular basement membrane nephritis. *Journal of the American Society of Nephrology* **5**, 161–168.

Disney, A. P. S. (1986). Tenth report of the Australian and New Zealand combined dialysis and transplant registry (ANZ-DATA). Queen Elizabeth Hospital, Adelaide, Australia.

Donaghy, M. and Rees, A. J. (1983). Cigarette smoking and lung haemorrhage in glomerulonephritis caused by autoantibodies to glomerular basement membrane. *Lancet* **ii**, 1390–1393.

Donald, K. J., Edwards, R. L., and McEvoy, J. D. (1975). Alveolar capillary basement membrane lesions in Goodpasture's syndrome and idiopathic pulmonary hemosiderosis. *American Journal of Medicine* **59**, 642–649.

Downie, G. H. *et al.* (1982). Experimental anti-alveolar basement membrane antibody-mediated pneumonitis. II. Role of endothelial damage and repair, induction of autologous phase, and kinetics of antibody deposition in Lewis rats. *Journal of Immunology* **129**, 2647–2652.

Drube, S., Maurin, N., and Sieberth, H. G. (1997). Coincidence of myasthenia gravis and antiglomerular basement membrane glomerulonephritis: a combination of two antibody-mediated autoimmune diseases on day 15. *Nephrology, Dialysis, Transplantation* **12**, 1478–1480.

Erwig, L. P., Kluth, D. C., and Rees, A. J. (2001). Macrophages in renal inflammation. *Current Opinion in Nephrology and Hypertension* **10**, 341–347.

Espinosa Melendez, E. *et al.* (1980). Goodpasture's syndrome treated with plasmapheresis. Report of a case. *Archives of Internal Medicine* **140**, 542–543.

Espinosa, G., Cervera, R., Font, J., and Asherson, R. A. (2002). The lung in the antiphospholipid syndrome. *Annals of the Rheumatic Diseases* **61**, 195–198.

Evan, A. P. *et al.* (1991). Shock wave lithotripsy-induced renal injury. *American Journal of Kidney Diseases* **17**, 445–450.

Ewan, P. W., Jones, H. A., Rhodes, C. G., and Hughes, J. M. (1976). Detection of intrapulmonary hemorrhage with carbon monoxide uptake. Application in Goodpasture's syndrome. *New England Journal of Medicine* **295**, 1391–1396.

Fawzi, A. *et al.* (2000). A peptide of the α3(IV) chain of type IV collagen modulates stimulated neutrophil function via activation of cAMP-dependent protein kinase and Ser/Thr protein phosphatase. *Cellular Signalling* **12**, 327–335.

Feintzeig, I. D. *et al.* (1986). Nephritogenic potential of sheep antibodies against glomerular basement membrane laminin in the rat. *Laboratory Investigation* **54**, 531–542.

Fervenza, F. C. *et al.* (1999). Recurrent Goodpasture's disease due to a monoclonal IgA-kappa circulating antibody. *American Journal of Kidney Diseases* **34**, 549–555.

Fillit, H. *et al.* (1985). Sera from patients with poststreptococcal glomerulonephritis contain antibodies to glomerular heparan sulfate proteoglycan. *Journal of Experimental Medicine* **161**, 2778–2779.

Fisher, M., Derry, C. J., Pusey, C. D., and Rees, A. J. (1994). T cells proliferating to the Goodpasture antigen show preferential expression of T cell receptor variable beta chain (TCR Vb) genes. *Journal of the American Society of Nephrology* **5**, 74–77.

Fivush, B., Melvin, T., Solez, K., and McLean, R. H. (1986). Idiopathic linear glomerular IgA deposition. *Archives of Pathology and Laboratory Medicine* **110**, 1189–1191.

Flores, J. C. *et al.* (1986). Clinical and immunological evolution of oliguric anti-GBM nephritis treated by haemodialysis. *Lancet* **i**, 5–8.

Fonck, C., Loute, G., Cosyns, J. P., and Pirson, Y. (1998). Recurrent fulminant anti-glomerular basement membrane nephritis at a 7-year interval. *American Journal of Kidney Diseases* **32**, 323–327.

Gallucci, S. and Matzinger, P. (2001). Danger signals: SOS to the immune system. *Current Opinion in Immunology* **13**, 114–119.

Garcia-Canton, C. *et al.* (2000). Goodpasture's syndrome treated with mycophenolate mofetil. *Nephrology, Dialysis, Transplantation* **15**, 920–922.

Goodpasture, E. W. (1919). The significance of certain pulmonary lesions in relation to the etiology of influenza. *American Journal of Medical Science* **158**, 863–870.

Gossain, V. V., Gerstein, A. R., and Janes, A. W. (1972). Goodpasture's syndrome: a familial occurrence. *American Review of Respiratory Disease* **105**, 621–624.

Guerin, V. *et al.* (1990). Anti-glomerular basement membrane disease after lithotripsy. *Lancet* **i**, 856–857.

Guillen, E. L., Ruiz, A. M., Fernandez, M. A., and Losa, A. M. (1995). Goodpasture syndrome: re-exacerbations associated with intercurrent infections. *Revista Clinica Española* **195**, 761–764.

Gunnarsson, A., Hellmark, T., and Wieslander, J. (2000). Molecular properties of the Goodpasture epitope. *Journal of Biological Chemistry* **275**, 30844–30848.

Gunwar, S. *et al.* (1991). Alveolar basement membrane: molecular properties of the noncollagenous domain (hexamer) of collagen IV and its reactivity with Goodpasture autoantibodies. *American Journal of Respiratory Cell Molecular Biology* **5**, 107–111.

Haramoto, T. *et al.* (1994). Ultrastructural localization of the three major basement membrane components—type IV collagen, heparan sulfate proteoglycan and laminin—in human membranous glomerulonephritis. *American Journal of Nephrology* **14**, 30–36.

Haworth, S. J. *et al.* (1985). Pulmonary haemorrhage complicating Wegener's granulomatosis and microscopic polyarteritis. *British Medical Journal* **290**, 1775–1778.

Heaf, J., Lokkegaard, H., and Larsen, S. (1999). The epidemiology and prognosis of glomerulonephritis in Denmark 1985–1997. *Nephrology, Dialysis, Transplantation* **14**, 1889–1897.

Heale, W. F., Matthiesson, A. M., and Niall, J. F. (1969). Lung haemorrhage and nephritis (Goodpasture's syndrome). *Medical Journal of Australia* **2**, 355–357.

Hellmark, T., Segelmark, M., and Wieslander, J. (1997). Anti-GBM antibodies in Goodpasture syndrome; anatomy of an epitope. *Nephrology, Dialysis, Transplantation* **12**, 646–648.

Henderson, R. D., Saltissi, D., and Pender, M. P. (1998). Goodpasture's syndrome associated with multiple sclerosis. *Acta Neurologica Scandinavica* **98**, 134–135.

Heptinstall, R. H. Schönlein–Henoch syndrome; lung hemorrhage and glomerulonephritis. In *Pathology of the Kidney* (ed. R. H. Heptinstall), pp. 761–791. Boston MA: Little, Brown, 1983.

Herody, M. *et al.* (1993). Anti-GBM disease: predictive value of clinical, histological and serological data. *Clinical Nephrology* **40**, 249–255.

Hind, C. R. K. *et al.* (1983). Prognosis after immunosuppression of patients with crescentic nephritis requiring dialysis. *Lancet* **i**, 263–265.

Hind, C. R., Bowman, C., Winearls, C. G., and Lockwood, C. M. (1984). Recurrence of circulating anti-glomerular basement membrane antibody three years after immunosuppressive treatment and plasma exchange. *Clinical Nephrology* **21**, 244–246.

Holdsworth, S., Boyce, N., Thomson, N. M., and Atkins, R. C. (1985). The clinical spectrum of acute glomerulonephritis and lung haemorrhage (Goodpasture's syndrome). *Quarterly Journal of Medicine* **55**, 75–86.

Jaeger, P. *et al.* (1995). Morphological and functional changes in canine kidneys following extracorporeal shock-wave treatment. *Urology International* **54**, 48–58.

James, S. H., Lien, Y. H., Ruffenach, S. J., and Wilcox, G. E. (1995). Acute renal failure in membranous glomerulonephropathy: a result of superimposed crescentic glomerulonephritis. *Journal of the American Society of Nephrology* **6**, 1541–1546.

Jampol, L. M., Lahov, M., Albert, D. M., and Craft, J. (1975). Ocular clinical findings and basement membrane changes in Goodpasture's syndrome. *American Journal of Ophthalmology* **79**, 452–463.

Jardim, H. M. P. F. *et al.* (1992). Crescentic glomerulonephritis in children. *Pediatric Nephrology* **6**, 231–235.

Jaskowski, T. D., Martins, T. B., Litwin, C. M., and Hill, H. R. (2002). Comparison of four enzyme immunoassays for the detection of immunoglobulin G antibody against glomerular basement membrane. *Journal of Clinical Laboratory Analysis* **16**, 143–145.

Jayne, D. R. W., Marshall, P. D., Jones, S. J., and Lockwood, C. M. (1990). Autoantibodies to glomerular basement membrane and neutrophil cytoplasm in rapidly progressive glomerulonephritis. *Kidney International* **37**, 965–970.

Jennings, L. *et al.* (1981). Experimental anti-alveolar basement membrane antibody-mediated pneumonitis. I. The role of increased permeability of the alveolar capillary wall induced by oxygen. *Journal of Immunology* **127**, 129–134.

Johansson, C., Hellmark, T., and Wieslander, J. (1994). Anti-type IV collagen antibodies in Goodpasture syndrome. *Contributions to Nephrology* **107**, 188–193.

Johnson, J. P., Whitman, W., Briggs, W. A., and Wilson, C. B. (1978). Plasmapheresis and immunosuppressive agents in antibasement membrane antibody-induced Goodpasture's syndrome. *American Journal of Medicine* **64**, 354–359.

Johnson, J. P. *et al.* (1985). Therapy of anti-glomerular basement membrane antibody disease: analysis of prognostic significance of clinical, pathologic and treatment factors. *Medicine (Baltimore)* **64**, 219–227.

Kalderon, A. E., Bogaars, H. A., and Diamond, I. (1973). Ultrastructural alterations of the follicular basement membrane in Hashimoto's thyroiditis. *American Journal of Medicine* **55**, 485–491.

Kefalides, N. A. *et al.* (1986). Antibodies to basement membrane collagen and to laminin are present in sera from patients with poststreptococcal glomerulonephritis. *Journal of Experimental Medicine* **163**, 588–602.

Kefalides, N. A., Ohno, N., and Wilson, C. (1993). Heterogeneity of antibodies in Goodpasture's syndrome reacting with type IV collagen. *Kidney International* **43**, 85–93.

Kelly, P. T. and Haponik, E. F. (1994). Goodpasture syndrome: molecular and clinical advances. *Medicine (Baltimore)* **73**, 171–185.

Kim, Y. *et al.* (1991). Differential expression of basement membrane collagen chains in diabetic nephropathy. *American Journal of Pathology* **138**, 413–420.

Klasa, R. J., Abboud, R. T., Ballon, H. S., and Grossman, L. (1988). Goodpasture's syndrome: recurrence after a five-year remission. Case report and review of the literature. *American Journal of Medicine* **84**, 751–755.

Klassen, J. *et al.* (1974). Evolution of membranous nephropathy into anti-glomerular-basement membrane glomerulonephritis. *New England Journal of Medicine* **290**, 1340–1344.

Kleinknecht, D. *et al.* (1980). Antiglomerular basement membrane nephritis after solvent exposure. *Archives of Internal Medicine* **140**, 230–232.

Kleppel, M. M. *et al.* (1989). Human tissue distribution of novel basement membrane collagen. *American Journal of Pathology* **134**, 813–825.

Komadina, K. H. *et al.* (1988). Goodpasture's syndrome associated with pulmonary eosinophilic vasculitis. *Journal of Rheumatology* **15**, 1298–1301.

Komatsu, T., Utsunomiya, K., and Oyaizu, T. (1998). Goodpasture's syndrome associated with primary biliary cirrhosis. *Internal Medicine (Tokyo)* **37**, 611–613.

Laczika, K. *et al.* (2000). Immunoadsorption in Goodpasture's syndrome. *American Journal of Kidney Diseases* **36**, 392–395.

Leatherman, J. W. (1987). Immune alveolar hemorrhage. *Chest* **91**, 891–897.

Leatherman, J. W., Davies, S. F., and Hoidal, J. R. (1984). Alveolar hemorrhage syndromes: diffuse microvascular lung hemorrhage in immune and idiopathic disorders. *Medicine (Baltimore)* **63**, 34361.

Lee, H. Y. and Stretton, T. B. (1975). The lungs in renal failure. *Thorax* **30**, 46–53.

Lerner, R. A., Glassock, R. J., and Dixon, F. J. (1967). The role of anti-glomerular basement membrane antibody in the pathogenesis of human glomerulonephritis. *Journal of Experimental Medicine* **126**, 989–1004.

Lerner, R. A., Glassock, R. J., and Dixon, F. J. (1999). The role of anti-glomerular basement membrane antibody in the pathogenesis of human glomerulonephritis (1967), reprinted with commentaries by R. J. Glassock and A. J. Rees. *Journal of the American Society of Nephrology* **10**, 1389–1404.

Levy, J. B., Turner, A. N., George, A. J., and Pusey, C. D. (1996). Epitope analysis of the Goodpasture antigen using a resonant mirror biosensor. *Clinical and Experimental Immunology* **106**, 79–85.

Levy, J. B., Turner, A. N., Rees, A. J., and Pusey, C. D. (2001). Long-term outcome of anti-glomerular basement membrane antibody disease treated with plasma exchange and immunosuppression. *Annals of Internal Medicine* **134**, 1033–1042.

Li, S., Holdsworth, S. R., and Tipping, P. G. (1997). Antibody independent crescentic glomerulonephritis in mu chain deficient mice. *Kidney International* **51**, 672–678.

Li, S. *et al.* (1998). Major histocompatibility complex class II expression by intrinsic renal cells is required for crescentic glomerulonephritis. *Journal of Experimental Medicine* **188**, 597–602.

Litwin, C. M. *et al.* (1996). Anti-glomerular basement membrane disease: role of enzyme-linked immunosorbent assays in diagnosis. *Biochemical and Molecular Medicine* **59**, 52–56.

Lockwood, C. M. *et al.* (1976). Immunosuppression and plasma-exchange in the treatment of Goodpasture's syndrome. *Lancet* **i**, 711–715.

Ma, K. W. *et al.* (1978). Glomerulonephritis with Hodgkins disease and herpes zoster. *Archives of Pathology and Laboratory Medicine* **102**, 527–529.

Maes, B. *et al.* (1999). IgA antiglomerular basement membrane disease associated with bronchial carcinoma and monoclonal gammopathy. *American Journal of Kidney Diseases* **33**, E3.

Maeshima, Y. *et al.* (2002). Tumstatin, an endothelial cell-specific inhibitor of protein synthesis. *Science* **295**, 140–143.

Masson, R. G., Rennke, H. G., and Gottlieb, M. N. (1992). Pulmonary hemorrhage in a patient with fibrillary glomerulonephritis. *New England Journal of Medicine* **326**, 369.

Mathew, T. H. *et al.* (1975). Goodpasture's syndrome: normal renal diagnostic findings. *Annals of Internal Medicine* **82**, 215–218.

Maxwell, A. P., Nelson, W. E., and Hill, C. M. (1988). Reversal of renal failure in nephritis associated with antibody to glomerular basement membrane. *British Medical Journal* **297**, 3334.

McIntosh, R. M. *et al.* (1975). The human choroid plexus and autoimmune nephritis. *Archives of Pathology* **99**, 48–50.

McPhaul, J. J., Jr. and Dixon, F. J. (1970). Characterization of human anti-glomerular basement membrane antibodies eluted from glomerulonephritic kidneys. *Journal of Clinical Investigation* **49**, 308–317.

McPhaul, J. J., Jr. and Mullins, J. D. (1976). Glomerulonephritis mediated by antibody to glomerular basement membrane. Immunological, clinical, and histopathological characteristics. *Journal of Clinical Investigation* **57**, 351–361.

Mehler, P. S., Brunvand, M. W., Hutt, M. P., and Anderson, R. J. (1987). Chronic recurrent Goodpasture's syndrome. *American Journal of Medicine* **82**, 833–835.

Merkel, F., Pullig, O., Marx, M., Netzer, K. O., and Weber, M. (1994). Course and prognosis of anti-basement membrane antibody-mediated disease: report of 35 cases. *Nephrology, Dialysis, Transplantation* **9**, 372–376.

Meyers, K. E. *et al.* (1998). Human Goodpasture anti-alpha3(IV)NC1 autoantibodies share structural determinants. *Kidney International* **53**, 402–407.

Milliner, D. S., Pierides, A. M., and Holley, K. E. (1982). Renal transplantation in Alport's syndrome: anti-glomerular basement membrane glomerulonephritis in the allograft. *Mayo Clinic Proceedings* **57**, 35–43.

Miner, J. H. (1999). Renal basement membrane components. *Kidney International* **56**, 2016–2024.

Miner, J. H. and Sanes, J. R. (1994). Collagen α3 chain, α4 chain, and α5 chain in rodent basal laminae—sequence, distribution, association with laminins, and developmental switches. *Journal of Cell Biology* **127**, 879–891.

Morello, R. *et al.* (2001). Regulation of glomerular basement membrane collagen expression by LMX1B contributes to renal disease in nail patella syndrome. *Nature Genetics* **27**, 205–208.

Morgan, P. G. and Turner-Warwick, M. (1981). Pulmonary haemosiderosis and pulmonary haemorrhage. *British Journal of Diseases of the Chest* **75**, 225–242.

Nakajima, I. *et al.* (1999). Goodpasture's syndrome initially presenting with alveolar hemorrhage. *Nihon Kokyuki Gakkai Zasshi—Journal of the Japanese Respiratory Society* **37**, 652–657.

Netzer, K. O., Merkel, F., and Weber, M. (1998). Goodpasture syndrome and end-stage renal failure—to transplant or not to transplant? *Nephrology, Dialysis, Transplantation* **13**, 1346–1348.

New Zealand Glomerulonephritis Study Group (1989). The New Zealand Glomerulonephritis Study: introductory report. *Clinical Nephrology* **31**, 239–246.

Nolasco, F. E. B. *et al.* (1987). Intraglomerular T cells and monocytes in nephritis: study with monoclonal antibodies. *Kidney International* **31**, 1160–1166.

O'Donoghue, D. J. *et al.* (1989). Sequential development of systemic vasculitis with anti-neutrophil cytoplasmic antibodies complicating anti-glomerular basement membrane disease. *Clinical Nephrology* **32**, 251–255.

Ortega, L. G. and Mellors, R. C. (1956). The role of localized antibodies in the pathogenesis of nephrotoxic nephritis in the rat. *Journal of Experimental Medicine* **104**, 151–170.

Paueksakon, P., Hunley, T. E., Lee, S. M., and Fogo, A. B. (1999). A 12-year-old girl with pulmonary hemorrhage, skin lesions, and hematuria. *American Journal of Kidney Diseases* **33**, 404–409.

Peces, R., Rodriguez, M., Pobes, A., and Seco, M. (2000). Sequential development of pulmonary hemorrhage with MPO-ANCA complicating anti-glomerular basement membrane antibody-mediated glomerulonephritis. *American Journal of Kidney Diseases* **35**, 954–957.

Pepys, E. O., Rees, A. J., and Pepys, M. B. (1982). Enumeration of lymphocyte populations in whole peripheral blood of patients with antibody-mediated nephritis during treatment with cyclosporin A. *Immunology Letters* **4**, 211–214.

Perez, G. O. *et al.* (1974). A mini-epidemic of Goodpasture's syndrome—clinical and immunological studies. *Nephron* **13**, 16173.

Peten, E. *et al.* (1991). Outcome of thirty patients with Alport's syndrome after renal transplantation. *Transplantation* **52**, 823–826.

Peters, D. K., Rees, A. J., Lockwood, C. M., and Pusey, C. D. (1982). Treatment and prognosis in antibasement membrane antibody-mediated nephritis. *Transplantation Proceedings* **14**, 513–521.

Phelps, R. G. and Turner, A. N. (2003). Anti-glomerular basement membrane disease. In *Principles of Nephrology* 2nd edn. Mosby (in press).

Phelps, R. G. *et al.* (1998). Presentation of the Goodpasture autoantigen to CD4 T cells is influenced more by processing constraints than by HLA class II peptide binding preferences. *Journal of Biological Chemistry* **273**, 11440–11447.

Phelps, R. G., Jones, V., Turner, A. N., and Rees, A. J. (2000). Properties of HLA class II molecules divergently associated with Goodpasture's disease. *International Immunology* **12**, 1135–1143.

Proskey, A. J. *et al.* (1970). Goodpasture's syndrome. A report of five cases and review of the literature. *American Journal of Medicine* **48**, 162–173.

Pusey, C. D. *et al.* (1987). A single autoantigen in Goodpasture's syndrome identified by a monoclonal antibody to human glomerular basement membrane. *Laboratory Investigation* **56**, 23–31.

Querin, S. *et al.* (1986). Linear glomerular IgG fixation in renal allografts: incidence and significance in Alport's syndrome. *Clinical Nephrology* **25**, 134–140.

Querin, S., Schurch, W., and Beaulieu, R. (1992). Cyclosporin in Goodpasture's syndrome. *Nephron* **60**, 353–359.

Rajaraman, S., Pinto, J. A., and Cavallo, T. (1984). Glomerulonephritis with coexistent immune deposits and antibasement membrane activity. *Journal of Clinical Pathology* **37**, 176–181.

Raya, A. *et al.* (2000). Goodpasture antigen-binding protein, the kinase that phosphorylates the goodpasture antigen, is an alternatively spliced variant implicated in autoimmune pathogenesis. *Journal of Biological Chemistry* **275**, 40392–40399.

Rees, A. J., Lockwood, C. M., and Peters, D. K. (1977). Enhanced allergic tissue injury in Goodpasture's syndrome by intercurrent bacterial infection. *British Medical Journal* **2**, 723–726.

Rees, A. J., Peters, D. K., Compston, D. A., and Batchelor, J. R. (1978). Strong association between HLA-DRW2 and antibody-mediated Goodpasture's syndrome. *Lancet* **i**, 966–968.

Rees, A. J., Lockwood, C. M., and Peters, D. K. Nephritis due to antibodies to GBM. In *Progress in Glomerulonephritis* (ed. P. Kincaid-Smith, A. J. F. dApice, and R. C. Atkins), pp. 347–370. New York: Wiley, 1979.

Rees, A. J., Demaine, A. G., and Welsh, K. I. (1984a). Association of immunoglobulin Gm allotypes with antiglomerular basement membrane antibodies and their titer. *Human Immunology* **10**, 213–220.

Rees, A. J. *et al.* (1984b). The influence of HLA-linked genes on the severity of anti-GBM antibody-mediated nephritis. *Kidney International* **26**, 445–450.

Relman, A. S., Dvorak, H. F., and Colvin, R. B. (1971). Case records of the Massachusetts General Hospital. Weekly clinicopathological exercises. Case 461971. *New England Journal of Medicine* **285**, 1187–1196.

Revert, F. *et al.* (1995). Phosphorylation of the Goodpasture antigen by type A protein kinases. *Journal of Biological Chemistry* **270**, 13254–13261.

Rowe, P. A., Mansfield, D. C., and Dutton, G. N. (1994). Ophthalmic features of fourteen cases of Goodpasture's syndrome. *Nephron* **68**, 52–56.

Sabnis, S. G., Nandedkar, M. A., and Antonovych, T. T. (1988). Antiglomerular basement membrane antibody-induced glomerulonephritis with glomerular multinucleated giant cell reaction: a case study. *American Journal of Kidney Diseases* **12**, 544–547.

Sado, Y., Naito, I., Akita, M., and Okigaki, T. (1986). Strain specific responses of inbred rats on the severity of experimental autoimmune glomerulonephritis. *Journal of Clinical and Laboratory Immunology* **19**, 193–199.

Salama, A. D., Chaudhry, A. N., Ryan, J. J., Eren, E., Levy, J. B., Pusey, C. D., Lightstone, L., and Lechler, R. I. (2001). In Goodpasture's disease, CD4(+) T cells escape thymic deletion and are reactive with the autoantigen $\alpha3$(IV)NC1. *Journal of the American Society of Nephrology* **12**, 1908–1915.

Salama, A. D. *et al.* (2002). Goodpasture's disease in the absence of circulating anti-glomerular basement membrane antibodies as detected by standard techniques. *American Journal of Kidney Diseases* **39**, 1162–1167.

Salama, A. D. *et al.* (2003). Regulation by CD25+ lymphocytes of autoantigen-specific T-cell responses in Goodpasture's (anti-GBM) disease. *Kidney International* **64**, 1685–1694.

Saraf, P., Berger, H. W., and Thung, S. N. (1978). Goodpasture's syndrome with no overt renal disease. *Mount Sinai Journal of Medicine (New York)* **45**, 451–454.

Saus, J. *et al.* (1988). Identification of the Goodpasture antigen as the $\alpha3$(IV) chain of collagen IV. *Journal of Biological Chemistry* **263**, 13374–13380.

Savage, C. O. S. *et al.* (1986). Antiglomerular basement membrane antibody mediated disease in the British Isles 19804. *British Medical Journal* **292**, 301–304.

Savage, C. O. S. *et al.* (1989). Hereditary nephritis: immunoblotting studies of the glomerular basement membrane. *Laboratory Investigation* **60**, 613–618.

Saxena, R., Bygren, P., Rasmussen, N., and Wieslander, J. (1991). Circulating autoantibodies in patients with extracapillary glomerulonephritis. *Nephrology, Dialysis, Transplantation* **6**, 389–397.

Scheer, R. L. and Grossman, M. A. (1964). Immune aspects of the glomerulonephritis associated with pulmonary hemorrhage. *Annals of Internal Medicine* **60**, 1009–1021.

Schena, F. P. (1997). Survey of the Italian Registry of Renal Biopsies. Frequency of the renal diseases for 7 consecutive years. The Italian Group of Renal Immunopathology. *Nephrology, Dialysis, Transplantation* **12**, 418–426.

Schindler, R. *et al.* (1998). Complete recovery of renal function in a dialysis-dependent patient with Goodpasture syndrome. *Nephrology, Dialysis, Transplantation* **13**, 462–466.

Schmidt, R. H. *et al.* (1999). Spontaneous remission of Goodpasture syndrome in a 21-year-old patient. *Deutsche Medizinische Wochenschrift* **124**, 1201–1203.

Segelmark, M., Butkowski, R., and Wieslander, J. (1991). Antigen restriction and IgG subclasses among anti-GBM autoantibodies. *Nephrology, Dialysis, Transplantation* **5**, 9916.

Sharma, S. (1998). Bilateral serous retinal detachments associated with Goodpasture's syndrome. *Canadian Journal of Ophthalmology* **33**, 226–227.

Short, A. K., Esnault, V. L., and Lockwood, C. M. (1995). Anti-neutrophil cytoplasm antibodies and anti-glomerular basement membrane antibodies: two coexisting distinct autoreactivities detectable in patients with rapidly progressive glomerulonephritis. *American Journal of Kidney Diseases* **26**, 439–445.

Simonsen, H. *et al.* (1982). Goodpasture's syndrome in twins. *Acta Medica Scandinavica* **212**, 425–428.

Simpson, I. J. *et al.* (1982). Plasma exchange in Goodpasture's syndrome. *American Journal of Nephrology* **2**, 301–311.

Srivastava, R. N. *et al.* (1992). Crescentic glomerulonephritis in children: a review of 43 cases. *American Journal of Nephrology* **12**, 155–161.

Stanton, M. C. and Tange, J. D. (1958). Goodpasture's syndrome (pulmonary haemorrhage associated with glomerulonephritis). *Australian and New Zealand Journal of Medicine* **7**, 132–144.

Steblay, R. W. and Rudofsky, U. H. (1983). Experimental autoimmune antiglomerular basement membrane antibody-induced glomerulonephritis. I. The effects of injecting sheep with human, homologous or autologous lung basement membranes and complete Freunds adjuvant. *Clinical Immunology and Immunopathology* **27**, 65–80.

Sundaramoorthy, M., Meiyappan, M., Todd, P., and Hudson, B. G. (2002). Crystal structure of NC1 domains. Structural basis for type IV collagen assembly in basement membranes. *Journal of Biological Chemistry* **277**, 31142–31153.

Takeuchi, K. *et al.* (1997). An autopsy case of Goodpasture syndrome preceded with membranous glomerulonephritis. *Ryumachi (Rheumatism)* **37**, 781–787.

Tan, S. Y. and Cumming, A. D. (1993). Vaccine related glomerulonephritis. *British Medical Journal* **306**, 248.

Teague, C. A. *et al.* (1978). Goodpasture's syndrome: an analysis of 29 cases. *Kidney International* **13**, 492–504.

Than, M. E. *et al.* (2002). The 1.9-A crystal structure of the noncollagenous (NC1) domain of human placenta collagen IV shows stabilization via a novel type of covalent Met-Lys cross-link. *Proceedings of the National Academy of Sciences of the USA* **99**, 6607–6612.

Timoshanko, J. R., Holdsworth, S. R., Kitching, A. R., and Tipping, P. G. (2002). IFN-gamma production by intrinsic renal cells and bone marrow-derived cells is required for full expression of crescentic glomerulonephritis in mice. *Journal of Immunology* **168**, 4135–4141.

Trpkov, K., Abdulkareem, F., Jim, K., and Solez, K. (1998). Recurrence of anti-GBM antibody disease twelve years after transplantation associated with de novo IgA nephropathy. *Clinical Nephrology* **49**, 124–128.

Turner, N. *et al.* (1992). Molecular cloning of the human Goodpasture antigen demonstrates it to be the $\alpha3$ chain of type IV collagen. *Journal of Clinical Investigation* **89**, 592–601.

Uezu, Y., Kiyatake, I., and Tokuyama, K. (1999). A case of Goodpasture's syndrome with massive pulmonary hemorrhage ameliorated by cyclophosphamide pulse therapy. *Nippon Jinzo Gakkai Shi* **41**, 499–504.

Umekawa, T. *et al.* (1993). Glomerular-basement-membrane antibody and extracorporeal shock wave lithotripsy. *Lancet* **341**, 55–56.

Vats, K. R. *et al.* (1999). Henoch–Schönlein purpura and pulmonary hemorrhage: a report and literature review. *Pediatric Nephrology* **13**, 530–534.

Verburgh, C. A., Bruijn, J. A., Daha, M. R., and van Es, L. A. (1999). Sequential development of anti-GBM nephritis and ANCA-associated pauci-immune glomerulonephritis. *American Journal of Kidney Diseases* **34**, 344–348.

von Vigier, R. O. *et al.* (2000). Pulmonary renal syndrome in childhood: a report of twenty-one cases and a review of the literature. *Pediatric Pulmonology* **29**, 382–388.

Wahls, T. L., Bonsib, S. M., and Schuster, V. L. (1987). Coexistent Wegener's granulomatosis and anti-glomerular basement membrane disease. *Human Pathology* **18**, 202–205.

Wakui, H. *et al.* (1992). Goodpasture's syndrome: a report of an autopsy case and a review of Japanese cases. *Internal Medicine* **31**, 102–107.

Walker, R. G. *et al.* (1985). Clinical and morphological aspects of the management of crescentic anti-glomerular basement membrane antibody (anti-GBM) nephritis/Goodpasture's syndrome. *Quarterly Journal of Medicine* **54**, 75–89.

Wick, G., von der Mark, H., Dietrich, H., and Timpl, R. (1986). Globular domain of basement membrane collagen induces autoimmune pulmonary lesions in mice resembling human Goodpasture disease. *Laboratory Investigation* **55**, 308–317.

Williams, P. S. *et al.* (1988). Increased incidence of anti-glomerular basement membrane antibody (anti-GBM) nephritis in the Mersey region, September 1984–October 1985. *Quarterly Journal of Medicine* **68**, 727–733.

Wilson, C. B. and Dixon, F. J. (1973). Anti-glomerular basement membrane antibody-induced glomerulonephritis. *Kidney International* **3**, 74–89.

Wilson, C. B. and Dixon, F. J. (1974). Diagnosis of immunopathologic renal disease. *Kidney International* **5**, 389–401.

Wilson, C. B. and Dixon, F. J. The renal response to immunological injury. In *The Kidney* (ed. B. M. Brenner and F. C. Rector), pp. 1237–1350. Philadelphia, PA: W.B. Saunders, 1981.

Wilson, C. B. and Smith, R. C. (1972). Goodpasture's syndrome associated with influenza A2 virus infection. *Annals of Internal Medicine* **76**, 91–94.

Wilson, C. B., Dixon, F. J., Evans, A. S., and Glassock, R. J. (1973). Anti-viral antibody responses in patients with renal disease. *Clinical Immunology and Immunopathology* **2**, 121–132.

Wong, D., Phelps, R. G., and Turner, A. N. (2001). The Goodpasture antigen is expressed in the human thymus. *Kidney International* **60**, 1777–1783.

Wu, J. *et al.* (2002). CD4(+) T cells specific to a glomerular basement membrane antigen mediate glomerulonephritis. *Journal of Clinical Investigation* **109**, 517–524.

Wu, M. J. *et al.* (1980). Vasculitis in Goodpasture's syndrome. *Archives of Pathology and Laboratory Medicine* **104**, 300–302.

Wucherpfennig, K. W. (2001). Mechanisms for the induction of autoimmunity by infectious agents. *Journal of Clinical Investigation* **108**, 1097–1104.

Wuthrich, R. P. (1994). Pernicious anaemia, autoimmune hypothyroidism and rapidly progressive anti-GBM glomerulonephritis. *Clinical Nephrology* **42**, 404.

Xenocostas, A. *et al.* (1999). Anti-glomerular basement membrane glomerulonephritis after extracorporeal shock wave lithotripsy. *American Journal of Kidney Diseases* **33**, 128–132.

Yaar, M. *et al.* (1982). The Goodpasture-like syndrome in mice induced by intravenous injections of anti-type IV collagen and anti-laminin antibody. *American Journal of Pathology* **107**, 79–91.

Yamamoto, T. and Wilson, C. B. (1987). Binding of anti-basement membrane antibody to alveolar basement membrane after intratracheal gasoline instillation in rabbits. *American Journal of Pathology* **126**, 497–505.

Yankowitz, J., Kuller, J. A., and Thomas, R. L. (1992). Pregnancy complicated by Goodpasture syndrome. *Obstetrics and Gynecology* **79**, 806–808.

Yaqoob, M., Bell, G. M., Percy, D. F., and Finn, R. (1992). Primary glomerulonephritis and hydrocarbon exposure: a casecontrol study and literature review. *Quarterly Journal of Medicine* **301**, 409–418.

3.12 Infection related glomerulonephritis

Philippe Lesavre and Alex M. Davison

General introduction

The effects of infections on the kidney are variable and depend on a number of factors relating to both the host and the infecting organism. The well-recognized association between a group A β-haemolytic streptococcal infection and the subsequent development of an acute nephritic illness has been used for many years to explain certain important immunological principles. The infecting organism releases antigens to which there is a subsequent antibody response with local or systemic immune complex formation and complement activation, and a resulting inflammatory response may occur in the glomerulus, leading to glomerulonephritis (GN). Many other infections are known to have similar consequences.

It is becoming increasingly recognized that infections may be associated with a variety of lesions in the kidney (Table 1). Septicaemia is frequently associated with significant toxin production which can result in an acute tubular necrosis (Mactier and Dobbie 1984) and acute renal failure. Severe *Escherichia coli* septicaemia may be associated with verocytotoxin production and the development of haemolytic uraemic syndrome, particularly in children. Other infections have a major influence on the interstitium: acute tubulointerstitial nephritis is well recognized in patients with hantavirus infection, together with many bacterial and other infectious agents, and a wide variety of lesions have been reported in AIDS patients, including glomerular changes, tubular necrosis, tubulointerstitial nephritis, granulomatous lesions due to opportunistic infections, nephrocalcinosis, and direct involvement of the kidney by Kaposi's sarcoma and lymphoma. Other viral infections may precipitate or cause a relapse of nephritis due to antiglomerular basement membrane antibodies (Goodpasture's syndrome) or may result in an haemolytic uraemic syndrome with renal involvement. Vasculitis has been described in association with hepatitis B virus infections. Finally, chronic bacterial infections, such as subacute bacterial endocarditis, infected ventriculoatrial shunts, and visceral abscesses, have been associated with the development of GN, particularly of the mesangiocapillary form. Other chronic bacterial infections, particularly bronchiectasis, oesteomyelitis, and tuberculosis, are associated with a chronic stimulation of the immune system which results in amyloid deposition. The complications of antibiotic therapy for infections have been shown to result in the development of an allergic type of eosinophilic tubulo-interstitial nephritis (Pusey *et al.* 1983). Thus, all compartments of the kidney may be involved as an indirect effect of infections (Table 1); here the focus is on the glomerular lesions. It is particularly important to remember that the same organism may produce different morphological appearances in different patients. For instance, membranous GN, mesangiocapillary GN, and IgA nephropathy have all been described in patients with persistent hepatitis B antigenaemia. In addition, different infections may produce the same glomerular morphological appearance in different patients (Boulton-Jones and Davison 1986). Furthermore, similar infections from different geographical regions may present completely different clinical features (see Chapters 3.14 and 10.7.3).

Table 1 Recognized renal consequences of infections

	Chapter no.
Blood vessels	
Vasculitis	4.5.1
Haemolytic uraemic syndrome	10.6.3
Glomeruli	
Glomerulonephritis	This chapter
Intravascular coagulation	10.2, 10.6.3
Amyloidosis	4.2
Tubules	
Acute tubular necrosis	10.2
Interstitium	
Tubulointerstitial nephritis	6.1
Infection-associated	10.6.2
Antibiotic-induced nephrocalcinosis	19.1
With granuloma formation	10.6.2
Kaposi's sarcoma	20.2, 20.5
Lymphoma	20.8

The glomerular response to infection appears to depend on both patient factors and characteristics of the infecting organism (see also Chapter 3.2). The immune response to infection may determine the resulting glomerular lesion through the type, quantity, and duration of antibody response, and localization of the antigen–antibody immune complexes in a subendothelial, subepithelial, and/or mesangial position. The immune response may be influenced by genetic factors, and this may explain the geographical differences which have been reported for certain infections; for instance, more than 80 per cent of patients with focal and segmental glomerulosclerosis associated with HIV infection are Black. Some forms of glomerular disease, such as IgA nephropathy, are common, and this will increase the possibility of a coincidental association with an infecting organism. Furthermore, organisms differ in their virulence, and this may be further affected by passage, resulting in either increased virulence or attenuation. Thus, the consequences of an infection in any given population is dependent on a number of variables, and this may well explain the wide variety of responses that are seen even within an epidemic of a single infection arising from the same strain of organism.

Socioeconomic status and environmental health are significant factors in explaining the changing clinical pattern of glomerular disease associated with infections. With increasing affluence the general health of a community improves and this is associated with an increased ability to deal with infection. Poststreptococcal GN is now relatively uncommon in Western and Northern Europe, although it remains epidemic in certain areas of the world. In a study of infection as a cause of renal disease leading to renal biopsy carried out in the United Kingdom, 21 per cent of patients with infection-associated renal disease were immigrants (Boulton-Jones and Davison 1986). Other factors such as a reduction in the virulence of the streptococcus may also partially explain the phenomenon. Many other factors can be implicated in the changing epidemiology of infection-associated glomerular disease. The eradication *of Plasmodium malariae* from British Guiana has been associated with a reduction in the incidence of nephropathy (see Chapter 3.14). However, the AIDS epidemic has been accompanied by an increasing number of reports describing an associated nephropathy and renal disease. Although many diseases cannot be eradicated, the development of effective antibiotic therapy has been associated with a reduction in infection-related complications. It is now relatively uncommon to encounter patients with renal amyloidosis secondary to tuberculosis or chronic osteomyelitis in the resident population of Western Europe, but this remains common in many other parts of the world (Chapter 4.2).

A causal relationship between infection and nephropathy was initially established by epidemiological studies in which epidemic or endemic infections were associated with specific glomerular abnormalities (Table 2). The link has been strengthened further by the clinical observation that in many instances the renal lesion resolves following effective treatment of the underlying infection; malaria and schistosomiasis are exceptions. In addition, there have been many experimental animal studies in which glomerular lesions have been induced by bacterial, viral, or parasitic infections. A direct causal relationship has been suggested by the detection of antigen arising from the infecting organism within the glomerulus, and from elution studies demonstrating specific antibody directed against bacterial or viral antigens also present in the lesions. A role for the humoral immune system has been suggested by the demonstration of immunoglobulins and complement components within glomerular deposits. Although many early reports are of doubtful significance, owing to the poor specificity of the antisera used, recent reports (particularly those using monoclonal antibodies) have demonstrated specific antigens, immunoglobulins, and complement within the glomerulus, thus confirming the immunological nature of the nephropathy (see Chapter 3.2).

Reports from the preantibiotic era frequently associated nephropathy with chronic infections such as tuberculosis. It is interesting that a recent re-examination of three of the kidneys which formed the original report by Richard Bright in the early nineteenth century revealed that one has amyloidosis, possibly associated with an underlying chronic tuberculosis (Weller and Nester 1972). The association between an infectious illness, scarlatina, and renal abnormalities was reported at about the same time (Miller 1849). Of course, detailed studies could not be undertaken until the nature of the infecting organism was elucidated.

Infections do not always produce an adverse effect on the glomerulus. It has been noted that measles may produce a remission in proteinuria in children with minimal change nephrotic syndrome, and primary

Table 2 Infection-associated glomerulonephritis

	Cross references
Viral infections	
Herpes viruses	
Cytomegalovirus	This chapter
Epstein–Barr virus	This chapter
Human herpes virus 8	This chapter
Paramyxoviruses	
Measles	This chapter
Mumps	This chapter
Parvoviruses	This chapter
Polyoma virus BK	This chapter
Hepatitis viruses	
Hepatitis B	Chapter 3.14
Hepatitis-B-associated polyarteritis nodosa	Chapter 4.5.3
Hepatitis C	Chapter 4.6
Retroviruses	
Human immunodeficiency virus	This chapter
HTLV-1	This chapter
Influenza viruses	This chapter
Bacterial infections	
Streptococcus	Chapter 3.9
Staphylococcus	This chapter
Streptococcus pneumoniae (pneumococcus)	This chapter
Salmonella	This chapter
Mycobacteria	
Tuberculosis	This chapter
Leprosy	Chapter 3.3
Other bacterial infections	
Brucella melitensis	This chapter
E. coli	This chapter
E. coli (sero type O157 : H7) and haemolytic uraemic syndrome	Chapter 10.6.3
Klebsiella pneumoniae	This chapter
Meningococcal meningitis	This chapter
Yersinia entercolitica	This chapter
Mycoplasma pneumoniae	This chapter
Bartonella henselae	This chapter
Spirochaete infections	
Treponema	This chapter
Leptospirosis	This chapter
Rickettsial infections	This chapter
Fungal infections	
Candida albicans	This chapter
Histoplasma capsulatum	This chapter
Protozoal infections	
Malaria	Chapter 3.14
Plasmodium malariae	Chapter 3.14
Plasmodium falciparum	Chapter 3.14
Toxoplasmosis	This chapter
Leishmaniasis (kala-azar)	This chapter
Trematode infections	
Schistosomiasis	Chapters 3.14 and 7.4
Nematode infections	
Filariasis	Chapter 3.14
Infections at particular sites	
Infective endocarditis	This chapter
Visceral abscesses	This chapter
Kimura's disease (angiolymphoid hyperplasia with eosinophilia)	This chapter

measles vaccination has been used therapeutically in this situation (Yuceoglu *et al.* 1969) (see Chapter 3.5). It is possible that measles virus infection has an inhibitory effect on T cells, suppressing lymphokine secretion and resulting in glomerular capillary wall changes which reduce proteinuria. Infections with varicella-zoster virus, *Salmonella typhi*, plasmodium, and pneumococcus have also occasionally been reported to have a similar effect. There has been an increased interest in the role of cellular immunity in infection-related glomerular disease following the reports of AIDS-associated nephropathy.

Many associations between infections and nephropathy are well accepted and well documented (see Levy 1988 for a comprehensive review). However, in many additional instances there are few or sporadic adequately documented reports. It is particularly difficult to establish a causal relationship if specific antigen has not been detected within the glomerulus and/or elution studies have not been undertaken. Increasing sophistication with respect to the detection of antigens in biopsy material, such as reverse transcription polymerase chain reaction and *in situ* hybridization techniques, have significantly enhanced the value of even single well-documented case reports. Despite this, caution is still needed before a particular infection is associated with a glomerular lesion unless (a) a specific antigen has been detected within the glomerulus, (b) elution studies have identified an immunoglobulin which reacts specifically with antigens of the affecting organism, and (c) epidemiological studies have excluded other compounding factors. Nevertheless, the possibility remains that the infection in some way generates the renal damage entirely though cell-mediated mechanisms (see Chapter 3.2), and no humoral immune reactants will be present.

In general, management is directed towards the identification of the infection and its subsequent treatment. In the majority of patients, treatment of the renal disease is symptomatic, aiming to control oedema, hypertension, and impaired kidney function. Effective treatment of the associated infection is commonly accompanied by resolution of the renal lesion. It must always be remembered that drugs, particularly antibiotic and diuretic agents, may be associated with a tubulointerstitial nephritis.

Viral infections

General remarks

Viral infection may produce glomerular effects by three different mechanisms: a direct cytopathic effect of the virus on glomerular cells, stimulation of an antibody response resulting in immune complex formation, and a direct effect on T cells altering the helper-to-suppressor ratio and affecting humoral immunity.

Viral infections resulting in immune-complex-mediated glomerular diseases occur naturally and in experimental animal diseases, including Aleutian disease in mink, spontaneous Gross leukaemia virus infection, and lymphocytic choriomeningitis virus infection. Hepatitis B virus, cytomegalovirus, and human immunodeficiency virus (HIV) have all been reported to cause glomerular lesions.

Viral infections are particularly common in the human, and it is surprising that so few patients with acute infections develop evidence of renal disease. There are many sporadic case reports of GN following viral diseases: varicella (Yuceoglu *et al.* 1967), measles virus (Lin and Hsu 1983), mumps (Hughes *et al.* 1966), subacute sclerosing encephalitis (O'Regan *et al.* 1979), Echo virus infection (Huang and Wiegenstein 1977), and Epstein–Barr virus infection (Lee and Kjellstrand 1978). Viral infections may also precipitate haemolytic uraemic syndrome, particularly in children (see Chapter 10.6.3).

Chronic infections, particularly those involving hepatitis B virus, cytomegalovirus, and HIV, have been associated with glomerular changes. Chronic hepatitis B infection has been associated with both GN (Kohler *et al.* 1974) and polyarteritis nodosa (Michalak 1978). GN associated with cytomegalovirus infection has been most commonly reported in patients following transplantation, but there is considerable doubt over whether this lesion is specific or represents a form of rejection. The HIV is associated with a focal–segmental glomerulosclerosis (FSGS), but the case reports include large numbers of intravenous drug abusers and patients with opportunistic infections, and a direct causal relationship is difficult to establish (see Chapter 4.12.1).

A direct causal relationship is also difficult to establish in other viral infections. An *in situ* hybridization study using DNA probes for herpes simplex and Epstein–Barr virus concluded that in some patients there may be coincidental rather than causal infection by the herpes group of viruses (Sinniah *et al.* 1993).

Herpes viruses

Cytomegalovirus

Cytomegalovirus infection has been associated with glomerular changes in two groups of patients: children with severe congenital or neonatal infection and immunosuppressed patients, particularly following transplantation. Circulating immune complexes are common in children with severe disease, but evidence of nephropathy is rare. Although granular deposits of IgG and C3 have been demonstrated in glomerular capillary walls in such patients, no cytomegalovirus antigen has been detected within glomeruli, casting doubt on the pathogenesis and specificity of the lesion. Conversely, human glomerular and tubular epithelial cells in culture are susceptible to infection with cytomegalovirus (Heieren *et al.* 1988).

The situation in adults remains unclear. Although the majority of the population will eventually become infected with cytomegalovirus, symptomatic infection is rare. Ozawa and Stewart (1979) reported a patient who developed proteinuria and haematuria during the course of fatal cytomegalovirus pneumonitis. The kidney showed mesangial proliferative GN with mesangial immune deposits containing cytomegalovirus. Detwiler *et al.* (1998) reported a patient with focal segmental glomerulosclerosis who developed necrotizing and crescentic GN with intraglomerular viral inclusions and cytomegalovirus by *in situ* hybridization. After 8 weeks of ganciclovir therapy, resolution of lesions and disappearance of the cytomegalovirus inclusions were observed. Andresdottir *et al.* (2000) reported a patient with idiopathic type I membranoproliferative glomerulonephritis (MPGN) who developed an acute exudative proliferative GN with immune deposits. After 3 weeks of ganciclovir therapy, the exudative lesions had disappeared.

Although it has been suggested that cytomegalovirus is involved in the pathogenesis of IgA nephropathy, there is no evidence that cytomegalovirus antigens are detected with any greater frequency in IgA nephropathy than in other types of GN (Park *et al.* 1994).

Cytomegalovirus infection is particularly common following transplantation (see Chapter 13.3.3). It is difficult to determine whether the lesions described in transplant recipients are due to cytomegalovirus infection (Richardson *et al.* 1981) or represent glomerular endothelial cell changes associated with rejection and precipitated by cytomegalovirus among other causes (Herrera *et al.* 1986; Boyce *et al.* 1988).

The balance of opinion at present would seem to favour the latter explanation (Browne *et al.* 2001) (see Chapter 13.3.3).

Epstein–Barr virus

The Epstein–Barr virus is associated with infectious mononucleosis and Burkitt's lymphoma. Renal complications are common in infectious mononucleosis, with proteinuria in 14 per cent of patients and haematuria in 11 per cent (Lee and Kjellstrand 1978). Some patients have macroscopic haematuria and there may be mild impairment of renal function (Woodroffe *et al.* 1974); some patients have been reported with severe impairment of renal function (Lee and Kjellstrand 1978). Renal biopsy shows a variety of glomerular changes, including IgA nephropathy and proliferative GN. An immune-complex-mediated GN associated with leucocytoclastic vasculitis has been reported in a girl (Lande *et al.* 1998). Renal abnormalities appear to resolve with resolution of the infections. On the other hand, the study of 33 patients with various forms of GN (IgA nephropathy, membranous nephropathy) showed that glomerular mesangial injury correlates with Epstein–Barr virus DNA detection, using polymerase chain reaction, in biopsies (Iwama *et al.* 1998). The use of molecular hybridization may be useful in patients with negative serology (Nadasdy *et al.* 1992). GN is uncommon in Burkitt's lymphoma, although a mesangiocapillary GN has been described. Detection of specific EBV antigens on kidney biopsy in a 14-year-old girl who presented with acute onset of SLE concurrently with infectious mononucleosis suggests a possible role of the virus in the pathogenesis of SLE (Dror *et al.* 1998).

Human herpes virus 8

Renal involvment in Crow–Fukase (POEMS) and in multicentric Castelman's disease (MCD) is common (see Chapter 3.13). Proteinuria and renal insufficiency are present in 25–50 per cent of patients. Renal histopathology is diverse: thrombotic microangiopathy and amyloidosis are frequent. MGN type I and membranous nephropathy are less frequently reported. Tubulointerstitial nephritis and type IV renal tubular acidosis have been reported in few cases (Rieu *et al.* 2000).

The role of human herpes virus-8 (HHV-8) in the pathogenesis of MCD (Oksenhendler *et al.* 1998) and Crow–Fukase (POEMS) syndrome (Belec *et al.* 1999; Papo *et al.* 1999) is not yet clear. HHV-8 may be a causative agent of a proportion of MCD with or without POEMS syndrome. Another hypothesis is that the infection with HHV-8 is favoured by the overproduction of cytokines, critical to its survival. HHV-8 infection may amplify the 'cytokine storm' of these syndromes and may be a factor of poorer prognosis (Rieu *et al.* 2000).

Paramyxoviruses

Measles

Measles is common and is frequently severe in malnourished children. Urinary epithelial cells from infected patients can be shown to contain measles antigen. However, glomerular involvement has only rarely been reported.

Lin and Hsu (1983) described a child who developed acute nephritis 2 weeks after exposure to measles and 4 days after the appearance of clinical measles. Renal biopsy showed mesangial proliferative GN, and electron microscopy revealed discrete granular electron-dense deposits within the basement membrane and also in a subepithelial position. Immunofluorescence revealed C3 and measles virus antigen within the mesangium. There was rapid resolution of the acute nephritis, and at follow-up 20 months later, renal function, urine analysis, and serum complement were all within normal limits. Partial lipodystrophy associated with C3 nephritic factor and dense deposits disease also may occur after measles infection (Peters *et al.* 1973).

Mumps

In an outbreak of mumps in Taiwan, of 124 children examined 36 had microscopic haematuria and eight had proteinuria. A renal biopsy in one of the patients with persistent haematuria revealed mumps virus antigen in the glomeruli associated with IgG, IgM, and complement (C3), suggesting a causal link between the mumps infection and the immune-complex-mediated GN (Lin *et al.* 1990). IgA nephropathy had been reported after mumps infection in a 5-year-old boy and confirmed by the detection of the mumps DNA virus in the renal biopsy specimen (Fujieda *et al.* 2000).

Parvoviruses

Wierenga *et al.* (1995) reported on seven patients homozygous for sickle cell disease who, following an aplastic crisis, developed proteinuria of sufficient degree to manifest nephrotic syndrome, in association with human parvovirus (B19) infection. Four of the patients who had a renal biopsy during the acute illness had a focal–segmental proliferative GN, and one who had a biopsy 4 months later had FSGS. The outcome in these patients was that one died from renal failure, one recovered completely, and the remainder continued to have impaired renal function. The relationship of the parvovirus infection and the aplastic crises to the glomerular lesions is not clear, as a cohort study of children without sickle cell disease identified 73 episodes of parvovirus B19 infection but none developed nephrotic syndrome. Isolated cases of acute GN secondary to parvovirus B19 infection have been reported (Schmid *et al.* 2000; Taylor *et al.* 2001; Iwafuchi *et al.* 2002). These cases, reviewed in Mori *et al.* (2002) are characterized by renal endocapillary and/or mesangioproliferative GN and spontaneous recovery. One case of Henoch–Schönlein purpura was associated with a parvovirus B19 infection (Diaz and Collazos 2000).

The DNA extracted from kidney tissue and amplified using nested polymerase chain reaction was studied in renal biopsy tissue from 40 patients with various glomerular diseases. Parvovirus B19 DNA was commonly found and the prevalence of parvovirus B19 DNA was significantly greater among patients with idiopathic focal segmental glomerulosclerosis and collapsing glomerulopathy compared with patients with other diagnoses (Tanawattanacharoen *et al.* 2000). The association between parvovirus B19 infection and collapsing glomerulopathy was analysed by polymerase chain reaction and by *in situ* hybridization of arcHIVed biopsies of patients with collapsing glomerulopathy. Parvovirus B19 was detected in renal biopsies of 18 out of 23 patients with collapsing glomerulopathy and only six out of 27 with idiopathic FSGS, and seven out of 27 controls. Parvovirus B19 was identified in glomerular parietal and visceral epithelial and tubular cells. These results suggests a specific association between Parvovirus B19 infection and collapsing glomerulopathy (Moudgil *et al.* 2001).

Polyoma virus BK

BK virus leads to tubular nephropathy in kidney graft recipients, responsible for kidney graft dysfunction and sometimes graft loss. BK virus had been also observed in glomeruli, in the nuclei of parietal epithelial cells (Nebuloni *et al.* 1999). BK-related polyomavirus vasculopathy with endothelial lesions involving glomeruli had been described in a renal-transplant recipient (Petrogiannis-Haliotis *et al.* 2001).

Hepatitis viruses

This important topic is extensively treated in other chapters:

Hepatitis B (see Chapter 3.14)

Hepatitis-B-associated polyarteritis nodosa (see Chapter 4.5.3)

Hepatitis C (see Chapters 3.14 and 4.6)

Retroviruses

HIV

When the first cases of human immunodeficiency virus HIV-associated nephropathy (HIVAN) were reported by Rao *et al.* 1984, the role of the HIV was not completely recognized as cause of AIDS. The clinical, histological characteristics and the evolution of a large variety of renal diseases were then rapidly established in patients with HIV infection. The glomerular, tubulointerstitial, and vascular compartments are affected. Tubulointerstitial injury predominates in most autopsy-based studies, whereas glomerular disease is most frequently identified in biopsy-based studies. The most common glomerular lesion is HIV-associated FSGS and related mesangiopathies (collectively termed HIVAN). Increasingly, a variety of immune-complex-mediated glomerular diseases such as MPGN, IgA nephropathy and 'lupus-like' GN, as well as haemolytic uraemic syndrome/thrombotic thrombocytopaenic purpura have been reported (D'Agati *et al.* 1989; D'Agati and Appel 1998).

The spectrum of tubulointerstitial lesions includes acute tubular necrosis, interstitial nephritis, drug-related interstitial nephritis, and neoplasms including lymphoma and Kaposi's sarcoma. Renal infections include pyelonephritis, and opportunistic infections such as aspergillosis (Halpern *et al.* 1992; Viale *et al.* 1994), *Pseudallescheria boydii* (Scherr *et al.* 1992), murcomycosis (Santos *et al.* 1994), and adenoviruses (Green *et al.* 1994).

Thus, clinical characteristics may provide diagnostic orientation, but a renal biopsy is necessary to differentiate HIVAN from the various other renal lesions observed in HIV infected patients. In fact, given the large variety of renal lesions and the frequent conjunction of opportunistic infections or intravenous drug abuse which may account for the glomerular changes, the term HIVAN should be restricted to patients presenting with proteinuria and progressive reduction of renal function and with a distinctive but not pathognomonic pathology (FSGS often coexisting with glomerular collapses and tubular microcystic dilations). The existence of this specific HIVAN, which may occur in patients with no associated heroin addiction or opportunistic infection, was debated in early reports and finally established (Pardo *et al.* 1987; Humphreys 1995).

Early reports

The first reported association of nephropathy in an AIDS patient was made from the United States by Collins *et al.* (1983), who reported hepatitis-B-associated nephropathy in a homosexual man with AIDS. The following year, Rao *et al.* (1984) reported from Brooklyn on a study of 92 AIDS patients. Renal histology was obtained by biopsy in eight patients, and at autopsy in a further three. On light microscopy, 10 patients exhibited a FSGS. One patient had mesangial proliferative GN with deposition of IgG and C3. Five of the patients were known intravenous drug abusers and all had opportunistic infections including herpes, candida, *Mycobacterium avium intracellulare*, pneumocystis, and cytomegalovirus. However, it was concluded that, although the lesion was similar to that found in intravenous drug abusers, it probably represented a discrete entity since drug abuse did not appear to be a factor in six of the 11 patients.

Pardo *et al.* (1984) reported a prospective study of 75 patients from Miami, of whom 32 had proteinuria in excess of 0.5 g/day. Seven of these had proteinuria in excess of 3 g daily. In addition, they reported an autopsy study of 36 patients, 18 Black and 18 White, of whom 18 were homosexual and 10 were intravenous drug abusers. At autopsy, 17 of the 36 patients had glomerular abnormalities; five had FSGS, of whom four also had tubulointerstitial disease, five had focal–segmental proliferative GN, four had mesangial proliferative GN, and three had diffuse proliferation. The glomeruli appeared normal in 19 patients. Although the FSGS seen in these patients was no different from that seen in intravenous drug abusers, only 10 of the patients examined were known drug addicts. Thirty-five of the 36 patients in this group had evidence of more than one opportunistic infection, with pneumocystis and cytomegalovirus being the most common.

Initial reports from Europe have not confirmed the North American findings. Brunkhorst *et al.* (1989), De Meyer *et al.* (1989), Strauss *et al.* (1993), and Casanova *et al.* (1995) indicated a very wide sprectrum of glomerular changes in HIV-infected adults and children, and the appearances described as 'typical' HIV nephropathy in the North American reports seemed to be rare. Later, typical HIV nephropathy as described initially in the North American reports became more frequent in Europe. A series from Paris (Nochy *et al.* 1993) reported on the renal biopsy findings of 60 HIV-infected patients admitted to departments of nephrology. Two distinct glomerular lesions were identified: focal and segmental glomerulosclerosis which occurred exclusively in Black patients; immune complex type GN which occurred in both black and white patients. Similar results were reported from London. In contrast with the series reported from North America (Pardo *et al.* 1984; Rao *et al.* 1984), none of the patients in the Paris and London (Connolly *et al.* 1995) series were intravenous drug abusers. Thus, the existence of a specific HIVAN became universally established. At the same time, a large variety of other glomerular lesions were reported in HIV-infected patients. The three main types of glomerular nephropathies observed in HIV-infected patients are presented in Table 3. The relative frequency of these three types differs from series to series, depending on clinical recruitment and particularly on ethnic background. This heterogeneity reflects the different pathogenetic links involved between acute or chronic nephropathies in HIV-1 infected patients.

HIV-associated nephropathy

HIVAN is a disease of progressive renal failure with both tubulointerstitial and glomerular lesions. Ocurring almost only in seropositive Black patients, HIVAN affects up to 10 per cent of HIV-positive Black adults and occasionally affects Caucasoids. A large proportion of HIVAN patients are intravenous drug users. HIVAN, the single most common cause of endstage renal failure in seropositive patients, has increased in incidence by 30 per cent each year since 1991 in the United States (Winston *et al.* 1998). Occurring almost exclusively in Blacks, HIVAN became the third leading cause of endstage renal disease (ESRD) in Blacks, ages 20–64, in 1995. During that year, the

Table 3 Types of HIV-associated glomerular nephropathies

Types of HIV associated glomerular nephropathies	Average frequency (%)	Histological renal lesions	Proposed pathogenetic links
HIV-associated nephropathy (HIVAN)	40–80	Focal glomerular sclerosis, 'collapsing nephropathy' Tubular atrophy, microcystic dilation	HIV infection of renal cells (epithelial tubular cells, podocytes, mesangial cells)
HIV-associated immune complexes nephropathy	20–50	Membranoproliferative glomerulonephritis, membranous nephropathy, IgA nephropathy, 'lupus like nephropathy', immunotactoid GN	HIV-associated immune complexes deposition, co-infections associated immune complexes deposition (HBV, HCV, intravenous drug use)
HIV-associated thrombotic microangiopathy	2–10	Glomerular microangiopathy, mesangiolysis	Endothelial cell injury (apoptosis, infection)

absolute number of new AIDS cases declined for the first time since the epidemic began. The decrease occurred predominantly in White males, whereas in Blacks with heterosexual exposures for risk factors, the incidence actually increased (Winston *et al.* 1998). Since the introduction of highly active antiretroviral therapy (HAART), the incidence of death due to AIDS had decreased in the United States for all ethnic groups, including African-American (Ross and Klotman 2002). However, the rate of decline in the incidence of ESRD due to HIV nephropathy has slowed and the number of new cases (in 1999, the most recent year for which datas are available) actually increased (Ross and Klotman 2002). The prevalence of HIVAN among HIV-1 seropositive Black patients has been estimated as low as 3.5 per cent in a cohort of HIV-1 patients screened for proteinuria (Ahuja *et al.* 1999) and as high as 12 per cent in an autopsy study (Shahinian *et al.* 2000).

By contrast, a Northern Italian study of 26 HIV-infected adults (Casanova *et al.* 1995), of whom 19 were intravenous drug addicts showed that none presented with the features which have been described as typical of HIVAN and the only case of HIVAN in a series of 239 autopsies performed on AIDS patients in Switzerland, before the introducion of HAART, was observed in one of the six African patients included in the study (Hailemariam *et al.* 2001). The reasons for this marked racial predilection are not known, but the role of genetic factors in the occurrence of HIVAN is suggested by the observation of a familial clustering of nephropathy in the uninfected relatives of index patients with HIV infection and renal disease. This familial aggregation of endstage renal failure appears to be independent of HIV infection. Although environmental factors cannot be excluded, it is possible that an inherited susceptibility to renal failure is present in many Blacks with HIV infection who subsequently develop nephropathy (Freedman *et al.* 1999).

In the early descriptions, the HIVAN was found to occur at any stage of the disease. In fact, in most patients HIVAN is a late, not early, manifestation of HIV-1 infection (Winston *et al.* 1999). However, HIVAN can some time occur early in the course of HIV infection, even during acute infection before seroconversion. Thus, a prolonged exposure to virus is not necessary for this renal involvement to occur in the susceptible host (Levin *et al.* 2001). The clinical course has changed very little from its early description (Bourgoignie 1990). Most patients present with proteinuria and progressive reduction of renal function. Hypertension is absent in most patients who are volume depleted. The proteinuria ranges from moderate to nephrotic levels. Suggestive features of HIVAN include the presence of renal tubular epithelial cells in the urinary sediment and normal or large echogenic kidneys despite significant renal insufficiency (Fig. 1). Even if the diagnosis of HIVAN may be clinically likely, biopsy confirmation is important in order to distinguish HIVAN from other forms of of renal disease in HIV-1 seropositive patients.

HIVAN has a remarkable, distinctive pathology involving all compartments of the kidney. FSGS is the most common lesion in adults with podocyte proliferation and loss of differentiation markers, often coexisting with glomerular collapses and tubular pathology including atrophy and microcystic dilations (D'Agati and Appel 1998). This microcystic dilation is responsible for increased kidney echogenicity and size. The interstitium shows infiltration by leucocytes, primarily $CD8^+$ T-lymphocytes and macrophages. Interstitial oedema and fibrosis is frequently noted. Diffuse mesangial hyperplasia associated with some degree of podocytes hypertrophy is more frequently observed in children and Caucasoids and has a less severe clinical presentation with non-nephrotic proteinuria and normal renal function (Strauss *et al.* 1993; Ray *et al.* 1998). Mesangial hyperplasia is considered by some authors as an early stage of FSGS (Bourgoignie *et al.* 1990). Conversely, idiopathic FSGS with predominantly collapsing features is not pathognomonic of HIVAN since it has been observed in patients lacking evidence of HIV-1 infection or intravenous drug use (Valeri *et al.* 1996).

Electron microscopy shows retraction of the glomerular basement membrane and frequently, tubular reticular inclusions in endothelial cells. The latter is not specific and thought to be induced by interferon-α. Indeed, the less frequent occurrence of tubular reticular inclusions observed recently may reflect the reduction of systemic interferon-α levels observed in patients treated by HAART. Multiple electron dense deposits observed in HIVAN may correspond to immune-complex-associated nephropathy superimposed on FSGF (D'Agati *et al.* 1989).

Physiopathology of HIV-associated nephropathy

The key role of the virus in HIVAN is now well established. Several studies demonstrated that HIV-1 is able to infect renal tubular and

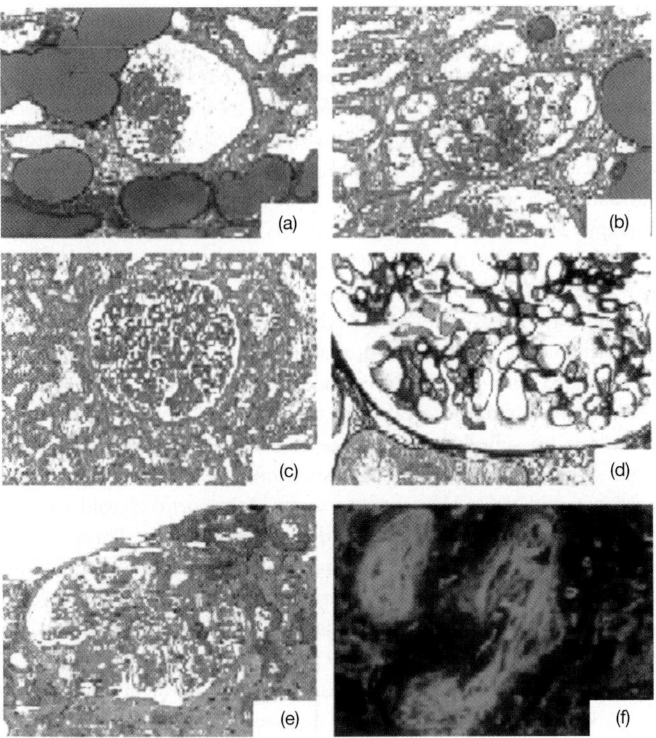

Fig. 1 HIV associated glomerular nephropathies. (a) Collapsing glomerulosclerosis: light microscopy showing few open loops, large urinary space in glomerulus and severe tubulointerstitial injury with microcyst formation and tubular degeneration. Masson's trichrome 160×. (b) Collapsing glomerulosclerosis: light microscopy showing micro- and macrovacuolization in podocytes and severe tubulointerstitial lesions. Masson's trichrome 160×. (c) MPGN: light microscopy showing mesangial proliferation and subendothelial deposits. Masson's trichrome 160×. (d) Membranous GN: light microscopy showing subepithelial deposits in red. Jones' staining 400×. (e) Thrombotic microangiopathy: light microscopy showing large endothelial cells in glomerulus and thrombosis in preglomerular arterioles. Masson's trichrome 200×. (f) Thrombotic microangiopathy: immunofluorescence study showing fibrinogen in arteriolar lumens 400× (with grateful acknowledgement to Dr Laure-Hélène Noël, INSERM U507, Hôpital Necker, Paris).

glomerular epithelial cells or podocytes, cells that are a critical part of the filtration barrier. The demonstration of HIV replication has been obtained in a human study of renal biopsy. Renal glomerular and tubular epithelial cells contain HIV-1 mRNA and DNA, indicating infection by HIV-1. In addition, circularized viral DNA, a marker of recent nuclear import of full-length, reverse-transcribed RNA, was detected in the biopsies, suggesting active replication in renal tissue. Thus, renal epithelium constitutes a unique and previously unrecognized reservoir and cell target for HIV-1 infection (Bruggeman *et al.* 2000). It was found that microcysts involve multiple nephron segments in both patients with HIVAN and HIV-1 transgenic mice. Furthermore, HIV-1 infection in HIVAN and HIV-1 transgene expression also occurs in multiple segments of the nephron, indicating a direct role for HIV-1 infection of renal epithelial cells in the pathogenesis of microcyst formation in patients with HIVAN (Ross *et al.* 2001). By contrast, HIV-1 RNA was not detected in intrinsic renal cells in a recent study. Thus, a role of productive HIV-1 infection of renal parenchymal cells in the pathogenesis of HIV-associated renal disease remain disputed (Eitner *et al.* 2000). However, increasing evidence supports a role for HIV-1 infection of renal epithelium in the pathogenesis of HIVAN. Marras *et al.* (2002) investigated whether renal epithelial cells were productively infected by HIV-1. Infected renal epithelial cells were removed by laser-capture microdissection from biopsies of two patients, DNA was extracted, and two particular HIV-1 sequences were amplified from individually dissected cells by nested PCR. Phylogenetic analysis of kidney-derived sequences as well as corresponding sequences from peripheral blood mononuclear cells of the same patients revealed evidence of tissue-specific viral evolution. These data, along with the detection of HIV-1-specific proviral DNA and mRNA in tubular epithelium cells, argue strongly for localized replication of HIV-1 in the kidney and the existence of a renal viral reservoir (Marras *et al.* 2002).

The normal differentiation of podocytes coincides with progressive expression of maturity markers, including WT-1, and synaptopodin. In collapsing forms of FSGS of HIVAN, podocytes undergo characteristic, irreversible ultrastructural changes together with the disappearance of the differentiation markers (Barisoni *et al.* 1999). In general, under pathological conditions, podocytes may undergo mitosis, but not cell division. Exceptions to this rule are collapsing glomerulopathies of HIVAN where podocytes undergo a dysregulation of their differentiated phenotype and proliferate. HIV-infection induces loss of contact inhibition (Schwartz *et al.* 2001) and loss of podocyte differentiation markers and increases podocyte proliferation (Kajiyama *et al.* 2000; Husain *et al.* 2002). In addition, HIVAN showed a marked reduction in the expression of cyclins and cyclin-dependent kinase inhibitors which may account for the activation of podocyte proliferation in collapsing nephropathy (Barisoni *et al.* 1999; Shankland *et al.* 2000). One HIV-1 gene responsible for proliferative changes was identified by using cultured podocytes *in vitro*. Deletion of nef markedly reduced proliferation and colony formation. Nef may therefore be an important gene in the pathogenesis of HIVAN. However, in the *in vivo* mice model nef is not required for the induction of renal disease (Kajiyama *et al.* 2000).

The genes responsible for the development of HIVAN have been mapped in transgenic animal models. Studies in HIV transgenic mice, bearing a gag–pol deleted HIV genome, strongly suggested that the HIV genes or proteins expressed in renal tissue cause a renal disease that is identical to HIVAN since these mice showed a rapidly progressive nephropathy similar to the human nephropathy. In this model, the HIVAN seems to be related to early states of intense viral replication rather than to later stages of the infection (Kopp *et al.* 1992; Bruggeman *et al.* 1997). In the rat HIV type 1 (HIV-1) transgenic (Tg) rat, the expression of a transgene, consisting of an HIV-1 provirus with a functional deletion of gag and pol led to viral transcripts expression in lymph nodes, thymus, liver, kidney, and spleen. The HIV-1 transgenic rat has many clinical and histopathological similarities (including renal lesions) to humans infected with HIV-1 (Reid *et al.* 2001). Therefore, it is unlikely that the genes gag and pol are required for HIVAN pathogenesis. Chimeric simian–human immunodeficiency viruses (SHIV) viruses containing tat, rev, vpu, and env from HIV-1 in a genetic background of simian immunodeficiency virus (SIV) have been produced. *In vivo* SHIV infection in rhesus macaques causes severe glomerulosclerosis analogous to HIVAN. The sclerosed glomeruli showed an active replication (Stephens *et al.* 2000).

The mode of penetration of the HIV is particular for renal cells since the usual viral receptors and coreceptors (CD4+, CXCR4, or

CCR5) are inconstantly found in renal cells. For example, the viral receptor CD4 has been found to be present on mesangial cells (Green *et al.* 1992) or absent (Alpers *et al.* 1992; Ray *et al.* 1998). The expression of other viral coreceptors has been studied (Green *et al.* 1992; Conaldi *et al.* 1998; Eitner *et al.* 2000) and the receptors CCR3, CXCR4, CCR5, and more recently CCR2b and GPR1 have been found on tubular and mesangial cells. In contrast, Eitner *et al.* studied renal biopsies from patients and found that chemokine receptors CCR5 and CXCR4 were undetectable in glomerular, tubular, and vascular cells and that in the presence of tubulointerstitial inflammation, CCR5 and CXCR4 expressions were localized to infiltrating mononuclear leukocytes (Eitner *et al.* 2000). Additionally, the HIV-1 infection of renal cells could be due to disruptions in nuclear envelope architecture and integrity induced by HIV-1 protein, Vpr (de Noronha *et al.* 2001).

Cytokines and growth factors imbalance secondary to HIV infection may amplify the renal lesions. TGF-β expression, increased in several progressive glomerular diseases, was particularly elevated in HIVAN (Bodi *et al.* 1995). In addition, renal cell production of IL-6 and TNF-α might provide a potent stimulus for HIV-1 expression in HIV-1-infected monocytes that infiltrate the kidney, and that this may play an important role in the pathogenesis of HIVAN (O'Donnell *et al.* 1998).

Treatment of HIV-associated nephropathy

The prognosis of patients with HIVAN is poor, particularly if interstitial changes are prominent. Although there is no evidence of effective therapy based on controlled studies, the efficiency of highly active antiretroviral therapy is likely since its introduction was accompanied, after 1995, by a decreased number of new cases of endstage renal failure caused by HIVAN in the United States (Ross and Klotman 2002). Corticosteroids and angiotensin-converting enzyme (ACE) inhibitors are also considered in the treatment of HIVAN.

The efficacy of antiretroviral medications has been evaluated in several studies. The efficacy of monotherapy with zidovudine is debated. Initial reports showed little benefit. However, some studies suggested that zidovudine is effective in preventing renal failure, particularly in compliant patients (Ifudu *et al.* 1995) and when started early in the course of HIVAN (Michel *et al.* 1992). Although not based on well-controlled trials, the efficacy of highly active antiretroviral therapy is almost certain since it had a beneficial effect on the incidence of HIVAN in the United States. A retrospective cohort study of 19 patients described the clinical course of HIV-related renal diseases and the effect of protease inhibitors on their progression. The cohort consisted of 16 African-Americans, two Caucasians, and one Native American. Longitudinal multivariate analyses demonstrated an association between protease inhibitors and prednisone and a slower decline in creatinine clearance (Szczech *et al.* 2002). In two case reports, treatment of patients with dialysis-dependent renal failure were sucessfully treated with HAART and repeat renal biopsies in both patients revealed resolution of the histological lesions including collapsing FSGS and tubular microcystic dilation (Wali *et al.* 1998; Winston *et al.* 2001).

Some patients with idiopathic FSGS may respond to corticosteroid therapy (Phinney *et al.* 1994). Smith *et al.* (1996) prospectively evaluated 20 consecutive HIV-infected adults with HIVAN ($n = 17$) and serum creatinine concentrations greater than 177 µmol/l (2 mg/dL) or proteinuria greater than 2.0 g/d or both, treated with prednisone at a dose of 60 mg/day for 2–11 weeks, followed by a tapering course of prednisone over a 2–26-week period. Two patients progressed to end stage renal disease in 4–5 weeks. In 17 patients serum creatinine levels decreased. Five patients relapsed after prednisone was discontinued and were retreated with partial response to the second course of prednisone. The 20 patients have been followed for a median of 44 weeks. Eight ultimately required maintenance dialysis. Eleven died from complications of HIV disease. Seven are alive and free from ESRD, a median of 25 weeks (range 8–81) from the initiation of prednisone therapy. Six patients developed serious infections while receiving prednisone, including Mycobacterium avium-complex infection in two (Smith *et al.* 1996). A retrospective cohort study of twenty one patients with biopsy-proven HIVAN and progressive azotaemia who were eligible for corticosteroid treatment. Thirteen selected patients were treated with 60 mg of prednisone for one month, followed by a several-month taper whereas eight had not. On long-term follow-up, there was no significant difference in the incidence of hospitalizations or of serious infections. At six months, only one of the non-corticosteroid-treated patients but seven of the corticosteroid-treated group continued to have independent renal function. Three of the corticosteroid-treated group continued to have independent function at two years of follow-up. Thus, a limited course of corticosteroid therapy in selected patients was beneficial and safe (Eustace *et al.* 2000). In the retrospective cohort study of 19 patients reported by Szczech *et al.* (2002), showing an effect of protease inhibitors on the progression of HIVAN, longitudinal multivariate analyses demonstrated an highly significant association between prednisone and a slower decline in creatinine clearance and corticosteroid-related side-effects were not prohibitive (Szczech *et al.* 2002). However, prospective, randomized controlled trials are required to confirm these results.

There is evidence that ACE inhibitors may be beneficial. Kimmel *et al.* (1996) showed in a retrospective study, using a Cox regression analysis, that captopril and antiretroviral therapy were associated with enhanced renal survival, while age, serum creatinine, urinary protein–creatinine ratio, and CD4 count were not. Burns *et al.* (1997) examined the effect of fosinopril (10 mg daily) in 20 patients with HIVAN and observed that treatment with ACE inhibitor stabilize serum creatinine and 24-h protein excretion for up to 24 weeks in patients with non-nephrotic-range proteinuria and for up to 12 weeks in patients with nephrotic-range proteinuria when initial serum creatinine is less or equal to 180 µmol/l. Such findings must be confirmed by randomized, double-blind, placebo-controlled trials.

Early reports indicated that survival on dialysis was limited and that peritoneal dialysis seemed to be preferable. The disparities in the demographic composition of the patient populations probably underlies differences in survival in dialysis patients reported from different centers. The course of therapy for dialysis patients is improving, but ultimately depends on the stage of the viral illness. Transplantation is currently a low-priority treatment option for HIV-infected patients with ESRD (Kimmel *et al.* 1998).

HIV-associated immune-complexes nephropathies

Although focal glomerulosclerosis is the most common renal disease, other proliferative glomerulonephritides are encountered in HIV-infected patients. Some HIV-infected patients with renal insufficiency, proteinuria, and proliferative GN, may have an immune-mediated nephropathy, related to deposition of immune complexes in multiple sites, mesangial, subendothelial, intra- and epimembranous. The complexes contain HIV antigen and antibody to gp 120 HIV (Kimmel *et al.* 1993). The histological lesions are characterized in most patients by endocapillary proliferation with parietal fibrinoid deposits in multiple sites. Deposits may be so intense that it resembles lupus nephropathy ('lupus like' GN). Deposits contain immunoglobulins, C1q and C3. Interstitial infiltrates are frequent with a higher frequency of B cells than in HIVAN and the progression to renal failure is slower than in HIVAN (Bodi *et al.* 1994). HIV-infected patients often have hepatitis C virus (HCV) coinfection. The clinical–pathological features and outcome of HCV-associated glomerular disease has been reported in 14 patients with HIV coinfection. All were intravenous drug users and all but one were African-Americans. Renal presentations included renal insufficiency, microscopic haematuria with active urine sediment, hypertension, and nephrotic syndrome or nephrotic-range proteinuria without hypercholesterolaemia. Hypocomplementaemia and cryoglobulinaemia were present in more than one third of patients. The predominant renal biopsy findings were MPGN and less frequently membranous glomerulopathy. The clinical course was characterized by rapid progression to renal failure requiring dialysis. In patients with HCV-associated GN, coinfection with HIV leads to an aggressive form of renal disease that can be easily confused with HIVAN. Although hypocomplementaemia, cryoglobulinaemia, and more prominent hypertension and microscopic haematuria may provide clues to the presence of HCV-related renal lesions, renal biopsy is essential to differentiate HCV-related renal lesions from HIVAN (Cheng *et al.* 1999).

A systematic study of kidney in 116 deceased AIDS patients showed diffuse mesangial IgA deposits in nine (7.75 per cent). Thus, IgA nephropathy related to HIV infection is not rare. Urinary abnormalities were mild in all cases. By light microscopy, glomerular lesions were absent or moderate (mesangial hypertrophy or some mesangial deposits) (Beaufils *et al.* 1995). Anti-idiotypic IgA reacting with anti-gp41 IgG were detected in circulating immune complexes in patients with HIV infection and IgA nephropathy (Kimmel *et al.* 1992).

Fibrillary/immunotactoid GN in HIV-positive patients was observed in three cases (Haas *et al.* 2000). Renal amyloidosis is rarely observed in HIV-infected patients (Joseph *et al.* 2000).

HIV-associated thrombotic microangiopathy

Boccia *et al.* (1984) reported the first observation of haemolytic uraemic syndrome in a man with AIDS treated with chemotherapy for Kaposi's sarcoma. Since that time, thrombotic microangiopathy (TMA) has been increasingly reported in HIV-infected humans over the past decade (Hymes and Karpatkin 1997; D'Agati and Appel 1998; Peraldi *et al.* 1999). TMA is an unfrequent cause of renal lesions in HIV-infected patients. Conversely, retroviral infections represent a significant cause in recent series of TMA. Eleven of 50 serum samples collected from patients with a diagnosis of TMA, from 1979 to 1991, tested positive for antiretroviral antibodies. Seven had HIV infection, and four had human lymphotrophic virus, type I (HTLV- I) infection (Ucar *et al.* 1994). Since the introduction of HAART, the incidence of TMA in HIV-infected patients had markedly diminished.

Renal insufficiency is constant and required haemodialysis in 20 per cent of cases. Haemolytic anaemia and thrombocytopaenia are present in all patients but shyzocytes are infrequently found (Peraldi *et al.* 1999). Severe hypertension is present in 50 per cent of cases. Neurological manifestations (convulsions, cerebellar signs, coma) are present in the majority of the cases. The course of TMA in HIV-infected patients is severe. Although short-term responses to plasma therapy in HIV-seropositive patients did not differ from other patients, no HIV-positive patient survived more than 2 years from diagnosis of TMA (Thompson *et al.* 1992). The typical histological TMA lesions (thrombi in glomerular capillary loops and small arteries, mesangiolysis) and electron microscopic lesions (mesangiolysis, subendothelial lucency, platelet thrombi in glomerular capillary lumina) may be associated with other renal lesions associated with AIDS. Multiple causes may be involved such as drugs, lymphomas, neoplasias, or infections. The pathogenesis is unknown, but is thought to be the result of endothelial injury. The role of HIV is unclear but its proapoptotic effect on endothelial cells may play a role (Laurence *et al.* 1996). The study of the renal pathology of macaques, acutely infected with a virulent strain of HIV-2. Typical lesions of human HIV-associated nephropathy were undetectable but about 25 per cent of macaques showed typical histological TMA lesions (Eitner *et al.* 1999). A complete deficiency of VWF-cleaving protease and the presence of a concentration-dependent IgG1 inhibitor in the plasma of a patient with AIDS (Sahud *et al.* 2002).

Other renal manifestations

Acute renal failure The coexistence of seropositivity for HIV-1 and/or AIDS with renal insufficiency is common. Patients with HIV infection may have acute or chronic renal failure. In a recent study in Paris, Peraldi *et al.* (1999) found the haemolytic uraemic syndrome to be the most frequent cause of acute renal failure in 35 per cent of the cases. In addition, 15 per cent of patients had HIVAN. In this study and in previous (Rao 1998), it was emphasized that acute elevation of serum creatinine was frequently due to others factors: volume depletion is frequent as a result of salt wasting, poor nutrition, or vomiting, obstructive uropathy and acute tubular necrosis due to recurrent infections and toxicity of medication or radiological contrast media. The nephrotoxicity of the medications used to treat bacterial, fungal, and viral complications of HIV infection (e.g. aminoglycosides, sulfamethoxazole/trimethoprim, amphotericin, pentamidine, and foscarnet) has been recognized for some time. The acute renal toxicity of antiretroviral drugs has been observed (Bourgoignie 1990; Rao 1998).

Crystalluria Indinavir, a protease inhibitor widely used to treat patients with HIV infection, has been associated with nephrolithiasis. Indinavir forms characteristic crystals in the urine and may be associated with dysuria and urinary frequency, with flank or back pain associated with intrarenal sludging, and with the classic syndrome of renal colic. Nineteen of the 240 patients receiving indinavir (8 per cent) developed urologic symptoms. Of these, seven (3 per cent) had nephrolithiasis and the other 12 (5 per cent) had previously undescribed syndromes: crystalluria associated with dysuria and crystalluria associated with back or flank pain (Kopp *et al.* 2002).

Electrolyte disorders Hyponatraemia is common (Glassock *et al.* 1990; Tang *et al.* 1993), occurring in 40 per cent of patients with AIDS or AIDS-related complex, and may be due to a variety of causes including gastrointestinal fluid loss, adrenal insufficiency, inappropriate ADH secretion associated with pulmonary and central nervous system infections, and acute renal failure. Hyponatraemia is mild in the majority of patients, but in a few it is severe and symptomatic. Hyperkalaemia is less common but may arise owing to adrenal insufficiency, pentamidine therapy, or acute renal failure, whereas hypokalaemia may result from gastrointestinal loss due to diarrhoea or metabolic alkalosis due to prolonged vomiting. Symptomatic hypocalcaemia and hypomagnesaemia due to renal magnesium wasting have been reported in a patient with AIDS treated with pentamidine (Shah *et al.* 1990).

HTLV-1

Two Jamaican children presented with infective dermatitis, GN, severe hypertension with hypertensive encephalopathy, renal failure, and human T-cell lymphotropic virus (HTLV-1) seropositivity. Histological findings from renal biopsy specimens in both cases revealed significant glomerulosclerosis with fibrosis, chronic inflammatory cell infiltrates in the interstitium, and arteriolar hypertensive changes. MPGN was demonstrable in case 1 and marked focal glomerulosclerosis in case 2. Both developed end-stage renal. A causal relationship between HTLV-1 infection and renal disease cannot be proven (Miller *et al.* 2001).

The anti-HTLV-1 antibody-positive rate in patients with primary GN in the Nagasaki district, an endemic area of HTLV-1, was evaluated. The antibody-positive rates in patients with primary GN (9.9 per cent) and in haemodialysis patients (18.4 per cent) were significantly greater than the rate in general blood donors (6.6 per cent). Of 142 patients with primary GN, 14 (9.9 per cent) were positive for the antibody; histological evaluation of these patients showed minor glomerular abnormality in one, mesangial proliferative glomerulonephritis in eight (IgA nephropathy in six and non-IgA nephropathy in two), membranous nephropathy in three, and crescentic GN in two (Namie *et al.* 1995).

Influenza viruses

Influenza

Although influenza is common and epidemics frequently occur, associated renal disease has only been reported occasionally. Goodpasture (1919) described a young man who died 6 weeks after contracting influenza and who had pulmonary haemorrhage and glomerulonephritis (see Chapter 4.11). Wilson and Smith (1972) described a patient who developed proteinuria and haematuria associated with haemoptysis following influenza. Renal biopsy revealed proliferative glomerulonephritis and a linear deposition of immunoglobulins on the glomerular capillary basement membrane. There was no impairment of renal function and the pulmonary and renal abnormalities resolved completely. However, Perez *et al.* (1974) reported a number of patients with rapidly progressive renal failure and typical Goodpasture's syndrome during an outbreak of influenza.

Haemolytic uraemic syndrome has also been reported in association with influenza A virus infection (Davison *et al.* 1973; Watanabe 2001). Clinical presentation was with acute renal failure requiring haemodialysis. Renal biopsy revealed endothelial cell changes and glomerular capillary fibrin deposition typical of disseminated intravascular coagulation. One patient recovered completely, whereas the other died from massive intrapulmonary haemorrhage.

Bacterial infections

General remarks

The association of bacterial infections with glomerulopathy has been accepted for many years. It is well established that the antibody response to bacterial antigens can result in the presence of immune complexes in the circulation and/or tissues. Whereas it was previously assumed that these immune complexes formed in the circulation and then became trapped in the glomerulus as a secondary event, it is now generally accepted that in the majority of cases the complexes are formed locally within the glomerular capillary wall or mesangium. There, they activate the complement and coagulation systems and induce an inflammatory response (see Chapters 3.2 and 3.3).

The pattern of glomerular response is not uniform. Even in epidemics not everyone who is infected develops glomerular disease, and the clinical picture and histological appearances of those who do are seldom uniform. This suggests that many other factors, possibly genetic and nutritional, have an important influence on the development of the glomerular lesion. The widespread use of antibiotic therapy, which has resulted in the prompt treatment of most infectious diseases, also has an effect. Chronic infections are much less of a problem than in the past and, as a result, complications such as amyloidosis are decreasing in frequency.

Streptococcus spp. (see Chapter 3.9)

The relationship between acute GN and epidemics of scarlatina has been recognized for over 200 years (see Miller 1849). However, there is no doubt that the epidemiology of poststreptococcal GN has changed significantly in the past century, in that there has been a significant decline in the incidence in developed countries, although sporadic cases continue to be reported. Epidemic poststreptococcal GN appears to occur mainly in developing countries such as Africa, the West Indies, and the Middle East. Reasons for this changing epidemiology relate to the nutritional status of the community, the more liberal use of antibiotics, and, possibly, changes in the nephritogenic potential of streptococcus.

Poststreptococcal GN is described in detail in Chapter 3.9.

Staphylococcus spp.

Glomerular lesions associated with staphylococcal infections arise mainly in two different clinical situations: most commonly after *Staphylococcus aureus* bacteraemia in patients with infective endocarditis but also after *Staphylococcus epidermidis* infection in patients with ventriculojugular shunt (see below).

Many organisms have been implicated in infective endocarditis (see below), but the most common is *S. aureus*. The first reports (Löhlein 1910) suggested that the glomerular lesion was due to bacterial embolization from the infected valve. This view is no longer supportable, and the lesion is considered to be immunologically mediated. Infective endocarditis is associated with high titres of circulating immune complexes, hypocomplementaemia and glomerular immunoglobulin deposition, and staphylococcal antigens are present within involved glomeruli. It is also possible that staphylococcal cell wall antigens may directly activate complement by the alternative pathway, resulting in glomerular damage, and this may explain the occurrence of glomerulonephritis after a short duration of endocarditis, in the absence of immune complexes and with no glomerular immunoglobulin deposition. On light microscopy, patients with acute fulminating endocarditis tend to have a diffuse proliferative GN, whereas those with a subacute form tend to have a focal segmental proliferative GN, which may show sclerosis in the late stages.

Koyama *et al.* (1995) have reported glomerulonephritis (mesangioproliferative with and without crescents, mesangiocapillary, and segmental necrotizing) in association with methicillin-resistant *S. aureus* (MRSA) infection. In the patients reported, there was a polyclonal increase in IgG and IgA with massive T-cell activation and cytokine release attributed to staphylococcal enterotoxin acting as a 'superantigen' (Koyama and Hirayama 2001). Patients who developed GN in association with MRSA infection showed a marked increase in

DR + CD4 + and DR + CD8 + subsets of T cells and in T cells expressing several TCR Vβ (Koyama *et al.* 1995), especially Vβ-5 family TCR. These patients also showed increased serum cytokines, including tumour necrosis factor-α (TNF-α), interleukin-1 β (IL-1 β), IL-2, IL-6, IL-8, and IL-10 suggesting that T cells activated by MRSA-derived staphylococcal enterotoxins and subsequent production of cytokines may play an important role in the pathogenesis of MRSA-associated GN (Yoh *et al.* 2000).

Staphylococcal septicaemia is associated with proliferative GN; an autopsy study demonstrated glomerular changes in 35 per cent of patients who died from staphylococcal septicaemia (Powell 1961). Septicaemia may also occur in association with intravenous drug abuse, and such patients have a high incidence of associated proliferative GN (Treser *et al.* 1974). Staphylococcal colonization of ventriculo-atrial and ventriculoperitoneal shunts, used in the treatment of hydrocephalus, is a relatively common problem (see below). These patients present with symptoms suggestive of recurrent bacteraemia such as fever, arthralgia, hepatosplenomegaly, and oedema. Infection most commonly occurs within 2 months of catheter insertion. Renal involvement is manifest by haematuria, which is occasionally macroscopic, and proteinuria, which results in a nephrotic syndrome in 25 per cent of patients. Circulating immune complexes, cryoglobulinaemia, hypocomplementaemia, and high titres of antistaphylococcal antibodies are well described. Renal biopsy most commonly reveals type I mesangiocapillary GN which may be associated with minor crescent formation. A few patients have diffuse exudative proliferative GN, minor mesangial proliferation, or segmental lesions.

Occasionally, other staphylococcal infections, such as osteomyelitis (Boonshaft *et al.* 1970; Griffin *et al.* 1997) and impetigo (Takaue and Tokumaru 1982) have been associated with GN; very occasionally, IgA nephropathy has been associated with staphylococcal infection (Levy *et al.* 1985).

Streptococcus pneumoniae (pneumococcus)

Historically, renal disease (mainly tubulointerstitial) was a common sequel to pneumococcal infections, but since the introduction of antibiotics only sporadic case reports have appeared. Clinical presentation is with haematuria, minimal proteinuria, and only mild impairment of renal function. Renal biopsy shows acute glomerulonephritis, with subepithelial humps and intramembranous deposits. Pneumococcal antigen has been detected within the mesangium (Hyman *et al.* 1975; Kaehny *et al.* 1978). In addition, cryoglobulins were detected in one patient and pneumococcal capsular antigen was demonstrated within the cryoprecipitate (Kaehny *et al.* 1978).

Disseminated intravascular coagulation may occur following pneumococcal infection, and one case has been described with focal membranous GN and granular deposition of pneumococcal capsular antigen along glomerular capillary walls (Rytel *et al.* 1974). Disseminated intravascular coagulation is thought to be precipitated by neuraminidase released by the bacterium.

Salmonella typhi

Typhoid fever is relatively common but is rarely associated with GN, even in endemic areas, presumably because of the predominance of the gastrointestinal symptoms. Renal involvement in typhoid fever may be manifest as cystitis or pyelonephritis. Acute renal failure may result from dehydration or as a result of intravascular coagulation and haemolysis, as in haemolytic uraemic syndrome; this occurs more commonly in patients with glucose 6-phosphate dehydrogenase deficiency. Glomerular involvement occurs in approximately 2–4 per cent of patients in endemic areas.

Typhoid fever rarely presents with renal manifestation although renal involvement may be relatively common. Microscopic (and occasionally macroscopic) haematuria, associated with moderate proteinuria and normal or slightly diminished renal function, are found on presentation. In a series of children reported from South Africa, oedema had been present for more than 1 month in 50 per cent of patients, and pyrexia and splenomegaly were common (Buka and Coovadia 1980). *Salmonella typhi* may be isolated from blood, stool, or urine culture, and there may be serological evidence of infection with the detection of O and H antibodies. C3 concentrations are frequently reduced, as is IgG and IgM, although IgA values are significantly elevated, presumably due to antigenic stimulation of plasma cells within the lamina propria of the gastrointestinal tract, which is the site of entry of the bacteria.

Renal biopsy has shown both mesangial proliferative GN (Musa *et al.* 1981) and IgA nephropathy (Amerio *et al.* 1972; Indrapasit *et al.* 1985); acute diffuse proliferative GN (Buka and Coovadia 1980) and crescentic IgA nephropathy in an HIV-positive patient with enteric salmonella infection have also been described (Hsieh *et al.* 1996). Most commonly, there is a proliferation of mesangial cells, and matrix and minor crescents may be present in a few glomeruli. Mesangial deposition of IgA, IgG, and C3 are common, and there are two reports on the detection of salmonella Vi antigen within glomeruli (Sitprija *et al.* 1974; Indrapasit *et al.* 1985). There is frequently a focal interstitial fibrosis. Histology reveals normal glomeruli in patients in whom haemolytic uraemic syndrome develops as a consequence of typhoid fever, but there is widespread tubular degeneration and interstitial mononuclear cell infiltration similar to that found in acute tubular necrosis.

Several reports from Egypt and Sudan have implicated chronic salmonella bacteraemia in the pathogenesis of acute nephrotic syndrome in patients with hepatosplenic schistosomiasis (Barsoum *et al.* 1977). Biopsy in these patients reveals acute diffuse proliferative GN. Resolution occurs on effective treatment of the typhoid fever, suggesting that salmonella, rather than the schistosomes, is responsible for the nephropathy in these patients.

The glomerular lesion is probably immune-complex mediated. The significantly elevated serum IgA may result from antigenic stimulation within the lamina propria of the gastrointestinal tract at the site of entry of the bacteria. The association of mesangial IgA deposition and the detection of the Vi antigen within the mesangium is further support for the conception of immune mediation. The glomerular disease is frequently mild and transient. Prognosis clearly depends on a number of factors; many patients are frequently malnourished. In the study of Buka and Coovadia (1980) the overall mortality of children with typhoid fever was between 3 and 8 per cent, but was 20 per cent in those complicated by GN. In adults, the mortality in typhoid glomerulonephritis may be as high as 30 per cent.

Mycobacteria

Mycobacterium tuberculosis

Glomerular involvement in tuberculosis usually results from amyloidosis arising from chronic infection (see Chapter 4.2). The decreasing incidence of tuberculosis associated with effective antituberculous chemotherapy has resulted in a significant decline in the incidence of such amyloidosis.

Chronic tuberculosis may also be associated with other types of glomerular disease, however. One patient with a dense deposit type mesanigocapillary GN was described by Hariprasad *et al.* (1979) and by Pecchini *et al.* (1997), and further case reports described patients with focal proliferative GN (Shribman *et al.* 1983) and also with IgA nephropathy (De Siati *et al.* 1999; Matsuzawa *et al.* 2002).

Tuberculous patients treated with rifampicin may develop acute tubular and interstitial nephritis and rarely rapidly progressive GN (De Vriese *et al.* 1998; Muthukumar *et al.* 2002).

Mycobacterium leprae

This is dealt with in Chapter 3.14.

Other bacterial infections

There are many reports of GN in patients with other bacterial infections. However, the frequency of the infections and the relative paucity of the reports must cast doubt on a causal relationship. Detection of an appropriate bacterial antigen has not been possible in the majority, and it is likely that glomerular disease is coincidental in a number of cases.

Brucellosis may be complicated by proteinuria and haematuria, particularly during acute infection. There are case reports of patients with acute *Brucella melitensis* infection who had IgA nephropathy (Nunan *et al.* 1984; Siegelmann *et al.* 1992) or mesangiocapillary GN (Sharivker *et al.* 2001; Altiparmak *et al.* 2002).

E. coli infection is common and a significant number of patients have septicaemia, but glomerular disease has been reported only in three patients. In two patients, renal involvement became manifest after *E. coli* septicaemia, in one as a severe nephrotic syndrome (Jacquot and Bariéty 1980) and in the other as acute renal failure due to acute proliferative GN (Zappacosta and Ashby 1977). Following antibiotic therapy, renal disease completely resolved in both patients. In the third patient acute proliferative GN occured after *E. coli* infection associated to vesicorenal malakoplakia (Yang *et al.* 2000). The association between infection with verocytotoxin-producing *E. coli* (sero type 0157 : H7) and haemolytic uraemic syndrome is described in Chapter 10.6.3.

Klebsiella pneumoniae has been described as an antecedent of GN in two patients, who developed a microscopic haematuria and minor proteinuria in association with severe glomerulonephritis. *K. pneumoniae* antigens were detected along glomerular basement membranes on immunofluorescence microscopy. In addition, immunoglobulins containing capsular polysaccharide antigens were eluted from the glomeruli (Forrest *et al.* 1977).

Yersinia enterocolitica has been associated with GN, particularly in reports from Scandinavia (Denneberg *et al.* 1981; Friedberg *et al.* 1981). Renal involvement is usually characterized by a variable degree of proteinuria, with occasional microscopic haematuria and, less frequently, impairment of renal function. Renal biopsy shows either proliferative or membranous GN. *Yersinia* antigen has been demonstrated in both the mesangium and the glomerular capillary wall, particularly in those patients with a membranous glomerulonephritis. One patient has been described whose renal biopsy revealed an IgA nephropathy 3 weeks after an acute *Y. enterocolitica* infection (Cusack *et al.* 1983).

Mycoplasma pneumoniae: there are a number of sporadic case reports of glomerular lesions in association with this infection. Renal biopsy has shown proliferative GN (Vitullo *et al.* 1978; Said *et al.* 1999), crescentic GN (Campbell *et al.* 1991), both type I and type II mesangiocapillary GN (von Bonsdorff *et al.* 1984; van Westrhenen *et al.* 1998), and IgA nephropathy (Kanayama *et al.* 1982). Mycoplasma antigen has been demonstrated in the mesangium and the capillary wall (Cochat *et al.* 1985). Acute tubulointerstitial nephritis has also been reported (Campbell *et al.* 1991).

Legionella: the most usual renal disease associated with legionnaires' disease is tubulointerstitial nephritis, but one patient has been reported in whom acute renal failure was associated with mesangial proliferative GN (Hariprasad *et al.* 1985).

Bartonella henselae: 'cat scratch' disease, which is currently considered to be due to infection with this agent has been described in association with GN (D'Agati *et al.* 1990).

Spirochaetal infections

Treponema pallidum

The association between syphilis and dropsy was reported early in the nineteenth century (Blackall 1818), although it is recognized as uncommon. Nephropathy may develop in either congenital syphilis or the secondary phase of an acquired infection.

Nephropathy is uncommon in *congenital syphilis*, but may become evident in the first few months of life, usually with other clinical signs of syphilis. Very occasionally, clinical evidence of congenital syphilis may be absent, and it is wise to undertake serological tests for syphilis in all nephrotic neonates. The most common mode of presentation is with nephrotic syndrome, which may be particularly severe. A few cases present as a nephritic illness. The typical findings on renal biopsy are membranous GN (Losito *et al.* 1979) with subepithelial deposition of IgG and complement (C1q and C3). Mesangial proliferation is variable and small crescents may be present in some cases. The glomerular lesion is immunologically mediated; treponemal antigens have been identified in the glomerular capillary wall deposits (O'Regan *et al.* 1976) and antitreponemal antibodies have been detected by elution studies (Losito *et al.* 1979). Associated tubulointerstitial nephritis is common and may be the dominant feature. Treatment with penicillin is accompanied by resolution of the proteinuria, usually within 2–6 weeks, and by recovery of the glomerular lesion. Further, courses of penicillin may be required for patients in whom significant proteinuria persists. Follow-up biopsies frequently demonstrate a significant percentage of hyalinized glomeruli.

Nephropathy is an uncommon complication of *acquired syphilis* but may become clinically apparent during the secondary phase of the infection. The majority of patients present with a nephrotic syndrome (O'Reagan *et al.* 1976) which becomes clinically manifest about the same time as the typical skin lesions develop. Microscopic haematuria, hypertension, and/or impairment of renal function occur only rarely. On light microscopy there is a membranous GN, frequently accompanied by a slight mesangial proliferation. Immunofluorescence demonstrates subepithelial electron-dense deposits containing IgG and complement (C3 and C1q). Following the institution of penicillin therapy, there is a rapid resolution of the nephropathy. Spontaneous improvement in nephrotic syndrome prior to penicillin therapy is also well recognized (Sterzel *et al.* 1974). This is presumably because the secondary phase of syphilis is a self-limiting immune-complex-mediated disease. Rare cases of rapidly progressive GN have resolved after penicillin therapy alone in one case and after plasma exchange, methylprednisolone, and penicillin in the second (Walker *et al.* 1984; Krane *et al.* 1987).

Leptospirosis

Leptospirosis (Weil's disease) is most commonly associated with acute oliguric renal failure with evidence of hepatic involvement. The renal lesion is usually acute tubulointerstitial nephritis, although some patients develop a mesangial proliferation associated with mesangial subepithelial and intramembranous deposits which contain immunoglobulins and complement (Lai *et al.* 1982).

Rickettsial infections

Rickettsial infections have a predilection for endothelium. Initial swelling of infected endothelial cells is followed by perivascular and intramural infiltration by lymphocytes and macrophages, resulting in a vasculitis.

Rickettsia rickettsii

The mortality from Rocky Mountain spotted fever remains at about 7 per cent despite effective early antibiotic therapy. Death is associated with multiorgan vasculitis involving the central nervous system, myocardium, and kidney. Acute renal failure is common in fatal cases, and is a consequence of systemic rickettsial vasculitis (Walker and Mattern 1979). In these patients, the kidneys show a multifocal perivascular interstitial nephritis of the intertubular capillaries and vessels of the other medulla and corticomedullary junction. Immunofluorescence studies reveal *Rickettsia rickettsii* antigens in intertubular capillaries and in the endothelium of arteries and veins. There are reports of an acute diffuse glomerulonephritis (Allen and Spitz 1945), while others describe a slight glomerular endothelial cell swelling associated with mesangial prominence (De Brito *et al.* 1968). However, none of the 10 cases reported by Walker and Mattern (1979) had evidence of glomerulonephritis. A case of acute oliguric renal failure that developed more than two weeks following the onset of Rocky Mountain spotted fever was reported. Renal biopsy showed acute glomerulonephritis with inflammatory cell infiltration and subendothelial immune deposits (Quigg *et al.* 1991).

Haemolytic uraemic syndrome has been described in a rickettsial infection also (Mettler 1969).

Fungal infections

Candida albicans

Candida infection is relatively common, but there has only been one report convincingly demonstrating an association with glomerular disease. Chesney *et al.* (1976) described a patient with mucocutaneous candidiasis associated with a type I mesangiocapillary GN. *Candida albicans* antigen was detected within both the mesangium and tubular basement membranes. A causal link between the candidiasis and the renal involvement was inferred from the improved renal function and diminution in proteinuria which followed improvement in the mucocutaneous candidiasis.

Histoplasma capsulatum

Renal involvement may occur in approximately one-third of patients with disseminated histoplasmosis and is thought to be immune complex mediated. Bullock *et al.* (1979) described a patient with disseminated histoplasmosis in whom the renal biopsy revealed mild diffuse mesangial proliferation with IgA, IgM, and C3 deposition within the mesangium. Unfortunately, histoplasma antigen could not be detected by indirect immunofluorescence. Nephrotic-range proteinuria and preserved renal function was observed in an HIV-infected patient in association with disseminated histoplasmosis. Immunohistochemical staining of renal biopsy tissue demonstrated immune complexes within the mesangium; *H. capsulatum* antigen was also demonstrated in the mesangium. Therapy with oral itraconazole resulted in marked clinical improvement (Burke *et al.* 1997).

Protozoal infections (see Chapter 3.14)

Protozoal infections are widespread, particularly in tropical areas. The many published reports linking such infections with specific glomerular lesions must be interpreted with caution since these patients frequently have multiple infections (protozoal, bacterial, and viral) and there is commonly associated malnutrition. However, malarial and schistosomal antigens have been detected within glomerular lesions, strongly supporting a causal link for these two parasitic infections.

Malaria-associated (*P. malariae, P. falciparum*) glomerular lesions are described in Chapter 3.14.

Toxoplasmosis

Toxoplasma gondii is an intracellular parasite which has a predilection for cells of the reticuloendothelial and nervous systems. Infection may be congenital or acquired, and in the latter case patients present with a clinical picture similar to that of infectious mononucleosis.

One child with *congenital* toxoplasmosis and glomerular disease presented with the nephrotic syndrome, and a renal biopsy revealed mesangial proliferative GN in which there was also a segmental area of sclerosis and a capsular adhesion. Immunofluorescence revealed IgM and toxoplasma antigen. Following remission a further biopsy was performed, and this revealed a significant number of hyalinized glomeruli; although IgM was still present, toxoplasma antigen could not be identified.

Renal involvement is extremely rare in *acquired* toxoplasmosis. Ginsburg *et al.* (1974) examined 150 biopsy specimens and detected only one patient in whom there was a simultaneous increase in circulating antitoxoplasma antibodies and glomerular deposition of toxoplasma antigen. Treatment with corticosteroids produced a gradual improvement in symptoms and subsequent resolution. A repeat renal biopsy revealed segmental sclerosis, but the toxoplasma antigen was no longer detectable.

Leishmaniasis (kala-azar)

Leishmania donovani: Leishmaniasis is a tropical disease which occurs in two clinical forms, visceral and cutaneous. A number of patients with visceral leishmaniasis, caused by *L. donovani*, have been reported to have associated nephropathy. De Brito *et al.* (1975) described increased mesangial matrix and cellularity and paramesangial electron-dense deposits in biopsy tissue from such patients, and mesangial IgG and C3 deposition have also been reported. The exact relationship between these findings and leishmaniasis is difficult to determine as the majority of patients have considerable malnutrition and intercurrent infections are common. Clinically, the nephropathy is manifested by microscopic haematuria and minor proteinuria. In a prospective study of 50 patients with visceral leishmaniasis, Dutra *et al.* (1985) found that renal involvement was not infrequent. Proteinuria and/or microscopic haematuria or pyuria were observed in 51 per cent of such cases. Of interest was the demonstration of tubulointerstitial involvement in the renal histology of all seven patients studied; also, in five of seven patients there was a proliferative GN, usually mild, on histological examination. Renal involvement was mild and seemed to revert with the cure of the leishmanial infection (Dutra *et al.* 1985). A case of collapsing focal segmental glomerulosclerosis associated with visceral leishmaniasis was observed (Leblond *et al.* 1994).

Trematode infections

Schistosomiasis is described in detail in Chapters 3.14 and 7.4.

Nematode infections

Filariasis is described in detail in Chapter 3.14.

Infections at particular sites

Infective endocarditis

Renal involvement in infective endocarditis is the result of immune-complex-mediated damage to glomeruli and small blood vessels. Tubulointerstitial changes are also common, and may arise as a direct consequence of the infective endocarditis or through a reaction to antibiotic therapy. The association between endocarditis and renal disease was reported early in the last century (Löhlein 1910) and was originally thought to be embolic in nature; the descriptive term 'flea-bitten' kidney was applied. However, the embolic nature of the glomerular lesion was questioned by Bell (1932), who suggested an immunological mechanism. This was further supported by the work of Barker (1949) in a study of endocarditis confined to the right side of the heart. However, the immune nature of the condition was not confirmed until the finding of hypocomplementaemia (Williams and Kunkel 1962), the demonstration of glomerular immune complex deposition (Gutman *et al.* 1972), the identification of circulating immune complexes in 97 per cent of patients (Bayer *et al.* 1976), and the elution from the kidney of antibody which specifically reacted with bacteria isolated from the blood (Levy and Hong 1973).

Clinically, endocarditis results from infection of valves which are congenitally abnormal or have been previously damaged by rheumatic heart disease or hypertension. Normal valves may also be infected, particularly following septicaemia with virulent bacteria such as *S. aureus*, group A β-haemolytic streptococci, or *S. pneumoniae*. Such infections may arise as a complication of central intravenous catheters or through the use of non-sterile needles in intravenous drug addicts. There is often a fulminant illness, leading to rapid destruction of the valves, associated with myocarditis and evidence of infection elsewhere, such as phlebitis, meningitis, and pneumonia. Less virulent organisms such as *Streptococcus viridans* produce a subacute form of endocarditis which has an insidious clinical onset and is more common in patients with previously damaged valves. Many different organisms have been isolated in patients with endocarditis and associated GN (Table 4).

The frequency with which renal disease occurs in endocarditis is not clear. O'Connor *et al.* (1978) showed abnormal urine analysis in 13 of 24 patients with infective endocarditis; a more recent post-mortem study (Neugarten *et al.* 1984) detected GN in 22 per cent of patients, most of whom had right-sided endocarditis complicating intravenous drug abuse.

Table 4 Organisms reported to be involved in endocarditis and associated glomerulonephritis

Organism	Reference
β-Haemolytic streptococci	Gutman *et al.* (1972)
α-Haemolytic streptococci	Perez *et al.* (1976)
Streptococcus viridans	Boulton-Jones *et al.* (1974)
Streptococcus mitis	Keslin *et al.* (1973)
Streptococcus mutans	Allen *et al.* (1982)
S. aureus	Tu *et al.* (1969); Gutman *et al.* (1972)[a]
S. epidermidis	Boulton-Jones *et al.* (1974)
Enterococcus	Levy and Hong (1973)
Gonococcus	Ebright and Komorowski (1980)
Pseudomonas aeruginosa	Beaufils *et al.* (1978)
Coxiella burnetti	Hall *et al.* (1975)
Chlamydia psittaci	Boulton-Jones *et al.* (1974)
Fungi	Roberts and Rabson (1975)

[a] Plus many subsequent reports.

The clinical presentation depends on the virulence of the infecting organism and the degree of cardiac involvement. Commonly, patients present with fever, malaise, arthralgia, and intermittent arthritis. The diagnosis can be made on clinical grounds by the finding of a changing cardiac murmur, splenomegaly, 'splinter' haemorrhages in the nail beds, and microscopic haematuria. Retinal and subconjunctival haemorrhages may occur, but are uncommon. There is also a normochromic normocytic anaemia associated with significant leucocytosis. Non-specific evidence of inflammation is provided by the finding of an increased erythrocyte sedimentation rate and increased C-reactive protein. On urine microscopy, haematuria is universal and red blood cell casts are seen, with varying amounts of proteinuria. Blood culture is positive in approximately 70 per cent of patients.

Rheumatoid factor, cryoglobulinaemia, and circulating immune complexes are variably present. During the acute phase of the illness, C3 and C4 are decreased, which is an indicator of (but not diagnostic of) renal involvement. The blood urea and serum creatinine values depend on the extent of the renal failure, which is frequently mild, but occasionally there is acute renal failure with a rapid deterioration in renal function.

The introduction of effective antibiotic therapy has produced a significant change in the pattern of the disease. *S. aureus* appears to be increasing in incidence, particularly in drug abusers, whereas *S. viridans* is becoming less common. The pathogenesis involves immune complex formation with complement activation, apparently by the classical pathway although there are reports of alternative pathway activation by *S. aureus* (O'Connor *et al.* 1978). The immune complexes arise as a result of prolonged antigenaemia and are frequently present in high titres in the circulation. The role of immune complexes has been confirmed by the detection of antibodies to infecting organisms in glomeruli (Perez *et al.* 1976). Further confirmation comes from the demonstration of staphylococcal antigen (Pertschuk *et al.* 1976; Yum *et al.* 1978) and streptococcal antigen (Perez *et al.* 1976) in glomeruli.

Renal biopsy reveals two distinct patterns of glomerular damage. The findings in acute fulminating infections are similar to those in acute poststreptococcal GN, with an acute diffuse exudative proliferation with or without crescents (Neugarten *et al.* 1984). In such patients, immunofluorescence demonstrates IgG, IgM, and C3 deposition, and dense subendothelial and subepithelial deposits may be present on ultrastructural examination. In the subacute form, focal–segmental proliferative GN is more common; those with a prolonged history may have evidence of sclerosis. Although the changes seen on light microscopy are focal in nature, immunofluorescence shows the deposits to be more diffuse and predominantly mesangial. As with many other forms of infection-associated GN, a wide variety of glomerular changes have been noted, and there are reports of type I mesangiocapillary GN and crescentic GN. Tubulointerstitial changes are common, consisting of a mononuclear cell infiltrate, tubular atrophy, and fibrosis (Morel-Maroger *et al.* 1972). The interstitial changes may be aggravated by antibiotic therapy prescribed for the cardiac lesion. A recent retrospective pathological study of 62 patients with infective endocarditis noted localized infarcts in 19 patients and acute GN in 16 patients. Thus, the most frequent type of glomerular lesion was vasculitis, without deposition of immunoglobulins or complement. Of the renal infarcts over half were due to septic emboli, mostly in patients infected with *S. aureus*. Acute interstitial nephritis was found in 6 patients and seemed attributable to antibiotics. Renal cortical necrosis was observed at necropsy in 6 cases (Majumdar *et al.* 2000).

The course and prognosis are very variable. No specific treatment is required for the renal lesion, which commonly improves following effective treatment of the endocarditis. In patients with significantly impaired renal function, recovery depends more on the outcome of the endocarditis than on the type of renal disease. Antibiotic therapy is essential, and must be given in a sufficient dose and for a sufficient length of time to eradicate the endocarditis completely. Although it has been advocated that antibiotic therapy should be given intravenously for 6 weeks, this is now disputed, and currently there is no consensus regarding the length of intravenous therapy or of overall treatment. Although corticosteroid therapy is generally not recommended, it should be considered for patients whose renal dysfunction secondary to GN does not improve with appropriate antimicrobial treatment, especially if the duration of the illness is long (Le Moing *et al.* 1999). Anecdotal case report indicates that infective endocarditis-induced crescentic GN dramatically improved by plasma exchange (Daimon *et al.* 1998; Kannan and Matoo 2001). In patients with known valvular disease, prophylactic antibiotic therapy to prevent endocarditis is essential in situations where significant bacteraemia may arise, such as tooth extraction.

'Shunt' nephritis

Surgical treatment for hydrocephalus consists in the insertion of a catheter into the distended ventricle and drainage to the atrium via either the jugular vein or the superior vena cava, or (more commonly today) the peritoneal cavity. A common complication of this procedure is colonization of the catheter by bacteria of low virulence. About 30 per cent of juguloatrial catheters become infected, and 70 per cent of these infections occur within 2 months of insertion. However, the development of nephritis is a late complication with a long time interval after insertion (Vernet and Rilliet 2001). Vella *et al.* (1995) reported on five patients with shunt nephritis in whom the average time from insertion to nephritis was 12.5 years. The time interval ranged from 0.3 to 4.5 years after the last shunt operation in the six patients reported by Haffner *et al.* (1997). Although infection seems to be relatively common, the subsequent development of GN may occur in less than 5 per cent of infected patients. A variety of shunts are available, but it appears that superadded infection can complicate all types. The first report of shunt nephritis (Black *et al.* 1965) described two patients who developed haematuria and a nephrotic syndrome after prolonged bacteraemia following the insertion of Spitz–Holter valves. Since then there have been many further reports confirming the association between ventriculoatrial shunts and the development of GN. A few reports indicate that ventriculoperitoneal shunts can also be associated with this complication, but this occurs much less frequently. The causal organism is *S. epidermidis (albus)* in approximately 70 per cent of patients and *S. aureus* in another 20 per cent. A wide variety of organisms have been reported from the remaining 10 per cent (Arze *et al.* 1983), in some instances as single case reports (Table 5).

Colonization of the shunt probably occurs at insertion or shortly thereafter. It appears that some subtypes of *S. epidermidis* produce an excess of a mucoid substance ('slime') which promotes adherence of the bacteria to smooth surfaces and may provide a protective layer against the action of lysozymes (Schena 1985). The glomerular lesion arises as a consequence of prolonged low-grade bacteraemia leading to antibody production and the formation of immune complexes. In screening for chronically infected ventriculoatrial shunts in 138 patients, Samtleben *et al.* (1993) found increased circulating immune complexes in 24 patients of whom 20 had infected shunts. Such complexes within the glomerulus activate complement by the classical pathway and lead to glomerular inflammation. A role for the bacterial antigen has been confirmed by the detection of specific bacterial antigens, including *S. epidermidis* (Kaufman and McIntosh 1971; Dobrin *et al.* 1975), *Proprionibacterium acnes* (Groenveld *et al.* 1982), *diphtheria* spp. (O'Regan and Makker 1979), and *Corynebacterium bovis* (Bolton *et al.* 1975), within glomerular deposits and also within circulating cryoprecipitates in some cases.

Evidence of infection always precedes the renal manifestations. Fever is universal and may be low grade or spiking. It is associated with symptoms such as arthralgia, purpura, rash, anorexia, malaise, and occasionally signs of increasing intracranial pressure. Very occasionally

Table 5 Microorganisms responsible for shunt nephritis

S. epidermidis (albus)	Lam *et al.* (1969)
S. aureus	Stickler *et al.* (1968)
C. bovis	Bolton *et al.* (1975)
Bacillus subtilis	Schoenbaum *et al.* (1975)
Bacillus cereus	Campbell *et al.* (1981)
Listeria monocytogenes	Strife *et al.* (1976)
P. acnes	Beeler *et al.* (1976)
P. aeruginosa	Zunin *et al.* (1977)
Serratia	Levy *et al.* (1981)
Peptococcus	Caron *et al.* (1979)
Diphtheroids	O'Regan and Makker (1979)
Propionibacterium acnes	Setz *et al.* (1994); Balogun *et al.* (2001)
Moraxella bovis	Bogdanovic *et al.* (1996)
Gemella morbillorum	Nagashima *et al.* (2001)

a patient may be asymptomatic, but have a profound anaemia. Anaemia and hepatosplenomegaly are common; haematuria is usually microscopic, but may occasionally be macroscopic. Proteinuria is variable, but is sufficient to result in a nephrotic syndrome in approximately 25 per cent of patients. There is evidence of infection with a leucocytosis associated with increased erythrocyte sedimentation rate, plasma viscosity, and C-reactive protein. Complement studies may indicate a reduced C3, C4, and C1q. Some patients produce rheumatoid factor, and mixed cryoglobulins may be detected. Blood cultures are positive, and, whilst *S. epidermidis* would be considered as a contaminant in normal clinical practice, it must always be taken as clinically significant in a patient with a ventriculoatrial shunt.

The most common appearance on renal biopsy is that of type I mesangiocapillary GN, in some cases with occasional crescent formation. Subendothelial electron-dense deposits are common, and immunofluorescence microscopy usually reveals IgM and C3. Some patients have a diffuse exudative proliferative GN, while others may have a minor mesangial proliferation or segmental lesions.

The association of serum antineutrophil cytoplasm antibodies (ANCA) with shunt nephritis has been reported in two patients; ANCA specific for proteinase 3 in a patient with shunt nephritis induced by *Gemella morbillorum* (Nagashima *et al.* 2001) and c-ANCA positive mesangiocapillary GN recovering after removal of a cystoatrial shunt infected by *P. acnes* (Bonarek *et al.* 1999).

Antibiotic therapy alone is usually insufficient and patients require shunt removal. Repeat renal biopsies have been performed in a number of successfully treated patients, and show a reduction in glomerular cellularity with disappearance of the electron-dense deposits (Zunin *et al.* 1977; Levy *et al.* 1981; Wakabayashi *et al.* 1985; Fukuda *et al.* 1993), but residual mild to moderate mesangial proliferative GN. The prognosis is variable, and whilst adequate antibiotic therapy and shunt removal will allow urinary abnormalities to resolve, these will persist in a few patients (Dobrin *et al.* 1975; Levy *et al.* 1981). In the series reported by Samtleben *et al.* (1993), eight of 20 patients had impaired renal function and four of these required dialysis; following removal of the infected shunt renal function improved in seven with only one patient continuing to require dialysis. Similar results were reported by Vella *et al.* (1995) who noted an improvement in renal function, with two of five patients returning to normal after antibiotic therapy and/or shunt removal. The clinical course and long-term outcome have been analysed in seven patients who received antibiotics intravenously. Complete recovery was observed in three of four patients in whom the shunt was totally removed, supported by transient external drainage of cerebrospinal fluid, and followed by placement of a ventriculoperitoneal shunt. One child with delayed diagnosis, presenting with a serum creatinine of 3.2 mg/dl, hypertension, and severe scarring on renal biopsy, rapidly progressed to irreversible ESRD within 5 months. Two patients without and only partial removal of the shunt died subsequently from sepsis (Haffner *et al.* 1997). Thus, the renal outcome of shunt nephritis is good if early diagnosis and treatment is provided including intravenous antibiotics and total removal of the infected shunt.

There are two reports of nephritis complicating infected ventriculoperitoneal shunts. Noe and Roy (1981) described a child who presented with microscopic haematuria, nephrotic syndrome, and deteriorating renal function; these resolved following removal of the shunt. Unfortunately, no specific organisms were isolated in this case. Patriarca and Lauer (1980) described a child with fever in whom *Haemophilus influenzae* was isolated; this organism was considered to be responsible for the subsequent development of proteinuria.

Visceral abscesses

GN has been associated with visceral abscesses in a variety of clinical situations. Multiple cutaneous abscesses (Pertschuk *et al.* 1976), severe pulmonary infection (Salyer and Salyer 1974; Danovitch *et al.* 1979), chronic granulomatous disease (van Rhenen *et al.* 1976; Cottin *et al.* 1982), infected arterial prostheses (Beaufils 1981; Coleman *et al.* 1983), and a variety of deep-seated abscesses (Beaufils *et al.* 1976) have all been described. A common feature is that of a severe infection which has been present for several months, unlike the situation in amyloidosis where the infection has been present for many years.

Clinical presentation is extremely variable and can range from mild urinary abnormalities (Salyer and Salyer 1974) to severe fulminating renal failure (Nydahl and Hall 1965; Beaufils *et al.* 1976). Impaired renal function is common (Pertschuk *et al.* 1976; Spector *et al.* 1980) but, interestingly, the nephrotic syndrome has been rarely described (Danovitch *et al.* 1979).

The most common infecting organism in visceral abscesses is *S. aureus* (Beaufils *et al.* 1976; Pertschuk *et al.* 1976), although there are instances of infections due to *Pseudomonas aeruginosa, E. coli, Proteus mirabilis*, and *C. albicans*.

As with many other forms of infection-related glomerular disease, a wide variety of histological appearances have been described. Proliferative GN (Nydahl and Hall 1965; Danovitch *et al.* 1979) or mesangial proliferative GN (Beaufils *et al.* 1976; Spector *et al.* 1980) are most common. Others have reported mesangiocapillary GN (Beaufils 1981), membranous GN (Cottin *et al.* 1982), a focal proliferative GN (Beaufils *et al.* 1976), and glomerulosclerosis (van Rhenen *et al.* 1976). Thus, no single histological entity is associated with visceral abscesses, although in the majority there are marked proliferative changes.

A series of 76 adult patients, living in a suburban borough of Paris with a below-average socioeconomic status, with infectious GN have been retrospectively studied. Thirty-four patients (45 per cent) were alcoholics, diabetics, or intravenous illicit-drug users. Sixty-six patients presented with acute nephritic and/or nephrotic syndrome. Acute renal failure was present in 56 (76 per cent) and required dialysis in 14. Initial renal biopsy disclosed endocapillary GN in 44 patients, crescentic GN in 26, and membranoproliferative GN in six. Ten patients had endocarditis. Staphylococci and Gram-negative strains, not streptococci, were the most common bacteria identified. The origin of sepsis was mainly the oropharynx (21), the skin (19), and the lung (14); 19 cases involved multiple sites of infection. Eight patients died (11 per cent) and 20 (26 per cent) recovered renal function, but GN followed a chronic course in 38 (50 per cent), rapidly requiring maintenance dialysis in six. Poor prognostic factors included age over 50 years, purpura, endocarditis, and glomerular extracapillary proliferation (Montseny *et al.* 1995).

The management of such patients is directed predominantly at the underlying infection, and culture of the infecting organism is particularly important. The majority of patients have some impairment of renal function and antibiotic therapy may need to be adjusted appropriately. Management of the renal failure is along conventional lines, although it is frequently complicated by the fact that many patients are malnourished because of their long-standing sepsis. The overall outcome depends on the severity of the underlying infection and whether it can be eradicated or controlled. Recovery with effective treatment occurs in a number of patients (Beaufils *et al.* 1976). Steroids for deep-infection-associated GN is a two-edged sword (Vanwalleghem *et al.* 1998). Patients presenting with acute renal failure clearly have a poor prognosis, although recovery has been described. A small number of patients may progress to a chronic impairment of renal function.

'Heroin' nephropathy (see also Chapter 4.12.1)

A variety of glomerular lesions have been reported in intravenous heroin addicts (Bakir and Dunea 1996; Crowe *et al.* 2000), including focal glomerulosclerosis (Rao *et al.* 1974), membranous nephropathy associated with chronic hepatitis B antigenaemia, and immune complex nephritis. Mesangiocapillary GN associated with mixed cryoglobulinaemia and hepatitis C infection has been described (Ramos *et al.* 1994). Most commonly patients present with nephrotic syndrome, hypertension, impaired renal function, and anaemia. Heroin addicts with nephropathy are usually young adult males who have been addicted for at least 6 months. Addicts may inject heroin intravenously (mainlining) or subcutaneously (skin popping), frequently sharing syringes with 'friends'.

Renal biopsy most commonly shows a focal segmental glomerulosclerosis with a variable degree of tubular injury. Progression to renal failure is rapid, although there are reports of stabilization of renal function in a few patients who have ceased heroin abuse. In addition to glomerulosclerosis, heroin addicts may develop other renal consequences such as acute renal failure associated with rhabdomyolysis and myoglobinuria as a consequence of overdose, a necrotizing angiitis, and infection-associated proliferative GN. Haemolytic uraemic syndrome has been reported in a heroin addict (Peces *et al.* 1998).

It is unlikely that heroin itself is causally related to the nephropathy. It is more than likely that adulterants and associated infections are responsible for what has been described as 'heroin-associated nephropathy'. The recent decline in the incidence of nephropathy in the absence of any reduction in heroin addiction may be due to an increase in the purity of 'street' heroin and the consequent reduced exposure to adulterants (Friedman and Rao 1995).

Kimura's disease (angiolymphoid hyperplasia with eosinophilia)

Kimura's disease, an angiolymphoid proliferative disorder of soft tissue with eosinophilia or eosinophilic folliculosis, is a syndrome found almost exclusively in Orientals, even in the few reported cases from outside the Orient (Whelan *et al.* 1988): most of the patients described have been Japanese (Yamada *et al.* 1982), although it has been reported in Chinese (Akosa *et al.* 1991; Chan *et al.* 1991), an Arab (Qunibi *et al.* 1988), a Turk (Uthgennant *et al.* 1991), and also from Israel (Atar *et al.* 1994). All the reported patients with renal disease have been males and the syndrome as a whole has a male–female ratio of 9 : 1. The age at onset has ranged from 5 to 71 years (Akosa *et al.* 1991), but the majority have been young adults.

The principal features of the syndrome are cutaneous lesions consisting of multiple red–brown papules, which arise from an eosinophilic folliculitis, together with subcutaneous nodules and enlargement of the lymph nodes, which show enlarged lymphoid follicles and infiltration with eosinophils and IgE-positive cells. Both features have a predilection for the head and neck including the orbit. Malignancy is frequently the initial suspected clinical diagnosis. There is a blood eosinophilia and the serum concentrations of IgE are often markedly elevated (Akosa *et al.* 1991) and the IgA concentrations less so.

Yamada *et al.* (1982) reviewed 175 cases reported up to 1981 and noted that 21 (12 per cent) had proteinuria, including their own patient; 13 of these had a nephrotic syndrome. In some patients, the onset of proteinuria preceded the other manifestations of the condition, occasionally by several years. Renal biopsy has shown membranous nephropathy (Yamada *et al.* 1982; Akosa *et al.* 1991; Matsuda *et al.* 1992), but minimal change nephropathy (Matsuda *et al.* 1992; Atar *et al.* 1994), IgM nephropathy (Chan *et al.* 1991), mesangial proliferative GN (Qunibi *et al.* 1988; Uthgennant *et al.* 1991), and FSGS (Cameron unpublished observation) have also been reported.

The pathogenesis is unclear and no infectious agent has been identified in any case, although an infectious aetiology appears likely. One patient suffered from tuberculous mastoiditis and IgE antibodies specific for Candida have been reported (Akosa *et al.* 1991). IL-5 mRNA is present in the peripheral lymphocytes of many cases (Enokihara *et al.* 1994), a finding otherwise confined to patients with parasitic diseases.

The overall prognosis is not clear from the limited number of reports available. In four patients, a response to corticosteroid therapy was reported (Qunibi *et al.* 1988; Whelan *et al.* 1988; Uthgennant *et al.* 1991; Atar *et al.* 1994); three patients had mild mesangial lesions with only IgM aggregates on renal biopsy, and one had minimal change nephropathy. Yamada *et al.*'s (1982) patient died of infection during treatment with corticosteroids and resistance to corticosteroid treatment has been recorded (Moriga *et al.* 1994). There is always the possibility of the two conditions being coincidental but Kimura's disease is not common and it is likely that the steriod-responsive nephropathy is causally linked.

General conclusions

Infection-associated GN is well established and has been recognized for almost two centuries. In that time there have been many significant advances, including the identification of microorganisms, the development of effective specific therapy in the form of antibiotics, antiviral drugs, and antifungal agents, the complete eradication of certain infections such as smallpox, and eradication of other infections from certain geographical regions (e.g. malaria from Guyana). There have also been very significant changes in the socioeconomic status of many communities, which have had an influence on the development of infection-associated nephropathy. There is no doubt that changes will continue to take place and it is likely that bacterial and parasitic infections will be less prominent, while viral infections are likely to be of more importance.

In the general management of a patient with GN, careful consideration should be given to the possibility of an associated underlying infection. In many, but not all, instances this will be obvious at clinical presentation. An investigation of potential infective causes will depend to a large extent on local factors, particularly where certain infections are endemic. A causal link can only be established by identification of antigen and elution of specific antibody and so, in the majority of instances, the link will be inferred from the satisfactory resolution of the renal abnormalities after successful eradication of the infection. Although this is the usual course, malaria and schistosomiasis are striking examples of the progression of renal disease despite effective treatment of the infection.

References

Ahuja, T. S. *et al.* (1999). Is the prevalence of HIV-associated nephropathy decreasing? *American Journal of Nephrology* **19**, 655–659.

Akosa, A. B., Sherif, A., and Maidment, C. G. (1991). Kimura's disease and membranous nephropathy. *Nephron* **58**, 472–474.

Allen, A. C. and Spitz, S. (1945). A comparative study of the pathology of scrub typhus (tsutsugamushi disease) and other rickettsial diseases. *American Journal of Pathology* **21**, 603–682.

Allen, D. B., Friedman, A. L., Croker, B., and Osofsky, S. G. (1982). Glomerulonephritis associated with infective endocarditis in a pediatric patient. *North Carolina Medical Journal* **43**, 113–117.

Alpers, C. E., McClure, J., and Bursten, S. L. (1992). Human mesangial cells are resistant to productive infection by multiple strains of human immunodeficiency virus types 1 and 2. *American Journal of Kidney Diseases* **19**, 126–130.

Altiparmak, M. R. *et al.* (2002). Brucella glomerulonephritis: review of the literature and report on the first patient with brucellosis and mesangiocapillary glomerulonephritis. *Scandinavian Journal of Infectious Diseases* **34**, 477–480.

Amerio, A., Campese, V., Coratelli, P., and Schena, F. P. (1972). Glomerulonephritis in typhoid fever. *Abstracts of the Fifth International Congress of Nephrology* p. 62.

Andresdottir, M. B. *et al.* (2000). Type I membranoproliferative glomerulonephritis in a renal allograft: a recurrence induced by a cytomegalovirus infection? *American Journal of Kidney Diseases* **35**, E6 (electronic file).

Arze, R. S. *et al.* (1983). Shunt-nephritis. Report of two cases and review of the literature. *Clinical Nephrology* **19**, 48–53.

Atar, S., Oberman, A. S., Ben-Izhak, O., and Flatau, E. (1994). Recurrent nephrotic syndrome associated with Kimura's disease in a young non-oriental male. *Nephron*, **68**, 259–261.

Bakir, A. A. and Dunea, G. (1996). Drugs of abuse and renal disease. *Current Opinion in Nephrology and Hypertension* **5**, 122–126.

Balogun, R. A. *et al.* (2001). Shunt nephritis from *Propionibacterium acnes* in a solitary kidney. *American Journal of Kidney Diseases* **38**, E18 (electronic file).

Barisoni, L. *et al.* (1999). The dysregulated podocyte phenotype: a novel concept in the pathogenesis of collapsing idiopathic focal segmental glomerulosclerosis and HIV-associated nephropathy. *Journal of the American Society of Nephrology* **10**, 51–61.

Barker, P. S. (1949). A clinical study of subacute bacterial infection confined to the right side of the heart. *American Heart Journal* **37**, 1054–1060.

Barsoum, R. S. *et al.* (1977). Renal disease in hepatosplenic schistosomiasis—a clinicopathological study. *Transactions of the Royal Society for Tropical Medicine and Hygiene* **71**, 287–291.

Bayer, A. S. *et al.* (1976). Circulating immune complexes in infective endocarditis. *New England Journal of Medicine* **295**, 1500–1505.

Beaufils, M. (1981). Glomerular disease complicating abdominal sepsis. *Kidney International* **19**, 609–618.

Beaufils, M. *et al.* (1976). Acute renal failure of glomerular origin during visceral abscesses. *New England Journal of Medicine* **295**, 185–189.

Beaufils, M. *et al.* (1978). Glomerulonephritis in severe bacterial infections with and without endocarditis. *Advances in Nephrology* **7**, 217–234.

Beaufils, H. *et al.* (1995). HIV-associated IgA nephropathy—a post-mortem study. *Nephrology, Dialysis, Transplantation* **10**, 35–38.

Beeler, B. A., Crowder, J. G., Smith, J. W., and White, A. (1976). *Proprionibacterium acnes*: pathogen in central nervous system shunt infection. Report of 3 cases including immune complex glomerulonephritis. *American Journal of Medicine* **61**, 935–938.

Belec, L. *et al.* (1999). Human herpesvirus 8 infection in patients with POEMS syndrome-associated multicentric Castleman's disease. *Blood* **93**, 3643–3653.

Bell, E. T. (1932). Glomerular lesions associated with endocarditis. *American Journal of Pathology* **8**, 639–664.

Black, J. A., Challacombe, D. N., and Ockenden, B. G. (1965). Nephrotic syndrome associated with bacteraemia after shunt operations for hydrocephalus. *Lancet* **ii**, 921–924.

Blackall, J. *Observations on the Nature and Cure of Dropsies, and Particularly on the Presence of the Coagulable Part of the Blood in Dropsied Urine*. London: Longmans Green, 1818.

Boccia, R. V. *et al.* (1984). A hemolytic–uremic syndrome with the acquired immunodeficiency syndrome. *Annals of Internal Medicine* **101**, 716–717.

Bodi, I., Abraham, A. A., and Kimmel, P. L. (1994). Macrophages in human immunodeficiency virus-associated kidney diseases. *American Journal of Kidney Diseases* **24**, 762–767.

Bodi, I., Abraham, A. A., and Kimmel, P. L. (1995). Apotosis in human immunodeficiency virus-associated nephropathy. *American Journal of Kidney Diseases* **26**, 286–291.

Bogdanovic, R. *et al.* (1996). Shunt nephritis associated with *Moraxella bovis*. *Acta Paediatrica* **85**, 882–883.

Bolton, W. K. *et al.* (1975). Ventriculojugular shunt nephritis with *Corynebacterium bovis*. *American Journal of Medicine* **59**, 417–423.

Bonarek, H. *et al.* (1999). Reversal of c-ANCA positive mesangiocapillary glomerulonephritis after removal of an infected cysto-atrial shunt. *Nephrology, Dialysis, Transplantation* **14**, 1771–1773.

Boonshaft, B., Maher, J. F., and Schreiner, G. E. (1970). Nephrotic syndrome associated with osteomyelitis without secondary amyloidosis. *Archives of Internal Medicine* **125**, 322–327.

Boulton-Jones, J. M. and Davison, A. M. (1986). Persistent systemic infection as a cause of renal disease in patients submitted to renal biopsy: a report from the Glomerulonephritis Registry of the United Kingdom MRC. *Quarterly Journal of Medicine* **58**, 123–132.

Boulton-Jones, J. M., Sissons, J. G. P., Evans, D. J., and Peters, D. K. (1974). Renal lesions of subsequent infective endocarditis. *British Medical Journal* **2**, 11–14.

Bourgoignie, J. J. (1990). Renal complications of human immunodeficiency virus type 1. *Kidney International* **37**, 1571–1584.

Boyce, N. W. *et al.* (1988). Cytomegalovirus infection complicating renal transplantation and its relationships to acute transplant glomerulopathy. *Transplantation* **45**, 706–709.

Browne, G. *et al.* (2001). Acute allograft glomerulopathy associated with CMV viraemia. *Nephrology, Dialysis, Transplantation* **16**, 861–862.

Bruggeman, L. A. *et al.* (1997). Nephropathy in human immunodeficiency virus-1 transgenic mice is due to renal transgene expression. *Journal of Clinical Investigation* **100**, 84–92.

Bruggeman, L. A. *et al.* (2000). Renal epithelium is a previously unrecognized site of HIV-1 infection. *Journal of the American Society of Nephrology* **11**, 2079–2087.

Brunkhorst, R. *et al.* (1989). Lack of clinical evidence for a glomerulopathy in 203 patients with HIV infection. *Nephrology, Dialysis, Transplantation* **4**, 433 (abstract).

Buka, I. and Coovadia, H. M. (1980). Typhoid glomerulonephritis. *Archives of Disease in Childhood* **55**, 305–307.

Bullock, W. E., Artz, R. P., Bhathena, D., and Tung, K. S. K. (1979). Histoplasmosis. Association with circulating immune complexes, eosinophilia and mesangiopathic glomerulonephritis. *Archives of Internal Medicine* **139**, 700–702.

Burke, D. G. *et al.* (1997). Histoplasmosis and kidney disease in patients with AIDS. *Clinical Infectious Diseases* **25**, 281–284.

Burns, G. C. *et al.* (1997). Effect of angiotensin-converting enzyme inhibition in HIV-associated nephropathy. *Journal of the American Society of Nephrology* **8**, 1140–1146.

Campbell, A., Futrakul, P., Musgrave, J. E., Surapathana, L. O., and Eisenberg, C. S. (1981). *Bacillus cereus* prosthesis nephritis. *Second International Symposium of Pediatric Nephrology*, Paris.

Campbell, J. H. *et al.* (1991). Rapidly progressive glomerulonephritis and nephrotic syndrome associated with *Mycoplasma pneumoniae* pneumonia. *Nephrology, Dialysis, Transplantation* **6**, 518–520.

Caron, C. *et al.* (1979). La glomerulonéphrite de shunt: manifestations cliniques et histopathologiques. *Canadian Medical Association Journal* **120**, 557–561.

Casanova, S. *et al.* (1995). Pattern of glomerular involvement in human immunodeficiency virus-infected patients: an Italian study. *American Journal of Kidney Diseases* **26**, 446–453.

Chan, T. M., Chan, P. C., Chan, K. W., and Cheng, I. K. (1991). IgM nephropathy in a patient with Kimura's disease. *Nephron* **58**, 489–490 (letter).

Cheng, J. T. *et al.* (1999). Hepatitis C virus-associated glomerular disease in patients with human immunodeficiency virus coinfection. *Journal of the American Society of Nephrology* **10**, 1566–1574.

Chesney, R. W., O'Regan, S., Guyda, H. J., and Drummond, K. N. (1976). Candida endocrinopathy syndrome with membranoproliferative glomerulonephritis: demonstration of glomerular candida antigen. *Clinical Nephrology* **5**, 232–238.

Cochat, P. *et al.* (1985). Glomérulonéphrite membranoproliférative et infection à *Mycoplasma pneumoniae. Archives Francaises de Pediatrie* **42**, 29–31.

Coleman, M., Burnett, J., Barrat, L. J., and Dupont, P. (1983). Glomerulonephritis associated with chronic bacterial infection of a Dacron arterial prosthesis. *Clinical Nephrology* **20**, 315–320.

Collins, B. *et al.* (1983). Hepatitis B immune complex glomerulonephritis: simultaneous glomerular deposition of hepatitis B surface and e antigens. *Clinical Immunology and Immunopathology* **26**, 137–153.

Conaldi, P. G. *et al.* (1998). HIV-1 kills renal tubular epithelial cells *in vitro* by triggering an apoptotic pathway involving caspase activation and Fas upregulation. *Journal of Clinical Investigation* **102**, 2041–2049.

Connolly, J. O., Weston, C. E., and Hendry, B. M. (1995). HIV-associated renal disease in London hospitals. *Quarterly Journal of Medicine* **88**, 627–634.

Cottin, X., Chopard, P., Cotton, J. B., and Larbre, F. (1982). Glomerulonéphrite extra-membraneuse, au cours d'une granulomatose septique chronique. *Pédiatrie* **37**, 299–304.

Crowe, A. V. *et al.* (2000). Substance abuse and the kidney. *Quarterly Journal of Medicine* **93**, 147–152.

Cusack, D. *et al.* (1983). IgA nephropathy in association with *Yersinia enterocolitica. Irish Journal of Medical Science* **152**, 311–312.

D'Agati, V. and Appel, G. B. (1998). Renal pathology of human immunodeficiency virus infection. *Seminars in Nephrology* **18**, 406–421.

D'Agati, V. *et al.* (1989). Pathology of HIV-associated nephropathy: a detailed morphologic and comparative study. *Kidney International* **35**, 1358–1370.

D'Agati, V., McEachrane, S., Dicker, R., and Neilsen, E. (1990). Cat scratch disease and glomerulonephritis. *Nephron* **56**, 431–435.

Daimon, S. *et al.* (1998). Infective endocarditis-induced crescentic glomerulonephritis dramatically improved by plasmapheresis. *American Journal of Kidney Diseases* **32**, 309–313.

Danovitch, G. M., Nord, E. P., Barki, Y., and Krugliak, L. (1979). Staphylococcal lung abscess and acute glomerulonephritis. *Israel Journal of Medical Science* **10**, 840–843.

Davison, A. M., Thomson, D., and Robson, J. S. (1973). Intravascular coagulation complicating influenza A virus infection. *British Medical Journal* **i**, 654–655.

De Brito, T., Tiriba, A., and Godoy, C. V. F. (1968). Glomerular response in human and experimental rickettsial disease (Rocky Mountain spotted fever group). A light and electron microscopy study. *Pathologia et Microbiologia* **31**, 365–377.

De Brito, T. *et al.* (1975). Glomerular involvement in human kala-azar. *American Journal of Tropical Medicine and Hygiene* **24**, 9–18.

De Meyer, M., Cosyns, J. P., and Van Ypersele De Strihou, C. (1989). Does HIV-related nephropathy exist in AIDS patients? *Nephrology, Dialysis, Transplantation* **4**, 434.

de Noronha, C. M. *et al.* (2001). Dynamic disruptions in nuclear envelope architecture and integrity induced by HIV-1 Vpr. *Science* **294**, 1105–1108.

De Siati, L. *et al.* (1999). Immunoglobulin A nephropathy complicating pulmonary tuberculosis. *Annals of Diagnostic Pathology* **3**, 300–303.

De Vriese, A. S. *et al.* (1998). Rifampicin-associated acute renal failure: pathophysiologic, immunologic, and clinical features. *American Journal of Kidney Diseases* **31**, 108–115.

Denneberg, T., Friedberg, M., Samuelsson, T., and Winblad, S. (1981). Glomerulonephritis in infections with *Yersinia enterocolitica* O-serotype 3. *Acta Medica Scandinavica* **209**, 97–101.

Detwiler, R. K. *et al.* (1998). Cytomegalovirus-induced necrotizing and crescentic glomerulonephritis in a renal transplant patient. *American Journal of Kidney Diseases* **32**, 820–824.

Diaz, F. and Collazos, J. (2000). Glomerulonephritis and Henoch–Schöenlein purpura associated with acute parvovirus B19 infection. *Clinical Nephrology* **53**, 237–238.

Dobrin, R. S. *et al.* (1975). The role of complement, immunoglobulin and bacterial antigen in coagulase-negative staphylococcal shunt nephritis. *American Journal of Medicine* **59**, 660–673.

Dror, Y. *et al.* (1998). Systemic lupus erythematosus associated with acute Epstein–Barr virus infection. *American Journal of Kidney Diseases* **32**, 825–828.

Dutra, M. *et al.* (1985). Renal involvement in visceral leishmaniasis. *American Journal of Kidney Diseases* **6**, 22–27.

Ebright, J. R. and Komorowski, R. (1980). Gonococcal endocarditis associated with immune complex glomerulonephritis. *American Journal of Medicine* **68**, 793–796.

Eitner, F. *et al.* (1999). Thrombotic microangiopathy in the HIV-2-infected macaque. *American Journal of Pathology* **155**, 649–661.

Eitner, F. *et al.* (2000). Chemokine receptor CCR5 and CXCR4 expression in HIV-associated kidney disease. *Journal of the American Society of Nephrology* **11**, 856–867.

Enokihara, H. *et al.* (1994). IL-5 mRNA expression in blood lymphocytes from patients with Kimura's disease and parasitic infections. *American Journal of Hematology* **47**, 69–73.

Eustace, J. A. *et al.* (2000). Cohort study of the treatment of severe HIV-associated nephropathy with corticosteroids. *Kidney International* **58**, 1253–1260.

Forrest, J. W., Jr. *et al.* (1977). Immune complex glomerulonephritis associated with *Klebsiella pneumoniae* infection. *Clinical Nephrology* **7**, 76–80.

Freedman, B. I. *et al.* (1999). Familial clustering of end-stage renal disease in blacks with HIV-associated nephropathy. *American Journal of Kidney Diseases* **34**, 254–258.

Friedman, E. A. and Rao, T. K. S. (1995). Disappearance of uremia due to heroin-associated nephropathy. *American Journal of Kidney Diseases* **25**, 689–693.

Friedberg, M. *et al.* (1981). Glomerulonephritis in infection with *Yersinia enterocolitica* O-serotype 3. *Acta Medica Scandinavica* **209**, 103–110.

Fujieda, M. *et al.* (2000). Mumps associated with immunoglobulin A nephropathy. *Pediatric Infectious Disease Journal* **19**, 669–671.

Fukuda, Y., Ohtomo, Y., Kaneko, K., and Yabuta, K. (1993). Pathologic and laboratory dynamics following removal of the shunt in shunt nephritis. *American Journal of Nephrology* **13**, 78–82.

Ginsburg, B. E., Wasserman, J., Huldt, G., and Bergstrand, A. (1974). Case of glomerulonephritis associated with acute toxoplasmosis. *British Medical Journal* **iii**, 664–665.

Glassock, R. J., Cohen, A. H., Danovitch, G., and Parsa, K. P. (1990). Human immunodeficiency virus (HIV) infection and the kidney. *Annals of Internal Medicine* **112**, 35–49.

Goodpasture, E. W. (1919). The significance of certain pulmonary lesions in relation to the etiology of influenza. *American Journal of Medical Science* **158**, 863–870.

Green, D. F., Resnick, L., and Bourgoignie, J. J. (1992). HIV infects glomerular endothelial and mesangial but not epithelial cells *in vitro. Kidney International* **41**, 956–960.

Green, W. R., Greaves, W. L., Frederick, W. R., and Taddesse-Heath, L. (1994). Renal infection due to adenovirus in a patient with human immunodeficiency virus infection. *Clinical Infectious Diseases* **18**, 989–991.

Griffin, M. D., Bjornsson, J., and Erickson, S. B. (1997). Diffuse proliferative glomerulonephritis and acute renal failure associated with acute staphylococcal osteomyelitis. *Journal of the American Society of Nephrology* **8**, 1633–1639.

Groeneveld, A. B. J. *et al.* (1982). Shunt nephritis associated with *Propionibacterium acnes* with demonstration of the antigen in the glomeruli. *Nephron* **32**, 365–369.

Gutman, R. A., Striker, G. E., Gilliland, B. C., and Cutler, R. E. (1972). The immune complex glomerulonephritis of bacterial endocarditis. *Medicine (Baltimore)* **51**, 1–25.

Haas, M. *et al.* (2000). Fibrillary/immunotactoid glomerulonephritis in HIV-positive patients: a report of three cases. *Nephrology, Dialysis, Transplantation* **15**, 1679–1683.

Haffner, D. *et al.* (1997). The clinical spectrum of shunt nephritis. *Nephrology, Dialysis, Transplantation* **12**, 1143–1148.

Hailemariam, S. *et al.* (2001). Renal pathology and premortem clinical presentation of Caucasian patients with AIDS: an autopsy study from the era prior to antiretroviral therapy. *Swiss Medical Weekly* **131**, 412–417.

Hall, G. H. *et al.* (1975). Glomerulonephritis associated with *Coxiella burnetii* endocarditis. *British Medical Journal* **ii**, 275.

Halpern, M. *et al.* (1992). Renal aspergilloma: an unusal cause of infection in a patient with acquired immunodeficiency syndrome. *American Journal of Medicine* **92**, 437–440.

Hariprasad, M. K., Dodelson, R., Eisinger, R. P., and Gary, N. E. (1979). Dense deposit disease in tuberculosis. *New York State Journal of Medicine* **79**, 2084–2085.

Hariparsad, D., Ramsaroop, R., Seedat, Y. K., and Patel, P. L. (1985). Mesangial proliferative glomerulonephritis with legionnaires' disease. A case report. *South African Medical Journal* **67**, 649–650.

Heieren, M. H., Kim, Y. K., and Balfour, H. H., Jr. (1988). Human cytomegalovirus infection of kidney glomerular visceral epithelial and tubular epithelial cells in culture. *Transplantation* **46**, 426–432.

Herrera, G. A. *et al.* (1986). Cytomegalovirus glomerulopathy: a controversial lesion. *Kidney International* **29**, 725–733.

Hsieh, W. S. *et al.* (1996). Crescentic IgA nephropathy and acute renal failure in an HIV-positive patient with enteric salmonella infection. *Nephrology, Dialysis, Transplantation* **11**, 2320–2323.

Huang, T. W. and Wiegenstein, L. M. (1977). Mesangiolytic glomerulonephritis in an infant with immune deficiency and echovirus infection. *Archives of Pathology* **101**, 125–128.

Hughes, W. T., Steigman, A. J., and Delong, H. F. (1966). Some implications of fatal nephritis associated with mumps. *American Journal of Disease in Children* **111**, 297–301.

Humphreys, M. H. (1995). Human immunodeficiency virus-associated glomerulosclerosis. *Kidney International* **48**, 311–320.

Husain, M. *et al.* (2002). HIV-1 Nef induces proliferation and anchorage-independent growth in podocytes. *Journal of the American Society Nephrology* **13**, 1806–1815.

Hyman, L. R. *et al.* (1975). Alternate C3 pathway activation in pneumococcal glomerulonephritis. *American Journal of Medicine* **58**, 810–815.

Hymes, K. B. and Karpatkin, S. (1997). Human immunodeficiency virus infection and thrombotic microangiopathy. *Seminars in Hematology* **34**, 117–125.

Ifudu, O. *et al.* (1995). Zidovudine is beneficial in human immunodeficiency virus associated nephropathy. *American Journal of Nephrology* **15**, 217–221.

Indrapasit, S., Boonpucknavig, V., and Boonpucknavig, S. (1985). IgA nephropathy associated with enteric fever. *Nephron* **40**, 219–222.

Iwafuchi, Y. *et al.* (2002). Acute endocapillary proliferative glomerulonephritis associated with human parvovirus B19 infection. *Clinical Nephrology* **57**, 246–250.

Iwama, H. *et al.* (1998). Epstein–Barr virus detection in kidney biopsy specimens correlates with glomerular mesangial injury. *American Journal of Kidney Diseases* **32**, 785–793.

Jacquot, C. and Bariéty, J. (1980). Syndromes glomérulaires aïgues révélateurs d'une infection bactérienne grave. *Nouvelle Presse Médicale* **9**, 1629–1631.

Joseph, A., Wali, R. K., and Weinman, E. J. (2000). Renal amyloidosis in AIDS. *Annals of Internal Medicine* **133**, 75.

Kaehny, W. D. *et al.* (1978). Acute nephritis and pulmonary alveolitis following pneumococcal pneumonia. *Archives of Internal Medicine* **138**, 806–808.

Kajiyama, W. *et al.* (2000). Glomerulosclerosis and viral gene expression in HIV-transgenic mice: role of nef. *Kidney International* **58**, 1148–1159.

Kanayama, Y. *et al.* (1982). *Mycoplasma pneumoniae* pneumonia associated with IgA nephropathy. *Scandinavian Journal of Infectious Diseases* **14**, 231–233.

Kannan, S. and Mattoo, T. K. (2001). Diffuse crescentic glomerulonephritis in bacterial endocarditis. *Pediatric Nephrology* **16**, 423–428.

Kaufman, M. B. and McIntosh, R. (1971). The pathogenesis of the renal lesion in a patient with streptococcal disease, infected ventriculoatrial shunt, cryoglobulinaemia and nephritis. *American Journal of Medicine* **50**, 262–268.

Keslin, M. H., Messner, R. P., and Williams, R. C. (1973). Glomerulonephritis with subacute bacterial endocarditis. *Archives of Internal Medicine* **132**, 578–581.

Kimmel, P. L. *et al.* (1992). Brief report: idiotypic IgA nephropathy in patients with human immunodeficiency virus infection. *New England Journal of Medicine* **327**, 702–706.

Kimmel, P. L. *et al.* (1993). Viral DNA in microdissected renal biopsy tissue from HIV infected patients with nephrotic syndrome. *Kidney International* **43**, 1347–1352.

Kimmel, P. L., Mishkin, G. J., and Umana, W. O. (1996). Captopril and renal survival in patients with human immunodeficiency virus nephropathy. *American Journal of Kidney Diseases* **28**, 202–208.

Kimmel, P. L., Bosch, J. P., and Vassalotti, J. A. (1998). Treatment of human immunodeficiency virus (HIV)-associated nephropathy. *Seminars in Nephrology* **18**, 446–458.

Kohler, P. F. *et al.* (1974). Chronic membranous glomerulonephritis caused by hepatitis B antigen–antibody immune complexes. *Annals of Internal Medicine* **81**, 448–451.

Kopp, J. B. *et al.* (1992). Progressive glomerulosclerosis and enhanced renal accumulation of basement membrane components in mice transgenic for human immunodeficiency virus type 1 genes. *Proceedings of the National Academy of Sciences USA* **89**, 1577–1581.

Kopp, J. B. *et al.* (2002). Indinavir-associated interstitial nephritis and urothelial inflammation: clinical and cytologic findings. *Clinical Infectious Diseases* **34**, 1122–1128.

Koyama, A. and Hirayama, K. (2001). Glomerulonephritis associated with Staphylococcus aureus infection. *Internal Medicine* **40**, 365–367.

Koyama, A. *et al.* (1995). Glomerulonephritis associated with MRSA infection: a possible role of bacterial superantigen. *Kidney International* **47**, 207–216.

Krane, N. K. *et al.* (1987). Renal disease and syphilis: a report of nephrotic syndrome with minimal change disease. *American Journal of Kidney Diseases* **9**, 176–179.

Lai, K. N., Arrons, I., Woodroffe, A. J., and Clarkson, A. R. (1982). Renal lesions in leptospirosis. *Australian and New Zealand Journal of Medicine* **12**, 276–279.

Lam, C. N., McNeish, A. S., and Gibson, A. M. M. (1969). Nephrotic syndrome associated with complement deficiency and staphylococcal albus bacteraemia. *Scottish Medical Journal* **14**, 86–88.

Lande, M. B. *et al.* (1998). Immune complex disease associated with Epstein–Barr virus infectious mononucleosis. *Pediatric Nephrology* **12**, 651–653.

Laurence, J. *et al.* (1996). Plasma from patients with idiopathic and human immunodeficiency virus-associated thrombotic thrombocytopenic purpura induces apoptosis in microvascular endothelial cells. *Blood* **87**, 3245–3254.

Leblond, V. *et al.* (1994). Collapsing focal segmental glomerulosclerosis associated with visceral leishmaniasis. *Nephrology, Dialysis, Transplantation* **9**, 1353.

Lee, S. and Kjellstrand, C. M. (1978). Renal disease in infectious mononucleosis. *Clinical Nephrology* **9**, 236–240.

Le Moing, V. *et al.* (1999). Use of corticosteroids in glomerulonephritis related to infective endocarditis: three cases and review. *Clinical Infectious Diseases* **28**, 1057–1061.

Levin, M. L. *et al.* (2001). HIV-associated nephropathy occurring before HIV antibody seroconversion. *American Journal of Kidney Diseases* **37**, E39.

Levy, M. Infection related proteinuria syndromes. In *The Nephrotic Syndrome* (ed. J. S. Cameron and R. J. Glassock), pp. 745–804. New York: Dekker, 1988.

Levy, M., Gubler, M. C., and Habib, R. Pathology and immunopathology of shunt nephritis in children: report of 10 cases. In *Proceedings of the Eighth International Congress of Nephrology, Athens* (ed. W. Zurukyoglu, M. Papadimitriou, M. Pyrpasopoules, M. Sion, and C. Zamboulis), pp. 290–296. Basel: Karger, 1981.

Levy, M. *et al.* (1985). Berger's disease in children. *Medicine (Baltimore)* **64**, 157–180.

Levy, R. L. and Hong, R. (1973). The immune nature of subacute bacterial endocarditis. *American Journal of Medicine* **54**, 645–652.

Lin, C.-Y. and Hsu, H.-C. (1983). Measles and acute glomerulonephritis. *Pediatrics* **71**, 398–401.

Lin C.-Y., Chen, W. P., and Chiang, H. (1990). Mumps associated nephritis. *Child Nephrology and Urology* **10**, 68–71.

Löhlein, M. (1910). Ueber hammorrhagische Nierenaffektionen bei chronischer ulzerözer Endocarditis. *Medinizische Klinik* **10**, 375–379.

Losito, A., Bucciarelli, E., Massi-Benedetti, F., and Lato, M. (1979). Membranous glomerulonephritis in congenital syphilis. *Clinical Nephrology* **12**, 32–37.

Mactier, R. A. and Dobbie, J. W. (1984). Acute infectious disease presenting as acute renal failure. *Scottish Medical Journal* **29**, 96–100.

Majumdar, A. *et al.* (2000). Renal pathological findings in infective endocarditis. *Nephrology, Dialysis, Transplantation* **15**, 1782–1787.

Marras, D. *et al.* (2002). Replication and compartmentalization of HIV-1 in kidney epithelium of patients with HIV-associated nephropathy. *Nature Medicine* **8**, 522–526.

Matsuda, O. *et al.* (1992). Long term effects of steroid treatment on nephrotic syndrome associated with Kimura's disease and a review of the literature. *Clinical Nephrology* **37**, 119–123.

Matsuzawa, N. *et al.* (2002). Nephrotic IgA nephropathy associated with disseminated tuberculosis. *Clinical Nephrology* **57**, 63–68.

Mettler, N. E. (1969). Isolation of a microtatobiote from patients with hemolytic–uremic syndrome and thrombotic thrombocytoponeic purpura and from mites in the United States. *New England Journal of Medicine* **281**, 1023–1027.

Michalak, T. (1978). Immune complexes of hepatitis B surface antigen in the pathogenesis of polyarteritis nodosa. A study of seven necropsy cases. *American Journal of Pathology* **90**, 619–632.

Michel, C. *et al.* (1992). Nephropathy associated with infection by human immunodeficiency virus: a report on 11 cases including 6 treated with zidovudine. *Nephron* **62**, 434–440.

Miller, J. (1849). Observations on scarlatinal albuminuria and a short notice on the sequela proper to that infection. *Lancet* **i**, 127–128.

Miller, M. E. *et al.* (2001). Human T-cell lymphotropic virus-1-associated renal disease in Jamaican children. *Pediatric Nephrology* **16**, 51–56.

Montseny, J. J. *et al.* (1995). The current spectrum of infectious glomerulonephritis. Experience with 76 patients and review of the literature. *Medicine (Baltimore)* **74**, 63–73.

Morel-Maroger, L., Sraer, J. D., Herrman, G., and Godeau, P. (1972). Kidney in subacute endocarditis. *Archives of Pathology* **94**, 205–213.

Mori, Y. *et al.* (2002). Association of parvovirus B19 infection with acute glomerulonephritis in healthy adults: case report and review of the literature. *Clinical Nephrology* **57**, 69–73.

Moriga, T. *et al.* (1994). Diffuse and broad podocyte detachment in a case of nephrotic syndrome associated with Kimura's disease. *Japan Journal of Nephrology* **36**, 69–75.

Moudgil, A. *et al.* (2001). Association of parvovirus B19 infection with idiopathic collapsing glomerulopathy. *Kidney International* **59**, 2126–2133.

Musa, A. M., Saleh, S. T., and Abu Asha, H. (1981). Transient nephritis during typhoid fever in five Sudanese patients. *Annals of Tropical Medicine and Parasitology* **75**, 181–184.

Muthukumar, T. *et al.* (2002). Acute renal failure due to rifampicin: a study of 25 patients. *American Journal of Kidney Diseases* **40**, 690–696.

Nadasdy, T. *et al.* (1992). Epstein–Barr virus infection-associated renal disease: diagnostic use of molecular hybridization technology in patients with negative serology. *Journal of the American Society of Nephrology* **2**, 1734–1742.

Nagashima, T. *et al.* (2001). Antineutrophil cytoplasmic autoantibody specific for proteinase 3 in a patient with shunt nephritis induced by *Gemella morbillorum*. *American Journal of Kidney Diseases* **37**, E38.

Namie, S. *et al.* (1995). Evaluation of anti-HTLV-1 antibody in primary glomerulonephritis. *Journal of International Medical Research* **23**, 56–60.

Nebuloni, M. *et al.* (1999). BK virus renal infection in a patient with the acquired immunodeficiency syndrome. *Archives of Pathology & Laboratory Medicine* **123**, 807–811.

Neugarten, J., Gallo, G. R., and Baldwin, D. S. (1984). Glomerulonephritis in bacterial endocarditis. *American Journal of Kidney Diseases* **5**, 371–379.

Nochy, D. *et al.* (1993). Renal disease associated with HIV infection, a multicentric study of 60 patients from Paris hospitals. *Nephrology, Dialysis, Transplantation* **8**, 11–19.

Noe, N. H. and Roy, S. (1981). Shunt nephritis. *Journal of Urology* **125**, 731–733.

Nunan, T. O., Eykyn, S. J., and Jones, N. F. (1984). Brucellosis with mesangial IgA nephropathy: successful treatment with doxycyline and rifampicin. *British Medical Journal* **288**, 1802.

Nydahl, B. C. and Hall, W. H. (1965). The treatment of staphylococcal infection with nafcillin with a discussion of staphylococcal nephritis. *Annals of Internal Medicine* **63**, 27–43.

O'Connor, D. T., Weisman, M. H., and Fierer, J. (1978). Activation of the alternate complement pathway in *Staphylococcus aureus* infective endocarditis and its relationship to thrombocytopaenia, coagulation abnormalities and acute glomerulonephritis. *Clinical and Experimental Immunology* **34**, 179–187.

O'Donnell, M. P. *et al.* (1998). Renal cell cytokine production stimulates HIV-1 expression in chronically HIV-1-infected monocytes. *Kidney International* **53**, 593–597.

Oksenhendler, E. *et al.* (1998). Transient angiolymphoid hyperplasia and Kaposi's sarcoma after primary infection with human herpesvirus 8 in a patient with human immunodeficiency virus infection. *New England Journal of Medicine* **338**, 1585–1590.

O'Regan, S. and Makker, S. P. (1979). Shunt nephritis: demonstration of diptheroid antigen in glomeruli. *American Journal of Medical Science* **278**, 161–165.

O'Regan, S. *et al.* (1976). Treponemal antigens in congenital and acquired syphilis. *Annals of Internal Medicine* **85**, 325–327.

O'Regan, S. *et al.* (1979). Subacute sclerosing panencephalitis associated glomerulopathy. *Nephron* **23**, 304.

Ozawa, T. and Stewart, J. A. (1979). Immune-complex glomerulonephritis associated with cytomegalovirus infection. *American Journal of Clinical Pathology* **72**, 103–107.

Papo, T. *et al.* (1999). Human herpesvirus 8 infection, Castleman's disease and POEMS syndrome. *British Journal of Haematology* **104**, 932–933.

Pardo, V. *et al.* (1984). Glomerular lesions in the acquired immunodeficiency syndrome. *Annals of Internal Medicine* **101**, 429–434.

Pardo, V. *et al.* (1987). AIDS-related glomerulopathy: occurrence in specific risk groups. *Kidney International* **31**, 1167–1173.

Park, J. S. *et al.* (1994). Cytomegalovirus is not specifically associated with immunoglobulin A nephropathy. *Journal of the American Society of Nephrology* **4**, 1623–1626.

Patriarca, P. A. and Lauer, B. A. (1980). Ventriculoperitoneal shunt-associated infection due to *Haemophilus influenzae. Pediatrics* **65**, 1007–1009.

Pecchini, F., Bufano, G., and Ghiringhelli, P. (1997). Membranoproliferative glomerulonephritis secondary to tuberculosis. *Clinical Nephrology* **47**, 63–64.

Peces, R. *et al.* (1998). Haemolytic–uraemic syndrome in a heroin addict. *Nephrology, Dialysis, Transplantation* **13**, 3197–3199.

Peraldi, M. N. *et al.* (1999). Acute renal failure in the course of HIV infection: a single-institution retrospective study of ninety-two patients and sixty renal biopsies. *Nephrology, Dialysis, Transplantation* **14**, 1578–1585.

Perez, G. O. *et al.* (1974). A mini epidemic of Goodpasture's syndrome. *Nephron* **13**, 161–173.

Perez, G. O., Rothfield, N., and Williams, R. C. (1976). Immune complex nephritis in bacterial endocarditis. *Archives of Internal Medicine* **136**, 334–336.

Pertschuk, L. P., Vuletin, J. C., Sutton, A. L., and Vesasquez, L. A. (1976). Demonstration of antigen and immune complex in glomerulonephritis due to *Staphylococcus aureus. American Journal of Clinical Pathology* **66**, 1027.

Peters, D. K. *et al.* (1973). Mesangiocapillary nephritis, partial lipodystrophy, and hypocomplementaemia. *Lancet* **2**, 535–538.

Petrogiannis-Haliotis, T. *et al.* (2001). BK-related polyomavirus vasculopathy in a renal-transplant recipient. *New England Journal of Medicine* **345**, 1250–1255.

Phinney, M. *et al.* (1994). Prednisolone improves renal function and proteinuria in HIV associated nephropathy. *Journal of the American Society of Nephrology* **5**, 358 (abstract).

Powell, D. E. B. (1961). Non-suppurative lesions in staphylococcal septicaemia. *Journal of Pathology and Bacteriology* **82**, 141–149.

Pusey, C. D. *et al.* (1983). Drug associated acute interstitial nephritis: clinical and pathological features and response to high dose steroids. *Quarterly Journal of Medicine* **52**, 194–211.

Quigg, R. J. *et al.* (1991). Acute glomerulonephritis in a patient with Rocky Mountain spotted fever. *American Journal of Kidney Diseases* **17**, 339–342.

Qunibi, W. Y., Al-Sibai, M. B., and Akhtar, M. (1988). Mesangio-proliferative glomerulonephritis associated with Kimura's disease. *Clinical Nephrology* **30**, 111–114.

Ramos, A., Vinhas, J., and Carvalho, M. F. (1994). Mixed cryoglobulinemia in a heroin addict. *American Journal of Kidney Diseases* **23**, 731–734.

Rao, T. K. (1998). Acute renal failure syndromes in human immunodeficiency virus infection. *Seminars in Nephrology* **18**, 378–395.

Rao, T. K. S., Nicastri, A. D., and Friedman, E. A. (1974). Natural history of heroin associated nephropathy. *New England Journal of Medicine* **290**, 19–23.

Rao, T. K. S. *et al.* (1984). Associated focal and segmental glomerulosclerosis in the acquired immunodeficiency syndrome. *New England Journal of Medicine* **310**, 669–673.

Ray, P. E. *et al.* (1998). Infection of human primary renal epithelial cells with HIV-1 from children with HIV-associated nephropathy. *Kidney International* **53**, 1217–1229.

Reid, W. *et al.* (2001). An HIV-1 transgenic rat that develops HIV-related pathology and immunologic dysfunction. *Proceedings of the National Academy of Sciences USA* **98**, 9271–9276.

Richardson, W. P. *et al.* (1981). Glomerulopathy associated with cytomegalovirus viremia in renal allografts. *New England Journal of Medicine* **305**, 57–63.

Rieu, P. *et al.* (2000). Glomerular involvement in lymphoproliferative disorders with hyperproduction of cytokines (Castleman, POEMS). *Advances in Nephrology from the Necker Hospital* **30**, 305–331.

Roberts, W. C. and Rabson, A. S. (1975). Focal glomerular lesions in fungal endocarditis. *Annals of Internal Medicine* **71**, 963–970.

Ross, M. J. and Klotman, P. E. (2002). Recent Progress in HIV-Associated Nephropathy. *Journal of the American Society of Nephrology* **13**, 2997–3004.

Ross, M. J. *et al.* (2001). Microcyst formation and HIV-1 gene expression occur in multiple nephron segments in HIV-associated nephropathy. *Journal of the American Society of Nephrology* **12**, 2645–2651.

Rytel, M. W., Dee, T. H., Ferstenfeld, J. E., and Hensley, G. T. (1974). Possible pathogenetic role of capsular antigens in fulminant pneumococcal disease with disseminated intravascular coagulation. *American Journal of Medicine* **57**, 889–896.

Sahud, M. A. *et al.* (2002). von Willebrand factor-cleaving protease inhibitor in a patient with human immunodeficiency syndrome-associated thrombotic thrombocytopenic purpura. *British Journal of Haematology* **116**, 909–911.

Said, M. H. *et al.* (1999). Mycoplasma pneumoniae-associated nephritis in children. *Pediatric Nephrology* **13**, 39–44.

Salyer, W. R. and Salyer, D. C. (1974). Unilateral glomerulonephritis. *Journal of Pathology* **113**, 247–257.

Samtleben, W. *et al.* (1993). Renal complications of infected ventriculoatrial shunts. *Artificial Organs* **17**, 695–701.

Santos, J. *et al.* (1994). Isolated renal mucormycosis in two AIDS patients. *European Journal of Clinical Microbiology and Infectious Diseases* **13**, 430–432.

Schena, F. P. (1985). Renal manifestations in bacterial infections. *Contributions to Nephrology* **48**, 125–134.

Scherr, G. R., Evans, S. G., Kiyabu, M. T., and Klatt, E. C. (1992). *Archives of Pathology and Laboratory Medicine* **116**, 535–536.

Schmid, M. L., McWhinney, P. H., and Will, E. J. (2000). Parvovirus B19 and glomerulonephritis in a healthy adult. *Annals of Internal Medicine* **132**, 682.

Schoenbaum, S. C., Gardner, P., and Shillito, J. (1975). Infections of cerebrospinal fluid shunts: epidemiology, clinical manifestations and therapy. *Journal of Infectious Diseases* **131**, 543–551.

Schwartz, E. J. *et al.* (2001). Human immunodeficiency virus-1 induces loss of contact inhibition in podocytes. *Journal of the American Society of Nephrology* **12**, 1677–1684.

Setz, U. *et al.* (1994). Shunt nephritis associated with *Propionibacterium acnes. Infection* **22**, 99–101.

Shah, G. M., Alvarado, P., and Kirschenbaum, M. A. (1990). Symptomatic hypocalcaemia and hypomagnesaemia with renal magnesium wasting associated with pentamidine therapy in a patient with AIDS. *American Journal of Medicine* **89**, 380–382.

Shahinian, V. *et al.* (2000). Prevalence of HIV-associated nephropathy in autopsies of HIV-infected patients. *American Journal of Kidney Diseases* **35**, 884–888.

Shankland, S. J. *et al.* (2000). Differential expression of cyclin-dependent kinase inhibitors in human glomerular disease: role in podocyte proliferation and maturation. *Kidney International* **58**, 674–683.

Sharivker, D., Vazan, A., and Varkel, J. (2001). Brucella endocarditis complicated by acute glomerulonephritis—early surgical intervention. *Acta Cardiologica* **56**, 399–400.

Shribman, J. H., Eatwood, J. B., and Uff, J. (1983). Immune complex nephritis complicating miliary tuberculosis. *British Medical Journal* **287**, 1593–1594.

Siegelmann, N. *et al.* (1992). Brucellosis with nephrotic syndrome, nephritis and IgA nephropathy. *Postgraduate Medical Journal* **68**, 834–836.

Sinniah, R., Khan, T. N., and Dodd, S. (1993). An *in situ* hybridization study of herpes simplex and Epstein Barr viruses in IgA nephropathy and non-immune glomerulonephritis. *Clinical Nephrology* **40**, 137–141.

Sitprija, V., Pipatanagul, V., Boonpucknavig, V., and Boonpucknavig, S. (1974). Glomerulonephritis in typhoid fever. *Annals of Internal Medicine* **81**, 210–213.

Smith, M. C. *et al.* (1996). Prednisone improves renal function and proteinuria in human immunodeficiency virus-associated nephropathy. *American Journal of Medicine* **101**, 41–48.

Spector, D. A., Millan, J., Zauber, N., and Buton, J. (1980). Glomerulonephritis and *Staphylococcus aureus* infections. *Clinical Nephrology* **14**, 256–261.

Stephens, E. B. *et al.* (2000). Simian–human immunodeficiency virus-associated nephropathy in macaques. *AIDS Research and Human Retroviruses* **16**, 1295–1306.

Sterzel, R. B., Krause, P. H., Zobl, H., and Kuhn, K. (1974). Acute syphilitic nephrosis: a transient glomerular immunopathy. *Clinical Nephrology* **2**, 164–168.

Stickler, G. B. *et al.* (1968). Diffuse glomerulonephritis associated with infected ventriculoatrial shunt. *New England Journal of Medicine* **279**, 1077–1082.

Strauss, J. *et al.* (1993). Human immunodeficiency virus nephropathy. *Pediatric Nephrology* **7**, 220–225.

Strife, C. F. *et al.* (1976). Shunt nephritis: the nature of the serum cryoglobulins and their relation to the complement profile. *Journal of Pediatrics* **88**, 403–413.

Szczech, L. A. *et al.* (2002). Protease inhibitors are associated with a slowed progression of HIV-related renal diseases. *Clinical Nephrology* **57**, 336–341.

Takaue, Y. and Tokumaru, M. (1982). Staphylococcal skin lesions and acute glomerulonephritis. *New England Journal of Medicine* **307**, 1213–1214.

Tanawattanacharoen, S. *et al.* (2000). Parvovirus B19 DNA in kidney tissue of patients with focal segmental glomerulosclerosis. *American Journal of Kidney Diseases* **35**, 1166–1174.

Tang, W. W. *et al.* (1993). Hyponatremia in hospitalized patients with the acquired immunodeficiency syndrome (AIDS) and the AIDS-related complex. *American Journal of Medicine* **94**, 169–174.

Taylor, G., Drachenberg, C., and Faris-Young, S. (2001). Renal involvement of human parvovirus B19 in an immunocompetent host. *Clinical Infections Diseases* **32**, 167–169.

Thompson, C. E. *et al.* (1992). Thrombotic microangiopathies in the 1980s: clinical features, response to treatment, and the impact of the human immunodeficiency virus epidemic. *Blood* **80**, 1890–1895.

Treser, G. *et al.* (1974). Renal lesions in narcotic addicts. *American Journal of Medicine* **57**, 687–694.

Tu, W. H., Shearn, M. A., and Lee, J. C. (1969). Acute diffuse glomerulonephritis in acute staphylococcal endocarditis. *Annals of Internal Medicine* **71**, 335–341.

Ucar, A. *et al.* (1994). Thrombotic microangiopathy and retroviral infections: a 13-year experience. *American Journal of Hematology* **45**, 304–309.

Uthgennant, D., Steinhoff, J., Barethon, G., and Sack, K. (1991). Morbus Kimura mit minimalische proliferatiren Glomerulonephritis. *Deutsche Medizinische Wohenschrift* **116**, 935–938.

Valeri, A. *et al.* (1996). Idiopathic collapsing focal segmental glomerulosclerosis: a clinicopathologic study. *Kidney International* **50**, 1734–1746.

van Rhenen, D. J. *et al.* (1976). Immune complex glomerulonephritis and chronic granulomatous disease. *Acta Medica Scandinavica* **206**, 233–237.

van Westrhenen, R., Weening, J. J., and Krediet, R. T. (1998). Pneumonia and glomerulonephritis caused by *Mycoplasma pneumoniae*. *Nephrology, Dialysis, Transplantation* **13**, 3208–3211.

Vanwalleghem, J. *et al.* (1998). Steroids for deep-infection-associated glomerulonephritis: a two-edged sword. *Nephrology, Dialysis, Transplantation* **13**, 773–775.

Vella, J. *et al.* (1995). Glomerulonephritis after ventriculoatrial shunt. *Quarterly Journal of Medicine* **88**, 911–918.

Vernet, O. and Rilliet, B. (2001). Late complications of ventriculoatrial or ventriculoperitoneal shunts. *Lancet* **358**, 1569–1570.

Viale, P., Di Matteo, A., Voltolini, F., Paties, C., and Alberici, F. (1994). Isolated kidney localisation of invasive aspergillosis in a patient with AIDS. *Scandinavian Journal of Infectious Diseases* **26**, 767–770.

Vitullo, B. B., O'Regan, S., de Chandarevian, J. P., and Kaplan, B. S. (1978). *Mycoplasma pneumoniae* associated with acute glomerulonephritis. *Nephron* **21**, 284–288.

von Bonsdorf, M., Ponka, A., and Torproth, T. (1984). *Mycoplasmal pneumoniae* associated with mesangiocapillary glomerulonephritis type II (dense deposit disease). *Acta Medica Scandinavica* **216**, 427–429.

Wakabayashi, Y., Kobayashi, Y., and Shigematsu, M. (1985). Shunt nephritis: histological dynamics following removal of the shunt. *Nephron* **40**, 111–117.

Wali, R. K. *et al.* (1998). HIV-1-associated nephropathy and response to highly-active antiretroviral therapy. Lancet **352**, 783–784.

Walker, D. H. and Mattern, W. D. (1979). Acute renal failure in Rocky Mountain spotted fever. *Archives of Internal Medicine* **139**, 443–448.

Walker, P. D. *et al.* (1984). Rapidly progressive glomerulonephritis in a patient with syphilis. Identification of antitreponemal antibody and treponemal antigen in renal tissue. *American Journal of Medicine* **76**, 1106–1112.

Watanabe, T. (2001). Hemolytic uremic syndrome associated with influenza A virus infection. *Nephron* **89**, 359–360.

Weller, R. O. and Nester, B. (1972). Histological re-assessment of three kidneys originally described by Richard Bright in 1827–1836. *British Medical Journal* **ii**, 761–763.

Whelan, T. V. *et al.* (1988). Nephrotic syndrome associated with Kimura's disease. *American Journal of Kidney Diseases* **11**, 353–356.

Wierenga, K. J. J. *et al.* (1995). Glomerulonephritis after human parvovirus infection in homozygous sickle cell disease. *Lancet* **346**, 475–476.

Williams, R. L. and Kunkel, H. C. (1962). Rheumatoid factor, complement and conglutinin aberrations in patients with subacture bacterial endocarditis. *Journal of Clinical Investigation* **41**, 666–675.

Wilson, C. B. and Smith, R. C. (1972). Goodpasture's syndrome associated with influenza A2 virus infection. *Annals of Internal Medicine* **76**, 91–94.

Winston, J. A., Burns, G. C., and Klotman, P. E. (1998). The human immunodeficiency virus (HIV) epidemic and HIV-associated nephropathy. *Seminars in Nephrology* **18**, 373–377.

Winston, J. A., Klotman, M. E., and Klotman, P. E. (1999). HIV-associated nephropathy is a late, not early, manifestation of HIV-1 infection. *Kidney International* **55**, 1036–1040.

Winston, J. A. *et al.* (2001). Nephropathy and establishment of a renal reservoir of HIV type 1 during primary infection. *New England Journal of Medicine* **344**, 1979–1984.

Woodroffe, A. J., Row, P. G., Meadows, R., and Lawrence, J. R. (1974). Nephritis in infectious mononucleosis. *Quarterly Journal of Medicine* **43**, 451–460.

Yamada, A. *et al.* (1982). Membranous glomerulonephritis associated with eosinophilic lymphofolliculosis of the skin (Kimura's disease): report of a case and review of the literature. *Clinical Nephrology* **18**, 211–215.

Yang, A. H. *et al.* (2000). Post-infectious glomerulonephritis in a patient with vesicorenal malacoplakia—coincidence or causal relationship? *Nephrology, Dialysis, Transplantation* **15**, 1060–1062.

Yoh, K. *et al.* (2000). Cytokines and T-cell responses in superantigen-related glomerulonephritis following methicillin-resistant *Staphylococcus aureus* infection. *Nephrology, Dialysis, Transplantation* **15**, 1170–1174.

Yuceoglu, A. M., Berkovich, S., and Minkowitz, S. (1967). Acute glomerulonephritis as a complication of varicella. *Journal of the American Medical Association* **202**, 879–881.

Yuceoglu, A. M., Berkovich, S., and Chiu, J. (1969). Effect of live measles vaccine on childhood nephrosis. *Journal of Pediatrics* **74**, 291–293.

Yum, M., Wheat, L. J., Maxwell, D., and Edwards, J. L. (1978). Immunofluorescent localisation of *Staphylococcus aureus* antigen in acute bacterial endocarditis nephritis. *American Journal of Clinical Pathology* **70**, 832–835.

Zappacosta, A. R. and Ashby, B. L. (1977). Gram-negative sepsis with acute renal failure. *Journal of the American Medical Association* **238**, 1389–1390.

Zunin, C. *et al.* (1977). Membranoproliferative glomerulonephritis associated with infected ventriculoatrial shunt; report of two cases recovered after removal of shunt. *Pathologica* **69**, 297–305.

3.13 Malignancy-associated glomerular disease

Alex M. Davison and Barrie Hartley

General introduction

Benign and malignant tumours, most commonly adenocarcinoma of the lung and gastrointestinal tract, and lymphoproliferative and myeloproliferative disorders, have been associated with nephropathy. This chapter is devoted to the glomerular consequences of solid tumours, lymphoproliferative and myeloproliferative disorders: those associated with plasma cell dyscrasias are detailed in Chapter 4.3.

The association between malignancy and glomerular disease was made by Galloway in 1922, who described a patient with Hodgkin's lymphoma and nephrotic syndrome. The association was either unrecognized or ignored until Lee *et al.* (1966) reported carcinoma in 11 of 101 patients with nephrotic syndrome. This paper suggested a high prevalence of carcinoma in adult patients with nephrotic syndrome, and that the most common glomerular appearance was membranous nephropathy. Since then, further series and many anecdotal reports have been published. It is now accepted that glomerular disease associated with malignancy usually presents as a nephrotic syndrome, that the majority of such patients have membranous nephropathy and that most patients are adult males; only very rarely are children involved.

Conversely, urinary abnormalities are common in patients with neoplasia and there are many possible reasons for this. Proteinuria is more common in patients with malignancy than in controls (Sawyer *et al.* 1988) and, interestingly, this indicates a poor prognosis with respect to the neoplasm. In addition, some studies suggest that mild glomerular pathology without extensive proteinuria is relatively common in patients with malignancy (Pascal *et al.* 1976; Helin *et al.* 1980).

Although the nephropathy most commonly found associated with malignant disease is membranous, many other glomerular changes have been reported. Similarly, although the most widely recognized association with Hodgkin's lymphoma is a minimal change nephropathy, other nephropathies have been described. Particular glomerular appearances are not specific for a particular tumour type, and there is no association between tumour load, as assessed by tumour size or the presence of metastases, and glomerulopathy.

Evidence for a causal relationship between malignancy and nephropathy

A number of conditions should be satisfied if a causal relationship between malignancy and nephropathy is to be established (Table 1).

Table 1 Evidence of a causal relationship

1. Close temporal relationship between the clinical appearance of the renal lesion and the tumour
2. Remission or complete removal of tumour should be associated with a remission of the nephropathy
3. Recurrence of the tumour should be accompanied by recurrence of the nephropathy
4. Demonstration of tumour antigen and appropriate antibody in glomeruli

The seminal paper of Lee *et al.* (1966) reported that in two-thirds of the patients the renal disease preceded the diagnosis of malignancy. Keur *et al.* (1989) found that the glomerulopathy was clinically apparent in the 6 months before or after recognition of the tumour in 63 per cent of the reported cases, and that the nephrotic syndrome and the tumour were recognized simultaneously in nearly 40 per cent. However, 15 patients developed the nephrotic syndrome more than 12 months before the tumour was diagnosed.

Improvement or remission of glomerulonephritis has been described after removal or treatment of a wide variety of tumours (Cantrell 1969; Barton *et al.* 1980; Yamauchi *et al.* 1985), and most reports indicate a very prompt response (Young *et al.* 1985; Beauvais *et al.* 1989). However, few follow-up biopsy studies have been reported, and these rather rare case reports need to be interpreted with caution as many patients have had therapy for the tumour, such as corticosteroids and immunosuppressive or cytotoxic drugs which may have benefited the glomerulopathy directly. Not all patients improve after remission or removal of the tumour (Couser *et al.* 1974; Row *et al.* 1975).

Recurrence of the tumour is usually associated with recurrence of the nephropathy, but this is not invariable. In a case reported by Cairns *et al.* (1978), there was a rapid resolution of proteinuria and haematuria with an increase in creatinine clearance following removal of a squamous cell carcinoma of the bronchus, but a local recurrence of the tumour was not associated with evidence of any recurrence of renal disease.

Renal involvement in malignancy

Malignant disease may involve the kidney in a variety of ways (Table 2), either direct or indirect. Renal disease may also be a result of therapy prescribed for either the tumour or its consequences.

Table 2 Renal involvement in carcinoma

Direct effects
Metastases
Infiltration
Ischaemia
Obstruction
Indirect effects
Electrolyte disorders
Hypokalaemia, hyponatraemia, hypercalcaemia
Acute renal failure
Disseminated intravascular coagulation
Renal vein thrombosis
Amyloidosis
Glomerulopathy
Nephrocalcinosis
Treatment associated
Drug nephrotoxicity
Tumour lysis syndrome
Radiation

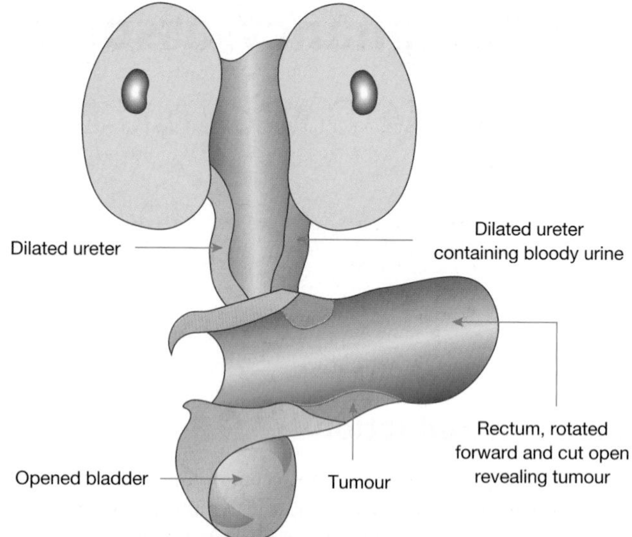

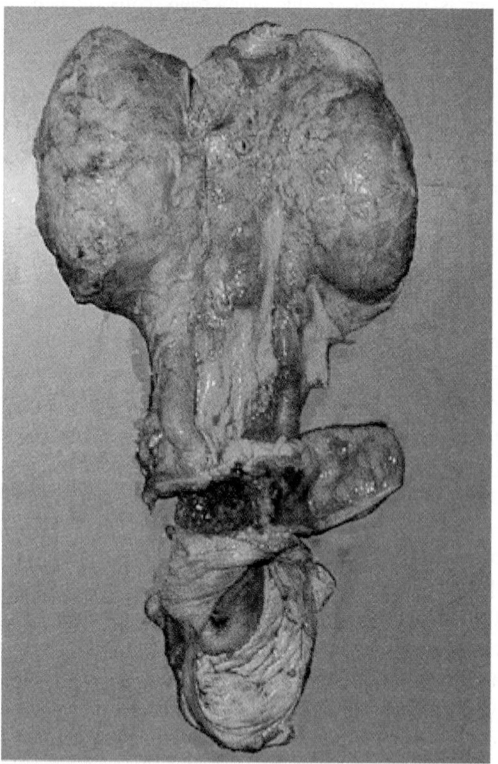

Fig. 1 Autopsy specimen showing a carcinoma at the recto-sigmoid junction which has extended laterally and resulted in obstruction of both ureters. The ureters are distended and one contains bloody fluid. The bladder has been opened and shows some erythema presumed to be due to an indwelling catheter.

Direct effects

Metastatic spread of a solid tumour to the kidney is relatively uncommon, despite the magnitude of renal blood flow. However, when present, metastases are usually multiple and often bilateral. They are usually manifested by either loin pain or haematuria; renal functional impairment is very rare. Lymphomatous and leukaemic infiltrates, diffuse or nodular, may occur and present with impaired renal function. Tumours at the hilum of the kidney, either metastatic or from lymphoma involving the para-aortic nodes, may compress the renal artery, resulting in ischaemia and subsequent hypertension. Although retroperitoneal tumours rarely cause obstruction, pelvic tumours, particularly of cervix or the rectosigmoid colon, may produce ureteric compression and eventually occlusion (Fig. 1).

Obstructive uropathy is most frequently produced by prostatic enlargement, which is benign in the majority of patients—less than 10 per cent of cases are due to carcinoma. Bladder cancer, particularly involving the trigone, can also lead to ureteric obstruction.

Indirect effects

Malignancy may have many indirect effects on the kidney, particularly in patients with advanced disease. Hypokalaemia may develop either from potassium loss, for example, in patients with prolonged diarrhoea or in those with a villous adenoma of the rectum (Roy and Ellis 1959), or from the profound metabolic alkalosis that accompanies prolonged vomiting. Hyponatraemia may occur in association with diarrhoea and vomiting, or from inappropriate antidiuretic hormone (ADH) secretion in patients with oat-cell carcinoma of the lung. Hypercalcaemia arises more commonly from marrow infiltration with myeloma than from metastatic disease, and may also be caused by release of parathyroid hormone (PTH)-like substances from certain tumours, such as oat-cell tumours of the lung, and by secretion of prostaglandins from tumours (Seyberth *et al.* 1975). Release of skeletal calcium following immobilization and, rarely, as a result of hormonal therapy for breast carcinoma can also cause hypercalcaemia (Swaroop and Krant 1973). In some patients, the hypercalcaemia causes nephrocalcinosis which may lead to papillary necrosis and to tubulointerstitial inflammation and fibrosis. Hypercalcaemia can also impair urinary concentration, by inhibition of sodium transport in the ascending limb of the loop of Henle, and through inhibition of the effect of ADH in collecting ducts. The net result is polyuria and polydipsia, with the risk of dehydration if the patient is unable to maintain an adequate fluid intake.

Table 3 Glomerular appearances most commonly associated with carcinoma

Membranous nephropathy
Mesangiocapillary glomerulonephritis
IgA nephropathy
Mesangial proliferative glomerulonephritis
Crescentic nephritis
Amyloidosis

Table 4 Pathogenesis of malignancy-associated glomerulonephritis

1. Tumour-associated antigen
2. Re-expressed fetal antigen
3. Viral antigen
4. Autologous non-tumour antigen
5. Disseminated intravascular coagulation
6. Amyloidosis

Acute renal failure may arise as an indirect effect of malignancy. This may be prerenal, as in patients with hypovolaemia from prolonged diarrhoea and vomiting, associated with hepatic failure due to metastatic tumours, or may be due to acute tubular necrosis caused by septicaemia as a consequence of the generalized immunosuppression of advanced malignancy. Impaired renal function may also occur in patients who develop disseminated intravascular coagulation as has been described in carcinoma of the pancreas, lung, and in trophoblastic tumours. Renal vein thrombosis may develop (De Swiet and Wells 1957) due to the generalized hypercoagulable state of malignancy.

A variety of glomerular changes (Table 3) have been reported in association with malignancy (see below).

Effects of therapy

Drug nephrotoxicity may occur due to drugs such as cisplatinum or from antibiotics and analgesics. Dosik *et al.* (1978) described three patients with malignant melanoma treated with *Cryptosporidium parvum* who developed an acute renal failure and in whom renal biopsy showed a mesangial proliferative glomerulonephritis. Although subendothelial deposits containing immunoglobulin and complement were found, no *C. parvum* antigen could be detected. A causal link is clearly tenuous, but the renal failure resolved on stopping *C. parvum* therapy. Although radiotherapy is widely used in the treatment of malignancies, radiation nephropathy (see Chapter 6.6) is now uncommon: recognition of the susceptibility of renal tubular cells to irradiation injury has led to the development of effective shielding during therapy. In some circumstances it is impossible to shield the whole kidney and acute and chronic radiation nephritis may result. Acute effects usually become manifest within 6–12 months, whereas chronic effects develop years later and may not be preceded by an acute syndrome.

Pathogenesis of glomerulopathy

Glomerular injury in malignancy may be immunologically mediated, resulting from disseminated intravascular coagulation, or amyloidosis (Table 4). Eagen and Lewis (1977) observed that the immunopathological features of the glomerular lesions associated with carcinoma were similar to those found in immune complex disease and suggested that they might result from (a) tumour associated antigens; (b) re-expressed fetal antigens; (c) viral antigens; or (d) the development of autoimmunity to autologous non-tumour antigens. Unfortunately, no suitable animal models exist to facilitate experimental studies.

Although malignancy can be associated with impaired cell-mediated immunity, tumours are able to stimulate both cellular and humoral responses.

Circulating immune complexes have been described in up to 80 per cent of patients with malignancy (Rossen *et al.* 1976) only a few develop nephropathy; this could, however, be due to variation in the size and/or charge of the complexes. The most common histological appearance in malignancy-associated nephropathy is membranous, and patients with idiopathic membranous glomerulonephritis rarely have circulating immune complexes. In addition, electron microscopy commonly shows subepithelial deposits, whereas in patients with glomerular disease associated with circulating immune complexes, and also in experimental animals given intravenous injections of preformed immune complexes, deposits are usually found within the subendothelial area of the glomerular capillary wall or in the mesangium (see Chapter 3.2). All these observations suggest that the immune deposits are more likely to have been formed *in situ* from antigen and antibody deposited separately. It is possible that some tumour antigens have a high affinity for basement membrane constituents and thus become 'planted' with subsequent antibody attachment.

Melanoma antigen and antibody have been demonstrated both directly and indirectly within glomerular deposits (Weksler *et al.* 1974; Olson *et al.* 1979), and eluates from glomeruli have been shown to cross-react with antigens on bronchogenic carcinoma (Lewis *et al.* 1971), colonic carcinoma (Couser *et al.* 1974), and gastric carcinoma (Wakashin *et al.* 1980) cells. One report describes a patient with metastatic prostatic carcinoma and acute renal failure who was found to have a crescentic glomerulonephritis at autopsy associated with glomerular deposition of prostate-specific acid phosphatase and prostate-specific antigen in a focal and segmental distribution (Haskell *et al.* 1990). Thus, although there have been no large studies, many reports involving small numbers of patients provide convincing evidence that malignancy-associated nephropathy is immune complex mediated.

Re-expressed fetal antigens have been demonstrated, both on tumours and within glomerular deposits. Carcinoembryonic antigen has been demonstrated in glomerular deposits (Costanza *et al.* 1973; Couser *et al.* 1974) and Pascal and Slovin (1980) described a patient with gastric carcinoma in whom carcinoembryonic antigen and antibodies could be detected within the glomerular capillary wall in a subendothelial and paramesangial position.

Viruses are being implicated as causal agents in an increasing number of malignancies, particularly in lymphoproliferative diseases: no such association has yet been demonstrated with human solid tumours. Pascal *et al.* (1980) described virus-like particles adjacent to the plasma membranes of numerous mesangial and epithelial cells in a patient with prostatic cancer and membranoproliferative glomerulonephritis. Antibodies to Epstein–Barr virus have been reported in patients with Burkitt's lymphoma and in a patient with membranous nephropathy associated with angiofollicular lymph node hyperplasia (Castleman's disease). The significance of these findings and, in particular, their relationship to the pathogenesis of the glomerular findings is unknown. Glomerular deposition of viral antigen and antibody has been demonstrated in mice with virus-induced mammary tumours (Pascal *et al.* 1975). Thus, although viruses may play a part in the glomerular lesions associated with lymphoma and leukaemia, there is currently little evidence that they play any part in the nephropathy associated with carcinoma.

Patients with malignancy seem more prone than controls to develop autoimmunity, with the formation of non-specific autoantibodies, and there are reports of glomerular deposition of autologous non-tumour antigens. One such antigen may be the p53 protein and mutations of this are known to occur in malignancy. This is supported by the finding that mutations are more common in carcinoma of the lung and less frequent in patients with carcinoma of the breast (Lubin *et al.* 1995) and this may explain why nephropathy is more frequently associated with lung than with breast cancer. Other endogenous antigens have been implicated, for instance, Higgins *et al.* (1974) described a patient with oat-cell carcinoma of the bronchus in whom large quantities of extracellular DNA in necrotic tumour tissue were associated with serum antinuclear antibody and the presence of Feulgen-positive material within glomerular capillary walls. The authors suggested that, in this patient, there was antibody formation against nuclear antigen released by tumour necrosis. Ozawa *et al.* (1975) described three patients with renal cell carcinoma in whom glomerular and tumour eluates reacted with normal proximal tubular brush border antigens as well as antigens on the tumour membrane supporting the concept that the renal tubular epithelial antigen is shed from renal cell carcinoma and that subsequent antibody leads to immune complex formation.

Cytokines may play a role in the pathogenesis of tumours and glomerulonephritis. Interleukin 6 (IL-6), a pleiotropic cytokine, has a central role in defence mechanisms and in particular has potent antitumour activity against certain tumours mediated by induction of tumour specific cytotoxic T-cells and by growth inhibitory activity. Abnormal expression of the IL-6 gene has been suggested to be involved in the pathogenesis of glomerulonephritis, myeloma, and sarcoma. An IL-6–IL-6-receptor autocrine loop has been implicated in oncogenesis. If IL-6 is confirmed to be implicated in the pathogenesis of malignancy-associated nephropathy then it may illustrate two separate consequences of a common cause rather than a direct causal link between one and the other.

Local intravascular coagulation may be responsible for glomerular lesions in a small number of cases. Young *et al.* (1985) described two patients with distinctive glomerular abnormalities consisting of occlusive eosinophilic deposits in glomerular capillary lumina in which immunofluorescence revealed fibrin-related antigens and IgM. It is possible that this lesion was initiated by the release of coagulant proteins from tumour cells.

Amyloidosis is a well-recognized complication of malignancy and is discussed fully in Chapter 4.2.1. It has been described particularly in association with renal cell carcinoma (Kimball 1961) and there is speculation that the tumour secretes a precursor of amyloid proteins, which is later cleaved and precipitates as amyloid. Alternatively, the tumour may secrete an enzyme which cleaves a precursor of amyloid already present in the circulation (Couser 1980). It has also occasionally been reported in association with Hodgkin's lymphoma.

Clinical features

The most common presentation of tumour-associated nephrosis in adults is the nephrotic syndrome, but this is influenced by whether the series is being reported by a nephrologist or an oncologist. Burstein *et al.* (1993) found that all patients in their series presented with nephrotic range proteinuria, but this was a study designed to look for malignancy in patients known to have membranous nephropathy. Nephrotic syndrome is manifested before the tumour in about 40 per cent of patients (Keur *et al.* 1989), and they are therefore likely to present to a nephrologist (Fig. 2). There is, however, no indication of the true incidence

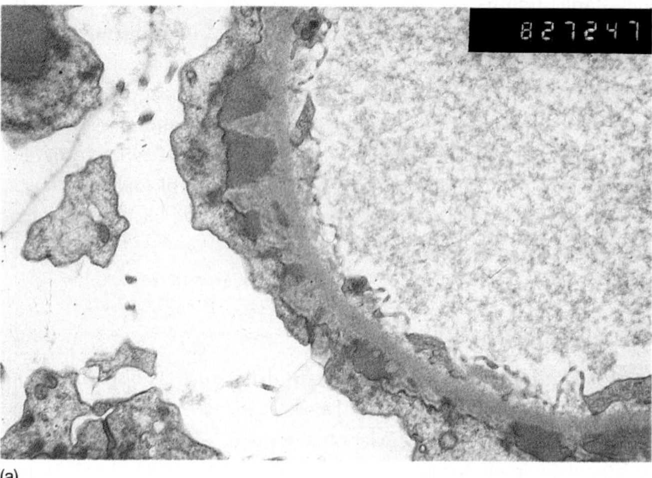

(a)

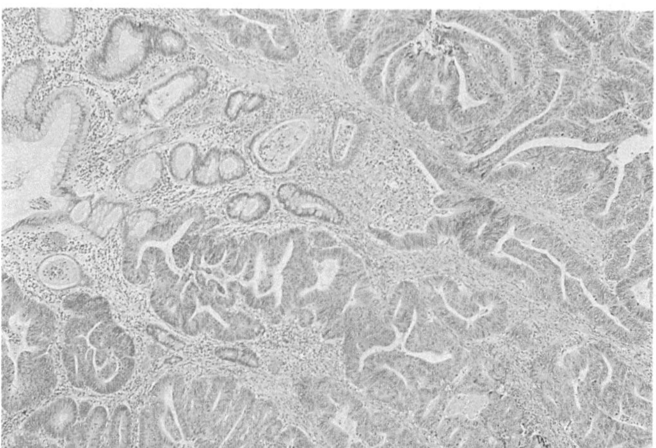

(b)

Fig. 2 A 60-year-old man who presented with nephrotic syndrome. Renal biopsy revealed a membranous type lesion. (a) Electron micrograph illustrating three finely granular subepithelial electron-dense deposits in the glomerular capillary wall (1325× reduced for publication). (b) Ten months later a well differentiated adenocarcinoma of the sigmoid colon was excised (haematoxylin and eosin, 212× reduced for publication) with subsequent resolution of the nephrotic syndrome. Illustrations by kind permission of Dr S.R. Aparicio, Department of Pathology, St James's University Hospital, Leeds.

of nephropathy in malignancy since many patients may have only minor degrees of proteinuria.

Microscopic haematuria or symptomless proteinuria are common, but a number of patients have proteinuria severe enough to produce a nephrotic syndrome. There is seldom significant renal functional impairment: Puolijoki *et al.* (1989) reported that three of 70 patients had a serum creatinine greater than 150 μmol/l, but in none was this greater than 190 μmol/l. There are a number of reports of patients in whom renal function improved after removal of the tumour (Cairns *et al.* 1978; Jermanovich *et al.* 1982). No reports have documented the rate of deterioration of renal function, but it is likely that progression of the tumour is faster than progression of the renal impairment.

Other less common forms of presentation have included steroid-resistant nephrotic syndrome in a child (Beauvais *et al.* 1989) and Henoch–Schönlein purpura (Cairns *et al.* 1978).

Incidence of glomerulopathy in neoplasia

The prevalence of tumour-associated nephropathy is unknown, but in view of the frequency of malignancy in the general population, the development of clinically-apparent nephropathy is rare. Glomerular lesions are most common in patients with carcinoma of the lung or gastrointestinal tract and are uncommon in patients with carcinoma of the breast or uterus. Most reports therefore show a male preponderance. Subclinical glomerular involvement is probably much more common. The majority of patients with advanced or incurable malignancy are not subjected to invasive renal investigations, and in many the rate of progression of the malignancy may well exceed that of the nephropathy. In an autopsy study of 303 patients with malignancy, Sutherland *et al.* (1974) found that two of 124 patients with solid tumours had deposition of IgG and complement in histologically normal glomeruli. The antigens were not identified, clinical details were not given and some of the patients had been treated with irradiation and chemotherapy. In another autopsy study, mesangial and/or subendothelial immune deposits were detected in 22 of 129 patients (17 per cent) with solid tumours, mainly of the gastrointestinal tract (Beaufils *et al.* 1985). Twenty of the patients had a mild increase in mesangial matrix, with occasional hypercellularity on light microscopy, and two had no glomerular changes. A greater incidence of immune deposits was reported by Pascal *et al.* (1976) who found mesangial and subendothelial deposits in 30 per cent of patients at autopsy. In a further autopsy study, Pascal (1980) detected overt glomerulonephritis in five of 314 patients with malignancy, giving an incidence of glomerular disease of about 1.5 per cent among patients with solid tumours. Thus, it appears that although immune deposits may be common, occurring in 17–40 per cent of patients with malignancy coming to autopsy, histologically obvious glomerular changes are rare.

Two studies have attempted to determine the incidence of urinary abnormalities in patients with carcinoma. Sawyer *et al.* (1988) found that 58 per cent of 504 patients with a variety of malignancies had urinary abnormalities consisting of either proteinuria and/or haematuria. In addition, actuarial analysis showed that patients with proteinuria had significantly shorter median survival than those without. A further retrospective study from Finland (Puolijoki *et al.* 1989) found proteinuria and haematuria in 15 per cent of 450 patients with lung cancer. This group also reported a prospective study of 150 patients, 23 of whom had proteinuria and/or haematuria. Exclusion of patients with renal metastases, anticoagulant therapy, nephrolithiasis, and hypertension gave an incidence of 12 per cent. In both studies, however, the threshold for the detection of proteinuria was within the normal range, which will thus result in an overestimate of the true incidence.

It is difficult to reconcile these major differences between autopsy and clinical studies. It is possible that the clinical studies detected a significant number of patients with mild proteinuria associated with little in the way of glomerular pathology. This is supported by Pascal *et al.* (1976) and Helin *et al.* (1980), who concluded that mild glomerulopathy without extensive proteinuria was relatively common in patients with solid tumours. It is likely that the autopsy series underestimated the frequency of deposits, since both electron microscopy and immunological tests are notoriously difficult to perform in post-mortem material.

Incidence of carcinoma in patients with glomerulopathy

Adults

The initial report of Lee *et al.* (1966) recorded that 11 of 101 patients with nephrotic syndrome had cancer. A series reported by Row *et al.* (1975) recorded evidence of malignancy in 10.9 per cent, a figure remarkably similar to the 10.3 per cent recorded by Burstein *et al.* (1993). This high incidence has not been reported in other series or reviews. Kaplan *et al.* (1976) reviewed 14 series, comprising a total of 1643 patients with nephrotic syndrome and found only six who were reported to have malignancy. Details of the 14 series are not recorded, but they could not have included the 11 patients reported by Lee *et al.* (1966). In a study of 76 patients with nephrotic syndrome and over the age of 60, Zech *et al.* (1982) showed that 7.9 per cent had an associated malignancy. Keur *et al.* (1989) reviewed nine reported series and identified 52 of 763 patients with an associated malignancy. This gives an overall incidence of 7 per cent, while the incidence in the individual series varied between 3 and 13 per cent.

It is likely that the incidence increases with increasing age, but this may be due to the fact that with age secondary causes of nephrotic syndrome become more common and malignancy increases in frequency.

Children

Glomerular disease has only very rarely been reported in children with malignancy. There were no cases of malignancy in 121 children with membranous glomerulonephritis (Kleinknecht *et al.* 1979; Latham *et al.* 1982; Ramirez *et al.* 1982). Cameron and Ogg (1975), however, recorded that three of 350 children with nephrotic syndrome had evidence of neoplasia, and one of their patients with Wilms' tumour and nephrotic syndrome was also reported by Row *et al.* (1975). A 1-year-old child with an abdominal neuroblastoma and membranous nephropathy was also described: the nephropathy apparently resolved after tumour removal and chemotherapy (Zheng *et al.* 1979). Similarly, steroid-resistant nephrotic syndrome in a 14-year-old girl with a benign ovarian tumour resolved after tumour removal (Beauvais *et al.* 1989).

Diffuse mesangial sclerosis has been reported in association with the Denis-Drash syndrome of Wilms' tumour, pseudohermaphroditism, and nephropathy (see Chapter 18.2) (Drash *et al.* 1970; Habib *et al.* 1985). Since the original two patients (Drash *et al.* 1970) there have been a number of reports confirming the association. Clinically, the patients present at a young age (from 2 months to 2 years old) with proteinuria which may be sufficient to cause the nephrotic syndrome, hypertension, and progressive renal failure.

Thus, the incidence of malignancy in patients with nephrotic syndrome is likely to be less than 7 per cent, but it may increase with increasing age. Nonetheless, it is advisable to seek an underlying malignancy in adults presenting with nephrotic syndrome due to a membranous glomerulonephritis, especially in those aged more than 50 years, as tumour removal may be curative. Enquiry should include a full history identifying risk factors and the presence of cancer in family members. Simple screening tests such as chest radiography, faecal occult blood, and carcinoembryonic antigen should be performed. Gastrointestinal contrast studies, however, are not justified as a routine investigation although colonoscopy and/or gastroscopy should be considered. Regular follow-up is required particularly in patients aged over 50 years.

Types of malignancy involved

A very wide variety of malignant and benign tumours has been implicated. The most common are adenocarcinomata of the lung and gastrointestinal tract (stomach, colon, rectum), but many other tumours have been associated with nephropathy, usually on the basis of single case reports (Table 5). Interestingly, the nephropathy is relatively rarely associated with carcinoma of the breast, despite the relatively high incidence of this tumour (Barton *et al.* 1980).

Benign tumours are only occasionally implicated, but there are two particularly striking reports. Membranous glomerulonephritis was associated with a benign teratoma in a child and the associated nephrotic syndrome resolved on removal of the tumour (Beauvais *et al.* 1989). In addition, a carotid body tumour was reported in association with a membranous glomerulonephritis in a 16-year-old girl (Lumeng and Moran 1966).

Angiomyolipoma is a benign congenital tumour which occurs in the kidney in patients with tuberous sclerosis, an autosomal dominant condition of variable expression. In this syndrome, hamartomata may involve the brain, retina, skin, heart, lungs, bone, and kidney. In the kidney, the angiomyolipomas are commonly multiple and bilateral and are frequently associated with cysts (Stillwell *et al.* 1987). Frequently, the renal lesions of tuberous sclerosis are asymptomatic, although some patients develop macroscopic haematuria, loin pain, and renal failure. Tumour embolization or surgical intervention, partial nephrectomy or tumour embolization, may be necessary for severe bleeding or severe pain (see also Chapter 18.1).

Table 5 Types of malignancy associated with nephropathy

Site	Type	Reference
Lung	Adenocarcinoma Squamous cell carcinoma Oat-cell carcinoma	Lewis *et al.* (1971) Cairns *et al.* (1978) Heaton *et al.* (1975) Mustonen *et al.* (1981)
Oesophagus	Squamous cell carcinoma	Heckerling *et al.* (1985)
Stomach	Adenocarcinoma	Cantrell (1969) Wakashin *et al.* (1980)
Colon	Adenocarcinoma	Costanza *et al.* (1973)
Rectum	Adenocarcinoma	Kitano (1984)
Bile duct	Adenocarcinoma	Brueggemeyer and Ramirez (1987)
Skin	Basal cell Squamous cell Melanoma	Lee *et al.* (1966) Lee *et al.* (1966) Weksler *et al.* (1974)
Breast	Adenocarcinoma	Lewis *et al.* (1971) Barton *et al.* (1980)
Thyroid	Adenocarcinoma	Castleman *et al.* (1963)
Adrenal	Phaeochromocytoma	Endoh (1984)
Ovary	Teratoma Adenocarcinoma	Beauvais *et al.* (1989) Lee *et al.* (1966)
Cervix	Adenocarcinoma	Lee *et al.* (1966)
Uterus	Trophoblastic	Young *et al.* (1985)
Kidney	Renal cell carcinoma Wilms' tumour	Ozawa *et al.* (1975) Kimball (1961) Drash *et al.* (1970)
Prostate	Adenocarcinoma	Stuart *et al.* (1986)
Bladder	Transitional cell carcinoma	Brueggemeyer and Ramirez (1987)
Palate	Adenocarcinoma	Borochovitz *et al.* (1982)

Glomerular appearances (Table 5)

Membranous nephropathy (see Chapter 3.7)

Membranous glomerulonephritis is by far the most common histological type observed, occurring in approximately 70 per cent of patients. It has been associated with both benign and malignant tumours, but most commonly with bronchogenic carcinoma, although there are also reports of colorectal, renal (Kerpen *et al.* 1978), and gastric adenocarcinomas. Other tumours have only been described in small numbers, the majority being single case reports. The histological appearances of membranous nephropathy associated with malignancy on light microscopy, immunofluorescence, and electron microscopy are no different from those of idiopathic membranous nephropathy.

The frequency of neoplasia in patients with membranous nephropathy is variable, Hopper (1974) reported an associated carcinoma in 6 per cent, Row *et al.* (1975) recorded evidence of malignancy in 10.9 per cent, a figure remarkably similar to the 10.3 per cent reported by Burstein *et al.* (1993). Not all series or reviews have recorded such incidences; in a review of 14 reported series of patients with nephrotic syndrome (Kaplan *et al.* 1976) only six patients with an associated malignancy were detected from a total of 1643 patients.

Mesangiocapillary glomerulonephritis (see Chapter 3.8)

Lee *et al.* (1966) describe one patient as having a 'lobular glomerulonephritis'. A subendothelial type mesangiocapillary glomerulonephritis was reported in a patient with carcinoma of the breast (Lewis *et al.* 1971) and in a patient with bronchogenic carcinoma (Heaton *et al.* 1975). Similar findings were reported by Robinson *et al.* (1984) in a patient with adenocarcinoma of the stomach. In addition, Olson *et al.* (1979)

reported three patients with malignant melanoma in whom glomerular deposits contained antigen which was also identified on the tumour: the appearance on light microscopy was that of mesangiocapillary glomerulonephritis. Walker *et al.* (1981) described a patient with squamous cell carcinoma of the oesophagus and membranoproliferative glomerulonephritis.

IgA nephropathy (see Chapter 3.6)

There are two reports of typical IgA nephropathy associated with malignancy. Cairns *et al.* (1978) reported two patients with bronchial squamous cell carcinoma who presented with clinical features of Henoch–Schönlein purpura and mesangial IgA deposition. Mustonen *et al.* (1981) also described two patients, one with recurrent haematuria during febrile illnesses who was found to have a bronchogenic carcinoma associated with IgA nephropathy, the second with purpura in a distribution similar to that of Henoch–Schönlein purpura associated with microscopic haematuria and mesangial IgA deposition. In a subsequent series, Mustonen *et al.* (1984) found that six of 26 patients aged over 60 years with IgA nephropathy had cancer whereas none of 158 patients less than 60 years old had malignancy. Thus, in patients aged over 60 with IgA nephropathy a search should be made for an underlying solid tumour particularly of the respiratory tract, buccal cavity, or nasopharynx.

Although IgA nephropathy is rarely associated with malignancy, Endo and Hara (1986) found that 17 per cent of patients with lung carcinoma had glomerular IgA deposits. Caution, however, is required as mesangial IgA deposits were reported at autopsy in some patients with gastrointestinal malignancy without previous evidence of renal disease (Puolijoki *et al.* 1989).

Mesangial proliferative glomerulonephritis

There is a single case report of a mesangial proliferative glomerulonephritis associated with an anaplastic small cell carcinoma of the lung (Jermanovich *et al.* 1982).

Crescentic nephritis

A number of reports have suggested an association between malignancy and crescentic glomerulonephritis. Biava *et al.* (1984) reviewed 80 patients with crescentic glomerulonephritis and found seven (9 per cent) to have a coexistent non-renal malignancy—six with carcinoma and one with lymphoma. This is a similar incidence to that reported by Whitworth *et al.* (1975), who found malignancy in four of 60 patients (7 per cent) with crescentic glomerulonephritis. Immunohistochemistry demonstrated glomerular fibrin deposition without immune reactants. In one patient with prostatic carcinoma, there was glomerular deposition of prostate specific antigen (Haskell *et al.* 1990). The clinical course appears to be similar to that of idiopathic crescentic glomerulonephritis, with the exception that tumour removal may be associated with improvement in renal function (Biava *et al.* 1984).

Minimal change nephropathy (see Chapter 3.5)

Minimal change nephropathy has only rarely been associated with solid tumours, in contrast to its frequent association with Hodgkin's lymphoma (see below). One of the 11 patients reported by Lee *et al.* (1966) had minimal change nephropathy and an adenocarcinoma of the colon. Other single cases have been reported, and the associated malignancies include carcinoma of the colon (Caruana and Griffin 1980), small cell carcinoma of the lung (Moorthy 1983), renal cell carcinoma (Dupond *et al.* 1980), and a mesothelioma (Schroeter *et al.* 1986).

Amyloidosis (see Chapter 4.2.1)

Vanatta *et al.* (1983) reviewed the literature and found 40 renal cell carcinoma patients with systemic amyloidosis, presumed to be of the AA type. The incidence of renal amyloidosis in carcinoma is not known, but in a study of 4033 autopsies, 16 patients were identified with amyloidosis, seven of whom also had carcinoma (Kimball 1961). A review by Glenner (1980) concluded that 24–33 per cent of all tumour-associated amyloidosis was associated with renal cell carcinoma. It is possible that circulating precursors are produced by epithelial cells in the renal cell carcinoma and lead to subsequent amyloid deposition.

Other glomerular pathology

Placental trophoblastic tumour has been associated with glomerular appearances identical to those of disseminated intravascular coagulation (Young *et al.* 1985).

Prognosis

In general, the prognosis of malignancy-associated nephropathy is determined more by the malignancy than by the glomerular findings. There are as noted above, several reports of improvement in the nephropathy or a remission of glomerulonephritis after removal or adequate treatment of the tumour (Cantrell 1969; Walker *et al.* 1981; Moorthy 1983; Yamauchi *et al.* 1985; Burstein *et al.* 1993) (Fig. 3). There is one interesting case report of a patient with renal cell carcinoma in whom systemic amyloidosis, as assessed by serial liver biopsies, showed a progressive reduction and was undetectable 22 months after nephrectomy (Paraf *et al.* 1970).

Few reports contain information obtained at follow-up biopsy, but Walker *et al.* (1981) described a patient with membranoproliferative glomerulonephritis who showed a marked regression of mesangial hypercellularity, a reduction in immunofluorescence and a disappearance of electron microscopic evidence of mesangial interposition in the glomerular capillary walls 5 months after oesophagectomy and 3 months after initial biopsy. Although some studies report no improvement after remission or removal of the tumour (Couser *et al.* 1974; Row *et al.* 1975), it is generally believed that complete resection or remission of the malignancy is associated with long-term remission of the nephropathy. If complete removal of the tumour is not possible there may be improvement in the nephropathy with reduction in tumour mass. Robinson *et al.* (1984) reported a patient in whom the nephrotic syndrome remitted on two occasions following irradiation of metastatic disease; the patient died from gastric cancer nearly 4 years after presentation with nephrotic syndrome. In other patients, however, in whom the tumour is unresponsive to treatment 50 per cent are dead within 3 months, usually from disseminated carcinomatosis.

Renal involvement in lymphoma and leukaemia

Introduction

Renal disease can arise in patients with lymphoma and leukaemia in a number of ways (Table 6).

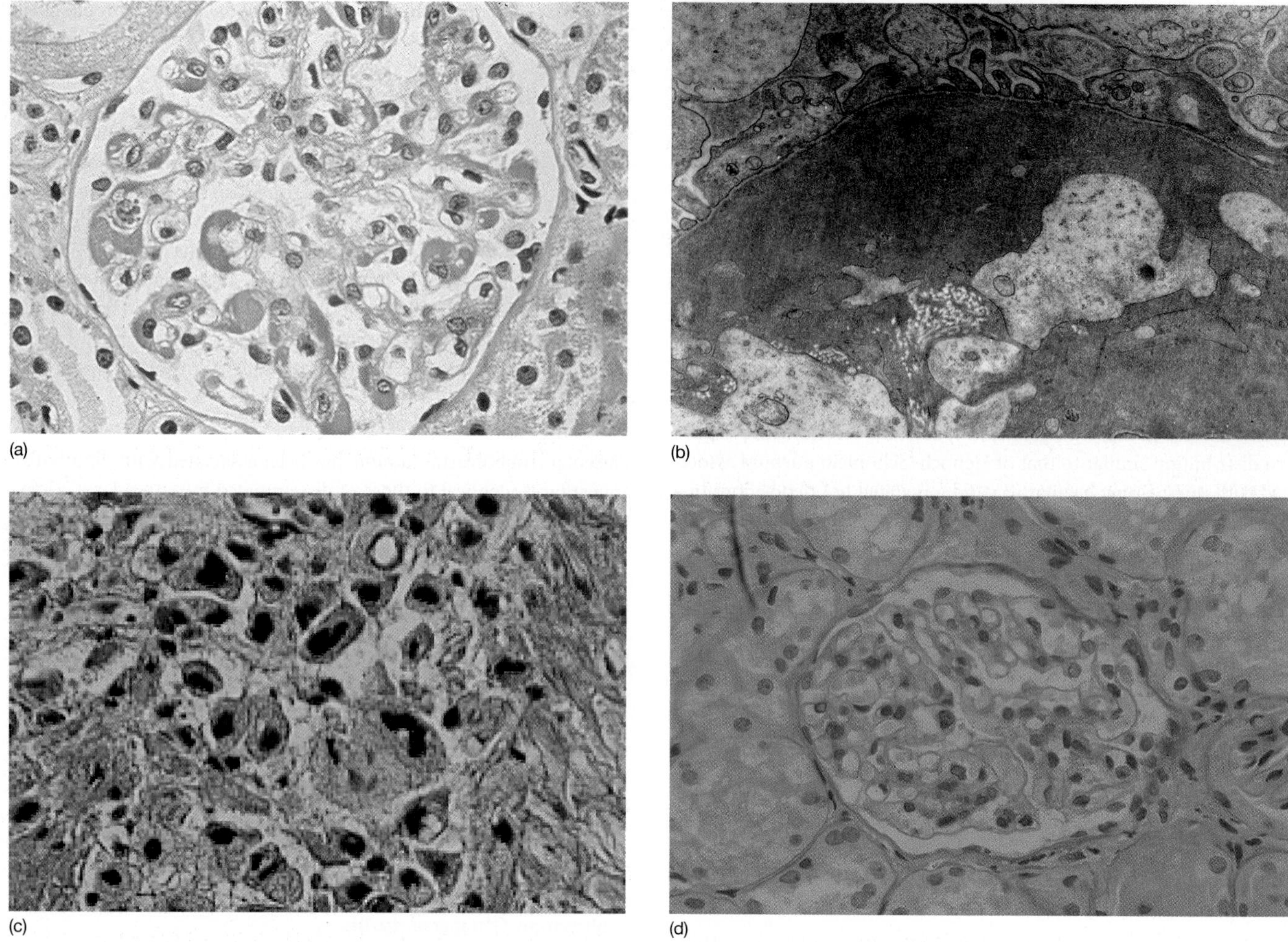

Fig. 3 A 26-year-old girl who presented with acute renal failure 2 weeks after delivery. The cause of the acute renal failure was not obvious and a renal biopsy was undertaken; this showed on light microscopy large intracapillary amorphous deposits which in some, occluded the capillary lumina (a) (haematoxylin and eosin 400×). Electron microscopy revealed large subendothelial deposits which had a granular character (b) (8160×). A uterine curettage suggested the presence of a choriocarcinoma and consequently hysterectomy was undertaken. On light microscopy strands of placental trophoblastic tumour were seen to be invading the myometrium (c) (haematoxylin and eosin 256×). Renal function promptly returned to normal and 6 months later a follow-up renal biopsy was undertaken. This showed resolution of the deposits although a minor increase in mesangial cells remained (d) (haematoxylin and eosin 400×).

Table 6 Renal involvement in lymphoma and leukaemia

1. Obstructive uropathy
2. Infiltration of renal parenchyma
3. Amyloidosis
4. Therapy associated
5. Urate nephropathy
6. Glomerulopathy
7. Disseminated intravenous coagulation

Obstructive uropathy may result from enlargement of hilar nodes or para-aortic nodes. Hydronephrosis due to ureteral obstruction was reported in 10 per cent of patients with lymphoma (Richmond *et al.* 1962), although it is likely that this is much less in present-day practice, because of earlier detection of lymphadenopathy by computed tomography (CT) scanning and more effective treatment regimens which limit lymph node enlargement.

Renal infiltration occurs in approximately one-third of patients with lymphoma and in 50 per cent of patients with leukaemia. The infiltration is usually nodular in patients with Hodgkin's lymphoma, but more diffuse in non-Hodgkin's lymphoma (Fig. 4). Although all types of leukaemia may infiltrate the kidney, this most commonly occurs with lymphoblastic leukaemia, when it is usually bilateral and diffuse throughout the cortex (Norris and Wiener 1961). Renal infiltration only rarely leads to significant impairment of renal function.

Amyloidosis is now rarely associated with lymphoma. Earlier reports described amyloidosis developing insidiously after many years of active disease. This late and previously frequently fatal complication is now uncommon due to the more recent development of successful therapeutic regimens.

As in patients with carcinoma, renal disease may arise as a complication of therapy of lymphoma, either directly, as in the tumour

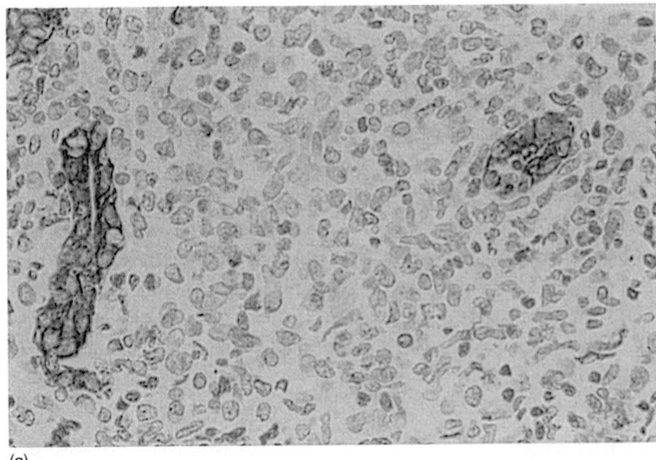
(a)

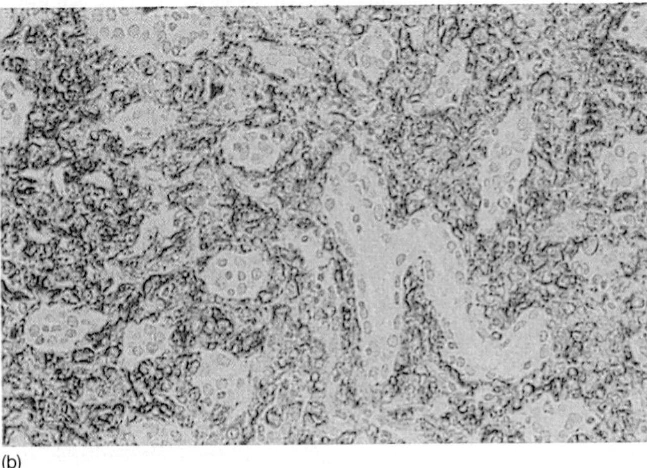
(b)

Fig. 4 B-cell non-Hodgkin's lymphoma of the kidney; tubules are widely separated by a dense interstitial infiltrate of small to medium sized lymphoma cells. (a) An antibody to cytokeratin shows positive staining of the tubular epithelium and negative staining of the tumour cells. (b) An antibody that recognizes B-lymphocytes (L26) shows the reverse pattern of staining (figure kindly provided by Dr Andrew Davison).

lysis syndrome (see below), or indirectly due to the development of intercurrent infection.

Hyperuricaemia (Chapter 6.4) is common in diseases associated with a rapid turnover of cells. Urinary uric acid excretion is increased by approximately 80 per cent in patients with leukaemia: this is sparingly soluble at a low pH and urinary precipitation may occur in the distal tubules where concentration and acidification are maximal. Effective chemotherapy increases the breakdown of cells and therefore increases nucleic acid catabolism; severe uric acid nephropathy may follow chemotherapy in up to 10 per cent of patients with acute lymphoblastic leukaemia. The so-called 'tumour lysis syndrome' is, in part, an acute urate nephropathy which occasionally occurs in patients with lymphoproliferative disorders treated with cytotoxic drugs (see Chapter 6.4). However, many other substances which could affect renal function are released from disintegrating tumour cells.

There is an interesting case report of a child presenting with non-oliguric acute renal failure, hyperuricaemia, and enlarged kidneys who on investigation was found to have acute lymphocytic leukaemia confined to the kidneys (Bunchman *et al.* 1994). In this paper this is called lymphocytic leukaemia, but it is almost certainly lymphoblastic.

Glomerulopathy is a rare complication of lymphoma or leukaemia. Ronco (1999), in a literature review of 1700 patients with Hodgkin's lymphoma, identified 0.4 per cent with minimal change nephropathy and 0.1 per cent with amyloidosis. Furthermore, from ten published reports he was able to identify 106 patients with glomerulopathy associated with Hodgkin's lymphoma and 45 with chronic lymphocytic leukaemia and other low grade B-cell non-Hodgkin's lymphoma. Hodgkin's lymphoma was most commonly associated with minimal change nephropathy, non-Hodgkin's lymphoma with crescentic nephritis and mesangiocapillary glomerulonephritis, and chronic lymphocytic leukaemia with mesangiocapillary glomerulonephritis. The incidence of amyloidosis is decreasing due to prompt effective therapy, most reports of amyloidosis are pre-1970 and involved patients at a late stage in the disease.

Pathogenesis

The pathogenesis of the minimal change nephropathy in Hodgkin's lymphoma is thought to be due to a T-cell disorder in which there is an abnormal T4/T8 ratio with a reduction in T4 (helper cells) and an increase in T8 (suppressor cells). It has been suggested that there is an alteration in T-cell function with increased secretion of lymphokines or of abnormal lymphokines producing increased vascular permeability and proteinuria (see Chapter 3.5). At present, however, it is not possible to determine which cell type or which particular lymphokine is responsible for increasing glomerular permeability.

An alternative hypothesis implicates a tumour related virus or an unrelated intercurrent viral infection as the cause of the glomerular lesion. This indeed may be the case in patients with chronic lymphocytic leukaemia as cryoglobulinaemia in those with nephropathy and is not present in patients without associated renal involvement. Experimentally, many New Zealand mice chronically infected with murine leukaemia virus develop lymphomas and glomerulonephritis, with immune deposits containing viral antigens and antibodies. Similarly, AKR mice develop leukaemia due to the Gross murine leukaemia virus and have a high incidence of glomerular deposition of immune complexes containing viral antigens.

Clinically, glomerular deposits of antibodies to Epstein–Barr virus have been demonstrated in Burkitt's lymphoma (Oldstone *et al.* 1974), and an oncornavirus has been implicated in two patients with an acute myelomonocytic leukaemia (Sutherland and Mardiney 1973). The involvement of an intercurrent viral infection is supported by the report of Hyman *et al.* (1973) who detected Herpes zoster viral antigen in a young child with Hodgkin's disease, Herpes zoster infection, and nephrotic syndrome.

Hodgkin's lymphoma

The association between nephropathy and Hodgkin's lymphoma, although well recognized, is rare: Kramer *et al.* (1981) and Plager and Stutzman (1971) report glomerular disease in only seven of more than 1700 patients with Hodgkin's lymphoma. Although a direct link has not been established there is considerable circumstantial evidence to link the two conditions: they can both present at the same time, they may relapse together, and effective treatment of the lymphoma is associated with remission of the nephrotic syndrome, even when this is confined to local radiotherapy and in patients not treated with corticosteroids.

Hodgkin's lymphoma presents before or at the same time as the nephrotic syndrome in 75 per cent of patients. It may occur at any age and has a male : female ratio of 2 : 1. Severe proteinuria with hypoproteinaemia and hypercholesterolaemia is common, but haematuria, hypertension, and impaired renal function are rare.

Prior to effective therapy for Hodgkin's lymphoma amyloidosis, mostly of AA type, was the most common glomerular lesion. All recent reports, however, indicate that minimal change nephropathy is now the most common histological finding and that this is more likely to develop in mixed cellularity forms of the lymphoma. Other lesions which have been reported include focal glomerulonephritis (Watson *et al.* 1983), membranous nephropathy (Eagen and Lewis 1977), mesangiocapillary glomerulonephritis (Morel-Maroger Striker *et al.* 1984), and crescentic nephritis (Wolf *et al.* 2001). A number of patients have been described who progressed from a minimal lesion nephropathy to a focal glomerulosclerosis (Hyman *et al.* 1973; Watson *et al.* 1983). Immunofluorescence microscopy may show IgG, IgM, and complement C3. Deposits have been described as being subendothelial (Hyman *et al.* 1973), intramembranous (Lokich *et al.* 1973), and/or subepithelial (Froom *et al.* 1972).

Effective treatment of Hodgkin's lymphoma is almost always associated with remission of the nephrotic syndrome (Froom *et al.* 1972) and recurrence of proteinuria may signal relapse of the Hodgkin's lymphoma.

Non-Hodgkin's lymphoma

Nephropathy has been described in patients with non-Hodgkin's lymphoma, but the association is extremely rare. In a review of the literature, Gonzalez *et al.* (1986) were able to identify only 22 patients with non-Hodgkin's lymphoma and a variety of glomerular diseases. The average age of the patients was 47 years (range 7–74) and there was a male preponderance. The nephropathy and lymphoma became apparent simultaneously in seven cases, and the majority had a nephrotic syndrome. Various glomerular appearances have been described (Harper and Adu 1997) including minimal change nephropathy (Ghosh and Muehrcke 1970; Muggia and Ultman 1971; Gagliano *et al.* 1976), mesangiocapillary glomerulonephritis, membranous nephropathy (Gluck *et al.* 1973; Rabkin *et al.* 1973), focal glomerulosclerosis (Belghiti *et al.* 1981), and crescentic glomerulonephritis (Biava *et al.* 1984; Rerolle *et al.* 1999). Cronin *et al.* (1990) reported an instance of a patient presenting with an acute renal failure, nephrotic syndrome due to minimal change nephropathy, and non-Hodgkin's lymphoma in whom antitumour therapy was associated with resolution of the renal failure and the nephrotic syndrome. In addition to the wide variety of glomerular histological changes, the associated lymphomas have been diverse (Ghosh and Muehrcke 1970; Gluck *et al.* 1973; Gonzalez *et al.* 1986). It is thus very much open to question as to whether these represent coincidental occurrences or whether there is any direct causal link.

Other lymphoid tumours

Immunoblastic lymphadenopathy, which would now be discussed as angioblastic T-cell lymphoma, is a prelymphomatous lymphoproliferative disorder that has been associated with acute renal failure in two patients (Wood and Harkins 1979).

Mycosis fungoides, a variant of T-cell lymphoma involving the skin, has been associated with IgA nephropathy in two patients (Ramirez *et al.* 1982).

Burkitt's lymphoma frequently involves the kidney and has been described by Abdurrahman *et al.* 1990.

Angiofollicular lymph node hyperplasia is a benign lymphoid tumour of unknown aetiology first described by Castleman *et al.* (1956) and now usually referred to as Castleman's disease. The tumour may be solitary or multifocal and usually occurs in the mediastinum or mesentery. Two distinct types are recognized, a plasma cell type and a hyaline vascular type. Nephrotic syndrome has been described associated with the plasma cell type due to membranous glomerulonephritis (Weisenburger 1979) and minimal change nephropathy (Humphreys *et al.* 1975). In the latter case removal of the tumour was associated with a prompt reduction in proteinuria and a brisk diuresis suggesting a causal link.

Leukaemia

Chronic lymphocytic leukaemia has been associated with the nephrotic syndrome in 46 patients (reviewed by Mc'Ligeyo *et al.* 1993). Most commonly, the nephropathy, usually manifest as nephrotic syndrome, and leukaemia have been detected simultaneously. In the series of Moulin *et al.* (1992), 10 of 13 patients had impaired renal function (creatinine > 120 μmol/l) which was severe in three (>400 μmol/l). This contrasts sharply with the apparent rarity of renal functional impairment seen in patients with solid tumour associated nephropathy. A variety of histological appearances have been described, mesangiocapillary glomerulonephritis being the most common (Mandalenakis *et al.* 1971; Feehally *et al.* 1981; Touchard *et al.* 1989; Moulin *et al.* 1992; Mc'Ligeyo *et al.* 1993) but focal proliferative/sclerosis (Dabbs *et al.* 1986), amyloidosis (Leonard 1957; Scott 1957), atypical membranous nephropathy (Brodovsky *et al.* 1968; Dathan *et al.* 1974), and minimal change nephropathy (Kerkhoven *et al.* 1973; Gagliano *et al.* 1976). There is at present no adequate explanation for the preponderance of mesangiocapillary glomerulonephritis in patients with chronic lymphatic leukaemia but cryoglobulinaemia is common in these patients raising the possibility of an associated viral infection. However there may also be a direct link between glomerulopathy and leukaemia because of the finding of circulating and deposited IgG k, or IgM k in a number of patients (Moulin *et al.* 1992). Improvement of the nephropathy after treatment for the leukaemia is well described (Brodovsky *et al.* 1968; Touchard *et al.* 1989; Moulin *et al.* 1992). Unfortunately, however, the therapy prescribed for the leukaemia (e.g. prednisolone or chlorambucil) may often have had a direct effect on the renal lesion.

An AA type amyloidosis has been described in association with hairy cell leukaemia (Linder *et al.* 1982).

Disseminated intravascular coagulation has been associated with a variety of neoplasms, particularly acute progranulocytic leukaemia.

Conclusions

An association between nephropathy and neoplasia is now generally accepted. In carcinoma, the pathogenesis in the majority of patients is thought to involve the formation, most commonly *in situ*, of immune complexes in a subepithelial position in the glomerular capillary wall producing a membranous nephropathy. The association has been demonstrated most commonly in adults and in patients with adenocarcinoma, particularly of the lung and gastrointestinal tract. Many other malignancies have been implicated, but usually on the basis of anecdotes. In adult patients with apparently idiopathic membranous glomerulonephritis, routine cancer screening tests are advisable to detect underlying malignancy, especially in those aged over 50. The prognosis depends more on the underlying malignancy than the type of renal disease. If tumour removal or therapeutic remission is achieved the nephropathy sometimes resolves, but when the tumour is uncontrollable the overall prognosis is particularly poor.

Glomerular disease also occurs in patients with lymphoma or leukaemia. The majority of patients with Hodgkin's lymphoma have an associated minimal change nephropathy, possibly mediated by concurrent T-cell abnormalities; the nephropathy resolves on successful treatment of the lymphoma. In non-Hodgkin's lymphoma, there are only a few reported cases, involving a wide variety of glomerular appearances and of lymphoma types, suggesting that the association may be fortuitous. In leukaemia, particularly chronic lymphocytic leukaemia, a number of patients have been reported, particularly with a mesangiocapillary or membranous nephropathy. While this association is probably not fortuitous, it is apparently rare.

References

Abdurrahman, M. B., Babaoye, F. A., and Aikhionbare, H. A. (1990). Childhood renal disorders in Nigeria. *Pediatric Nephrology* **4**, 88–93.

Barton, C. H., Vaziri, N. D., and Spear, G. S. (1980). Nephrotic syndrome associated with adenocarcinoma of the breast. *American Journal of Medicine* **68**, 308–312.

Beaufils, H., Jouanneau, C., and Chomette, G. (1985). Kidney and cancer: results of immunofluorescence microscopy. *Nephron* **40**, 303–308.

Beauvais, P., Vaudour, G., Boccon Gibod, L., and Levy, M. (1989). Membranous nephropathy associated with ovarian tumour in a young girl: recovery after removal. *European Journal of Paediatrics* **148**, 624–625.

Belghiti, D., Vernant, J. P., Hirbec, G., Gubler, M. C., Andre, C., and Sobel, A. (1981). Nephrotic syndrome associated with T-cell lymphoma. *Cancer* **47**, 1878–1881.

Biava, C. G., Gonwa, T. A., Naughton, J. L., and Hopper, J., Jr. (1984). Crescentic glomerulonephritis associated with non-renal malignancies. *American Journal of Nephrology* **4**, 208–214.

Borochovitz, D., Kam, W. K., Nolte, M., Graner, S., and Kiss, J. (1982). Adenocarcinoma of the palate associated with nephrotic syndrome and epimembranous carcinoembryonic antigen deposition. *Cancer* **49**, 2097–2102.

Brodovsky, M. H., Samuels, M. L., Migliore, P. J., and Howe, C. D. (1968). Chronic lymphocytic leukaemia, Hodgkin's disease and the nephrotic syndrome. *Archives of Internal Medicine* **121**, 71–75.

Brueggemeyer, C. D. and Ramirez, G. (1987). Membranous nephropathy: a concern for malignancy. *American Journal of Kidney Diseases* **9**, 23–26.

Bunchman, T. E., Gale, G. B., O'Conner, D. M., Salinas-Madrigal, L., and Chu, J.-Y. (1994). Renal biopsy diagnosis of acute lymphocytic leukemia. *Clinical Nephrology* **38**, 142–144.

Burstein, D. M., Korbet, S. M., and Schwartz, M. M. (1993). Membranous glomerulonephritis and malignancy. *American Journal of Kidney Diseases* **22**, 5–10.

Cairns, S. A., Mallick, N. P., Lawler, W., and Williams, G. (1978). Squamous cell carcinoma of bronchus presenting with Henoch–Schönlein purpura. *British Medical Journal* **2**, 174–175.

Cameron, J. S. and Ogg, C. S. (1975). Neoplastic disease and the nephrotic syndrome. *Quarterly Journal of Medicine* **44**, 630–631.

Cantrell, E. G. (1969). Nephrotic syndrome cured by removal of gastric carcinoma. *British Medical Journal* **2**, 739–740.

Caruana, R. J. and Griffin, J. W. (1980). Nephrotic syndrome in a patient with ulcerative colitis and colonic carcinoma. *American Journal of Gastroenterology* **74**, 525–528.

Castleman, B., Iverson, L., and Menedex, V. (1956). Localised mediastinal lymph node hyperplasia resembling thymoma. *Archives of Pathological and Laboratory Medicine* **103**, 591–594.

Castleman, B., Nichols, G., and Roth, S. I. (1963). Case records of the Massachusetts General Hospital. *New England Journal of Medicine* **268**, 943–953.

Costanza, M. E., Pinn, V., Schwartz, R. S., and Nathanson, L. (1973). Carcinoembryonic antigen–antibody complexes in a patient with colonic carcinoma and nephrotic syndrome. *New England Journal of Medicine* **289**, 520–522.

Couser, W. G. (1980). Renal cell cancer with amyloid disease. Case records of the Massachussets General Hospital. *New England Journal of Medicine* **303**, 985–995.

Couser, W. G., Wagonfeld, J. B., Spargo, B. H., and Lewis, E. J. (1974). Glomerular deposition of tumour antigen in membranous nephropathy associated with colonic carcinoma. *American Journal of Medicine* **57**, 962–970.

Cronin, C., Carmody, E., Ryan, F., and Carmody, M. (1990). Acute renal failure and non-Hodgkins lymphoma in a patient with minimal change glomerulonephritis. *Journal of Internal Medicine* **228**, 65–68.

Dabbs, D. J., Morel-Maroger, S. L., Mignon, F., and Striker, G. (1986). Glomerular lesions in lymphomas and leukaemias. *American Journal of Medicine* **80**, 63–67.

Dathan, J. R. E., Heyworth, M. F., and MacIver, A. G. (1974). Nephrotic syndrome in chronic lymphocytic leukaemia. *British Medical Journal* **3**, 655–675.

De Swiet, J. and Wells, A. L. (1957). Nephrotic syndrome associated with renal venous thrombosis and bronchial carcinoma. *British Medical Journal* **1**, 1341–1343.

Dosik, G. M., Guterman, J. V., Hersh, E. M., Akhtar, M., Sonoda, T., and Horn, R. G. (1978). Nephrotoxicity from cancer immunotherapy. *Annals of Internal Medicine* **89**, 41–46.

Drash, A., Sherman, F., Hartman, W., and Blizzard, R. M. (1970). A syndrome of pseudohermaphroditism, Wilms' tumour hypertension and degenerative renal diseases. *Journal of Pediatrics* **76**, 585–593.

Dupond, J. L. *et al.* (1980). Renal cancer disclosed by a nephrotic syndrome with minimal glomerular lesion. *Presse Medicale* **9**, 884–885.

Eagen, J. W. and Lewis, E. J. (1977). Glomerulopathies of neoplasia. *Kidney International* **11**, 297–306.

Endo, Y. and Hara, M. (1986). Glomerular IgA deposition in pulmonary diseases. *Kidney International* **29**, 557–562.

Endoh, M. (1984). Focal segmental glomerulonephritis associated with pheochromocytoma. *Tokai Journal of Experimental and Clinical Medicine* **9**, 191–197.

Feehally, J., Hutchinson, R. M., MacKay, E. H., and Walls, J. (1981). Recurrent proteinuria and chronic lymphatic leukaemia. *Clinical Nephrology* **16**, 51–54.

Froom, D. W., Franklin, W. A., Hano, J. E., and Potter, E. V. (1972). Immune deposits in Hodgkin's disease with nephrotic syndrome. *Archives of Pathology* **94**, 547–553.

Gagliano, R. G., Costanzi, J. J., Beathard, G. A., Sarles, H. E., and Bells, J. D. (1976). The nephrotic syndrome associated with neoplasia: an unusual paraneoplastic syndrome. *American Journal of Medicine* **60**, 1026–1031.

Galloway, J. (1922). Remarks on Hodgkin's disease. *British Medical Journal* **2**, 1201.

Ghosh, L. and Muehrcke, R. C. (1970). The nephrotic syndrome: a prodrome to lymphoma. *Annals of Internal Medicine* **72**, 379–382.

Glenner, G. G. (1980). Amyloid deposits and amyloidosis. *New England Journal of Medicine* **302**, 1283–1292.

Gluck, M. C., Gallo, G., Lowenstein, J., and Baldwin, D. S. (1973). Membranous glomerulonephritis: evolution of clinical and pathologic features. *Annals of Internal Medicine* **78**, 1–12.

Gonzalez, J. A. G., Bango, M. Y., Morales, F. M., Caro, J. L. M., Marin, F. J. D., and Martinez, A. D. (1986). The association of non-Hodgkin's lymphoma with glomerulonephritis. *Postgraduate Medical Journal* **62**, 1141–1145.

Habib, R. *et al.* (1985). The nephropathy associated with male pseudohermaphroditism and Wilms' tumour (Drash syndrome): a distinctive glomerular lesion—report of 10 cases. *Clinical Nephrology* **24**, 269–278.

Harper, L. and Adu, D. (1997). Glomerulonephritis and non-Hodgkin lymphoma. *Nephrology, Dialysis, Transplantation* **12**, 1520–1525.

Haskell, L. P., Fusco, M. J., Wadler, S., Sablay, L. B., and Mennemeyer, R. P. (1990). Crescentic glomerulonephritis associated with prostatic carcinoma: evidence of immune-mediated glomerular injury. *American Journal of Medicine* **88**, 189–192.

Heaton, J. M., Menzin, M. A., and Carney, D. N. (1975). Extra-renal malignancy and the nephrotic syndrome. *Journal of Clinical Pathology* **28**, 944–946.

Heckerling, P. S. *et al.* (1985). Oesophageal carcinoma with membranous nephropathy. *Annals of Internal Medicine* **103**, 474.

Helin, M., Pasternack, A., Hakala, J., Penttinen, K., and Wager, O. (1980). Glomerular electron-dense deposits and circulating immune complexes in patients with malignant tumours. *Clinical Nephrology* **14**, 23–30.

Higgins, M. R., Randall, R. E., and Still, W. J. S. (1974). Nephrotic syndrome with oat-cell carcinoma. *British Medical Journal* **3**, 450–451.

Hopper, J. (1974). Tumour-related renal lesions. *Annals of Internal Medicine* **81**, 550–551.

Humpherys, S. R., Holley, K. E., Smith, L. H., and McIlrath, D. C. (1975). Mesenteric angiofollicular lymph node hyperplasia (lymphoid hamartoma) with nephrotic syndrome. *Mayo Clinic Proceedings* **50**, 317–321.

Hyman, L. R., Burkholder, P. M., Joo, P. A., and Segar, W. E. (1973). Malignant lymphoma and nephrotic syndrome. *Journal of Pediatrics* **82**, 207–217.

Jermanovich, N. B., Giammarco, R., Ginsberg, S. J., Tinsley, R. W., and Jones, D. B. (1982). Small cell anaplastic carcinoma of the lung with mesangial proliferative glomerulonephritis. *Archives of Internal Medicine* **142**, 397–399.

Kaplan, B. S., Klassen, J., and Gault, M. H. (1976). Glomerular injury in patients with neoplasia. *Annual Reviews of Medicine* **27**, 117–125.

Kerkhoven, P., Briner, J., and Blumberg, A. (1973). Nephrotisches Syndrome als Erstmanifestation maligner Lymphoma. *Schweizer Medizinische Wochenschrift* **103**, 1706–1709.

Kerpen, H. O., Ganesh Bhat, J., Felner, H. D., and Baldwin, D. S. (1978). Membranous nephropathy associated with renal cell carcinoma. *American Journal of Medicine* **64**, 863–867.

Keur, I., Krediet, R. T., and Arisz, L. (1989). Glomerulopathy as a paraneoplastic phenomenon. *Netherlands Journal of Medicine* **34**, 270–284.

Kimball, K. G. (1961). Amyloidosis in association with neoplastic disease: report of an unusual case and clinicopathological experience at the Memorial Center for Cancer and Allied Diseases during eleven years (1948–1958). *Annals of Internal Medicine* **55**, 58–74.

Kitano, S. (1984). Poorly differentiated adenocarcinoma of rectum in a nephrotic patient with focal segmental glomerulosclerosis. *Japanese Journal of Surgery* **14**, 155–158.

Kleinknecht, C., Levy, M., Gagnadoux, M. F., and Habib, R. (1979). Membranous glomerulonephritis with extra-renal disorders in children. *Medicine* **58**, 219–228.

Kramer, P., Sizoo, W., and Twiss, E. E. (1981). Nephrotic syndrome in Hodgkin's disease. *Netherlands Journal of Medicine* **24**, 114–119.

Latham, P., Poucell, D., Koresaar, A., Arbus, G., and Baumal, R. (1982). Idiopathic membranous glomerulopathy in Canadian children: clinicopathologic study. *Journal of Pediatrics* **101**, 682–685.

Lee, J. C., Yamauchi, H., and Hopper, J. (1966). The association of cancer and the nephrotic syndrome. *Annals of Internal Medicine* **64**, 41–51.

Leonard, B. J. (1957). Chronic lymphatic leukaemia and the nephrotic syndrome. *Lancet* **i**, 1356–1357.

Lewis, M. G., Loughbridge, L., and Phillips, T. M. (1971). Immunological studies in nephrotic syndrome associated with extra-renal malignant disease. *Lancet* **ii**, 134–135.

Linder, J., Silberman, H. R., and Croker, B. P. (1982). Amyloidosis complicating hairy cell leukaemia. *American Journal of Clinical Pathology* **78**, 864–867.

Lokich, J. J., Galvanek, E. G., and Moloney, W. C. (1973). Nephrosis of Hodgkin's disease. *Archives of Internal Medicine* **132**, 597–600.

Lubin, R. *et al.* (1995). p53 Antibodies in patients with various types of cancers: assay, identification and characterization. *Clinical Cancer Research* **1**, 1463–1469.

Lumeng, J. and Moran, J. F. (1966). Carotid body tumour associated with mild membranous glomerulonephritis. *Annals of Internal Medicine* **65**, 1266–1270.

Mandalenakis, N., Mendoza, N., Pirani, C. L., and Pollak, V. E. (1971). Lobular glomerulonephritis and membranoproliferative glomerulonephritis: a clinical and pathologic study based on renal biopsies. *Medicine* **50**, 319–355.

McLigeyo, S. O., Notghi, A., Thomson, D., and Anderton, J. L. (1993). Nephrotic syndrome associated with chronic lymphatic leukaemia. *Nephrology, Dialysis, Transplantation* **8**, 461–463.

Moorthy, A. V. (1983). Minimal change glomerular disease: a paraneoplastic syndrome in two patients with bronchogenic carcinoma. *American Journal of Kidney Diseases* **3**, 58–62.

Morel-Maroger Striker, L., Mignon, F., Dabbs, D., and Striker, G. E. Glomerular lesions in lymphomas and leukaemias. In *Nephrology* (ed. R. R. Robinson *et al.*), pp. 905–915. New York: Springer-Verlag, 1984.

Moulin, B., Ronco, P. M., Mougenot, B., Francois, A., Fillastre, J. P., and Mignon, F. (1992). Glomerulonephritis in chronic lymphocytic leukemia and related B-cell lymphomas. *Kidney International* **42**, 127–135.

Muggia, F. M. and Ultmann, J. E. (1971). Glomerulonephritis or nephrotic syndrome in malignant lymphoma, reticulum-cell type. *Lancet* **i**, 805.

Mustonen, J., Henn, H., and Pasternack, A. (1981). IgA nephropathy associated with bronchial small cell carcinoma. *American Journal of Clinical Pathology* **76**, 652–656.

Mustonen, J., Pastrnack, A., and Helin, H. (1984). Mesangial nephropathy in neoplastic diseases. *Contributions to Nephrology* **40**, 283–291.

Norris, H. J. and Weiner, J. (1961). The renal lesions in leukaemia. *American Journal of Medical Science* **241**, 512–517.

Oldstone, M. B. A., Theofilopoulos, A. N., Gunven, P., and Klein, G. (1974). Immune complexes associated with neoplasia: presence of Epstein–Barr virus antigen–antibody complexes in Burkitt's lymphoma. *Intervirology* **4**, 292–302.

Olson, J. L., Philips, T. M., Lewis, M. G., and Solez, K. (1979). Malignant melanoma with renal dense deposits containing tumour antigens. *Clinical Nephrology* **12**, 74–82.

Ozawa, T. *et al.* (1975). Endogenous immune complex nephrology associated with malignancy. 1. Studies on the nature and immunopathogenic significance of glomerular bound antigen and antibody. Isolation and characterisations of tumour specific and antibody circulating immune complexes. *Quarterly Journal of Medicine* **44**, 523–541.

Pascal, R. R. (1980). Renal manifestations of extra-renal neoplasms. *Human Pathology* **11**, 7–17.

Pascal, R. R. and Slovin, S. G. (1980). Tumour directed antibody and carcinoembryonic antigen in the glomeruli of a patient with gastric carcinoma. *Human Pathology* **11**, 679–682.

Pascal, R. R. *et al.* (1975). Glomerular immune complex deposits associated with mouse mammary tumour. *Cancer Research* **35**, 302–304.

Pascal, R. R., Innaccone, P. M., and Rollwagen, F. M. (1976). Electron microscopy and immunofluorescence of glomerular immune complex deposits in cancer patients. *Cancer Research* **36**, 43–47.

Pascal, R. R., Finney, R. P., Rifkin, S. I., and Kahana, L. (1980). Glomerulonephritis and virus like particles associated with prostatic cancer. *Human Pathology* **11**, 391–395.

Paraf, A., Coste, T., Rautureau, J., and Texier, J. (1970). La régression de l'amylose: disparition d'une amylose hépatique massive après nephrectomie pour cancer. *Presse Medicale* **78**, 547–548.

Plager, J. and Stutzman, J. (1971). Acute nephrotic syndrome as a manifestation of active Hodgkin's disease. *American Journal of Medicine* **50**, 56–66.

Puolijoki, H., Mustonen, J., Pettersson, E., Pasternack, A., and Lamdensuo, A. (1989). Proteinuria and haematuria and frequently present in patients with lung cancer. *Nephrology, Dialysis, Transplantation* **4**, 947–950.

Rabkin, R., Thatcher, G. N., Diamond, L. H., and Eales, L. (1973). The nephrotic syndrome, malignancy and immunosuppression. *South African Medical Journal* **14**, 605–606.

Ramirez, F., Brouhard, B. H., Travis, L. B., and Ellis, E. N. (1982). Idiopathic membranous nephropathy in children. *Journal of Pediatrics* **101**, 677–681.

Rerolle, J.-P. *et al.* (1999). Crescentic glomerulonephritis and centrocytic lymphoma. *Nephrology, Dialysis, Transplantation* **14**, 1744–1745.

Richmond, J. *et al.* (1962). Renal lesions associated with malignant lymphomas. *American Journal of Medicine* **32**, 184–207.

Robinson, W. L., Mitas, J. A., Haerr, R. W., and Cohen, I. M. (1984). Remission and exacerbation of tumour-related nephrotic syndrome with treatment of the neoplasm. *Cancer* **54**, 1082–1084.

Ronco, P. M. (1999). Paraneoplastic glomerulopathies: new insights into an old entity. *Kidney International* **56**, 355–377.

Rossen, R. D., Reisberg, R. A., Hersh, E. M., and Gutterman, J. U. (1976). Measurement of soluble immune complexes: a guide to prognosis in cancer patients. *Clinical Research* **24**, 462A.

Row, P. G. *et al.* (1975). Membranous nephropathy, long term follow up and association with neoplasia. *Quarterly Journal of Medicine* **44**, 207–239.

Roy, A. D. and Ellis, M. (1959). Potassium secreting tumour of the large intestine. *Lancet* **i**, 759–760.

Sagel, J., Muller, H., and Logan, E. (1971). Lymphoma and the nephrotic syndrome. *South African Medical Journal* **45**, 79–80.

Sawyer, N., Wadsworth, J., Winnen, M., and Gabriel, R. (1988). Prevalence, concentration and prognostic importance of proteinuria in patients with malignancies. *British Medical Journal* **296**, 295–298.

Schroeter, N. J., Rushing, D. A., Parker, J. P., and Beltaos, E. (1986). Minimal change nephrotic syndrome associated with malignant mesothelioma. *Archives of Internal Medicine* **146**, 1834–1836.

Scott, R. B. (1957). Chronic lymphatic leukaemia. *Lancet* **i**, 1162–1167.

Seyberth, K. W., Segre, G. V., Morgan, J. L., Sweetman, B. J., Potts, J. T., and Oaes, J. A. (1975). Prostaglandins as mediators of hypercalcaemia associated with certain types of cancer. *New England Journal of Medicine* **293**, 1278–1283.

Stillwell, T. J., Gomez, M. R., and Kelalis, P. P. (1987). Renal lesions in tuberous sclerosis. *Journal of Urology* **138**, 477–481.

Stuart, K., Fallon, B. G., and Cardi, M. A. (1986). Development of the nephrotic syndrome in a patient with prostatic carcinoma. *American Journal of Medicine* **80**, 295–298.

Sutherland, J. C. and Mardiney, M. R. (1973). Immune complex disease in the kidneys of lymphoma-leukaemia patients: the presence of an oncornavirus-related antigen. *Journal of the National Cancer Institute* **50**, 633–644.

Sutherland, J. C., Markham, R. V., and Mardiney, M. R. (1974). Subclinical immune complexes in the glomeruli of kidneys postmortem. *American Journal of Medicine* **57**, 536–541.

Swaroop, S. and Krant, M. J. (1973). Rapid estrogen-induced hypercalcaemia. *Journal of the American Medical Association* **223**, 913–914.

Touchard, G. *et al.* (1989). Nephrotic syndrome associated with chronic lymphocytic leukaemia: an immunological study. *Clinical Nephrology* **31**, 107–116.

Vanatta, P. R., Silva, F. G., Taylor, W. E., and Costa, J. C. (1983). Renal cell carcinoma and systemic amyloidosis. *Human Pathology* **14**, 195–201.

Wakashin, M., Wakashin, Y., and Iesato, K. (1980). Association of gastric cancer and nephrotic syndrome. An immunologic study in three patients. *Gastroenterology* **78**, 749–756.

Walker, J. F., O'Neill, S., and Campbell, E. (1981). Carcinoma of the oesophagus associated with membranoproliferative glomerulonephritis. *Postgraduate Medical Journal* **57**, 592–596.

Watson, A., Stachura, I., Fragola, J., and Bourke, E. (1983). Focal and segmental glomerulosclerosis in Hodgkin's disease. *American Journal of Nephrology* **3**, 228–232.

Weisenburger, D. D. (1979). Membranous nephropathy, its association with multicentric angiofollicular lymph node hyperplasia. *Archives of Pathological and Laboratory Medicine* **103**, 591–594.

Weksler, T. C., Day, N., Susin, M., Sherman, R., and Becker, C. (1974). Nephrotic syndrome in malignant melanoma: demonstration of melanoma antigen–antibody complexes in kidney. *Kidney International* **6**, 112A.

Whitworth, J. A., Unge, A., and Cameron, J. S. (1975). Carcinoembryonic antigen in tumour-associated membranous nephropathy. *Lancet* **ii**, 611.

Wolf, G. *et al.* (2001). Necrotizing glomerulonephritis associated with Hodgkin's disease. *Nephrology, Dialysis, Transplantation* **16**, 187–188.

Wood, W. G. and Harkins, M. M. (1979). Nephropathy in angioimmunoblastic lymphadenopathy. *American Journal of Clinical Pathology* **71**, 58–63.

Yamauchi, M., Linsey, M. S., Biava, C. G., and Hopper, J. (1985). Cure of membranous nephropathy after resection of carcinoma. *Archives of Internal Medicine* **145**, 2061–2063.

Young, R. H., Scully, R. E., and McCluskey, R. T. (1985). A distinctive glomerular lesion complicating placental site trophoblastic tumour: report to two cases. *Human Pathology* **16**, 35–42.

Zech, P., Colon, S., Pointet, P. L., Deteiz, P., Labeevu, M., and Leitienne, P. L. (1982). The nephrotic syndrome in adults aged over 60: etiology, evolution and treatment of 76 cases. *Clinical Nephrology* **17**, 232–236.

Zheng, H. L., Maruyama, T., Matsuda, S., and Satomura, K. (1979). Neuroblastoma presenting with the nephrotic syndrome. *Journal of Paediatric Surgery* **14**, 414–419.

3.14 Glomerular disease in the tropics

Vivekanand Jha and Kirpal S. Chugh

Glomerulonephritis is the commonest cause of endstage renal failure in most part of the tropics. Reliable statistics on the pattern and natural history of glomerular diseases encountered in tropical countries are sparse because of the lack of national or regional registries, but it has been estimated that out of every million population living in the tropical countries, about 100–250 people develop endstage renal disease (ESRD) annually (Chugh and Jha 1995). Chronic glomerular diseases constitute about 30–60 per cent of all ESRD cases reported from different geographic regions (Jha and Chugh 1996). The data are based mostly on individual experiences and suggest a significant difference in the epidemiology, aetiology, and natural history of glomerulonephritis between populations living in countries with tropical and temperate climates. Hospital-based surveys from South Africa, Zimbabwe, Senegal, Uganda, Nigeria, Yemen, and Papua New Guinea show that nephrotic syndrome forms 0.2–4 per cent of all hospital admissions (Chugh and Sakhuja 1998; Okoro *et al.* 2000). If the prevalence of nephrotic syndrome were to be extrapolated from this data, it would turn out to be 60–100 times greater than that in the United Kingdom, Europe, and the United States. An important factor that appears to account for this difference is the high prevalence of infection-related glomerular diseases in the tropical regions (Chugh and Sakhuja 1990).

Malnutrition increases susceptibility to severe peripheral oedema and serous effusions with relatively lower degree of protein loss compared to those with adequate nutritional status. Glomerulonephritis often remains undiagnosed and untreated for long periods due to lack of access to healthcare, culminating in higher morbidity and mortality. There are enormous variations in the standards of living, sanitation, healthcare delivery systems, and vaccination policies amongst different countries of the tropical region. Combined with a wide variation in the prevalence of endemic infections, this leads to differences in the aetiologic factors and the rate of progression of glomerulonephritis even within different regions of the same country.

Primary glomerular diseases constitute over two-thirds of all cases of glomerulonephritis in most tropical countries, with some notable exceptions like Malaysia, Zimbabwe, and Jamaica where secondary causes are responsible for 40–55 per cent of cases of nephrotic syndrome (Morgan *et al.* 1984; Seggie *et al.* 1984a,b; Zainal *et al.* 1995; Diallo *et al.* 1997; Chugh and Sakhuja 1998). Over 80 per cent of all glomerulonephritides in paediatric population in Zimbabwe is estimated to be secondary to hepatitis B and streptococcal infections (Seggie *et al.* 1984b). The HBsAg positivity rate amongst Nigerian adults with glomerulonephritis was 33 per cent, compared to an overall population prevalence of 9 per cent (Akinsola *et al.* 1984).

Primary glomerular diseases

The relative frequency of various primary glomerulonephritides amongst adult and paediatric populations in the tropical countries and the rest of the world is shown in Fig. 1(a) and (b). Minimal-change disease (Chapter 3.5) is the most common cause of nephrotic syndrome during childhood (Lai *et al.* 1987; Choi *et al.* 2001), and is seen in 20–35 per cent of adult nephrotics in China and India. However, the disease appears to be much less frequent amongst the Blacks in the African continent. Contrasting clinicopathological patterns were noted in a study of 130 South African children with nephrotic syndrome (Seedat 1978). Minimal change disease was responsible for nephrotic syndrome in 75 per cent of children of Indian ancestry, but only 13.5 per cent of Black children showed this lesion. In another report from Nigeria, minimal change disease was encountered in less than 10 per cent of all children with glomerulonephritis (Asinobi *et al.* 1999). In published studies from Nigeria, Tunisia, and amongst the South African Black population, minimal-change disease is observed in less than 4 per cent of adults; and is not seen at all in Senegal and Malawi (Morel-Maroger *et al.* 1975; Brown *et al.* 1977; Hachicha *et al.* 1992; Habte 1993; Kadiri *et al.* 1993; van Buuren *et al.* 1999). Another difference is the high incidence of steroid resistance amongst African Blacks with biopsy-proved minimal change disease (Kadiri *et al.* 1993; Bhimma *et al.* 1997; Gbadoe *et al.* 1999).

The incidence of focal–segmental glomerulosclerosis (FSGS) (Chapter 3.5) has shown a rise over the last 20 years throughout the tropics, mostly at the expense of mesangiocapillary glomerulonephritis (MCGN) (Bodaghi *et al.* 1989; Pakasa *et al.* 1993; Yahya *et al.* 1998; Hurtado *et al.* 2000). It is the commonest cause of chronic renal failure requiring transplantation amongst Black South African children (Thomson 1999). There was an over-representation of Blacks amongst FSGS patients in the Bahia province of Brazil (Lopes *et al.* 1999). An unusually high incidence of FSGS has also been reported amongst adult nephrotics in Ghana (Adu *et al.* 1981) and children from Senegal (Morel-Maroger *et al.* 1975). A distinctive fibrillary splitting of the capillary walls with intrusion of basement membrane-like material into the capillary lumen has been described in the Senegalese children. Though these lesions are morphologically similar to those of quartan malarial nephropathy, no evidence of malaria was seen in these patients.

Membranous nephropathy (Chapter 3.7) is encountered frequently with an increased frequency in Africa and South-East Asian countries with high hepatitis B carrier rate. It is the commonest cause of nephrotic syndrome amongst the paediatric population in parts of Africa

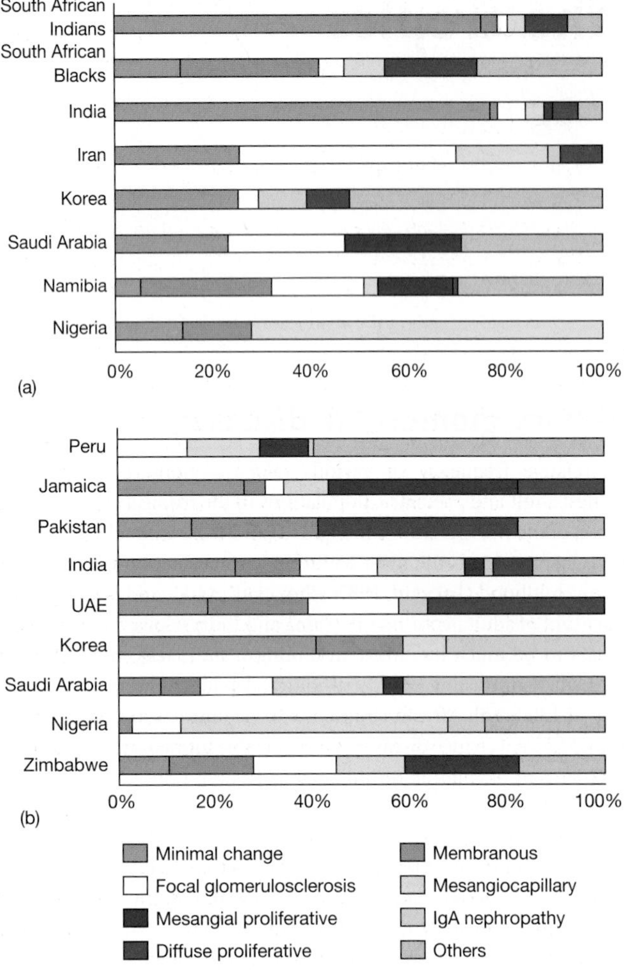

Fig. 1 Prevalence of different types of glomerular disease amongst children (a) and adults (b) submitted to renal biopsy in different parts of the tropical world. Please note: these were not necessarily nephrotic syndrome. (Data from Srivastava *et al.* 1975; Sadiq *et al.* 1978; Coovadia *et al.* 1979; Akinsola *et al.* 1984; Morgan *et al.* 1984; Bodaghi *et al.* 1989; Kadin *et al.* 1993; Al-Rasheed *et al.* 1996; Borok *et al.* 1997; Chugh and Sakhuja 1998; Yahya *et al.* 1998; Al-Homrany 1999; Asinobl *et al.* 1999; van Buuren *et al.* 1999; Hurtado *et al.* 2000; Choi *et al.* 2001; Shin *et al.* 2001.)

(Adhikari *et al.* 1983). In Taiwan, Japan, and Hong Kong, childhood membranous nephropathy is almost universally associated with HBsAg positivity (Takekoshi *et al.* 1978; Hsu *et al.* 1989; Lai *et al.* 1989; Wong *et al.* 1993; Chen *et al.* 1995). About 86 per cent of all South African children with membranous nephropathy show evidence of this infection (Bhimma *et al.* 1997). Clearance of hepatitis B virus (HBV) antigens, especially HBeAg, is strongly correlated with disease remission in children with HBV-associated membranous nephropathy (Bhimma *et al.* 1998). Immunohistochemical studies have shown HBV antigens in 68 per cent of all Chinese adults with membranous nephropathy; with HBsAg in two-thirds (Chen *et al.* 1995). A variant of membranous nephropathy associated with hypocomplementaemia has been described from Senegal.

IgA nephropathy (Chapter 3.6) has emerged as the commonest primary glomerular disease in many parts of the world, including the Far Eastern countries. It constitutes 25–45 per cent of all glomerulonephritides in Hong Kong, Taiwan, and Singapore (Woo *et al.* 1999), around 18–22 per cent in Malaysia and South Korea (Choi *et al.* 2001), and 8 per cent in Thailand. The frequency is estimated at 1–15 per cent in the Indian subcontinent, South America, and the Middle East (Abu-Romeh *et al.* 1989; Bodaghi *et al.* 1989; Al-Rasheed *et al.* 1996; Hurtado *et al.* 2000), and 0–3 per cent amongst the Black population of Africa (Levy and Berger 1988; Borok *et al.* 1997; Diouf *et al.* 1999). The prevalence rates of IgA nephropathy are different between people of Indian and African ancestry living in the same geographic regions of South Africa, suggesting that a genetic basis for the disease is probably more important (Seedat *et al.* 1988; Swanepoel *et al.* 1989). Since immunofluorescence microscopy is required for diagnosis, the reported differences in prevalence may be partly related to the lack of facilities for this investigation in many tropical centres. In a Japanese study, IgA nephropathy was documented in 47 per cent of all biopsies that were examined by immunofluorescence microscopy (Research Group on Progressive Chronic Renal Disease 1999). High dietary fibre intake has been suggested to protect Blacks from IgA nephropathy (Seedat *et al.* 1988). The prevalence of hepatitis B surface antigenaemia is significantly increased amongst patients with IgA nephropathy in certain geographic regions (Lai *et al.* 1988). IgA nephropathy has also been described following hepatitis A infection (Al-Homrany 2001).

Postinfectious glomerulonephritis (Chapter 3.9) due to streptococcal and non-streptococcal organisms continues to be encountered in a significant proportion of patients in tropical countries (Chugh *et al.* 1987). Thomson (1997) found poststreptococcal rapidly progressive glomerulonephritis to be the second commonest cause of ESRD amongst Black South African children.

A consistent decline has been observed in the incidence of membranoproliferative glomerulonephritis (MPGN) (Chapter 3.8) in most tropical countries over the last two decades. Some notable exceptions are Nigeria and Kuwait, where MPGN continues to be encountered with a high frequency (Al-Homrany 1999; Asinobi *et al.* 1999). A significant association has been noted between MPGN and hepatitis C infection in some countries (Yamabe *et al.* 1995). The hepatitis C-associated MPGN is similar to idiopathic MPGN in all respects.

Secondary glomerular diseases specific to the tropics

The tropical countries, with vast populations and poor economic resources, are not only exposed to diseases commonly seen in temperate climates but are also heavily burdened with those caused by infectious agents specific to the tropics (Table 1). The conditions caused by organisms encountered in temperate climates are described elsewhere (Chapter 3.13). Glomerular diseases due to infections seen almost exclusively in the tropics are described here. These tropical infections vary considerably from country to country. The causal relationship between these infections and glomerulonephritis was initially based on epidemiological studies and demonstration of resolution of renal lesions following treatment of infection. More recently, improved diagnostic techniques and well-designed experimental studies have provided concrete evidence in favour of cause-and-effect relationship. Confirmatory evidence is obtained by demonstration of specific antigens, immunoglobulins, and complement within the lesions, pointing to the immunological origin of glomerular disease.

Table 1 Tropical infections associated with glomerulonephritis

Protozoal
Plasmodium malariae and P. falciparum
Leishmania donovani
Toxoplasma gondii
Trypanosoma cruzei, T. brucei
Toxocara canis[a]
Strongloides stercoralis[a]
Helminthic
Schistosoma mansoni, S. japonicum, S. haematobium
Wuchereria bancrofti
Brugia malayi
Loa loa
Onchocerca volvulus
Trichinella spiralis[a]
Bacterial
Mycobacterium leprae, M. tuberculosis
Treponema pallidum
Salmonella typhi, S. paratyphi, S. typhimurium
Streptococcus pneumoniae
Leptospira species[a]
Yersinia enterocolitica[a]
Neisseria meningitidis, N. gonorrhoeae[a]
Corynebacterium diphtheriae[a]
Coxiella burnettii[a]
Brucella abortus[a]
Listeria monocytogenes[a]
Viral (also seen in other parts of the world)
Hepatitis B and C
Human immunodeficiency virus
Epstein–Barr virus
Coxsackie B
ECHO virus
Cytomegalovirus
Varicella-zoster
Mumps
Rubella
Influenza
Fungal
Histoplasma capsulatum[a]
Candida[a]
Coccidiodes immitis[a]

[a] Only case reports documented.

Malarial nephropathy

Malaria, caused by the protozoan *Plasmodium*, is endemic in the Indian subcontinent, Middle and Far Eastern Asia, sub-Saharan Africa, and Central America. The hot and humid tropical climate is conducive to multiplication of the disease vector, the *Anopheles* mosquito. According to the World Health Organization, over 2.5 billion people living in 103 endemic countries are at risk, of which about 300–500 million are infected annually. Malaria is responsible for approximately 1–3 million deaths every year. About 90 per cent of these occur in Africa, with children being the most affected. Of the four pathogenic species, *Plasmodium vivax, Plasmodium ovale, Plasmodium malariae,* and *Plasmodium falciparum*, only the latter two are associated with clinically significant glomerular disease. Glomerulonephritis has been reported most commonly following *P. malariae* infection (quartan malarial nephropathy) and only in some cases after *P. falciparum* malaria.

Quartan malarial nephropathy

Although malarial nephropathy finds a mention in Hipprocratic writings, the first recorded case in the modern medical literature dates back to 1884. A definite cause-and-effect relationship between *P. malariae* and nephrotic syndrome was established by Giglioli (1930) during surveys carried out in British Guyana. Several reports subsequently supported his observations, most notable being that by Gilles and Hendrickse (1963) who recorded increased prevalence of *P. malariae* parasitaemia amongst nephrotic children in western Nigeria.

The exact incidence of glomerulonephritis associated with quartan malaria is not known, but the frequency of nephrotic syndrome in areas endemic for this infection is 20–60 times higher compared to non-endemic areas (Chugh and Sakhuja 1998). In northern Nigeria, quartan malarial nephropathy is observed in 25–33 per cent of children with nephrotic syndrome (Abdurrahman *et al.* 1990). In a survey conducted in primary schools in Kenya (Johansen *et al.* 1994), a significant correlation between prevalence of malaria and proteinuria was found. The admission rate for the nephrotic syndrome declined dramatically in Guyana after the elimination of endemic *P. malariae* infection (Giglioli 1972). A malarial aetiology has been suspected in a significant proportion of patients with otherwise 'idiopathic' glomerulonephritis (Pakasa *et al.* 1993).

Clinical features

Quartan malarial nephropathy is rare during the first 2 years of life. Incidence increases with age and the peak is seen between 5 and 8 years. Most patients are poor and malnourished. Fever, peaking once every 72 h, is the initial manifestation. Renal involvement is indicated by the appearance of proteinuria, which typically develops after several weeks of fever. Oedema and ascites are prominent features and are further accentuated by concomitant protein energy malnutrition. A full-blown nephrotic syndrome is seen in about half of the cases with non-selective proteinuria in 80 per cent (Hendrickse *et al.* 1972). Gross haematuria is not seen, but microscopic haematuria is noted occasionally. The blood pressure is normal at onset of disease, but increases once renal failure sets in. Anaemia is universal and enlargement of liver and/or spleen is noted in over 75 per cent cases. Hypoalbuminaemia is usually profound, and serum albumin values of 1–2 gm/dl are noted frequently. In contrast to other causes of nephrotic syndrome, serum cholesterol tends to be normal or low, reflecting concomitant malnutrition. Serum creatinine is usually normal. Serum complement (C3) is within normal range. *P. malariae* parasitaemia is detected in early stages in about 75 per cent cases (Chugh and Sakhuja 1986).

Pathology

The predominant light microscopic abnormality is segmental thickening of glomerular capillary walls. The wall thickening is focal in early stages, but the number of affected glomeruli increases as the disease progresses. The thickening is due to subendothelial deposition of periodic acid-Schiff reagent (PAS) and silver stain positive fibrils arranged in a plexiform manner (Sinniah *et al.* 1988). Laying down of new basement membrane material on the opposite side of the deposits gives rise to the classical 'double contouring'. Eventually the capillary lumina become obliterated and mesangial sclerosis extends to involve all components. Proliferative lesions are more common in adults, and include mesangial hypercellularity, neutrophilic infiltration, and small fibroepithelial crescents. The tubulointerstitial changes include tubular atrophy and infiltration with lymphomononuclear cells.

Hendrickse *et al.* (1972) divided the histological lesions into three grades of increasing severity. In Grade I, less than one-third glomeruli show localized capillary-wall thickening and segmental sclerosis; in Grade II, 30–75 per cent of glomeruli are affected, often with diffuse thickening of capillary walls and sclerosis producing a 'honeycomb' appearance; and in Grade III more than 75 per cent of glomeruli are involved with prominent tubular atrophy and interstitial inflammation.

Immunofluorescence shows deposits of IgG, IgM_2, C3, and rarely, IgA. Three patterns of immune deposit have been described. The most common is a coarse, granular deposition of IgG3 (with or without other immunoglobulins and complement) along the capillary walls. A smaller number shows diffuse, fine, and homogeneously distributed IgG2 deposits without complement, and a mixed pattern is observed in the remaining cases. *P. malariae* antigen is detected in about 25 per cent cases (Ward and Kibukamusoke 1969; Houba *et al.* 1971; Houba 1979). IgG, IgM, and *P. malariae* antigen can also be demonstrated along the proximal tubules. Electron microscopy reveals subendothelial deposits of basement membrane-like material. Intramembranous deposits are noted occasionally. Hendrickse *et al.* (1972) described mesangial lacunae of electron-dense material with a density similar to the basement membrane.

Pathogenesis

Demonstration of malarial antigen in the deposits and binding of specific antibody to circulating malarial antigens with serum components of affected individuals suggest an immunological basis for this entity. Rhesus monkey (*Macaca mulatta*) infected with *P. inui* develops an immune complex glomerulonephritis. Subendothelial location of the immune complexes indicates deposition of circulating immune complexes rather than *in situ* formation. In mice infected with *Plasmodium berghei*, malarial antigen first appears in circulation 3 days after infection, either in free-floating form or within erythrocytes. From the seventh day onwards, the antigen, along with immunoglobulins and complement, can be detected along the glomerular capillary walls and in mesangium (Boonpucknavig *et al.* 1973). A similar sequence of events has been observed in rhesus monkeys infected with *P. cynomolgi* (Ward and Conran 1966) and in *Aotus nancymai* monkeys with *P. malariae* infection (Voller *et al.* 1971). These findings suggest the need for processing of parasitic antigen after its release from the erythrocytes before it can form immune complexes and get deposited in glomeruli.

The reason why only a small proportion of patients with *P. malariae* infection develop renal lesions, and the factors that determine its progressive nature are not well understood, but a permissive role of environmental factors such as malnutrition and co-infection with Epstein–Barr virus (EBV) have been suggested. Wedderburn *et al.* (1988) demonstrated proteinuria and oedema due to glomerulonephritis in common marmosets (*Callithrix jacchus*) infected with *Plasmodium brasilianum* and EBV but not with *P. brasilianum* alone. Since *P. malariae* can persist for long periods in the liver, continuous supply of antigen from the liver may contribute to perpetuation of renal lesions. Another possibility is the formation of autoantibodies to autologous antigens that are normally hidden, and are exposed as a result of the damage produced by plasmodium. Cross-reactivity of antibodies against plasmodial antigens with autologous antigen (molecular mimicry) has also been suspected. Voller (1974) showed an increased prevalence of antinuclear antibody positivity amongst people living in endemic areas.

The molecular mechanisms of injury involved in malaria-associated glomerulonephritis have not been clearly defined. Sinniah *et al.* (1999) showed elevated mRNA levels along with progressively increasing glomerular staining of tumour necrosis factor (TNF)-α, interleukin (IL)-1α, IL-6, IL-10, and granulocyte macrophage-colony stimulating factor (GM-CSF) in C57BL/6J mice infected with *P. berghei*. Increased IL-6 production in experimental murine malaria could be completely abolished by anti-TNFα antibody (Grau *et al.* 1990). Romero Alvira *et al.* (1995) have speculated about the role of free oxygen radicals in the genesis of glomerular lesions in malaria.

Management

Treatment of quartan malarial nephropathy is highly unsatisfactory. Once established, the disease follows an inexorably progressive course, culminating in renal failure in 2–4 years. Antimalarial drugs such as chloroquine and pyrimethamine have been ineffective (Gilles and Hendrickse 1963). Corticosteroids too are ineffective in inducing remissions and may lead to secondary infections and worsening of hypertension. Good response to corticosteroids, however, can be expected in those with highly selective proteinuria, who may in some cases have coincidental minimal change disease. Cyclophosphamide can induce a complete or partial remission of proteinuria in steroid resistant patients with mild histological lesions, but there is no improvement in overall survival (Adeniyi *et al.* 1979). Although patients showing a satisfactory response are more likely to have Grade I lesions (Hendrickse *et al.* 1972), no difference in overall outcome has been observed between the three grades. Renal failure, infections, and malnutrition are the commonest causes of death. In one study, disappearance of immune deposits was seen on repeat biopsies in children who showed good response to corticosteroids, azathioprine, or cyclophosphamide.

Falciparum malaria

In contrast to the persistent and progressive course of quartan malarial nephropathy, the glomerulonephritis associated with falciparum malaria is mild and transient. Autopsy studies reveal glomerular lesions in about 18 per cent but urinary abnormalities such as proteinuria, microhaematuria, and casts are noted in 20–50 per cent of cases of falciparum malaria (Boonpucknavig and Sitprija 1979; Rabenantoandro *et al.* 1994). Children are involved more frequently than adults. Proteinuria is non-selective and usually less than 1 g/24 h. Full-blown nephrotic and acute nephritic syndromes are seen occasionally. There is no correlation between the height of fever and the degree of proteinuria or the type of urinary sediment. Hypocomplementaemia (low C3 and C4) is common, and circulating immune complexes along with *P. falciparum* antigen can be demonstrated during the acute phase (Barsoum 1998). The glomerulonephritis usually resolves within 4–6 weeks of eradication of infection.

Pathology

Histological descriptions of glomerular pathology in falciparum malaria are scarce. Spitz (1946) found histological abnormalities in nine out of 50 autopsies of patients dying of falciparum infection. The histological lesions are characterized by mesangial hypercellularity and a modest increase in mesangial matrix. Basement membrane changes are usually absent. An eosinophilic granular material is present in capillary walls, mesangium, and Bowman's capsule along with pigment-laden macrophages in the capillary lumina. Parasitized erythrocytes can be seen in peritubular capillaries and interlobular veins but are rarely detected in the glomerular capillaries. Tubules show swelling and necrosis of cells and casts in the lumina. Interstitial infiltration and oedema are commonly seen. Immunofluorescence shows finely granular IgG3, IgM, and C3 in the mesangial area. Malarial antigen can be demonstrated in some cases. Electron microscopy reveals subendothelial and mesangial deposits along with diffuse foot process effacement. El-Shoura (1994) showed irregular thickening of the glomerular basement membrane along with subendothelial humps. The severity of deposits correlated with the degree of parasitaemia.

Pathogenesis

Transient glomerular lesions akin to those in falciparum malaria can be induced in BALB/c mice and Sprague–Dawley rats infected with *P. berghei* and *P. falciparum* infected squirrel monkeys (*Saimiri sciureus*) (Aikawa *et al.* 1988). The latter model shows endocapillary proliferation in addition to mesangial hypercellularity. *P. falciparum* antigen can be demonstrated in these lesions. Recent studies have suggested that CD4 cell subpopulations, in particular Th2 cells, may be playing a significant role in the genesis of glomerular lesions in falciparum malaria. Activation of these cells leads to increase in production of immunoglobulins. The role of concomitant infection, especially with HBV, is under investigation.

Schistosomal nephropathy

Schistosomiasis (*syn.* Bilharziasis) is a chronic infection by trematodes (blood flukes) and affects over 200 million people in 74 countries of Asia, Africa, and South America (Chitsulo *et al.* 2000). Five species are pathogenic to humans, with *Schistosoma haematobium* (sub-Saharan Africa and Middle East), *Schistosoma mansoni* (South America and Africa), and *Schistosoma japonicum* (China and Far East) being the most prevalent. At a time when concerted efforts are being undertaken by several organizations to eradicate this infection, environmental changes induced by the construction of dams over rivers and consequent migration of population has led to spread of the disease to new geographical areas in Africa and China (Ross *et al.* 2002).

Infection follows direct contact with larval forms (cercariae) floating freely in fresh water. They penetrate the skin, turn into schistosomulae by shedding their tails, enter the capillaries, and travel via the pulmonary circulation to the liver where they mature into adult worms. The worms then migrate to the mesenteric veins (*S. mansoni* and *S. japonicum*) or the veins draining the ureters and bladder (*S. haematobium*) where they reside and lay eggs. Disease manifestations result from the host's immune response to the schistosomes and the granulomatous reaction to the egg antigens, and hence are determined by the site of maximal accumulation of eggs. *S. haematobium* primarily involves the lower urinary and genital tracts. Involvement of bladder wall and ureters leads to reduced bladder capacity and ureteral stenosis, causing hydroureter, hydronephrosis, and progressive renal failure (Chugh *et al.* 1986). *S. mansoni* and *S. japonicum* involve the gastrointestinal tract and portal system, producing a granulomatous inflammation in the gut wall. In about 4–8 per cent of infected individuals, this leads to development of a typical form of hepatic fibrosis, called clay-pipe-stem fibrosis and portal hypertension.

Although both *S. mansoni* and *S. japonicum* have been shown to cause glomerular lesions in experimental studies, clinical glomerular disease has been described most frequently in association with hepatosplenic schistosomiasis due to *S. mansoni*. The initial reports came in 1964 from autopsies on patients dying with hepatosplenic disease due to *S. mansoni* in Brazil (Lopes 1964). In the subsequent years, clinical observations from endemic areas and several experimental studies have confirmed the cause and effect relationship of *S. mansoni* infection with glomerulonephritis (Andrade *et al.* 1971; Rocha *et al.* 1976; Musa *et al.* 1980; Chandra Shekhar and Pathmanathan 1987; Sobh *et al.* 1987; Abu Romeh *et al.* 1989).

Lack of systematic epidemiological studies prevents an exact estimate of the incidence of this entity. The prevalence and pattern vary depending upon nature of the study (clinical or histological), and on the stage of the infection. Essamie *et al.* (1995) found schistosomiasis to be the commonest cause of ESRD in the young population of rural Egypt. In clinical studies, overt proteinuria has been seen in 1–10 per cent in those with *S. mansoni* and 2–5 per cent in *S. haematobium* infections, and microalbuminuria is found in about 22 per cent of patients with hepatosplenic schistosomiasis (Barsoum *et al.* 1992; Barsoum 1993). Sobh *et al.* (1990) documented asymptomatic proteinuria in 20 per cent patients with 'active' *S. mansoni* infection. A field study in an endemic area of Brazil revealed a low (1 per cent) incidence of proteinuria as measured by the protein/creatinine ratio (Rabello *et al.* 1993).

Histological studies have documented glomerular lesions in a much higher proportion of patients. In one study, glomerular abnormalities were detected on renal biopsy in 40 per cent of patients who underwent splenectomy, though none had evidence of clinical renal disease (Rocha *et al.* 1976). Autopsies on patients with hepatosplenic schistosomiasis dying of various causes revealed glomerular changes in 12 per cent (Andrade *et al.* 1971). Sobh *et al.* (1990) documented glomerular lesions in over 50 per cent of asymptomatic patients with *S. mansoni* infection. Thus the true extent of subclinical glomerular involvement in schistosomiasis is unknown. Recent studies have shown a drastic reduction in the number of cases with schistosomal glomerulopathy associated with a decline in the incidence of severe *S. mansoni* infection following the widespread use of oxamniquine in the endemic population (Correia *et al.* 1997).

Clinical features

Though described at all ages, glomerulonephritis is most common in young adults, and males are affected twice as frequently as females. The hepatosplenic disease and portal hypertension are usually overt. Peripheral oedema and ascites are the hallmarks of clinical glomerular involvement. Proteinuria is poorly selective and haematuria is uncommon in the absence of lower urinary tract involvement. Eosinophiluria can be documented in 65 per cent of cases with schistosomal glomerulopathy (Eltoum *et al.* 1989). The presenting features depend upon the histopathological pattern of glomerular changes (see below). About 30 per cent of patients exhibit hypergammaglobulinaemia, and the serum cholesterol is not elevated in an equal proportion whilst serum complement (C3) concentrations are usually low. Some patients with schistosomiasis and proteinuria have been shown to have coexistent *Salmonella* infection. These patients present with prolonged fever, bloody diarrhoea, splenomegaly, vasculitic skin lesions, and a rapidly developing nephrotic syndrome with normal blood pressure and cholesterol levels (Martinelli *et al.* 1992). Serum C3 is uniformly low, but the C4 levels are normal. Non-specific antibody production is demonstrated by false positive rheumatoid factor, antinuclear antibody or venereal disease research laboratory test (VDRL), especially in those with concomitant *Salmonella* infection.

The diagnosis of schistosomiasis is made by demonstrating viable eggs in stool. Egg-shedding is extremely variable, and a number of sedimentation and concentration techniques have been used to increase the diagnostic yield. Demonstration of egg-containing granulomas in rectal or liver biopsies may be needed in patients who fail to exhibit eggs in stools but where the clinical suspicion is high. Several serologic techniques are under evaluation, and an immunoblot assay for adult worm antigen is quite promising (Wang *et al.* 1999). It is important to exclude other causes of nephrotic syndrome before attributing the lesions to schistosomiasis. Presence of concomitant *Salmonella* infection can be confirmed by blood, urine, or bone marrow culture.

Pathology

Several patterns of glomerular pathology have been described (Table 2). Class I (mesangioproliferative) lesion (Fig. 2) is the earliest and most frequent, and is seen with equal frequency in all three types of schistosomal infection (Andrade and Rocha 1979; Chandra Shekhar and Pathmanathan 1987; Barsoum 1993). About two-thirds of the patients are asymptomatic, and the rest exhibit occult proteinuria (Barsoum *et al.* 1992). Blood pressure and renal function are usually normal. It is also the principal lesion in renal allografts with recurrent schistosomal nephropathy (Azevedo *et al.* 1987). In contrast to the other classes, this type has been reported with all the three schistosoma species. As opposed to the idiopathic minimal change disease, the light microscopically unremarkable Class IA (minimal lesion) lesion of schistosomal glomerulopathy exhibits immune deposits, and responds poorly to steroids.

Class II (diffuse proliferative) lesion is more frequent in patients with concomitant *Salmonella* infection (Lambertucci *et al.* 1988). Light microscopy reveals endocapillary proliferation, and infiltration with neutrophils, monocytes, platelets, and fibrin deposition.

The frequency of Class III (mesangiocapillary) lesion varies from 20 per cent in asymptomatic patients to over 80 per cent in those with overt renal disease (Barsoum 1993). Hepatic fibrosis is an essential prerequisite for the development of this lesion. In certain parts of the world, it is the commonest histological lesion (Abensur *et al.* 1992). Over 90 per cent of patients are classified under Class IIIA, which resembles type I idiopathic MCGN on light microscopy. Class IIIB shows more marked membrane thickening along with epimembranous deposits. The mesangial proliferation is less marked in this type. Some authors have described a 'pure' membranous nephropathy in association with schistosomiasis; but the existence of this entity is doubted (Barsoum 1993). In both classes, immunofluorescence shows

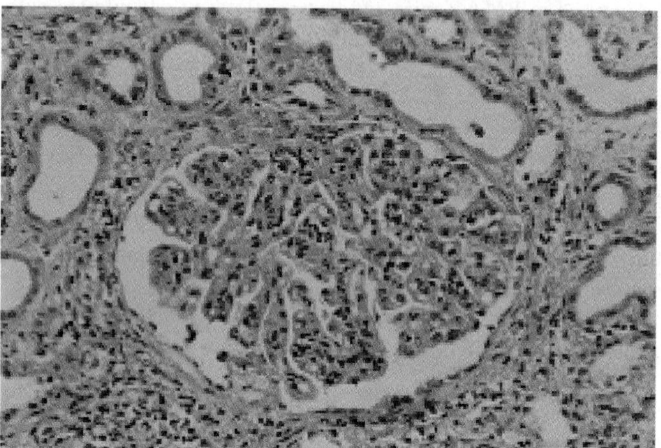

Fig. 2 Microphotograph showing diffuse mesangial proliferation in *Schistosoma mansoni* infection (original magnification 250×, haematoxylin and eosin).

Table 2 Clinicopathological classification of schistosomal glomerulopathy (adapted from Barsoum 1993)

Class	Light microscopic pattern	Immunofluorescence	Asymptomatic proteinuria	Nephrotic syndrome	Hyper-tension	Progression to ESRD	Response to treatment
I	Mesangioproliferative A. Minimal lesion B. Focal proliferative C. Diffuse proliferative	Mesangial IgM, C3, schistosomal gut antigens	+++	+	+/−	?	+/−
II	Exudative	Endocapillary C3, schistosomal antigens	−	+++	−	?	+++
III	A. Mesangiocapillary type I	Mesangial IgG, C3, schistosomal gut antigen (early), IgA (late)	+	++	++	++	−
	B. Mesangiocapillary type III	Mesangial and subepithelial IgG, C3, schistosomal gut antigen (early), IgA (late)	+	+++	+	++	−
IV	Focal and segmental glomerulosclerosis	Mesangial IgG, IgM, IgA	+	+++	+++	+++	−
V	Amyloidosis	Mesangial IgG	+	+++	+/−	+++	−

IgG and C3 and less commonly, IgM and IgA. Schistosomal antigen is detected in a minority of cases. Most patients present with a full-blown nephrotic syndrome, and about half have hypertension. Some authors have suggested a role for hepatitis B infection in the genesis of Class IIIB lesions. This speculation is primarily based on the demonstration of a high prevalence of hepatitis B in patients with hepatosplenic schistosomiasis (Bassily *et al.* 1983), but its exact significance needs further evaluation.

Class IV (focal and segmental glomerulosclerosis) lesion are seen in 15–40 per cent cases, and cannot be distinguished from idiopathic focal segmental glomerulosclerosis on the basis of light microscopy (Musa *et al.* 1980; Sobh *et al.* 1988b). In addition to the segmental hyalinosis, light microscopy reveals focal mesangial proliferation. Immunofluorescence, however, reveals IgA deposition in 11–38 per cent of cases (Barsoum *et al.* 1988). As in Class III, this lesion is also seen in patients with fibrotic livers. Clinically, this class is characterized by severe proteinuria, and a high incidence of hypertension.

Prevalence of amyloidotic Class V lesions varies from 15 to 40 per cent, with a higher frequency in African patients (Musa *et al.* 1980). This form is seen with equal frequency in *S. mansoni* and *S. haematobium* infections and is usually not affected by the presence or absence of hepatic fibrosis (Barsoum 1993). Nephrotic syndrome is the commonest presentation. Involvement of extrarenal tissues like liver and spleen has been described. The amyloid is of the secondary (AA) variety. Some authors have suggested a role for chronic pyogenic infection in the genesis of this lesion.

Schistosomal nephropathy (see also Chapter 7.5) is primarily caused by immunological reaction to specific parasitic antigens, which is discussed in Chapter 7.5. The portal blood carrying the primary load of worm antigen is diverted to the systemic circulation without undergoing degradation by the hepatic macrophages as a result of hepatic fibrosis and portacaval shunting. This, and an immunoglobulin isotype 'switch' from IgM to IgA producing B-cells, lead to generation of IgA antibodies that predominate in the circulation and glomerular deposits of patients with schistosomal glomerulonephritis. Activation of monocyte–macrophage system leading to release of cytokines which in turn activate Th1 and Th2 lymphocytes has also been shown.

Racial and genetic factors may be important in the development and progression of schistosomal glomerulopathy. Fujiwara *et al.* (1988) were able to induce glomerulonephritis in female BXSB but not in C57BL/6 (B6) mice following infection with *S. mansoni*, confirming the role of genetic background. Hassan (1982) showed an increased frequency of HLA-A28 in those with glomerular disease. Furthermore, Class V lesions are more common in certain geographic areas, and males are more prone to this lesion, suggesting a genetic influence in the generation and/or disposal of amyloid fibrils.

The exact role of *Salmonella* infection in the genesis of this entity is not clear. Epidemiological studies have shown disappearance of urinary abnormalities following anti-*Salmonella* therapy alone, suggesting that at least in some cases, the overt renal disease could have been precipitated by the *Salmonella* infection superimposed on a subclinical schistosomal glomerulopathy (Bassily *et al.* 1976; Lambertrucci *et al.* 1988; Martinelli *et al.* 1992). *Salmonella* receptors have been identified on adult schistosomes. Once attached to the receptor, the bacteria escape recognition by the host cells. The presence of *Salmonella* endotoxins has been confirmed on immunofluorescence studies. The endotoxin induces alternate pathway complement activation, which explains the depressed C3 and normal C4 concentrations.

Management

Praziquantel, given in a dose of 20 mg/kg three times a day, is effective in curing 60–90 per cent patients with schistosomiasis. Oxamniquine is the only alternative for *S. mansoni* infection, whereas metrifonate is useful for *S. haematobium* infection (Ross *et al.* 2002). Successful treatment helps in amelioration of hepatic fibrosis if reinfection can be avoided. Established schistosomal glomerulopathy, however, does not respond to any of these agents.

The role of corticosteroids, cytotoxic agents, and cyclosporin is unclear (Martinelli *et al.* 1995). In one recent trial, an 8-week-course of 60 mg/day of prednisolone, given in combination with praziquantel and oxamniquine induced more remissions, and was associated with significant increase in plasma albumin when compared with praziquantel and oxamniquine administered alone or in combination with cyclosporin (Sobh *et al.* 1989). The remissions, however, were of short duration; and repeat biopsies failed to show disease regression. A combination of antischistosomal therapy, steroids, and azathioprine has been shown to be effective in 2/3 of patients with Class I lesions (Barsoum 1993). Several reports have now confirmed that the proteinuria responds to anti-*Salmonella* therapy in some cases (Lambertucci *et al.* 1988; Martinelli *et al.* 1992). Hence, it is imperative to look for and treat this infection in all patients with schistosomiasis and proteinuria.

The prognosis is relatively good in Class I and II lesions, provided sustained eradication of schistosoma and *Salmonella* infection can be achieved, whereas Classes IV and V lesions usually progress to ESRD (Sobh *et al.* 1988a, 1993; Martinelli *et al.* 1995). Colchicine, when given with antischistosomal treatment, led to reduction in the amyloid deposits and proteinuria in experimental animals (Sobh *et al.* 1995), but this therapy has not been tried in humans.

Transplantations on some patients with ESRD due to schistosomal nephropathy have been successful (Azevedo *et al.* 1987). Compared to controls, there was no difference in the incidence of rejections, cyclosporine toxicity, urinary tract infection, or other urological complications in these cases (Mahmoud *et al.* 2001). Recurrent glomerular disease can occur in the graft.

Glomerulonephritis in *S. japonicum* and *S. haematobium* infections

Prospective studies in patients with *S. japonicum* infection in the Philippines have not shown any increase in the incidence of renal disease when compared with a control population (Watt *et al.* 1987). In a study carried out in rural Egypt, Ezzat *et al.* (1974) documented proteinuria in 40–55 per cent people living in areas with high prevalence of *S. haematobium* infection, with 2–5 per cent showing proteinuria of 1–5 g/day. However, neither *S. mansoni* nor concomitant chronic *Salmonella* infection were ruled out in these cases. In another study (Rasendramino *et al.* 1998b), 75 per cent of 574 patients with urinary bilharziasis showed dipstick positive proteinuria, with 6 per cent showing heavy (>5 g/day) proteinuria. Greenham and Cameron (1980) reported two instances of nephrotic syndrome due to MCGN in the absence of salmonellosis. Although the association may have been purely coincidental, remission of the nephrotic state following a course of niridazole suggested a cause-and-effect relationship between the infection and glomerulonephritis. In an autopsy study of 268 subjects from Egypt, no correlation could be found between glomerular abnormalities and the presence or intensity of *S. haematobium* infestation (Sadigursky *et al.* 1976). On the other hand, Soliman *et al.* (1987)

performed renal biopsies in 16 asymptomatic patients and found glomerular changes in 19 per cent. IgG and IgM deposits were found in over 50 per cent while schistosomal antigens were detectable in 25 per cent. It was concluded that *S. haematobium* infestation may infrequently cause a glomerulopathy that is not clinically apparent. In an interventional study, Rasendramino *et al.* (1998a) showed a significant decrease in the prevalence of proteinuria in areas endemic for *S. haematobium* following praziquantel therapy. In another case report, Turner *et al.* (1987) showed complete resolution of proteinuria and haematuria in a patient with biopsy-proved minimal change glomerulonephritis in association with *S. haematobium* infection.

Filarial nephropathy

Filarial worms are nematodes that are transmitted to humans through arthropod bites. They dwell in the subcutaneous tissues and lymphatics of their vertebrate hosts, and clinical manifestations depend upon the location of microfilariae and adult worms in the tissues. Of the eight filarial species that infect humans, *Loa loa, Onchocerca volvulus, Wuchereria bacrofti*, and *Brugia malayi* are associated with glomerular disease. An association between filariasis and glomerular disease has been reported from Africa and some Asian countries (Bariéty *et al.* 1967; Pillay *et al.* 1973; Chugh *et al.* 1978; Date *et al.* 1979; Ngu *et al.* 1985).

Loiasis is prevalent in west and central Africa, and characteristically manifests with localized areas of allergic inflammation and Calabar swellings. Onchocerciasis (river blindness) is characterized by subcutaneous nodules, pruritic skin rash, sclerosing lymphadenitis, and ocular lesions. Bancroftian and Brugia infections cause febrile episodes associated with acute lymphangitis and lymphadenitis, leading ultimately to lymphoedema manifesting as hydrocoele and elephantiasis. This form of filariasis is endemic in Africa and South-East Asia.

Clinical features

The frequency of glomerular involvement in filariasis is difficult to estimate. Asymptomatic urinary abnormalities have been reported in 11–25 per cent of patients with loiasis and onchocerciasis and nephrotic syndrome is seen in 3–5 per cent of cases. Ngu *et al.* (1985) showed a 5.5 greater prevalence of proteinuria amongst Cameroonians living in an area hyperendemic for onchocerciasis when compared to a control population. In another population study, proteinuria 2+ or more was demonstrated in 11 per cent and nephrotic syndrome in 2.7 per cent of patients. Haematuria and nephrotic range proteinuria were documented in 25 per cent and 5 per cent of patients with loiasis. Nephrotic syndrome has been described more commonly in those with polyarthritis and chorioretinitis (Hall *et al.* 2001). Renal function may be impaired in an occasional case of onchocerciasis associated glomerulonephritis.

The available data concerning the incidence of glomerulonephritis in Wucherarian and Bancroftian filariasis are scanty. Earlier studies indicated an increased incidence of proteinuria in patients infected with *B. malayi* compared to controls, but no correlation could be found with the severity of filariasis. Proteinuria and/or haematuria was detected in over 50 per cent of cases with filariasis, 25 per cent showed glomerular proteinuria (Dreyer *et al.* 1992). Langhammer *et al.* (1997) found a high prevalence of proteinuria in *B. malayi* infected patients with obstructive disease compared to those with filarial fever or microfilaraemia with the former showing glomerular pattern compared to purely tubular and mixed patterns, respectively, in the other two groups. Microhaematuria and hypertension were also more common in this form of filariasis than the other two groups. False positive rheumatoid factor, both of IgG and IgM type, anti-DNA and antiphospholipid antibodies, and autoantibodies against a variety of cytoplasmic proteins were also noted. Chaturvedi *et al.* (1995) found antibodies to microfilarial ES antigen using stick enzyme-linked immunosorbent assay (ELISA) test in about 68 per cent patients with nephrotic syndrome and 38 per cent patients with acute nephritic syndrome in a region endemic for lymphatic filariasis.

Pathology

Light microscopy reveals a gamut of lesions consistent with diffuse and mesangial proliferative, mesangiocapillary, minimal change and chronic sclerosing glomerulonephritides, and the collapsing variant of focal segmental glomerulosclerosis (Pakasa *et al.* 1997). A diffuse basement membrane thickening and mild increase in number of endocapillary cells are the commonest findings. There are a large number of eosinophils amongst the infiltrating cells. Small number of crescents may also be noted. Mononuclear interstitial infiltration and microinfarcts around blood vessels have been demonstrated in patients with loiasis. Microfilariae may be found in the arterioles, glomerular and peritubular capillary lumina, tubules, and interstitium (Pakasa *et al.* 1997). Electron microscopy shows widely spaced subepithelial, subendothelial, and intramembranous deposits, basement membrane spikes, and podocyte effacement (Ormerod *et al.* 1983). Sheaths and cuticular ridges of *L. loa* may also be identified. Immune deposits containing IgM, IgG, and C3 are seen in the mesangium and along the capillary loops. *O. volvulus* and *B. malayi* antigens have been demonstrated in about 50 per cent cases. Those with loiasis-associated glomerulonephritis exhibit cross-reactivity with hyperimmune anti-Onchocerca serum, raising the possibility of a shared antigen.

Pathogenesis

An immune complex mechanism is widely accepted to be responsible for filarial glomerulopathies. Dogs infected with *Dirofilaria immitis* develop glomerular lesions similar to human filariasis, and the circulating immune complex levels correlate with the adult worm burden (Katner *et al.* 1984; Nakagaki *et al.* 1990). Kamiie *et al.* (2000) performed ultrastructural studies on the distribution of anionic sites on the glomerular basement membrane in control and *D. immitis* infected dogs. These sites were present only in the lamina rara externa of controls, but were found in a thickened lamina densa in the infected dogs. They also found extensive subendothelial dense deposits. Immune complexes can also form *in situ*, as shown in one study where glomerular lesions were induced after selective catheterization and infusion of renal arteries with *D. immitis*. The contralateral kidneys remained either uninvolved or showed minor lesions (Grauer *et al.* 1989). Diethylcarbamazine (DEC) or ivermectin treatment may lead to antigen release into circulation by killing the parasite and exacerbate the immune process (Ngu *et al.* 1980; Cruel *et al.* 1997; Langhammer *et al.* 1997).

Treatment

A good response to antifilarial therapy with DEC is observed in patients with non-nephrotic proteinuria and/or haematuria. The response is inconsistent in those with nephritic syndrome and renal function deterioration may continue despite clearance of microfilariae with treatment. Therapeutic apheresis has been utilized to reduce the microfilarial load before starting DEC therapy to prevent antigen release, which may otherwise exacerbate the renal disease (Abel *et al.* 1986).

Mycobacterial infections

Leprosy

Leprosy is a chronic, granulomatous, multisystem disorder caused by *Mycobacterium leprae*. The disease primarily involves peripheral nerves and skin. The clinical presentation depends upon the immunological status of the host, and may take one of the two forms. The paucibacillary (*syn.* tuberculoid, non-lepromatous) form is characterized by preserved cell mediated immunity and well-formed epitheoid cell granulomas. The second type is multibacillary disease (*syn.* lepromatous), where the immune protection mechanisms fail leading to widespread dissemination of bacilli and poor granuloma formation. The prevalence of leprosy has declined in recent years, and the WHO estimates that there are about 640,000 patients around the world. About 70 per cent of these are in India, where the prevalence is 5.0 per 10,000. Leprosy is also endemic in Brazil, China, Africa, and other countries of South-East Asia and South America.

Mitsuda and Ogawa were the first to describe the renal histological changes in 1937. Renal disease continued to be an important cause of death in leprosy until the 1950s. Renal lesions in leprosy can involve the glomerular as well as the tubular and the interstitial compartments, and may present as glomerulonephritis, secondary amyloidosis, interstitial nephritis, lepromas, and isolated renal tubular defects.

Glomerulonephritis

The incidence of glomerulonephritis varies from less than 2 per cent on clinical evaluation to over 60 per cent on histology (Weiner and Northcutt 1989). Interpretation of studies is confounded by bias in referral patterns, patient selection, and variations in indications for biopsies. Date *et al.* (1977) recorded glomerulonephritis on renal biopsies in 63 per cent of patients who had clinical evidence of renal disease. In studies on unselected cases, Chugh *et al.* (1983) and Gupta *et al.* (1977) found histopathological changes in 8 and 6 per cent of cases, respectively. Chopra *et al.* (1991) observed glomerular lesions in 13 out of 50 biopsies. In autopsy studies, the prevalence has been reported to vary from 5 to 14 per cent (Jayalakshmi *et al.* 1987; Nakayama *et al.* 2001). Kirztajn *et al.* (1993) found microalbuminuria in 16 per cent and microscopic haematuria in 22 per cent of patients, over 2/3 of them showing dysmorphic RBCs. Another study documented proteinuria and/or microhaematuria in 35 per cent of consecutive leprosy patients (Ponce *et al.* 1989). Most studies have found the frequency of renal involvement to be equal in both lepromatous and non-lepromatous forms of leprosy (Ng *et al.* 1981). Chopra *et al.* (1991), on the other hand, observed that patients showing glomerular lesions on histology were three times more likely to have lepromatous leprosy. Glomerulonephritis is more common during episodes of erythema nodosum leprosum (ENL).

Clinical features

Most patients have symptomless urinary abnormalities but several studies have reported the occurrence of nephrotic syndrome, acute nephritic syndrome, and rapidly progressive renal failure (Chopra *et al.* 1991; Kirsztajn *et al.* 1993). Hypertension is uncommon. Reduced creatinine clearance is noted in patients with ENL. Chopra *et al.* (1991) noted reduced creatinine clearance in 20 of 70 patients with various types of leprosy. Hypocomplementaemia is common. Impairment of urinary acidification and concentration abilities are observed frequently (Ponce *et al.* 1989). Circulating cryoglobulins are present in a significant proportion of cases. Rapidly progressive renal failure due to crescentic glomerulonephritis has been observed *de novo* (Chugh *et al.* 1998) or may develop following treatment with rifampicin (Muthukumar *et al.* 2003).

Pathology

The histological lesion observed on light microscopy include those of mesangial proliferative (Fig. 3a), diffuse proliferative, and MCGN, and less commonly, chronic sclerosing and crescentic glomerulonephritis (Fig. 3b) (Al-Mohaya *et al.* 1988; Sinniah *et al.* 1988; Madiwale *et al.* 1994; Ahsan *et al.* 1995). Acid fast bacilli are rarely seen (Ahsan *et al.* 1995). In addition to the glomerular changes, Matsuo *et al.* (1997) showed lesions suggestive of vasculitis, including fibrinoid necrosis, afferent arteriolar microaneurysms, and strictures of efferent arterioles. Rarely, granulomata typical of mycobacterial infection can be seen (Al-Mohaya *et al.* 1988). Electron microscopy reveals electron-dense deposits in mesangial and subendothelial regions, focal foot process widening, reduplication of glomerular capillary basement membrane with mesangial interposition, and endothelial cytoplasmic vacuolation. Immunofluorescence reveals granular deposits of IgG, C3, and less frequently, IgM, IgA, and fibrin in the mesangium and along capillary walls.

Pathogenesis

The glomerular lesions are manifestations of an immune complex process. Circulating immune complexes are observed in one-third of those with lepromatous disease, and in more than 75 per cent of patients with active ENL. Hypocomplementaemia is common, especially during episode of ENL (Shwe 1972). Though antigen is suspected to be a product of *M. leprae*, the demonstration of glomerulonephritis with equal frequency in both pauci- and multibacillary forms of leprosy raises the possibility of involvement of non-mycobacterial antigens, such as HBV and HCV, bacteria like staphylococci and streptococci, and other parasites. The role of disordered immunity was suggested by Freire *et al.* (1998) who showed presence of antibodies against neutrophilic cytoplasmic antigens (ANCA) in about 30 per cent of patients with all forms of leprosy. There was no correlation between ANCA positivity and the duration of disease. Patients at the lepromatous end of the spectrum and those with reactions had a higher prevalence. Since these antibodies do not react with the common ANCA antigens, for example proteinase-3 or myeloperoxidase, the exact nature of antigens against which these antibodies are directed remains uncertain. The development of antidapsone antibodies during treatment suggest that dapsone–antidapsone immune complexes could contribute to the pathogenesis of glomerular lesions (Das *et al.* 1980). Alternate pathway complement activation by cryoprecipitates can also exacerbate the glomerular injury. Cryoglobulin containing deposits have been identified in the glomeruli (Weiner and Northcutt 1989). Agnihotri *et al.* (1995) showed evidence of increased lipid peroxidation and increased excretion of brush border enzymes in mice infected with *M. leprae*. The precise role of cell-mediated immunity in the genesis of glomerulonephritis in leprosy has not been fully investigated.

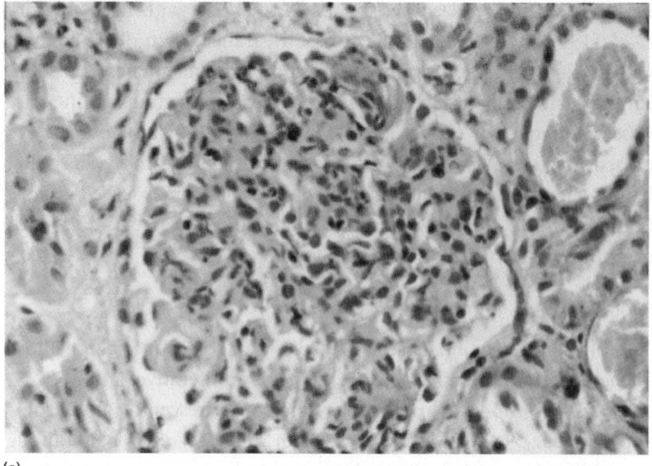

(a)

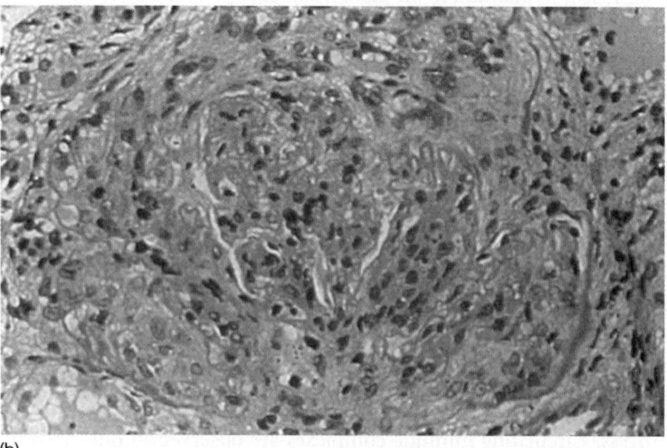

(b)

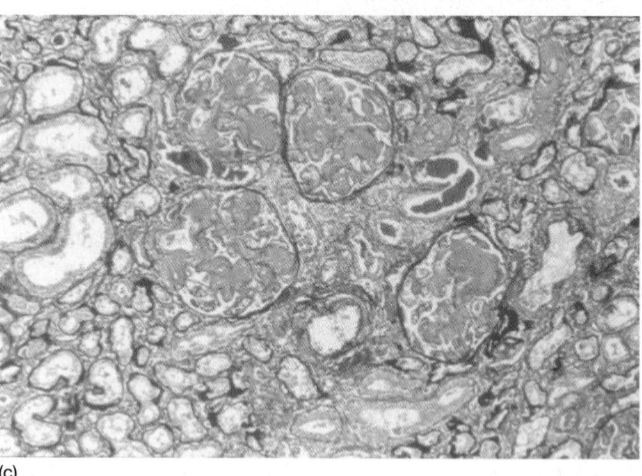

(c)

Fig. 3 (a) Lepromatous leprosy: the glomerulus shows diffuse proliferative glomerulonephritis (haematoxylin and eosin, magnification 235×). (b) Lepromatous leprosy: renal biopsy showing crescentic glomerulonephritis (haematoxylin and eosin, magnification 310×). (c) Lepromatous leprosy: a 35-year-old patient with nephrotic proteinuria. The renal biopsy showed massive deposits of amyloid. Periodic acid–silver methanamine, 280×.

Amyloidosis

The incidence of renal amyloidosis (see Chapter 4.2.1) in leprosy has been reported to vary from 2 to 55 per cent in different studies. Nakayama *et al.* (2001) found renal amyloidosis in 31 per cent of 199 leprosy autopsies over a 16-year period. In contrast, reports from Mexico, Panama, Malaysia, Papua New Guinea, Malawi, Africa, and India put the incidence at less than 10 per cent. Of 203 consecutive patients of secondary amyloidosis seen in a North Indian centre, only 2.5 per cent were due to lepromatous leprosy (Fig. 3c) (Chugh *et al.* 1981) whereas in Papua New Guinea, 60 per cent of all cases of amyloidosis are secondary to leprosy (Cooke and Champness 1967). The difference is probably related to genetic and nutritional factors, differences in numbers of lepra reactions and different standards of management in different countries. No correlation has been shown between the duration of disease and the development of amyloidosis. The latter may supervene as early as 2–3 years after the diagnosis of leprosy. The amyloid is of AA type. The occurrence of amyloidosis is far more frequent in lepromatous compared to non-lepromatous leprosy. Nakayama *et al.* (2001) documented amyloid in only 6 per cent of patients with non-lepromatous leprosy, compared to 36 per cent in those with the lepromatous form. ENL reactions increase the risk of amyloid, as each episode is associated with a marked and persistent elevation of serum amyloid A protein (Nakayama *et al.* 2001). The hepatic synthesis of this protein is increased by IL-1 and IL-6 released during the inflammatory episodes. The ability of monocytes to clear AA protein is also lowered, favouring its deposition in tissues. Patients with tuberculoid leprosy who have long-standing and infected trophic ulcers can also develop this complication.

In contrast to glomerulonephritis, patients with amyloidosis usually present with a full-blown picture of nephrotic syndrome, with prominent oedema and profound hypoalbuminaemia. Serum cholesterol concentrations are usually not elevated, reflecting a state of malnutrition and hepatic involvement by the amyloid. Renal insufficiency is evident at presentation in over 50 per cent cases, and progresses to ESRD over 2–5 years. Renal failure is the most frequent cause of death in these cases.

Management

In general, corticosteroids or antileprosy drugs have no effect on the course of glomerular disease. Amyloidosis can be prevented by early and aggressive anti-leprosy treatment with particular attention to preventing ENL reactions. Use of dapsone alone is associated with increased risk of ENL, and hence combination chemotherapy with clofazimine and rifampicin should be used in patients with multibacillary leprosy. Prednisolone may hasten the recovery of renal function in those who develop renal failure during episodes of ENL (Weiner and Northcutt 1989). Patients with ESRD can undergo dialysis or kidney transplantation. Renal transplant recipients are exposed to increased risk of recrudescence on immunosuppressive therapy.

Tuberculosis

Renal involvement in tuberculosis may take the form of granuloma formation, interstitial nephritis, or caseous destruction. An association between glomerulonephritis and tuberculosis was postulated in the preantibiotic era, but only stray reports have documented such an association in recent times (Somvanshi *et al.* 1989; O'Brien *et al.* 1990). The lesions include diffuse proliferative glomerulonephritis, dense-deposit disease, and IgA nephropathy (De Siati *et al.* 1999; Matsuzawa *et al.* 2002). De Siati *et al.* (1999) described a case of IgA nephropathy with pulmonary tuberculosis in whom the elevated serum IgA concentrations fell, creatinine clearance normalized, and proteinuria disappeared following antitubercular chemotherapy alone. Several reports have documented the presence of circulating ANCA in patients with tuberculosis. The cause-and-effect relationship between tuberculosis and glomerulonephritis remains speculative, and a chance association cannot be excluded. Renal amyloidosis, however, is still seen in a significant proportion of patients who remain untreated for long periods of time in poor countries. Tuberculosis is responsible for about 70–80 per cent cases of secondary amyloidosis in India (Chugh *et al.* 1981; Mehta *et al.* 1990; Shah *et al.* 1996). A few cases of regression of renal amyloidosis have been documented following treatment of underlying tuberculosis (Chugh *et al.* 1981; Sunga *et al.* 1989). Crescentic glomerulonephritis can develop in patients on rifampicin (De Vriese *et al.* 1998; Yoshioka *et al.* 2002; Muthukumar *et al.* 2003). Circulating antirifampicin antibodies have been demonstrated in some cases (De Vriese *et al.* 1998). In contrast to rifampicin-induced acute interstitial nephritis (AIN) typically seen after intermittent rifampicin regimens, rapidly progressive glomerulonephritis (RPGN) develops following continuous therapy, and shows a good response to steroid pulses (De Vriese *et al.* 1998; Yoshioka *et al.* 2002; Muthukumar *et al.* 2003).

Typhoid

Typhoid (*syn.* enteric fever), common in the tropical and subtropical regions, presents with intermittent fever, splenomegaly, and gastrointestinal symptoms. Complications involving the urinary tract include cystitis, pyelitis, and acute renal failure. Overt glomerular involvement is seen in less than 2 per cent of all cases, but haematuria and subnephrotic proteinuria can be detected in 25–40 per cent of cases. In a series reported from South Africa, oedema of more than 1-month duration was detected in more than half of all children with typhoid fever. Patients with hepatic dysfunction are more predisposed to develop this complication (Khan *et al.* 1999). Familial clustering of patients with typhoid nephritis has been reported by Katz *et al.* (1987), though no HLA link could be demonstrated. The diagnosis is made by demonstrating the organism in blood, stool, or urine cultures, or by rising titres in the Widal test. C3 levels are frequently depressed, and IgA levels may be elevated, probably secondary to the intestinal mucosal involvement.

A variety of histological lesions have been described. These include diffuse exudative proliferative and mesangial proliferative glomerulonephritis and IgA nephropathy (Sankaran *et al.* 1981; Indraprasit *et al.* 1985). Variable number of crescents may be observed. The interstitium shows localized small cell infiltration. Electron microscopy reveals electron-dense deposits in the paramesangial areas, and thickening of the lamina rara interna. Immunofluorescence microscopy reveals IgM, IgG, and C3 in the mesangium and along the capillary loops. Dense granular mesangial IgA deposits may be seen in some cases. *Salmonella* Vi antigen has been demonstrated in the affected glomeruli. The glomerular involvement is transient and does not require any specific therapy. The prognosis usually depends upon the extent of systemic disease.

Pneumococcal infections

Streptococcus pneumoniae (Pneumococcus) is a common cause of community acquired pneumonia in the developing countries. Nephritis following this infection was well described in the preantibiotic era, but the incidence came down drastically following the widespread availability of effective antibiotics (Berkowitz 1981; Brzeski *et al.* 1991; Lawlor *et al.* 1992). Clinical manifestations include microhaematuria and moderate proteinuria. Renal failure is seen in an occasional case. Sporadic reports have documented mesangiocapillary or mesangioproliferative lesions. Ultrastructural studies reveal electron-dense deposits in the subepithelial, mesangial, and intramembranous regions and immunofluorescence shows immunoglobulin and complement components. The demonstration of pneumococcal antigen (especially type 14) in the deposits provides the proof for immune complex nature of the disease. The polysaccharide capsular antigen activates the alternate complement pathway as in the case of post-streptococcal glomerulonephritis. A limited activation of classical pathway has also been demonstrated. A role of pneumococcal antigen in the genesis of IgA nephropathy has also been proposed (Drew *et al.* 1987; Kukuminato *et al.* 1993). The disease is self limiting, and the urinary findings disappear following successful treatment of infection.

Syphilis

Syphilis, caused by *Treponema pallidum*, used to be a common cause of nephrotic syndrome in the developing countries. Mass treatment campaigns have effectively eradicated the infection from large parts of the world, although it still occurs in parts of Africa, Asia, and Oceania.

Nephropathy has been observed in both congenital and acquired forms of the disease. Renal disease may manifest at birth or may appear in the first few months in congenital syphilis (Sarkar *et al.* 1992). In one report, urinary abnormalities were detected in 45 per cent of patients with congenital syphilis (Sanchez-Bayle *et al.* 1983). Nephropathy is seen in approximately 0.3 per cent of all patients with acquired syphilis. Renal involvement becomes apparent in the secondary phase, but may also be noticed during the latent phase (Hruby *et al.* 1992). Nephrotic syndrome is the commonest form of presentation, but some patients develop an acute nephritic illness, with microhaematuria, azotaemia, and hypertension (Hunte *et al.* 1993). Rarely, glomerulonephritis may occur in association with syphilitic hepatitis. The commonest histological lesion is a membranous nephropathy with mild mesangial proliferation. Other lesions include endo- and extracapillary proliferative glomerulonephritis and MPGN with or without crescents (Cahen *et al.* 1989; Hruby *et al.* 1992). Interstitial compartment frequently reveals inflammatory cell infiltration. Electron microscopy reveals subepithelial deposits and immunofluorescence shows IgG, C3, and C1q along the basement membranes. Treponema antigen has been identified in these deposits and elution studies have yielded antitreponemal antibodies (Chen *et al.* 1988/1989). Penicillin treatment leads to a prompt and complete disappearance of abnormalities (Chen *et al.* 1988/1989; Sarkar *et al.* 1992). Repeated courses may be required. Spontaneous remission has been reported in some cases. Methylprednisolone and plasmapheresis produce a favourable response in RPGN.

Glomerulopathy following syphilitic infection is presumed to be immune complex mediated. The *T. pallidum* haemagglutination titre is usually very high. *T. pallidum*-specific antigens have been detected by radioimmunoblot techniques in the circulating immune complexes from patients with secondary syphilis (Jorizzo *et al.* 1886), which diminish quickly following penicillin therapy. Immunological studies show high CD4+ and low level of CD8+ cells (Chen *et al.* 1988/1989).

Toxoplasmosis

Toxoplasma gondii is an intracellular parasite involving reticuloendothelial and nervous systems. Infection may be congenital or may develop later in life. Congenital toxoplasmosis may be asymptomatic or present with hydrocephalus, raised intracranial pressure, visual impairment, and neonatal hypoglycaemia. In adults, the commonest presentation is with infectious mononucleosis-like illness, but immunocompromised patients may develop severe systemic disease.

Renal involvement has been reported in a few cases (Beale *et al.* 1979; Haskell *et al.* 1989). Congenital toxoplasmosis generally presents with a nephrotic syndrome, and renal biopsy shows a mesangial proliferative glomerulonephritis. Toxoplasma antigen and IgM can be demonstrated on immunofluorescence. Disappearance of the antigen following treatment of the infection has been documented on renal biopsy. Glomerulonephritis has been documented rarely in acquired toxoplasmosis. Most patients present with a nephrotic syndrome and moderate renal failure. The light microscopic picture is consistent with MCGN, and immunofluorescence shows IgG, IgA, IgM, C3, and fibrinogen along the glomerular capillary walls and in the mesangial region. The histological abnormalities are known to reverse after treatment with pyrimethamine and sulfafurazole along with prednisolone.

Leishmaniasis (kala-azar)

Leishmaniasis is seen in various parts of the world in endemic, epidemic, or sporadic forms. The cutaneous form, caused by *L. tropica*, is seen mostly in the Middle East and Mediterranean regions and the visceral form (caused by *L. donovani*) is reported from India and East Africa. The usual features include prolonged fever, weight loss, anaemia, and splenomegaly. Mild-to-moderate proteinuria and/or microscopic haematuria are observed in over 50 per cent of patients (Dutra *et al.* 1985). Renal dysfunction, however, is exceptional. Histology reveals diffuse proliferative, mesangial proliferative, or membranous glomerulonephritis. A collapsing form of glomerulosclerosis has also been reported (Leblond *et al.* 1994). Basement membrane thickening has been shown in a few patients at autopsy. Tubulointerstitial lesions and amyloidosis have also been reported. Electron microscopy shows paramasangial as well as subepithelial electron-dense deposits along with thickening and irregularities of lamina densa. Experimental studies have documented similar lesions in dogs and hamsters infected with Leishmania. Immunofluorescence shows mesangial immunoglobulin deposits. Leishmania antigen has been demonstrated in the glomeruli of dogs and hamsters infected with *L. donovani* (Costa *et al.* 2000), but not in kala-azar patients. The infiltrating cells include both $CD4^+$ and $CD8^+$ T-cells. A cause-and-effect relationship has not been proved beyond doubt and it has been suggested that the renal lesions could be due to concomitant malnutrition and other infections. Indirect proof, however, comes from complete disappearance of urinary abnormalities following successful treatment of the disease (Dutra *et al.* 1985).

Trypanosomiasis

Trypanosoma is a haemoflagellate transmitted to humans through insect bites. Two forms of trypanosomiasis are known. The American form (Chagas' disease), seen in Southern United States and Latin American countries, is caused by *Trypanosoma cruzei*, transmitted by the faeces of reduviid bugs. Clinical manifestations consist of cardiac rhythm disturbances and gut dysmotility leading to megaesophagus and megacolon, and usually appear several years after the initial infection. The African form is caused by *Trypanosoma brucei*, transmitted through bites of tsetse flies. The symptoms are mainly related to the nervous system (sleeping sickness). The disease is seen typically in the non-immune tourists upon their return home after a brief sojourn to an endemic area.

Experimental studies have shown that BALB/c mice develop a moderate to severe proliferative glomerulonephritis or MCGN after infection with *T. brucei* or *T. cruzei* (van Velthuysen *et al.* 1992a,b); but an association between either form of trypanosomiasis and nephropathy has not been confirmed in human beings. In experimental animals, the lesions are seen typically 4–6 months after the infection. There is a relationship with genetic background, since all strains are not equally susceptible (van Velthuysen *et al.* 1993). Immunoglobulin and complement deposits are observed in the mesangial, subendothelial, and subepithelial regions. Although the trypanosomal antigen has not been demonstrated in the deposits, specific antitrypanosoma antibodies have been found in the glomerular eluates. Antibodies against glomerular basement membrane, laminin and gp-330 have been demonstrated both in circulation and in the eluates (Bruijn *et al.* 1987; van Velthuysen *et al.* 1992a,b). This is thought to be secondary to molecular rearrangement of the basement membrane components after *in situ* binding of the immune complexes.

Fungal infections

Out of the large number of fungi that cause human disease, glomerulonephritis has been described in only a few. About one-third of all patients with disseminated histoplasmosis exhibit urinary abnormalities, but glomerular lesions have been documented histologically in only two patients (Bullock *et al.* 1979; Papo *et al.* 1993). A mesangial proliferative glomerulonephritis was documented in one patient with mucocutaneous candidiasis (Chesney *et al.* 1976). Candida antigen was demonstrated in the glomeruli and urinary abnormalities improved following therapy. Given the rarity with which glomerular involvement has been noted, the aetiological relationship remains speculative.

Other secondary diseases with glomerular involvement in the tropics

Common systemic diseases that produce glomerular involvement in tropical countries include diabetes mellitus (Chapter 4.1), systemic lupus erythematosus (Chapter 4.7.2), systemic vasculitis (Chapters 4.5.1–4.5.3), and other collagen vascular diseases (Chapters 4.8 and 4.11).

As in the rest of the world, the incidence of diabetic nephropathy is rising rapidly throughout the tropics. This is related to an overall improvement in the standard of living, changes in lifestyle and increased life expectancy. Diabetic nephropathy has now emerged as the commonest cause of chronic renal failure amongst the elderly and in the affluent sections of the society (Sakhuja *et al.* 1994). The distribution of systemic lupus erythematosus varies throughout the tropics. It is common amongst Chinese patients in Malaysia and Singapore (Frank 1980; Prathap and Looi 1982; Feng 1986) and in Jamaica (Morgan *et al.* 1984). However, the disease appears to be rare in Africa. Lupus nephritis accounts for 11 per cent of all patients with secondary glomerular disease in India (Chugh and Sakhuja 1984).

Sickle-cell disease is discussed separately in Chapter 4.11.

References

Abdurrahman, M. B. *et al.* (1990). Clinicopathological features of childhood nephrotic syndrome in northern Nigeria. *Quarterly Journal of Medicine* **75**, 563–576.

Abel, L., Ioly, V., Jeni, P., Carbon, C., and Bussel, A. (1986). Apheresis in the management of loiasis with high microfilariaemia and renal disease. *British Medical Journal* **292**, 24.

Abensur, H. *et al.* (1992). Nephrotic syndrome associated with hepatointestinal schistosomiasis. *Revista do Instituto Medical Tropical Sao Paulo* **34**, 273–276.

Abu-Romeh, S. H. *et al.* (1989). Renal diseases in Kuwait. Experience with 244 renal biopsies. *International Urology and Nephrology* **21**, 25–29.

Adeniyi, A., Hendrickse, R. G., and Soothill, J. F. (1979). A controlled trial of cyclo-phosphamide and azathioprine in Nigerian children with the nephrotic syndrome and poorly selective proteinuria. *Archives of Disease in Childhood* **54**, 204–207.

Adhikari, M., Coovadia, H. M., and Chrystal, V. (1983). Extramembranous nephropathy in black South African children. *Annals of Tropical Paediatrics* **3**, 17–24.

Adu, D. *et al.* (1981). The nephrotic syndrome in Ghana: clinical and pathological aspects. *Quarterly Journal of Medicine* **50**, 297–306.

Agnihotri, N. *et al.* (1995). Role of reactive oxygen species in renal damage in experimental leprosy. *Leprosy Reviews* **66**, 201–209.

Ahsan, N., Wheeler, D. E., and Palmer, B. F. (1995). Leprosy-associated renal disease: case report and review of the literature. *Journal of American Society of Nephrology* **5**, 1546–1552.

Aikawa, M. *et al.* (1988). Glomerulopathy in squirrel monkeys with acute *Plasmodium falciparum* infection. *American Journal of Tropical Medicine and Hygiene* **38**, 7–14.

Akinsola, A., Olusanya, O., Iyun, A. O., and Mbanefo, C. O. (1984). Role of hepatitis Bs antigen in chronic glomerulonephritides in Nigerians. *African Journal of Medical Sciences* **13**, 33–39.

Al-Homrany, M. A. (1999). Pattern of renal diseases among adults in Saudi Arabia: a clinicopathologic study. *Ethnic Diseases* **9**, 463–467.

Al-Homrany, M. (2001). Immunoglobulin A nephropathy associated with hepatitis A virus infection. *Journal of Nephrology* **14**, 115–119.

Al-Mohaya, S. A., Coode, P. E., Alkhder, A. A., and Al-Suhaibani, M. O. (1988). Renal granuloma and mesangial proliferative glomerulonephritis in leprosy. *International Journal of Leprosy and Other Mycobacterial Diseases* **56**, 599–602.

Al-Rasheed, S. A., al-Mugeiren, M. M., al-Salloum, A. A., and al-Sohaibani, M. O. (1996). Childhood renal diseases in Saudi Arabia. A clinicopathological study of 167 cases. *International Urology and Nephrology* **28**, 607–613.

Andrade, Z. A. and Rocha, H. (1979). Schistosomal glomerulopathy. *Kidney International* **16**, 23–29.

Andrade, Z. A., Andrade, S. G., and Sadigursky, M. (1971). Renal changes in patients with hepatosplenic schistosomiasis. *American Journal of Tropical Medicine and Hygiene* **20**, 77–83.

Asinobi, A. O. *et al.* (1999). The predominance of membranoproliferative glomerulonephritis in childhood nephrotic syndrome in Ibadan, Nigeria. *West African Journal of Medicine* **18**, 203–206.

Azevedo, L. S. *et al.* (1987). Renal transplantation and schistosomiasis mansoni. *Transplantation* **44**, 795–798.

Bariéty, J. *et al.* (1967). Proteinurie et loase. Étude histologique, optique et electronique d'un cas. *Bulletin et Mémoires de la Société Médicale des Hôpitaux de Paris* **118**, 1015–1125.

Barsoum, R. S. (1993). Schistosomal glomerulopathies. *Kidney International* **44**, 1–12.

Barsoum, R. S. (1998). Malarial nephropathies. *Nephrology, Dialysis, Transplantation* **13**, 1588–1597.

Barsoum, R. S. *et al.* (1988). Hepatic macrophage function in schistosomal glomerulopathy. *Nephrology, Dialysis, Transplantation* **3**, 612–616.

Barsoum, R. S. *et al.* Patterns of glomerular injury associated with hepato-splenic schistosomiasis. In *Proceedings of XII Egyptian Congress of Nephrology*, Cairo, 1992.

Bassily, S. *et al.* (1976). Renal biopsy in Schistosoma–salmonella associated nephrotic syndrome. *Journal of Tropical Medicine and Hygiene* **79**, 256–258.

Bassily, S. *et al.* (1983). Chronic hepatitis-B in patients with *Schistosoma mansoni. Journal of Tropical Medicine and Hygiene* **86**, 67–71.

Beale, M. G., Strayer, D. S., Kissane, J. M., and Robson, A. M. (1979). Congenital glomerulosclerosis and nephrotic syndrome in two infants. Speculations and pathogenesis. *American Journal of Diseases of Children* **133**, 842–845.

Berkowitz, F. E. (1981). Pneumococcal bacteraemia—a study of 75 black children. *Annals of Tropical Paediatrics* **1**, 229–235.

Bhimma, R., Coovadia, H. M., and Adhikari, M. (1997). Nephrotic syndrome in South African children: changing perspectives over 20 years. *Pediatric Nephrology* **11**, 429–434.

Bhimma, R., Coovadia, H. M., and Adhikari, M. (1998). Hepatitis B virus-associated nephropathy in black South African children. *Pediatric Nephrology* **12**, 479–484.

Bodaghi, E. *et al.* (1989). Glomerular diseases in children. 'The Iranian experience'. *Pediatric Nephrology* **3**, 213–217.

Boonpucknavig, V. and Sitprija, V. (1979). Renal disease in acute *Plasmodium falciparum* infection in man. *Kidney International* **16**, 44–52.

Boonpucknavig, V., Boonpucknavig, S., and Bhamarapravati, N. (1973). *Plasmodium berghei* infection in mice. An ultrastructural study of immune complex nephritis. *American Journal of Pathology* **70**, 89–108.

Borok, M. Z., Nathoo, K. J., Gabriel, R., and Porter, K. A. (1997). Clinicopathological features of Zimbabwean patients with sustained proteinuria. *Central African Journal of Medicine* **43**, 152–158.

Brown, K. G. E., Abrahams, C., and Meyers, A. M. (1977). The nephrotic syndrome in Malawian blacks. *South African Medical Journal* **52**, 275–278.

Bruijn, J. A. *et al.* (1987). Anti-basement membrane glomerulopathy in experimental trypanosomiasis. *Journal of Immunology* **139**, 2482–2488.

Brzeski, M. *et al.* (1991). Pneumococcal septic arthritis after splenectomy in Felty's syndrome. *Annals of Rheumatic Diseases* **50**, 724–726.

Bullock, W. E., Artz, R. P., Bhathena, D., and Tung, K. S. (1979). Histoplasmosis. Association with circulating immune complexes, eosinophilia, and mesangiopathic glomerulonephritis. *Archives of Internal Medicine* **139**, 700–702.

Cahen, R. *et al.* (1989). Aetiology of membranous glomerulonephritis: a prospective study of 82 adult patients. *Nephrology, Dialysis, Transplantation* **4**, 172–180.

Chandra Shekhar, K. and Pathmanathan, R. (1987). Schistosomiasis in Malaysia. *Review of Infectious Diseases* **9**, 1026–1037.

Chaturvedi, P. *et al.* (1995). Filarial antibody detection in suspected occult filariasis in children in an endemic area. *Journal of Tropical Pediatrics* **41**, 243–245.

Chen, G., Zhang, Y., and Zou, W. (1995). Hepatitis B virus, the main cause of membranous nephropathy in China. *Zhonghua Yi Xue Za Zhi* **75**, 540–542 (see also 574–575).

Chen, W. P., Chiang, H., and Lin, C. Y. (1988/1989). Persistent histological and immunological abnormalities in congenital syphilitic glomerulonephritis after disappearance of proteinuria. *Childhood Nephrology Urology* **9**, 93–97.

Chesney, R. W., O'Regan, S., Guyda, H. J., and Drummond, K. N. (1976). Candida endocrinopathy syndrome with membranoproliferative glomerulonephritis: demonstration of glomerular candida antigen. *Clinical Nephrology* **5**, 232–238.

Chitsulo, L., Engels, D., Montresor, A., and Savioli, L. (2000). The global status of schistosomiasis and its control. *Acta Tropica* **77**, 41–51.

Choi, I. J. *et al.* (2001). An analysis of 4,514 cases of renal biopsy in Korea. *Yonsei Medical Journal* **42**, 247–254.

Chopra, N. K. *et al.* (1991). Renal involvement in leprosy. *Journal of Association of Physicians of India* **39**, 165–167.

Chugh, K. S. and Jha, V. (1995). Differences in the care of ESRD patients worldwide: required resources and future outlook. *Kidney International Supplement* **50**, s7–s13.

Chugh, K. S. and Sakhuja, V. Renal disease in northern India. In *Tropical Nephrology* (ed. J. W. Kibukamusoke), pp. 428–440. Canberra: Citiforge, 1984.

Chugh, K. S. and Sakhuja, V. (1986). Renal involvement in malaria. *International Journal of Artificial Organs* **9**, 391–392.

Chugh, K. S. and Sakhuja, V. (1990). Glomerular diseases in the tropics. *American Journal of Nephrology* **10**, 437–450.

Chugh, K. S., and Sakhuja, V. Glomerular disease in the tropics. In *Oxford Textbook of Clinical Nephrology* 2nd edn. (ed. A. M. Davison, J. S. Cameron, J. P. Grunfeld, D. N. S. Kerr, E. Ritz, and C. G. Winearls), pp. 703–719. Oxford, UK: Oxford University Press, 1998.

Chugh, K. S., Singhal, P. C., and Tewari, S. C. (1978). Acute glomerulonephritis associated with filariasis. *American Journal of Tropical Medicine and Hygiene* **27**, 630–631.

Chugh, K. S. *et al.* (1981). Pattern of renal amyloidosis in Indian patients. *Postgraduate Medical Journal* **57**, 31–35.

Chugh, K. S. *et al.* (1983). Renal lesions in leprosy amongst North Indian patients. *Postgraduate Medical Journal* **59**, 707–711.

Chugh, K. S. *et al.* (1986). Urinary schistosomiasis in Maiduguri, North East Nigeria. *Annals of Tropical Medicine and Parasitology* **80**, 593–599.

Chugh, K. S. *et al.* (1987). Progression to end-stage renal disease in post-streptococcal glomerulonephritis. *International Journal of Artificial Organs* **10**, 189–194.

Cooke, R. A. and Champness, L. T. (1967). Amyloidosis in Papua and New Guinea. *Papua and New Guinea Medical Journal* **10**, 43–48.

Correia, E. I., Martinelli, R. P., and Rocha, H. (1997). Is glomerulopathy due to schistosomiasis mansoni disappearing? *Revista da Sociedade Brasilero de Medicina Tropical* **30**, 341–343.

Costa, F. A. *et al.* (2000). CD4 (+) T cells participate in the nephropathy of canine visceral leishmaniasis. *Brazilian Journal of Medical and Biological Research* **3**, 1455–1458.

Cruel, T. *et al.* (1997). Nephropathy and filariasis from *Loa loa*. Apropos of 1 case of adverse reaction to a dose of ivermectin. *Bulletin de la Societe de Pathologie Exotique* **90**, 179–181.

Das, P. K. *et al.* (1980). Dapsone and anti-dapsone antibody in circulating immune complexes in leprosy patients. *Lancet* **1**, 1309–1310.

Date, A., Thomas, A., Mathai, R., and Johny, K. V. (1977). Glomerular pathology in leprosy. An electron microscopic study. *American Journal of Tropical Medicine and Hygiene* **26**, 266–272.

Date, A., Gunasekaran, V., Kirubakaran, M. G., and Shastry, J. C. M. (1979). Acute eosinophilic glomerulonephritis with Bancroftian filariasis. *Postgraduate Medical Journal* **55**, 905–907.

De Siati, L. *et al.* (1999). Immunoglobulin A nephropathy complicating pulmonary tuberculosis. *Annals of Diagnostic Pathology* **3**, 300–303.

De Vriese, A. S. *et al.* (1998). Rifampicin-associated acute renal failure: pathophysiologic, immunologic, and clinical features. *American Journal of Kidney Diseases* **31**, 108–115.

Diallo, A. D., Nochy, D., Niamkey, E., and Yao Beda, B. (1997). Etiologic aspects of nephrotic syndrome in Black African adults in a hospital setting in Abidjan. *Bulletin de la Societe de Pathologie Exotique* **90**, 342–345.

Diouf, B. *et al.* (1999). First case of primary IgA glomerulonephritis (Berger's disease) in Senegal. *Dakar Medicine* **44**, 140–142.

Drew, P. A., Nieuwhof, W. N., Clarkson, A. R., and Woodroffe, A. J. (1987). Increased concentration of serum IgA antibody to pneumococcal polysaccharides in patients with IgA nephropathy. *Clinical and Experimental Immunology* **67**, 124–129.

Dreyer, G. *et al.* (1992). Renal abnormalities in microfilaremic patients with Bancroftian filariasis. *American Journal of Tropical Medicine and Hygiene* **46**, 745–751.

Dutra, M. *et al.* (1985). Renal involvement in visceral leishmaniasis. *American Journal of Kidney Diseases* **6**, 22–27.

El-Shoura, S. M. (1994). Falciparum malaria in naturally infected human patients: X. Ultrastructural pathological alterations of renal glomeruli. *Parasite* **1**, 205–210.

Eltoum, I. A. *et al.* (1989). Significance of eosinophiluria in urinary schistosomiasis. A study using Hansel's stain and electron microscopy. *American Journal of Clinical Pathology* **92**, 329–338.

Essamie, M. A. *et al.* (1995). Serious renal disease in Egypt. *International Journal of Artificial Organs* **18**, 254–260.

Ezzat, E., Osman, R. A., Ahmet, K. Y., and Soothill, J. F. (1974). The association between *Schistosoma haematobium* infection and heavy proteinuria. *Transactions of the Royal Society of Tropical Medicine and Hygiene* **68**, 315–318.

Feng, P. H. (1986). Lupus nephritis—the Asian connection. *Philippines Journal of Nephrology* **1**, 30–31.

Frank, A. O. (1980). Apparent predisposition to systemic lupus erythematosus in Chinese patients in West Malaysia. *Annals of the Rheumatic Diseases* **39**, 266–269.

Freire, B. F. *et al.* (1998). Anti-neutrophil cytoplasmic antibodies (ANCA) in the clinical forms of leprosy. *International Journal of Leprosy and Other Mycobacterial Diseases* **66**, 475–482.

Fujiwara, M., Makino, M., and Watanabe, H. (1988). *Schistosoma mansoni*: induction of severe glomerulonephritis in female BXSB mice following chronic infection. *Experimental Parasitology* **65**, 214–221.

Gbadoe, A. D. *et al.* (1999). Primary nephrotic syndrome in the black African child. *Archives of Pediatrics* **6**, 985–989.

Giglioli, G. (1930). Malarial nephritis: epidemiological and clinical notes on malaria. In *Blackwater Fever, Albuminuria and Nephritis in the Interior of British Guiana, Based on Seven Years' Continual Observation*. London: Churchill, 1930.

Giglioli, G. (1972). Changes in the pattern of mortality following the eradication of hyperendemic malaria from a highly susceptible community. *Bulletin of the World Health Organization* **46**, 181–202.

Gilles, H. M. and Hendrickse, R. G. (1963). Nephrosis in Nigerian children: role of *Plasmodium malariae*, and effect of anti-malarial treatment. *British Medical Journal* **1**, 27–31.

Grau, G. E. *et al.* (1990). Interleukin 6 production in experimental cerebral malaria: modulation by anticytokine antibodies and possible role in hypergammaglobulinemia. *Journal of Experimental Medicine* **172**, 1505–1508.

Grauer, G. F. *et al.* (1989). Experimental Dirofilaria immitis-associated glomerulonephritis induced in part by in situ formation of immune complexes in the glomerular capillary wall. *Journal of Parasitology* **75**, 585–593.

Greenham, R. and Cameron, A. H. (1980). *Schistosoma haematobium* and nephrotic syndrome. *Transactions of the Royal Society of Tropical Medicine and Hygiene* **74**, 609–613.

Gupta, J. C. *et al.* (1977). A histopathological study of renal biopsies in 50 cases of leprosy. *International Journal of Leprosy* **45**, 167–170.

Habte, B. (1993). Pattern of glomerular diseases in adult Ethiopians. *Proceedings of the XII International Congress of Nephrology*, Jerusalem, p. 601 (abstract).

Hachicha, J. *et al.* (1992). Primary glomerular nephropathies in southern Tunisia. *Presse Médicale* **21**, 1914.

Hall, C. L., Stephens, L., Peat, D., and Chiodini, P. L. (2001). Nephrotic syndrome due to loiasis following a tropical adventure holiday: a case report and review of the literature. *Clinical Nephrology* **56**, 247–250.

Haskell, L., Fusco, M. J., Ares, L., and Sublay, B. (1989). Disseminated toxoplasmosis presenting as symptomatic orchitis and nephrotic syndrome. *American Journal of Medical Sciences* **298**, 185–190.

Hassan, A. A. (1982). Schistosomal nephropathy and HLA association. Thesis, Cairo University.

Hendrickse, R. G. *et al.* (1972). Quartan malarial nephrotic syndrome: collaborative clinicopathological study in Nigerian children. *Lancet* **i**, 1143–1149.

Houba, V. (1979). Immunologic aspects of renal lesions associated with malaria. *Kidney International* **16**, 3–8.

Houba, V., Allison, A. C., Adeniyi, A., and Houba, J. E. (1971). Immunoglobulin classes and complement in biopsies of Nigerian children with the nephrotic syndrome. *Clinical and Experimental Immunology* **8**, 761–774.

Hruby, Z. *et al.* (1992). The variety of clinical and histopathologic presentations of glomerulonephritis associated with latent syphilis. *International Urology and Nephrology* **24**, 541–547.

Hsu, H. C. *et al.* (1989). Membranous nephropathy in 52 hepatitis B surface antigen (HBsAg) carrier children in Taiwan. *Kidney International* **36**, 1103–1107.

Hunte, W., al-Ghraoui, F., and Cohen, R. J. (1993). Secondary syphilis and nephrotic syndrome. *Journal of American Society of Nephrology* **3**, 1351–1355.

Hurtado, A. *et al.* (2000). Distinct patterns of glomerular disease in Lima, Peru. *Clinical Nephrology* **53**, 325–332.

Indraprasit, S., Boonpucknavig, V., and Boonpucknavig, S. (1985). IgA nephropathy associated with enteric fever. *Nephron* **40**, 219–222.

Jayalakshmi, P., Looi, L. M., Lim, K. J., and Rajogopalan, K. (1987). Autopsy findings in 35 cases of leprosy in Malaysia. *International Journal of Leprosy and Other Mycobacterial Diseases* **55**, 510–514.

Jha, V. and Chugh, K. S. (1996). Dialysis in developing countries: priorities and obstacles. *Nephrology* **2**, 65–71.

Johansen, M. V. *et al.* (1994). A survey of *Schistoma mansoni* induced kidney disease in children in an endemic area of Machakos District, Kenya. *Acta Tropica* **58**, 21–28.

Jorizzo, J. L. *et al.* (1986). Role of circulating immune complexes in human secondary syphilis. *Journal of Infectious Diseases* **153**, 1014–1022.

Kadiri, S., Osobamiro, O., and Ogunniyi, J. (1993). The rarity of minimal change disease in Nigerian patients with the nephrotic syndrome. *African Journal of Medical Sciences* **22**, 29–34.

Kamiie, J. *et al.* (2000). Abnormal distribution of anionic sites in the glomerular basement membrane in glomerulonephritis of dogs infected with *Dirofilaria immitis*. *Journal of Veterinary Medical Science* **62**, 1193–1195.

Katner, H., Beyt, B. E., Jr., and Krotoski, W. A. (1984). Loiasis and renal failure. *Southern Medical Journal* **77**, 907–908.

Katz, Y., Azizi, E., Eshel, G., and Mundel, G. (1987). Familial occurrence of typhoid acute glomerulonephritis. *Israel Journal of Medical Sciences* **23**, 199–201.

Khan, M. *et al.* (1999). Clinical significance of hepatic dysfunction with jaundice in typhoid fever. *Digestive Disease and Science* **44**, 590–594.

Kirsztajn, G. M. *et al.* (1993). Renal abnormalities in leprosy. *Nephron* **65**, 381–384.

Ko, K. W. *et al.* (1987). Childhood renal diseases in Korea. A clinicopathological study of 657 cases. *Pediatric Nephrology* **1**, 664–669.

Kukuminato, Y., Hamamoto, M., and Kataura, A. (1993). Role of serum antibodies to streptococci in patients with IgA nephropathy. *Acta Otolaryngologia Supplement* **508**, 6–10.

Lai, F. M. *et al.* (1987). Pattern of glomerulonephritis in Hong Kong. *Pathology* **19**, 247–252.

Lai, K. N., Lai, F. M., Tam, J. S., and Vallance-Owen, J. (1988). Strong association between IgA nephropathy and hepatitis B surface antigenemia in endemic areas. *Clinical Nephrology* **29**, 229–234.

Lai, K. N. *et al.* (1989). High prevalence of hepatitis B surface antigenaemia in nephrotic syndrome in Hong Kong. *Annals of Tropical Paediatrics* **9**, 45–48.

Lambertucci, J. R. *et al.* (1988). Glomerulonephritis in *Salmonella–Schistosoma mansoni* association. *American Journal of Tropical Medicine and Hygiene* **38**, 97–102.

Langhammer, J., Birk, H. W., and Zahner, H. (1997). Renal disease in lymphatic filariasis: evidence for tubular and glomerular disorders at various stages of the infection. *Tropical Medicine and International Health* **2**, 875–884.

Lawlor, M. T., Crowe, H. M., and Quintiliani, R. (1992). Cellulitis due to *Streptococcus pneumoniae*: case report and review. *Clinical Infectious Disease* **14**, 247–250.

Leblond, V. *et al.* (1994). Collapsing focal segmental glomerulosclerosis associated with visceral leishmaniasis. *Nephrology, Dialysis, Transplantation* **9**, 1353.

Levy, M. and Berger, J. (1988). Worldwide perspective of IgA nephropathy. *American Journal of Kidney Diseases* **12**, 340–347.

Lopes, A. A., Martinelli, R. P., Silveira, M. A., and Rocha, H. (1999). Racial differences between patients with focal segmental glomerulosclerosis and membranoproliferative glomerulonephritis from the State of Bahia. *Revista da Asocidade Medicina Brasilera* **45**, 115–120.

Lopes, M. (1964). Aspectos renais da Sindrome hepato-splenica da Esquistossomose mensonica. Thesis University of Minas Gerais School of Medicine, Brazil, Belo Horizonte.

Madiwale, C. V., Mittal, B. V., Dixit, M., and Acharya, V. N. (1994). Acute renal failure due to crescentic glomerulonephritis complicating leprosy. *Nephrology, Dialysis, Transplantation* **9**, 178–179.

Mahmoud, K. M. *et al.* (2001). Impact of schistosomiasis on patient and graft outcome after renal transplantation: 10 years' follow-up. *Nephrology, Dialysis, Transplantation* **16**, 2214–2221.

Martinelli, R., Pereira, L. J., Brito, E., and Rocha, H. (1992). Renal involvement in prolonged Salmonella bacteremia: the role of schistosomal glomerulopathy. *Revista do Istituto Medicina Tropical de Sao Paulo* **34**, 193–198.

Martinelli, R., Pereira, L. J., Brito, E., and Rocha, H. (1995). Clinical course of focal segmental glomerulosclerosis associated with hepatosplenic schistosomiasis mansoni. *Nephron* **69**, 131–134.

Matsuo, E. *et al.* (1997). Hansen's disease and nephropathy as its sequence. *Nihon Hansenbyo Gakkai Zasshi* **66**, 103–108.

Matsuzawa, N., Nakabayashi, K., Nagasawa, T., and Nakamoto, Y. (2002). Nephrotic IgA nephropathy associated with disseminated tuberculosis. *Clinical Nephrology* **57**, 63–68.

Mehta, H. J. *et al.* (1990). Pattern of renal amyloidosis in western India. A study of 104 cases. *Journal of Association of Physicians of India* **38**, 407–410.

Mitsuda, K. and Ogawa, M. (1937). A study of one hundred and fifty autopsies on cases of leprosy. *International Journal of Leprosy* **5**, 53–60.

Morel-Maroger, L. *et al.* (1975). Tropical nephropathy and tropical extramembranous glomerulonephritis of unknown aetiology in Senegal. *British Medical Journal* **1**, 541–544.

Morgan, A. G., Shah, D. J., Williams, W., and Forrester, T. E. (1984). Proteinuria and glomerular disease in Jamaica. *Clinical Nephrology* **21**, 205–209.

Musa, A. M., Abu Asha, H., and Veress, B. (1980). Nephrotic syndrome in Sudanese patients with schistosomiasis mansoni infection. *Annals of Tropical Medicine and Parasitology* **74**, 615–618.

Muthukumar, T., Jayakumar, M., Fernando, E. M., and Muthusethupathi, M. A. (2002). Acute renal failure due to rifampin—a study of 25 patients. *American Journal of Kidney Diseases* **40**, 690–696.

Nakagaki, K., Hayasaki, M., and Ohishi, I. (1990). Histopathological and immunopathological evaluation of filarial glomerulonephritis in *Dirofilaria immitis* infected dogs. *Japanese Journal of Experimental Medicine* **60**, 179–186.

Nakayama, E. E., Ura, S., Fleury, R. N., and Soares, V. (2001). Renal lesions in leprosy: a retrospective study of 199 autopsies. *American Journal of Kidney Diseases* **38**, 26–30.

Ng, W. L., Scollard, D. M., and Hua, A. (1981). Glomerulonephritis in leprosy. *American Journal of Clinical Pathology* **76**, 321–329.

Ngu, J. L., Adam, M., Leke, R., and Titanji, V. (1980). Proteinuria associated with diethylcarbamazine treatment of onchocerciasis. *Lancet* **i**, 254–255.

Ngu, J. L. *et al.* (1985). Nephropathy in Cameroon: evidence for filarial derived immune complex pathogenesis in some cases. *Clinical Nephrology* **24**, 128–134.

O'Brien, A. A. *et al.* (1990). Immune complex glomerulonephritis secondary to tuberculosis. *Irish Journal of Medical Sciences* **159**, 187.

Okoro, B. A., Okafor, H. U., and Nnoli, L. U. (2000). Childhood nephrotic syndrome in Enugu, Nigeria. *West African Journal of Medicine* **19**, 137–141.

Ormerod, A. D., Petersen, J., Hussey, J. K., Weir, J., and Edward, N. (1983). Immune complex glomerulonephritis and chronic anaerobic urinary tract infection: complication of filariasis. *Postgraduate Medical Journal* **59**, 730–733.

Pakasa, M., Mangani, N., and Dikassa, L. (1993). Focal and segmental glomerulosclerosis in nephrotic syndrome: a new profile of adult nephrotic syndrome in Zaire. *Modern Pathology* **6**, 125–128.

Pakasa, N. M., Nseka, N. M., and Nyimi, L. M. (1997). Secondary collapsing glomerulopathy associated with Loa loa filariasis. *American Journal of Kidney Diseases* **30**, 836–839.

Papo, T. *et al.* (1993). Disseminated histoplasmosis with glomerulonephritis mimicking Wegener's granulomatosis. *American Journal of Kidney Diseases* **21**, 542–544.

Pillay, V. K. G., Kirch, E., and Kurtzman, N. A. (1973). Glomerulopathy associated with filarial loiasis. *Journal of the American Medical Association* **255**, 179 (letter).

Ponce, P. *et al.* (1989). Renal involvement in leprosy. *Nephrology, Dialysis, Transplantation* **4**, 81–84.

Prathap, K. and Looi, L. M. (1982). Morphological patterns of glomerular disease in renal biopsies from 1000 Malaysian patients. *Annals of the Academy of Medicine (Singapore)* **21**, 52–56.

Rabello, A. L. *et al.* (1993). Evaluation of proteinuria in an area of Brazil endemic for schistosomiasis using a single urine sample. *Transactions of Royal Society of Tropical Medicine and Hygiene* **87**, 187–189.

Rabenantoandro, R., Rakotondrajao, R., Rakotondranaivo, S., and Rasamindrakotroka, A. J. (1994). Renal glomerular lesions and *Plasmodium falciparum* infection. *Archives de l' Institut Pasteur Madagascar* **61**, 111–114.

Rasendramino, M. H. *et al.* (1998a). Effect of praziquantel on the uro-nephrologic complications of urinary bilharziasis. *Néphrologie* **19**, 347–351.

Rasendramino, M. H. *et al.* (1998b). Prevalence of uro-nephrologic complications of urinary bilharziasis in hyperendemic focus in Madagascar. *Néphrologie* **19**, 341–345.

Research Group on Progressive Chronic Renal Disease (1999). Nationwide and long-term survey of primary glomerulonephritis in Japan as observed in 1,850 biopsied cases. *Nephron* **82**, 205–213.

Rocha, H., Cruz, T., Brito, E., and Susin, M. (1976). Renal involvement in patients with hepatosplenic schistosomiasis mansoni. *American Journal of Tropical Medicine and Hygiene* **25**, 108–115.

Romero Alvira, D., Guerrero Navarro, L., Gotor Lazaro, M. A., and Roche Collado, E. (1995). Oxidative stress and infectious pathology. *Anales de Medicina Interna (Madrid)* **12**, 139–149.

Ross, A. G. P. *et al.* (2002). Schistosomiasis. *New England Journal of Medicine* **346**, 1212–1220.

Sadigursky, M. *et al.* (1976). Absence of schistosomal glomerulopathy in *S. haematobium* infection in man. *Transactions of the Royal Society of Tropical Medicine and Hygiene* **70**, 322–332.

Sakhuja, V. *et al.* (1994). Chronic renal failure in India. *Nephrology, Dialysis, Transplantation* **9**, 871–873.

Sanchez-Bayle, M. *et al.* (1983). Incidence of glomerulonephritis in congenital syphilis. *Clinical Nephrology* **20**, 27–31.

Sankaran, K. *et al.* (1981). Typhoid glomerulitis. *Journal of Association of Physicians of India* **29**, 835–836.

Sarkar, A. K. *et al.* (1992). Glomerulonephritis in congenital syphilis. *Indian Pediatrics* **29**, 1563–1565.

Seedat, Y. K. (1978). Nephrotic syndrome in the Africans and Indians of South Africa. A ten year study. *Transactions of the Royal Society of Tropical Medicine and Hygiene* **72**, 506–512.

Seedat, Y. K. *et al.* (1988). IgA nephropathy in blacks and Indians of Natal. *Nephron* **50**, 137–141.

Seggie, J., Davies, P. G., Ninin, D., and Henry, J. (1984a). Pattern of glomerulonephritis in Zimbabwe. Survey of disease characterised by nephrotic proteinuria. *Quarterly Journal of Medicine* **53**, 109–118.

Seggie, J., Nathoo, K., and Davies, P. G. (1984b). Association of hepatitis B antigenemia and membranous glomerulonephritis in Zimbabwean children. *Nephron* **38**, 115–119.

Shah, V. B. *et al.* (1996). Renal amyloidosis—a clinicopathologic study. *Indian Journal of Pathology and Microbiology* **39**, 179–185.

Shin, J. H. *et al.* (2001). Renal biopsy in elderly patients: clinicopathological correlation in 117 Korean patients. *Clinical Nephrology* **56**, 19–26.

Shwe, T. (1972). Serum complement [C3] in leprosy. *Leprosy Review* **42**, 268–272.

Sinniah, R. *et al. Renal Disease Classification and Atlas of Infectious and Tropical* Diseases (WHO). ASCP Press, Chicago (USA), 1988.

Sinniah, R., Rui-Mei, L., and Kara, A. (1999). Up-regulation of cytokines in glomerulonephritis associated with murine malaria infection. *International Journal of Experimental Pathology* **80**, 87–95.

Sobh, M. *et al.* (1990). Nephropathy in asymptomatic patients with active *Schistosoma mansoni* infection. *International Urology and Nephrology* **22**, 37–43.

Sobh, M., Moustafa, F., Hamed, S., and Ghoneim, M. (1995). Effect of colchicine on schistosoma-induced renal amyloidosis in Syrian golden hamsters. *Nephron* **70**, 478–485.

Sobh, M. A. *et al.* (1987). Schistosomal specific nephropathy leading to end-stage renal failure. *Kidney International* **31**, 1006–1011.

Sobh, M. A. *et al.* (1988a). Effect of anti-schistosomal treatment on schistosomal-specific nephropathy. *Nephrology, Dialysis, Transplantation* **3**, 744–751.

Sobh, M. A. *et al.* (1988b). Characterisation of kidney lesions in early schistosomal-specific nephropathy. *Nephrology, Dialysis, Transplantation* **3**, 392–398.

Sobh, M. A. *et al.* (1989). A prospective, randomized therapeutic trial for schistosomal specific nephropathy. *Kidney International* **36**, 904–907.

Sobh, M. A., Moustafa, F. E., Hamed, S. M., and Ghoneim, M. A. (1993). Infectious glomerulopathy induced by a defined agent (*Schistosoma mansoni*): progression despite early elimination of the causal agent. *Experimental Nephrology* **1**, 261–264.

Soliman, M. *et al.* Schistosomiasis haematobium glomerulopathy: a clinical or pathological entity. *Proceedings of the Xth International Congress of Nephrology*, p. 362 (abstract), 1987.

Somvanshi, P. P., Patni, P. D., and Khan, M. A. (1989). Renal involvement in chronic pulmonary tuberculosis. *Indian Journal of Medical Sciences* **43**, 55–58.

Spitz, S. (1946). The pathology of acute falciparum malaria. *Military Surgeon* **99**, 555–572.

Sunga, M. N., Jr., Reyes, C. V., Zvetina, J., and Kim, T. W. (1989). Resolution of secondary amyloidosis 14 years after adequate chemotherapy for skeletal tuberculosis. *Southern Medical Journal* **82**, 92–93.

Swanepoel, C. R. *et al.* (1989). IgA nephropathy—Groote Schuur Hospital experience. *Nephron* **53**, 61–64.

Takekoshi, Y. *et al.* (1978). Strong association between membranous nephropathy and hepatitis-B surface antigenaemia in Japanese children. *Lancet* **2**, 1065–1068.

Thomson, P. D. (1997). Renal problems in black South African children. *Pediatric Nephrology* **11**, 508–512.

Turner, I. *et al.* (1987). Minimal change glomerulonephritis associated with *Schistosoma hematobium* infection—resolution with praziquantel treatment. *Australian and New Zealand Journal of Medicine* **17**, 596–598.

van Buuren, A. J., Bates, W. D., and Muller, N. (1999). Nephrotic syndrome in Namibian children. *South African Medical Journal* **89**, 1088–1091.

van Velthuysen, M. L., Bruijn, J. A., van Leer, E. H., and Fleuren, G. J. (1992a). Pathogenesis of trypanosomiasis-induced glomerulonephritis in mice. *Nephrology, Dialysis, Transplantation* **7**, 507–515.

van Velthuysen, M. L. *et al.* (1992b). Phagocytosis by glomerular endothelial cells in infection-related glomerulopathy. *Nephrology, Dialysis, Transplantation* **9**, 1077–1083.

van Velthuysen, M. L. *et al.* (1993). Susceptibility for infection-related glomerulopathy depends on non-MHC genes. *Kidney International* **43**, 623–629.

Voller, A. (1974). Immunopathology of malaria. *Bulletin of the World Health Organization* **50**, 177–186.

Voller, A., Draper, C. C., Shwe, T., and Hutt, M. S. (1971). Nephrotic syndrome in monkey infected with human quartan malaria. *British Medical Journal* **4**, 208–210.

Wang, X., Li, S., and Zhou, Z. (1999). A rapid one-step method of EIA for detection of circulating antigen of *Schistosoma japonicum*. *Chinese Medical Journal* **112**, 124–128.

Ward, P. A. and Conran, P. B. (1966). Immunopathology of renal complications in simian malaria and human quartan malaria. *Military Medicine* **134**, 1228–1236.

Ward, P. A. and Kibukamusoke, J. W. (1969). Evidence for soluble immune complexes in the pathogenesis of the glomerulonephritis in quartan malaria. *Lancet* **i**, 281–285.

Watt, G., Long, G. W., Calubaquib, C., and Ranoa, C. P. (1987). Prevalence of renal involvement in *Schistosoma japonicum* infection. *Transactions of the Royal Society of Tropical Medicine and Hygiene* **81**, 339–342.

Wedderburn, N. *et al.* (1988). Glomerulonephritis in common marmosets infected with *Plasmodium brasilianum* and Epstein–Barr virus. *Journal of Infectious Diseases* **158**, 789–794.

Weiner, I. D. and Northcutt, A. D. (1989). Leprosy and glomerulonephritis: case report and review of the literature. *American Journal of Kidney Diseases* **13**, 424–429.

Wong, S. N., Yu, E. C., and Chan, K. W. (1993). Hepatitis B virus associated membranous glomerulonephritis in children—experience in Hong Kong. *Clinical Nephrology* **40**, 142–147.

Woo, K. T. *et al.* (1999). The changing pattern of glomerulonephritis in Singapore over the past two decades. *Clinical Nephrology* **52**, 96–102.

Yahya, T. M., Pingle, A., Boobes, Y., and Pingle, S. (1998). Analysis of 490 kidney biopsies: data from the United Arab Emirates Renal Diseases Registry. *Journal of Nephrology* **11**, 148–150.

Yamabe, H. *et al.* (1995). Hepatitis C virus infection and membranoproliferative glomerulonephritis in Japan. *Journal of American Society of Nephrology* **6**, 220–223.

Yoshioka, K. *et al.* (2002). Rapidly progressive glomerulonephritis due to rifampicin therapy. *Nephron* **90**, 116–118.

Zainal, D., Riduan, A., Ismail, A. M., and Norhayati, O. (1995). Glomerulonephritis in Kelantan, Malaysia: a review of the histological pattern. *Southeast Asian Journal of Tropical Medicine and Public Health* **26**, 149–153.

Index

Page numbers in **bold** refer to major sections of the text.
Page numbers in *italics* refer to pages on which tables may be found.